Illustrated

Study Guide for the

NCLEX-RN® EXAM

SEVENTH EDITION

Study Guide for the
NCLEX-RN® EXAM

Editors

JoAnn Zerwekh, EKH, MSN, EdD, RN

Jo Carol Claborn, MS, RN

MOSBY

ELSEVIER

MOSBY
ELSEVIER

3251 Riverport Lane
St. Louis Missouri 63043

Notices

Knowledge and best practice in this field are constantly changing. As new research and experience
broaden our understanding, changes in research methods, professional practices, or medical treatment may
become necessary.

Practitioners and researchers must always rely on their own experience and knowledge in evaluating
and using any information, methods, compounds, or experiments described herein. In using such
information or methods, they should be mindful of their own safety and the safety of others, including
parties for whom they have a professional responsibility.

With respect to any drug or pharmaceutical products identified, readers are advised to check the most
current information provided (i) on procedures featured or (ii) by the manufacturer of each product to be
administered, to verify the recommended dose or formula, the method and duration of administration,
and contraindications. It is the responsibility of practitioners, relying on their own experience and
knowledge of their patients, to make diagnoses, to determine dosages and the best treatment for each
individual patient, and to take all appropriate safety precautions.

To the fullest extent of the law, neither the Publisher nor the authors, contributors, or editors, assume
any liability for any injury and/or damage to persons or property as a matter of products liability,
negligence or otherwise, or from any use or operation of any methods, products, instructions, or ideas
contained in the material herein.

International Standard Book Number: 978-0-323-05664-9

Managing Editor: Nancy L. O'Brien   *Design Direction:* Amy Buxton
Publishing Services Manager: Anne Altepeter   *Multimedia Producer:* Dave Rushing
Senior Project Manager: Cheryl A. Abbott

Printed in The United States of America

Last digit is the print number: 9 8 7 6 5 4 3 2 1

Working together to grow
libraries in developing countries

www.elsevier.com | www.bookaid.org | www.sabre.org

ELSEVIER   BOOK AID International   Sabre Foundation

Contributors

Joanna G. Barnes, MSN, RN
Grayson County Community College
Denison, Texas

Jeannette Gloria Brown, MSN, RNC-OB,
C-EFM, RN
Virginia Commonwealth University
Richmond, Virginia

Marianne Call, MN, RN
Geriatric Behavioral Health
East Jefferson General Hospital
Metairie, Louisiana

Sharon I. Decker, RN, PhD, ACNS-BC, ANEF
Professor and Director of Clinical Simulations
Covenant Health System Endowed Chair in Simulation
    and Nursing Education
Texas Tech University Health Science Center
Lubbock, Texas

Barbara S. Devitt, MSN, RN
Lecturer
Louise Herrington School of Nursing
Baylor University
Dallas, Texas

Ashley Garneau, MS, RN
Nursing Faculty
Gateway Community College
Phoenix, Arizona

Lt. Col. (Ret.) Michael W. Hutton, MSN, RN
Instructor
Blinn College
Bryan, Texas

Susan B. Priest, MSN, RN, CNS
Director, Health and Medical Programs
Continuing Education Workforce Development
Adjunct Faculty, Associate Degree Nursing
Alvin Community College
Alvin, Texas

Catherine Rosser, EdD, CNA-BC, RN
Undergraduate Program Director
Louise Herrington School of Nursing
Baylor University
Dallas, Texas

Linda Stevenson, PhD, RN
Assistant Professor
Louis Herrington School of Nursing
Baylor University
Dallas, Texas

Mary Ann Yantis, BS, MS, PhD, RN
Associate Professor of Nursing
Louis Herrington School of Nursing
Baylor University
Dallas, Texas

Reviewers

Judy Cole, MSN, RNC
Maternal Child Educator
Saint Francis Hospital, Memphis
Memphis, Tennessee

Faith Darilek, MSN, RN
Nursing Professor
The Victoria College
Victoria, Texas

Mary M. Fabick, MEd, MSN
Associate Professor of Nursing
Milligan College
Milligan College, Tennessee

Cene' Gibson, MSN, ARNP
Family Nurse Practitioner
Family Healthcare and Minor Emergency Clinic
Yukon, Oklahoma

Margaret M. Gingrich, MSN, RN
Professor
Harrisburg Area Community College
Harrisburg, Pennsylvania

Sarah M. Howell, MSN, RN
Assistant Professor of Nursing
Mississippi University for Women
Columbus, Mississippi

Jolee M. Preston, MSN, RN
Assistant Professor
Jefferson College of Health Sciences
Roanoke, Virginia

Sharon Redding, MN, RN, CNE
Associate Professor of Nursing
College of Saint Mary
Alegent Bergon Mercy Medical Center
Omaha, Nebraska

Katherine Roberts
Assistant Professor
Joann Gay Dishman Department of Nursing
Lamar University
Beaumont, Texas

Donna Wilsker, MSN, BSN, RN
Assistant Professor
Lamar University
Beaumont, Texas

Connie S. Wilson, EdD, RN, CNE
Professor
University of Indianapolis
Indianapolis, Indiana

Preface

This seventh edition of *Illustrated Study Guide for the NCLEX-RN® Exam* continues to provide an up-to-date review book illustrated with graphics, pictures, and cartoon images to enhance your review and retention of critical nursing information. The book contains information specifically designed to assist you in preparing for the National Council Licensure Examination for Registered Nurses (NCLEX-RN®). This text emphasizes the integrated approach to nursing practice that the NCLEX-RN is designed to test. The book's primary purpose is to assist you to thoroughly review facts, principles, and applications of the nursing process. It should alleviate many of the concerns you may have about what, how, and when to study.

We have spent a great deal of time studying the NCLEX-RN test format and have incorporated that information into this book. We have included discussion and examples of the alternate format questions. In our review courses, which we have taught across the country, we have identified specific student needs and have correlated this information with the test plan in order to develop this study guide. Study questions are at the end of each chapter to help you check your level of comprehension. In addition, there is a CD-ROM in the back of this text that contains questions for practicing your testing skills.

We have designed graphics that highlight important information to make the book more visually appealing:

ALERT Alert! identifies important concepts that are reflected on the RN Practice Analysis from the National Council of State Boards of Nursing, Inc.

❗ Nursing Priority assists to distinguish priorities of nursing care.

📋 Adult disease conditions are easily located by this design element.

🎈 Pediatric disease conditions are easily located by this design element.

❋ Self-Care and Home Care can be found under the Nursing Interventions section.

℞ Medication information is easily found in chapter appendixes.

▲ High-Alert Medications identified by The Joint Commission and the Institute for Safe Medication Practices are noted by this symbol.

The comments from our review course participants, as well as extensive faculty reviews on our sixth edition, have helped to shape the development of this seventh edition. We hope this text will prove to be even more beneficial to nursing faculty, students, and graduate nurses. Thank you for allowing us to be part of your success in nursing.

JoAnn Zerwekh
Jo Carol Claborn

Acknowledgments

We wish to express our appreciation to our children—Tyler Zerwekh and Ashley Garneau, Mike Brown, Kimberley Aultman, and Jaelyn Conway—for their continuing support as their mothers wrote, rewrote, and put together another edition of this book. To Robert and John, thank you for your tolerance, love, and willingness to continue to share and support us in the midst of our hectic professional lives.

A special note of thanks to C.J. Miller, RN, BS, our cartoonist, who has worked with us from the beginning of the *Memory Notebooks of Nursing* and the past few editions of *Nursing Today: Transition and Trends*, and more recently with the *Mosby's Memory Notecard* series. She continues to brighten our day and bring to all of our books images and cartoons that are so unique.

The revision of a book offers the opportunity to be responsive to nursing faculty and students who have utilized the book. We appreciate their comments and suggestions for the production of this seventh edition. It is our pleasure to express an appreciation to the individuals who assisted us in the technical preparation and production of this edition. Our sincere appreciation to:

Elaine Nokes, our administrative assistant, who keeps everything organized and running smoothly for our business.

Kristin Green, senior editor, whose calm demeanor and flexibility with our schedules supported us as we worked all the way to the last possible minute.

Cheryl Abbott, senior project manager, who monitored the production of this book and kept us on schedule.

Thank you to all!

Contents

9 Psychiatric Nursing Concepts, 145

10 Psychiatric Disorders, 165

11 Integumentary System, 197

25 Intrapartum and Postpartum, 525

26 Newborn, 551

CHAPTER ONE

Testing Strategies for the NCLEX-RN® Examination

One of the first steps to be being successful on the NCLEX® (National Council Licensure Examination) is to understand how the test is developed. An important step in preparing for the examination is to find out as much as possible about the test; this will help to reduce stress and anxiety. During each of your nursing classes, you were given a syllabus with course objectives and provided with presentations to guide you through the information that would be included on the next test. In most academic settings, the faculty member who teaches the course is also responsible for the development and construction of examinations—thus you are being taught by the same person who prepares the tests, which can be a great advantage. As you begin to prepare for the NCLEX, it is important to consider who determines the content of the test plan and constructs the questions based on the test plan.

The National Council of State Boards of Nursing (NCSBN) is responsible for the development of the content and the construction of questions or items for the NCLEX examination. A practice analysis is conducted by the NCSBN every 3 years to validate the test plan and to determine currency of nursing practice. Content experts are consulted to assist in the creation of the practice analysis. The activity performances and knowledge identified by the content experts are analyzed with consideration given to frequency, as well as importance of the nursing activity. The percentage of test items on the test plan does not specifically address specialty areas. However, on review of the nursing activities, many of the test plan areas address specialty areas of nursing practice. This analysis provides the basis for development of the content to be included in the NCLEX Test Plan.

The content experts are practicing nurses who work with or supervise new graduates in the practice setting. These content experts represent all geographic areas and are selected according to their area of practice; therefore all areas of nursing practice are addressed in the development of the test plan. Item writers are selected to create questions based on the content identified in the test plan. All new test items or questions are reviewed by item reviewers who are also nurses in current practice and who have been directly involved with supervision of new graduate nurses. Not only do content experts and item reviewers create new items, they

are also involved in the continual review of items in the NCLEX test pool to ensure all items reflect current practice.[1]

So, what does this all mean? It means that nurses in current practice and nursing faculty work together to identify the content and to develop questions for the NCLEX-RN. All geographic areas, as well as all areas of nursing practice, are included. The purpose of the examination is to assure the public that each candidate who passes the examination can practice safely and effectively as a newly licensed, entry-level RN.

The NCLEX-RN is used by every U.S. state to determine entry into nursing practice as an RN. Each state is responsible for the testing requirements, retesting procedures, and entry into practice within that state. Each state requires the same competency level or passing standard on the NCLEX; there is no variation in the passing standard from state to state.

TEST PLAN

The test plan is based on research conducted by the NCSBN every 3 years. The purpose of this research is to determine the most important and frequent activities of nurses who were successful on the NCLEX and who have been working after successful completion of the NCLEX. The research indicates that the majority of graduate nurses are working in an acute care environment and are responsible for caring for adult and elderly adult clients. Each question will reflect a level of the nursing process or an area of client needs, and each question will be categorized according to a validated level of difficulty. The exam consists of questions that are designed to test the candidate's ability to apply the nursing process and to determine appropriate nursing responses and interventions to provide safe nursing care.

Integrated Processes

Integrated throughout the test plan are principles that are fundamental to the practice of nursing.

Nursing Process

The nursing process is a scientific approach to problem solving; it has been a common thread in your nursing curriculum since the beginning of school. There is nothing new about the nursing process on the NCLEX. Assessment data are obtained, analysis of those data occurs, a plan is formulated, nursing actions are implemented, and the results of that intervention are evaluated. It is important to keep the steps of the nursing process in mind when you are critically evaluating an NCLEX question.

Caring

The interaction of the client and the nurse occurs in an atmosphere of mutual respect and trust. To achieve the desired outcome, the nurse provides hope, support, and compassion to the client.

Communication and Documentation

Events and activities—both verbal and nonverbal—that involve the client, the client's significant others, and the health care team are documented in handwritten or electronic records. These records reflect quality and accountability in the provision of client care. Principles of documentation and provision of client confidentiality are important considerations in any area of nursing practice.

Teaching and Learning

Nurses provide or facilitate knowledge, skills, and attitudes that promote a change in clients' behavior through teaching and learning. Nurses provide education to clients and to their significant others in a variety of settings. Identifying critical learning needs for clients and their significant others and providing information in a manner that promotes the health and safety of clients are important across all levels of nursing practice.[2]

Areas of Client Needs

The National Council Examination Committee has identified four primary areas of client needs, which provide a structure to define nursing actions and competencies across all practice settings and for all clients. These areas reflect an integrated approach to the testing content; no predetermined number of questions or percentage of questions pertain to any particular area of practice (e.g., medical-surgical, pediatric, obstetric).

Table 1-1 lists the areas of client needs, along with the subcategories and the specific percentages associated with each subcategory. The range of percentages for each

Table 1-1	NCLEX-RN® TEST PLAN—EFFECTIVE APRIL 2010 TO APRIL 2013*
Safe and Effective Care Environment	
Management of Care (16%-22%)	Concepts of management of nursing care—supervision, delegation, establishing priorities in client care; legal and ethical responsibilities; client rights; confidentiality
Safety and Infection Control (8%-14%)	Prevention of errors and accidents, implementation of standard precautions, asepsis, use of restraints, disaster planning, handling hazardous materials
Health Promotion and Maintenance (6%-12%)	
Aging process and developmental stages, lifestyle choices, high-risk behaviors; principles of learning and teaching; ante/intra/postpartum and newborn; health promotion and disease prevention, techniques of physical assessment	
Psychosocial Integrity (6%-12%)	
Mental health concepts and interventions, end-of-life care, grief and loss, sensory and perceptual alterations, religious and spiritual influences; behavioral intervention/crisis intervention, chemical dependency, abuse and neglect, therapeutic communication	
Physiologic Integrity	
Basic Care and Comfort (6%-12%)	Assistive devices, mobility, nutrition, personal hygiene, elimination, nonpharmacologic comfort measures
Pharmacologic and Parenteral Therapies (13%-19%)	Medication administration; expected medication actions, adverse effects/contraindication; nursing implications; dosage calculation; blood administration, parenteral/IV therapy, central venous access devices, pain control, parenteral nutrition
Reduction of Risk Potential (10%-16%)	Pathophysiology, nursing implications for and nursing care to minimize potential complications of diagnostic tests/procedures/surgery; potential for alterations in body systems (tubes, pacemakers, hyper/hypoglycemia, specimens, bleeding, immobility, wounds, positions); laboratory values; changes in and/or abnormal vital signs; system specific assessments
Physiologic Adaptation (11%-17%)	Pathophysiology/alterations in body systems: fluid and electrolyte imbalances, hemodynamics, medical emergencies (CPR, airway, hemorrhage), unexpected response to therapies (seizures, changes in vital signs); nursing management of illness

Adapted from the *NCLEX-RN® Test Plan for the National Council Licensure Examination for Registered Nurses,* Chicago, 2009, National Council of State Boards of Nursing.

*Test plan information is presented as examples only and is not intended to be a complete or thorough representation of information included in any specific category.

category reflects how important that area is on the test plan. Management of care, pharmacologic and parenteral therapies, and reduction of risk potential are the subcategories with the highest emphasis on the test plan.[2] When you are studying for the NCLEX, these are concepts that should be identified across the scope of nursing practice. This table has been adapted and summarized; it does not reflect the entire test plan content. The National Council's Detailed Test Plan for the NCLEX-RN may be obtained from the NCSBN, Inc. (www.ncsbn.org). What was great new information in last month's nursing journals will not be immediately reflected on the NCLEX. New information or new practices must be established as a standard of practice across the nation before being included on the NCLEX. Throughout this book are ALERT boxes that call your attention to areas of the test plan. Pay attention to these boxes and think about how each concept or principle can apply to different types of clients.

> **ALERT** The NCLEX-RN is a test that requires utilization of the nursing process and application of nursing concepts and principles across the life span.

As client conditions or nursing principles are presented, the NURSING PRIORITY boxes call your attention to critical information regarding a client with a specific condition or situation being presented.

> **! NURSING PRIORITY** This is critical information to consider in providing safe nursing care for a client with a specific problem.

Classification of Questions

The majority of questions on the NCLEX are written at the level of application or higher level of cognitive ability. This means a candidate must have the knowledge and understand concepts to be able to apply the nursing process to the client situation presented in the question. NCLEX questions are based on critical thinking concepts that demonstrate a candidate's ability to make decisions and solve problems. NCLEX questions are not fact, recall, or memory-level questions. Nurses who have taken the NCLEX have stated that the NCLEX questions were not like any questions they had on nursing school examinations; however, the nursing content and principles needed to determine the answer *were* provided in their nursing school curriculum. The questions and answers have been thoroughly researched and validated. The standardization of information is important because the NCLEX is administered nationwide to determine entry level into nursing practice. This ensures that regional differences in nursing care will not be a factor in the exam.

All questions presented to a candidate taking the NCLEX have been developed according to the test plan and the integrated processes fundamental to nursing practice and have been categorized according to their level of difficulty. The questions have been researched and documented as pertaining to entry-level nursing behaviors.[2,3]

WHAT IS COMPUTER ADAPTIVE TESTING?

Computer adaptive testing provides a method for generating an examination according to each candidate's ability. Each time a candidate answers a question, the computer then selects the next question based on the candidate's answer to the previous question. The examination continues to present test items based on the test plan and identified level of difficulty and provides an opportunity for each candidate to demonstrate competency. The NCLEX-RN is graded in a manner different from the grading of conventional school exams. A candidate's score is not based on the number of questions answered correctly, but rather on the standard of competency as established by the NCSBN (Figure 1-1).

A test bank of questions is loaded into the candidate's computer at the beginning of the examination. Different candidates receive different sets of questions, but all test banks contain questions that are developed according to the same test plan. For example, standard precautions are a critical element of the test plan. Many situations and clients can be presented to test this concept: one candidate may have a question based on standard precautions required for a client in labor; someone else, a situation with implications for a client with a respiratory problem; and still someone else, a situation involving a newborn. All the questions are different, but they are all based on the test plan's critical element of standard precautions.

The questions to be presented to the candidate are determined by the candidate's response to the previous questions. When a question is answered correctly, the next question presented to the candidate may have a higher level of difficulty. The more higher-level questions a candidate answers correctly, the closer he or she is to passing (Figure 1-2). A candidate cannot skip questions or go back to previously answered questions. As the examination progresses, it is interactively assembled. As questions are answered correctly, the next question is selected to test another area of the test plan, and it may be at a higher level of difficulty. When a question is answered incorrectly, the computer will select an easier question. This helps to prevent a candidate from being bombarded with very difficult questions and becoming increasingly frustrated. The computer will continue to present questions that are based on the test plan and on the level of ability of the candidate until a level of competency has been established (see Figure 1-2)[3].

FIGURE 1-1 Competency level.

FIGURE 1-2 Plateau to establish pass or fail.

TAKING THE NCLEX® EXAMINATION

Application

An application must be submitted to the state board of nursing in the state in which the candidate wants to be licensed. The contact information for the state boards of nursing is available on the National Council website. After the candidate's application and registration fees have been received and approved by the state, the candidate will receive an **a**uthorization **t**o **t**est (ATT) from the NCSBN. After the examination fee has been paid, it will not be refunded, regardless of how the candidate registered.[3] The candidate may register for the NCLEX at the NCLEX Candidate website (listed in the ATT) or by regular mail or by telephone (also listed in the ATT). The Candidate Bulletin (CB) is available on the National Council website—be sure to print this bulletin for future reference. The CB provides critical information, including addresses and phone numbers for registration and specific details regarding the registration process.

Scheduling the Examination

After you have been declared eligible to take the NCLEX and have received an ATT, you may schedule an examination date. You *must have an ATT* before you can schedule your examination. The CB lists the phone number to call to schedule the examination. Once the ATT has been issued, the state stipulates a period of time within which you must take the examination. This ranges from 60 to 365 days, with the average being 90 days; this period *cannot* be extended. You must test within the validity dates noted on your ATT. The ATT must be presented at the testing site before you can be admitted to take the examination. You are encouraged to call and schedule the appointment to take the examination as soon as possible after receiving the ATT, even if you do not plan to take the test immediately. This will increase the probability of getting the testing date you want.

Pearson Vue is the company that provides the testing facility and computers for the examination. A tutorial on how to use the computer on NCLEX is available at *www.pearsonvue.com/nclex/*. Go to the site and review the tutorial. It should be very familiar to you when you see it on NCLEX. This same tutorial will be presented to you at the beginning of your examination.

Testing Center Identification

Photo identification with a signature and the ATT will be required at the testing site. The name printed on the ATT must match the identification presented at the course site. Identification must be in English and cannot be expired. Acceptable forms of identification are a U.S. driver's license, a passport, or a U.S. state-issued identification, or a U.S. military issued identification. At the testing site before testing, each candidate will be digitally fingerprinted, a photo will be taken, and a signature will be required. Beginning in 2009, a new type of identity verification will be used in some testing locations. A Palm Vein Reader may be used at some testing sites, in addition to the digital fingerprinting, to validate identity on reentering the testing area.

Day of the Examination

You should plan on arriving at the center about 30 minutes before scheduled testing time. If you arrive more than 30 minutes late, the scheduled testing time will be canceled and you will have to reapply and repay the examination fee. An erasable note board will be available at your computer terminal. You are not allowed to take any type of books, personal belongings, hats, coats, blank tablets, or scratch paper into the testing area. A fingerprint scan will be required to reenter the testing area after each break.

Testing

You will have a maximum of 6 hours to complete the examination. After 2 hours of testing, you have an optional 10-minute break; another optional break occurs after 3 1/2 hours of testing. If you need a break before that time, notify one of the attendants at the testing center. The computer will automatically signal when a scheduled break begins. All of the break times and the tutorial are considered part of the total 6 hours of testing time.

The examination will stop when one of the following occurs:

1. Seventy-five questions have been answered, and a minimum level of competency has been established; or a lack of minimum competency has been established (see Figure 1-2).
2. The candidate has answered the maximum number of 265 questions.
3. The candidate has been testing for 6 hours, regardless of the number of questions answered.

Each candidate will receive between 75 and 265 questions. The number of questions on the NCLEX is not indicative of the level of competency. The majority of candidates who complete all 265 questions will have demonstrated a level of minimum competency and therefore pass the NCLEX. A mouse will be used for selecting answers, so candidates should not worry about different computer keyboard function keys. An onscreen calculator will also be available to use for math problems. If any problems occur with the environment or with the equipment, someone will be available to provide assistance.

In each candidate's examination, there will be 15 pretest or unscored items or questions. The statistics on these items will be evaluated in order to determine whether the item is a valid test item to be included in future NCLEX test banks. All of the items that are scored, or counted, on a candidate's examination have been pretested and validated. It is impossible to determine which questions or items are scored items and which are pretest items. It is important to treat each question as a scored item.

The CB from the NCSBN is very important; read it carefully and keep it until the results from NCLEX have been received. This bulletin will provide directions and will answer more of your questions regarding the NCLEX. The CB is available online (from the NCSBN at *www.ncsbn.org* or from Pearson Vue at *www.pearsonvue.com/nclex*).

Test Results

Each examination is scored twice, once at the testing center and again at the testing service. The test results are electronically transferred to the state boards of nursing. Test results are *not* available at the testing center, from Pearson Vue, or from the NCSBN. Check the information received from the appropriate state board of nursing to determine how and when your results will be available. Test results may be available online. In some states, results may be available within 2 to 3 days; in others, the results will be mailed, which will require a longer notification period. Do *not* call the Pearson Professional Center, NCLEX Candidate Services, the National Council, or the individual state board of nursing for test results. Follow the procedure found in the information from the state board of nursing where the license will be issued.[3]

SUCCESSFUL TEST TAKING ON THE NCLEX® EXAM

ALERT Practicing test-taking skills is critical if a candidate is going to be able to effectively use them on the NCLEX. Practice test taking should be a component of NCLEX preparation.

Being able to effectively apply test-taking strategies on an examination is almost as important as having the basic knowledge required to answer the questions correctly. Everyone has taken an examination only to find, on review of the exam, that questions were missed because of poor test-taking skills. Nursing education provides the graduate with a comprehensive base of knowledge; how effectively the graduate can *demonstrate* the use of this knowledge will be a major factor in the successful completion of the examination.

The NCLEX-RN is designed to evaluate minimum levels of competency. The exam does not test total knowledge, knowledge of specialty areas, or any degree of professionalism. The purpose of the examination is to determine whether a candidate has the knowledge, skills, and ability required for safe and effective entry-level nursing practice. Throughout the examination, questions are described as being based on clinical situations common in nursing; uncommon situations are not emphasized. NCLEX questions are not fact, recall, or memory-level questions; they are questions that require critical thinking to determine the correct answer. Critical thinking will require an analysis of client data, an understanding of the client's condition or disease, and the ability to determine the best action or nursing judgment that will most effectively meet the client's needs.

Practice testing is an excellent method of studying for the NCLEX. After taking a practice test, use the results to determine whether you need additional review in certain areas or whether you are missing questions because of poor test-taking strategies.

NCLEX® TEST-TAKING STRATEGIES

The NCLEX questions are different from those used in nursing schools. One of the biggest problems candidates encounter is that two or more answers may appear to be correct. Sometimes a candidate believes that more information is necessary to answer the question. However, the answer must be determined from the information provided; no one is going to clarify or provide additional information regarding a specific question or content. The strategies described below are critical in evaluating and successfully answering NCLEX questions.

- **The NCLEX Hospital:** What a great place to work! Remember, on the NCLEX, all clients are being cared for in an ideal environment—the NCLEX Hospital. Questions ask for nursing care and decisions based on situations in which everything is available for client care.

NCLEX questions are based on textbook practices, not necessarily on the real world. It must be assumed that clients will respond just as the textbooks indicate they will. Candidates who have a lot of clinical experience will have problems on the test if they answer questions based on the possibility that there may not be adequate staff or equipment or if they believe the option for the nursing care presented is not "realistic." Nursing care provided on the examination is performed in the NCLEX Hospital, where the nurse always has adequate staff, supplies, and anything else required to provide the safest care for the client. This approach is necessary because this is a nationally standardized examination.

- **Calling the Doctor (or anyone else):** Be cautious about passing the responsibility for care of the client to someone else. This is an exam on nursing care; evaluate the question carefully and see what nursing action should to be taken before consulting or calling someone else. This includes the social worker, respiratory therapist, and hospital chaplain, as well as the physician. After you have carefully evaluated the question, if the client's condition is such that the nurse cannot do anything to resolve the problem, then calling for assistance may be the best answer. Frequently, there is a nursing action to be taken before contacting someone for assistance. A specific item on the test plan states that the nurse will identify client data that must be reported immediately.[2]

- **Doctor's Orders:** It should be assumed that a doctor's order is available to provide the nursing care in the options presented in the question. If the question asks for administration of a specific medication for the client's problem, then assume that there is an order for it. If the focus of a question is to determine if a nursing action is a dependent or an independent nursing action, then it will be stated in the stem of the question. For example, the question may ask what would be an independent nursing action to provide pain relief for a specific client.

- **Focus on the Client:** Look for answers that focus on the client. Identify the significant or central person in the question. Most often, this is going to be the client. Wrong choices would be those that focus on maintaining hospital rules and policies, dealing with equipment, or solving the nurse's problems. Evaluate the status of the client first, and then deal with the equipment problems, or concerns. Other questions may ask the nurse to respond to a client's family or significant others. Determine the person to whom the question is directed.

- **Client's Age:** Consider a client to be an adult unless otherwise stated. If the age of a client is important to the question, it will be stated in years or in months. Descriptions such as "elderly adult" and "geriatric client" are not commonly used. These terms have been established as negative descriptors of older clients. The description of such a client may be "older adult," or a specific age may be given.

- **Laboratory Values:** It is important to know normal values for the common laboratory tests. Be able to identify lab values and/or diagnostic procedures that indicate a client's progress or lack of progress or indicate whether or not a client's status is getting better or worse. Determine whether specific nursing actions are required based on the abnormal values or diagnostic results. For example, when a client's blood glucose level is 50 mg/mL and he or she is awake and alert, the client will need something to eat, preferably a complex carbohydrate. If a client has a hemoglobin value of 8.5 g/dL, nursing care will involve avoidance of unnecessary physical activities, and the client will need to be kept warm.

- **Positions:** Positioning a client may be an option to consider in the implementation of care. If a specific position for the client appears in the stem of the question, then consider whether the position is for comfort, for treatment, or to prevent a complication. Evaluate the question: What is to be accomplished by placing the client in the position, and why is the position important for this client? Sometimes a client position will appear in the options. Consider whether positioning is important to the care of the client presented. For example, the semi-Fowler's position is very important to a client who is having difficulty breathing, and the supine position or low Fowler's position may provide the most comfort for a client after surgery. Determine why a client is placed in a specific position and then determine whether this is a priority in planning or intervention. See Appendix 3-1 for a further description of positions.

- **Mathematic Computations:** Mathematic computations may include calculations of intravenous (IV) rate and drip factors, calculations of medication dosages, conversion of units of measurement, as well as calculation of intake and output. You should be able to apply the appropriate formula to the situation. Some of the questions may call for two computations, as in a question in which all items must be converted to one unit of measurement before a dosage is calculated. There will be an onscreen calculator; find the "calculator" button when you do the NCLEX Tutorial. The mathematic calculations may be presented in a multiple-choice format or in an alternate format question in which you are asked to fill in the blank. For fill-in-the-blank questions, calculate your answer and then type the answer into the box provided. The unit of measurement will be provided in the box.

Management of Client Care

As the role of the RN has expanded, management of client care has become increasingly important. Nursing care assignments should take into consideration the nurse who is educationally prepared, experienced, and most capable of caring for the client. Unlicensed assistive personnel (UAP), patient care attendants (PCA), and/or nursing assistants must be directly supervised in the provision of safe nursing care. Licensed practical nurses (LPNs or licensed vocational nurses [LVNs]) have more independence in providing nursing care. They may direct the care of the nursing assistants. However, LPNs are ultimately under the supervision of a registered nurse. Don't panic and pull out all your management textbooks to review. Evaluate such questions in terms of general guidelines for delegation and supervision. Pay close attention to the person to whom the nurse is assigning the care or nursing activity: Is it to another RN, is it to a less qualified person (LVN or LPN), or is a specific activity (bathing, ambulating, etc.) being delegated to an unlicensed nursing assistant?

- **Don't assign steps of the nursing process or nursing judgment to anyone except an RN.** The implementation of the nursing process and the judgments based on the nursing process must be performed by an RN.
- **Don't delegate teaching assignments to anyone except another RN.** This is another area that is the primary responsibility of the RN.
- **Keep in mind the NCLEX Hospital.** Adequate staff is available to provide client care; don't worry about staff shortages. Focus on the needs of the client in the question; what is happening in the rest of the unit is not a consideration unless it is part of the actual question. The only client to consider in each question is the one involved in that question, not the other clients the nurse may have been assigned.
- **Identify the most stable client.** The most stable client is the one who has the *most predictable outcome* and is *least likely* to have abrupt changes in condition that would require critical nursing judgments. For stable clients, some nursing care activities can be delegated to a nursing assistant or assigned to an LPN. When determining the stability of clients, Maslow's hierarchy of needs must be considered (see Chapter 3, Figure 3-1). Very carefully assess and identify clients who are in a changing unstable situation, especially those clients with a potential for respiratory compromise. These are clients for whom an RN should provide the care.
- **Delegate tasks that have specific guidelines.** Those tasks that have specific guidelines that are unchanging and are used in the care of a stable client can often be delegated. Bathing, collecting urine samples, feeding, providing personal hygiene, and assisting with ambulation are just a few examples of these activities. Remember you are in the NCLEX Hospital, so carefully evaluate the question and select an answer that has the RN delegating tasks to the assistive personnel and making appropriate assignments for other licensed health care personnel.
- **Identify your priority client.** The priority client is the one who is most likely to experience problems or ill effects if not taken care of first. Priority clients include those with respiratory compromise, those whose conditions are unstable and changing, and those who are at high risk for developing complications. NCLEX questions may present a typical nursing care assignment and ask which client the nurse would care for first; or a situation with a client may be presented, and you will be asked to select the first nursing action. Review the testing strategies regarding priority questions. It is important to identify the most unstable client, to see him or her first, and to determine what is necessary to do first for this client.

Establishing Nursing Priorities

Almost all nurses will agree that the NCLEX is full of priority questions. These questions may be worded in a variety of ways:

"What is the priority nursing action?"

"What should the nurse do first?"

"What is the best nursing action?"

In other words, the NCLEX wants to know whether the nurse can identify the most important nursing action to be taken in order to provide safe care for the client in the situation presented. In such cases, three or four of the options are frequently correct actions; however, one of the actions needs to be performed before the others. This is where critical thinking is necessary—*think like a nurse!* There are three areas to consider when determining priority nursing actions: Maslow's hierarchy of needs, the nursing process, and client safety.

- **Maslow's Hierarchy of Needs:** And you thought this was just for fundamentals! *Always consider Maslow's hierarchy of needs and remember that physiological needs must come first.* When evaluating options, identify client needs that are physiologic and those that are psychosocial. Physiologic needs are a higher priority than psychosocial or teaching needs. A client's physical needs must be met before his or her psychosocial or teaching needs are considered. Also remember that the ABCs (airway, breathing, and circulation) are the critical physiologic needs because these are at the base of Maslow's pyramid. However, be cautious— don't always select "airway" as the best answer. Sometimes the client does not have an airway problem, so don't read that into the question and give the client an airway problem! Maslow's hierarchy of needs also applies to psychosocial questions (see the section in this chapter regarding answering psychosocial questions).
- **Nursing Process:** The first step in the nursing process is *assessment.* However, do not automatically select an option that includes the word *assess* or an option that involves assessment. Assessment must be done to analyze and construct a nursing diagnosis, to develop a plan of care, and to determine the priority of nursing care implementation. If the assessment data are provided in the stem of the question, then it will be important to consider Maslow's hierarchy of needs when planning or selecting the best nursing action or implementation. If a nursing action has been implemented, then the question may focus on evaluating the effectiveness of the nursing action. Read the question carefully and determine what is being asked.
- **Safety Issues:** These issues may include situations in the hospital or in the client's home environment. The first

issue to consider is meeting basic needs of survival: oxygen, hydration, nutrition, elimination. Reduction of environmental hazards is also a concern and may include prevention of falls, accidents, and medication errors. Environmental safety also includes the prevention and spread of disease. This may include how to avoid contagious diseases or even activities such as handwashing. When you are critically evaluating questions that involve a client's safety and multiple options appear to be correct, determine what activity will be of most benefit to the client.

Example Questions for Management and Priority Setting

Question 1

An RN who has been working in the labor and delivery area has been reassigned to a step-down telemetry unit for the afternoon shift. Which clients would reflect the most appropriate assignment for this nurse?
1. Client who has undergone cardioversion and a client who was admitted during the night for possible myocardial infarction (MI).
2. Client who had a cardiac catheterization this morning and a client admitted for 24-hour observation for first-degree heart block.
3. Client who is currently in third-degree heart block and a client who had a hypertensive crisis with congestive heart failure 48 hours ago.
4. Client who had an MI 72 hours ago and is experiencing an increase in premature ventricular contractions (PVCs) and a newly admitted client with paroxysmal onset of atrial fibrillation.

Answer: 2. The labor and delivery RN needs to be assigned the most stable clients and the ones with the most predictable prognoses—these are the clients in option 2. Do not read into the situation and give the client who has had cardiac catheterization more problems. In option 1, the client who had a possible MI 16 hours ago is at risk for complications, as is the client who underwent cardioversion. In option 3, the client with third-degree heart block is most likely very unstable and may need a pacemaker. In option 4, the client who has had an MI is demonstrating signs of ventricular irritability, and the client with atrial fibrillation will need to be evaluated.

Question 2

The nurse is assigned a group of clients for care. Which client would the nurse assess first?
1. A client who had surgery 2 days ago and who is complaining of pain.
2. An older adult client reported to have increasing confusion and lethargy.
3. A newly admitted client with a serum blood urea nitrogen (BUN) level of 32 mg/dL.
4. A hypertensive client complaining of epigastric discomfort and midsternum chest pain.

Answer: 4. The client with chest pain is at greatest risk of experiencing immediate problems. This client needs to be evaluated immediately. Option 1, the client who had surgery, is experiencing pain. This is important but not alarming. Pain control needs to be addressed as soon as possible. In option 2, the client with increased lethargy and confusion needs to be evaluated. The confusion and lethargy are increasing; therefore, they were present prior to this time. These are psychosocial needs that need to be addressed; however, with the information presented, they do not represent an immediate physical problem. The newly admitted client in option 3 has a slightly elevated BUN level. This could be related to hydration problems, but the client is not presented in an unstable situation.

Question 3

A cardiac client turns on his call light and tells the nurse he is experiencing chest pain. What is the first nursing action?
1. Administer oxygen to the client at 4 L/min through a nasal cannula.
2. Assess heart sounds for the presence of ectopic beats.
3. Auscultate breath sounds and maintain airway.
4. Determine what the client was doing before the onset of pain.

Answer: 1. When a client complains of chest pain, oxygen should be started immediately and then vital signs should be further assessed. In the stem of the question, a cardiac client with chest pain is presented; that is enough critical assessment information for a nursing action. It is assumed that the nurse has an order for the oxygen. Further assessment will determine the status of the vital signs, and options 2 and 4 can be completed. Listening for ectopic beats and determining breath sounds are assessment activities; however, this does not provide further definitive information for determining immediate nursing care. In option 4, whether physical exertion was a factor in the occurrence of the chest pain can be determined later, but this is not an immediate concern. Option 3 gives this client airway problems, and there is no indication in the stem that the airway is an issue at this time.

Question 4

A client has returned from abdominal surgery, and the nurse is assessing the incisional area. The dressing has some bright red blood on it, and on closer inspection, the nurse determines that there is a loop of bowel protruding. What is the best nursing action?
1. Remove the dressing and place a sterile dressing soaked in saline on the wound with dry reinforcement dressings on top.
2. Remove the dressing and with sterile gloves apply very gentle pressure to replace the exposed bowel.
3. Leave the dressing in place and apply an abdominal pressure dressing to prevent further exposure of the bowel.
4. Immediately notify the health care provider and then cleanse the wound area with sterile saline solution and replace the dressing.

Answer: 1. The best nursing action is to cover the exposed bowel with a sterile dressing soaked in saline to prevent drying and tissue damage to the exposed bowel; then the surgeon or health care provider should be notified. Option 2 should not be done, because there may be vascular impairment to the bowel below the surface. In option 3, the dressing needs to be replaced with a moist one to protect the bowel. In option 4, the wound needs to be covered with the moist dressing before notifying the doctor. The wound should not be cleansed, because it is not a dirty wound.

Strategies for Evaluating Multiple-Choice Questions

Test-taking strategies are very beneficial during nursing school, as well as on the NCLEX. Start using them on current exams. Implementing testing strategies now will help to increase test scores in school, in addition to being one more step toward success on the NCLEX (Box 1-1).

Question Characteristics

The majority of questions on the NCLEX, as well as on nursing school exams, are multiple-choice format. This is the type of test question that is the most familiar to candidates.

Stem of the Question

The *stem* presents information or describes a client situation. The part of the stem that asks the question will present a problem or situation. The question may be presented as complete or an incomplete sentence. One of the options presented will most correctly answer the question or complete the sentence. (Figure 1-3)

Box 1-1 APPLYING TESTING STRATEGIES

Check Out the Question!
1. Read the question from beginning to end.
2. Check for words that establish the question as asking for a priority: *first action, priority nursing action, most important,* or *best.*
3. Is the answer going to be a true or positive statement? Or is the question asking for an answer that is a negative or false statement? Words such as *not working, contraindication,* and *avoid* indicate answers that are giving negative or false statements.
4. Rephrase the question in your own words. Do you understand what the question is asking?

Now Go for the Options ...
- Look at option 1: Is it true or false? Does it answer what the question is asking?
- Go through every option: Eliminate it if it is not a correct answer; keep it around if it is a possible right answer.
- If option 2 is a good option, but option 3 is better, then eliminate option 2! After all options have been evaluated, what is left? If you are left with only one option, great, that is the answer!
- If you are left with two options, go back and reread the question; decide which of the two options is best, select it, and move on.

Options

There are four options from which to choose an answer.
- Three options are distracters; they are designed to create a distraction from the correct answer.
- One option correctly answers the question asked in the stem.
- There is only one correct response; no partial credit is given for another answer.

FIGURE 1-3 Multiple-choice question.

Specific Strategies and Examples of Multiple-Choice Questions

1. **Read the question carefully before ever looking at or considering the options.** If you glance through the options before understanding the question, you may pick up key words that will affect the way you perceive the question.

   It is important to understand the question and not formulate an opinion about the answer before you understand the question. On a paper-and-pencil test, cover the answers with your hand or a note card. If you practice this strategy before taking the NCLEX, you will be able to focus on the question without physically covering the answers when taking a test on the computer.

2. **Do not read extra meaning into the question.** The question is asking for specific information; if it appears to be simple "common sense," then assume it is simple. Do not look for a hidden meaning in a question. Avoid asking yourself "what if …?" or speculating about the future ("maybe the client will …"). Don't make the client any sicker then he or she already is!

Example: A bronchoscopy was performed on a client at 7:00 AM. The client returns to his room, and the nurse plans to assist him with his morning care. The client refuses the morning care. What is the best nursing action regarding the morning care for this client?
1. Perform all of his morning care to prevent him from becoming short of breath.
2. Avoid morning care and continue to monitor vital signs and assess swallowing reflexes.
3. Postpone the morning care until client is more comfortable and can participate.
4. Cancel all of the morning care because it is not necessary to perform it after a bronchoscopy.

The correct answer is 3. The question is asking for a nursing judgment regarding morning care. Do not read into the question and make it more difficult by trying to put in information relating to respiratory care, such as checking for gag and swallowing reflexes.

3. **Read the stem correctly.** Make sure you understand exactly what information the question is asking. Determine whether the question is stated in a positive (true) or negative (false) format.

   Watch for words that provide direction to the question. A positive or true stem may include the following: "indicates the client understands," "the best nursing action is," "the preoperative teaching would include," or "the best nursing assignment is." Also watch for words in the stem that have a

negative meaning so that the question is asking for a response that is *not* accurate or is false. Phrases such as "is contraindicated," "the client should *avoid*," "indicate the client *does not understand*," "does not occur," and "indicates [medication, equipment, nursing action] is *not working*" are negative indicators. The question is asking for information that is not accurate or actions the nurse would not take. The following words or phrases change the direction of the question: *except, never, avoid, least, contraindicated, would not occur.* It may help to rephrase the question in your own words to better understand what information is being requested.

Example: Clients with arteriosclerotic heart disease (ASHD) go through several stages before becoming severely compromised. In considering the pathophysiology of heart disease, the nurse would identify what physical response that **does not occur** in the early stages of ASHD?
1. Decreased urine output
2. Dyspnea on exercise
3. Anginal pain relieved by rest
4. Increased serum triglyceride levels

Rephrase the question: What is not a characteristic finding in the early stages of ASHD? It is important to identify the key point "early stages of ASHD" and the key words "does not occur." If you miss these essential points, you do not understand the question, and chances are you will not choose the correct answer. The correct answer is option 1; a decrease in urine output occurs when cardiac disease is advanced enough to cause a severe decrease in cardiac output and renal perfusion. All the other options occur earlier in ASHD.

4. **Watch where the client is in the disease process or condition he or she is experiencing.** Examples of this are phrases such as "immediately postoperatively," "the first postoperative day," and "experienced a myocardial infarction this morning."

Example: A client had a cardiac catheterization through the left femoral artery. During the first few hours after the cardiac catheterization procedure, which nursing action would be most important?

*Rewording: What is the **most important** nursing care in the **first few hours** after a cardiac catheterization?*
1. Check his temperature every 2 hours and monitor catheter insertion site for inflammation.
2. Elevate the head of his bed 90 degrees and keep affected extremity straight.
3. Evaluate his blood pressure and respiratory status every 15 minutes for 4 to 6 hours.
4. Check his pedal and femoral pulses every 15 minutes for first hour, and then every 30 minutes.

The correct answer is 4. The phrase, "during the first few hours after the procedure," is important in answering this question correctly. The danger of hemorrhage and hematoma at the punc-

ture site is greatest during this time. The question also asks for the most important nursing care. Option 3: it is important to evaluate vital signs, but it is not required that they be evaluated every 15 minutes for 4 to 6 hours if client is stable. Option 4 is critical in the first few hours following a cardiac catheterization.

> 5. **Before considering the options, think about the characteristics of the condition and critical nursing concepts.** What are the nursing priorities in caring for a client with this condition/procedure/medication/problem?

Example: A woman who gave birth 3 days ago returns to the clinic with complaints of soreness and fullness in her breasts and states that she wants to stop breastfeeding her infant until her breasts feel better. What is the best nursing response?

This is a positive question. The answer will be a true statement. Think about breastfeeding and the common discomforts and problems the client encounters. Don't look at the options yet. Think, "Is it normal to have fullness and soreness in the breasts during the first 3 days of lactation, and what happens if she stops breastfeeding the infant?" Now evaluate the options:

1. Show the client how to apply a breast binder to decrease the discomfort and the production of milk.
2. Tell the client that breast fullness may be a sign of infection and she will not be able to continue breastfeeding.
3. Suggest to the client that she decrease her fluid intake for the next 24 hours to temporarily suppress lactation.
4. Explain to the client that the breast discomfort is normal and that the infant's sucking will promote the flow of milk.

In this question, option 4 is correct. Initially, breast soreness may occur for about 2 to 3 minutes at the beginning of each feeding until the let-down reflex is established. Options 1, 2, and 3 would decrease her milk production; the question did not state that she wanted to quit breastfeeding permanently.

> 6. **Identify the step in the nursing process being tested.** Remember, you must have adequate *assessment* data before you move through the steps of the nursing process. Is there adequate information presented in the stem of the question to determine appropriate nursing planning or intervention? Is the correct nursing action to obtain further assessment data? Look for key words that can assist you in determining what type of information is being requested.

Example: An 85-year-old client from a residential care facility is brought into the emergency department. Numerous bruises and abrasions in various stages of healing are present on the client's face and arms. The attendant from the residential facility explains that the client fell down. What is the priority nursing action?

1. Call the residential facility and ask for an incident report.
2. Put ice on the bruises and cover the abrasions with protective gauze.
3. Notify the supervisor regarding the possibility of an abusive situation.
4. Perform a head-to-toe assessment and determine the extent of the injuries.

The correct answer is 4, to determine or assess the extent of injuries. The stem of the question did not present adequate information with which to make a nursing judgment, and the client's physiologic needs are the priority. Option 1 does not immediately alleviate pain or assist the client. Options 2 and 3 relate to nursing actions that may be done after the immediate injuries and needs have been assessed. Focus on the client; priority setting and physiologic needs must be addressed first.

> 7. **Confused at this point? What if, after reading the question, you aren't sure what the question is even asking?** Take a deep breath, reread the question, and ask yourself, "What is the main topic of the question?" Now read the option choices, not to eliminate options or select a correct answer, but to get a clue as to the *direction* of the question. It might be helpful to read the options from the bottom up (start with option 4, rather than option 1) to help your brain focus on the options.

Example: A mother brings in a toddler with pediculosis capitis. A prescription of 1% permethrin (Nix) is given to her. What is important for the nurse to teach the mother?

Ask yourself: Is the question asking about prevention of pediculosis, complications, prevention of spread of the disease, or treatment? Check out the options. Is there an indication in the options as to the direction of the question?

1. Medication should be applied daily for 1 week with an additional follow-up treatment in 7 days.
2. Clothing, toys, and personal belongings of other family members do not require any special care.
3. Solution should be applied today and be applied again if nits are still visible in 24 hours.
4. Allow the medication to remain in contact with the scalp for 10 minutes and then thoroughly rinse.

After checking out the options, it appears that the question is asking for teaching implications for the mother regarding the use of the medication, Nix. Now that you have determined what you need to identify, you can begin the process of elimination of the options until you have found the correct answer.

The correct answer is 4. The Nix solution needs to remain on the scalp for 10 minutes before the hair is rinsed. Option 1 is too frequent for the medication to be used. Option 2 is incorrect, because the child's clothing and toys, as well as clothing and toys of the siblings, will need to be treated. Option 3 is not correct because medication should be reapplied in 7 days.

8. **Don't focus on predicting a right answer!** Frequently, the answer you anticipate is not going to be an option! Keep in mind the characteristics and concepts of nursing care for a client with the condition or problem in the situation presented. Eliminate options: every time you eliminate an option, you increase your chance of selecting a correct answer. If all of the options are plausible, then rank the options. The first one is the highest priority, and the fourth one is the lowest priority. Which one is the first action or answers the question?

Example: A client has an ulcer (2 in × 2 in) on the calf of his right leg. The area around the ulcer is inflamed, and the ulcer is draining purulent fluid. The vital signs are pulse, 114 beats/min; respiration, 22 breaths/min; temperature, 101° F. Which order will the nurse implement first?

Reword the question: The client has an infection in the ulcer on his leg. His temperature is elevated, and so is his pulse; this is a normal response to infection. Of the orders listed here, what nursing actions do I need to do first?

1. Administer ceftriaxone (Rocephin), 1 g, intravenously every 4 hours.
2. Perform blood cultures ×2, 20 minutes apart and drawn from different sites.
3. Apply polysporin (Bacitracin) ointment topically to leg ulcer three times a day.
4. Administer acetaminophen (Tylenol), 650-mg suppository, every 4 hours for temperature above 101.8° F.

Rank the options:

1st—Option 2; blood cultures must be obtained prior to antibiotic.

2nd—Option 1 needs to done after the blood cultures have been drawn.

3rd—Option 4 will not produce any immediate response or assistance in treating the problem, although it will make the client more comfortable.

4th—Option 3 will help to reduce the infection, but the priority is to obtain the culture and then for the antibiotic to be started.

Here is another approach to the options:

Consider option 1—This is an antibiotic that will begin to fight the infection.

Consider option 2—This is important to do to identify the causative bacteria. This is more important now than option 1; eliminate option 1.

Consider option 3—This is treating the infection topically. It will cause a decrease in the surface bacteria, but the blood cultures are still a priority. Eliminate this option because both options 1 and 2 are more important.

Consider option 4—This is treating the symptoms rather than the cause of the problem, which is not as important as option 1 or option 2; eliminate it.

All of these options are feasible for treating this client; however, obtaining the blood culture is the most important (option 2). If

you had approached this question with a specific answer in mind (give an antibiotic), you would have found that answer; however, it would have been wrong.

9. **Evaluate all of the options in a systematic manner.** After you understand the question, read all options carefully. Remember, distracters are designed to be plausible to the situation and thus to "distract" you from the correct answer. All the options may be correct, but only one will be the best answer.

Example: A client has just returned to his room from the recovery room after a lumbar laminectomy and is in stable condition. In considering possible complications the client might experience in the next few hours, what nursing action is most important?

1. Monitor vital signs every 4 hours.
2. Assess breath sounds every 2 hours.
3. Evaluate every 2 hours for urinary retention.
4. Check when he last had a bowel movement.

All of these options are plausible for the situation. However, consider that this is the client's operative day, he is currently stable, and the question is asking for complications he might encounter in the next few hours after lumbar laminectomy. Options 1 and 4 are not appropriate at this period of postoperative recovery; vital signs should be checked more often, and constipation can be more effectively addressed at a later time— eliminate these from consideration. Option 2 would be appropriate if respiratory problems were anticipated; however, there is no indication of respiratory compromise. (Remember, don't always select airway-related answers.) The correct answer is 3, because this is a common problem in the immediate postoperative period after a lumbar laminectomy.

10. **As you read the options, eliminate those that you know are not correct.** Consider each option as true or false. This will help narrow the field of choice. When you select an answer or eliminate an option, you should have a specific reason for doing so. Correctly eliminating options will increase your chances of selecting the correct answer.

Example: A client is in her third trimester of pregnancy and she is scheduled for an abdominal ultrasonogram. The nurse explains to the client that results of this exam will reveal what information regarding the fetus?

1. Maturity of the fetus's lungs *(No, this is false; the ultrasound does not show any evidence of surfactant or maturational level of the lungs.)*
2. Presence of congenital heart defect *(No, this is false; the ultrasound is not specific enough to reveal congenital heart defects, but will show fetal cardiac movement.)*

3. Gestational age *(Yes, this is true; ultrasonography gives an overall picture of bone formation [biparietal diameter (BPD)], thereby indicating gestational age.)*
4. Rh factor antibody level *(No, this is false; this level must be determined by a blood test to evaluate for isoimmunization or hemolytic disease of the newborn.)*

After a systematic evaluation of the options, option 3 is the correct answer.

---

11. **Identify similarities in the options.** Frequently, the options will contain similar information, and sometimes you can eliminate similar options. If three options are similar, the different one may be the correct answer. When two of the options are very similar and one of those options is not any better than the other, both of them are probably wrong, so start looking for another answer. Sometimes three of the options have very similar characteristics; the option that is different may be the correct answer.

Example: The nurse is assisting a client to identify foods that would meet the requirements for a high-protein, low-residue diet. Which foods would represent correct choices for this diet?
1. Roast beef, slice of white bread.
2. Fried chicken, green peas.
3. Broiled fish, green beans.
4. Cottage cheese, tomatoes.

Options 1, 2, and 3 all contain a meat or fish that would be needed for a high-protein diet; therefore option 4 can be eliminated. Options 2, 3, and 4 all contain a vegetable that has a skin, making these high-residue choices. The correct answer is option 1, for both high-protein and low-residue qualities. Note that the NCLEX will not focus on dishes that contain a mixture of foods, in which you would need to know the recipe to answer correctly. Also, unless specified, do not attribute special characteristics to a food; if a food has a special characteristic, it will be stated (e.g., "low sodium" soup or "low fat" yogurt).

---

12. **Identify words in the options that are "qualifiers."** *Every, none, all, always, never,* and *only* are words that have no exceptions. Options containing these words are frequently incorrect. Seldom in health care is anything absolute with no exceptions; thus you can often eliminate these options. In some situations the qualifiers are correct, especially when a principle or policy is described. For example, the nurse *always* establishes positive client identification before administering medications. This would be a correct statement. Carefully evaluate qualifiers; they are clues to the correct answer.

Example: The nurse is obtaining a specimen from a client's incisional area for a wound culture and sensitivity. What client information will the sensitivity part of the procedure reflect?
1. Presence and characteristics of all bacteria present in the client's wound
2. Which antibiotics will effectively treat the bacteria present
3. Differentiation of the bacteria and viruses present in the wound
4. All the treatments to which the bacteria are responsive

Options 1 and 4 contain the word "all." If you did not know the answer, you could eliminate options 1 and 4. Identifying all the bacteria and all the treatments is not feasible from a culture and sensitivity. This would give you a 50% chance of finding the right answer, which is option 2.

---

13. **Select the most comprehensive answer.** All of the options may be correct, but one option may *include* the other three options or need to be considered first.

Example: The nurse is planning to teach a client with diabetes about his condition. Before the nurse provides instruction, what is most important to evaluate? The client's:
1. Required dietary modifications.
2. Understanding of the exchange list.
3. Ability to administer insulin.
4. Present understanding of diabetes.

Options 1, 2, and 3 are certainly important considerations in diabetic education. However, they cannot be initiated until the nurse evaluates the client's knowledge of his or her disease state. When two options appear to say the same thing, only in different words, then look for another answer; that is, eliminate the options that you know are incorrect. Options 1 and 2 both refer to the client's understanding of nutrition.

---

14. **Some questions may have options that contain several items to consider.** After you are sure you understand what information the question is requesting, evaluate each part of the option. Is the option appropriate to what the question is asking? If an option contains one incorrect item, the entire option is incorrect. All of the items listed in the option must be correct if that option is to be the correct answer to the question.

Example: In evaluating the lab data of a client experiencing renal failure, the nurse would identify what findings as indicative of increasing renal failure?
1. Increased BUN level, hyperkalemia, decreased creatinine clearance
2. Increased hemoglobin, hyponatremia, increased urine electrolytes

3. High fasting blood glucose level, increased prothrombin time
4. Increased platelets, increased urine specific gravity, proteinuria

Option 1 is correct. In a methodic evaluation of the items in the options, you can eliminate options. The item "increased hemoglobin and urine electrolytes" in option 2 and the item "increased urine specific gravity" in option 4 make these two options incorrect. Option 3 has nothing to do with renal failure; the blood glucose level is associated more with diabetes and endocrine problems.

---

15. **After you have selected an answer, reread the question.** Does the answer you chose give the information the question is asking for? Sometimes the options are correct but do not answer the question.

Example: A client is 88 years of age and has previously been alert, oriented, and active. The nursing assistant reports that on awakening this morning, the client was disoriented and confused. What initial action would the nurse take to determine the possible cause of this change in the client's behavior?
1. Review the history for any previous episodes of this type of behavior.
2. Call the health care provider and discuss the changes in the client's behavior.
3. Do a thorough neurologic evaluation to evaluate the specific changes in behavior.
4. Evaluate for the presence of a urinary tract infection and for adequate hydration.

Option 4 is the only answer that supplies what the question asked for ("determine the possible cause of this change"). The most common cause of a sudden change in the behavior of an older adult client is a significant physiologic change, often an infection (commonly in the urinary tract) or dehydration. Options 1 and 3 relate more to the gradual behavior changes seen in the progression of dementia and do nothing "to determine the possible cause ..." Option 2 also does not provide any assistance in determining the cause of the behavior change; further nursing assessment needs to be conducted before calling for assistance.

Alternate Format Questions

In an effort to improve and more effectively assess the entry-level nurse, the NCSBN has introduced "alternate format questions" to the examination. These questions were included on the NCLEX beginning in April 2003. There is no established percentage of alternate format items a candidate will receive. The alternate format questions that have been previously validated are placed in the test item pools and are randomly selected to meet the items on the test plan and the established level of difficulty. The NCSBN has not specified a number of alternate format questions that will be included in a candidate's test bank. A candidate should expect several alternate format questions. It is important to consider that there will be 15 pretest or unscored items in the first 75 questions on every candidate's examination. Within those 15 items, there may be several unscored alternate format items. It is important to answer all the questions to the very best of your ability because you do not know which questions are scored items and which are unscored items.[3,4]

The alternate format questions should not have any impact on what you study or how you study. The content on the alternate format questions is from the same test plan as the other questions. The test-taking strategies are essentially the same with minor modifications. In other words, there is no reason to be alarmed about the alternate format questions; they are testing the same information, just in a different type of question.

Multiple Response

[NCLEX-RN]

Candidate Name   Section time remaining: 3:15.20

The nurse is caring for an 85-year old client who has a diagnosis of *Mycoplasma* pneumonia. What precautions will the nurse implement in assisting the client with morning care?

Select all that apply:

☑ 1.   Wear clean gloves.
☐ 2.   Remove all extra suctioning supplies from the room.
☐ 3.   Dispose of the gown and mask in container outside client's door.
☑ 4.   Wear face mask when working within 3 feet of the client.
☑ 5.   Put on a gown prior to entering the room.
☐ 6.   Remove the stethoscope from the room if it did not come in contact with the client.

Select the best response. Click the Next (N) button or the Enter key to confirm answer and proceed.   ITEM 21

Next (N)   Calculator (O)

Answer: The answer is based on standard precautions, plus respiratory precautions for the pneumonia. Nothing should be removed from the room and the gown should be removed prior to leaving the room, not outside the room.

FIGURE 1-4 Alternate format question—multiple response.

Multiple-Response Items

Multiple-response items require you to select all of the options that apply to the question. The items have more than four options from which to select and will clearly state "Select all that apply." Using the mouse, you will select each item to be included in the answer—consider each item and make a decision whether it is to be included in the correct answer. The options are preceded by square boxes, and you can check more than one box. You must select all the answers that are correct to the question. If you do not select all of the correct options that apply to the question, the answer will be considered wrong.

Testing Strategy: Think about the question presented in Figure 1-4. Standard plus droplet precautions will be used for this client. What is added to standard precautions when droplet precautions are included? Go through all of the options and decide which options are true and are something the nurse should do; then select all of the true options that apply to this client.

Answer: Options 1, 4, and 5. In option 1, yes (true), the nurse is going to provide morning care and have direct contact with the client; therefore gloves should be worn. Option 2, no (false), the suctioning supplies should be left in the room. Option 3, no (false), the gown and mask are disposed of in the client's room. Option 4, yes (true), a mask is necessary if the nurse is to come within 3 feet of the client, which the nurse can expect to do when providing or assisting with morning care. Option 5, yes (true), a gown should be worn because the nurse is going to be close to and have direct contact with the client. Option 6, no (false), the stethoscope should not be taken into the client's room; if it is taken into the room, it should be left in the room.

Fill-in-the-Blank

Fill-in-the-blank questions are frequently presented for medication dosage calculations, IV drip calculations, or intake and output calculations—just to name a few (Figure 1-5). A drop-down calculator is provided on the computer screen. With calculation questions, the final unit of measurement will always be provided. Only the number will be placed in the answer box. Check the items necessary to make this calculation. For example, is it necessary to make conversions from grams to milligrams? from liters to milliliters? Make sure all of the units of measure needed in the final answer are in the same system of measurement.

Memorize the formulas necessary to calculate the drug dosages and conversions. The number of decimal places to be included in the answer will be indicated in the question. Do not round any numbers until you have the final answer. You should not enter any other characters except those necessary to form a number.[3]

Hot Spot Questions

In a hot spot question, you will be presented with a graphic and asked to identify a specific item, area, or location on the graphic. Look at Figure 1-6. Find the requested area on the graphic and then you would click on it with the mouse.

Answer: The "hot spot" (in this case, the correct area to assess the apical heart rate) is at the PMI, or point of maximum impulse, which is located at the fifth intercostal space, just to the left of the sternal border. In this situation, you would place the mouse over the area and click on that area.

Drag and Drop

In a drag-and-drop question, several steps or actions are listed, and your job is to place them in a correct sequence (Figure 1-7). All of the options will be used, but you must place them in the correct order. The first thing to do is to decide in what order you want to place the options or rank the actions. After you have determined your answer, click on the option you want to place first, "drag" that option over, and place it in the first box. Then select the option you want to place second, drag that option over, and place it in the next box. Continue this process until you have used all of

Fill in the Blank

[NCLEX-RN]

Candidate Name   Section time remaining: 2:25.40

The physician calls the unit and leaves an order for cefaclor (Ceclor) 0.1 gm PO, every 6 hours. The dose available in the unit is 125 mg/5 mL. How many milliliters will the nurse give?

What is the Apgar score?

Answer: 4 mL

Select the best response. Click the Next (N) button or the Enter key to confirm answer and proceed.   ITEM 20

Next (N)   Calculator (0)

Answer - 4 mL: Rationale: 1 gm = 1000 mg, therefore 0.1 gm = 100 mg   125 mg : 5 mL :: 1000 mg : x mL
Formula: 125 x X = 125X (Note: Multiply the two outside numbers of the ratio equation together, then the two inside numbers; solve for X by dividing the total of the inside numbers by the outside numbers.)
5 x 100 = 500   X = 500/125 = 4 mL

FIGURE 1-5 Alternate format question—fill-in-the-blank.

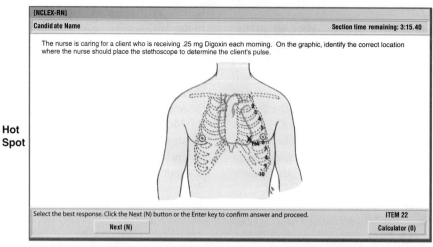

Hot Spot

Answer: To evaluate the apical pulse the stethoscope should be placed on the area of the PMI - left midclavicular line, 5th intercostal space. To answer this question, you would simply click the area on the graphic. The correct location is noted in the figure.

FIGURE 1-6 Alternate format question—hot spot.

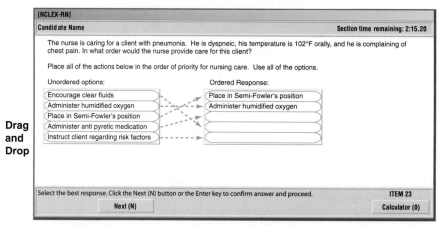

Drag and Drop

Need to know: Review each of the items in the list. Determine what is the most important action to take first, then second, etc. This question is asking you to provide care for a client who is experiencing difficulty breathing and has chest pain. The dyspnea and chest pain are most likely a result of the client's pneumonia. Position is the first thing that you can do that will benefit the client the most, then begin the oxygen, administer the antipyretic medication, encourage clear liquids, and teaching is last. Remember Maslow when setting priorities.

FIGURE 1-7 Alternate format question—ordered response (drag and drop).

the options present. Practice by considering how you would answer the question in Figure 1-7.

Answer: The client should be placed in a semi-Fowler's position before oxygen administration is started; an antipyretic medication should then be given. This action addresses current needs. Next, encourage intake of clear liquids to decrease viscosity of secretions. Finally, provide instruction regarding risk factors (psychosocial need).

Chart or Exhibit Items

In this type of question, a client situation or problem and client information are provided in a chart or an exhibit (Figures 1-8 through 1-12). To begin, click on the tab on the bottom of the screen to see the exhibit; then click on the tabs within the exhibit to find the information needed to answer the question. There may be several tabs to click on, check the information included within each tab, and determine if it is pertinent to the situation.

Interpretation of information: Client received morphine 10 mg IM at 11:00 AM; became lethargic and slept for the next 5 hours. He received hydrocodone PO at 4:00 PM and was com-

fortable for the next 4 hours. The doctor's orders are current for both the IM and the PO medication for pain.

Answer: 4. Give the hydrocodone, PO, for pain at this time. It is preferable to give a client a PO pain medication than a parenteral pain medication. The hydrocodone provided effective pain relief for 4 hours when it was administered the last time, and the doctor's order is current.

Audio Questions

Beginning in 2010. "audio" questions will be included on the NCLEX. The screen will tell the candidate to place the head phones on to listen to the information. The information may be replayed if necessary. After listening to the information, the candidate will select an answer from the options presented.

Therapeutic Nursing Process: Principles of Communication

Throughout the examination there will be questions requiring use of the principles of therapeutic communication. In therapeutic communication questions, do not assume

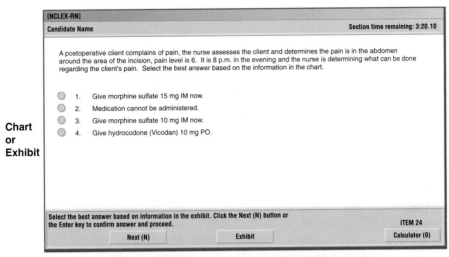

FIGURE 1-8 Alternate format question—exhibit item.

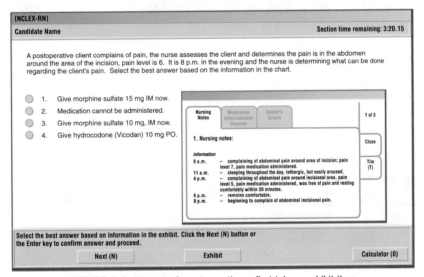

FIGURE 1-9 Alternate format question—first tab on exhibit item.

[NCLEX-RN]

Candidate Name   Section time remaining: 3:20.20

A postoperative client complains of pain, the nurse assesses the client and determines the pain is in the abdomen around the area of the incision, pain level is 6. It is 8 p.m. in the evening and the nurse is determining what can be done regarding the client's pain. Select the best answer based on the information in the chart.

  1. Give morphine sulfate 15 mg, IM now.
  2. Medication cannot be administered.
  3. Give morphine sulfate 10 mg, IM now.
  4. Give hydrocodone (Vicodan) 10 mg PO.

| Nursing Notes | Medication Administration Records | Doctor's Orders | | 2 of 3 |

2. Medication administration record (MAR):

Morphine sulfate 10 mg IM administered at 8 a.m.

Hydrocodone 10 mg, PO administered at 4 p.m.

Close

Tile (T)

Select the best answer based on information in the exhibit. Click the Next (N) button or the Enter key to confirm answer and proceed.

ITEM 24

Next (N)   Exhibit   Calculator (0)

FIGURE 1-10 Alternate format question—second tab on exhibit item.

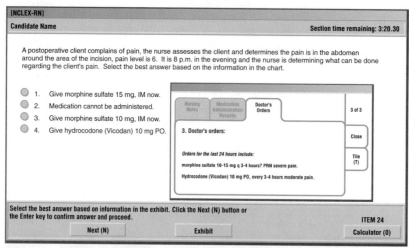

FIGURE 1-11 Alternate format question—third tab on exhibit item.

FIGURE 1-12 Alternate format question—analysis and selection of an answer for exhibit item.

the client is being manipulative or is in control of how he or she feels. Psychosocial problems or mental health problems are most often not under the conscious control of the client.

ALERT Use therapeutic communication techniques to provide support to client and the family; establish a trusting nurse-client relationship; assess psychosocial, spiritual, cultural and occupational factors affecting care; allow time to communicate with client/family and significant others; provide therapeutic environment.

- **Situations requiring use of therapeutic communication are not always centered around a psychiatric client.** Frequently, these questions are centered on the client experiencing stress and anxiety. There may be questions relating to therapeutic communication in the care of

clients experiencing stress, anxiety related to a specific client situation, or a change in body image as a result of physiologic problems.

- **Look for responses that focus on the concerns of the client.** Do not focus on the concerns of the nurse, hospital, or physician. Determine whether the client is the central focus of the question or whether the question pertains to a spouse or significant other.

- **Watch for responses that are open-ended and encourage the client to express how he or she feels.** Clients frequently experience difficulty in expressing their feelings. Focus on responses that encourage a client to describe how he or she feels. These are frequently open-ended statements made by the nurse.

- **Eliminate responses that are not honest and direct.** In order to build trust and promote a positive relationship, it is important to be honest with the client. Options that include telling the client "don't worry," or "everything is going to be all right," or "your doctor knows best" will be wrong answers.

- **Look for responses that indicate an acceptance of the client.** Regardless of whether the client's views or moral values are in agreement with yours, it is important to respect his or her views and beliefs. Responses that involve telling clients what they *should* or *should no*t be doing are often wrong answers (e.g., telling an alcoholic that she should quit drinking or telling a depressed client that he should not feel that way).

- **Be careful about responses that give opinions or advice on the client's situation.** Do not assume an authoritarian position. You should not insist that the client follow your advice (e.g., quit drinking, exercise more, quit smoking).

- **Do not select options or responses that block further interaction.** These options are frequently presented as closed statements or questions that encourage a yes-or-no answer from the client. Better responses are those that indicate an expectation of a more revealing verbal response from the client. **Examples:** "Are you feeling better today?" The client can just answer no to this question. It is better to ask, "How are you feeling today as compared to yesterday?" Likewise, it is better to ask, "How did you feel when your family visited today?" rather than "Did your family visit today?"

- **Look for responses that reflect, restate, or paraphrase feelings the client expressed.** Look for responses that encourage the client to describe how he or she feels— responses that reflect, restate, or paraphrase feelings the client expresses. An option such as "You should not feel that way" is bound to be a wrong answer. It is better to ask, "How did that make you feel?"

- **Do not ask "why" a client feels the way he or she does.** Most of the time, if a client understood why he or she felt a certain way, the client would be able to do something about it. The most common answer when a nurse asks a client why he or she feels a certain way is "I don't know," which does not help anyone.

- **Do not use coercion to achieve a desired response.** Do not tell clients that they can't have their lunch until they get out of bed or bribe children to take their medicine with a promise of candy.

- **See examples of therapeutic and nontherapeutic communication in Chapter 9 (Table 9-3).**

TIPS FOR TEST-TAKING SUCCESS

- **Do not indiscriminately change answers.** On a paper-and-pencil test, if you go back and change an answer, you should have a specific reason for doing so. Sometimes you do remember information and realize you answered the question incorrectly. However, students often "talk themselves out" of the correct answer and change it to the incorrect one. The good news is that you cannot go back to previously answered questions on the NCLEX. At the point at which the examination asks you to confirm your answer, review the strategies used to answer

the question, confirm your answer, and move on to the next question.

- **Watch your timing. Do not spend too much time on one question.** It is very important to track your timing on practice exams. This will help you be more comfortable with timing on computer testing. The NCLEX will allow you a total of 6 hours to complete the examination. When you are taking a practice test, plan to spend about a minute on each question. Some questions you will answer quickly; others may take some time. Do not spend more than 2 minutes deliberating the answer to a question. If you do not have a good direction for the right answer in 2 minutes, then you probably don't know the answer. Eliminate all of the options you can, pick the best one, and move on. (Remember, you are not supposed to know *all* of the right answers.) Plan for an hour of practice testing, select 60 questions, and answer the questions using testing strategies. After answering the questions, review the correct answers and focus on what and why you missed questions. Practice your timing and application of test strategies so you will be comfortable with timing and the progression of questions on the NCLEX.

- **The NCLEX is a nursing competency examination, and the correct answer will focus on nursing knowledge and the provision of nursing care.** The examination does not focus on medical management or making a medical diagnosis.

- **Eliminate distracters that include the assumption that the client would not understand or would be ignorant of the situation and those distracters that protect clients from worry.** For example, "The client should not be told she has cancer because it would upset her too much" would almost certainly be an incorrect answer.

- **There is no pattern of correct answers.** The exam is compiled by a computer, and the position of the correct answers is selected at random. So, do not believe those who say to pick option 3 when you are guessing.

STUDY HABITS

Study Effectively

1. **Use memory aids, mind mapping, and mnemonics.** Memory aids and mind mapping are tools that assist you in drawing associations from other ideas with the use of visual images (Figure 1-13). Mnemonics are words, phrases, or other techniques that help you remember information. Images, pictures, and mnemonics will stay with you longer than written text information.

2. **Develop 3 × 5 cards with critical information.** Do not overload the card; put a statement or question on one side and answers or follow-up information on the other side. For example, on one side you might write "low potassium," and on the other side you would list the relevant values. Another card might say "nursing care for hypokalemia" on the front, and on the back, you could

FIGURE 1-13 Peritonitis: "Hot Belly." (From Zerwekh J, Claborn J: *Memory notebook of nursing,* vol 1, ed 4, Ingram, Texas, 2008, Nursing Education Consultants.)

list the nursing care. These cards are much easier for you to carry than a load of books or class notes. When you have developed and studied your set of cards with priority information, trade them with friends, and see what they have put on their cards. Sets of cards can be used whenever you have only 15 to 20 minutes of study time. Take 20 cards with you to soccer practice, the doctor's office, or anywhere you are going where you will to have to sit and wait for a few minutes. This is quick, easy, and very effective.

3. **Review class notes the next day.** A very effective study habit to develop during school is to review your class notes the day after the class. Set aside about an hour on the day after the class and spend about 30 to 45 minutes reviewing the notes from class. Do the notes make sense to you, or are you unclear on the meaning of some of the areas? Correlate the notes and the visuals the instructor presented with the information in the textbook. It is important to take the time now to understand the information presented the previous day because it is fresher in your mind and you are more receptive to learning. By reviewing the information after the class presentation, you more effectively and positively reinforce the learning process.

4. **Plan your study time when you are most receptive to learning.** Do not wait until the end of the day when you have finished everything else. It is difficult to get up at 6:00 AM, work all day, deal with family activities, and finally realize at 10:30 PM that you are just too tired to study. You may feel guilty that you were not able to study for the intended 2 hours that evening. Schedule your study time—it may be easier for you to study for 2 hours before leaving school than it may be to study for 2 hours when you get home.

5. **Set a schedule and let everyone know the schedule.** For example, when you set aside 1 hour for review on the day after your class, make sure everyone knows this is your study time. Do not expect your family to leave you alone while you study; this is frequently too much to ask, especially of children or a spouse. Go to the library, nursing school, or someone's house where there are no disturbances.

6. **Start planning your NCLEX preparation at the beginning of your last semester in school or 2 to 3 months before you will take the NCLEX.** Do not wait until the week before the exam to start preparing. Even if you were an A student, you still need to review. Information that was presented at the beginning of school, last year, or even last semester may not be current in your knowledge base.

Set a Study Goal

1. Decide on a study method.
2. Divide the review material into segments.
3. Prioritize the segments; review first the areas in which you feel you are deficient or weak. Leave those areas you are the most comfortable with and most knowledgeable about for last.
4. Practice testing, or an end of the semester assessment examination, will help you to identify areas in which you need additional review. Review this information in an NCLEX Review book, and then if it is not clear or if you need further explanation and information, consult your nursing textbooks.
5. Establish a realistic schedule and follow it. Planning for 8 hours of studying on your day off does not work. Instead, plan for 2 to 4 hours each day (in 20- to 30-minute chunks of time) and maybe 3 to 4 hours

on your days off. Let everyone know when you are planning to study and how important it is for you to study.

6. Plan on achieving your study goal several days before the examination.

Group Study

1. Limit the group to four or five people.
2. Group members should be mature and serious about studying.
3. The group should agree on the planned study schedule.
4. If the group makes you anxious or you do not feel it meets your study needs, do not continue to participate.
5. Group study is very effective with the right mix of participants.

Testing Practice

1. Include testing practice in your schedule.
2. Structure your practice testing.
   - Plan to answer one question per minute. Set aside 10 questions and answer them in 10 minutes; then review the answer and rationale for the question. This will allow you to focus on testing strategies and not break your train of thought by checking the right answers.
   - Evaluate your comfortable pace for answering questions; this will keep you on target with your timing as you practice answering test questions.
   - Do not answer a question and then stop to look up the correct answer. Answer all of the questions in the section you have set aside; then review the correct answers. This will reinforce your test-taking strategies and your test timing.
3. Try to answer the questions as if you were taking the real exam.
4. Use the testing strategies and practice on the questions included at the end of each chapter in the book and on the CD that accompanies this book.
5. Evaluate your practice exams for problem areas.
   - Test-taking skills: Did you know the material but answer the question incorrectly? In this case, a test-taking strategy can be applied; go back and review the strategies. Can you identify what strategy you should have used to identify the correct answer? By becoming aware of your test-taking habits, you will become more aware of the strategies you need to implement and you can begin to practice them more effectively.
   - Knowledge base: You did not know the material. Make a note of these areas and see whether the content begins to show trends or clusters of information in areas you need to study/review.
6. Evaluate the questions you answered incorrectly. Review the rationale for the right answer and understand why you missed it.
7. Reuse the questions at a later point to review the information again.
8. A CD with additional practice questions can be found in the back of this book. The more questions you practice

answering, the more effectively you will implement test-taking strategies.

DECREASE ANXIETY

Your activities on the day of the examination will strongly influence your level of anxiety. By carefully planning ahead, you can eliminate some anxiety-provoking situations.

1. Review the NCLEX tutorial at the Pearson Vue website. This same tutorial will be your orientation to the computer and the testing process. It should seem like an old friend when you see it.
2. Visit the examination site before the day of the exam. Consider travel time, parking, and time to get to the designated area. Get an early start to allow extra time; you need to arrive at the site 30 minutes before your scheduled testing time.
3. If you have to travel some distance to the examination site, try to spend the night in the immediate vicinity. Don't cram four or five people in one room. Everyone needs his or her own space!
4. Do something pleasant the evening before the examination. This is not the time to cram.
5. Anxiety is contagious. If those around you are extremely anxious, avoid contact with them before the examination.
6. Carefully consider whether you want to go to the testing site with anyone else. If the other person finishes before you do, will it put increased pressure on you to hurry up and finish? You don't need any additional pressures on the day of the exam or while you are taking it.
7. Make sure your meal before the test is a light, healthy one. Avoid eating highly spiced or different foods. This is not the time for a gastrointestinal upset.
8. Wear comfortable clothes. This is not a good time to wear tight clothing or new shoes.
9. Wear clothing of moderate weight. It is difficult to control the temperature to keep everyone comfortable. Wear layers of clothes that can be removed if you get too warm.
10. Wear soft-soled shoes; this decreases the noise in the testing area.
11. Make sure you have the ATT papers and photo ID that are required to gain admission to the examination site.
12. Do not take study material to the examination site. You are not allowed to take it into the testing area, and it is too late to study.
13. Do not panic when you encounter a clinical situation you have not heard of or a situation that increases your anxiety. Take a deep breath, close your eyes, and take a "mini" vacation to one of your very favorite places. Give yourself about 30 to 45 seconds and then return to the question. You may have gained a different perspective. Use good test-taking strategies, select an answer, and move on.
14. Reaffirm to yourself that you know the material. This is not the time for self-defeating behavior or negative

self-talk. **YOU WILL PASS!!** Build your confidence by visualizing yourself in 6 months as an RN working in the area you desire. Create that mental picture of where you want to be and who you want to be—an RN. Use your past successes to bring positive energy and "vibes" to your NCLEX exam. **WE KNOW YOU CAN DO IT!**

REFERENCES

1. Smith J, Crawford L: *Report of findings from the 2005 RN Practice Analysis, NCSBN research brief,* vol 9, Chicago, 2006, National Council of State Boards of Nursing.

2. Wendt A, Kenny L, Anderson J: *2007 NCLEX RN Detailed Test Plan* (Item writer, item reviewer, nurse educator version), Chicago, 2007, National Council of State Boards of Nursing.

3. *2009 NCLEX Examination Candidate Bulletin.* Chicago, National Council of State Boards of Nursing. Available at www.ncsbn.org. Accessed April 2009.

4. *Fast facts about alternate item formats and the NCLEX examination.* National Council of State Boards of Nursing. Available at www.ncsbn.org. Accessed April 2009.

CHAPTER TWO

Health Implications Across the Life Span

GROWTH AND DEVELOPMENT

A. Normal growth and development progress in a steady, predictable pattern across the life span.

B. When assessing the growth and development of a child or an adult, it is important to consider the characteristics of the developmental stage.
  1. Development progresses in a cephalocaudal (head to tail) manner.
  2. Development progresses from proximal to distal, with a progression from gross to fine motor skills.

C. Psychosocial, cognitive, moral, and spiritual development can be observed to occur in specific patterns as an infant matures.

D. The developmental age of a client is critical to the planning of care in the hospital.
  1. Nurses need to be aware of the major developmental milestones.
  2. Nursing care is planned around the child's developmental level, not his or her chronologic age.
  3. If an infant displays head lag at 6 months or cannot sit with support at 9 months, this is considered a significant developmental lag and the infant needs to have further developmental/neurologic evaluation (Table 2-1).

> **ALERT** Assess developmental stage of client. Evaluate client and/or family achievement of expected developmental level—especially with consideration to the developmental milestones.

Anticipatory Guidance for the Family of an Infant

A. Use an infant car seat, facing backwards.

B. Put the baby on his or her back or side to sleep.

C. By 3 to 4 months, infants sleep approximately 15 hours per day.

D. Safety.
  1. Keep one hand on the baby when he or she is on a high surface; baby rolls over around age 3 to 4 months.
  2. Never leave baby alone with young children or pets.
  3. Baby-proof your home: prevent access to stairs and cabinets; practice pool and tub water safety.
  4. After feeding, place infant on right side.

E. Immunization schedule (Figure 2-1).

> **NURSING PRIORITY** General contraindications to receiving an immunization include a moderate to severe illness with or without fever and an anaphylactic reaction to a previously administered immunization or to a substance in the immunization.

F. Talk and read to infant; provide visual and auditory stimulation; toys should stimulate hand-eye coordination, as well as provide sensory stimulation.

G. To prevent bottle tooth decay, do not put infant to bed with a bottle; offer juice in a cup at around 4 to 6 months when infant can put his or her lips to the rim of the cup.

H. For colds, fevers, and reactions to immunizations, administer infant-strength acetaminophen (Tylenol) and/or ibuprofen (Advil); increase fluids; do not administer aspirin products. Tepid baths also help to reduce fever.

I. Separation anxiety is a major stress for hospitalized child from middle infancy through the preschool years.
  1. Protest: loud crying and screaming for parent; child refuses attention from anyone else.
  2. Despair: crying stops and there is less activity; child is not interested in play and withdraws.
  3. Detachment (denial): child appears to have adjusted to hospitalization. Behavior is due to resignation, not a sign of contentment. This is not a positive reaction to hospitalization.

> **ALERT** Assist client/family to identify and participate in activities fitting the child's age, preference, physical capacity, and developmental level. Provide care that meets the special needs of the preschool client ages 1 month to 4 years.

Anticipatory Guidance for the Family of a Toddler

A. Continue to emphasize safety; discuss medications, poisons, car seats, latches on doors, falls, and water safety.

B. Toilet training usually begins around 2 years; accidents are common.

C. Sibling rivalry is common if there is a new baby in the family.

D. Temper tantrums are attention-seeking behavior and are not uncommon for a toddler.

Table 2-1	GROWTH AND DEVELOPMENT	
Birth-4 months	Consistently gains weight (5-7 oz per week) Posterior fontanel closes Responds to sounds and begins vocalizing Gains head control → lifts chest → rolls over one way Smiles responsively → smiles when spoken to	Teething may begin Coordination progresses from jerky movement to grasping objects Provide toys that increase hand-eye coordination
4-9 months	Doubles birth weight (gains 3-5 oz per week) Teething begins with lower incisors Sits with support; begins crawling Turns over in both directions Laughs aloud	Reaches for objects and grasps them Begins "stranger anxiety" Begins vocalizing with single consonants Provide brightly colored toys that are easy to grasp Enjoys noisemakers and mirrors; plays pat-a-cake
9-12 months	Birth weight triples Head and chest circumferences are equal Anterior fontanel begins to close Teething: has 6-8 teeth Sits alone → moves from prone to sitting position Crawling→ pulling up → walks holding on to furniture	May stand alone Has developed crude to fine pincer grasp Transfers objects from one hand to another Recognizes own name Enjoys playing alone (solitary) Explores objects by putting them in mouth
Toddler (12-24 months)	50% of height at 2 years Exaggerated lumbar curve Mobile: walks, runs, jumps Walks up and down stairs, one foot at a time Begins using eating utensils Obeys simple commands Begins to develop vocabulary	Speech becomes understandable Thumb sucking may be at peak Solitary play at 12 months; parallel play at 18 months Beginning to develop bladder and bowel control Attention-seeking behavior: temper tantrums Enjoys activities that provide mobility: riding vehicles, wagons, pull toys
Preschool (3-5 years)	Birth length doubles at 4 years Coordination continues to improve Rides tricycle, throws a ball Walks up and down stairs with alternating feet	Begins to demonstrate self-care abilities Knows own name Good verbalization: talks about activities Plays "dress up"; plays with cars, dolls, grooming aids
School-age (6-10 years)	Growth spurts begin Increasingly active Very concerned with body image Need for conformity: rules and rituals	Increasing importance of peer groups Plays with groups of same sex Competes for attention
Adolescence (11-17 years)	Beginning and completing puberty Girls mature earlier than boys Very conscious of changes in body Rapid growth	Moves from concrete to abstract thinking Increased independence Strong peer group association Increased interest in opposite sex
Young adult (18-30 years)	Physical maturity Full mental capacity Assumes responsibility for own learning Adult relationship with parents	Launches career Selects a mate, begins own family Begins involvement in community
Adult (30-60 years)	Physiologic processes begin slow decline Cognitive skills peak Creativity at maximum Increase in community involvement Increase in concern for future of society	Family tasks Assist children to responsible adulthood Role reversal with aging parents Defines role of grandparenting
Older adult (60+ years)	Decline of physiologic status Demineralization of bones ↓ Cardiac output ↓ Respiratory vital capacity ↓ Glomerular filtration rate ↓ Serum albumin ↓ Glucose tolerance	Maintains reasoning ability and abstract thinking Thinking slows Restructure in family roles Retirement Reorganization of activities Continues with community involvement and politics

Recommended Immunization Schedule for Persons Aged 0 Through 6 Years—United States • 2009
For those who fall behind or start late, see the catch-up schedule

Vaccine ▼ Age ▶	Birth	1 month	2 months	4 months	6 months	12 months	15 months	18 months	19–23 months	2–3 years	4–6 years	
Hepatitis B[1]	HepB	HepB		see footnote 1		HepB						Range of recommended ages
Rotavirus[2]			RV	RV	RV[2]							
Diphtheria, Tetanus, Pertussis[3]			DTaP	DTaP	DTaP	see footnote 3	DTaP				DTaP	
Haemophilus influenzae type b[4]			Hib	Hib	Hib[4]	Hib						
Pneumococcal[5]			PCV	PCV	PCV	PCV				PPSV		Certain high-risk groups
Inactivated Poliovirus			IPV	IPV		IPV					IPV	
Influenza[6]						Influenza (Yearly)						
Measles, Mumps, Rubella[7]						MMR		see footnote 7			MMR	
Varicella[8]						Varicella		see footnote 8			Varicella	
Hepatitis A[9]						HepA (2 doses)				HepA Series		
Meningococcal[10]										MCV		

This schedule indicates the recommended ages for routine administration of currently licensed vaccines, as of December 1, 2008, for children aged 0 through 6 years. Any dose not administered at the recommended age should be administered at a subsequent visit, when indicated and feasible. Licensed combination vaccines may be used whenever any component of the combination is indicated and other components are not contraindicated and if approved by the Food and Drug Administration for that dose of the series. Providers should consult the relevant Advisory Committee on Immunization Practices statement for detailed recommendations, including high-risk conditions: http://www.cdc.gov/vaccines/pubs/acip-list.htm. Clinically significant adverse events that follow immunization should be reported to the Vaccine Adverse Event Reporting System (VAERS). Guidance about how to obtain and complete a VAERS form is available at http://www.vaers.hhs.gov or by telephone, 800-822-7967.

FIGURE 2-1 Recommended Immunization Schedule for Persons Aged 0-6 Years, 2009. For recent updates and a full explanation of footnotes, refer to the Centers for Disease Control and Prevention website, *http://www.cdc.gov/vaccines/recs/schedules/child-schedule.htm#printable*. (From Centers for Disease Control and Prevention, Advisory Committee on Immunization Practices [ACIP], United States, 2009. Available at *www.cdc.gov*.)

E. Need to start regular dental checkups.
F. Establish and maintain consistency in discipline.
G. Toddler enjoys motion toys such as pull toys, riding toys, and wagons.
H. Finger paints, interlocking blocks, and large-piece puzzles increase fine motor skills.
I. May regress to previous level of development in time of stress and illness, especially with toilet training.
J. Has no concept of death; primary reaction is to separation and loss.
K. See separation anxiety under anticipatory guidance for the infant.

ALERT Identify expected physical, cognitive, psychosocial and moral stages of development.

Anticipatory Guidance for the Family of a Preschooler

A. Safety: discuss use of car seat/seat belts, precautions for swimming pools, pedestrian and street safety skills, proper use of playground equipment.
B. Preschool activities: reading, puzzles, coloring large pictures. Toys include building blocks, cars, and dolls.
C. Control time spent watching TV; screen programs for suitability.
D. Encourage socialization with other children.
E. Household chores: picking up clothes, straightening room, etc.
F. Structured learning environment: Mother's Day Out, Head Start, Sunday school.

G. School readiness (attention span, easy separation from mother) begins around 5 years.
H. Should know full name and address by age 5 years.
I. Curious about fire, matches, firearms; keep such items out of reach and locked up.
J. Sees death as temporary and reversible, much like going to sleep. May view death as a punishment; fears the separation and abandonment.
K. Can tolerate brief periods of hospitalization; may trust other significant adults. Stress of illness may cause regression of previously attained levels of behavior, and separation anxiety may become an issue.

ALERT Provide care that meets the needs of the school-age client ages 5-12 years.

Anticipatory Guidance for the Family of a School-Age Child

A. Safety: water, seat belts, skateboard, bicycle, fire safety. Establish a plan for child if approached by stranger (stranger danger).
B. Encourage good dental hygiene habits.
C. Encourage good eating habits.
D. Regular physical activity (group and team activities); make sure child wears protective sports gear.
E. Encourage peer relationships and communication.
F. Maintain consistency in limit setting.
G. Parental role-model behaviors: using seat belts, avoiding tobacco, eating properly, exercising regularly.

Recommended Immunization Schedule for Persons Aged 7 Through 18 Years—United States • 2009
For those who fall behind or start late, see the schedule below and the catch-up schedule

Vaccine ▼ Age ▶	7-10 years	11-12 years	13-18 years
Tetanus, Diphtheria, Pertussis[1]	see footnote 1	Tdap	Tdap
Human Papillomavirus[2]	see footnote 2	HPV (3 doses)	HPV Series
Meningococcal[3]	MCV	MCV	MCV
Influenza[4]	Influenza (Yearly)		
Pneumococcal[5]	PPSV		
Hepatitis A[6]	HepA Series		
Hepatitis B[7]	HepB Series		
Inactivated Poliovirus[8]	IPV Series		
Measles, Mumps, Rubella[9]	MMR Series		
Varicella[10]	Varicella Series		

Range of recommended ages

Catch-up immunization

Certain high-risk groups

This schedule indicates the recommended ages for routine administration of currently licensed vaccines, as of December 1, 2008, for children aged 7 through 18 years. Any dose not administered at the recommended age should be administered at a subsequent visit, when indicated and feasible. Licensed combination vaccines may be used whenever any component of the combination is indicated and other components are not contraindicated and if approved by the Food and Drug Administration for that dose of the series. Providers should consult the relevant Advisory Committee on Immunization Practices statement for detailed recommendations, including high-risk conditions: http://www.cdc.gov/vaccines/pubs/acip-list.htm. Clinically significant adverse events that follow immunization should be reported to the Vaccine Adverse Event Reporting System (VAERS). Guidance about how to obtain and complete a VAERS form is available at http://www.vaers.hhs.gov or by telephone, 800-822-7967.

FIGURE 2-2 Recommended Immunization Schedule for Persons Aged 7-18 Years, 2009. For recent updates and a full explanation of footnotes, refer to the Centers for Disease Control and Prevention website, *http://www.cdc.gov/vaccines/recs/schedules/child-schedule.htm#printable.* (From Centers for Disease Control and Prevention, Advisory Committee on Immunization Practices [ACIP], United States, 2009. Available at *www.cdc.gov.*)

H. Teaching: avoid drugs, alcohol, and tobacco.

I. Provide age-appropriate sex education materials.

J. Injury prevention: Around ages 8 to 10 years, child may begin to engage in dangerous risk-taking behavior (dares, smoking, drinking).

K. Maintain yearly health checkups and immunizations as indicated (Figure 2-2).

L. Develop independence: give allowance, choice of when to complete household chores; child tests rules and questions authority.

M. Avoid high noise levels (e.g., music headsets).

N. Physical development and puberty changes may begin in girls as early as 10 years.

O. Strong influence and dependence on peer group.

P. Spends less time with family.

Q. In early childhood, begins to see death as irreversible; may interpret it as destructive, scary, and/or violent.

R. In later childhood, views death as final and irreversible. May become interested in details regarding biologic death and funerals.

S. The hospitalized child fears being away from the family, peers, and usual activities. May exhibit feelings of loneliness, boredom, and isolation.

ALERT Evaluate incorporation of healthy behaviors into lifestyle by the client /family (screening exams, immunizations, limiting risk-taking behaviors).

Anticipatory Guidance for the Family of an Adolescent

A. Establish realistic expectations for family rules.

B. Minimize criticism, nagging, and derogatory or demeaning comments.

C. Respect child's need for privacy.

D. Recognize positive behavior and achievement.

E. Establish clear limits: curfew, work hours.

F. Strives for independence from parents and acceptance by peers.

G. Begins to exhibit a mature understanding of death; may deny own mortality by increased risk taking. May have difficulty coping with death of significant other.

H. Maintain yearly physical checkups and immunizations as indicated (see Figure 2-2).

I. Hospitalized adolescents may exhibit rejection, uncooperativeness, or withdrawal because of the loss of control. Are frequently labeled by caregivers as difficult, unmanageable clients.

ALERT Modify approaches to care in accordance with client developmental stage. Provide care that meets the special needs of the adult client ages 19 to 64 years.

Anticipatory Guidance for the Adolescent

A. Learn techniques to protect self from physical, emotional, and sexual abuse, including rape.

B. Seek help if physically or sexually abused.

C. If sexually active, obtain information about safe sex and pregnancy prevention (e.g., condoms, sexually transmitted diseases, contraceptives).

D. Avoid smoking, drugs, and alcohol.

Health Implications and Guidance for Adults and Older Adults (Box 2-1)

ALERT Provide care to meet the special needs of older clients ages 65 to 85 years and adult clients over 85 years old.

Box 2-1 OLDER ADULT CARE FOCUS
Age-Related Factors Influencing Older Adult Care

- Frequent absence of social and financial support
  Examples: Disease and/or loss of spouse, inadequate income from pension
- Presence of significant concurrent illness
  Examples: Dementia, chronic obstructive disease, congestive heart failure, depression, diabetes
- Altered pain perception
  Example: Increased incidence of referred pain
- Impaired homeostatic mechanisms
  Examples: Increased problems with dehydration, incontinence, impaired defecation, altered immune status
- Impaired mobility
  Examples: Dependence on walkers, need for assistance with bed transferring, change in use of transportation, presence of Parkinsonism or degenerative joint disease
- Increased frequency of adverse reactions to drugs
- Impaired equilibrium, resulting in falls

A. Assist in identifying health care resources within community.

B. Encourage health screening, regular physical examination, and immunizations as indicated (Figure 2-3).

C. Encourage healthy living style: exercise, good nutrition, decreased stress, decreased alcohol intake, and no tobacco use.

D. Response to hospitalization will reflect moral and cultural values.

E. Hospitalization causes increased stress because of family and job responsibilities, as well as threat to client's well-being.

F. Concepts of death follow common sequence.
1. Shock, anger, denial, disbelief.
2. Development of an awareness, bargaining; may experience depression.
3. Acceptance, reorganization, restitution.

G. Adults ages 18 to 65 years tend to have an abstract and realistic concept of death.

H. Older adult clients (65 and older) have frequently lost a spouse, a child, or close friends. Death is very realistic, but older adults tend to have a more philosophic concept of death.

COMMUNICABLE DISEASES

ALERT Understand communicable diseases and modes of organism transmission (airborne, droplet, contact). Apply principles of infection control.

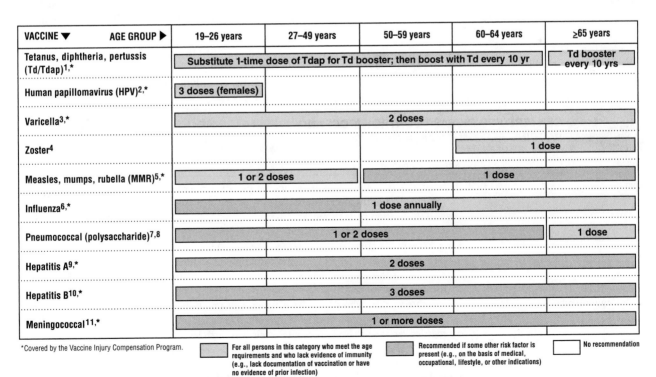

VACCINE ▼ AGE GROUP ▶	19–26 years	27–49 years	50–59 years	60–64 years	≥65 years
Tetanus, diphtheria, pertussis (Td/Tdap)[1],*	Substitute 1-time dose of Tdap for Td booster; then boost with Td every 10 yr				Td booster every 10 yrs
Human papillomavirus (HPV)[2],*	3 doses (females)				
Varicella[3],*	2 doses				
Zoster[4]				1 dose	
Measles, mumps, rubella (MMR)[5],*	1 or 2 doses		1 dose		
Influenza[6],*	1 dose annually				
Pneumococcal (polysaccharide)[7,8]	1 or 2 doses				1 dose
Hepatitis A[9],*	2 doses				
Hepatitis B[10],*	3 doses				
Meningococcal[11],*	1 or more doses				

*Covered by the Vaccine Injury Compensation Program.

For all persons in this category who meet the age requirements and who lack evidence of immunity (e.g., lack documentation of vaccination or have no evidence of prior infection)

Recommended if some other risk factor is present (e.g., on the basis of medical, occupational, lifestyle, or other indications)

No recommendation

FIGURE 2-3 Recommended Adult Immunization Schedule, 2009. For recent updates and a full explanation of footnotes, refer to the Centers for Disease Control and Prevention website, *http://www.cdc.gov/vaccines/recs/schedules/adult-schedule.htm#print.* (From Centers for Disease Control and Prevention, Advisory Committee on Immunization Practices [ACIP], United States, 2009. Available at *www.cdc.gov.*)

A. Incubation period: time from exposure to the pathogen until clinical symptoms occur.

B. Communicability: period of time in which an infected person is most likely to pass the pathogens to another person.

C. Prodromal period: begins with early manifestations of the disease or infection and continues until there are overt clinical symptoms characteristic of the disease.

D. Vaccinations for health care workers (Table 2-2).

 Varicella (Chicken Pox)

Characteristics

A. Herpes virus: varicella zoster; highly contagious, usually occurs in children under 15 years of age.

B. Maculopapular rash with vesicular scabs in multiple stages of healing.

C. Incubation period: 14 to 16 days.

D. Transmission: contact, airborne.

E. Communicability: 1 day before lesions appear to time when all lesions have formed crusts.

Assessment

A. Prodromal: low-grade fever, malaise.

B. Acute phase: red maculopapular rash, which turns almost immediately to vesicles, each with an erythematous base; vesicles ooze and crust.

C. New crops of vesicles continue to form for 3 to 5 days, spreading from trunk to extremities.

D. All three stages are usually present in varying degrees at one time; pruritus.

E. Complications: secondary infection may lead to sepsis, abscess, cellulitis, or pneumonia.

Health Care Interventions

A. Preventive: varicella immunization (see Figure 2-1, Figure 2-2, Figure 2-3).

B. Skin care to decrease itching.
   1. Antihistamines, antipruritics, calamine lotion, and acetaminophen and/or ibuprofen for fever.
   2. Acyclovir decreases the number of lesions and shortens duration of clinical symptoms.
   3. Cool baths.
   4. Paste of baking soda and/or calamine lotion may decrease irritation.

C. Keep child's fingernails short; apply mittens if necessary.

D. Isolate affected child from other children until vesicles have crusted.

E. Provide quiet activities to keep child occupied to lessen pruritus and prevent scratching.

F. Avoid use of aspirin.

G. Check with health care provider before administering vaccine to immunocompromised children. Vaccine should not be given to pregnant women.

 Parotitis (Mumps)

Characteristics

A. An acute viral disease characterized by tenderness and swelling of one or both of the parotid glands and/or the other salivary glands.

B. Incubation period: 14 to 21 days.

C. Transmission: direct contact and droplet.

D. Communicability: most commonly occurs immediately before and after swelling begins.

Assessment

A. Prodromal: headache, fever, malaise.

B. Acute phase: swelling of salivary glands (peaks in 3 days), leading to difficulty in swallowing, earache.

C. Complications.
   1. Postinfectious encephalitis.
   2. Sensorineural deafness.
   3. Orchitis, epididymitis.

Table 2-2	CENTERS FOR DISEASE CONTROL (CDC) AND PREVENTION HEALTH CARE PERSONNEL (HCP) VACCINE RECOMMENDATIONS

Disease	Recommendation
Hepatitis B	Three-dose series of hepatitis B vaccine for preexposure protection and anti-HBs serologic testing 1-2 months after third dose.
Influenza	Annual vaccination with current vaccine. Give live attenuated influenza vaccine (LAIV) intranasally. Give trivalent (inactivated) influenza vaccine (TIV) intramuscularly.
Tetanus/diphtheria/pertussis	Booster dose of tetanus and diphtheria toxoid every 10 years after primary series of diphtheria and tetanus toxoids; give 1-time dose of DTaP to all personnel younger than 65 who have direct patient contact.
Measles/mumps/rubella (MMR)	Health care workers who do not have evidence of immunity to measles (physician-diagnosed measles or laboratory evidence of immunity) should have documentation of two doses of measles vaccine received on or after their first birthday; vaccine can be given as MMR. A single dose of live attenuated rubella vaccine received on or after the first birthday is sufficient; vaccine can be given as MMR.
Varicella	Give 2 doses of varicella vaccine, 4 weeks apart, if there is no reliable history of varicella or evidence of immunity.

From Centers for Disease Control and Prevention: *Healthcare personnel vaccine recommendations, Atlanta,* 2008, Center for Disease Control and Prevention. Available at *www.immunize.org/catg.d/p2017.pdf.* Accessed December 2008.

Health Care Interventions

A. Preventive: measles, mumps, and rubella (MMR) immunization (see Figure 2-1, Figure 2-2, Figure 2-3). MMR vaccine should not be given to pregnant or severely immunocompromised clients.
B. Bed rest until swelling subsides.
C. Fluids and soft, bland food.
D. Orchitis: warm or cold packs; light support to scrotum.
E. Cool compresses applied to swollen neck area.

Rubeola (Measles, Hard Measles, Red Measles)

Characteristics

A. An acute viral disease characterized by fever and a rash.
B. Incubation: 10 to 20 days.
C. Transmission: direct contact with respiratory droplet.
D. Communicability: 4 days before rash to 5 days after rash appears.

Assessment

A. Prodromal: fever, malaise, cold-like symptoms.
B. Koplik's spots: small, irregular red spots noticed on the buccal mucosa opposite the molars; usually appear 2 days before rash.
C. Acute phase: begins 3 to 4 days after prodromal symptoms; maculopapular rash begins on face and gradually spreads downward from head to feet.
D. Photophobia, conjunctivitis, and bronchitis.
E. Complications: otitis media, pneumonia, laryngotracheitis, and encephalitis.

Health Care Interventions

A. Preventive: MMR immunization (see Figure 2-1, Figure 2-2). MMR should not be given to pregnant or severely immunocompromised clients.
B. Bed rest until fever subsides, acetaminophen or ibuprofen for fever control.
C. Dim lights to decrease photophobia.
D. Tepid baths and lotion to relieve itching.
E. Encourage intake of fluids to maintain hydration; temperature may spike 2 to 3 days after rash appears.

Rubella (German Measles, Three-Day Measles)

Characteristics

A. An acute, mild systemic viral disease that produces a distinctive 3-day rash and lymphadenopathy.
B. Incubation: 14 to 21 days.
C. Transmission: nasopharyngeal secretions, direct contact.
D. Communicability: from up to 7 days before rash until 5 days after rash.

Assessment

A. Prodromal: low-grade fever, headache, malaise, and symptoms of a cold.
B. Rash first appears on face and spreads down to neck, arms, trunk, and then legs.

C. Diagnostics: persistent rubella antibody titer of 1:8 usually indicates immunity.
D. Complications: can have teratogenic effects on fetus.

Health Care Interventions

A. Primarily symptomatic; bed rest until fever subsides.
B. Preventive: MMR immunization (see Figure 2-1, Figure 2-2). MMR should not be given to severely immunosuppressed clients.
C. Pregnant women should avoid contact with children who have rubella. If not immunized before pregnancy, vaccination should not be given until completion of pregnancy.

Roseola Infantum (Exanthema Subitum)

Characteristics

A. A common, acute benign viral infection, usually occurring in infants and young children (ages 6 months to 3 years), characterized by sudden onset of a high temperature, followed by a rash.
B. Incubation period: usually 5 to 15 days.
C. Transmission: unknown, generally limited to children age 6 months to 3 years.
D. Communicability: unknown.

Assessment

A. Sudden onset of high fever.
B. As fever drops, a maculopapular, nonpruritic rash appears abruptly; rash blanches or fades under pressure and disappears in 1 to 2 days.
C. Complications: febrile seizures.

Health Care Interventions

A. Symptomatic: provide tepid baths, offer fluids frequently, dress child in cool clothing.
B. Acetaminophen and/or ibuprofen for fever control.

Diphtheria

Characteristics

A. An infection caused by *Corynebacterium diphtheriae*.
B. Incubation period: 3 to 6 days.
C. Transmission: direct contact, contaminated articles (fomites).
D. Communicability: variable, usually 2 weeks, but may be longer; three negative cultures required.

Assessment

A. Nasal discharge, anorexia, sore throat, low-grade fever.
B. Smooth, white or gray membrane over tonsillar region; hoarseness and potential airway obstruction.
C. Frequently, tachypnea, dyspnea, stridor, or airway obstruction may occur if condition goes untreated.
D. Complications: myocarditis, neuritis.

Health Care Interventions

A. Maintain isolation from other children.
B. Antibiotic and IV diphtheria antitoxin are common medications.

C. Humidified oxygen with respiratory problems; have tracheostomy set available.

D. Provide adequate humidification to allow for liquefaction of secretions.

E. Preventive: diphtheria, tetanus, and pertussis (DTaP) immunization (see Figure 2-1, Figure 2-2, Figure 2-3).

 Pertussis (Whooping Cough)

Characteristics

A. An acute inflammation of the respiratory tract caused by *Bordetella pertussis*; is most severe in children under 2 years of age.

B. Incubation period: 6 to 20 days; average, 7 days.

C. Transmission: air droplet.

D. Communicability: highly contagious; greatest during the catarrhal stage before the onset of paroxysms of coughing.

Assessment

A. Catarrhal stage: usually begins with symptoms of an upper respiratory tract infection, fever.

B. Paroxysmal stage.
  1. Cough occurs primarily at night; consists of a series of short rapid coughs, followed by a sudden inspiration that is a high-pitched, crowing sound or a "whoop."
  2. Paroxysms of coughing may continue until thick mucus plug is expelled.

C. Convalescent stage: paroxysms of coughing are less frequent.

D. Diagnostics: culture and sensitivity of nasopharyngeal secretions; identification of organism.

E. Complications: pneumonia, atelectasis, convulsions.

Health Care Interventions

A. Respiratory isolation during catarrhal stage; continue bed rest as long as fever is present.

B. Administer pertussis immunoglobulin and antibiotic therapy (erythromycin).

C. Provide oxygen and humidification and observe for signs of increasing respiratory distress.

D. Avoid exposure to environmental precipitants of paroxysms of coughing such as cold air, smoke, dust, etc.

E. Maintain nutrition by small frequent feedings.

F. Avoid use of cough suppressants and sedatives.

 Tetanus (Lockjaw)

Characteristics

A. An acute, very serious, potentially fatal disease characterized by painful muscle spasms and convulsions caused by the anaerobic gram-positive bacillus *Clostridium tetani*.

B. Incubation period: generally from 2 days to 2 months; average is 10 days.

C. Transmission: through a puncture wound that is contaminated by soil, dust, or excreta that contain *Clostridium tetani* or by way of burns and minor wounds (e.g., infection of the umbilicus of a newborn).

Assessment

A. Progressive stiffness and tenderness in the muscles of the neck and jaw (trismus or lockjaw).

B. Progressive involvement of trunk muscles causes opisthotonos positioning.

C. Paroxysmal contractions occur in response to stimuli (noise, touch, light).

D. Client remains alert; mental status is not affected.

E. Complications: laryngospasm and tetany of the respiratory muscles cause contractions that may precipitate atelectasis and pneumonia.

Health Care Interventions

A. Preventive.
  1. Careful cleansing and debridement of wounds.
  2. Immunization: DTaP for child (Figure 2-1, Figure 2-2); adult tetanus toxoid (Td) every 10 years (see Figure 2-3).

B. Administration of tetanus immune globulin and/or tetanus antitoxin for inadequate immunization in child who receives a tetanus-prone injury/wound.

C. Maintain seizure precautions: quiet, nonstimulating environment; monitor vital signs, muscle tone, etc.

D. Dose of tetanus antitoxin is not necessary for clean minor wounds in immunized clients.

 Poliomyelitis

Characteristics

A. An acute, contagious disease affecting the central nervous system.

B. Incubation period: 5 to 35 days; average, 7 to 14 days.

C. Transmission: fecal-oral or pharyngeal-oropharyngeal contact.

D. Communicability: virus in throat for 1 week after onset; in feces, intermittently for 4 to 6 weeks.

Assessment

A. Abortive or inapparent type.
  1. Fever, sore throat, headache, malaise, nausea, vomiting, abdominal pain.
  2. Lasts a few hours to a few days.

B. Nonparalytic type: same symptoms as abortive type but more severe, with pain and stiffness in the neck, back, and legs.

C. Paralytic type: initial symptoms are similar to those of nonparalytic poliomyelitis, followed by recovery, then signs of central nervous system paralysis.

Health Care Interventions

A. Preventive: inactivated polio virus vaccine (see Figure 2-1, Figure 2-2).

B. Bed rest during acute phase.

C. Physical therapy with warm moist packs and range of motion.

D. Position to maintain body alignment.

E. Complications: teach family and client early symptoms of respiratory distress.

Scarlet Fever (Scarlatina)

Characteristics

A. Group A beta-hemolytic streptococcal infection that often follows acute streptopharyngitis.

B. Incubation period: 1 to 7 days; average, 3 days.

C. Transmission: direct contact or droplet of nasopharyngeal secretions.

D. Communicability: variable, approximately 10 days.

Assessment

A. Sudden onset of high fever and tachycardia.

B. Enlarged edematous tonsils covered with exudate; nausea, vomiting; "strawberry" tongue.

C. Diffuse, fine erythematous rash that resembles a sunburn with goose bumps; rash is more intense in folds and joints but is often absent from the face.

D. Desquamation of the skin, which usually begins by end of first week and is often seen on the palms and soles of the feet during the convalescent period.

E. Diagnostics: history of a recent streptococcal infection, positive antistreptolysin-O (ASO) titer, and a throat culture positive for group A beta-hemolytic streptococci.

F. Complications: otitis media, tonsillar abscess, glomerulonephritis.

Health Care Interventions

A. Administration of a full course of penicillin (or erythromycin in penicillin-sensitive clients).

B. Administration of antipyretics and anesthetic throat sprays or gargles to relieve sore throat.

C. Encourage intake of fluids to prevent dehydration during febrile phase.

D. Assess for, and teach family to observe for, early symptoms of complications.

Infectious Mononucleosis

Characteristics

A. An acute, self-limiting infectious disease caused by the Epstein-Barr virus; member of the herpes group of viruses, occurring most often among young persons under 25 years of age; often called the "kissing disease."

B. Incubation period: 30-50 days.

C. Transmission: direct or indirect contact with oral secretions—intimate contact, sharing same drinking cup, hand to mouth; probably oral pharyngeal route.

Assessment

A. Onset of symptoms occurs anytime from 10 days to 6 weeks after exposure; may be acute or insidious.

B. Malaise, sore throat, fever with generalized lymphadenopathy.

C. Diagnostic: a positive heterophil antibody test (titer of 1:160 is considered diagnostic); positive Monospot test result.

D. Complications: spleen involvement; pneumonitis, pericarditis, and neurologic involvement.

Health Care Interventions

A. Bed rest, anesthetic throat gargles, antipyretics.

B. Provide adequate nutrition: soft foods, fluids.

> **ALERT** Provide information about health maintenance (e.g., physician visits, immunizations, screening exams).

POISONING

General Principles (Remember *SIRES*)

A. *S*tabilize the client's condition.
  1. Assess the condition and provide respiratory support; obtain IV access site.
  2. Terminate exposure to the toxic substance: remove pills from mouth, flush eyes, remove contaminated clothing, etc.

B. *I*dentify the toxic substance.
  1. Obtain accurate history and retrieve any available poison.
  2. Notify local poison control center, emergency facility, or physician for immediate care and advice regarding treatment.

C. *R*emove the substance to decrease absorption.
  1. Shower or wash off radioactive substances.
  2. Antidotes: for heroin or other drug overdose.
  3. Ingested substances: lavage, absorbents (activated charcoal), or cathartics.

D. *E*liminate the substance from the client's body.
  1. Activated charcoal may be administered to absorb the toxic substance. Inducing emesis by administering syrup of ipecac is no longer routinely recommended for home or emergency treatment.

E. *S*upport the client both physically and psychologically.
  1. If intentional overdose or suicide attempt, refer for psychiatric evaluation.
  2. If accidental poisoning occurs with a child, parents often demonstrate guilt and self-reproach in regard to their parenting role.

> **ALERT** Educate client/family on home safety issues

Salicylate Poisoning

A. Toxic dose levels: 300-500 mg/kg of body weight. For a 30-lb child (13.6 kg), 12 adult-strength aspirin or 48 baby aspirin would be toxic.

B. In severe toxic overdose, metabolic activity increases; this results in an increased consumption of oxygen, increased temperature, and increased production of carbon dioxide. Metabolic acidosis eventually occurs as a result of the change in body processes.

C. Chronic overdose causes a deficiency in platelets, leading to bleeding tendencies.

Assessment

A. Clinical manifestations.
   1. Hyperventilation, nausea, vomiting.
   2. Increased temperature, tinnitus.
   3. Altered consciousness, oliguria.
   4. Metabolic acidosis, seizures (severe toxicity).
   5. Diaphoresis and dehydration.
   6. Bleeding tendencies in chronic poisoning.
B. Diagnostics.
   1. Serum salicylate level.
   2. Electrolytes.

Treatment

A. Administer activated charcoal.
B. Administer vitamin K to decrease bleeding tendencies.
C. Oxygen and ventilatory support for respiratory depression. Provide IV fluids and sodium bicarbonate to treat the acidosis.
D. Cooling activities and treatments for hyperthermia.
E. In severe cases, hemodialysis may be performed.

Nursing Interventions

Goal: To provide initial stabilization of the child.
A. Administer activated charcoal to reduce systemic absorption. Dose of charcoal should be 10 times the amount of drug ingested; frequently difficult to get this amount down the child.
B. Administer a cathartic (magnesium sulfate) with charcoal to hasten elimination of the drug.
C. Ongoing assessment of vital signs, level of consciousness, and urine output.
Goal: To prevent salicylate poisoning and provide teaching to family.
A. Educate family regarding safe storage of medications: childproof caps, locked medicine cabinets, etc.
B. Teach parents to read labels on medications; other medications frequently contain salicylate.
C. Advise parents that activated charcoal will cause the child's stool to be black.

Acetaminophen Poisoning

A. Definition of toxicity in children is 150 mg/kg or greater.
B. Primary toxic effects are on the liver.
C. Antidote: N-acetylcysteine (Mucomyst).
D. Most common poisoning in children.

Assessment

A. Clinical manifestations: four stages.
   1. Stage 1 (2 to 4 hours).
      a. Nausea and vomiting.
      b. Sweating and pallor.
   2. Stage 2 (latent stage, 24 to 36 hours); child improves.
   3. Stage 3 (hepatic involvement).
      a. Right, upper quadrant pain.
      b. Coagulation defects.
      c. Jaundice.
   4. Stage 4 (recovery if hepatic damage is not severe).

Treatment

A. Early administration of activated charcoal—preferably within 30 minutes to 1 hour after ingestion.
B. N-acetylcysteine: one loading dose and multiple maintenance doses.

Nursing Interventions

See Salicylate Poisoning.

Lead Poisoning

A. Ingestion of lead from hand to mouth and exposure to lead-contaminated dust, eating from improperly glazed glassware (leaded glass) or lead-based pottery or chewing on furniture with lead based paint.
B. Increased risk in children under 6 years of age because they absorb 40% to 50% of lead, whereas adults absorb only 5% to 10%.

Assessment

A. Clinical manifestations.
   1. Renal: problem in adults with occupational exposure; renal impairment will delay excretion of the lead from the body.
   2. Hematologic.
      a. Anemia.
      b. Iron deficiencies increase lead absorption; serum ferritin level is sensitive indicator of iron status.
      c. Chronic: blue lead line on gums and "lead lines" on x-rays of the long bones.
   3. Neurologic.
      a. Hyperactivity.
      b. Increased distractibility.
      c. Possible encephalopathy to mental retardation.
      d. Seizures.
B. Diagnostics.
   1. Blood lead level (BLL) is used for screening and for diagnostic. A BLL greater than 10 mcg/dL requires follow-up investigation, BLL greater than 20 mcg/dL requires treatment.

Treatment

A. Chelation therapy process for removing lead from the circulating blood; aids in secretion by the kidneys.
   1. Calcium disodium edetate (EDTA) administered by deep intramuscular injection or by IV; do not give in absence of adequate urine output.
   2. Dimercaprol (BAL): administered by deep intramuscular injection.
   3. Succimer (Chemet): an oral chelator.

Nursing Interventions

Goal: To identify lead poisoning and assist with the elimination of lead from the body.
A. Identify high-risk groups such as children who engaged in pica or those living in environment containing old lead-based paint.

1. Monitor children with lead levels greater than 10 mcg/dL.
2. Treat children at 6 to 12 months of age.

B. Administer chelating agents: compliance is critical; important to support the child who will be receiving multiple injections.

C. Encourage high fluid intake.

D. Seizure precautions.

Goal: To educate parents and child as to the nature of the disease and provide instruction in ways to maintain homeostasis and reduce lead exposure.

A. Educate parents about the dangers and sources of lead ingestion, including 12 to 24 months being the age of greatest risk.

B. Assist parents in identifying measures to prevent occurrence or recurrence of the problem.

LONG-TERM CARE

Long-term care includes those services provided in institutional settings, such as a nursing home, rehabilitation center, or adult day care program after the acute phase of an illness has passed. Often involves restorative care for clients with chronic health care problems.

A. Types of long-term care facilities.

1. Nursing home: provides services ranging from maintenance to restorative care with skilled nursing, use of certified nursing assistants, licensed practical nurses, and registered nurses.

2. Adult day care facility: client lives at home during the evening and night and spends the day in a facility that provides a range of care from skilled nursing to restorative care.

3. Hospice care: end-of-life care provided in the home and/or client care settings. See End-of-Life Care, Chapter 3.

4. Respite care: a type of short-term care provided to give the primary caregiver (often a family member) a rest from the daily responsibilities of taking care of the client.

5. Rehabilitation center: facility that provides multiple services for the client and family to make adjustments to daily living. Assists the client in achieving as much independence as possible in activities of daily living (ADLs).

6. Home care: nursing care provided in the home to clients who do not need hospitalization but do need additional assistance with medical problems.

7. Adult housing or assisted living centers: facilities for clients to live as independently as possible but still receive supervision, meals, and other services.

CHRONIC ILLNESS

A chronic illness may be defined as an illness or condition that is present for more than 3 months in a year and interferes with daily function and lifestyle. As medical technology continues to increase the life spans of individuals with chronic illnesses, the nurse's role continues to expand, including providing initial health care and assisting with planning, as well as providing long-term care.

> **ALERT** Help client cope with life transitions. Help client and significant others adjust to role changes; assess a family's emotional reaction to a client's illness; determine ability of family/support system to provide care for client.

Nursing Considerations

A. The majority of clients with extended health care needs have at least two chronic health conditions. These conditions may or may not be interrelated.

B. The focus of care for chronically ill clients is on assisting them to control their health problems and disease symptoms and manage their lifestyle.

1. Prevention and management of medical crises.
2. The control of disease symptoms, which may focus on pain control and comfort measures.
3. Implementation of the prescribed therapeutic regimens.
4. Psychosocial implications and adjustments to lifestyle; frequently, client must deal with social isolation.
5. Adjustments to lifestyle as disease or condition changes.
6. Financial strain caused by paying for medical care and supplies.
7. Coping with strain on marriage and family structure.

C. The majority of clients with chronic health care needs are over 65 years old. The developmental level of these individuals, according to Erikson, is ego integrity versus despair. The feeling of powerlessness is a common problem in the older adult.

D. The nursing process is directed toward identification of nursing actions to assist the older adult to maintain independence and to be as functional as possible.

> **! NURSING PRIORITY** In planning home health care for a client with a chronic disease, remember that the goal is to *assist the client in maintaining control* over his or her condition and lifestyle. Frequently, health care providers and family tend to take control of the situation, thus increasing the feeling of powerlessness in the individual.

 Chronically Ill Pediatric Client

The diagnosis of a child's chronic illness is a major situational crisis in the family. Available support systems, perception of the problem, and coping mechanisms will ultimately determine the resolution of the crisis.

A. Focus care on the child's developmental age rather than chronological age. Emphasis should be placed on the child's strengths rather than disabilities.

B. Assist the child and the family in returning to or establishing a normal pattern of living.

C. Promote the child's maximum level of growth and development. Current trend is to promote education within child's peer group.

D. Assess the family's response to the child's illness and evaluate for parental overprotection. Overprotection by the parents prevents the child from developing self-esteem, independence, and self-control over the disease and ADLs. Observe for the following parental characteristics that will impede development.

1. Inconsistency in discipline; disciplinary measures often differ from those used with other children in the family.

2. Attempts to protect the child from every discomfort, both physical and psychosocial. Frequently restricts play with peers based on fear of injury and/or rejection by peers.

3. Makes decisions for the child without involving the child.

4. Does not allow the child the opportunity to learn self-care; frequently, afraid the child cannot handle the requirements for self-care (e.g., a child with diabetes becoming responsible for administration of his or her own insulin).

5. Continues to do things for the child, even when child is capable of doing them on his or her own.

6. Self-sacrifice and isolation of family from social interactions.

> ❗ **NURSING PRIORITY** Determine the needs of the family regarding ability to provide home care after discharge. A pediatric situation may include questions regarding the parents' or family's response to the child's chronic illness.

It is frequently the nurse who assesses the family and the client regarding their immediate needs. The appropriateness of the nurse's response depends on the nurse-client-family relationship and the environment. Priorities of care must be established, with goals and nursing interventions to meet the client's immediate health care needs. In an acute care environment, it is difficult to even *attempt* to meet long-term needs of the client and family. It is important to assist them in identifying community resources and to determine the availability of counseling and home health care to meet the ever-changing needs encountered in dealing with a chronic health condition.

REHABILITATION

> **ALERT** Assist and intervene in client's performance of instrumental activities of daily living. Provide support to client and/or family in coping with life changes. Determine client's ability to perform self-care (ADLs, hygiene, resources); plan with client to meet self-care needs.

Rehabilitation means the restoration of an individual to his or her optimum level of functioning. This includes physical, mental, social, vocational, and economic parameters.

A. Rehabilitation: this term is used when an individual has lost functional ability because of illness or injury.

B. Habilitation: this term is used when an individual has congenital problems or deficiencies.

Goals of Rehabilitation

> ❗ **NURSING PRIORITY** Rehabilitation is an area that affects all levels of nursing care. Primary goals in planning any client's care are prevention of complications and promotion of independence.

For the rehabilitation client to achieve the highest level of productivity, the rehabilitation process must begin when the condition becomes evident or when the disease is diagnosed.

A. Prevention of deformities and complications.

1. Maintain function and prevent deterioration of unaffected organs or areas.

2. Prevent further injury to affected area or organ.

3. Prevent or reduce complications of immobility.

B. Assist client in performing ADLs with minimum or no assistance, depending on his or her level of disability. *Examples of ADLs: eating, dressing, bathing.*

C. Assist client with independent activities of daily living (IADLs). *Examples of IADLs: shopping for groceries, paying bills, lawn care.*

D. Promote continuity of care when the client is discharged or transferred.

1. Consult with other rehabilitation team members to determine appropriate placement.

2. Assist client and family through the transitional process.

> ❗ **NURSING PRIORITY** Client needs to be actively involved in setting goals for his or her care.

Psychologic Responses to Disability

Not every client will progress through all stages of grief in an orderly fashion. Clients will fluctuate between emotional crises.

A. Initial responses of confusion, disorganization, and denial represent a state of internal conflict.

B. A period of depression may occur as the client mourns for the loss of or change in body function.

C. An anger stage may occur as client projects blame and hostility on family and health care providers.

D. Adaptation and adjustment will come as the client begins to redirect his or her energy toward coping with the disability.

E. New situations (going home, new job, etc.) may precipitate emotional outbursts and trauma.

F. Some clients will refuse to accept their disability and will not put forth any effort to adapt to everyday living.

HOME HEALTH CARE

Home health care is the provision of health care to clients in the home environment.

A. Levels of home health care.
   1. Intensive: clients with serious health care problems requiring the expertise of skilled nursing care.
   2. Intermediate: clients with stable health care problems who require a professional level of care to promote rehabilitation through restorative nursing.
   3. Maintenance: clients who require assistance with ADLs; the underlying health care problem is stable.
B. Guidelines for home health care personnel.
   1. Respect client's religious, cultural, and ethnic background.
   2. As a caregiver/guest in the client's home, your behavior should reflect sensitivity to the client and family; a pleasant attitude and sense of humor are helpful.
   3. Develop family members and significant others as your advocates.
   4. Communication with other health care team members is vital to the maintenance of the client's well-being.
   5. Working with more autonomy without immediate hospital support is challenging and requires an increased level of nursing competence for decision making.
   6. A Patient's Bill of Rights is applicable in the home health care setting (i.e., client has the right to disclosure of information concerning his or her condition and care and the right to refuse or stop treatment, etc).

NUTRITION

> **ALERT** Monitor client's nutritional and hydration status.

Dietary Considerations Throughout the Life Span

Infant

> **NURSING PRIORITY** A newborn will lose weight for the first few days but should not lose more than 10% of his or her birth weight or take longer than 10 to 14 days to regain it.

A. Growth.
   1. Birth weight doubles at 6 months, and triples by 1 year.
   2. Infant gains only another 4 to 6 lb until 2 years of age.
      Birth weight 7 lb; at 4 months, should be 14 lb; at 1 year, another 7 lb gained = 21 lb (birth weight tripled).
B. Diet.
   1. Ideal food is breast milk, because it is nutritionally superior to alternatives, is easier to digest, and contains maternal antibodies.
   2. Bottle-fed infants need to be on a formula that is iron-fortified.
   3. Breastfed infants do not need additional water.

> **NURSING PRIORITY** A newborn has a higher fluid requirement in relation to body size than an adult.

   4. Whole cow's milk, low-fat cow's milk, skim milk, and imitation milks are not recommended for infants younger than 12 months of age.
   5. Iron fortified cereal, usually rice, is the first solid food introduced and is recommended around age 4 to 6 months.
   6. Strained vegetables and fruits are introduced one at a time to determine infant's tolerance of each food.
   7. Chopped foods are introduced at 6 to 9 months.
   8. Strained meats are usually added last because of the difficulty the infant may encounter swallowing.

> **NURSING PRIORITY** Breastfed infants may gain weight at a slower rate than formula-fed infants. Breastfed infants are leaner and often have less body fat than formula fed infants.

   9. Formula consumption.
      a. 1 month old: up to 22 oz per day.
      b. 4 months old: up to 30 oz per day.
      c. 6 months old: up to 28 oz per day; solid foods are introduced.
      d. 12 months old: up to 23 oz per day with intake of solid food.
C. Implications for family teaching.

> **ALERT** Assist client with infant feeding. Provide discharge instructions (postpartum and newborn care).

   1. Newborns cannot swallow voluntarily until 10 to 12 weeks of age.
   2. Extrusion reflex (pushing food out of mouth with tongue) lasts until 4 months; therefore solids are not introduced until around 6 months.
   3. When solids are being introduced, offer only one new food per week; avoid multigrain cereals until tolerance is established.
   4. Usual progression of food textures is strained to mashed to minced to chopped to cut-up table foods.
   5. Increase the use of small-sized finger foods as pincer grasp develops (9 months).
   6. Texture of food becomes increasingly important from 6 months to 1 year, but the food must be easily dissolved, (e.g., crackers or zwiebacks).
   7. Teach parents *not* to warm frozen breast milk in the microwave; this may change the composition of the milk.

Toddler

A. Diet.
   1. Needs 16 oz of milk daily; more than 24 oz can lead to refusal of other foods and development of a milk anemia (peak incidence at 18 months).
   2. Prefers finger foods (e.g., vegetables he or she can pick up, crackers, macaroni).
   3. Tends to refuse casseroles, salads, and mixed dishes.

4. After 2 years of age, a child may be given fat-free milk if fat intake is a concern.
5. Struggle for autonomy may be manifested by refusal of food, mealtime negativism, and ritualism.
6. Bribery and rewards for eating should be avoided.
7. Around 18 months of age, a decreased appetite is normal; toddler may become a very picky eater. Don't mix foods on plate or overfill the plate.
8. Ritualistic behavior frequently carries over into eating habits (e.g., same dish, same spoon, etc.).

Preschooler

A. Diet.
   1. *Food jags* are common; may refuse to eat anything except one food at each meal.
   2. Continues to refuse casseroles and mixed food items.
   3. Finger foods remain popular.
   4. Do not bribe child to eat or tell child to "clean your plate." Serve smaller portions; if sufficient amounts are not eaten during mealtimes, eliminate snacks.
   5. Recognize that refusing to eat is a way to attract attention.

School-Age Child

A. Diet.
   1. Food intake is more varied.
   2. Child enjoys most foods, with vegetables being the least favorite.
B. Implications for family teaching.
   1. After-school snack: encourage healthy choices such as fruits, raw vegetable sticks, and peanut butter sandwiches.
   2. Appetite is usually good, but a child often does not want to take the time to eat. Sometimes it is helpful to spend a specific amount of time at the table (15 to 20 minutes) to prevent the child from forming the habit of gulping food down.
   3. Avoid using food as a reward for behavior.
   4. Influence of media and peers regarding fast food is increased.
   5. Begin teaching child to recognize high-fat foods.

Adolescent

A. Rapid growth rate and maturation changes make the adolescent vulnerable to nutritional deficiencies. Diets in general are deficient in iron, calcium, and vitamin C.
B. Girls' peak growth occurs between 10 and 14 years of age.
C. Boys' peak growth occurs between 12 and 15 years of age.
D. Six out of ten girls eat only two-thirds of the nutrients required. Girls tend to be deficient in iron, whereas boys tend to be deficient in thiamine (Table 2-3).

Adult

A. Diet.
   1. Energy requirements decrease with age.
      Example: A 55-year-old man requires 2400 kcal; at age 76, he requires only 2050 kcal.
      Example: A 55-year-old woman requires 1800 kcal; at age 76, she requires only 1600 kcal.
   2. Improved financial status during middle adulthood tends to promote an increased intake of rich foods and frequency of dining out.
B. Nursing implications.
   1. Adherence to a prudent diet pattern.
   2. Promotion and continued maintenance of a regular exercise program.
   3. Reduce sodium intake to 3 to 6 g daily.
   4. Maintain serum cholesterol level below 200 mg/dL.

Older Adult

A. Diet.
   1. Encourage a diet low in fat and high in fiber, iron, vitamin C, and thiamine with adequate sources of calcium (see Table 2-3).
   2. If bed rest is prescribed, fluid intake should be as high as 3 to 4 L/day to prevent kidney stones, unless client has fluid restrictions (e.g., client with congestive heart failure).
   3. Because the older adult often has impaired renal function, protein and potassium intake should be evaluated.

Table 2-3	VITAMINS AND MINERALS		
Name	**Function**	**Food Sources**	**Nursing Implications**
Vitamins: Fat-Soluble			
Vitamin A: Retinol	Vision adaptation, night vision, normal bone and tooth formation	Liver, whole milk, egg yolk, yellow/green vegetables	If child eats excessive amounts of yellow vegetables, he or she will have yellow skin color. Important in preterm infants. Children with reduced fat absorption may have deficiency (CF, hepatitis, etc).
Vitamin D: Cholecalciferol	Promotes normal absorption of calcium and phosphorus	Fish, direct sunlight, enriched foods (e.g., milk products, cereals)	Breastfed infants may need supplement. Expose infant to short periods of mild sunlight.
Vitamin E: Tocopherol	Production of normal red blood cells, antioxidant	Milk, meat, egg yolks, whole grains, legumes, spinach, broccoli	Preterm infant may need supplement.

Table 2-3	VITAMINS AND MINERALS—cont'd

Name	Function	Food Sources	Nursing Implications
Vitamins: Fat-Soluble			
Vitamin K: Aqua-Mephyton	Necessary for production of clotting factors	Pork, liver, green leafy vegetables, tomatoes, egg yolks, cheese	Administer vitamin K prophylactically to newborns. Intake may be decreased in clients receiving warfarin and dicumarol anticoagulants.
Vitamins: Water-Soluble			
Vitamin B_1: Thiamine	Necessary for healthy nervous system, coenzyme for carbohydrate metabolism	Pork, beef, legumes, whole grains, enriched cereals, green vegetables	Clients with increased metabolic rate need more vitamin B_1 (e.g., clients with fever, clients who are pregnant, clients receiving long-term IV therapy). Increase intake in alcoholic clients.
Vitamin B_6: Pyridoxine	Stimulates heme production for red blood cells, necessary for antibody formation	Organ meats, wheat and corn cereal grains, soybeans, tuna, chicken, salmon	Be aware of drug-induced deficiencies: isoniazid, oral contraceptives.
Vitamin B_{12}: Cobalamin	Formation of normal red blood cells, nerve function	Meat, liver, fish, poultry, milk, eggs, cheese	Supplement necessary for clients with gastric resection; must have intrinsic factor for normal absorption.
Vitamin C: Ascorbic acid	Increases absorption of iron for hemoglobin formation, necessary for collagen formation, antioxidant	Citrus fruits, tomatoes, strawberries, potatoes, cabbage, broccoli, melons, spinach	Cook vegetables with a lid and minimum water added. Clients taking aminoglycosides and anticoagulants need increased intake. Need is increased during growth or conditions that cause an increase in metabolism.
Minerals			
Iron (Fe)	Normal formation of hemoglobin, essential part of enzymes	Red meat such as liver, pork, and beef; poultry; beans; whole grains; enriched infant formula; enriched cereals and bread	Administer iron between meals; avoid use of antacids; stool will be black. Increase iron intake for clients with iron-deficiency anemias, those on vegetarian diets, pregnant women, infants consuming excessive amounts of milk.
Calcium (Ca)	Normal formation of bone and teeth; muscle contraction, especially the heart; clotting factors; normal nerve conduction	Dairy products, egg yolks, dark-green leafy vegetables (except spinach)	Adequate intake is needed for normal bone and tooth formation. Administer IV preparations with caution because of effects on heart. Increase supplements during pregnancy and lactation and after menopause.
Potassium (K)	Acid-base balance, nerve conduction, cardiac muscle contraction	Dried fruits, bananas, citrus fruits	Supplement when client is taking diuretics. Decreased potassium increases effects of digitalis.
Sodium (Na)	Acid-base balance, fluid balance	Table salt, prepared foods	Sodium deficiency is rare; focus is on decreasing intake except in situations of significant sodium loss (e.g., CF, diaphoresis).

B. Nursing implications.
1. Alteration in taste and reduced digestive function occur.
2. Logical sequence of eating food is biting, chewing, and swallowing. New denture wearers should be encouraged to reverse this order: swallow a liquid diet first, then chew soft foods, and finally, bite into regular foods.
3. The older adult may intentionally restrict fluids because of nocturia or stress incontinence.
4. Constipation is a chronic problem caused by decreased peristalsis; encourage increased intake of fluids and a high-fiber diet.
5. Loneliness and depression are often associated with poor appetite.

⚠ OLDER ADULT PRIORITY It usually takes more time for an older person to eat, and satiety is reached more quickly. Encourage frequent small meals rather than three large meals; providing liquid supplements is also beneficial.

Nutritional Assessment

A. Assess nutritional needs.
B. Create client profile: age, sex, height, weight, socioeconomic status, culture.
C. Determine nutritional status: note food habits; observe for physical signs indicative of nutritional status.
D. Determine disease or pathophysiologic process.
E. Be alert to high-risk clients: those who are overweight or underweight; those with congenital anomalies of GI tract; those who have had surgery of the GI tract; those who have problems with ingestion, digestion, absorption; and those receiving IV therapy for 10 days or more.

ALERT Intervene with the client who has an alteration in nutritional intake (adjust diet, change delivery to include method, tine and food preferences.)

Diet Therapy for High-Level Wellness

A. MyPyramid Plan (Figure 2-4).
B. Prudent diet.

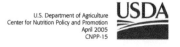

FIGURE 2-4 MyPyramid food guide. (From the U.S. Department of Agriculture Center for Nutrition Policy and Promotion, April 2005. Available at www.mypyramid.gov).

1. Increased amounts of fresh fruits, vegetables, and whole grains.
2. Reduced amounts of animal fats, cholesterol, refined sugar, salt, and alcohol.
3. Adaptations to MyPyramid (see Figure 2-4).
   a. Meat: includes fish, chicken, turkey, beef, legumes, eggs, nuts, and seeds as a source of protein.
   b. Milk: includes milk, yogurt, and cheese (select low-fat).
   c. Oils: selected fish, nut, and vegetable oils; limit butter, margarine, shortening, and lard.
   d. Fruits and vegetables: eat a variety; go easy on fruit juices.
   e. Vegetables: eat more dark green and orange vegetables.
   f. Grains, breads, and cereals: select whole-grain products and eat at least 3 oz every day.
C. Body mass index (BMI): measures weight as corrected for height.
   1. Divide the client's weight in kilograms by height in meters squared.

2. A client who weighs 165 lb, (75 kg) and is 5 ft 9 in tall (1.8 m) has a BMI of 23.15 (75 divided by $1.8^2 = 23.15$).
3. A client is considered overweight if the BMI is 25 to 30. A BMI greater than 30 is considered as obesity.

ALERT Apply knowledge of mathematics to client nutrition (body mass index, BMI). Evaluate and monitor client height and weight.

Therapeutic Meal Plans

A therapeutic meal plan or prescription diet is a modification of an individual's normal nutritional requirements based on the changes in his or her physiologic needs as a result of an illness or disease state (Table 2-4).

ALERT Consider client choices regarding meeting nutritional requirements and/or maintaining dietary restrictions, including mention of specific food items. Provide/maintain special diets based on the client diagnosis/nutritional needs and cultural considerations.

Table 2-4	THERAPEUTIC MEAL PLANS		
Diet	**Purpose/Use**	**Foods Allowed**	**Foods Restricted**
Clear liquid	To begin introduction of food after removal of NG tube, after GI surgery. Prior to GI diagnostics.	Liquids that are clear	Milk products, juice with pulp, any solid food; anything that is not liquid at room temperature
Full liquid	To begin introduction of food; used after removal of NG tube or after GI surgery	Any food that is liquid at room temperature	Any solid food
Soft diet	To progress diet as tolerated; food should be easy to chew and swallow	Soft, tender foods easy to swallow and digest	Highly seasoned foods, whole grains, fruits, vegetables, nuts, fried foods
Mechanical soft diet	To assist clients who cannot chew effectively	Soft foods that are easy to chew and swallow	Tough foods that are difficult to chest and swallow
Bland diet	To eliminate foods irritating to the digestive system; used in clients after GI surgery and those with peptic ulcer disease and GI inflammatory problems	Milk, custards, refined cereals, creamed soups, potatoes (baked or broiled); all foods are white; no bright-colored food	Highly seasoned or strong-flavored foods; tea, colas, coffee, fruits, whole grains, raw fruit
Low-residue diet	To decrease fiber or stool in GI tract; acute episodes of enteritis, diarrhea; before and/or after GI surgery	Clear liquids, meats, fats, eggs, refined cereals, white bread, peeled white potatoes, small amount of milk	Cheeses; whole grains; raw fruits and vegetables; high-carbohydrate foods, which are usually high in residue and fiber
High-residue diet	To prevent constipation and prevent acute diverticulitis	Raw fruits and vegetables; whole grains; high-carbohydrate foods, which are high in residue and fiber	Indigestible fibers: celery, whole corn; seeds such as sesame and poppy; foods with small seeds
Lactose-free diet	To prevent GI effects of lactose intolerance	Nonmilk products, yogurt	Milk and milk products, processed foods that may have dried milk as filler

Continued

Table 2-4	**THERAPEUTIC MEAL PLANS—cont'd**		
Diet	*Purpose/Use*	*Foods Allowed*	*Foods Restricted*
PKU diet	To control intake of phenylalanine, an essential acid; affected children cannot metabolize it	Specially prepared infant formula if infant is not breastfed, vegetables, fruits, juices, some cereals, and breads; may allow 20-30 mg of phenylalanine per kilogram of body weight to fulfill normal growth needs	Most high-protein foods, including meat and dairy products, are significantly reduced
Low-fat/low-cholesterol diet	To prevent gall bladder spasms, clients with increased cholesterol levels, or problems with malabsorption of fat (cystic fibrosis)	Low-fat or fat-free milk, fruits, vegetables, breads, cereals, reduced amounts of red meat	Egg yolks, whole milk, fried foods, processed cheese, shrimp, avocados, pastries, butter
Low-sodium diet	To reduce sodium intake to decrease retention of fluids, especially in clients with cardiac disease or hypertension	Salt-free preparations, fresh fruits, vegetables with no added salt	Processed foods, smoked or salted meats, prepared foods, frozen and canned vegetables, breads and pastries
High-potassium diet	To replace lost potassium in clients taking diuretics and/or digitalis	Dried fruits, fruit juices, fresh fruits (e.g., bananas, apricots, grapefruit, oranges, and tomatoes)	No specific restrictions
Renal diet	Control potassium, sodium, and protein levels in clients with renal problems	High biological protein (limited intake): eggs, milk, meat; decreased sodium products and decreased potassium (cabbage, peas, cucumbers are low in potassium)	High-potassium foods (dried fruits), high-sodium foods (processed foods), salt substitutes with high-potassium content
Low-purine diet	To decrease serum levels of uric acid; prescribed for clients with gout and high levels of uric acid	Vegetables, fruits, cereals, eggs, fat-free milk, cottage cheese	Glandular meats, fish, poultry, nuts, beans, oatmeal, whole wheat, cauliflower

GI, Gastrointestinal; *NG,* nasogastric; *PKU,* phenylketonuria.

Appendix 2-1	**DEVELOPMENTAL TASKS**		
STAGE OF DEVELOPMENT	ERIKSON'S DEVELOPMENTAL TASKS	PLAY/SOCIAL ACTIVITIES	HEALTH PROMOTION/MAINTENANCE
Infancy (birth to 1 year)	*Trust versus mistrust.* Parent-child bonding is crucial to the foundation for building a basic sense of trust. It is essential for primary needs to be gratified promptly.	Involved in solitary play activities. Provide toys that are soft, cuddly, and colorful; mobiles are very popular.	Encourage routine immunizations. Teach safety precautions related to burns, poisonings, accidents, and drowning.
Toddler (1 year to 3 years)	*Autonomy versus shame and doubt.* Child relies heavily on parental responses for support.	Toilet training is the major developmental accomplishment. Involved in parallel play activities. Provide toys that can be pulled, stacked together.	Continue to monitor safety by "childproofing" the home. Increased incidence of respiratory tract and ear infections.
Early childhood (3 years to 6 years)	*Initiative versus guilt.* Child uses imagination and creativeness.	Follows rules, compares self to others.	Progresses from solitary play to more cooperative play with others in a group.
Middle childhood (6 years to 12 years)	*Industry versus inferiority.* "Chum" period; progresses from self-centered to more other-directed behavior. Reality testing improves.	Younger child plays by assuming roles as a fireman, doctor, nurse, teacher, etc. Older child involved with bicycle riding, table games, sports, etc.	Respiratory tract infections are common illnesses as child goes to school. Booster immunizations are important.

Appendix 2-1   DEVELOPMENTAL TASKS—cont'd

STAGE OF DEVELOPMENT	ERIKSON'S DEVELOPMENTAL TASKS	PLAY/SOCIAL ACTIVITIES	HEALTH PROMOTION/ MAINTENANCE
Adolescence (12 years to 18 years)	*Identity versus role confusion.* Completion of previous tasks successfully will lead to a secure sense of self.	Peer groups are most important, with behavior being defined more by group members. Social activities include dating.	Mood swings common. Accidents associated more with driving cars and motorcycles.
Young adulthood (18 years to 44 years)	*Intimacy versus isolation.* Disturbances in sex role identity may occur because of inadequate resolution of identity crisis.	Involvement with social network of peers from community, work, etc. Appraisals by others affects sense of identity and self.	Stress-related illnesses and drug and alcohol abuse are common during this period. Another health issue is pregnancy.
Middle adulthood (45 years to 64 years)	*Generativity versus stagnation.* Reassessment of life goals. Mutuality among peers.	Leisure time becomes more of a concern. Key socializing agents are lovers, spouses, and close friends. Retirement occurs.	Menopause occurs, along with chronic health problems (e.g., diabetes, cancer).
Older adulthood (65 years and older)	*Ego integrity versus despair.* If person viewed life as worthwhile, will be better equipped to deal with aging.	Central process is introspection with the favorable outcome of wisdom along with a detached yet active concern with life in the face of death.	Safety concerns reoccur because of impaired sensory input. Alterations in all major body systems occur.

Study Questions Health Implications Across the Life Span

More questions on companion CD!

1. Which behavior indicates that an 18-month-old infant is developing a nonadaptive reaction to hospitalization?
   1   Cries when the mother leaves
   2   Ignores mother when she arrives to visit
   3   Eats using fingers rather than utensils
   4   Is afraid of the dark
2. An 8-month-old infant is sitting contentedly on the mother's lap. The nurse is preparing to perform a well-baby checkup. Which of the following steps should the nurse do first?
   1   Measure the head circumference.
   2   Obtain body weight and height.
   3   Auscultate heart and lung sounds.
   4   Check pupil response to light.
3. When obtaining a health history from an older client, the nurse must take which characteristics of the older client into consideration?
   1   The older client responds to pain sensation with the same intensity as a young client.
   2   Auditory acuity is the most common sensory loss in the older adult population and may hinder the interview.
   3   The older client requires a lot of repetition because the IQ declines with the aging process.
   4   An older client's response time to answering a question is just as quick as that of a young client.

4. Which of the following actions would the nurse recommend to provide a 12-month-old infant with nutrients for growth?
   1   Exclude milk from the infant's diet until he or she begins to like other foods.
   2   Offer the infant small amounts of meat and vegetables before offering milk.
   3   Withhold desserts until the infant has eaten his or her vegetables.
   4   Mix strained meat and vegetables into the milk given to the infant.
5. What are appropriate toys for an 18-month-old infant to have for play while in a croup tent?
   1   Rattles
   2   Stacking rings
   3   Crayons and coloring book
   4   Soap bubbles
6. The nurse is discussing nutrition with a woman who is 55-years-old and has a history of hypertension. What food choices would be best to help meet the dietary needs of this client?
   1   Cheese and macaroni, fresh fruit, and milk shake
   2   Cottage cheese, glass of skim milk, and fresh spinach salad
   3   Roast beef with whole wheat bread, potato, and lettuce salad
   4   Cheeseburger, french fries, and milk shake

7. The nurse is serving a food tray to a client who has glomerulonephritis and azotemia. Which food selection would the nurse question?
   1. Bread and rice
   2. Dried peaches and apricots
   3. Bran muffin and eggs
   4. Apples and cucumbers

8. Planning anticipatory guidance is an important nursing function. Considering the teaching for the family of an 18-month-old, which comment by the mother indicates she understands safety concerns?
   1. "I will keep an eye on her all of the time; I will not let her out of my sight."
   2. "When she says 'no-no,' then she understands right and wrong."
   3. "I will need to be sure that the locks on the medicine cabinet are secure."
   4. "I'll be sure to give her syrup of ipecac if she swallows any poison."

9. The nurse is assisting in the discharge preparation of a new mother and her infant. The mother asks when the immunizations will begin for her infant. What is the best nursing response?
   1. The first series of the DTaP vaccine will be given prior to her discharge.
   2. DTaP and varicella vaccines will be administered around 3 months of age.
   3. The series of infant immunizations will begin around 6 months of age.
   4. Immunizations are recommended to begin at 2 months old.

10. The nurse is assessing an infant on the first office visit after birth. The mother asks the nurse when the chicken pox vaccination should be given. What is the best nursing response?
    1. The infant received this vaccination at the hospital when he was born.
    2. The varicella vaccination will be given at the infant's 1-month checkup.
    3. The infant should receive the immunization immediately if he is exposed to varicella.
    4. The varicella vaccination is administered after 12 months.

11. A mother brings her 5-year-old daughter to the wellness clinic complaining of a rash covering the child's body. The nurse recognizes the rash as chicken pox (varicella), which is characterized by:
    1. Clusters of small blisters
    2. Raised, reddened areas on the upper trunk
    3. A maculopapular rash
    4. Petechiae

12. A client comes to the emergency department with a deep penetrating wound he received in his garden. What is an important nursing action?
    1. Rinse the wound with antibiotic solution.
    2. Administer gamma globulin intramuscularly.
    3. Anticipate notifying poison control for plant toxicology.
    4. Determine when the client received his last tetanus injection.

13. An infant with a diagnosis of acquired immunodeficiency disease syndrome (AIDS) has a nursing diagnosis of altered growth and development on the nursing care plan. Which nursing measure would enhance growth and development in the infant?
    1. Provide opportunities for the family to participate in the infant's care.
    2. Stimulate the infant with a mobile in the crib.
    3. Weigh the infant daily and count diapers for estimation of fluid loss.
    4. Provide nutritional supplements throughout the day.

14. In clients 65 years and older, how is death most commonly viewed?
    1. As a romanticized situation
    2. As a time of disassociation
    3. As a part of life
    4. As a time of denial

15. A client who is scheduled for a colonoscopy is instructed to take nothing except clear liquids for 6 hours before the procedure. What comment by the client would indicate to the nurse that the client does not understand the concept of clear liquids?
    1. "I can have beef or chicken broth."
    2. "Lemon-, orange-, or lime-flavored gelatin is okay."
    3. "I can have a small amount of vanilla ice cream."
    4. "I can have tea and coffee with sugar."

16. Which of the following is an appropriate teaching topic for the parents of a school-age child?
    1. Using a night light to allay night terrors
    2. Encouraging the child to dress without help
    3. Explaining the components of a healthy diet
    4. Reviewing information about accident prevention

Answers and rationales to these questions can be found in the section at the end of the book titled Chapter Study Questions: Answers and Rationales.

CHAPTER THREE

Concepts of Nursing Practice

BASIC HUMAN NEEDS

A. Maslow's hierarchy of basic human needs.
1. Human behavior is motivated by a system of needs.
2. Clients will focus or attempt to satisfy needs at the base of the pyramid before focusing on those higher up (Figure 3-1).
3. Human needs are *universal*; however, some may be modified by cultural influence.
4. The nursing process is always concerned with physiologic needs first; it then progresses to teaching, decreasing anxiety, etc. This is also true for the client with psychosocial needs; the client's physiologic needs must be met before he or she can progress to the next level.

❗ NURSING PRIORITY Maslow's hierarchy of needs is very useful in answering test questions related to setting priorities. Always remember that the physiologic needs at the base of the pyramid must be satisfied first in order to focus on other needs—and remember that oxygenation is always the first physiologic need or priority.

HEALTH ASSESSMENT

Subjective Health Assessment

ALERT Obtain a health history and conduct a risk assessment; perform a complete physical assessment.

❗ NURSING PRIORITY Ensure proper identification of client when providing care. Maintain client confidentiality.

Health History

A. Demographic data.
1. Name, address, phone, age, sex, marital status.
2. Race, religion, usual source of medical care.
B. Chief complaint/reason for visit.
1. Chief complaint: main reason client sought health care.
2. Chief complaint is recorded in client's own words. *Example: "I have been vomiting blood since this morning."*

C. History of the present illness.
1. Chronologic narrative.
2. *Areas of investigation* to evaluate the symptom.
   a. Sequence, chronology, and frequency.
   b. Bodily location and radiation.
   c. Character of the complaint: intensity or severity.
   d. Associated phenomena or manifestations.
   e. Aggravating or alleviating factors.
3. Includes relevant family history.
D. Medical history.
1. Perception of illness.
2. Previous illnesses: hospitalization, surgery, chronic illnesses.
3. Allergies, status of immunizations.
4. Accidents and injuries.
5. Current medications—prescribed and nonprescribed, including herbs and any complementary therapy.
6. Prenatal, labor and delivery, or neonatal history (recorded for all children under age of 5 and older children with a congenital or developmental problem).
7. Psychosocial history: sources of stress, coping mechanisms.

ALERT Perform a mental status assessment on nonpsychiatric client (see Chapter 10 for Mental Status Exam).

8. Activities of daily living.
   a. Nutrition and elimination routine.
   b. Rest/sleep.
   c. Personal habits (alcohol, smoking, exercise, etc.).
9. Developmental level: school/education, work, family activities, social activities.
   a. Denver II (or DDST-R): a developmental screening test for young children; not an IQ test, but a test to determine what a child can do at a particular age.
   b. Mental Status Exam: purpose is to evaluate the client's current cognitive processes (see Chapter 10.)
E. Review of systems.
1. Brief account from the client regarding any recent signs or symptoms associated with the body systems.

Maslow's Hierarchy of Basic Human Needs

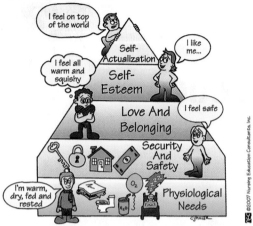

FIGURE 3-1 Maslow's hierarchy of needs. (From Zerwekh J, Claborn J: *Memory notebook of nursing,* vol 1, ed 4, Ingram, Texas, 2008, Nursing Education Consultants.)

2. Contains subjective data given by the client; *does not* contain information from the physical examination.
3. When a symptom or problem is encountered in the review of systems, the following information should be determined:
   a. Location: In what area of the body does the symptom occur?
   b. Character: Quality of the problem, feeling, or sensation. Is pain sharp or dull, constant or intermittent?
   c. Intensity: Severity of symptom or feeling. Does it interfere with activities of daily living?
   d. Timing: When does the problem occur (onset, duration, frequency)? Does anything precipitate the problem?
   e. Aggravating/alleviating factors: What activities make the problem better or worse?
4. Review of system's progress is from head to toe. The pertinent information to include is located in the assessment section at the beginning of each system.

Nursing Assessment

Comprehensive Physical Assessment

ALERT Perform comprehensive health assessment—physical, psychosocial, and health history. Choose physical assessment equipment and technique appropriate for client.

A. General guidelines.
   1. If examiner is right-handed, examination should be conducted from the right side of the bed.
   2. Position bed or examining table at appropriate height.
   3. Adequately expose areas being examined.
   4. Explain each part of the examination to client as examination proceeds.
   5. Establish rapport by asking non-personal questions before the physical examination.

B. Techniques of physical assessment.
   1. Inspection.
      a. Careful examination and observation of area are important parts of the assessment.
      b. Each anatomic area is inspected *before* it is touched by examiner's hands or instruments.
   2. Palpation.
      a. Parts of the hand used during palpation.
         (1) Fingertips for fine, tactile discrimination (e.g., lymph nodes, skin texture).
         (2) Dorsa of hands for skin temperature (dorsal skin is thinner and more sensitive).
         (3) Palmar and ulnar surfaces for vibratory sensation.
         (4) Grasping position (pinching) of fingers for tissue consistency.
      b. Light palpation identifies areas of tenderness and muscle resistance.
      c. Deep palpation is essentially the same as light palpation; however, examiner uses two hands to press more deeply into the client's abdomen. If there is any tenderness present, perform deep palpation last.
   3. Percussion.
      a. Technique of striking body surface lightly but sharply to produce sounds.
      b. Indirect percussion.
         (1) Middle finger of the nondominant hand *(pleximeter)* is placed against the body surface, with palm and other fingers raised off the skin. Tip of middle finger of dominant hand *(plexor)* strikes the base of the distal phalanx of the pleximeter in a quick, sharp stroke.
      c. Direct percussion.
         (1) Gentle, direct striking of the body with one or more fingers or with the ulnar surface of the clenched fist.
         (2) Useful in assessing sinuses, kidneys, or the liver.
      d. Percussion sounds.
         (1) Resonance: loud, low note heard over normal lung tissue.
         (2) Hyperresonance: louder, lower, and longer note heard over emphysematous lung.
         (3) Tympany: loud, musical note with drum-like quality, heard over air-filled viscera (e.g., stomach or bowel).
         (4) Flat: soft, high-pitched, short note heard, for example, over the thigh.
         (5) Dull: medium-pitched note of intensity and duration heard over the liver.
   4. Auscultation.
      a. Bell of stethoscope is used for low-pitched sounds, such as murmurs and bruits.
      b. Diaphragm of stethoscope is used for high-pitched sounds such as wheezes and crackles.

C. Sequence of the physical examination (Table 3-1).

Table 3-1	SEQUENCE OF PHYSICAL EXAMINATION

Client Position	Areas Assessed
Supine, seated, and standing	Blood pressure and other vital signs
Seated	Head, face, eyes, ears, nose, mouth, neck, chest, breasts, hands
Supine	Breasts, heart, abdomen, inguinal region, anus and rectum, female genitourinary system (lithotomy position), hips, knees, ankles, feet
Seated	Reflexes, hands, arms, shoulders (muscle strength), cerebellum (rapid, alternating movements, sensory function [stereognosis])
Standing	Spine, ROM, varicose veins, cerebellum, gait, male genitourinary system

ROM, Range of motion.

D. When a client indicates a problem or symptom during the physical examination, that area should be investigated (see Review of systems above).

E. Detailed assessment findings for each body system are discussed at the beginning of each chapter.

Focused Assessment

> **ALERT** Perform a focused assessment (GI, respiratory, sensory, etc.). Perform a risk assessment (falls, mobility, ADLs).

A. An assessment that is limited to the particular need, health care problem, or health risk the client is experiencing.

B. Frequently used for bedside assessments.
1. Assess the specific characteristics of the problem.
2. Determine what type of nursing intervention is necessary.
3. Determine when the intervention should be done: immediately, later in shift, before client's discharge, etc.

C. An ongoing assessment is frequently focused on a client's current health problems. This type of assessment is most often done at the beginning of each shift by the nurse responsible for the care of the client.
1. Focus on client's current status; determine whether it correlates with the report the nurse received.
2. Monitor or determine the client's response to previous nursing interventions.
3. Evaluate client's response to current plan of care and determine whether any changes are necessary.
4. Evaluate for any evidence of development of complications. (Systems focused assessment is found at the beginning of each of the system chapters.)

> **ALERT** Implement measures to manage/prevent/lessen complications of client condition.

5. Determine whether there are any other problems the client is experiencing that have not been addressed.

HEALTH PROMOTION

Levels of Prevention

Preventive health care is more dynamic than health maintenance; it focuses on health enhancement and health promotion, whereas health maintenance is concerned with maintaining the status quo.

A. Primary: prevention of disease.
1. Goal is to achieve maximum functioning in each health potential area.
Examples: Stop smoking, practice safe sex, maintain body weight, limit alcohol intake, follow a regular exercise program and a healthy diet.

B. Secondary: early diagnosis and treatment.
1. Emphasis is on determining intervention priorities.
Examples: Screening for tuberculosis; glaucoma test, Pap smear, colon-rectal cancer, and testicular self-examination.

C. Tertiary: prevention of complications.
1. Focus is on the prevention of complications and rehabilitation after the disease or condition has already occurred.
Examples: Have blood drawn for a complete blood count before chemotherapy; initiate speech therapy after a cerebrovascular accident; start cardiac rehabilitation after a heart attack.

> **ALERT** Provide information regarding health maintenance recommendations, teach client actions to maintain health and prevent disease (immunizations, screening, etc.).

HEALTH TEACHING

Principles of Client Education (Box 3-1)

Box 3-1 STEPS IN CLIENT EDUCATION

1. Assessment—What needs to be taught? How does the client perceive the need to learn? Are there any physical or psychosocial learning barriers? Consider the client's age.
2. Planning—Establish learning objectives and content to be discussed. Determine how it will best be delivered.
3. Implementation—Determine whether the client is comfortable (physiologic needs are always first). Present the information in a manner the client can understand; provide opportunity for client feedback; provide written information and review it with the client; provide positive feedback.
4. Evaluation—Plan for a return demonstration if skill was taught; follow up with family; plan home visits, etc. to determine client's use of information.

> **❗ NURSING PRIORITY** Consider client's background and culture when preparing teaching materials and determine when client is ready to learn.

A. Common characteristics of the adult learner.
 1. Self-directed.
 2. Client's background of experience, skills, attitudes, and culture form the basis for any new information received.
 3. Level of psychosocial development affects readiness to learn. If a client is in a midlife transition, it may be very difficult for the client to learn new attitudes and skills that threaten his or her self-image. *Example: A man in his early forties may have difficulty accepting any education regarding his colostomy.*
 4. Client wants to apply the learning immediately.

> **❗ OLDER ADULT PRIORITY** Older clients tend to be solitary learners; the nurse needs to consider ill health and sensory deficits that tend to occur (e.g., provide large-type books for reading); encourage wearing prescription eyeglasses and hearing aids.

B. Factors contributing to the teaching-learning process.
 1. Readiness to learn.
  a. Belief that material is relevant.
  b. Mental capacity to learn and physical ability to perform the skills.
  c. Must have physical and safety needs met.
  d. Comfort.
   (1) Physical comfort: discomforts such as pain, nausea, hunger, and the need to void are distractions that affect the learning process.
   (2) Psychologic comfort: anger, frustration, fear, and guilt severely hamper the learning process.

> **❗ NURSING PRIORITY** The first step in the education process is to make sure the client's physiologic needs are met; then determine what the client already knows about his or her condition.

  e. Client and nurse need to discuss and agree on specific long-term and short-term goals.
C. Factors relating to the presentation.

> **ALERT** Assess readiness to learn, learning preferences, and barriers to learning. Use age-appropriate explanations of procedures and treatments. Evaluate client understanding of information presented.

 1. State the specific objective of each teaching session; identify exactly what the client is to gain.
 2. Use vocabulary and terminology appropriate to client's understanding and to his or her developmental level. Use correct terms for body parts.

 3. Try to stimulate as many senses as possible. Use charts, handouts, and pieces of equipment when appropriate.
 4. Repetition is an integral part of learning.
 5. The more active the client is in the process, the better he or she will retain the information.
 6. Plan short sessions; do not overwhelm the client with too much information at one time.
 7. Actively involve the family and significant others, when appropriate.
 8. Be generous with positive reinforcement.
D. Pediatric factors influencing the learning process.
 1. Intellectual development moves from the concrete to the abstract.
 2. Nurse needs to assess the developmental level of a child before planning the educational approach.

> **❗ NURSING PRIORITY** A typical "no" response from a toddler being taught a new activity (e.g., combing hair) is usually an assertion of the child's independence, not an indication that he or she will not learn.

  a. Preschooler.
   (1) Frequently experiences fear of injury.
   (2) If under 4 years:
    (a) Generally does not benefit from anatomy and physiology information.
    (b) Needs clarification of reality and fantasy.
    (c) Separation anxiety is a problem; include parents in teaching session.
   (3) Preschoolers are aware of the physical and mechanical causes of problems they can see; unaware of physical and mechanical forces they cannot see.

> **❗ NURSING PRIORITY** It is important to emphasize to the preschooler that treatment is not punishment.

  b. School-age child.
   (1) Benefits from tours, drawings, anatomically correct dolls.
   (2) Cooperates with treatment and expresses feelings in words.
   (3) Learns well from role playing and puppets.
   (4) Needs to have parents included in teaching session for reinforcement and consistency.
  c. Adolescent.
   (1) Needs to be as independent as possible in management of health problem.
   (2) Present information with a scientific rationale rather than by giving specific directions.
   (3) Needs assistance in coping with loss of independence and self-direction.
   (4) Focus programs to deal with changes in body image and maintaining ego.

E. Special needs of the older client.
1. Determine functional losses (e.g., hearing or vision impairment, memory loss).
2. Identify social support to aid the older adult; this often increases compliance with instructions.

END-OF-LIFE CARE

A. Provide psychosocial support to client and family.

ALERT Provide end-of-life care to clients and families. Assist client and family to cope with end-of-life interventions.

1. Assist client and family to participate in treatment decisions, prepare advance directives.
2. Promote spiritual comfort—encourage/assist client to contact spiritual advisors.
3. Protect client from feeling abandoned or isolated—respond quickly to call lights, check on client often.
4. Encourage family to participate in care—assisting with food, hygiene measures, physical contact.

B. Promote culturally competent care—acknowledge and respect cultural differences and needs.
C. Assist client to understand terms.

NURSING PRIORITY It is important that clients understand that full comfort and physical assistance will continue to be provided regardless of their choice to be resuscitated or not.

1. Do not resuscitate or allow natural death (AND): maintain comfort measures, hygiene and pain control; order must be written on chart.
2. Full code: full CPR and resuscitation actions, including medications.
3. Chemical code: medications but no CPR.
4. Hospice care or palliative care.
   a. Does not refer to a place, but rather to a concept of care that provides support for the client who is dying.
   b. Care may be provided in long-term care facility, hospital, or at home.
   c. Criteria for hospice care includes the client's desire for the service and a physician's statement that the client will probably not survive beyond the next 6 months (the allowed time frame is somewhat flexible since actual amount of time cannot be predicted).

Physical Management of Symptoms

A. Physical symptoms of impending death.
1. Sensory.
   a. Hearing is usually the last sense to disappear.
   b. Taste, smell are diminished.
   c. Vision is often blurred, blink reflex may be absent.
2. Integumentary: skin is often cool and clammy; mottling occurs on extremities; cyanosis occurs around mouth and nose and on nail beds.

3. Respiratory.
   a. Respirations become shallow and irregular; Cheyne Stokes—periods of apnea alternating with deep rapid breathing.
   b. Increased mucus in upper airway causing gurgling, noisy respirations.
   c. Inability to cough or clear airway.
4. Cardiovascular.
   a. Heart rate may vary from a regular, increased rate to a slowing and irregular heartbeat before death.
   b. Decreased blood pressure and tissue perfusion.
5. Elimination.
   a. Urinary: output decreases, incontinence occurs.
   b. Bowel: monitor for constipation; bowel incontinence may occur.
6. Musculoskeletal.
   a. Gradual loss of ability to move, loss of facial muscle tone.
   b. Difficulty speaking, unaware of body position.
7. Neurologic.
   a. Decreased level of consciousness.
   b. Decreased reflexes: gag, cough, swallow.

B. Nursing interventions.
1. Provide palliative pain management—the prevention or relief of pain when a cure for the client's illness is not feasible.

ALERT Assess client symptoms related to end of life; ensure client receives appropriate end-of-life symptom management; assess client for nonverbal signs of pain/discomfort; assess, intervene, educate client and family regarding pain management.

   a. Pain medication is frequently administered on an around-the-clock schedule to maintain therapeutic levels of medication; do not delay or deny pain relief measures to a dying client.
   b. Moderate to large amounts of opioids may be required to maintain client's comfort.
   c. Administer analgesics based on client's level of pain; medication is increased as client's pain increases.
   d. Adjuvant medications to increase effectiveness of analgesics—antiemetics, antidepressants, corticosteroids.
   e. A nurse's or family's fear that the client will become dependent on, addicted to, or tolerant to the pain medication is inappropriate in provision of pain control in palliative care.
2. Dehydration: maintain oral hygiene; do not force the client to eat or drink. The option to withhold artificial nutrition or hydration should be made by the client in the advance directive, or by the person designated in advance directive.
3. Respiratory distress: elevate the head of the bed, offer oxygen, provide medications to decrease apprehension.

4. Elimination.
   a. Utilize incontinence pads, prevent skin irritation, follow facility protocol for indwelling catheters.
   b. Monitor bowel function, assess for impaction, promote normal function within client limitations.
5. Anorexia, nausea and vomiting.
   a. Assess for precipitating cause and administer medications to decrease nausea.
   b. Offer small, frequent meals, but do not focus on client's need to eat.
6. Determine client's personal preferences and cultural implications regarding death. Provide family care regarding cultural needs.

Postmortem Care

ALERT Provide postmortem care.

A. Determine whether there are any tissues or organs to be donated.
B. Determine whether the client's death should be reported and whether the client's death necessitates an autopsy and/or release from autopsy.
   1. Death resulting from foul play, homicide, suicide, or accident.
   2. Unattended death; death occurring at a workplace or during incarceration.
   3. Determine legal implications in the state of residence or in the state in which the client died.
C. Perform postmortem care as soon as possible.
   1. Determine whether family wants to participate in post mortem care.
   2. Unless client is to have an autopsy, remove all equipment according to facility policy.
   3. Cleanse the body and cover with a clean sheet. Place a pillow under the head and leave the arms on the outside of the sheet. Deodorize room if necessary.
   4. Offer the family an opportunity to be with the client. Provide privacy in an unrushed atmosphere.
   5. Return all personal belongings to the family. Document what items were taken and by whom.
   6. Attach identifying name tag to the body and to the shroud. Shroud the body according to facility policy.

BASIC NURSING SKILLS

Body Alignment and Range of Motion

A. Characteristics of correct body alignment in bed.
   1. Head up with eyes looking straight forward.
   2. Neck and back straight.
   3. Arms relaxed and supported at sides.
   4. Legs parallel to hips with knees slightly flexed.
   5. Feet separated and parallel to the legs with the toes pointed upward and slightly outward.

ALERT Perform a risk assessment for problems with mobility. Maintain correct body alignment.

B. ROM.
   1. Active ROM.
      a. Client performs exercise without assistance.
      b. Used for client who independently performs activities of daily living but for some reason is immobilized or limited in terms of activity.
      c. Purpose is to maintain muscle tone, decrease venous stasis, prevent muscle atrophy, and prevent contracture.
   2. Passive ROM.
      a. Client cannot actively move.
      b. Cannot contract muscles; therefore muscle strengthening *cannot* be accomplished.
      c. Purpose is to maintain joint flexibility, prevent contractures, and promote venous return.
C. Principles of ROM exercises.
   1. Stretch muscles by moving the body part; avoid movement to the point of discomfort.
   2. Perform ROM at least twice daily for immobile clients, with a minimum of 4 to 5 repetitions of each exercise.
   3. Always support extremity above and below the joint when performing passive ROM on extremities.
   4. Involve the client in planning the exercise program.
D. Client positions (see Appendix 3-1).

Asepsis

ALERT Always apply principles of infection control (handwashing, room assignment, isolation, aseptic/sterile technique, standard precautions).

A. Medical asepsis.
   1. Designed to reduce the number of pathogens in an area and decrease the likelihood of their transfer (e.g., by handwashing).
   2. Often referred to as *clean technique*; wash hands between visits with individual clients.
   3. Included in this category are daily hygiene practices and administration of oral medications, enemas, and tube feedings.
B. Surgical asepsis.
   1. Designed not simply to *reduce* the number of pathogens but to make the object *free* of all microorganisms.
   2. Also known as *sterile technique*.
   3. Surgical asepsis is reserved primarily for sterile dressing changes, sterile catheterizations, and surgical procedures in the operating room (Box 3-2).

ALERT Set up a sterile field. Use appropriate supplies to maintain asepsis (gloves, mask, sterile supplies); evaluate whether aseptic techniques are performed correctly.

Box 3-2 STERILE TECHNIQUE: PROCEDURES AND GUIDELINES

Procedures Requiring Sterile Technique

- Surgical procedures in the operating room (e.g., transurethral prostatectomy [TURP], appendectomy)
- Biopsies in the operating room, treatment room, or client's room
- Catheterizations of the heart, bladder, or other body cavities
- Injections: intramuscular (IM), subcutaneous (subQ), intradermal
- Infusions: IV, instillations or infusions of medication or radioactive isotopes into body cavities
- Dressing changes:
  - Usually, first postoperative dressing change done by using sterile technique
  - Dressings over catheters inserted into body cavities (e.g., Hickman catheter, subclavian lines, dialysis access sites)
  - Dressings of clients with burns, immunological disorders, and skin grafts

Guidelines for Sterile Field

- Never turn your back on a sterile field.
- Avoid talking.
- Keep all sterile objects within view (e.g., below waist is not within sterile field).
- Moisture will carry bacteria across/through a cloth or paper barrier.
- Transfer of objects from sterile to contaminated (not sterile) = contaminated.

Wound Care

A wound is a disruption in normal tissue caused by traumatic injury or created surgically.

> **ALERT** Provide wound care (irrigations, dressings). Monitor wounds for signs of infection.

A. Primary goals.
  1. Promote healing.
  2. Prevent further damage.
  3. Prevent infection.
B. Types of wounds.
  1. Black wounds.
    a. Necrotic devitalized tissue; high risk for infection.
    b. Frequently require sharp or surgical debridement of tissue for healing to occur.
  2. Yellow wounds.
    a. Contain devitalized tissue; require cleaning for healing to occur.
    b. Mechanical debridement requires irrigations and dressing changes. A 19F intravenous (IV) catheter on a 30-mL syringe provides safe pressure for irrigation and removal of devitalized tissue.
    c. Wet-to-dry dressings, wet-to-moist dressings, wound packing, and enzymatic debridement may be used to cleanse yellow wounds.
    d. Hydrocolloidal dressings to retain moisture.

  3. Red wounds.
    a. Require protection of fragile granulation tissue.
    b. Topical antibiotic ointment and nonadhering dressings may be used on shallow wounds.
    c. Wounds should be kept moist (moisture-retention dressings); dry dressings will damage the new granulation tissue.
C. Wound healing.
  1. Primary intention: wound margins are well approximated, as in a surgical incision or a repaired laceration.
  2. Secondary intention.
    a. Traumatic, infected wounds with exudates and wide, irregular margins and extensive tissue loss.
    b. Healing occurs by granulation from the edges inward and/or from the bottom up.
    c. Larger scar formation than with primary healing.
  3. Tertiary intention.
    a. Delayed suturing of the wound after infection is cleared and granulation tissue has been established.
    b. Occurs when a primary wound is infected and left open to heal by secondary intention; then the wound is sutured.
D. Wound healing affected by:
  1. Nutritional status.
    a. Adequate calories and protein are necessary for tissue healing.
    b. The obese client is at increased risk for poor wound healing and effective wound approximation.
  2. Tissue perfusion and oxygenation to wound.
  3. Excessive wound drainage: impairs tissue regeneration and will harbor bacteria.
  4. Diseases: cancer, renal disease, diabetes, and hepatic disease can delay wound healing.
  5. Medications: corticosteroids.
  6. Aging: slowing of tissue regeneration.
  7. Infection: prolongs inflammation and delays wound granulation.

> **ALERT** Promote client wound healing (nutrition, prevention of infection); identify factors that result in delayed wound healing.

E. Nursing intervention.

> **NURSING PRIORITY** When cleansing an area, always start at the cleanest area and work away from that area. Never return to an area you have previously cleaned; discard cleansing swab after each horizontal or vertical stroke.

  1. Cleansing of wound (Figure 3-2).
    a. Horizontal wound: cleansed from center of incision outward, then laterally.
    b. Vertical wound: cleansed from top to bottom, then laterally.
    c. Drain or stab wound: cleansed in a circular motion (Figure 3-3).

FIGURE 3-4 Penrose drain. (From Potter P, Perry A: *Fundamentals of nursing,* ed 7, St. Louis, 2009, Mosby).

FIGURE 3-2 Methods for cleansing a wound site. (From Potter P, Perry A: *Fundamentals of nursing,* ed 7, St. Louis, 2009, Mosby.)

FIGURE 3-3 Cleansing a drain site. (From Potter P, Perry A: *Fundamentals of nursing,* ed 7, St. Louis, 2009, Mosby).

FIGURE 3-5 Jackson-Pratt drain. (From Perry A, Potter P: *Clinical nursing skills and techniques,* ed 6, St. Louis, 2006, Mosby).

2. Penrose drain: soft, flexible drain inserted into an open wound to prevent the accumulation of secretions and exudate; frequent dressing changes are preferable to reinforcement of the same dressing (Figure 3-4).

> **⚠ NURSING PRIORITY** Avoid pooling of excessive drainage under saturated dressing; this can lead to skin irritation and infection.

3. Montgomery straps: used when frequent dressing changes are needed; help to prevent skin irritation that could occur with tape removal.
4. Elasticized abdominal binders.
5. Jackson-Pratt catheter or drainage system: bulb must be compressed to allow air to escape and then recapped to maintain suction (Figure 3-5).
6. Hemovac: evacuator must be compressed at least every 4 hours to provide suction; be sure to empty drainage from pouring spout; keep drainage spout sterile when emptying.

> **ALERT** Monitor and maintain devices and equipment used for drainage. Manage wound care (irrigations, dressings, wound suction devices).

7. Negative pressure wound therapy: a device is used to apply localized negative pressure to the wound to assist in closing the wound.
   a. Measure appropriate size foam to cover the wound.
   b. Apply transparent dressing over foam, sealing the wound.
   c. Secure tubing from the vacuum source to the port on transparent dressing.
   d. Dressing and foam are changed every 24 hours to several days.
8. Wet-to-dry dressings.
   a. Purpose is to trap necrotic or nonviable tissue in the dressing as it dries.
   b. Dressing should be moist when applied and allowed to dry for 4 to 6 hours.
   c. When dressing is changed, the packed dressing should be gently removed along with absorbed

drainage and nonviable tissue. Do not soak packing before removal; this will decrease the removal of non viable tissue.

9. Moisture retention dressings.
   a. Maintain moisture to promote healing and prevent damage to healing tissue.
   b. Dressing is coated with gel, colloids, or antibacterial preparations to prevent skin maceration and promote healing.
   c. May be used to assist in debridement of wounds or to protect healthy tissue during healing process.
10. Obtain a specimen of wound drainage.
    a. Gently roll a sterile swab in the purulent drainage.
    b. Obtain wound specimen before any medication or antimicrobial agent is applied to wound area or administered to client.

Specimen Collection

A. General principles.
   1. Use sterile equipment.
   2. Use the correct container for each specimen; preservatives, anticoagulants, or chemicals may be required.
   3. Always observe standard precautions when obtaining specimens; keep outside of container clean to prevent contamination in transfer to the laboratory.
   4. Properly label the specimen. Collect the correct amount at the correct time.

ALERT Obtain specimens for diagnostic testing (e.g., wound cultures, stool, urine).

B. Types of specimen (refer to appendixes in chapters listed).
   1. Urine (see Chapter 23).
   2. Stool (see Chapter 18).
   3. Sputum and throat (see Chapter 15).
   4. Blood (see Chapter 14).

ALERT Obtain blood specimens peripherally or through a central line.

   5. Wound specimen.

Heat and Cold Applications

A. Heat applications.
   1. Purposes: to soften exudate, increase vasodilatation, promote healing, decrease pain.
   2. General principles.
      a. Moist heat penetrates more deeply than dry heat.
      b. Unless a physician orders continuous heat applications, treatment time is usually 20 to 30 minutes.
      c. Caution client regarding hot baths and vasodilating effect that may cause postural hypotension.
   3. Do not use heat on an area that is being treated with radiation, is bleeding, has been injured within the last 24 hours, or has decreased sensation.

4. Types of heat application.
   a. Moist heat pack.
   b. Pad that circulates warmed water to distribute dry heat to body parts. Cover the source to protect the skin.
   c. Heat lamp or heat cradle.
   d. Sitz bath.
B. Cold applications.
   1. Purposes: to promote vasoconstriction, decrease edema or temperature, stop bleeding, or stop pain by numbing pain receptors.
   2. Do not use cold applications on areas of decreased circulation, open wounds, or area treated with radiation therapy.
   3. Types of cold applications.
      a. Ice bag, ice collar, cold compress, or cold pack.
      b. Hypothermia blanket.
      c. Always cover the source with a cloth or towel to protect the skin.
   4. Reduces edema, if applied immediately after an injury.

NURSING PRIORITY Do not use hot or cold applications with conditions of impaired circulation (e.g., peripheral vascular disease or diabetes).

Vital Signs

ALERT Assess client's vital signs. Intervene when vital signs are abnormal (hypotension, hypertension, bradycardia, etc). Be able to compare client's current vital signs with baseline and know the range of normal for vital signs at different age levels. This is critical in identifying abnormal findings, as well as in evaluating response to treatment and specific criteria for medication administration.

A. Normal values (Table 3-2).
B. Assessment.
   1. Respirations.
      a. Evaluate an infant's respiratory pattern before stimulating him or her.
      b. Check thoracic cavity for symmetrical excursion.
      c. Breath sounds: evaluate with adult client in sitting position.
      d. Compare breath sounds on each side of client's chest.
   2. Pulse.
      a. Irregular radial pulse, weak volume, or low rate should be assessed by taking an apical pulse for a full minute.
      b. Apical pulse: auscultated at the fifth intercostal space at the midclavicular line (point of maximal impulse).
      c. Apical-radial pulse: determined by two people counting both the apical and radial pulses at the same time; provides the *pulse deficit*, which is the difference in the two values.

Table 3-2	NORMAL VITAL SIGNS

Neonate

Respiration	30-60 breaths/min
Pulse	120-140 beats/min

Child 2 to 4 years

Respiration	24-32 breaths/min
Pulse	90-130 beats/min

Child 6 to 10 years

Respiration	15-26 breaths/min
Pulse	70-110 beats/min
Blood pressure	90/40-110/60 mm Hg

Adult

Respiration	12-18 breaths/min
Pulse	60-100 beats/min
Blood pressure	100/60-120/80 mm Hg

d. Weak peripheral pulse: evaluate by means of Doppler ultrasonography.
e. Check apical pulse in neonates, infants, and small children.
3. Temperature.
   a. Temperature affected by mouth-breathing and temperature of oral intake.
   b. Oral temperature is taken unless otherwise indicated.
4. Blood pressure assessment (Box 3-3).

ALERT Apply knowledge of client's pathophysiology when measuring and assessing vital signs.

IMMOBILITY

Immobility is the therapeutic or unavoidable restriction of a client's physical activity.

A. Causes of restricted movement.
   1. Spinal cord injury or neurologic damage.
   2. Presence of severe pain (e.g., from arthritis, surgery, or injury).
B. Therapeutic reasons for restricted movement.
   1. To decrease pain.
   2. To immobilize a wound.
   3. To limit exercise and activity for clients with cardiac problems.
   4. To reduce effects of gravity on the vascular bed and reduce edema formation.

Adverse Physical Effects of Immobility

ALERT Identify complications of immobility. Provide measures to prevent complications of immobility.

Box 3-3	BLOOD PRESSURE ASSESSMENT

Procedure: Client should be in a sitting position without legs crossed. The inflatable cuff is wrapped snugly around the upper half of the arm. The cuff is inflated 20 to 30 mm Hg above the point at which radial pulsation disappears. As the cuff is deflated, a sound is produced within the brachial artery just below the cuff and is audible with the stethoscope. The sounds (Korotkoff sounds) coincide with each pulse beat. Usually, when the cuff pressure is below diastolic, the sounds will cease or become muffled.

❗ NURSING PRIORITY *It is important to ascertain and record when the sounds become muffled. If there is any doubt, the blood pressure (BP) may be recorded as a tripartite pressure (120/70/50 mm Hg), implying that the sound became muffled at 70 mm Hg and disappeared at 50 mm Hg.*

Nursing Implications: Size of cuff should be 20% wider than the diameter of the limb. If the cuff is too large (e.g., on a child's arm), the BP obtained will be substantially lower than the true BP. If the cuff is too small (e.g., on an obese person's arm), the BP obtained will be higher than the true BP. The difference in BP between the right and left arms is normally 5 to 10 mm Hg.

Goal: To prevent complications.
A. Cardiovascular system.
   1. Assessment of physical effects.
      a. Orthostatic hypotension.
      b. Decrease in cardiac reserve.
      c. Venous stasis.
      d. Formation of thrombi.
      e. Increase in cardiac workload.
   2. Nursing implications.
      a. Position body to decrease venous stasis.
      b. Change position frequently.
      c. Passive and active ROM.
      d. Begin activity gradually; allow client to sit before standing.
      e. Have client use bedside commode when possible to decrease effects of Valsalva maneuver.
B. Respiratory system.
   1. Assessment of physical effects.
      a. Decrease in thoracic excursion.
      b. Decrease in ability to mobilize secretions.
      c. Decrease in oxygen/carbon dioxide exchange.
      d. Increase in pulmonary infections.
   2. Nursing implications.
      a. Elevate head of bed.
      b. Maintain adequate hydration: 2400-3000 mL/day if tolerated.
      c. Have client turn, cough, and breathe deeply at regular intervals (every 2 hours while awake).
      d. Promote increase in activity as soon as possible: have client sit up in chair at bedside.
      e. Evaluate pulmonary secretions for infection.

C. Urinary system.
  1. Assessment of physical effects.
     a. Urinary stasis.
     b. Increased calcium level, stasis, and infection precipitate stone formation.
     c. Urinary tract infections.
  2. Nursing implications.
     a. Have client sit or stand to void if possible.
     b. Establish/maintain voiding schedule.
D. Musculoskeletal system.
  1. Assessment of physical effects.
     a. Demineralization of bones: decrease in bone strength.
     b. Muscle weakness and atrophy.
     c. Loss of motion in joints leads to fibrosis and contractures.
  2. Nursing implications.
     a. Perform ROM exercises.
     b. Active contraction and relaxation of large muscles.
     c. Position body to maintain proper alignment.
     d. Encourage daily weight-bearing exercise when possible.
E. Gastrointestinal system.
  1. Assessment of physical effects.

ALERT Identify factors that interfere with elimination.

     a. Anorexia.
     b. Ineffective movement of feces through colon: constipation and fecal impaction.
     c. Diarrhea caused by impaction.
  2. Nursing implications.
     a. Establish bowel program: every other day or three times a week.
     b. Encourage diet with adequate protein, fiber, and liquids.
     c. Check for impaction.
F. Integumentary system.
  1. Assessment of physical effects.

ALERT Identify client with potential for skin breakdown; maintain client skin integrity; manage client with impaired skin integrity.

     a. Decrease in tissue perfusion leading to decubitus ulcer.
     b. Decrease in sensation in area of increased pressure.
  2. Nursing implications.
     a. Maintain cleanliness.
     b. Promote circulation through frequent repositioning.
     c. Protect bony prominences when turning.
     d. Prevent creation of pressure areas by tight clothing, cast, braces.
     e. Perform frequent visual inspection of pressure areas.

Adverse Psychologic Effects of Immobility

A. Assessment of psychologic effects.
  1. Depression, increased anxiety.
  2. Feelings of helplessness.
  3. Intellectual and sensory deprivation.
  4. Change in body image.
B. Nursing implications.
  1. Maintain sensory stimulation.
  2. Encourage family, social contact.
  3. Promote reality orientation.
  4. Encourage family to bring items from home such as pictures, bed clothes, toys.
  5. Encourage verbalization of feelings.
  6. Provide opportunities for client to make choices and participate in care.
  7. Arrange counseling as appropriate: vocational, sexual, financial.

ALERT Evaluate client's response to immobility and response to interventions to prevent complications of immobility.

PAIN

- Clients have the right to appropriate assessment and pain management.
- Physiologic and behavioral signs of pain should not replace the client's ability to report the pain unless client is unable to communicate.
- Pain can exist even when there is no identifiable physical cause; it is a totally subjective personal experience.
- Different clients experience different pain levels, even in response to same type of pain stimulus.
- Pain is an early warning system; its presence triggers awareness that something is wrong in the body.
- Unrelieved pain causes adverse physical and psychologic response.

ALERT Plan measures to care for clients with anticipated or actual alterations in comfort.

Classification of Pain

- Acute pain: has an identifiable cause; is protective; short, predictable duration (lasting less than 3 months); immediate onset; reversible or controllable with treatment. Most often has an identifiable source such as postoperative pain that disappears as the wound heals.
- Chronic pain: lasts more than 6 months; continual or persistent and recurrent. Pain may not go away; periods of decreased and increased pain. Origin of pain may not be known.
- Nociceptive pain: *somatic* pain affecting skeletal muscles, joints, and ligaments; generally diffuse and less localized; *visceral* pain arises from internal organs and may be caused by a tumor or obstruction.
- Neuropathic pain: caused by damage or peripheral nerves or to the CNS; can result from trauma, metabolic disease, or neurologic disease.

- Referred pain: pain that does not occur at the point of injury. For example, pain related to myocardial ischemia may be felt in the left arm or shoulder; cholecystitis may be felt as shoulder pain.
- Phantom pain: pain that follows the amputation of a body part; may be described as throbbing, cramping, or burning in the body part amputated.

Pain Characteristics (Figure 3-6, Box 3-4)

> **ALERT** Assess and document client's discomfort and pain levels.

A. Pattern of pain.
  1. Pain onset and duration: when it started, precipitating causes, and how long it lasts.
  2. Breakthrough pain: transient; may be moderate to severe and occurs beyond current analgesic treatment; usually rapid onset and very intense.
B. Area of pain.
  1. Ask the client to identify the pain site.
  2. Pain may be referred from the precipitating site to another location—shoulder pain with cholecystitis, left arm pain with MI.
  3. Sciatica pain follows a nerve pathway of the sciatic nerve, generally down the back of the thigh and inside the leg.
C. Intensity of pain: use a pain scale to help the client communicate the pain intensity.

Box 3-4   MNEMONIC TO EVALUATE PAIN

P: Provoking or palliative factors
Q: Quality
R: Region
S: Severity
T: Timing

D. Pain quality/type.
  1. Neuropathic pain may be burning, numbing, shooting.
  2. Visceral and somatic pain may be sharp, throbbing, cramping.
E. Determine any activities and situations that increase the level of the pain—movement, ambulation, coughing.
F. Client responses to pain (Box 3-5; see Figure 3-6).
  1. Increased blood pressure, pulse, and respirations.
  2. Diaphoresis, increased muscle tension, nausea and vomiting.
  3. Client's interpretation and meaning of the pain experience.

> **NURSING PRIORITY** In addition to the pain and discomfort associated with a surgical procedure, it is important to assess other possible sources of discomfort, such as a full bladder, occluded catheter or tube, gas accumulation, IV infiltration, or compromised circulation caused by position or pressure.

Cultural Implications of Pain

A. Cultural beliefs and values affect how a client responds to pain.

Box 3-5   ASSESSING THE HARMFUL EFFECTS OF PAIN

Acute Pain	**Chronic Pain**
Disturbs sleep	Fatigue
Appetite decreases	Weight gain
Fluid intake decreases	Poor concentration
Nausea and vomiting	Job loss
	Divorce
	Depression

> **NURSING PRIORITY** The nurse should administer pain medication to clients experiencing acute pain without fear of addicting the client to the medication.

PHYSIOLOGIC FACTORS

Organic origin
Integrity of nervous system, including endogenous opioids
Concomitant physical influences (stress, fatigue)
Age
Type of pain
Location
Intensity
Duration
Frequency
Quality
Threshold
Tolerance
Genetics

AFFECTIVE FACTORS

Distress of pain
Depression
Mood
Anxiety, fear, worry

PSYCHOSOCIAL INFLUENCES

Family and occupational roles
Personal beliefs
Spiritual belief system
Cultural/societal influences
Sexual identity and stereotypes
Demographic factors

COGNITIVE

Past experience
Meaning of pain experience
Attention paid to sensation/distraction
Expectations
Coping mechanisms
Knowledge
Values/attitudes
Communication skills

FIGURE 3-6 Considerations of the pain experience. (From Black J, Hawks J: *Medical-surgical nursing: clinical management for positive outcome,* ed 7, Philadelphia, 2005, Saunders.)

B. Assess attitudes and beliefs that may affect effective treatment of the pain. Some clients may believe that taking pain medications will cause "addiction"; other clients may believe that complaining of pain is a sign of weakness.

C. Avoid stereotyping clients by assuming that members of a specific cultural group will or will not exhibit more or less pain.

D. Nursing considerations of pain control associated with a client's culture.
1. Identify what the pain means to the client; for example, a woman in labor will perceive the pain differently than a client who experiences pain as an indication of advanced disease.
2. Identify cultural implications regarding how a client responds to or expresses pain; some clients moan and complain loudly; others may be very quiet and stoic.
3. Individualize pain control based on client's response to pain.
4. Establish a communication method for the client to express the level of pain and effectiveness of pain control (e.g., pain rating scale, FACES scale, pictures, images).
5. Expression of pain is subjective; accept client's perception of pain and expression of pain and facilitate nursing care to meet client's cultural needs when providing pain control.

> **ALERT** Assess importance of client culture/ethnicity when planning/providing/evaluating care.

Non-Drug Pain Relief Measures

A. Relaxation techniques.

> **! NURSING PRIORITY** Low levels of anxiety or pain are easier to reduce or control than higher levels. Consequently, pain relief measures should be used *before* pain becomes severe.

1. Relaxed muscles result in a decreased pain level.
2. Relaxation response requires quiet environment, comfortable position, and a focus of concentration.
3. Identify relaxation method that is most effective for client—music, imagery meditation for progressive muscle relaxation.
4. Meditation: focuses attention away from pain.

> **ALERT** Assess client need for pain management and intervene using nonpharmacologic comfort measures. Recognize differences in client perception and response to pain. Evaluate client response to nonpharmacologic comfort measures.

B. Hypnosis: produces a state of altered consciousness characterized by extreme responsiveness to suggestion.

C. Biofeedback: provides client with information about changes in bodily functions of which he or she is usually unaware (e.g., blood pressure, pulse).

D. Cutaneous stimulation: alleviates pain through stimulation of skin.
1. Use of pressure, massage, bathing, and heat or cold therapy to promote relaxation.
   a. Applied to different areas of the body.
   b. Contralateral stimulation: when stimulation of the skin near the pain site is ineffective, the side *opposite* the painful area is stimulated for pain relief.

E. Therapeutic touch: holistic approach in which touch is used to realign energy fields (laying on of hands).

F. Transcutaneous electric nerve stimulation (TENS).
1. Delivers an electrical current through electrodes applied to the skin surface of the painful region or to a peripheral nerve.
2. Instruct client to adjust TENS unit intensity until it creates a pleasant sensation and relieves the pain.

G. Acupuncture: most common complementary therapy.
1. Requires insertion of thin metal needles into the body at designated points to relieve pain.
2. Is effective in pain management, as well as nausea and vomiting associated with postoperative and chemotherapy.
3. Encourage client to review the credentials of the practitioner, who should have a master's degree in oriental medicine and be registered to practice in the state.

H. Nursing intervention for pain relief (nonpharmacologic).
1. Change positions frequently and support body parts.
2. Encourage early ambulation after surgery.
3. Elevate swollen body parts.
4. Check drainage tubes to ensure that they are not stretched, kinked, or pulled.

Medications for Pain Relief

A. Nurse-administered as-needed (PRN) analgesic medications (see Appendixes 3-2 and 3-3).

> **! NURSING PRIORITY** Plan pain medication administration schedule. Use a preventive approach to pain relief by giving analgesics before the pain occurs—or at least before it reaches severe intensity.

1. Steps in administering PRN medications.
   a. Assess client to determine source, quality, and characteristics of pain.
   b. Analyze nursing assessment data; determine most appropriate nursing intervention.
   c. Check client's chart.
      (1) Determine the last medication received and how it was administered.
      (2) The time administered.
      (3) Client's response to previous medication.
   d. Select appropriate medication.
      (1) Use nonopioid analgesics for mild to moderate pain.
      (2) Avoid combinations of opioids for older adults.

(3) IV medications act more rapidly for acute pain relief.

(4) Avoid IM injections in older adults.

(5) Sustained-release and extended-release oral medications work well for chronic pain management and will provide pain management over a longer period of time.

e. Decrease stimuli in room; determine other factors influencing discomfort.

f. Assess client's response to pain intervention at regular intervals and document nursing actions.

> **ALERT** Determine client's need for PRN medications; review pertinent data before medication administration (vital signs, lab results, allergies, potential interactions); evaluate appropriateness/accuracy of medication order for client. Provide pharmacologic pain management appropriate for age and diagnosis; evaluate and document client's use of and response to pain medication.

2. Types of medications.
   a. Narcotic analgesics (opioids) are used for relieving severe pain (see Appendix 3-2).
   b. Nonnarcotic analgesics act at peripheral sites to reduce pain (see Appendix 3-3).

B. Patient-controlled analgesia (PCA).
   1. Client controls pain by delivery of IV infusion of medication through a PCA pump.

> **⊞ OLDER ADULT PRIORITY** Analgesics tend to last longer in older adults; there is an increased risk for side effects and toxic effects. Recommendation from the American Geriatric Society is to "start low" and "go slow"—but provide adequate pain relief for older adults.

2. Confused clients are not good candidates; surgical clients should be oriented to PCA procedure before surgery.
3. PCA is effective in pediatrics; ability to comprehend the procedure is more important than the age.
4. PCA pump procedure.
   a. Pain should be under control when PCA is initiated.
   b. Delivers a specific amount of medication as controlled by client.
   c. Parameters for bolus dose of medication should be available for episodes of increased pain (dressing changes, chest tube insertion, etc.) as well as for the client who goes to sleep and awakens with severe pain unrelieved by PCA.
   d. Dose interval is usually 6 to 8 minutes with lockout time of 1 hour.
   e. Only one dose can be administered over 6 to 8 minutes for a lockout time of 10 mg in 1 hour. Even though the client may push the button several times in succession, only 1 dose will be given every 6 to 8 minutes and a total of only 10 mg can be give in 1 hour.

f. Example: PCA morphine 1 mg/1 mL, 1.5 mg of morphine every 8 minutes with a lockout of 10 mg over 1 hour.

g. Check the PCA pump every 4 hours for correct settings and to determine how much pain medication is being used.

h. Instruct any family member or significant others *not* to administer medication (document that you have done this). Explain that PCA works on the principle that when the client is uncomfortable, he or she will use the PCA.

> **⊞ NURSING PRIORITY** PCA pumps are part of the High-Alert Medications ▲ and Patient Safety protocols from The Joint Commission. PCA protocols include double-checks of the drug, pump setting, and dosage. Watch the decimals! An order for morphine 0.5 mg could be mistakenly entered in the PCA pump as 5 mg.

5. Advantages of PCA.
   a. More effective pain control.
   b. Decreased client anxiety (no waiting for medication).
   c. Increased client independence.
   d. Decreased level of sedation.
   e. Clients tend to use fewer narcotics.

C. Patient-controlled epidural analgesia (PCEA).
   1. Injection of medication through a small catheter into the epidural space of the spinal cord; common pain medications are morphine and fentanyl.
      a. Relieves pain without causing sympathetic and motor nerve block.
      b. May be an intermittent (patient- or nurse-controlled) or constant infusion.
      c. Client may experience numbness, tingling and coolness when analgesia is initiated.
      d. Requires the use of High-Alert Medications. ▲
   2. Complications.
      a. Opioid medications: nausea and vomiting, constipation, respiratory depression, and pruritus.
      b. Urinary retention may occur: palpate suprapubic area; client may require urinary catheterization.
      c. Catheter dislodgement and migration: client begins to experience pain even with additional medication; catheter should be securely taped and labeled.
      d. Lower extremity motor or sensory deficits can be the result of a hematoma or infection; notify the health care provider.
   3. Monitor every 15 minutes for initial response; then every hour after stabilization.

D. Perineural local anesthetic infusion.
   1. Utilizes an infusion pump, which provides local anesthetic (bupivacaine or ropivacaine) to a nerve root or a group of nerves.
      a. Catheter or tubing may be placed in a surgical wound and positioned near the nerve root; catheter is usually not sutured.

b. May be continuous or on demand; usually left in place for about 48 hours.

2. May be used in conjunction with oral analgesics.

Barriers to Pain Management

A. Addiction: the need to take pain medication for reason other than therapeutic relief of pain.

B. Physical dependence: the occurrence of withdrawal syndrome when the medication is abruptly decreased. When opioid medications are no longer needed for pain relief, a tapering schedule should be initiated to decrease the symptoms of the withdrawal syndrome.

C. Tolerance: characterized by the need to increase the medication to achieve the same reduction of pain. If opioid tolerance is suspected, use of another type of opioid is recommended.

> **! OLDER ADULT PRIORITY** Analgesics tend to last longer in older adults; this increases the risk for side effects and toxic effects.

Palliative Pain Relief

A. The prevention or relief of pain when a cure for the client's illness is not feasible.

> **ALERT** Palliative/comfort care: assess client for nonverbal signs of pain/discomfort. Assess, intervene, and educate client/family about pain management.

B. Administer analgesics based on client's level of pain; medication is increased as client's pain increases.

C. Adjuvant medications to increase effectiveness of analgesics.
   1. Antiemetics, antidepressants.
   2. Corticosteroids.
   3. Nonsteroidal antiinflammatory drugs (NSAIDs).

D. Pain medication is frequently administered on an around-the-clock schedule rather than a PRN schedule to maintain therapeutic levels of medication. Pain medication is administered in the absence of pain.

E. A nurse's or client's fear that the client will become dependent on, addicted to, or tolerant to medication is inappropriate in the provision of pain control in palliative care.

F. Breakthrough pain: occurs frequently in clients with cancer.
   1. Transient, moderate to severe pain that may occur with clients who have adequate pain control with dosing schedule.
   2. Develops quickly and intensifies rapidly.
   3. May occur spontaneously, may be precipitated by coughing, may occur at any time during the dosing interval, or may occur toward the end of the dose.
   4. Rescue medication should be available—a strong opioid with a rapid onset and short duration is preferred.

G. Fear that opioids will hasten death is unsubstantiated, even in clients at the very end of life. It is important that nurses provide adequate pain relief for the terminally ill client.

PERIOPERATIVE CARE

Preoperative Care

> **ALERT** Determine whether client is prepared for a procedure or surgery.

A. Client profile.
   1. Age: older adult clients are more likely to have chronic health problems, as well as age-related factors; infants have more difficulty maintaining homeostasis than adults and children (Box 3-6).

> **! OLDER ADULT PRIORITY** Older clients have less physiologic reserve (the ability of an organ to return to normal after a disturbance in its equilibrium) than younger clients.

   2. Obesity predisposes client to postoperative complications of infection and wound dehiscence.
   3. Preoperative interview.
      a. Chronic health problems and previous surgical procedures and experiences.
      b. Past and current drug therapy, including over-the-counter medications (vitamins, herbal remedies, homeopathic medications).

Box 3-6 OLDER ADULT CARE FOCUS

Preoperative and Postoperative Considerations

Older clients are at increased risk for developing postoperative complications because of the decreased response of the immune system (which delays healing) and the increased incidence of chronic disease.

- Cardiovascular: decreased cardiac output and peripheral circulation, along with arrhythmias and increased incidence of arteriosclerosis and atherosclerosis, can lead to hypotension or hypertension, hypothermia, and cardiac problems.
- Respiratory: decreased vital capacity, reduced oxygenation, and decreased cough reflex can lead to an increased risk for atelectasis, pneumonia, and aspiration.
- Renal: decreased renal excretion of wastes and renal blood flow along with increased incidence of nocturia can lead to fluid overload, dehydration, and electrolyte imbalance.
- Musculoskeletal: increased incidence of arthritis and osteoporosis can lead to trauma on bones and joints with positioning in the operating room if pressure points and limbs are not padded.
- Sensory: decreased visual acuity and reaction time can lead to safety problems associated with falls and injuries.

The older client may require repeated explanation, clarification, and positive reassurance. Older clients often have a poor nutritional status, which can directly influence healing and postoperative recovery.

c. History of drug allergies and dietary restrictions.

d. Client's perception of illness and impending surgery.

e. Discomfort or symptoms client is currently experiencing.

f. Religious affiliation.

g. Family or significant others.

4. Psychosocial needs: fear of the unknown is the primary cause of preoperative anxiety.

> **! OLDER ADULT PRIORITY** The older client may require repeated explanation, clarification, and positive reassurance.

5. Medications: may predispose client to operative complications.

a. Anticoagulants: potentiate bleeding.

b. Antidepressants: monoamine oxidase inhibitors increase hypotensive effects of anesthetic agents.

c. Tranquilizers: increase the risk for hypotension; may be used to enhance anesthetic agent.

d. Thiazide diuretics: create electrolyte imbalance, particularly in potassium level.

e. Steroids: prolonged use impairs the physiologic response of the body to stress and decrease wound healing and decreases the inflammatory response necessary for wound healing.

6. Check results of routine diagnostic laboratory studies.

a. Complete blood count: serum electrolytes, coagulation studies, serum creatinine, blood urea nitrogen, and fasting glucose.

b. Urinalysis.

c. Chest x-ray.

d. Electrocardiogram for clients over 40 years of age.

e. Coagulation studies for clients with known problems or to establish a baseline.

B. Preoperative teaching: goal is to decrease the client's anxiety and prevent postoperative complications.

> **ALERT** Provide pre- and/or postoperative education.

1. Preoperative teaching content.

a. Deep breathing and coughing exercises.

b. Turning and extremity exercises.

c. Pain medication administration policy.

d. Adjunct equipment used for breathing: nebulizer, oxygen mask, spirometer.

e. Explanation of NPO (nothing by mouth) policy.

f. Antiembolism stockings and/or pneumatic compression device to decrease venous stasis.

2. Pediatric implications in preoperative teaching.

a. Plan the teaching content around the child's developmental level and previous experiences.

b. Use concrete terms and visual aids.

c. Plan teaching session at a time in the child's schedule when he or she will be most receptive to learning.

d. Use correct terms for body parts and clarify terms with which the child is unfamiliar.

e. Introduce anxiety-provoking information last (increased anxiety may decrease comprehension).

f. Use role playing to either explain procedures to the child or to allow the child to do a return demonstration.

g. Fear of anesthesia is very common in children.

h. Include the parents in the teaching process.

C. Physical preparation of client.

1. Skin preparation: purpose is to reduce bacteria on the skin (may be done in surgical suite or in the preoperative holding area).

a. Area of preparation is always longer and wider than area of incision.

b. Antiseptic soap is used to cleanse area.

2. Gastrointestinal preparation.

a. Food and fluid restriction: NPO orders may be individualized for each client. Client may be NPO for 6 to 8 hours before surgery or NPO from midnight on the night before surgery. Trend is to allow clear liquids up to 2 hours preoperatively. Always check physician orders and agency policy.

b. Enemas or cathartics: may be administered the evening before surgery to prevent fecal contamination in the peritoneal cavity.

3. Promote sleep and rest: sleep-aid medication may be given to promote rest (e.g., barbiturate).

4. In older adults, evaluate status of teeth, presence of bridges and dentures; in children, evaluate for presence of loose teeth.

D. Legal implications (see Chapter 4).

1. Each surgical procedure must have the voluntary, informed, and written consent of the client or the person legally responsible for the client.

> **ALERT** Provide written materials in client's spoken language if possible. Describe components of informed consent (purpose of procedure, risks of procedure). Participate in obtaining informed consent. Ensure that client has given informed consent for treatment.

2. Physician: gives the client a full explanation of the procedure, including complications, risks, and alternatives.

3. Client's informed consent record (permit) must be signed by the client or guardian. A witness signs to validate this is the client's signature. The witness is frequently a staff nurse. Depending on facility policy, the surgeon may also be required to sign the consent form.

> **! NURSING PRIORITY** Determine that the client understands relevant information before procedure/surgery; do not witness the client's signature on an informed consent form until you verify that the client has received the relevant information.

4. The signed consent record (permit) is part of the permanent chart record and must accompany the client to the operating room.

Day of Surgery

ALERT Monitor a client before, during, and after a procedure/surgery.

A. Nursing responsibilities.
1. Routine hygiene care.
2. Vital signs within 1 hour before "on call" to surgery, or per agency policy.
3. Remove jewelry; wedding bands may be taped on finger.
4. Remove contact lenses, fingernail polish, depending on agency policy.
5. Dress client in patient gown.
6. Determine whether dentures and removable bridge work need to be removed before surgery.
7. Continue NPO status.
8. Check client's identification for two identifiers.
    a. The first identifier should reliably identify the client for whom service or treatment is intended, for example, the client's name.
    b. The second identifier is used to match the service or treatment to that individual—for example, the client's hospital identification number.
9. Identify family and significant others who will be waiting for information regarding client's progress.
10. Check the chart for completeness regarding laboratory reports, consent form, significant client observations, history, and physical exam records.
11. Allow parent to accompany child as far as possible.
B. Preoperative medications (see Appendix 3-4).

! **NURSING PRIORITY** Explain to client the purpose of preoperative medications and advise client not to get out of bed. Side rails should be up and the call light within reach.

1. Purpose.
    a. Induce anesthesia rapidly.
    b. Reduce anxiety.
2. Nursing responsibilities.

! **NURSING PRIORITY** The operative permit or informed consent record must be signed before the client receives the preoperative medication.

    a. Confirm that all consent forms are signed and that the client understands the procedure.
    b. Ask client to void before administration of medication.
    c. Obtain baseline vital signs.
    d. Administer medication 45 minutes to 1 hour before surgery or as ordered.

    e. Raise the side rails and instruct the client not to get out of bed.
    f. Observe for side effects of medication.
C. The "time out" or protocol for preventing wrong site, wrong procedure, wrong person surgery must occur in the location where the procedure is done. The surgical team are involved in the positive identification of the client, the intended procedure, and the site of the procedure.

ALERT Prepare client for surgery or procedure, monitor client before, during and after surgery or procedure; assess client's response to surgery and/or treatment.

Anesthesia

A. General anesthesia.
1. Intravenous anesthesia: used as an induction agent before the inhalation agent is administered.
2. Inhalation anesthesia: used to progress client from stage II to stage III of anesthesia.
B. Regional anesthesia: used to anesthetize one region of the body; client remains awake and alert throughout the procedure.
1. Topical: anesthetizing medication applied to mucous membrane or skin; blocks peripheral nerve endings.
2. Local infiltration: injection of anesthetic agent; only blocks peripheral nerves around area.
3. Peripheral nerve block: anesthetizes individual nerves or nerve plexuses (digital, brachial plexus); does not block the autonomic nerve fiber; medication is injected to block peripheral nerve fibers.
4. Spinal anesthesia: local anesthetics are injected into the subarachnoid space; may be used with almost any type of major procedure performed below the level of the diaphragm.
5. Epidural anesthesia: anesthetic agent is introduced into the epidural space; cerebral spinal fluid cannot be aspirated.
C. Nursing considerations for regional anesthesia (spinal/epidural) (Table 3-3).
D. Conscious sedation: the administration of an IV medication to produce sedation, analgesia, and amnesia.
1. Characteristics.
    a. Client can respond to commands, maintains protective reflexes, and does not need assistance in maintaining an airway.
    b. Amnesia most often occurs after the procedure.
    c. Slurred speech and nystagmus indicate the end of conscious sedation.

ALERT Determine that client and family understand relevant information before administration of conscious sedation.
Assist with preparing client for conscious sedation. Monitor client physiologic response during and after conscious sedation.

Table 3-3	NURSING CARE OF THE CLIENT UNDERGOING REGIONAL ANESTHESIA
Problem	*Nursing Interventions*
Preparation for procedure	1. Explain procedure. 2. Do preoperative preparation and have surgical client sign consent form. 3. Assess client for effectiveness as anesthesia is initiated. 4. Client will remain awake throughout procedure.
Hypotension	1. Report BP less than 100 mm Hg systolic or any significant decrease. 2. Place client flat. 3. Administer oxygen. 4. Increase IV rate if client is not prone to heart failure.
Respiratory paralysis	1. Avoid extreme Trendelenburg position before level of anesthesia is set. 2. Evaluate client's respiratory status. 3. Have ventilatory support equipment available.
Nausea and vomiting	1. Antiemetics. 2. Anticipate nausea if client becomes hypotensive. 3. Suction, or position client to prevent aspiration.
Loss of bladder tone	1. Evaluate for bladder distention.
Trauma to extremities	1. Support extremity during movement. 2. Remove legs from stirrups simultaneously.
Headache	1. Ensure adequate hydration before, during, and after procedure. 2. Maintain recumbent position 6 to 12 hr after procedure. 3. Administer analgesics.

BP, Blood pressure.

2. Nursing implications.
a. Perform baseline assessment before procedure; implications for care are the same as those for a client receiving general anesthesia.
b. Client is assessed continuously; vital signs are recorded every 5 to 15 minutes.
c. Monitor level of consciousness; client should not be unconscious, but relaxed and comfortable.
d. Client should respond to physical and verbal stimuli; protective airway reflexes should remain intact.
e. Potential complications include loss of gag reflex, aspiration, hypoxia, hypercapnia, and cardiopulmonary depression.
3. Does not require extensive postoperative recovery time.

Immediate Postoperative Recovery

ALERT Provide postoperative care.

A. Admission of client to recovery area.
1. Position client to promote patent airway and prevent aspiration.
2. Perform baseline assessment.
a. Vital signs, quality of respirations, pulse oximetry, pulse rate and rhythm, general skin color.
b. Type and amount of fluid infusing.
c. Special equipment; status of dressings.
3. Determine specifics regarding the operation from the operating room nurse.

a. Client's overall tolerance of surgery.
b. Type of surgery performed, type of anesthetic agents used.
c. Results of procedure: Was the condition corrected?
d. Any specific complications to watch for.
e. Status of fluid intake and urinary output.
f. Common postoperative complications (Table 3-4).

ALERT Assess client's response to surgery; evaluate client's response to postoperative interventions to prevent complications; intervene to prevent aspiration.

B. Nursing management during recovery.
Goal: To maintain respiratory function.

NURSING PRIORITY The client's respiratory status is a priority concern on admission to the postoperative recovery area and throughout the postoperative recovery period.

1. Leave airway in place until pharyngeal reflex (gag reflex) has returned.
2. Position client on side (lateral Sims' position) or on the back with the head turned to the side to prevent aspiration.
3. Suction excess secretions and prevent aspiration.
4. Encourage coughing and deep breathing.
5. Administer humidified oxygen.
6. Auscultate breath sounds.

Table 3-4	COMMON POSTOPERATIVE COMPLICATIONS	
Complication	*Signs and Symptoms*	*Nursing Intervention*
Atelectasis	Dyspnea, decreased or absent breath sounds over affected area, asymmetrical chest expansion, hypoxia	Prevention: have client turn, cough, and breathe deeply; provide adequate hydration; encourage ambulation. Position client on unaffected side. Maintain humidification, oxygen (see Chapter 15).
Shock	Decreasing blood pressure, weak pulse, restless, confusion, oliguria	Initiate IV access, keep NPO, maintain bed rest. Position supine with legs elevated and knees straight. Monitor ventilation and vital signs frequently (see Chapter 16).
Wound infection	Poor wound healing, redness, tenderness, fever, tachycardia, leukocytosis, purulent drainage	Prevention: identify high-risk clients; maintain sterile technique with dressing changes. Culture incision to determine organism. Evaluate progress and prevent spread of infection. **ALERT** Monitor wounds for signs and symptoms of infection.
Wound dehiscence	Unintentional opening of the surgical incision	Evaluate for hemorrhage; use measures to prevent further pressure at incision site.
Wound evisceration	Protrusion of a loop bowel through the surgical wound	Cover bowel with sterile saline solution–soaked dressing. Do not attempt to replace loop of bowel. Notify physician; client will most likely return to surgery for further exploration.
Urinary retention	Inability to void after surgery; bladder may be palpable; voiding small amounts, dribbling	Determine preoperative risks: medications, length of surgery, history of prostate problems. Determine amount of fluid intake and when to anticipate client to void—generally within 8 hr. Palpate suprapubic area, run tap water, provide privacy. Catheterize if necessary.
Gastric dilatation, paralytic ileus	Nausea, vomiting, abdominal distension, decreased bowel sounds	Prevention: Older adult clients are at increased risk; encourage activity as soon as possible; maintain nasogastric tube suction and NPO status; if NG tube is not present, may begin early feeding of clear liquids to increase intestinal motility; maintain IVs with hydrating solution. See Chapter 18.

IV, Intravenous; *NPO,* nothing by mouth; *NG,* nasogastric.

Goal: To maintain cardiovascular stability.

ALERT Plan and implement interventions to prevent complications after surgery. Intervene to manage potential circulatory complications; monitor for signs of bleeding; intervene to manage potential circulatory complications (hemorrhage, embolus, shock).

1. Check vital signs every 15 minutes until condition is stable.
2. Report blood pressure that is continually dropping 5 to 10 mm Hg with each reading.
3. Report increasing consistent bradycardia or tachycardia.
4. Evaluate quality of pulse and presence of dysrhythmia.
5. Evaluate adequacy of cardiac output and tissue perfusion.

Goal: To maintain adequate fluid status.

❗ NURSING PRIORITY Antidiuretic hormone secretion is increased in the immediate postoperative period. Administer fluids with caution; it is easy to cause fluid overload in a client.

1. Evaluate blood loss in surgery and response to fluid replacement.
2. Maintain rate of IV infusion; maintain I&O record.
3. Monitor urine output and possible bladder distention.
4. Evaluate hydration and electrolyte status.
5. Observe amount and character of drainage on dressings or drainage in collecting containers.
6. Assess amount and character of gastric drainage if nasogastric tube is in place.
7. Evaluate amount and characteristics of any emesis.

> ⚠ **NURSING PRIORITY** When client is vomiting, prevent aspiration by positioning client on the left side and suction, if not contraindicated.

Goal: To maintain incisional areas.
1. Evaluate amount and character of drainage from incision and drains.
2. Check and record status of Hemovac, Jackson-Pratt, Penrose, or any other wound drains.

Goal: To maintain psychologic equilibrium.
1. Speak to client frequently in calm, unhurried manner.
2. Continually orient client; it is important to tell client that surgery is over and where he or she is.
3. Maintain quiet, restful atmosphere.
4. Promote comfort by maintaining proper body alignment.
5. Explain all procedures, even if client is not fully awake.
6. In the anesthetized client, sense of hearing is the last to be lost and the first to return.

Goal: Client meets criteria to return to room.
1. Vital signs are stable and within normal limits.
2. Client is awake and reflexes have returned.
3. Dressings are intact with no evidence of excessive drainage.
4. Client can maintain a patent airway without assistance.

General Postoperative Care

> **Alert** Anticipate situations with questions regarding basic postoperative nursing care, as well as questions that are for a specific surgical condition or procedures. Nursing implications for specific surgical procedures may be found under the major systems in the care of the medical-surgical patient.

Goal: To maintain cardiovascular function and tissue perfusion.
1. Monitor vital signs every 4 hours.
2. Evaluate skin color and nail beds for pallor and cyanosis.
3. Monitor level of hematocrit.
4. Assess client's tolerance to increasing activity.
5. Encourage early activity and ambulation.

Goal: To maintain respiratory function.
1. Have client turn, cough, and breathe deeply every 2 hours.
2. Use incentive spirometry to promote deep breathing.
3. Administer nebulizer treatment and bronchodilator.
4. Maintain adequate hydration to keep mucus secretions thin and easily mobilized.
5. Encourage deep breathing with ambulation.

Goal: To maintain adequate nutrition and elimination.
1. Assess for return of bowel sounds, normal peristalsis, and passage of flatus.
2. Assess client with a nasogastric tube for return of peristalsis.
3. Assess client's tolerance of oral fluids; usually begin with clear liquids.
4. Encourage intake of fluids, unless contraindicated.
5. Progress diet as client's condition and appetite indicate or as ordered.
6. Record bowel movements; normal bowel function should return on the second or third postoperative day (provided that the client is eating).
7. Assess urinary output.
   a. Client should void 8 to 10 hours after surgery.
   b. Assess urine output; should be at least 30 mL/hr.
   c. Promote voiding by allowing client to stand or use bedside commode.
   d. Avoid catheterization if possible.

Goal: To maintain fluid and electrolyte balance.
1. Assess for adequate hydration.
   a. Moist mucous membranes.
   b. Adequate urine output with normal urine specific gravity.
   c. Good skin turgor.
2. Assess lab reports of serum electrolytes.
3. Assess character and amount of gastric drainage through the nasogastric tube.
4. Assess urine output as it correlates with fluid intake; maintain good intake and output records.
5. Evaluate lab data for indications of decreased renal function.

Goal: To promote comfort.
1. Determine nonpharmacologic pain relief measures.
2. Administer analgesics and or monitor patient controlled analgesia.

Appendix 3-1 POSITIONING AND BODY MECHANICS

POSITION	PLACEMENT	USE
Fowler's	Head of bed at 45- to 60-degree angle; hips flexed	The height may be determined by client preference or tolerance; frequently used for client with respiratory compromise.
Semi-Fowler's	Head of bed at 30- to 45-degree angle; hips flexed	Cardiac, respiratory, neurosurgical conditions.
Low Fowler's	Head of bed at 15- to 30-degree angle; hips may or may not be flexed	Postoperative, gastrointestinal conditions.
Trendelenburg	Head of bed lowered and foot raised; knee gatch straight	Thoracic percussion, vibration, and drainage procedure. Compromises respiratory function; client should not be left in position for extended time.
Modified Trendelenburg	Head of bed flat or slightly elevated; legs elevated about 20 degrees; knees should be straight	May be used for client in shock: promotes movement of fluids from lower extremities into circulation. Minimizes respiratory compromise.
Lateral (side-lying)	Head of bed lowered; pillows under arm and legs and behind back; flex knee of anterior side	For client comfort; increases uterine and renal perfusion in pregnancy and prevents supine vena cava syndrome during labor.
Semi-prone (Sims')	Head of bed lowered; client placed on side with dependent shoulder lifted out and lying partially on abdomen; place pillow under flexed arm and under upper flexed knees	Prevents pressure ulcer; used for comfort.
Lithotomy	On back with thigh flexed against abdomen and legs supported by stirrups	For examination of female reproductive tract and rectum, cystoscopy, and surgical procedures.
Prone	Head of bed flat, client on abdomen, head turned to side	To promote drainage after tonsillectomy; to prevent contractures in clients with above-the-knee amputation, to protect client with imperforate anus, or spina bifida.
Supine	Bed in flat position, small pillow under head	For client comfort.

ALERT Position client to prevent complications after tests, treatments, or procedures.

Body Mechanics—Prevention of Injury

- Use lift equipment and ask for adequate assistance.
- Manual lifting of a client should be avoided. If it is necessary to manually lift most or all of the client's weight, obtain adequate assistance or use safe client handling equipment.
- Ergonomics of lifting:
  1. Avoid twisting; keep your head and neck aligned with your spine.
  2. Place feet wide apart for good base of support; knees should be flexed.
  3. Position yourself close to the bed or close to the client.
  4. Use arms and legs to assist in lifting client, not your back.
- Use pull sheet or slide board to move client to side of bed and/or to move up in bed.

✓ KEY POINTS: Assisting the Client to Move Up in Bed

- Lower the head of the bed so that it is flat or as low as the client can tolerate; raise the bed frame to a position that does not require leaning.
- If more than one person is needed for assistance, obtain a lifting device.
- Determine the client's strong side and have him or her assist with the move.
- Instruct the client to bend legs, put feet flat on bed, and push.

- Use a draw sheet or a lift sheet.
- Never pull a client up in bed by his arms or by putting pressure under his arms.

✓ KEY POINTS: Logrolling the Client

- Spinal immobilization—use a team approach.
- Maintain proper alignment on head and back areas while turning.
- Before moving client, place a pillow between client's knees.
- Move client in one coordinated movement, using a turn/lift sheet.

✓ KEY POINTS: Moving From Bed to Chair

- Move client to the side of the bed (bed wheels locked) closest to the edge where the client will be getting up.
- Assist client out of bed on his strongest side.
- Raise head of bed to assist client in pivoting to the side of the bed.
- Move client to edge of bed and place hands under his legs and shift his weight forward, pivot his body so he is sitting position and his feet are flat on the floor.
- Have client reach across chair and grasp arm.
- Stabilize client by positioning your foot at the outside edge of client's foot.

Continued

Appendix 3-1 POSITIONING AND BODY MECHANICS—cont'd

- Pivot client into chair using your leg muscles instead of your back muscles.
- Assist client to move back and up in the chair for better position.

ALERT Maintain correct body alignment.

Tips for Moving Clients

- Use a turn sheet to provide more support for client.
- Encourage client to assist in move by using the side rails and strong side of his or her body.

- No-lift policy: use of equipment and assistance whenever a client requires most of his weight to be supported or lifted by someone.
- Obtain additional assistance and/or use lift equipment to help in moving the client.
- Use trochanter roll made from bath blankets to align the client's hips to prevent external rotation.
- Use foam bolsters to maintain side-lying positions.
- Use folded towels, blankets, or small pillows to position client's hands and arms to prevent dependent edema.

Appendix 3-2 ANALGESICS

General Nursing Implications

— Assess pain parameters, blood pressure, pulse, and respiratory status before and periodically after administration.
— Administer before pain is severe for better analgesic effect.
— Elderly or debilitated clients may require decreased dosage.

MEDICATIONS	SIDE EFFECTS	NURSING IMPLICATIONS

Narcotic Analgesics: Bind to opiate receptors in the central nervous system (CNS), altering the perception of and emotional response to pain; controlled substances (Schedule II)

MEDICATIONS	SIDE EFFECTS	NURSING IMPLICATIONS
Strong Opioid Analgesics ▲ Morphine sulfate: PO, subQ, IM, IV, epidural analgesia Meperidine (**Demerol**): PO, subQ, IM Fentanyl (**Fentanyl, Sublimaze, Duragesic**): IM, IV, PO, transdermal	Respiratory depression Orthostatic hypotension Sedation, dizziness, lightheadedness, dysphoria Constipation Tolerance, physical and psychological dependence May decrease awareness of bladder stimuli Seizure with Demerol **‼ NURSING PRIORITY** Advise clients using fentanyl patches not to expose patch to heat (hot tub, heating pad) since this will accelerate the release of the fentanyl. **‼ OLDER ADULT PRIORITY** Prevent problems with constipation.	1. Morphine is most commonly used for PCA. 2. Demerol: Not commonly used for control of chronic pain due to neurotoxic effect; use with caution in children and older adult clients because of increased risk for toxicity and seizures. 3. Morphine is not commonly used following biliary tract surgery. 4. All opioids: Use with caution in clients who have respiratory compromise. 5. Pediatric implications: Medication dosage is calculated according to body surface area and weight. 6. Assess voiding and encourage client to void every 4 hours. 7. Requires documentation as indicated by Controlled Substance Act. 8. Instruct client to change position slowly to minimize orthostatic hypotension.
Moderate to Strong Opioid Analgesics Codeine: PO, subQ Hydromorphone (**Dilaudid**): PO, subQ, IM, IV, suppository Oxycodone (**Percodan**, combination with ibuprofen; **Percocet, Tylox** combinations with acetaminophen; **OxyContin**): PO Hydrocodone (**Vicodin, Lorcet** combinations with acetaminophen; **Vicoprofen**, combination with ibuprofen): PO Propoxyphene (**Darvon, Darvocet**): PO	Sedation, euphoria, respiratory depression, constipation, urinary retention, cough suppression **‼ NURSING PRIORITY** Concurrent administration with nonnarcotic analgesics may enhance pain relief because they act at different sites.	1. Usually administered by mouth. 2. Codeine is an extremely effective cough suppressant. 3. Do not confuse hydromorphone with morphine. 4. Warn client to avoid activities requiring alertness until effects of drug are known. 5. Medications are often in various strength combinations with acetaminophen and/or ibuprofen. Advise client not to take additional acetaminophen or ibuprofen.

Appendix 3-2	ANALGESICS—cont'd	

MEDICATIONS	SIDE EFFECTS	NURSING IMPLICATIONS
Moderate Opioids		
Butorphanol (**Stadol**): IM, IV, nasal spray Nalbuphine (**Nubain**): subQ, IV, IM	Dizziness, drowsiness	1. Monitor client for effective pain control. 2. Abrupt withdrawal after prolonged use may produce symptoms of withdrawal.

Narcotic Antagonist: Antagonist that competitively blocks the effect of narcotics, without producing analgesic effects

Naloxone (**Narcan**): IV, IM, subQ	Hypotension, hypertension, dysrhythmias	1. Assess respiratory status, blood pressure, pulse, and level of consciousness until narcotic wears off. Repeat doses may be necessary if effect of narcotic outlasts the effect of the narcotic antagonist. 2. Remember that narcotic antagonists reverse analgesia along with respiratory depression. Titrate dose accordingly and monitor pain level. 3. *Uses:* Used to reverse CNS and respiratory depression in narcotic overdose. 4. *Contraindications and precautions:* Use with caution in narcotic-dependent clients; may cause severe withdrawal symptoms.

CDC, Centers for Disease Control and Prevention; *CNS,* central nervous system; *IM,* intramuscularly; *IV,* intravenously; *PCA,* patient-controlled analgesia; *PO,* by mouth (orally); *subQ,* subcutaneously

Appendix 3-3	NONSTEROIDAL ANTIINFLAMMATORY DRUGS (NSAIDs) AND ACETAMINOPHEN

General Nursing Implications
— Give with a full glass of water, either with food or just after eating.
— Store in childproof containers and out of reach of small children.
— Do not exceed recommended doses.
— Discontinue 1-2 weeks before elective surgery.
— NSAIDs prolong bleeding time by decreasing platelet aggregation; may increase anticoagulant activity of warfarin products.
— Avoid in clients with history of peptic ulcer disease or bleeding problems.
— May compromise renal blood flow and precipitate renal impairment.
— Do not crush enteric-coated tablets; if available, administer as enteric or buffered tablets.

Uses: Fever: acetaminophen, aspirin, ibuprofen; Inflammation: aspirin, naproxen; Arthritis: aspirin, ibuprofen, naproxen, piroxicam, sulindac; Dysmenorrhea: ibuprofen, naproxen

MEDICATIONS	SIDE EFFECTS	NURSING IMPLICATIONS
Nonsteroidal Antiinflammatory Drugs (NSAIDs) and Acetaminophen: Inhibit the enzyme cyclooxygenase, which is responsible for the synthesis of prostaglandins; suppress inflammation, relieve pain, and reduce fever		
Acetylsalicylic acid (**Aspirin, ASA**): PO ⚑ **NURSING PRIORITY:** Advise client that CDC warns against giving aspirin to children or adolescents with a viral infection or influenza.	Salicylism: skin reactions, redness, rashes, ringing in the ears, GI upset, hyperventilation, sweating, and thirst Long-term use: erosive gastritis with bleeding; increases anticoagulant properties of warfarin ⚑ **NURSING PRIORITY:** Aspirin is the only NSAID used to protect against MI and stroke.	⚑ 1. Most common agent responsible for accidental poisoning in small children. ⚑ 2. Associated with Reye's syndrome in children. 3. Assess for bleeding tendencies. 4. Prophylactic use for colon cancer. 5. Prophylactic use for cardiovascular problems due to the antiplatelet aggregation properties.

Continued

MEDICATIONS	SIDE EFFECTS	NURSING IMPLICATIONS
Ibuprofen **(Motrin, Nuprin, Advil)**: PO	Dyspepsia (heartburn, nausea, epigastric distress) Dizziness, rash, dermatitis	1. Do not exceed 3.2 g per day in adults and older adult clients. 2. Avoid taking with aspirin.
Naproxen **(Naprosyn)**; Naproxen sodium **(Anaprox, Aleve)**: PO	Headache, dyspepsia, dizziness, drowsiness	1. Avoid tasks requiring alertness until response is established. 2. Take with food to decrease GI irritation. 3. Primarily used for pain control.
Acetaminophen **(Tylenol, Datril, Tempra)**: PO	Anorexia, nausea, diaphoresis Toxicity: vomiting, RUQ tenderness, elevated liver function tests Antidote: acetylcysteine (Mucomyst, Acetadote) ⚠ **NURSING PRIORITY:** Frequently used in combination with OTC medications. Teach client to read labels to prevent overdosing.	1. Maximum dose of acetaminophen, 4 g per day. 2. Does not have antiinflammatory properties. 3. Overdose can cause severe liver injury; client should consult physician if he or she drinks more than 3 alcoholic beverages every day. 4. Has not been conclusively linked to bleeding problems.
Piroxicam **(Feldene)**: PO Sulindac **(Clinoril)**: PO	Dyspepsia, nausea, dizziness, diarrhea, nephrotoxicity	

GI, Gastrointestinal; *PO*, by mouth (orally); *RUQ*, right upper quadrant

MEDICATIONS	SIDE EFFECTS	NURSING IMPLICATIONS
Benzodiazepines: Decrease anxiety and promote amnesia before or during surgery		
Lorazepam **(Ativan)**: PO, IM, IV	Drowsiness, ataxia, confusion, fatigue May produce paradoxical effects in elderly	1. Decrease stimuli in the room after administration. 2. Offer emotional support to the anxious client. 3. Maintain bed rest after administration to reduce effects of hypotension. 4. A Schedule IV drug.
▲ Midazolam hydrochloride **(Versed)**: PO, IM, IV	Decreased respirations; pain at IM or IV site; nausea, vomiting	1. Commonly used for conscious sedation and amnesia prior to procedures. 2. Continuous monitoring during parenteral administration.
Diazepam **(Valium)**: PO, IM, IV	Same as for Ativan	
Histamine (H₂ Receptor Antagonists): Decrease gastric acid secretion, increase gastric pH		
Cimetidine **(Tagamet)** Famotidine **(Pepsid)** Ranitidine **(Zantac)**	See Appendix 18-5	
Anticholinergic: Prevent bradycardia, decrease secretions		
Atropine: PO, IM, IV Scopolamine: PO, IM Glycopyrrolate **(Robinul)**: PO, IM, IV	Flushed face Dilated pupils Increased cardiac rate Urinary retention	1. Children and older adult are at increased risk for side effects. 2. Advise clients regarding atropine flush. 3. Administer with caution to clients with glaucoma, MI, or CHF. 4. Postural hypotension may result if client ambulates after administration. 5. Monitor for urinary retention and decreased bowel sounds.

CHF, Congestive heart failure; *IV*, intravenously; *IM*, intramuscularly; *MI*, myocardial infarction; *PO*, by mouth (orally).
▲ High-Alert Medication.

Study Questions Concepts of Nursing Practice

More questions on companion CD!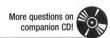

1. The nurse is preparing to take a blood pressure on a client who is obese. What is the most effective method for obtaining an accurate blood pressure reading from this client?
   1 Obtain a cuff that covers the upper one-third of the client's arm.
   2 Position the cuff approximately 4 inches above the antecubital space.
   3 Use a cuff that is wide enough to cover the upper-two thirds of the client's arm.
   4 Identify the Korotkoff sounds, and take a systolic reading at 10 mm Hg after the first sound.

2. The nurse is caring for a client who is dying. How will the nurse provide psychosocial comfort for the family and the client in the period before death?
   1 Encourage family to sit at the bedside, touch, and talk to the client.
   2 Discourage more that one family member at a time in the room.
   3 Discuss with the family the importance of not upsetting the client by talking to him.
   4 Administer pain medication so the client will not be upset by family visits.

3. The nurse is preparing a client for surgery. Which of the following items on the client's presurgery lab results would indicate a need to contact the surgeon?
   1 Platelet count of 325,000 mm^3
   2 Total cholesterol of 325 mg/dL
   3 Blood urea nitrogen (BUN) 17 mg/dL
   4 Hemoglobin 9.5 g/dL

4. The nurse has received a report on assigned clients. In planning the initial assessment of each client, what is the best approach?
   1 A thorough history of the hospitalization should be reviewed for trends in care, responses to therapy, and currency of medication orders.
   2 An assessment should be done to determine the client's current status, the development of complications, and whether any changes in nursing care are necessary.
   3 A complete head-to-toe physical examination should be conducted with emphasis on current health care problems.
   4 All laboratory results for the past 24 hours should be reviewed to determine changes that have occurred in the client's condition and to plan effective nursing care.

5. Which of the following clients would be at an increased risk for the development of a pulmonary embolus?
   1 A man with a fractured femur who is in balanced skeletal traction
   2 An elderly woman with a fractured hip who is in physical therapy
   3 A woman who gave birth 2 days ago and is going home
   4 A man who had a lung resection 3 days ago

6. In the recovery room, the postoperative client suddenly becomes restless with circumoral cyanosis. What is the first nursing action?
   1 Begin administration of oxygen through a nasal cannula.
   2 Call for assistance.
   3 Reposition the head and determine patency of airway.
   4 Insert an oral airway and suction the nasopharynx.

7. A 1-year-old infant has ibuprofen (Advil) ordered every 6 hours. It has been 6 hours since the last dose, and his parent has requested that the child receive his pain medication. When the nurse enters the room, the child is asleep. The parent requests that the pain medication be given because the child is still restless in sleep. What is the best nursing action?
   1 Refuse to awaken the child.
   2 Wake the child and give the medication.
   3 Tell the parent to call as soon as the child awakens.
   4 Explain the purpose and use of pain medications to the parent.

8. The nurse is preparing the preoperative client for surgery. Which of the following statements indicate to the nurse that the client is knowledgeable about his impending surgery? Select all that apply:
   _____ 1 "After surgery, I will need to wear the pneumatic compression device while sitting in the chair."
   _____ 2 "The skin prep area is going to be longer and wider than the anticipated incision."
   _____ 3 "I cannot have anything to drink or eat after midnight on the night before the surgery."
   _____ 4 "To ensure my safety, a time-out for identification will be conducted in the operating room before surgery."
   _____ 5 "I will be given the consent form, and I will sign it after I get to the operating room."

9. The nurse is designing a teaching plan for a 3-year-old in preparation for a surgical procedure. What teaching strategies should be included in the plan of care? Select all that apply:
   _____ 1 Include the child's parents in the teaching.
   _____ 2 Intellectual development moves from abstract to concrete.
   _____ 3 Prevent separation anxiety.
   _____ 4 Provide anatomy and physiology information.
   _____ 5 A "no" response from the child means he or she is not ready to learn.

10. A client is scheduled for major surgery. What is most important for the nurse to do before surgery?
    1 Remove all jewelry or tape wedding rings.
    2 Verify that all laboratory work is complete.
    3 Inform family or next of kin of recovery procedure.
    4 Check that consent forms are signed.

11. A client is admitted with a diagnosis of terminal cancer, and he is experiencing severe pain. The doctor has written an order for pain medication every 3 hours PRN. How will the nurse plan to administer the pain medication?
    1. Wait until the client complains of pain; then administer medication.
    2. Evaluate the client and determine need for pain medication every 3 hours.
    3. Administer the pain medication every 3 hours.
    4. Try to increase time between injections during the night.

12. The nurse is caring for a first-day postoperative surgical client. Prioritize the client's desired dietary progression by numbering the following from 1 to 4 (with 1 being the first step and 4 being the last step).
    1. _____ Full liquid
    2. _____ NPO
    3. _____ Clear liquid
    4. _____ Soft

13. The nurse is admitting a woman who is scheduled for a total hip replacement. What is the most effective way to initiate the health interview?
    1. Sit quietly until the client initiates the conversation.
    2. Start the interview with easy questions to build a rapport.
    3. Determine whether there are any family available to assist her.
    4. Do not dwell on the diagnosis and its effect on the client.

14. At the beginning of the shift, the nurse receives a report on a client. He is receiving IV therapy at 125 mL/hr. The nasogastric tube is patent and draining green drainage at about 75 mL/hr. New physician orders include the following:

    Vancomycin (Vancocin) 500 mg IVPB in 50 mL D₅W over 60 minutes, every 8 hours.

    Metoclopramide (Reglan) 10 mg IVPB in 50 mL D₅W over 30 minutes, every 8 hours.

    One unit packed red blood cells to run concurrent with the IV; infuse unit over 4 hours.

    Irrigate the nasogastric tube with 30 mL NS every 2 hours.

    How many milliliters should the nurse document as the intake for the 8-hour shift?

    Answer: _____ mL

15. A postoperative patient receives a dinner tray with gelatin, pudding, and vanilla ice cream. Based on the foods on the client's tray, what would the nurse anticipate the client's current diet order to be?
    1. Bland diet
    2. Soft diet
    3. Full liquid diet
    4. Regular diet

16. What is important for the nurse to do in order to obtain a comprehensive medical history?
    1. Ask a family member to be present.
    2. Ask the most difficult questions first.
    3. Ask about the family dynamics last.
    4. Document events and dates in chronologic order.

17. The nurse is conducting a teaching session for a client with a new diagnosis of diabetes. At the beginning of the session, what is most important for the nurse to do?
    1. Make sure the client understands the purpose and objectives of the teaching session.
    2. Determine whether the client is comfortable or needs to go to the bathroom before teaching begins.
    3. Introduce the client to the equipment that will be discussed during the teaching session.
    4. Review with the client the importance of learning how to manage his or her diabetic condition.

18. To prevent complications of immobility, what would be the most effective activities to implement for a client on the first postoperative day after a colon resection?
    1. Turn, cough, and deep-breathe every 30 minutes around the clock.
    2. Get the client out of bed and ambulate to a bedside chair.
    3. Provide passive range of motion three times a day.
    4. Immobility is not a concern on the first postoperative day.

19. A client has requested medication for his incisional pain. He had an exploratory laparotomy 12 hours ago. What would be the first nursing action?
    1. Check the medication administration record (MAR) for the last time he received something for pain.
    2. Check the physician's orders for the currency of the pain medication order.
    3. Determine from the nurses' notes the level of pain control over the past 12 hours.
    4. Assess the client's pain and determine whether the pain is appropriate to his surgical procedure.

Answers and rationales to these questions are in the section at the end of the book titled Chapter Study Questions: Answers and Rationales.

CHAPTER FOUR

Control Functions and Management

LEGAL ASPECTS

Nursing Practice Regulations

A. Elements of a nurse practice act.
  1. Establishes and authorizes a regulatory agency; each state has a regulatory agency.
  2. Defines nursing practice within the jurisdiction.
  3. Mission: to protect the public by ensuring that any individual holding a license is competent to practice entry-level nursing safely.
  4. Provides the method and the requirements of licensure.
     a. Examination: successful completion of the National Council Licensure Examination for Registered Nurses (NCLEX-RN).
     b. Endorsement: applying for a license in a state or jurisdiction when already licensed in another state.
     c. Compact states: as of July 2009, 24 states have adopted a compact licensure agreement whereby the state recognizes the nurse's license from another compact state. The license to practice must be issued from the state of primary residence (visit *www.ncsbn.org/158.htm* for specific state information).
     d. Requirements for foreign graduates.
        (1) Information on the federal screening process may be obtained from the Commission on Graduates of Foreign Nursing Schools (CGFNS, *www.cgfns.org*).
        (2) Individual states may require completion of the CGFNS test *before* a candidate can take the NCLEX-RN.
        (3) Complete state requirements for NCLEX-RN.
B. How to protect your license (Box 4-1).
C. Good Samaritan laws: enacted by individual states with the purpose of protecting health care providers who assist at accidents and emergencies.
  1. Care provided in good faith.
  2. Care must be gratuitous; no compensation is received for the care rendered.
  3. Care provided should not be negligent.
  4. Know the status in your state.

D. Standard of care.
  1. The American Nurses Association's "Standards of Nursing Practice" and "Code for Nurses," the American Hospital Association's "A Patient's Bill of Rights," and the individual state nurse practice acts provide the guidelines for safe, ethical nursing practice.
  2. Determining standard of care involves the legal concept of a fictional, reasonable, prudent individual of the same education and profession against which another professional's performance is judged.
  3. The guidelines are used to determine whether the nurse provided care in a reasonable, prudent manner.
  4. Expert nurse witnesses may be used to establish whether a nurse's performance met or was below the standard of care.
E. External forces regulating nursing practice.
  1. The Joint Commission (TJC): evaluates and accredits health care programs.
     a. Purpose is to improve the safety and quality of care provided by health care organizations.
     b. Sets standards for health care organization licensure and accreditation. These standards are frequently used to determine the standard of care for nurses working in the facility.
  2. Occupational Safety and Health Administration (OSHA): goal is to ensure a safe and healthy workplace and to prevent injury to employees in the United States.
  3. Health Insurance Portability and Accountability Act of 1996 (HIPAA): provides protection for the privacy and security of client's health information.

Liability for Actions

A. Individual liability: each person is liable for his or her own conduct; liability may be shared by another person or group (e.g., the doctor, another nurse, or the hospital), but it cannot be removed by the statements or actions of another.
B. Vicarious liability: liability is shared, but individual liability is not lessened.
  1. Respondent superior: employer can be held liable for the actions of an employee.

2. Supervisory negligence—supervisors can share liability if:
   a. Assignments are not within the capabilities of the health care giver (RN, LPN/LVN, UAP).
   b. Assignments are not appropriate for educational level of health care giver (RN, LPN/LVN, UAP).
   c. Assignments are not within legal limitations of practice.
   d. Supervision of the activities assigned does not reflect actual limits and abilities of that individual.
3. Physician may share liability but *cannot* alter an individual nurse's personal liability by a statement of *agreement to assume liability*.

Civil Torts

A. Torts: intentional or unintentional civil wrongs against individuals or groups. Compensation may be awarded to the victim.
B. Negligence: unintentional harm to a client that occurs through failure to act in a reasonable and prudent manner.
C. Malpractice: professional practice that injures a client through failure to meet the proper standard of care.
   1. Elements of a malpractice suit.
      a. A nurse-client relationship must exist; the nurse must owe a duty to the client.
         (1) Assignment to specific nursing team or client.
         (2) Nursing care given to client regardless of formal assignment.
      b. A professional must breach the duty by not conforming to the established standards of care.
      c. Harm must occur to client.
      d. Direct cause-and-effect relationship must exist between the breach (nurse's action) and the harm (injury to the client), which may be pecuniary or emotional.
      e. Foreseeability: a professional could reasonably expect injury to occur as a result of the breach of duty.
   2. It is the responsibility of the client's (plaintiff's) attorney to prove that each element occurred.
D. Invasion of privacy: protection of the constitutional right to be free from undesired publicity and exposure to public view.

> **ALERT** Provide care within legal scope of practice. Client confidentiality is a nursing legal and ethical responsibility.

1. Medical records.
   a. Records should be released only with written client consent.
   b. Release for medical "need to know" limited to caregivers only.
   c. Client has right to inspect and receive a copy of records.
   d. Electronic medical records are password-protected; never give another individual access to your password.
2. Belongings must be protected and may not be searched without specific authorization. The nurse should document the client's belongings. The list of belongings should be reviewed by the client and/or family and signed.
3. Confidentiality.
   a. Conversations are confidential; care should be taken to prevent conversations from being overheard.
   b. Photographs and viewing of procedures require consent of client.
   c. Control visitor access to client and client information: includes family and/or friends.
   d. Client information may not be released without client consent (family member, press, friend). Many institutions are establishing codes for family members or significant others to identify themselves to health care personnel in order to receive client information.
   e. Protect the medical record from being read by unauthorized individuals. Do not leave charts or computer screens open where visitors can read them.
   f. Health professionals are obligated to maintain confidentiality of client's health information in accordance with the HIPAA regulations.

> **ALERT** Assess staff member, client, and family understanding of confidentiality requirements (HIPAA). Maintain client confidentiality. Intervene when confidentiality has been breached by staff members.

4. Physical privacy.
   a. Properly cover the body during procedures or examination.
   b. Close curtains or doors when procedures are performed.
   c. Individuals may not observe a procedure without permission from the client.
5. Exceptions to privacy requirements: some information is required by law to be reported.
   a. Certain communicable diseases.
   b. Injuries that are, or could be, caused by physical violence (gunshot and knife wounds).
   c. Child or adult abuse.
   d. Deaths occurring under suspicious circumstances.
   e. Animal bites.
   f. Others defined by individual state statute.
6. Confidentiality rights may be waived by the client. Obtain written consent to photograph client or to have others present during treatment or procedure.

ALERT Comply with state and/or federal regulations on reporting client conditions (abuse/neglect, communicable disease, death by accident, gunshot wounds).

E. Defamation of character: written or oral communication to other persons concerning matters that may injure an individual's reputation.
   1. Slanderous or libelous statements made about client, staff, and/or co-workers.
   2. Defenses to defamation action.
      a. Truth: the communication is true; however, be aware that truth may be a matter of perspective.
      b. Privilege: statements that are legally protected from a defamation action—e.g., lawyer/client information.
F. False imprisonment: unlawfully restraining personal liberty; unlawful detention.
   1. Actual: use of physical force to prevent departure of client; inappropriate use of restraints.
   2. Implied: use of words, threats, or gestures to restrain client.
      a. Refusing to allow client to leave hospital, with or without signing against medical advice (AMA) form.
      b. Refusing to release newborn.
   3. Exceptions: depend on state laws.
      a. Refusing to allow departure of individual with communicable disease.
      b. Refusing to allow departure of incompetent or mentally ill client if there is imminent threat of serious injury to self or other.
G. Assault and battery: nonconsensual threat (assault) or actual touching (battery).
   1. For a client seeking health care, touching is usually expected. However, the client in the hospital does not surrender his or her rights to refuse treatment or to refuse to be touched.

2. The nurse cannot threaten the client with bodily harm to coerce him or her into a procedure or activity.
3. The nurse may not physically restrain or touch a client in a manner to prevent him or her from leaving the institution or to force the client to undergo a procedure.

ALERT Recognize the client's right to refuse treatments and/or procedures. Educate client and family about client rights and responsibilities. Identify legal issues affecting client, family member, and/or significant others (refusing treatment).

Protective Procedures

A. Documentation: written record of events surrounding client's hospital stay.
   1. Protects client by promoting good communication among health care providers.
   2. Provides evidence in court of care given.
      a. Courts will not assume care is given unless it is recorded.
      b. Demonstrates meeting of standard of care.
      c. Demonstrates decision making of nurse.
B. Effective documentation (Box 4-2).
   1. Documentation, either on paper chart or electronically, should follow the format required by the agency.
   2. Electronic documentation.
      a. Do not give your access code or password to anyone. Any documentation entered will have your entry code on it.
      b. Do not print pages or share pages from the chart; this could be interpreted as a breach of confidentiality or privacy.
      c. Follow the institution guidelines for making corrections in charting, as well as policies for correct documentation.
   3. Use descriptive, objective information based on what is seen, heard, felt, and smelled.
   4. Complete an honest record of events.
      a. Record all events, even unusual events, factually.
      b. Give all appropriate information about each documentation note (e.g., intravenous [IV] site, location, color, temperature, size [swelling, etc.], dressing, and condition).
      c. Do not include any reference to "incident report" filed.
      d. Do not alter record at any time.
      e. Explain omissions in care.
      f. Enter exception documentation as necessary to provide accurate picture of client's situation.
   5. Do not skip lines; do not leave any blank spaces on the paper chart for additional information to be entered.
   6. Correct errors properly.
      a. On paper charting, draw a straight line through error; date and initial.

Box 4-2 GUIDELINES FOR EFFECTIVE DOCUMENTATION

- All entries should be accurate.
- Make corrections appropriately and according to agency or hospital policies. Do not obliterate any information that is written on the paper chart.
- If there is information that should have been charted and was not, make a "late entry," indicating the time the charting actually occurred and the specific time the charting reflects. *Example:* 10/13/09. 10:00 a.m. late entry, charting to reflect 10/12/09.
- All identified client problems, nursing actions taken, and client responses should be noted. Do not describe a client problem and leave it without including nursing actions taken and the client's response.
- Be as objective as possible in charting. Rather then charting "The client tolerated the procedure well," chart the specific parameters checked to determine that conclusion. A chart entry worded "ambulated, tolerated well" would be more effective if charted "ambulated complete length of hall, no shortness of breath noted, pulse rate at 98, respirations at 22."
- Each page of the paper chart or each computer entry should contain the current date and time. Each time you enter information on a new page, make sure it reflects the current time of charting.
- Document who saw the client and what measures were initiated. Particularly note when the doctors visited; if you had to call a doctor because of a problem, record the doctor's response. If orders were received, be sure they are signed according to policy. This is especially important if you had to make several calls to the doctor.
- Make sure your notes on the paper chart are legible and clearly reflect the information you intended. It is a good idea to read over your nurse's notes from the previous day to see whether they still make sense and accurately portray the status of the client. If the notes do not make sense to you the next day, imagine how difficult it would be to decipher the information at a later date.
- Charting by exception may be available on electronic charts, as well as paper charts. In this case, the nurse may be required to document only significant findings or exceptions. It is important that exception notes are entered and provide a clear picture of the client's care or status.

Modified from Irvin J: Legal issues. In Zerwekh J, Claborn J, editors: *Nursing today: transitions and trends*, ed 6, St. Louis, 2009, Saunders.

b. Add omitted information by means of an "addendum" or "late entry": give date and time of original note *and* date and time of addendum.
7. Use meaningful, specific language. Do not use words you do not understand or unaccepted abbreviations.
8. Use standardized abbreviations as defined by the institution and by TJC.

ALERT Use documents to record and communicate client information (medical record, referral and transfer form). Enter computer documentation accurately, completely, and in a timely manner.

C. Incident reports.
1. Only the person directly involved in the incident should document the facts in the report.
2. Do not complete an incident report for someone else.
3. Document the facts.
   a. *Do not* draw conclusions or speculate on who caused or who was responsible for the incident.
   b. *Do not* state opinions or make judgments.
4. Report does not replace the documentation of the incident in the chart.
5. Do not document any reference to the incident report in the chart; the same factual information filed on the incident report should be included on the chart.
6. Failure to complete an incident report could be considered a cover-up.
7. Follow the line of authority within the institution for reporting an incident.
D. Know your limits.

ALERT Recognize task/assignments you are not prepared to perform and seek assistance.

1. Physical-emotional: be aware of fatigue and exhaustion and compensate for them.
2. Practice competency.
   a. Do not perform procedures without adequate preparation, knowledge, and experience. Request supervision if you are unsure of your skills.
   b. Report unsafe practices to your supervisor.
   c. Report evidence of Medicare fraud.
   d. Do not allow anyone to talk you into doing something you are not sure of by letting him or her agree to take the liability or telling you that you should do it.

ALERT Report unsafe practice of health care personnel to internal/external entities (emotional or physical impairment, substance abuse, improper care). Intervene appropriately when unsafe practice by staff member has been observed.

3. Floating.
   a. Floating (assigning nurses to work in areas outside their primary area of practice) is common in hospitals to reduce staffing costs and to enhance efficiency.
   b. When floating to another area, the nurse is not permitted to perform a task or render a service for which he or she lacks the skill or knowledge to perform competently.
   c. Negotiate with the unit supervisor regarding task(s) you are capable of performing, and determine those tasks you are not capable of performing.
   d. Ask the supervisor for assignment of a "backup resource" nurse to be available for assistance.
   e. The nurse's right to refuse a floating assignment has not been supported in all situations. The best

solution is to negotiate with the supervisor for an acceptable compromise.

Responsibility for Professional Practice

A. To maintain the standards of nursing care and to protect the client, the nurse should report anyone in the health care setting who engages in illegal, unethical, or incompetent practices.

B. Examples of unethical care include:
   1. Medication errors that are made and not reported/corrected.
   2. Physical and verbal abuse of client.
   3. Providing care while under the influence of alcohol or drugs.
   4. Breach of client confidentiality and privacy.
   5. Jeopardizing a client's well-being by withholding treatment.

> **ALERT** Identify ethical issues affecting staff or client/family. Intervene to promote ethical practice. Review outcomes of interventions to promote ethical practice.

C. Challenge inappropriate orders.
   1. Identify the problem; obtain current, accurate information; and contact the health care provider.
   2. Follow institution's policy and chain of command if provider is not available or if there is not an appropriate resolution to the situation.
   3. Document the nursing action taken regarding the order.

> **ALERT** Verify appropriateness and/or accuracy of a treatment order.

D. Provide safe environment.
   1. Restraints: may be physical or chemical and are used only to protect the physical safety of the client and others.
      a. Should be adequate and appropriate for the purpose.
      b. Use of a restraint on a client requires a physician's order that includes:
         (1) Type and location of restraint.
         (2) Type of behavior for which restraint is to be used.
         (3) Time frame that the order for the restraint covers.
      c. In an emergency situation, physical restraints may be used without a doctor's order for a very limited period of time.
      d. Safe nursing practice for the care of a client in restraints includes:
         (1) Check restrained client every 30 minutes and provide for physiologic needs.
         (2) Remove restraints and provide range of motion every 2 hours.
         (3) Document the time of each check and the neurovascular status of client's extremities.
      (4) Remove restraints as soon as possible.
      (5) Secure restraints to the bed frame, not to the side rails.
      (6) Discuss with family the rationale for and purpose of restraints.
      (7) Investigate all alternatives to restraints: family involvement, methods to increase client orientation, scheduled toileting activities.

> **ALERT** Apply and maintain prescribed restraints/bed alarms/safety devices according to facility policy. Monitor client response to restraints. Evaluate appropriateness of the type of restraint used.

   2. Prevention of falls.
      a. Educate the staff on fall-reduction protocol.
      b. Perform appropriate assessment of client at increased risk.
      c. Orient client to call light, bathroom; give instructions about calling for assistance.
      d. Keep bed in low position.
      e. Advise all personnel of clients at high risk for falling.
      f. Use side rails appropriately.
      g. Obtain adequate assistance for ambulation.
      h. Remove all obstacles or dangers on floor or in path.
      i. Check and use locks on wheelchairs, beds, stretchers.
      j. Establish toileting schedule.

Specific Situations of Risk

> **ALERT** Ensure proper identification of client when providing care.

A. Client identification—The Joint Commission requirements:
   1. Two identifiers are required; for example, the hospital identification number and the client's name on the armband or other person-specific identifier.
   2. The methods of identification should be appropriate to the care setting and individuals served; the room number is not considered an identifier.
   3. If client does not have an armband, then the individual's stated name would be one identifier; the client's date of birth, social security number, address, or phone number could serve as the second identifier.
   4. Client's current photograph or visual recognition may be used as one identifier in long-term care facilities, home care settings, or behavioral care facilities. For short-term clients, facilities with unstable staffing, and/or high-risk medications, the two-identifier requirement is necessary.
   5. The client does not have to state his or her name as an identifier.

> **⚠ NURSING PRIORITY** Always check client identification according to The Joint Commission guidelines.

B. Medication errors (see Chapter 5).
C. Telephone and other verbal orders.
  1. Write down the telephone order and read it back; receive confirmation that the order is correct.
  2. Do not take verbal orders with the physician present when it is not an urgent situation.
  3. Orders left on voice mail are not acceptable; the nurse must call the health care provider to obtain the order directly.
  4. Verbal orders left with clients or family members are not acceptable; the nurse must call the health care provider and obtain the order directly.
  5. Obtain needed signature promptly.
D. Changes in client's condition.

> **ALERT** Follow up on unresolved issues regarding client care. Evaluate and revise plan of care as needed (change in client condition).

  1. Notify appropriate individuals: supervisor, physician, health care provider.
  2. Challenge failure to provide appropriate care after notification of significant change in client condition.
  3. Document changes and events surrounding the change in the client's status.
  4. The nurse is responsible for assessing and evaluating client care and for taking action, obtaining assistance, or notifying appropriate individuals of the change in client condition.
  5. Follow up on assessments of client problems and what nursing action was taken to resolve the problem. For example, the nurse may very carefully document the events surrounding a client's fall, but it is also critical to follow up on what was done to provide care and to protect the client after the fall.
  6. Have all information necessary when you contact the physician regarding a client problem. Follow good communication guidelines for telephone communications (Box 4-3).
E. Hand-off (shift) report: purpose is to provide accurate information and safe quality care throughout the client's hospitalization.
  1. Use an interactive communication method understandable for all interdisciplinary teams—***SBAR***:
    *S*ituation—What is happening at the present time?
    *B*ackground—What are the circumstances leading up to this situation?
    *A*ssessment—What do I think the problem is?
    *R*ecommendation—What should we do to correct the problem?
  2. The oncoming nurse is responsible for the nursing care required on his or her shift.

Box 4-3   TIPS FOR COMMUNICATING WITH PHYSICIANS ON THE TELEPHONE

- Say who you are right away.
- Do not apologize for phoning.
- State your business briefly but completely.
- If you want the doctor to assess the patient, say so.
- If the doctor is coming, ask when to expect him or her.
- If you get disconnected, call back.
- Document attempts to reach a doctor.
- If a doctor is rude or abusive, tell him or her so and report it to the nursing manager.
- If you cannot reach a doctor or get what you need, always tell your nursing manager.

From Rosser C: Building Nursing Management Skills. In Zerwekh J, Claborn J, editors: *Nursing today: transitions and trends*, ed 6, St. Louis, 2009, Saunders, p 228.

---

    a. Status of IVs and amount of fluid to count.
    b. Any abnormal conditions (vital signs, pain, special treatments).
    c. Status of client with regard to diagnosis. For examples, cardiac client—presence or absence of chest pain and dysrhythmias; surgical client—voiding, incision status; orthopedic client—circulation distal to cast or traction.
    d. Psychosocial status of the client.

> **ALERT** Provide and receive report on assigned clients.

F. Do not resuscitate (DNR) orders.
  1. Written by the physician based on the client's written medical directives.
  2. Nurses are obligated to respect and observe the DNR order.
  3. Health care personnel should be advised of the DNR order.

Legal Documents

A. Client's medical record or chart.
B. Advance medical directive: a written document regarding a client's desires for provision of medical care if that person is unable to make his or her own choices or decisions.
  1. Patient Self-Determination Act (1990): ensures that clients know about advance directives (ADs); requires facilities receiving Medicare or Medicaid funds to ask adult clients whether they have ADs and to advise clients of their rights.
    a. Living will (natural death act): a written document describing the client's wishes and special instructions regarding life support measures in the event that the client is incapacitated.
    b. Medical power of attorney for health care.
      (1) Identifies the person designated by the client to ensure that previously agreed ADs are carried out according to the client's direction.

(2) Identifies the person designated to make health care decisions for the client if the client is incapacitated.
   c. ADs may be changed or revoked by the client at any time.

C. Consent forms.
   1. Informed consent (Box 4-4).
   2. A minor may not give consent; consent must be obtained from the parent or legal guardian.

EMERGENCY RESPONSE PLANS

A. Internal disasters occur within the health care facility (e.g., fire).
   1. Know the agency's fire policy and evacuation plan; immediately return to the unit if a fire code is announced.
   2. Know where to locate fire extinguishers, alarms, and exits.

Box 4-4 INFORMED CONSENT

Informed consent is the process whereby the client is informed of the risks, benefits, and alternatives of certain procedures and gives consent for a procedure to be done.
- Nurses witness signatures to determine client competency, validate the signature, and ensure that the consent is voluntary.
- Witnessed signature: Do not witness unless you know the client has all information needed to make informed decision.
- Procedure specified in terms the client can understand.
- Client understands the benefits of the procedure.
- Client understands significant risks of procedure.
- Client understands alternatives to procedure.
- Client is informed of the health care provider performing the procedure.
- Signed while client is free from mind-altering drugs or conditions.
- Consents are legal documents.

Withdrawal of Consent
- Can be written or verbal.
- Can occur at any time, even after the procedure has begun.

Exceptions
- Life-threatening emergencies or urgent situations.
- Minors: For clients up to age 18, a parent's signature is generally required for consent.
- Emancipated minor: Definition may vary, but usually this is a minor who is self-supporting and living away from home.
- Mentally incapacitated individual: Consent required of legal guardian or person specified in medical power of attorney.

3. Fire intervention guidelines—remember **RACE:**
   Rescue—remove all clients in immediate danger.
   Alert—initiate the alarm.
   Confine—close all doors and windows; turn off oxygen valves and electrical equipment.
   Extinguish—use the appropriate extinguisher for type of fire.
4. Know the types of fire extinguishers:
   Class A: water or solution for paper or linens.
   Class B: foam extinguisher for grease, chemical, or electrical fires.
   Class C: multipurpose extinguisher for paper or linens or electrical fires.
5. Using a fire extinguisher—remember **PASS:**
   Pull the pin.
   Aim at the base of the fire.
   Squeeze the trigger.
   Sweep from side to side.
6. If you need to evacuate your unit because of an immediate danger to staff and clients, evacuate clients in this order to provide for the most rapid removal of the most clients in a short period of time:
   a. First, ambulatory clients, because they can move most quickly.
   b. Next, clients in wheelchairs or walkers.
   c. Then, clients who are bedridden.
B. External disasters occur outside the health care agency (plane crashes, hurricanes, bombings).
   1. Level I: a disaster that involves a minimal level of damage (auto accidents, house fires); requires local emergency and community health support.
   2. Level II: a disaster affecting more people and involving state health and emergency management services (building collapses, train derailment, tornado); regional response agencies become involved.
   3. Level III: a disaster that consumes state and federal resources and requires an extended response from community health facilities (hurricanes, earthquakes, foreign attacks).
C. Triage—remember **START: S**imple **T**riage **A**nd **R**apid **T**reatment (Box 4-5).
   1. Emergency department (ED): objective of triage is to sort clients according to their injury and their need for medical attention when there are not enough resources available for all clients to be treated.
      a. Divides injured clients into groups according to level of injury.
      b. Bed availability is a problem; the ED nurse may request assistance to determine which hospitalized clients can be discharged in order to admit severely injured clients.
   2. Disaster triage: triage in the field or at the site of the disaster.
      a. **START** system (see Box 4-5) is combined with color-coded tags to identify clients according to level of injury.

Box 4-5　THE START SYSTEM

The START system (Figure 4-1) divides injured personnel into four separate groups:

- **Deceased (Black)**—Injured persons who are beyond the scope of medical assistance. Persons are tagged Deceased only if they are not breathing and attempts to resuscitate have been unsuccessful.
- **Immediate (Red)**—Injured persons who can be assisted or their health aided by advanced medical care immediately or within 1 hour of care.
- **Delayed (Yellow)**—Injured persons who can be assisted after Immediate-tagged persons are medically cared for first. Delayed persons are medically stable but require medical assistance.
- **Minor (Green)**—Injured persons who can be assisted after Immediate- and Delayed-tagged persons have been medically tended to. Minor-tagged persons will not need medical care for at least several hours and can usually walk with assistance mainly comprising of bandages and acute first aid.

Developed by Newport Beach Fire Department. Used with permission.

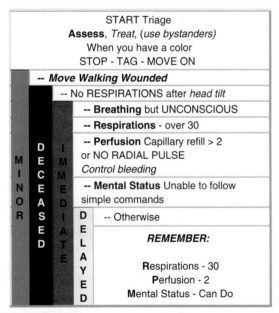

FIGURE 4-1 Simplified flowchart for START triage. (Developed by Newport Beach Fire Department, available at www.start-triage.com.)

ALERT Identify nursing roles in disaster planning. Determine which client(s) to recommend for discharge in disaster situation. Implement emergency response plans. Use clinical decision making for emergency response plan.

　　b. **IdMe** .
　　　Immediate—red.
　　　Delayed—yellow.
　　　Minimal—green.
　　　Expectant—black.
　　c. Clients involved in a mass casualty incident (MCI) are sorted into groups—remember **MASS** (**M**ove, **A**ssess, **S**ort, and **S**end).

(1) **M**ove those who can walk and follow directions to a designated area (green tags).
(2) **A**ssess and **S**ort clients based on level of injury and attach a color-coded tag to each client.
(3) **S**end, evacuate, and transport red-tagged clients first, then yellow, then green, and then black.

D. Do not enter a disaster scene until directed to do so by the people designated to secure the scene (police or fire department). Protect yourself and team members; then direct your attention to the injured.

ETHICAL CONCERNS

A. Resources.
　1. International Council of Nurses Code for Nurses (2006).
　2. American Nurses Association Code of Ethics (2008): provides direction for ethical decisions and behavior emphasizing the obligations and responsibilities of the nurse-client relationship.
B. Ethical decision making.
　1. Determine the facts of the situation; legal versus ethical.
　2. Identify the ethical issues of the situation: is the client's autonomy being respected? A client is free to form his or her own judgments and is entitled to whatever actions he or she chooses.
　3. Determine the possible courses of action and the potential outcomes.
　4. After a course of action has been implemented, evaluate the outcome.
C. Interdisciplinary ethics committee: usually consists of physicians, clergy, social workers, attorneys, and nurses. Any member of the health care team should have access to the committee. The committee may offer unbiased opinions, clarify issues, offer support, and suggest a course of action.
D. Advocacy: the nurse serves as an advocate for the client by respecting the client's rights and facilitating communication between the client and the health care team.

ALERT Intervene to promote ethical practice; inform client, family, significant others, and health care team members of ethical issues regarding client care.

MANAGEMENT CONCEPTS

Client Care Assignments and Delegation

A. The registered nurse (RN) is responsible for delegating client care and for supervision of the implementation of care (Figure 4-2).
B. Guidelines for making assignments, delegation, and supervision (Boxes 4-6 and 4-7).

ALERT Ensure appropriate education skills and experience of personnel performing assigned or delegated tasks.

FOUR Cs OF INITIAL DIRECTION

Is it **concise**? Have I confused the direction by giving too much unnecessary information?

Is it **clear**? Is what I am saying understood?

Is it **correct**? Do the directions follow policy, procedure, job description and the law?

Is it **complete**? Does it give all the information necessary to complete the task?

©2007 Nursing Education Consultants, Inc.

FIGURE 4-2 Four Cs of initial direction. (From Zerwekh J, Claborn J: *Memory notebook of nursing*, vol 2, ed 3, Ingram, Texas, 2007, Nursing Education Consultants.)

Box 4-6 DELEGATION TERMS

Delegation: "... the act of transferring to a competent individual the authority to perform a selected nursing task in a selected situation, the process for doing the work. Assignment describes the distribution of work that each staff member is to accomplish in a given time period." (NCSBN, p 1)*

Supervision: "The purpose of (supervision) surveillance and monitoring is related to nurse's responsibility for client care within the context of a client population. The nurse supervises the delegation by monitoring the performance of the task or function and assures compliance with standards of practice, policies, and procedures. Frequently, level and nature of monitoring vary with needs of client and experience of assistant." (NCSBN, p 12)*

Accountability: "Being responsible for what one has done, and standing behind that decision and/or action." (Hanston and Jackson)†

Assignment: "... To assign is to direct an individual to do activities within an authorized scope of practice. Assignment (noun) describes the distribution of work that each staff member is to accomplish in a given work period." (NCSBN, p 1)*

*National Council of State Boards of Nursing: Working with others: a position paper, Chicago, 2005, National Council of State Boards of Nursing.
†Hansten R, Jackson M: *Clinical delegation skills: a handbook for professional practice*, ed 3, Sudbury, Mass, 2004, Jones & Bartlett, p 68.

C. Assignments are based on the RN determining the client needs, the availability of qualified staff, the scope of practice of the available staff, (RN, LVN, UAP), and the job descriptions of the institution.
   1. Unlicensed assistive personnel (UAP) (client care assistant, nurse's aide, certified nursing assistant): del-

---

Box 4-7 THE FIVE RIGHTS OF DELEGATION

Right Task
One that is delegable for a specific patient.
Right Circumstances
Appropriate patient setting, available resources, and other relevant factors considered.
Right Person
Delegating the right task to the right person to be performed on the right person.
Right Direction/Communication
Clear, concise description of the task, including its objective, limits, and expectations.
Right Supervision
Appropriate monitoring, evaluation, intervention (as needed), and feedback.

Modified from National Council of State Boards of Nursing: *Delegation: concepts and decision-making process*, Chicago, 1995, National Council of State Boards of Nursing.

egate activities that have very specific guidelines—for example, bed making, bathing, feeding, ambulating, general activities of daily living (see Box 4-7).
   2. A licensed practical nurse (LPN) or licensed vocational nurse (LVN): performs nursing actions (e.g., suctioning, catheterization) requiring knowledge of sterile technique, medication administration; gathers data regarding client progress and provides information to RN.
   3. RN: implements the nursing process, develops nursing care plan, implements teaching plan, and plans for client discharge.

> **NURSING PRIORITY** Initial client assessment, provision of care to unstable clients requiring nursing judgment, discharge planning, and planning for client education are responsibilities of the RN.

   a. Performs the nursing assessment and analyzes data for client plan of care.
   b. Determines appropriate nursing diagnoses and nursing actions.
   c. Assigns most ill or unstable clients to RNs.
   d. Responsible for making decisions regarding client care; uses nursing judgment to determine care required of unstable clients.
   4. The nurse who delegates tasks and activities to a UAP and makes assignments to other nursing personal is responsible for supervision or periodic inspection to determine whether the task has been accomplished.
   5. Nurse practice acts of each state may dictate the specific activities of LPNs and RNs.
D. Considerations for assigning client rooms.
   1. Clients who need frequent nursing assessment or intervention should be assigned rooms near the nurses' station.

2. Group client assignments geographically together to assist in the organization of the work schedule of the nurse.

3. Consider the client diagnosis in planning assignments of care and client room assignments. Refer to the CDC website (*www.cdc.gov*) for additional guidelines for client placement.

   a. Consider the needs of immunosuppressed clients: do not put them at increased risk for opportunistic infections.

   b. Do not put clients at increased risk: a client with human immunodeficiency virus (HIV) infection should not share a room with a client with an upper respiratory tract infection; a client with wound infection should not share a room with a client who has an open lesion caused by poor circulation.

   c. Be aware of clients who will require additional levels of standard precautions and private rooms—for example, children with rotavirus or respiratory syncytial virus; clients with methicillin-resistant *Staphylococcus aureus* (MRSA) infections.

   d. When a group of clients is assigned to one nurse, consider the potential for cross-infections.
      Example: A client who is immunosuppressed and a client with an MRSA infection should not be assigned to the same nurse.

ALERT Make client room assignments.

E. Prioritizing client care assignments.

   1. Identify the most ill or unstable client on your assignment; assess and care for that client first.

      a. Determine which of the client's needs is most urgent.

      b. Determine which of the client's conditions is most unstable.

   2. Guidelines for prioritization of client needs.

      a. Physiologic needs are a priority (Maslow; see Figure 3-1): of the physiologic needs, airway, breathing, and circulation (ABCs) are the priority. Education, communication, and psychosocial needs can wait until physiologic needs have been met.

         (1) Client needs that are life-threatening are the first priority—for example, dysrhythmias, airway obstruction.

         (2) Clients who have changing needs and are likely to experience harm if their needs are not met immediately—for example, elderly client who is vomiting; client with difficulty breathing, incisional evisceration, or chest pain.

      b. Nursing process: assessment is the first step; adequate assessment must be done before nursing intervention can be determined.

      c. Considering time and resources, what can be done to benefit the client in the most expedient manner? For example:

         (1) Client with difficulty breathing—sit client up, clear the airway, begin administering oxygen.

         (2) Client with evisceration—put client flat, cover the incision with sterile dressing soaked in normal saline solution, notify physician.

ALERT Assess and triage a group of clients to prioritize the order of care to be delivered.

Quality Management

ALERT Participate in a quality assurance program and/or peer review.

A. Continuous quality improvement (CQI): constantly and continuously looking for opportunities to improve client care.

   1. Results from CQI audits are used to identify problem areas and to improve client care.

   2. CQI evaluates all aspects of nursing care (e.g., nutrition services, radiology).

B. Quality assurance process.

   1. Professional standards: use of general standards of care (e.g., American Nurses Association's *Standards of Nursing Practice*), along with the standards of each institution and each client care unit.

   2. Determining criteria to meet standards.

      a. Provides a measurable indicator to evaluate performance—for example, "Nursing care plan is to be developed and written by an RN within 10 hours of admission."

   3. Evaluating performance or how well the criteria have been met.

      a. Usual method is reviewing documented records (chart)—for example, checking the chart to see whether care plan is in place within the 10-hour time period.

   4. Following up on how effective changes were.

      a. Checking to see whether changes were made—for example, after the first audit of charts is done and suggested changes are made, a second audit of 20 charts determines whether an improvement in getting the care plan on the chart in 10 hours has occurred.

C. Methods of monitoring nursing care.

   1. Nursing audit: examination of the client's records, either retrospectively (after discharge) or concurrently (while client is receiving care).

   2. Peer review: practicing nurses evaluating peer performance based on standards and criteria.

   3. Utilization review: mandated by The Joint Commission to determine appropriate allocation of resources.

   4. Client satisfaction: questionnaire is given to clients to determine satisfaction regarding the care they received.

Study Questions Control Functions and Management

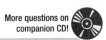

1. The nurse enters data on a paper chart and then discovers he or she has written on the wrong chart. How is this error best corrected?
   1 White-out the wrong information and write over it.
   2 Recopy the page with the error so that the chart will be neat.
   3 Draw a straight line through the error, initial, and date.
   4 Obliterate the error so that it will not be confusing.

2. Most states have reporting laws that require health care workers to report certain situations and behavior to authorities. Which is *not* usually a reportable matter?
   1 Child abuse
   2 Communicable disease
   3 Gunshot wounds
   4 Attempted suicide

3. Which of the following would *not* be considered a violation of HIPAA?
   1 Providing client information to an individual who claims to be a family member
   2 Allowing a student nurse, who is taking care of the client, to make copies of laboratory results
   3 Discussing the client's condition on the telephone with a family member who has provided the client information code
   4 Reviewing the client's chart with the CEO of the hospital, who is the client's brother-in-law

4. Which of the following would the nurse identify as an indication that the client understands the informed consent document?
   1 The client states that the physician has explained the procedure to him.
   2 The nurse finds the informed consent form already signed.
   3 The client can give a return verbal explanation of the informed consent document.
   4 The client states that his wife read it and said it was okay.

5. While caring for an 8-year-old child with a broken wrist, the nurse notices red, raised streaks on the child's back. The child's father enters the room and the child becomes quiet and distant, leaning away from the father as he approaches. What is the best nursing action?
   1 Chart that the child was probably beaten by the father.
   2 Notify the supervisor to report possible child abuse.
   3 Disregard suspicions and care for the immediate needs of the child.
   4 No action is required; there is no actual proof of abuse to the child.

6. What is the nurse's best approach to avoid claims of negligence?
   1 A strong and binding contract for services
   2 Adherence to all hospital policies
   3 Competent practice of nursing
   4 Keeping a current license

7. The nurse is involved in a legal case against the hospital. Which judgment error by the nurse would be considered most damaging?
   1 Making illegal changes in the chart
   2 Arguing with the plaintiff over the case
   3 Withholding information from the hospital attorney
   4 Being argumentative while on the witness stand

8. The nurse stopped on the highway at a multiple fatal accident to provide assistance. Immediately after the incident, the family members were appreciative of the help the nurse provided. They offered to replace the nurse's soiled clothes, which she accepted. The nurse was in violation of which rights?
   1 ANA Code of Ethics
   2 HIPAA
   3 Patient Self-Determination Act
   4 Good Samaritan Act

9. The physician asks the nurse to give a client a medication that the nurse knows the client is allergic to. When the nurse tries to point this out to the physician, the physician threatens to tell the nurse's supervisor. What is the best response?
   1 Tell the physician to give the medication himself.
   2 Walk away and ignore him.
   3 Agree to give the medication but do not initial the dose.
   4 Suggest a meeting between the nurse, supervisor, and physician.

10. A Code Red (fire alarm) is sounding on the nursing unit. The nurse determines there is a fire. In what sequence would the nurse implement the fire emergency steps? Number the following steps from 1 to 6 to show the proper sequence (with 1 being the first action and 6 being the last action.
    1 _____ Activate the alarm.
    2 _____ Pull the pin on the extinguisher.
    3 _____ Remove any victims from the fire.
    4 _____ Aim the extinguisher to the base of the fire.
    5 _____ Contain the fire.
    6 _____ Extinguish the fire from side to side.

11. Which of the following most clearly represents a situation of assault?
    1 In the emergency department, a client is intoxicated and verbally abusive; the nurse tells him she will put him in restraints if he does not quit talking.
    2 A client is in labor and has not received any medication for pain; she tells the nurse she does not want

anything for pain; the nurse administers the pain medication ordered.

3 The client advises the nurse that he is leaving; the nurse tells the client he cannot leave and threatens to restrain him if necessary.

4 A pastor calls regarding a client's condition; the nurse provides the pastor with detailed information regarding the client's condition.

12. The nurse receives a hand-off communication report for the change of shift. Which client should the nurse see first?

1 A 50-year-old woman who is scheduled for a breast biopsy this morning and is crying

2 An 85-year-old man admitted during the night because of increasing confusion who remains disoriented this morning

3 A 65-year-old woman who had a thoracotomy the previous day and has two midline chest tubes

4 A 40-year-old man who is complaining of chills and painful urination is scheduled for a colon resection in 2 hours

13. The charge nurse is planning assignments for the nursing staff. One of the staff nurses is pregnant. Which client would *not* be appropriate to assign to this nurse?

1 Child with a brain tumor being treated with radiation

2 Infant with respiratory syncytial virus receiving ribavirin

3 Toddler who is HIV-positive and has an opportunistic respiratory tract infection

4 Child with leukemia who is receiving vincristine (Oncovin) and allopurinol (Zyloprim)

14. A nurse manager has been notified to obtain a bed for a client. Of the following clients, which one would the nurse anticipate being able to discharge?

1 A client who had a myocardial infarction (MI) 2 days ago. She has the following vital signs: blood pressure (BP) 150/94 mm Hg, pulse 84 beats/min and irregular, respiration 28 breaths/min, minimal chest pain.

2 A client who underwent an abdominal aortic aneurysm resection 3 days ago. He has the following vital signs: BP 130/88 mm Hg, pulse 88 beats/min, respiration 22 breaths/min, and oral temperature 101° F. He is beginning oral intake without problems.

3 A client who has a subdural hematoma. He is lethargic; his pulse is 60 beats/min, BP is 150/90 mm Hg, respiration is 28 breaths/min, and temperature is 99° F.

4 A client who had abdominal exploratory surgery for a bowel obstruction 4 days ago. He has bowel sounds, is taking fluids orally, has an abdominal Penrose drain, and is continuing to experience abdominal pain.

15. The nurse is preparing to send a client to the radiation department for his scheduled radiation therapy. What action will the nurse take to determine the correct identification of the client?

1 Ask the client his name and check his armband to verify that the information correlates.

2 Check client's armband against the identification records on the client's chart for the correct name and hospital number.

3 Ask the client his name and the name of his doctor and compare his response with identification records on the client's chart.

4 Check the doctor's order on the client's chart and to determine whether he is to receive any medications before the treatment.

16. The nurse is planning assignments. Which task can be safely delegated to a nursing assistant?

1 Obtain a stool specimen from a client with diarrhea.

2 Help a client with a new colostomy in practicing his first colostomy irrigation.

3 Evaluate the voiding pattern for a client who had a urinary retention catheter removed.

4 Obtain a dietary history from a client with peptic ulcer disease.

17. The nurse received a report on the assigned clients for the shift. Which client should the nurse see first?

1 A client who underwent thoracotomy 3 days ago; his vital signs are as follows: temperature 101° F, pulse 100 beats/min, and respiration 28 breaths/min; he is complaining of chest pain when he coughs

2 An 85-year-old client who has a fractured hip and is in traction; she is complaining of pain and she is scheduled for surgery in 4 hours

3 An adult male client admitted 3 hours ago for dehydration; the vital signs are temperature 99° F, pulse 100 beats/min and irregular, respiration 24 breaths/min, and BP 118/80 mm Hg

4 A cardiac client whose cardiac monitor is beginning to show multifocal, trigeminal premature ventricular contractions

Answers and rationales to these questions are in the section at the end of the book titled Chapter Study Questions: Answers and Rationales.

RESOURCES

Commission on Graduates of Foreign Nursing Schools (CGFNS), 3600 Market St, Suite 400, Philadelphia, PA 19104.

The Joint Commission, One Renaissance Blvd, Oakbrook Terrace, IL 60181.

National Council of State Boards of Nursing (NCSBN), 111 Wacker Dr, Suite 2900, Chicago, IL 60601.

CHAPTER FIVE

Pharmacology

GENERAL CONCEPTS OF PHARMACOLOGY

No medication has a single action; all medications have the potential to alter more than one body function.

> ❗ **NURSING PRIORITY** Many medications have several desirable actions. Carefully evaluate the question as to what the desired response of the medication is for the specific client situation. Example: Aspirin is used to prevent platelet aggregation to prevent strokes and cardiac disease, but it is also used as an antipyretic and for pain control in arthritis.

A. Drug names: Drug Amendments of 1962 made it mandatory that each medication have one official name.
   1. Generic name (nonproprietary): the official designated name under which the medication is listed in official publications (e.g., acetaminophen).
   2. Chemical name: designates the specific chemical composition of the medication; usually quite long and complicated to pronounce and spell (e.g., *N*-acetyl-*para*-aminophenol).
   3. Trade name (proprietary, brand name): the name designated and registered by a specific manufacturer (e.g., Tylenol).

> ❗ **NURSING PRIORITY** Typically, the medications on the NCLEX-RN examination will be identified with both the generic and trade name—for example: diazepam (Valium).

B. Abuse potential: Controlled Substances Act, 1970, defines rules for the manufacture and distribution of drugs that are considered to have a potential for abuse.
   1. Defines drugs in five categories: Schedules I, II, III, IV, V—potential for abuse becomes lower with each subsequent category; thus the higher the schedule number, the lower the potential for abuse.
   2. Schedule I drugs are highly addictive (e.g., heroin) and are not used for medicinal purposes in the U.S. Schedule V drugs (e.g., diphenoxylate hydrochloride [Lomotil]) pose the lowest risk for abuse and represent the lowest level of pharmacokinetics.
C. Pharmacokinetic process: consists of four phases, acting together to determine the concentration of a drug at its site of action. Use the acronym **ADME** to remember these processes.
   1. **A**bsorption: movement of the drug from site of administration to the blood.
      a. Drug action may be increased or decreased by altering gastric emptying time, changing gastric pH, or forming drug complexes.
      b. Method of administration affects absorption: for example, IV versus oral.
   2. **D**istribution: movement of the drug throughout the body.
      a. Based on blood flow of drug to tissue, ability of the drug to leave the vascular system, and ability of the drug to enter the tissue cells.
      b. Albumin (protein) always remains in the bloodstream; drugs that are protein-bound restrict the drug distribution.
   3. **M**etabolism: the enzymatic alteration of the drug structure; most drug metabolism occurs in the liver.
      a. The most important action of drug metabolism is promotion of the renal excretion of the drug.
      b. Converts drugs to inactive compounds; also increases or decreases toxicity.
   4. **E**xcretion: the removal of drugs from the body.
      a. Kidney is the most important organ for excretion of a drug; in renal failure, the duration and the intensity of drug action may increase.
      b. Kidney of a newborn is not fully developed; infants have a limited ability to excrete drugs.
      c. Drugs are also excreted in breast milk, bile and the lungs.

> ❗ **OLDER ADULT PRIORITY** Creatinine clearance should be monitored to evaluate renal function, not serum creatinine levels. The source of serum creatinine (lean muscle mass) decreases with the decline in renal function, which may reveal normal serum creatinine levels even though renal function is decreased.

Drug Actions

A. Desired action: the desired, predictable response for which the medication is administered.
B. Adverse drug reactions (ADR).

❗ OLDER ADULT PRIORITY ADRs are 7 times more common in older adults than in young adults.

1. Side effects: undesirable drug effects, ranging from mild untoward effects to severe responses that occur at normal drug dosages.
2. Toxicity: drug reactions that primarily occur as a result of receiving an excessive dose (e.g., medication error, poisoning). However, this may also include severe reactions (anaphylaxis) that occur regardless of the dose.
3. Allergic reactions: drug reaction that occurs as a result of prior sensitization and results in an immune response. Intensity can range from very mild to very severe.
4. Idiosyncratic effect: an uncommon drug response.

ALERT Assess client for actual or potential side effects and adverse effects of medications; identify symptoms/evidence of allergic reactions to medications; implement procedures to counteract adverse effects of medications; evaluate and document client response to actions taken to counteract side effects and adverse effects of medications.

C. Factors influencing dose-response relationships.
   1. Age: young infants and the older adult client are generally more sensitive to medications.
   2. Medication history: a new medication may produce an interaction with one of the medications the client is currently taking.
   3. Drug half-life: the time required for the amount of the drug in the body to be decreased by 50%.
      a. Some drugs have short half-lives; they leave the body quickly. Drugs with long half-lives leave the body more slowly. For example, morphine has a very short half-life (approximately 3 hours), whereas levothyroxine (Synthroid) has a half-life of 7 days.
      b. The half-life of the drug will determine the dosing intervals.
   4. Presence of disease process, specifically kidney and liver problems.
   5. Method of administration.
   6. Adequate cardiac output.
   7. Emotional factors: clients are more likely to respond to a medication in a positive manner if they have confidence in the physician and anticipate therapeutic effects.
   8. Pregnancy: always ask a woman of childbearing age if she is pregnant.
   9. Breastfeeding: advise women who are lactating to always advise their health care provider; medications may be excreted in breast milk.
D. Tolerance: increased dose required to maintain expected drug response. For example, when a client with chronic pain requires higher doses of a strong opioid agonist (morphine sulfate) to achieve pain relief.

E. Dependence: an expected response to repeated use of a drug, resulting in physical signs and symptoms of withdrawal when the serum drug level decreases suddenly. For example, when a client abruptly stops taking a strong opioid agonist (methadone) and develops irritability, nausea, vomiting, muscle spasm, and musculoskeletal pain.
F. Addiction: the continued use of a psychoactive substance regardless of physical, psychologic, or social harm.

Drug Interactions

A. Potentiation effect (synergistic effect): if two or more drugs are given together and this increases the therapeutic effects, it is beneficial; if it increases adverse effects, it may be detrimental.
   Example: A desirable potentiation effect occurs when a diuretic and a beta blocker are given for hypertension. An undesirable effect can occur when warfarin and aspirin (both anticoagulants) are given together, because this increases the risk for spontaneous bleeding.
B. Antagonistic or inhibitory effect: if two or more drugs are given together, one may inhibit the effect of the other; this may be beneficial or detrimental.
   Example: When you administer an adrenergic beta blocker propranolol (Inderal) with an adrenergic beta stimulant isoproterenol (Isuprel), the action of each drug is canceled. However, the use of naloxone (Narcan) to suppress the effects of morphine results in a desirable inhibitory effect.
C. Unique response effect: this occurs when two drugs are given together and the effect creates a new response not seen when each drug is used alone.
   Example: When you administer disulfiram (Antabuse) and the client has ingested alcohol or is using products containing alcohol, the effects are undesirable.
D. Drug incompatibility: a chemical or physical reaction that occurs when two or more drugs are combined in vitro (outside the body).
   1. Do not combine two or more drugs in the same container unless it has been established that an interaction will not occur.
   2. When intravenous (IV) drugs are combined, they may form a precipitate. Do not give an IV solution in which a precipitate has formed after mixing drugs.

ALERT Use critical thinking skills when considering the effects and/or outcomes of medications; identify any contraindications to administration of a prescribed or OTC medication.

E. Drug-food interactions.
   1. Food can bind with drugs and delay drug absorption.
      Example: Tetracyclines bind with dairy products, leading to a decrease in the plasma tetracycline level.
   2. Food increases the absorption of nitrofurantoin (Macrodantin), an antiinfective; metoprolol (Lopressor), a beta blocker; and lovastatin (Mevacor), an antilipemic.

Example: Grapefruit juice can raise drug levels of calcium channel blockers because it decreases metabolism of the drug by inhibiting an intestinal isoenzyme, CYP3A4, which is needed for drug metabolism in the intestines.

3. Monoamine oxidase inhibitors (e.g., Marplan): antidepressants, which when taken with tyramine-rich foods (e.g., cheese, wine, organ meats, beer, yogurt), may lead to a hypertensive crisis.

F. Drug-laboratory value interactions.
　1. Abnormal plasma or serum electrolyte levels can affect drugs.
　Example: Digitalis toxicity can occur when a client's serum potassium and magnesium levels are decreased and the serum calcium level is increased.

> **⚠ NURSING PRIORITY** The **peak** drug level is the highest plasma concentration of a drug at a specific time. The **trough** level is the lowest plasma concentrations of a drug and measures the rate at which the drug is eliminated. Trough levels are determined a few minutes before the drug is to be given, regardless of whether it is administered orally or intravenously. These levels are determined for drugs that have a narrow therapeutic index and are considered toxic (e.g., aminoglycosides and other antibiotics).

Drug Therapy Considerations Across the Life Span

A. Pediatric implications (Table 5-1).
B. Older adult implications (Table 5-2).
　1. Avoiding adverse drug reactions.
　　a. Obtain a complete drug history that includes over-the-counter drugs and herbs.
　　b. Monitor client responses and drug levels.
　　c. Keep dosing regime as simple as possible, use daily dosing when possible rather than twice a day.

　　d. Emphasize to clients the importance of disposing of medications they are no longer taking.
　2. Promoting compliance: intentional underdosing (by clients) is the most common reason for nonadherence to drug regimen.
　　a. Provide written instructions to clients regarding medication administration, as well as why they are taking the medication.
　　b. Ask the pharmacist to label drug containers with large type.
　　c. Provide drug containers that can be opened easily.
　　d. Encourage clients to use a system to record or track their drug doses (calendar, pill organizer).
　　e. Determine whether clients can afford their medications.
C. Food and Drug Administration pregnancy risk categories (Table 5-3).

Herbal Supplements

A. Herbal medicine can be defined as the use of plant-derived products to promote health and relieve symptoms of disease.
B. Herbal medicine is the most common form of alternative medicine, which can be defined as treatment practices that are not widely accepted or practiced by mainstream clinicians in a given culture.
C. The word *natural* is not synonymous with *safe!* Remember, poison ivy and tobacco are natural too.
D. Some commonly used medicinal herbs (Table 5-4).

> **⚠ NURSING PRIORITY** Unlike conventional drugs, herbal and other dietary supplements can be marketed without any proof of safety or efficacy. Dietary supplements are not regulated by the FDA.

| Table 5-1 | PEDIATRIC PHARMACOLOGY AND NURSING IMPLICATIONS |

Pharmacokinetics	Body Effects and Possible Drug Responses
Absorption	Gastric emptying time is prolonged and irregular until about 6 months; delayed gastric emptying enhances drug absorption.
	Drugs administered IM to newborns may be poorly absorbed; by early infancy drugs are absorbed more rapidly.
	Topical drugs may be absorbed more quickly than in adults because infants have a proportionally greater body surface area; infant's skin is thin and drugs pass through more readily.
Distribution Phase	Protein-binding capacity does not reach adult values for 10-12 months; dosages for protein bound medications may need to be reduced in infants.
	Blood-brain barrier is not fully developed in infants; therefore it is easier for drugs and chemicals to enter the CNS.
	Infants and children have lower blood pressure.
	The liver and brain are proportionally larger and receive more blood flow.
Metabolism	Drug metabolizing is decreased in the infant due to an immature liver. Liver does not develop to full capacity until about 1 year.
Excretion	Blood flow volume through the kidneys is less than in adults, and glomerular filtration rate is significantly lower.
	At birth there is a significant decrease in drug excretion by the kidney.
	Adult level of renal excretion occurs around 1 year.

| Table 5-2 | OLDER ADULT PHARMACOLOGY AND NURSING IMPLICATIONS |

Pharmacokinetics	*Body Effects and Possible Drug Responses*
Absorption	Slowed due to decreased gastric motility and blood flow; drug responses may be delayed; absorption is slowed but not decreased. Decreased peristalsis with delayed intestinal emptying time. Gastric acidity is reduced and may alter the absorption of some drugs.
Distribution	Decreased serum protein and albumin. Drugs with a high affinity for protein compete for protein-binding sites with other drugs. Drug interactions result due to a lack of protein sites and an increase in free drugs intensifying drug effects.
Metabolism	Decreased hepatic blood flow, enzyme function, and total liver function results in reduction in drug metabolism. With a reduction in metabolic rate, the half-life of drugs increases and drug accumulation can result. Drug toxicity may occur when the half-life is prolonged.
Excretion	Decrease in renal function, therefore a decrease in drug excretion, and drug accumulation results. Continual assessment for drug toxicity while the client is taking the drug.

!! NURSING PRIORITY Adverse drug reactions secondary to a decrease in renal function is the primary cause of adverse drug reactions in the older client.

| Table 5-3 | FOOD AND DRUG ADMINISTRATION PREGNANCY RISK CATEGORIES |

Category	Description
A	*Remote Risk of Fetal Harm:* Adequate and well-controlled studies in pregnant women have not shown an increased risk of fetal abnormalities.
B	*Slightly More Risk Than A:* Animal studies have revealed no evidence of harm to the fetus; however, there are no adequate and well-controlled studies in pregnant women. *or* Animal studies have shown an adverse effect, but adequate and well-controlled studies in pregnant women have failed to demonstrate a risk to the fetus.
C	*Greater Risk Than B:* Animal studies have shown an adverse effect, and there are no adequate and well-controlled studies in pregnant women. No animal studies have been conducted, and there are no adequate and well-controlled studies in pregnant women.
D	*Proven Risk of Fetal Harm:* Studies—adequate well-controlled or observational—in pregnant women have demonstrated a risk to the fetus. However, the benefits of therapy may outweigh the potential risk.
X	*Proven Risk of Fetal Harm:* Studies—adequate well-controlled or observational—in animals or pregnant women have demonstrated positive evidence of fetal abnormalities. The use of the product is contraindicated in women who are or may become pregnant.

Modified from Lehne RA: *Pharmacology for nursing care,* ed 7, St. Louis, 2010, Saunders; and Meadows M: Pregnancy and drug dilemma, *FDA Consumer Magazine,* May-June 2001. Available at www.fda.gov/fdac/features/2001/301_preg.html.

MEDICATION ADMINISTRATION

!! NURSING PRIORITY The nurse's responsibility in administering medication is influenced by three primary factors: nursing guidelines for safe medication administration, pharmacologic implications of the medication, and the legal aspects of medication administration.

Nursing Responsibilities in Medication Administration

A. Follow the "6 Rights" of medication administration.
1. Right medication.
2. Right dosage.
3. Right route of administration.
4. Right time.
5. Right client.
6. Right charting (documentation).

ALERT Administer medications according to the "6 Rights" of medication administration. Refer to Chapter 4 for responsibilities and legal implications.

B. A nurse should administer *only* those medications that he or she has prepared.
C. Be familiar with medication.
1. General purpose for which the client is receiving the medication.
2. Common side effects.
3. Average dose or range of safe dosage.
4. Any specific safety precautions that apply before administration (e.g., digitalis: check apical pulse; heparin: check clotting times).
D. Check the medication against the health care provider's orders and document according to policy.

Table 5-4	COMMONLY USED MEDICINAL HERBS

Medicinal Herb	Drug Interactions
• **Aloe** is used for topical skin ailments with little or no topical side effects. Oral aloe is used for constipation and can cause severe diarrhea. Fresh aloe is more effective than stored product.	None noted with topical therapy.
• **Black cohosh** is a popular treatment for acute symptoms of menopause and premenstrual syndrome (PMS). Minor side effect of upset stomach may occur.	May potentiate hypotensive effects of antihypertensive drugs, as well as hypoglycemic action of insulin and oral hypoglycemics.
• **Echinacea** is used orally to stimulate the immune functions and suppress inflammation. Side effects include unpleasant taste, fever, nausea, and vomiting.	May oppose effects of immunosuppressant drugs.
• **Feverfew** for treatment of migraine, fever; stimulates menstruation and suppresses inflammation.	May suppress platelet aggregation and increase risk for bleeding in clients on anticoagulant medications (aspirin, warfarin, heparin).
• **Garlic** reduces levels of triglycerides and cholesterol and decreases formation of atherosclerotic plaque.	Increases risk for bleeding in clients taking antiplatelet drugs (aspirin) or anticoagulants (warfarin, heparin).
• **Ginger root** used for nausea and vomiting caused by motion sickness and perhaps nausea caused by chemotherapy.	Increases risk for bleeding in clients taking antiplatelet drugs (aspirin) or anticoagulants (warfarin, heparin).
• **Ginkgo biloba** is used for increased circulation, memory, clear thinking, and impotence. May cause stomach upset and dose-related headache.	Increases risk for bleeding in clients taking antiplatelet drugs (aspirin) or anticoagulants (warfarin, heparin).
• **Goldenseal** is used for bacterial, fungal, and protozoal infections of mucous membranes in the respiratory, gastrointestinal, and genitourinary tracts. Also used to treat inflammation of the gallbladder. Well tolerated but toxic in high doses.	Contraindicated in pregnancy.
• **Kava** is used to relieve anxiety, promote sleep, and relax muscles. Long-term use and high doses cause CNS depression, skin problems, and liver damage.	Intensifies the effects of CNS depressants. Should not be taken with alcohol.
• **Ma huang** (ephedra) reduces appetite, increases energy, and relieves bronchospasms. Increases blood pressure and heart rate. Potentially dangerous to the cardiovascular system with long-term use or in high doses.	Potentiates the effects of CNS stimulants; can counteract the effects of antihypertensive drugs. May cause hypertensive crisis if taken with MAO inhibitors.
• **St. John's wort** is used for depression. Potential interactions with other drugs.	May interfere with oral contraceptives; reduced anticoagulation in clients taking warfarin; decreased effectiveness of cyclosporine. Caution in use with antidepressants.
• **Saw palmetto** is used to relieve urinary symptoms related to benign prostatic hypertrophy (BPH) and is well tolerated. May cause a false-negative result on PSA test.	Avoid use in pregnancy. Should not use with finasteride (Proscar) in treatment of BPH.
• **Valerian** is a sedative to promote sleep and reduce restlessness. One possible side effect is daytime drowsiness. With high doses and long-term use, headache, nervousness, or cardiac abnormalities can occur.	

E. Evaluate client's overall condition and assess for changes that may indicate the medication is contraindicated (e.g., morphine would be contraindicated in a client who has increased intracranial pressure).

F. Evaluate compatibility with other medications the client is receiving.

G. Use appropriate aseptic technique in preparing and administering medication.

H. Do not leave medications at the client's bedside without a doctor's order to do so.

I. If client is to administer his or her own medication, review the correct method of administration (e.g., eye drops) with the client.

ALERT Evaluate appropriateness/accuracy of medication order; review pertinent data before medication administration; identify potential and actual incompatibilities of prescribed client medications.

Nurse's Legal Responsibilities in Administration of Medication

A. The nurse administers a medication only by order of a physician or health care provider and according to provisions of the specific institution.

B. The nurse should not automatically carry out an order if the dosage is outside the normal range or if the route of administration is not appropriate; he or she should consult the physician.

C. The nurse is legally responsible for the medication he or she administers, even when the medication is administered according to a physician's order.

D. The nurse is responsible for evaluating the client before and after the administration of an as-needed (PRN) medication.

E. The medication should be charted as soon as possible after administration.

F. When taking oral orders on the phone, the nurse should carefully repeat all the orders to verify they are correct (see Chapter 4, Box 4-3 for additional tips).

G. Medication errors.

1. If an error is found in a drug order, it is the nurse's responsibility to question the order.

2. Always report medication errors to the appropriate health care provider immediately.

3. It is the nurse's responsibility to carefully assess the client for effects of the erroneous medication.

4. Medication errors should be documented in an incident report and on the client's chart.

5. The U.S. Pharmacopeia and the Institute for Safe Medical Practices (ISMP) have developed a nation-wide medication errors reporting program called *Medication Errors Reporting (MER) Program.* Reporting is confidential and can be done via Internet, phone, or fax.

ALERT Identify situations in which the reporting of an incident/event/irregular occurrence/variance is appropriate; report the incident/error/event/occurrence per protocol.

▲ H. High-Alert Medications.

1. The Joint Commission (TJC) and the Institute for Safe Medication Practices (ISMP) have identified specific medications for which errors could have devastating effects on clients.

2. These medications are identified within the medication tables throughout this book.

3. TJC requires:

a. Institution or facility to develop processes to manage High-Alert Medications. ▲

b. A specific process of communication among health care workers to reconcile medications across the continuum of care. This includes a process for reconciling the list of medications during transfer, at discharge, and after major procedures.

4. Nursing Implications for High-Alert Medications (Box 5-1). ▲

Methods of Medication Administration

Note: This section on medications should not be used as a procedure guideline. The purpose is to point out specific characteristics of each method. All medications should be administered according to previously discussed nursing responsibilities in medication administration.

Box 5-1   NURSING IMPLICATIONS FOR HIGH-ALERT MEDICATIONS

- Maintain good communication and locate easily found information regarding the administration of pain medications to prevent overdose. You may use a visual pain scale. Limit the number of opiates and narcotics that are housed as floor stock. Store narcotics in individual client areas rather than as floor stock.
- Do not store together medications that have the same type of measurements. For example, heparin and insulin are both administered in units.
- Use only accepted abbreviations (see Appendixes 5-2, 5-3, 5-4).
- Establish a *check sy*stem where one nurse prepares the medication and another nurse reviews it.
- Infusion pump rates and concentrations must have an independent check system.
- Identify and exercise caution with medications that have similar names. For example, hydromorphone (Dilaudid) and morphine; potassium phosphate and potassium chloride; methyldopa (Aldomet) with levodopa or L-dopa.
- Increase the use of standardized concentrations and pre-mixed solutions (potassium chloride, sodium chloride or normal saline) on the nursing unit; decrease the premixing and calculation of medications on the nursing unit.
- Do not store vials or containers of saline in concentrations above 0.9% on the nursing unit.
- Use single-dose vials when possible.

ALERT Administer and document medications given by common routes (e.g. oral, topical), administer and document medications given by parenteral routes (intravenous, intramuscular, subcutaneous), and determine the need for administration of PRN medications.

A. Oral medication.

1. Assess level of consciousness and ability to follow directions.

2. Evaluate swallow reflex.

B. Topical medications.

1. Skin application: evaluate condition of the skin in the area that the medication is to be applied; if appropriate, rotate sites to prevent irritation.

2. Sublingual: allow medication to dissolve under the tongue; client should not chew or swallow.

3. Nasal: position client to allow nose drops or spray to enter nares directly without contaminating the eyes. Position should foster the movement of the medication to the affected area.

4. Eyes: medication must be specifically indicated for ophthalmic use.

a. Instill 1 or 2 drops in the middle of the lower conjunctival sac.

b. Do not allow tip of applicator to come in contact with the eye.

c. Do not drop medication directly on the cornea.

FIGURE 5-1 Injection routes. Needle insertion angles for intramuscular, subcutaneous, and intradermal injections. (From Lilley L, Harrington S, Snyder J: *Pharmacology and the nursing process,* ed 5, St. Louis, 2007, Mosby.)

d. Direct client to close his or her eyes gently to distribute the medication.

e. Make sure you administer the correct medication in the correct eye.

5. Ears: medication is instilled into the auditory canal.

   a. Position client with affected ear upward.

   b. Children under 3 years: pull pinna down and backward.

   c. Older children and adults: pull pinna up and backward.

   d. Administer solution at room temperature.

   e. Keep client in the same position for appropriate time to prevent medication from coming out.

6. Suppositories.

   a. Rectal: absorption of medication from rectal mucosa is slower and less predictable than that of medications administered systemically.

     (1) Frequently given for constipation or for nausea and vomiting.

     (2) May be preferred route for infant.

   b. Vaginal: absorption across vaginal mucous membranes.

     (1) Insert suppository about 3 to 4 inches into vagina; maintain supine position after insertion.

     (2) Should not douche unless advised to do so; maintain good perineal hygiene.

C. Transdermal medication: medication is stored in a patch or is measured on a dose-determined applicator placed on the skin; absorption occurs through the skin.

1. Provides more consistent blood levels and avoids gastrointestinal problems.

2. Patch sites should be rotated. Old patch should be removed and area should be cleansed after use.

3. Patch should *not* be applied over inflamed areas.

4. Do not allow transdermal medications to come in contact with your skin, because medication could be absorbed.

5. Patch must come in contact with skin; excessive body hair may need to be removed. Do not shave the area; use scissors to clip hair from area.

D. Inhalation medication: medication is in an aerosol or powder form and is inhaled and absorbed throughout the respiratory tract (see Chapter 15).

FIGURE 5-2 Needle gauges and lengths. (From Lilley L, Harrington S, Snyder J: *Pharmacology and the nursing process,* ed 5, St. Louis, 2007, Mosby.)

1. Place client in semi-Fowler's position.

2. Check instructions for use of inhaler and make sure client understands.

E. Parenteral medications: administration of medications by some method of injection.

1. Injection routes (Figure 5-1).

2. Selection of a syringe (Figure 5-2): select a syringe and type of needle that is appropriate for the type of parenteral medication to be administered.

3. Intradermal injection: administered just below the skin surface.

   a. Use a syringe with appropriate calibrations because amount is very small in volume (0.01 to 0.1 mL).

   b. Use a tuberculin or 1-mL syringe with a small-gauge (25- or 27-gauge) needle, $\frac{3}{8}$ to $\frac{5}{8}$ inch long.

   c. Select area where skin is thin (e.g., inner surface of forearm, middle of back).

   d. Insert needle bevel edge up at a 5- to 15-degree angle.

   e. Frequently used for tuberculin testing, administration of local anesthetic, allergy testing.

4. Subcutaneous injection: medication is injected into fatty tissue, just below the dermis.

   a. Medication should be small in volume (0.5 to 1 mL) and nonirritating.

   b. Areas on outer surface of upper arm, anterior surface of the thigh, and the abdomen are frequent sites.

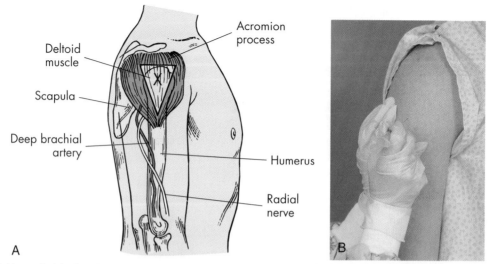

FIGURE 5-3 Deltoid muscle injection site in the upper arm. (From Potter P, Perry A: *Fundamentals of nursing*, ed 7, St. Louis, 2008, Mosby.)

FIGURE 5-4 Ventrogluteal intramuscular injection site. Place the palm of your hand over the greater trochanter, with your middle finger pointed toward the iliac crest, your index finger toward the anterosuperior iliac spine, and your thumb toward the client's groin. Administer the injection in the center of the triangle formed by your fingers. (From Lilley L, Harrington S, Snyder J: *Pharmacology and the nursing process*, ed 5, St. Louis, 2007, Mosby.)

c. Use a 25-gauge needle that is ⅝ inches long and insert at a 45-degree angle; or a 25-gauge needle that is ½ inch long and insert at a 90-degree angle.

5. Intramuscular injection: injection of medication into the muscle.
   a. The amount of medication is usually 0.5 to 3.0 mL.

   b. Appropriate sites.
      (1) Deltoid (Figure 5-3).
      (2) Ventrogluteal (Figure 5-4) and vastus lateralis muscles (Figure 5-5).
   c. Use a 1-inch to 1½-inch needle; gauge of needle depends on viscosity of medication; insert needle at 90-degree angle.

FIGURE 5-5 Vastus lateralis intramuscular injection site on the right thigh. Place one hand above the knee and the other hand below the greater trochanter. Locate the midline of both the anterior thigh and the lateral side of the thigh. Give the injection within the rectangular area. (From Lilley L, Harrington S, Snyder J: *Pharmacology and the nursing process,* ed 5, St. Louis, 2007, Mosby.)

(1) For oil-based or viscous medications use an 18- to 22-gauge needle.

(2) For less viscous medications use a 20- to 22-gauge needle.

d. Aspirate when needle is in place; if no blood returns, administer medication at a rate of 1 mL every 10 seconds.

e. Z-track technique is used to prevent medication from leaking back through the needle track and irritating or staining subcutaneous tissue.

(1) After medication is drawn up, change the needle.

(2) Pull skin over to one side at the injection site.

(3) Inject medication into taut skin at site selected.

(4) Remove the needle and release the skin. As the stretched skin returns to its original position, the needle track is sealed.

(5) The preferable site is the ventrogluteal area.

f. Intramuscular injections in children.

(1) Vastus lateralis (see Figure 5-5) muscle is common site in infants.

(2) Ventrogluteal (see Figure 5-4) site is the preferred site in children.

(3) A 22-gauge 1-inch needle is appropriate for an IM injection in most children.

(4) See **Calculation of Medication Dosages** section for pediatric calculations.

6. IV administration: injection of medication into the blood (Table 5-5).

a. Administration of large volumes of liquid by infusion.

b. Administration of irritating medications by piggyback method.

(1) Dilute medication according to directions, usually 25 to 250 mL of a compatible intravenous fluid-like normal saline (NS).

(2) Assess patency of primary infusion.

(3) Connect medication and adjust flow rate for the time designated, usually 30 to 45 minutes.

(4) Administration of medications through IV piggyback method enhances the action of the medication.

c. Administration of a specific medication into an already present IV infusion by *IV push* or *bolus* method.

(1) Clamp tubing of primary IV line, inject the medication slowly, and observe the client's response.

(2) Be aware of the institution's policy regarding guidelines for IV push medications.

d. Retrograde IV administration: medication is mixed with diluent, the port closest to client is clamped and medication is injected into the port and allowed to fill (retrograde) into the IV tubing. The clamp closest to the client is opened and the medication is allowed to infuse at the prescribed flow rate.

Forms of Medication Preparations

A. Solids.

1. Capsule: medication is placed in cylindrical gelatin container.

Table 5-5	INTRAVENOUS MEDICATION ADMINISTRATION	
Method	*Injection Rate*	*Nursing Implications*
Push or bolus	Rate of administration is determined by the amount of medication that can be given each minute based on each drug's protocol.	1. Drug is not diluted and is injected directly into the client's venous system. 2. Access is most often through an existing IV infusion. Use the access port closest to the client. 3. Has a rapid effect on the CNS and cardiopulmonary systems. 4. IV push or bolus is the most dangerous delivery method. Extreme care should be taken in following the drug protocol. If in doubt, do not deliver the bolus.
Intermittent infusion or piggyback (IVPB)	Medication is diluted in 25 to 100 mL and infused over 15 to 60 minutes.	1. Drug is diluted to decrease toxicity and hypertonicity of the solution. 2. Method of choice for multiple daily doses, especially antibiotics. 3. Concentrated medications require higher dilution and longer infusion time.
Constant and variable-rate infusion	Pump is set to deliver constant rate of infusion based on dose of medication and dilution of medication.	1. Method for medications that need to be highly diluted (chemotherapeutic drugs). 2. Provides for continuous medication infusion.

CNS, Central nervous system; *IV* intravenous.

2. Pills, tablets: medication is pressed into solid form in various shapes and colors.
   a. Enteric-coated: prevents medication from being released in stomach; dissolves in intestine. Do not crush enteric-coated, extended-release (ER), or sustained-release (SR) tablets.
   b. Lozenge: flavored tablet is held in the mouth for slow release of medication.
3. Suppositories: generally keep these in cool area; will melt at body temperature; may produce local or systemic effects.
   a. Rectal.
   b. Vaginal.
4. Ointments: used for external application.
5. Powders: finely ground medications that are stable only in dry form; frequently mixed with solution before administration.
B. Solutions.
   1. Syrups: medication prepared in an aqueous sugar solution.
   2. Elixirs: solutions containing alcohol, sugar, and water.
   3. Suspensions: finely ground particles of medication dispersed in a liquid; shake all suspensions well before preparing dose (antacids).
   4. Emulsions: medication is dispersed in an oil or fat solution; shake all emulsions well before preparing dose.
   5. Liniments, lotions: medication dispersed in a mixture of oil, soap, alcohol, water; used for external application.

Calculation of Medication Dosages

Occasionally, medications are ordered by the physician in amounts not supplied by the pharmacy. In these situations, the nurse must calculate the correct dosage. Another important area of calculation is in the administration of IV solutions. Thus it is essential that the nurse have a good working knowledge of the fundamental principles of mathematics to calculate medication dosages correctly.

Oral Medication Calculations

Dose desired ÷ Dose on hand = Amount to give

Example: Order reads to give Keflex 500 mg. Dose on hand is 250-mg capsules.

$$500 \div 250 = 2 \text{ capsules}$$

Dose desired ÷ Dose on hand ×
Quantity = Amount to give

Example: Order reads to give ampicillin 350 mg. Dose on hand is 250 mg in 5 mL.

$$350 \div 250 \times 5 = x$$

$$350 \div 250 = 14$$

$$14 \times 5 \text{ mL} = 7 \text{ mL}$$

The problem can also be set up in algebraic proportion:

$$350/x = 250/5 \text{ mL}$$

$$250x = 1750$$

$$x = 7 \text{ mL}$$

Parenteral Medication Calculations

Dose desired ÷ Dose on hand ×
Quantity of solution = Amount to give

Example: Order reads Gentamycin 60 mg IM. On hand is 80 mg in 1 mL.

$$60 \text{ mg} \div 80 \text{ mg} \times 1 \text{ mL} = x$$

$$60 \div 80 = 0.75$$

$$0.75 \times 1 \text{ mL} = \tfrac{3}{4} \text{ mL or } 0.75 \text{ mL}$$

Set up in algebraic proportion, the equation reads:

$$60 \text{ mg}/x = 80 \text{ mg}/1 \text{ mL}$$

$$60x = 75$$

$$x = 0.75 \text{ mL or } \tfrac{3}{4} \text{ mL}$$

Intravenous Medication Calculation

- To determine how long an infusion will run, divide the total number of milliliters to infuse by the hourly infusion rate.

$$\text{Amount to infuse} \div \text{Hourly rate} = \text{Number of hours}$$

Example: Order reads 1000 mL at 125 mL per hour. How long will it take the 1000 mL to infuse?

$$1000 \div 125 = x$$

$$1000 \div 125 = 8 \text{ hours}$$

- To determine the rate in milliliters per hour at which an infusion will run, divide the total number of milliliters to infuse by the infusion time.

$$\text{Amount to infuse} \div \text{Total infusion time} = \text{Rate(mL/hr)}$$

Example: Order reads 1000 mL to run every 8 hours. At what rate in milliliters per hour will the medication be infused?

$$1000 \text{ mL} \div 8 \text{ hours} = 125 \text{ mL/hr}$$

- Calculating drop factors: Check the IV equipment to determine how many drops are delivered in 1 mL. For example purposes, a drop factor of 10 gtt per 1 mL is used. The following are two formulas with which to calculate this factor.

$$\text{Total mL/Time in min} = \text{mL per min} \times$$
$$\text{Drop factor} = \text{gtt per min}$$

Example: 1000 mL is ordered to infuse in 8 hours. Set drop factor is 10 gtt/mL.

$$1000 \text{ mL} \div 480 \text{ min} = 2.08 \text{ mL/min}$$

$$2.08 \times 10 = 20.8 \text{ or } 21 \text{ gtt/min}$$

Example: 500 mL is ordered to infuse in 2 hours. Set calibration is 10 gtt/mL.

$$500 \text{ mL} \div 120 \text{ min} = 4.16 \times 10 = 41.6 \text{ or } 42 \text{ gtt/min}$$

- Determine the number of milliliters per hour and divide by 60 (60 minutes in 1 hour). This equals the number of milliliters per minute. Multiply by set calibration of number of drops per milliliter.

$$\text{Number of milliliters per hour} \div 60 = \text{mL/min}$$

$$\text{Rate(mL/min)} \times \text{Set calibration} = \text{gtt/min}$$

Example: 500 mL is ordered to infuse in 2 hours. Set calibration is 10 gtt/mL (250 mL/hr to infuse).

$$250 \text{ mL} \div 60 = 4.16 \text{ mL/min}$$

$$4.16 \text{ mL} \times 10 = 41.6 \text{ or } 42 \text{ gtt/min}$$

Note: There may be a difference of 2 to 4 gtt when different formulas are used.

Determining Safe Pediatric Dosages

Calculations for pediatric dosage should be considered as an approximation of the safe dose range. These calculations can be used as a guide when evaluating the appropriateness of a medication dose order.

$$\text{Safe dose/kg} \times$$
$$\text{child's weight in kg} = \text{approximation of safe dose}$$

Example: Order reads to give cefaclor (Ceclor) 50 mg qid. The child weighs 9.1 kg. Is this a safe dose?

Safe dose range is 20-40 mg/kg/day in divided doses.

$$20 \text{ mg} \times 9.1 \text{ kg} = 182 \text{ mg}$$

$40 \text{ mg} \times 9.1 \text{ kg} = 364 \text{ mg/day}$ is the approximate upper limits for maximum safe dose.

The child is receiving 50 mg $\times$ 4 doses (qid) = 200 mg/day. This dose is within the approximate safe range for a pediatric client.

The safest formula for evaluating drug dosages in children is to calculate the proportional amount of the body surface area (BSA) to the body weight. This requires the use of the West Nomogram (Figure 5-6) for estimation of body surface area.

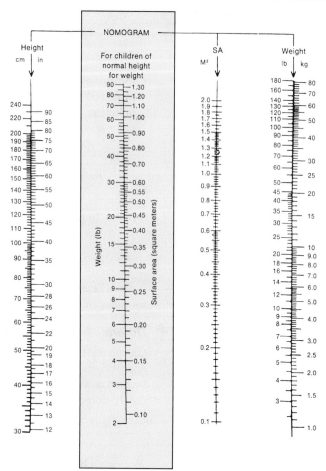

FIGURE 5-6 West Nomogram for Estimation of Body Surface Area. Surface area is indicated where a straight line connecting height and weight intersects surface area (SA) column or, if patient is approximately of normal proportion, from weight alone (yellow area). (Nomogram modified from data of E Boyd by CD West: From Behrman RE, Kliegman RM, Jenson HB, editors: *Nelson textbook of pediatrics,* ed 17, Philadelphia, 2000, Saunders).

Appendix 5-1   CONVERSIONS

CELSIUS AND FAHRENHEIT

Fahrenheit reading = 9/5 × Celsius reading + 32

Example: Temperature is 50° Celsius
Fahrenheit = 9/5 × 50 + 32
90 + 32 = 122° Fahrenheit

POUNDS AND GRAMS

1 pound = 454 grams
To convert pounds to grams, multiply the number of pounds by 454.

7.5 × 454 = 3405 g
To convert grams to pounds, divide the number of grams by 454.
Example: An infant weighs 3405 g
3405/454 = 7.5 lb, or 7 lb 8 oz

Appendix 5-2 COMMON ABBREVIATIONS AND SYMBOLS

ac	before meals	mcg	micrograms
ad lib	as desired	N	nitrogen
bid	twice daily	Na	sodium
$\bar{c}$	with	NPO	nothing by mouth
Ca	calcium	OOB	out of bed
CBC	complete blood count	pc	after meals
Cl	chloride	po	by mouth
gm	gram	prn	as needed
gtt	drops	qid	four times a day
H_2O	water	q2h	every 2 hours
H_2O_2	hydrogen peroxide	q3h	every 3 hours
K	potassium	$\bar{s}$	without
L	liter	stat	immediately
mL	milliliter	tab	tablet
Mg	magnesium	tid	three times a day

Appendix 5-3 LIST OF "DO NOT USE" ABBREVIATIONS, ACRONYMS, AND SYMBOLS APPROVED BY THE JOINT COMMISSION (TJC)

ABBREVIATION	POTENTIAL PROBLEM	PREFERRED TERM
U (unit)	Mistaken for "0" (zero), the number "4" (four) or "cc"	Write "unit"
IU (International Unit)	Mistaken for IV (intravenous) or the number 10 (ten)	Write "International Unit"
Q.D., QD, q.d., qd (daily)	Mistaken for each other	Write "daily"
Q.O.D., QOD, q.o.d, qod (every other day)	Period after the Q mistaken for "I" and the "O" mistaken for "I"	Write "every other day"
Trailing zero (X. 0 mg)*	Decimal point is missed	Write X mg
Lack of leading zero (.X mg)		Write 0.X mg
MS	Can mean morphine sulfate or magnesium sulfate	Write "morphine sulfate"
MSO_4 and $MgSO_4$	Confused for one another	Write "magnesium sulfate"

From Joint Commission on Accreditation of Healthcare Organizations: *The Official "Do Not Use" List Updated—March 2009*. Available at www.jointcommission.org/PatientSafety/DoNotUseList/. Accessed August 5, 2009. © The Joint Commission, 2009. Reprinted with permission.
*Exception: A "trailing zero" may be used only where required to demonstrate the level of precision of the value being reported, such as for laboratory results, imaging studies that report size of lesions, or catheter/tube sizes. It may not be used in medication orders or other medication-related documentation.

Appendix 5-4 ABBREVIATIONS AND SYMBOLS THAT ARE RECOMMENDED BUT NOT YET MANDATED BY THE JOINT COMMISSION (TJC) FOR INCLUSION IN THE OFFICIAL "DO NOT USE" LIST

ABBREVIATION	POTENTIAL PROBLEM	PREFERRED TERM
> (greater than)	Misinterpreted as the number "7" (seven) or the letter "L"	Write "greater than"
< (less than)	Confused for one another	Write "less than"
Abbreviations for drug names	Misinterpreted due to similar abbreviations for multiple drugs	Write drug names in full
Apothecary units	Unfamiliar to many practitioners Confused with metric units	Use metric units
@	Mistaken for the number "2" (two)	Write "at"
cc	Mistaken for U (units) when poorly written	Write "mL" or "ml" or milliliters" ("mL" is preferred)
μg	Mistaken for mg (milligrams) resulting in one thousand-fold overdose	Write "mcg" or "micrograms"

From Joint Commission on Accreditation of Healthcare Organizations: *The Official "Do Not Use" List Updated—March 2009*. Available at www.jointcommission.org/PatientSafety/DoNotUseList/. Accessed August 5, 2009. © The Joint Commission, 2009. Reprinted with permission.

Study Questions Pharmacology

More questions on companion CD!

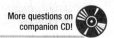

1. The nurse is preparing to administer an intramuscular injection to an infant who is 8 months old. Which muscle would be the most appropriate injection site?
   1 Biceps.
   2 Dorsogluteal.
   3 Vastus lateralis.
   4 Ventrogluteal.

2. The doctor has indicated that ampicillin and gentamicin are to be given piggyback in the same hour, every 6 hours (12-6-12-6). How would the nurse administer these drugs?
   1 Give both drugs together IV push.
   2 Give each drug separately, flushing between drugs.
   3 Retrograde both drugs into the tubing.
   4 Give one drug every 4 hours and one every 6 hours.

3. At the shift hand-off report, a nurse is told that one of her clients is becoming tolerant to his pain medication. What nursing observation would be in agreement with this conclusion?
   1 The current medication order, which has previously been effective, is no longer providing adequate pain relief.
   2 The client becomes irritable and confused before the next scheduled dose of medication.
   3 Pain medication is being administered every 3-4 hours around the clock for adequate pain relief.
   4 The client is sleeping, arouses with physical and verbal stimulation, but is very lethargic.

4. What should the nurse take into consideration when giving medication to an older adult client?
   1 Multiple simultaneous drugs can be dangerous.
   2 The older adult client metabolizes and excretes the drugs differently than do younger clients.
   3 Medication affects the older adult client during the early hours of the morning.
   4 Medication has an effect on the respiratory system of the older adult client.

5. What is the first step the nurse should take to ensure that the right medication is being given to a client?
   1 Check the client's ID band.
   2 Read the information insert for directions as to correct administration.
   3 Check the order with the medication administration sheet.
   4 Check the expiration date on the medication.

6. The nurse prepares a liquid medication and then finds that the client no longer needs the medication. What is the most appropriate nursing action?
   1 To keep the count correct, record that the dose was taken.
   2 Charge for the dose because it must be paid for.
   3 Record the medication as "not taken" and discard the poured dose.
   4 Pour the medication back into the container.

7. The nurse is working in the pediatric unit and receives a phone order from the doctor for a 10-year-old client who weighs 40 kg. The order is for ceftibuten (Fortaz) 1 g every 8 hours IV. The therapeutic dosage range is 100 to 150 mg/kg/24 hr. What would be the best nursing action?
   1 Administer the medication because it is within the therapeutic dosage range.
   2 Call the doctor to clarify the order since it is outside the therapeutic dosage range.
   3 Call the hospital pharmacist and ask them to calculate the dosage.
   4 Notify the nursing supervisor and request assistance.

8. The nurse is caring for a client who had a stroke (brain accident) 3 months ago and is taking Coumadin. The client tells the nurse she has started taking some herbal and vitamin supplements. She gives the nurse a list of the supplements she is taking. What supplements would cause concern for the client who is on Coumadin? Select all that apply:
   _____ 1 Garlic.
   _____ 2 Cyanocobalamin (vitamin B_{12}).
   _____ 3 St John's wort.
   _____ 4 Vitamin E (alpha tocopherol).
   _____ 5 Saw palmetto.
   _____ 6 Ginkgo biloba.

9. The nurse is preparing medications for a client. The medication order is for cefaclor (Ceclor) 0.1 g PO. The dose available in the unit is 125 mg/5 mL. How many milliliters will the nurse need to give?
   Answer: _____ mL

10. A client is receiving IV antibiotic therapy. The order is for methicillin 750 mg IV. The nurse has a vial on hand that contains 1g. The instructions for reconstitution say to add 1.5 mL sterile water. Reconstituted solution will contain 500 mg methicillin per milliliter. How much will the nurse give?
    Answer: _____ mL

11. The nurse is verifying whether to give a medication to a client. What would be the first nursing action?
    1 Check the client's name and hospital number.
    2 Validate the expiration date of the drug.
    3 Determine the appropriate route of delivery.
    4 Review the orders on the medication administration record.

Answers and rationales to these questions are in the section at the end of the book titled Chapter Study Questions: Answers and Rationales.

Homeostasis

Homeostasis, **for the purposes of this chapter, is defined as the mechanism for maintaining a steady state in the body.**

FLUID AND ELECTROLYTES

Physiology

A. Basic concepts of body fluid.
  1. Water is a primary body fluid. It is used to transport nutrients as well as to remove waste products.
      a. Infant: 70% to 80% of body weight is water.
      b. Adult: 50% to 60% of body weight is water.
      c. Older adult: 45% to 55% of body weight is water.
  2. Intracellular fluid: provides the cell with internal fluid necessary for cellular function.
      a. Approximately 40% to 50% of body weight.
      b. Electrolytes: potassium (primary), magnesium, phosphate.
  3. Extracellular (intravascular and interstitial) fluids: transport system for cellular waste, oxygen, electrolytes, and nutrients; help regulate body temperature; lubricate and cushion joints.
      a. Approximately 20% to 30% of body weight.
      b. An infant maintains a larger percentage of extracellular fluids than does an older child or adult.
      c. Vascular: circulating plasma volume.
      d. Interstitial: fluid surrounding tissue cells.
      e. Electrolytes: sodium (primary), chloride, bicarbonate.
B. Dynamic transport of fluid and electrolytes.
  1. Osmosis: movement of water between two compartments separated by a semipermeable membrane; from an area of low-solute concentration to an area of high-solute concentration.
      a. Oncotic pressure: the osmotic pressure created by plasma proteins; proteins pull fluid from the tissue space to the vascular space.
      b. Osmotic pressure is the amount of pressure required to stop the flow of water. It is determined by the concentration of solutes in solution.
  2. Hydrostatic pressure: the pressure created by the fluid volume in the vascular bed.
C. Fluid movement in capillaries.
  1. Filtration occurs in the arterial end of the capillaries because the hydrostatic pressure is higher than the oncotic pressure. Fluid then moves out of the vascular bed into the tissue.
  2. Capillary hydrostatic pressure and interstitial oncotic pressure move water out of the capillaries. At the venous end of the capillaries, the oncotic pressure is greater and the fluid moves back into the vascular volume.
  3. Osmolality refers to the concentration of the dissolved particles in a solution; osmolality controls the movement of fluid in each of the compartments.
      a. Hyperosmolar (hypertonic): fluids in which the concentration of solutes is higher than in the cells.
      b. Hypo-osmolar (hypotonic): fluids in which the concentration of solutes is less than in the cells.
      c. Iso-osmolar (isotonic): fluids with the same osmolality as the cell normal distribution of solutes and water in body fluid.
D. Fluid shifts.
  1. Plasma to interstitial fluid shift (edema).
      a. Edema: accumulation of fluid in interstitial spaces.
          (1) Venous hydrostatic pressure increases (client with fluid overload in heart failure).
          (2) Decrease in oncotic pressure, as in a client with excessive protein loss (renal disease).
          (3) Increased interstitial oncotic pressure, as in trauma and burns where the capillary wall has been damaged and plasma protein moves to the interstitial space.
      b. Hypovolemia may occur as a result of excessive fluid shift into the interstitial spaces, resulting in circulatory collapse (client with burns).
  2. Interstitial to plasma fluid shift: movement of fluid back into the circulatory volume, as in client with mobilization of burn edema; or in the case of excessive administration of hypertonic solution, causing the interstitial water to be returned to the plasma; client may demonstrate symptoms of circulatory overload.
  3. Fluid spacing.
      a. First spacing: normal distribution of fluids.
      b. Second spacing: abnormal accumulation of interstitial fluid—edema.
      c. Third spacing: fluid that is trapped and cannot easily move back into ECF—for example, edema associated with burns and ascites.

E. Homeostatic mechanisms.
  1. Endocrine system.
     a. Hypothalamus secretes antidiuretic hormone, which regulates the water reabsorption by the kidneys.
     b. Adrenal cortex secretes aldosterone, which promotes sodium retention and potassium excretion, thereby causing an increase in plasma volume.
  2. Lymphatic system: assists in the return of excessive protein and fluid, which escapes into the tissue, to the plasma volume.
  3. Cardiovascular system maintains blood pressure to ensure adequate renal perfusion.
  4. Kidneys maintain fluid volume and concentration of urine via the glomerular filtration rate.

ALERT Understand general principles of pathophysiology.

Fluid Imbalances

A. Fluid deficit: extracellular fluid volume deficit hypovolemia results from vascular fluid volume loss.
  1. Sensible fluid loss: fluid loss of which an individual is aware, as in urine.
  2. Insensible fluid loss: fluid loss of which an individual is not aware (approximately 600-900 mL of fluid is lost every 24 hours through the skin and lungs in a healthy adult).
  3. Causes of fluid deficit (all result from loss of both water and sodium).
     a. Decreased fluid intake.
     b. Loss of fluid through the gastrointestinal tract, as in vomiting, nasogastric suctioning, diarrhea.
     c. Excessive excretion due to renal disease; inappropriate antidiuretic hormone secretion.
     d. Iatrogenic loss due to overuse of diuretics or inadequate replacement of fluid loss.
     e. Increased insensible fluid loss through skin and lungs due to febrile state.
     f. Impaired integrity of the skin as in burns, wounds, and hemorrhage.

! NURSING PRIORITY Sodium is the major electrolyte that affects fluid balance. "Where goes the sodium, so goes the water."

  4. Clinical manifestations.
     a. Restlessness, lethargy, confusion.
     b. Dry skin and thirst (dry mucous membranes).
     c. Decreased skin turgor.
        (1) Assess skin turgor on the abdomen or the inner thigh in children (unless abdominal distention is present).
        (2) Assess skin turgor on the forehead or sternum in older adult clients.
        (3) Assess skin turgor on the sternum, abdomen, and anterior forearm in adults.

     d. Weight loss.
     e. Oliguria, concentrated urine.
     f. Postural hypotension.
     g. Increased respiratory and cardiac rate.
     h. Decreased central venous pressure (CVP).
     i. Infants and children: poor perfusion, poor capillary refill resulting in mottled skin color changes.
     j. Weakness, confusion, speech difficulty in the older adult client.
  5. Laboratory findings.
     a. Increased urine specific gravity.
     b. Increased blood urea nitrogen (greater than 25 mg/dL) without increase in creatinine.
     c. Increased hematocrit (the normal ratio of hematocrit to hemoglobin is 3:1)—for example, 12 grams hemoglobin to 36% hematocrit.

ALERT Identify signs and symptoms for client with fluid and/or electrolyte balance.

B. Extracellular fluid volume excess (circulatory overload): the retention of sodium and water in the intravascular and interstitial spaces.
  1. Causes of fluid excess.
     a. Excessive oral fluid intake.
     b. Failure to excrete fluids, as in renal disease and cardiac failure.
     c. Iatrogenic: fluid increase due to excessive infusion of hypotonic or isotonic fluids.
     d. Excess hypotonic and/or hypotonic IV fluids.
  2. Clinical manifestations.
     a. Pitting edema, sacral edema.
     b. Dyspnea, crackles, possible pulmonary edema.
     c. Bounding pulse, weight gain.
     d. Lethargy, dizziness, headache, confusion.
     e. Variable urine volume.
     f. Increased CVP, jugular vein distention.
     g. Increased blood pressure.
  3. Laboratory findings: based on the area of the body in which the shift occurs.
     a. Decreased specific gravity of urine (less than 1.010).
     b. Decreased hematocrit.
     c. Decreased serum sodium secondary to dilution.
     d. Vascular to interstitial space shift due to tissue damage such as blisters, sprains.
     e. Large fluid shifts occur in severe injuries, burns, intestinal perforations and obstruction, and lymphatic obstruction.
  4. Clinical manifestations.
     a. Decreased circulating volume, resulting in symptoms of hypovolemia.
     b. Localized symptoms when the fluid is obstructing an organ, as in the intestinal tract.

ALERT Implement interventions to restore client fluid and/or electrolyte balance.

C. Nursing management of client with fluid imbalances.
  1. Assessment.
    a. Evaluate client's history and predisposing factors contributing to the problem.
    b. Assess for direction of fluid problem: fluid excess or deficit.
    c. Evaluate appropriate lab data.
    d. Evaluate client's ability to tolerate and correct the problem.
    e. Older adult clients are more likely to develop extracellular fluid volume excess due to chronic diseases (renal, cardiac).
  2. Nursing intervention.
    a. Maintain accurate intake and output records.
    b. Obtain accurate daily weight.

> **! NURSING PRIORITY** Daily weight is the most reliable indicator of fluid loss or gain in all clients, regardless of age. Accurate daily weight: same time each day (preferably before breakfast), same scales, same clothing. 1 liter of fluid equals 2.2 lb or 1 kg.

    c. Evaluate for presence of edema.
    d. Maintain intravenous (IV) replacement fluids at prescribed flow rate.
    e. Monitor cardiovascular changes.
      (1) Central venous pressure, status of jugular vein.
      (2) Changes in blood pressure (blood pressure is not a reliable indicator of early problems of fluid balance in infants and children).
    f. Monitor for changes in respiratory status.
    g. Maintain good skin care: practice good oral hygiene, elevate edematous extremities, avoid soap, use measures to prevent skin breakdown.
    h. Assess lab data for changes in the problem.
    i. Carefully monitor older adult and pediatric clients and clients with cardiac disease for tolerance of fluid replacement.

> **! NURSING PRIORITY** Increased urine specific gravity, dark urine, decreased urine output and postural hypotension are very objective clues to ECF volume deficit.

  3. See Appendixes 6-1 through 6-6 for more on electrolyte imbalances and replacement.

INTRAVENOUS FLUID REPLACEMENT THERAPY

Isotonic Solutions

A. Used to expand extracellular fluid volume and for intravascular dehydration.
B. Solutions.
  1. D_5W: 5% dextrose in water (physiologically hypotonic).
  2. 0.9% NaCl (normal saline solution).
  3. Lactated Ringer's solution.
C. May be used to dilute medications or to keep the vein open.

> **! NURSING PRIORITY** In D_5W the dextrose is metabolized rapidly, leaving free water to be absorbed. It does not replenish electrolytes; it is contraindicated for clients with head injuries and should be used with caution in children because of the potential for increase in intracranial pressure.

Hypotonic Solutions

A. Solutions containing more water and less basic electrolytes.
B. 0.45% or half-strength NaCl (normal saline solution).
C. May be used to replenish cellular fluid.
D. Monitor closely for intravascular fluid loss, hypotension, changes in level of consciousness, and edema.

Hypertonic Solutions

A. Administered slowly; can cause intravascular volume overload; carefully monitor serum sodium, lung sounds, and blood pressure.
B. Solutions.
  1. Dextrose 5% in 0.45% or half-strength NaCl (normal saline).
  2. Dextrose 5% in 0.9% NaCl (normal saline).
C. Used to treat situations of hyponatremia and hypovolemia.

Nursing Implications in Administration of Intravenous Fluid

> **ALERT** Apply knowledge of nursing procedures and motor skills when caring for a client receiving intravenous and parenteral therapy.

Selection of Site and Equipment

A. Vein selection (Figure 6-1).
  1. Distal veins of the upper extremities should be used first. Subsequent venipuncture should be proximal to or higher than the previous site.
  2. Veins above or below an area of flexion.
  3. Try to select a site on the client's nondominant extremity.
  4. Select a vein large enough to accommodate the catheter.
B. Infants: scalp veins are frequently used because of easy access and less movement in the area; it is also easier to stabilize the insertion site.
C. Children: veins on the dorsal surface of the foot are frequently used (these should *not* be used as an access site in *adults* because of the risk for developing thrombophlebitis).

> **ALERT** Know which veins should be accessed for various therapies.

D. IV sites to avoid.
  1. Areas of flexion, especially the antecubital area.
  2. Veins previously injured by infiltration or phlebitis.
  3. Veins of an affected extremity: mastectomy, dialysis access.

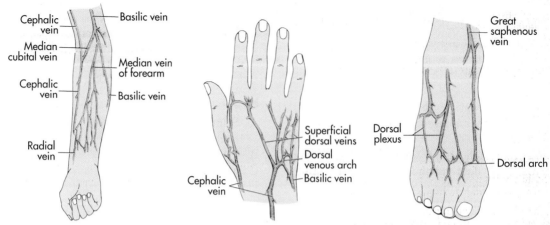

FIGURE 6-1 Common IV sites. A, Inner arm. B, Dorsal surface of hand. C, Dorsal surface of foot (infants and children). (From Potter PA, Perry AG: *Fundamentals of nursing,* ed 7, St. Louis, 2009, Mosby.)

4. Veins of an extremity affected by stroke or neurologic trauma.
5. Veins in the lower extremities and sclerosed or irritated veins.
6. Avoid previous venipuncture sites, areas of inflammation or bruising.

E. Venous access devices (Figure 6-2).
1. Butterfly needle: has wings for stabilization of needle; used for short-term infusions and for saline/heparin locks.
2. Plastic cannula/catheter: tubing threaded over a needle; used for infusions over several days and often with IV antibiotics.
3. Needle: used for short-term infusions.
4. Select the smallest-gauge needle or cannula for the type of fluid infused. The larger the gauge of the needle or cannula, the *smaller* the needle or cannula.
   a. 22-gauge needle or catheter most common for IV fluids.
   b. 18- or 20-gauge needle or catheter for blood or rapid administration of fluids.
   c. May convert a cannula into a saline/heparin lock if continuous fluids are not infusing.
5. Central line (see Appendix 6-10).
6. Implantable or tunneled ports (see Appendix 6-10).

ALERT Access implanted venous access devices.

7. Heparin or saline lock: may be an IV cannula or a butterfly needle.
   a. Used for intermittent access.
   b. May be flushed with a heparin solution, 100 units per 1 mL (depending on institution policy), or saline flush solution at regular intervals to maintain patency and prevent clot formation of line.
8. Site may be converted to fluid infusion if necessary.

! NURSING PRIORITY If the institution is using heparin for flushing locks and tubing, make sure the heparin flush solution (Hep-Lock)—1 mL per 100 units or 1 mL per 10 units—is used. It is easy to mistake the heparin 1-10,000 units as a flush solution.

FIGURE 6-2 IV access options. (From Potter PA, Perry AG: *Fundamentals of nursing,* ed 7, St. Louis, 2009, Mosby.)

ALERT Monitor and maintain infusion site(s) and rate(s).

Starting an Intravenous Infusion

! NURSING PRIORITY Always check the IV fluid for expiration date, color, and clarity.

A. Cleanse site thoroughly; re-cleanse the site if area was palpated before insertion.
B. Wear gloves during insertion of the needle and as long as there is possibility of skin contact with the client's blood.
C. Apply the tourniquet 4 to 6 inches above the site and insert the needle with the bevel up at a 15-degree to 30-degree angle.

D. After the needle has advanced into the vein and there is good blood return, release the tourniquet.

E. If the stylet has been removed (IV catheter or cannula), do not attempt to reinsert the stylet into the catheter shaft.

F. Always obtain a new catheter or needle if the insertion attempt was unsuccessful.

G. Cover the insertion site (transparent dressing or sterile gauze); do not place tape directly over the insertion site.

H. Label the site with time, date, catheter/needle size, and initials of nurse.

I. Label the infusion container with:
1. Time container was hung; rate of infusion.
2. Any medications that were added.

J. Do not encircle the arm with tape; this can restrict circulation to the extremity.

> **ALERT** Insert/remove peripheral intravenous line.

Maintenance of Intravenous Infusions

A. Factors influencing rate of fluid administration.
1. Type of fluid, age of client, and client's response to fluids.
2. Cardiac and renal status.
3. Size of the vein and gauge of catheter or needle.

> **ALERT** Monitor and maintain infusion site(s) and rate(s).

B. Maintain accurate intake and output records.

C. Average maintenance fluid rate is 3000 mL over 24 hours.

D. Peripheral IV infusion sites are changed every 72 to 96 hours (3-4 days, depending on institution policy) unless complications (inflammation, irritation, or fluid extravasation) occur at the site.

E. Carefully monitor the infusion rate: control with either a roller clamp or an infusion pump.

> **!** **NURSING PRIORITY** Always monitor the rate of infusion by evaluating the amount of fluid that has actually been infused and by checking the pump or IV control settings.

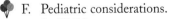

F. Pediatric considerations.
1. Children are very susceptible to rapid fluid shifts; cerebral edema may occur with infusion of D_5W. Most common IV solutions are a combination of normal saline (0.22%-0.3%) and 5% dextrose to decrease the possibility of an untoward fluid shift.
2. Volume chambers holding no more than a 3- to 4-hour supply of fluid or controlled infusion devices (pumps) should be used for children to prevent the inadvertent rapid infusion of too much fluid.
3. Always make sure infants and young children are voiding before beginning IV infusion of fluids containing added potassium.

> **ALERT** Evaluate client response to interventions used to correct fluid and electrolyte balance.

Indications for Use of Infusion Control Devices

A. To deliver a medication that requires a precise rate of administration (vasopressor agents, PCA).

B. To deliver fluids that would precipitate adverse effects if administered too rapidly (hyperalimentation).

C. To deliver fluids in controlled amounts to clients very sensitive to volume administered (infants, children under 10 years old, older adult clients, clients with pulmonary edema, and clients with decreased renal function).

> **ALERT** Operate and monitor the use of an infusion pump.

Complications of Peripheral Intravenous Therapy (Figure 6-3)

Infiltration

A. Common causes: dislodging of the needle by client movement or obstruction of fluid flow.

B. Signs and symptoms: edema, *blanching of skin*, discomfort at site, fluid that is flowing slowly or has stopped, *cooler skin temperature.*

C. Preventive nursing management: use the smallest gauge of catheter possible; use an arm board to stabilize catheter, especially for restless, confused clients or those with catheters placed in the antecubital fossa area; check frequently for coolness of skin around site; avoid looping tubing below bed level; check IV flow rate at least every 2 hours.

FIGURE 6-3 Complications of peripheral IV therapy. (From Zerwekh J, Claborn J, Gaglione T: *Mosby's fluids and electrolytes memory notecards: visual, mnemonic, and memory aids for nurses,* ed 2, St. Louis, 2010, Mosby.)

D. Nursing interventions.
1. Discontinue IV solution and remove catheter.
2. Apply warm, moist heat for 20 minutes to increase fluid absorption (if not contraindicated); may reapply warm, moist heat 3-4 times throughout the day; raise affected extremity to increase venous return and reduce swelling.
3. If infiltrated solution contains an irritating medication (chemotherapy, vasoconstrictive fluids), call the physician for orders to counteract effects of medication in the subcutaneous tissue.

Phlebitis

A. Common causes: overuse of a vein; irritating infusion solutions or medications; catheter left in vein for too long; use of large-gauge catheters.
B. Signs and symptoms: tenderness, pain along the course of the vein, edema, redness at insertion site, red streak along course of vein, extremity with IV feels warmer than other extremity.
C. Preventive nursing management.
1. Change IV site every 72-96 hours.
2. Use large veins to administer irritating solutions.
3. Stabilize cannula.
4. Dilute medications adequately and infuse at prescribed rates.
5. Choose the smallest-gauge catheter possible to administer solutions.
D. Nursing interventions: apply warm, moist compresses to stimulate circulation and promote absorption.

ALERT Evaluate client response to parenteral fluid therapy.

E. Prevention of infections related to IV therapy (Box 6-1).

ACID-BASE BALANCE

Basic Concepts of Acid-Base Balance

A. Terms used to describe acid-base balance.
1. pH: the chemical abbreviation for negative logarithm of hydrogen ion concentration.
2. CO_2: carbon dioxide.
3. $Paco_2$: pressure of dissolved CO_2 gas in the blood.
4. O_2: oxygen.
5. PaO_2: pressure of dissolved O_2 gas in the blood.
6. HCO_3^-: bicarbonate.
7. mm Hg: millimeters of mercury.
8. H^+: hydrogen ion concentration.
B. Normal blood gas values.
1. pH: 7.4 (7.35-7.45).
2. PaO_2: 80 to 100 mm Hg.
3. $Paco_2$: 35 to 45 mm Hg.
4. HCO_3^-: 22 to 26 mEq/L.
C. The hydrogen ion (H^+) concentration determines the acidity or alkalinity of a solution (pH); the higher the H^+ concentration, the more acidic the solution. An inverse relationship exists between pH and H^+ concentration: increased pH has fewer H^+ ions and is more

alkaline; decreased pH has more H^+ ions and is more acid (Figure 6-4).
D. Acid-base ratio is determined by sampling arterial blood. This provides a reliable index of overall body function.
E. The body maintains a normal or neutral state of acid-base balance. The stable concentration of H^+ balance is reflected in arterial blood with a relatively constant pH of 7.35 to 7.45.
F. It is necessary for the pH to remain relatively constant for the various enzyme systems of all body organs to function correctly.
G. O_2 saturation levels reflected in blood gas readings do not have a direct effect on the acid-base balance but are used to identify status of oxygenation.
H. A state of acid-base decompensation exists when the acid-base levels are either below 7.35 or above 7.45.

Box 6-1   GUIDELINES TO DECREASE INFECTION RELATED TO IV THERAPY

- Practice good hand hygiene (even when gloves are worn): before and after insertion, palpating, removing, or dressing any IV site.
- Replace and rotate peripheral catheters no more often than every 72-96 hours or when complications (infiltration, phlebitis, infection) occur.
- Pediatrics: do not replace peripheral catheters unless clinically indicated.
- Replace dressing on peripheral lines, PICC lines, or CVP lines if the dressing is damp, loosened or soiled.
- For peripheral catheters with large bulky dressings that prevent visualization or prevent palpation of the area, remove the dressing and visually inspect the site at least daily and apply new dressing.
- CVP, PICC lines: replace gauze dressings every 2 days and transparent dressing every 7 days, or when inspection of site is necessary.
- Transparent dressings are recommended because they permit continuous visual inspection of the catheter site, permit patients to bathe and shower without saturating the dressing, and require less frequent changes than do standard gauze and tape dressings.
- Peripheral IV, CVP, and PICC lines: replace intravenous tubing and add-on devices no more frequently than 72-hour intervals.
- Serious catheter-related infections are more frequently associated with central venous catheters (CVCs).
- There are no specific recommendations regarding the use of antibiotic ointments and/or iodine ointment.
- Avoid the use of steel needles (butterfly or needles) for the administration of fluids and medication that might cause tissue necrosis if extravasation occurs.
- A PICC catheter is recommended if the IV therapy is likely to exceed 6 days.

From Centers for Disease Control and Prevention (CDC) and *Morbidity and Mortality Weekly Report (MMWR)*: Recommendations and Reports Guidelines for the Prevention of Intravascular Catheter-Related Infections August 9, 2002 / 51(RR10), 1-26. Available at: *www.cdc.gov/ mmwr/preview/mmwrhtml/rr5110a1.htm*

FIGURE 6-4 Acid-base balance. (From Zerwekh J, Claborn J, Gaglione T: *Mosby's fluid and electrolyte memory notecards: visual, mnemonic, and memory aids for nurses*, ed 2, St. Louis, 2010, Mosby.)

I. Compensation: the system not primarily affected is responsible for returning the pH to a more normal level.

J. Full compensation: the problem in the system primarily affected is corrected, thereby returning the pH to a more normal level.

K. $Paco_2$ imbalance: the origin or primary system is respiratory, or it is compensating for a metabolic problem.

L. HCO_3^- imbalance: the origin or primary system is metabolic, or it is compensating for a respiratory problem.

M. The major clinical manifestations of an acid-base imbalance are indicative of central nervous system (CNS) involvement. The severity of the symptoms will depend on the length of time the imbalance exists, as well as the severity of the deviation.
   1. Acidosis (metabolic or respiratory): symptoms are indicative of depression of the CNS; this is common.
   2. Alkalosis (metabolic or respiratory): symptoms are indicative of increased stimulation of the CNS; death is a rare occurrence.

N. The normal ratio of HCO_3^- to $Paco_2$ is 20:1; when this ratio is maintained, the pH is normal.

Regulation of Acid-Base Balance

A. Buffer system: the most rapid-acting of the regulatory systems. The buffer system is activated when there is an excess acid or base present.
   1. A buffer is a chemical that helps maintain a normal pH.
   2. The buffer system chemicals are paired. The primary buffer chemicals are sodium HCO_3^- and carbonic

acid. The buffers are capable of absorbing or releasing H^+ ions as indicated.
   3. The body buffers an acid more effectively than it neutralizes a base.
   4. An effective buffer system depends on normal-functioning respiratory and renal systems.

B. Respiratory system: the second most rapid response in the regulation of acid-base balance. Carbonic acid is transported to the lungs, where it is converted to CO_2 and water, then excreted.
   1. The amount of CO_2 in the blood is directly related to the carbonic acid concentrations.
   2. Increased respirations will decrease CO_2 levels, thus decreasing the carbonic acid concentration and resulting in decreased H^+ concentration and an increase in the pH.
   3. Decreased respirations will cause retention of CO_2, increasing the carbonic acid concentrations and resulting in increased H^+ concentration and a decrease in the pH.
   4. With excessive acid formation, the respiratory center in the medulla is stimulated, which results in an increase in the depth and rate of respirations. This causes a decrease in the CO_2 levels and returns the pH to a more normal point.
   5. With excessive base formation, the respiratory rate slows to promote retention of CO_2 and decrease the alkalotic state. CO_2 is considered an acid substance because it combines with water to form carbonic acid. The $Paco_2$ levels are influenced only by respiratory causes.
   6. If the respiratory system is the source of the pH alteration, then it loses the ability to correct the problem.

C. Renal system: the slowest, but very effective, mechanism of acid-base regulation.
   1. The kidneys reabsorb sodium (Na) and produce and conserve sodium bicarbonate ($NaHCO_3^-$).
   2. In acidosis the H^+ concentration is increased; therefore the H^+ ions are excreted before the potassium (K^+) ions, thereby precipitating hyperkalemia. When the acidosis is corrected, the potassium moves back into the cell.
   3. In alkalosis the H^+ concentration is decreased; there is an augmented renal excretion of K^+ ions, thereby precipitating hypokalemia.
   4. If the renal system is the source of the pH alteration, it loses the ability to correct the problem.

Alterations in Acid-Base Balance

ALERT Know laboratory values for ABGs, evaluate results of diagnostic testing, and intervene as needed.

A. **Respiratory acidosis:** characterized by excessive retention of CO_2 due to hypoventilation; therefore an increased carbonic acid concentration produces an increase in H^+ ions and a decrease in the pH (decreases below 7.35).

1. Causes.
   a. Depression of the respiratory center.
      (1) Head injuries.
      (2) Oversedation with sedatives and/or narcotics.
   b. Conditions affecting pulmonary function.
      (1) Obstructive pulmonary diseases.
      (2) Pneumonia.
      (3) Atelectasis.
   c. Conditions that interfere with chest wall excursion.
      (1) Thoracic trauma: flail chest.
      (2) Diseases affecting innervation of thoracic muscle (Guillain-Barré syndrome, myasthenia gravis, polio).
      (3) Mechanical hypoventilation.
2. Clinical manifestations.
   a. Rapid, shallow respirations (hypoventilation).
   b. Disorientation, decreased level of consciousness.
   c. Decreased blood pressure.
   d. Ventricular irritability related to hyperkalemia.
   e. Hypoxemia secondary to respiratory depression.
3. Blood gas values.
   a. pH decreases below 7.35.
   b. $Paco_2$ increases above 45 mm Hg.
   c. HCO_3^- remains normal, unless compensated.
4. Compensation/correction.
   a. Compensation: renal system will compensate by retaining HCO_3^- and excreting increased amounts of H^+ ions.
   b. Correction: vigorous pulmonary hygiene to improve ventilation and decrease $Paco_2$ levels; may require mechanical ventilation.
5. Nursing management.
   a. Preventive management.
      (1) Have client turn, cough, and deep-breathe every 2 hours after surgery.
      (2) Use narcotics judiciously in the immediate postoperative period.
      (3) Maintain adequate hydration.
   b. Use semi-Fowler's position to facilitate deep breathing.
   c. Thoroughly assess client's pulmonary function.
   d. Perform postural drainage and percussion, followed by suction, to remove excessive pulmonary secretions.
   e. Anticipate the need for mechanical ventilation if client does not respond to pulmonary hygiene.
   f. Anticipate use of bronchodilator.
   g. Administer O_2 with caution, because it may precipitate CO_2 narcosis.
   h. Evaluate for hyperkalemia.
   i. Support renal system to promote adequate compensation.

ALERT Identify changes in respiratory status; provide pulmonary hygiene. The concept of respiratory acidosis may be tested in a variety of situations.

B. **Respiratory alkalosis:** characterized by a low $Paco_2$ due to hyperventilation. An excessive amount of CO_2 is exhaled, resulting in a decrease in H^+ concentration and an increase in pH (above 7.45).
1. Causes of respiratory alkalosis.
   a. Primary stimulation of CNS: hyperventilation.
      (1) Emotional origin (anxiety, fear, apprehension).
      (2) CNS infection (encephalitis).
      (3) Salicylate poisoning.
   b. Reflex stimulation of CNS.
      (1) Hypoxia stimulates hyperventilation (heart failure, pneumonia, pulmonary emboli).
      (2) Fever.
   c. Mechanical hyperventilation, resulting in "over breathing."
2. Clinical manifestations.
   a. Deep, rapid breathing (hyperventilation).
   b. CNS stimulation, resulting in confusion, lethargy, seizures.
   c. Hypokalemia.
   d. Hyperreflexia, muscle weakness, tingling of extremities.
3. Blood gas values.
   a. pH increases above 7.45.
   b. $Paco_2$ decreases below 35 mm Hg.
   c. HCO_3^- remains normal.
4. Compensation/correction.
   a. Compensation: renal system will compensate by increasing HCO_3^- excretion and retaining H^+ ions, thus returning pH to a more normal level.
   b. Correction: prevent loss of CO_2 from respiratory systems.
5. Nursing management.
   a. Identify and eliminate (if possible) causative factor.
   b. Evaluate need for sedation.
   c. Use rebreathing mask or techniques to increase CO_2 levels.
   d. Remain with client to decrease anxiety levels.
C. Metabolic alkalosis: characterized by an increase in the HCO_3^- levels in the serum, leading to a decrease in the H^+ concentration and an increase in the pH (increase above 7.45).
1. Causes (either an increase in serum HCO_3^- or a decrease in serum H^+ concentration).
   a. Diuretic therapy: loss of H^+, chloride (Cl^-), K^+ precipitates an increase in the HCO_3^- level in the serum.
   b. Excessive loss of H^+ ions.
      (1) Prolonged nasogastric suctioning without adequate electrolyte replacement.
      (2) Excessive vomiting, resulting in loss of hydrochloric acid and K^+.
   c. Prolonged steroid therapy: loss of H^+, Cl^-, and K^+ ions, leading to an increased retention of HCO_3^- by the kidneys.
   d. Excessive intake of bicarbonate (baking soda).
   e. Hypokalemia.

2. Clinical manifestations.
   a. Nausea, vomiting.
   b. Increased irritability, disorientation, restlessness.
   c. Muscle cramping, tremors, seizures.
   d. Shallow, slow respirations (hypoventilation).
   e. Dysrhythmias (tachycardia) related to hypo-kalemia.
3. Blood gas values.
   a. pH increases above 7.45.
   b. $Paco_2$ remains normal.
   c. HCO_3^- increases above 26 mEq/L.
4. Compensation/correction.
   a. Compensation: respiratory system will compensate by retaining CO_2 (hypoventilation) to compensate for the alkalosis.
   b. Correction: replacement of electrolytes and fluids lost due to excessive renal excretion or due to excessive gastric loss of acid.
5. Nursing management.
   a. Preventive.
      (1) Provide foods high in potassium and chloride for client receiving diuretics.
      (2) Administer potassium supplement to client receiving long-term diuretic therapy.
      (3) Administer IV solution with replacement electrolytes.
   b. Maintain accurate intake and output records.
   c. Evaluate the lab values for a decrease in serum potassium levels.

D. Metabolic acidosis: characterized by a decrease in HCO_3^- level in the serum, leading to an increase in H^+ concentration and a decrease in pH (below 7.35).
   1. Causes (deficit of a base or an increase in acid).
      a. Incomplete oxidation of fatty acids.
         (1) Diabetic ketoacidosis.
         (2) Starvation.
         (3) Shock, resulting in lactic acidosis.
      b. Abnormal loss of alkaline substances.
         (1) Deep, prolonged vomiting may cause excessive loss of base products.
         (2) Severe diarrhea and loss of pancreatic secretions.
      c. Renal insufficiency and failure: kidneys lose ability to compensate for acid overload; thus H^+ ions are not excreted, nor is HCO_3^- retained in normal amounts.
      d. Salicylate poisoning due to accumulation of ketone bodies produced as a result of the increased metabolic rate.
   2. Clinical manifestations.
      a. Drowsiness, confusion, headache, disorientation.
      b. Deep, rapid respirations (Kussmaul) compensatory action by the lungs.
      c. GI problems: nausea, vomiting, diarrhea.
      d. Dysrhythmias related to hyperkalemia.
      e. Decreased blood pressure.
   3. Blood gas values.
      a. pH decreases below 7.35.

   b. PCO_2 remains normal.
   c. HCO_3^- decreases below 22 mEq/L.
4. Compensation/correction.
   a. Compensation: respiratory system compensates by increasing rate and depth of respirations to blow off CO_2 and increase the pH.
   b. Correction: identification of the underlying problem and promotion of optimal function.
5. Nursing management.
   a. Assist in identification of underlying problem.
   b. In severe acidosis, HCO_3^- may be given intravenously to neutralize acid and return pH to normal.
   c. In clients with diabetes, evaluate for ketoacidosis and administer insulin accordingly.
   d. Assess renal function and hydration status.
   e. Maintain accurate intake and output records.
   f. Evaluate lab values for hyperkalemia.
   g. Support respiratory system to promote compensation.

INFLAMMATION

Inflammation is the tissue response to localized injury or trauma. It is an expected response to tissue injury.

Basic Concepts of Inflammation

A. Acute.
   1. Occurs rapidly.
   2. Neutrophils (white blood cells) are usually the predominant cell.
   3. Essential for normal tissue repair.
B. Chronic.
   1. Characterized by pain, redness, and swelling.
   2. Persists longer than 2 weeks; has a damaging course that lasts for weeks, months, or even years.
   3. Examples: rheumatoid arthritis, tuberculosis, chronic glomerulonephritis.
C. Inflammatory response.
   1. Vascular response.
      a. Initial local vasoconstriction caused by tissue injury.
      b. Vasodilatation in area of injury.
      c. Hyperemia and increased capillary permeability lead to changes in osmotic pressure and a leakage of fluid (exudate).
   2. Systemic response.
      a. Fever.
      b. Leukocytosis (increased numbers of neutrophils in circulation).
      c. Weight loss and nausea.
      d. Increased pulse and respiration.
      e. Increased sedimentation rate.
D. Cardinal signs of inflammation (Table 6-1).
E. Healing process (see Wound Care in Chapter 3).

■ **NURSING PRIORITY** Inflammation is necessary for normal healing to occur. A decrease in the normal inflammatory response will result in a decreased ability to heal.

Table 6-1	CARDINAL SIGNS OF INFLAMMATION
Clinical Symptom	**Pathophysiology**
Redness	Hyperemia from vasodilation
Heat	Increased metabolism at site and local vasodilation
Pain	Pressure from fluid exudate on adjacent nerve endings, which leads to nerve stimulation; change in local pH
Edema	Fluid shift and accumulation in interstitial spaces
Loss of function	Decreased movement due to swelling and pain

INFECTION

Infection is the process by which an organism (pathogen, pathogenic agent) invades the host and establishes a parasitic relationship. Infection may be localized or systemic.

A. Healthcare associated infections (HAIs, nosocomial infections): infections acquired from exposure to pathogens in a hospital setting or health care setting.

B. Iatrogenic infections are HAIs that result from a diagnostic or therapeutic procedure (urinary tract infection from urinary catheterization).

C. Emerging infection is an infectious disease that has increased over past 20 years.

D. Development of multiple drug-resistant organisms (MDRO) has further complicated treatment of infections (they are resistant to antibiotics).

Chain of Transmission

A. Pathogens.
  1. Incubation period: the period of time from exposure to the pathogen until symptoms of infection occur in the host.
  2. A person can be asymptomatic and still transmit a pathogen that will produce an infection in someone else.
  3. Toxigenicity refers to the destructive potential of the toxin that is released by the pathogen.

B. Reservoir.
  1. Environment within which the organism can live and multiply; provided by some organic substance, human or animal.
  2. A carrier provides an environment in which the pathogen can grow and multiply but shows no symptoms of the infection.

C. Portal of exit.
  1. How the infection leaves the host.
  2. Common ports of exit include skin, mucous membranes, respiratory tract, feces, and body fluids.
  3. Understanding port of exit is necessary to prevent transmission of pathogens.

D. Route of transmission.
  1. Method by which the pathogen moves to another host.
  2. Direct transmission occurs by immediate transfer from one host to another, as in sexually transmitted diseases, or by inhalation of contaminated droplets from respiratory tract infections.
  3. Indirect transmission occurs via an intermediate carrier (e.g., health care workers, mosquitoes, contaminated water, contaminated food).

E. Port of entry into susceptible host.
  1. May enter the host by inhalation or ingestion, through the mucous membranes, or percutaneously.
  2. Biologic and personal characteristics of the new host will determine the lines of defense that the host will have against the invading pathogen.

F. Control of transmission.
  1. Transmission of a contagious disease can be broken by interfering with any link of the transmission chain.
  2. Treatment is aimed at breaking the transmission chain at the most vulnerable and cost-effective point.
    a. Barrier precautions: gloves, gowns, condoms.
    b. Proper handling of food and water supplies.
    c. Avoidance of high-risk behavior: unsafe sex, IV drug use.
    d. Good hand hygiene technique and good personal hygiene (Box 6-2).
    e. Identification of carriers: skin test for tuberculosis, cultures for *Staphylococcus*.
  3. Host susceptibility can be greatly reduced through immunizations (see Chapter 2).

Prevention of Transmission of Infection in the Health Care Setting

A. Maintain standard precautions (see Appendix 6-8), especially good hand hygiene.

B. Consider all blood and body fluids from all clients to be contaminated.

Box 6-2   HAND HYGIENE

Hand Hygiene With Soap and Water
- Handwashing should be done under flow of water.
- Wet hands and wrists under running water: keep hands and forearms lower than elbows.
- Using antibacterial soap, lather and wash hands using friction for at least 15 seconds.
- Rinse hands thoroughly under running water, keeping hands lower than elbows.
- Do not allow washed hands to touch inside of sink.
- Use soap and water any time the hands are visibly soiled.

Hand Hygiene With Antiseptic Cleanser
- Rub hands together covering all surfaces of the hands and fingers with cleanser.
- Rub hands together until cleanser is dry.
- Use if hands are not visibly soiled.

❗ NURSING PRIORITY Hand hygiene is the most important and most basic action to prevent transmission of infections. Hand hygiene must be performed before and after the use of gloves.

C. Avoid contaminating outside of container when collecting specimens.

D. Do not recap needles and syringes.

E. Cleanse work surface areas with appropriate germicide (household bleach in concentrations of 1:100 to 1:10 is effective).

F. Clean up spills of blood and body fluid immediately. Remove as much of the body fluid as possible, then wash the area with a germicide solution.

G. Follow Centers for Disease Control and Prevention (CDC) recommendations for immunization of health care workers (see Table 2-2).

ALERT Apply principles of infection control; understand incubation periods for infectious diseases; evaluate client response to treatment.

Nursing Interventions

Goal: To prevent infection.

A. Handwashing is the single most effective mechanism for preventing spread of infection (see Box 6-2).

B. Monitor vital signs: increase in pulse, respiration, and temperature occurring 4 to 5 days after surgery may indicate infectious process.

C. Monitor for *Staphylococcus* and *Pseudomonas* pathogens (produce purulent, draining wounds).

D. Maintain aseptic technique in dressing changes and wound irrigations.

E. Maintain standard precautions (see Appendix 6-8).

F. Administer antibiotic medications (see Appendix 6-9).

G. Identify clients at increased risk for infections.
  1. Older adults (Box 6-3).
  2. Immunocompromised clients.
  3. Clients compromised by chronic health care problems.
  4. Poorly nourished clients.
  5. Client with high-risk lifestyle (IV drug use, unprotected sex).

Goal: To promote healing.

A. Encourage high fluid intake when client has a fever: 2000-3000 mL daily for adults.

B. Encourage a diet high in protein, carbohydrates, and vitamins—specifically vitamins A, C, and B complex.

C. Immobilize an injured extremity with a cast, splint, or bandage.

Box 6-3   OLDER ADULT CARE FOCUS

Infections

- May be manifested by changes in behavior: confusion, disorientation.
- May not exhibit fever or pain.
- Closely monitor client response to antibiotics, especially with regard to renal function.
- Maintain adequate hydration.
- Monitor gastrointestinal function; diarrhea is common with antibiotics.

Box 6-4   SIGNS OF INFECTION

Generalized
- Fever, localized inflammation, joint pain, fatigue, and increased white blood cells

Gastrointestinal Tract
- Diarrhea, nausea, and vomiting

Respiratory Tract
- Purulent sputum, sore throat, chest pain, and congestion

Urinary Tract
- Urgency and frequency, hematuria, purulent discharge, dysuria, and flank pain

---

D. Administer antipyretic medications (see Appendix 3-3).

E. Identify early signs of infection to facilitate treatment (Box 6-4).

Goal: To decrease pain.

A. Cold packs applied after initial trauma may help decrease swelling and pain.

B. Heat may be used later to promote healing and to localize the inflammatory agents.

C. Elevate the injured area to decrease edema and promote venous return.

ALERT Use correct hand hygiene techniques—soap and water or an antimicrobial cleanser.

Goal: To prevent complications.

A. Increase surveillance for clients with leukopenia or impaired circulation, clients receiving steroids or drugs that depress bone marrow, and clients exposed to a communicable disease.

B. Protect healing wounds from injury that could be caused by pulling or stretching.

C. Identify clients with compromised immune response; they are at high risk for opportunistic infection.

ALERT Protect immunocompromised clients.

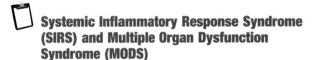

Systemic Inflammatory Response Syndrome (SIRS) and Multiple Organ Dysfunction Syndrome (MODS)

SIRS is a systemic inflammatory response secondary to a major body insult or trauma. MODS is the failure of two or major organ systems and occurs as a result of SIRS.

A. Characteristics.
  1. Risk factors.
    a. Systemic inflammatory response syndrome (SIRS) occurs as a result of tissue injury.
      (1) Tissue trauma: burns, crush injuries, surgery.
      (2) Ischemic or necrotic tissue: infarctions (myocardial, intestinal), pancreatitis, vascular disease.
      (3) Invasion of pathogens (bacterial, viral, fungal infection).
      (4) Infection from gram-negative bacteria.

b. SIRS characterized by overwhelming inflammation of organs involved.

c. Transition from SIRS to MODS is not clearly understood.

d. Organ perfusion is compromised secondary to hypertension, decreased perfusion, microemboli, and shunting of blood flow.

B. Clinical manifestations.

1. Precipitating event.

2. Respiratory: increased vascular permeability leads to alveoli collapse and development of adult respiratory distress syndrome (ARDS).

3. Cardiac compromise, decreased systemic vascular resistance (SVR) and vasodilation lead to severe hypotension and decreased cardiac output.

4. Neurologic problems of confusion, agitation, and lethargy.

5. Acute renal failure secondary to decreased renal perfusion.

6. GI tract problems are abdominal distention and paralytic ileus.

7. Hypermetabolic response with hyperglycemia and insulin resistance.

8. Failure of the coagulation system leads to development of disseminated intravascular coagulopathy (DIC).

Treatment

A. Prevention.

1. Prevent development of infections.

2. Surgical removal or debridement of necrotic or damaged tissue.

3. Maintain positive nitrogen balance for wound healing.

B. Aggressive treatment of existing infection.

C. Support of involved organs.

Nursing Interventions

Goal: Prevention and/or early detection of infection.

A. Identify clients at increased risk for development of SIRS and MODS.

B. Strict asepsis for clients with urinary catheter, IV sites, endotracheal tube, arterial line, and wound care.

C. Aggressive pulmonary hygiene.

D. Strict adherence to standard precautions (Appendix 6-8).

Goal: Maintain tissue oxygenation (Chapter 15).

A. Monitor for respiratory failure and hypoxia.

B. Decrease oxygen demand and increase oxygen delivery: supplemental oxygen, adequate hemoglobin level, sedation, mechanical ventilation.

Goal: Support nutritional needs.

A. Provide protein and calories to support hypermetabolic state.

B. Provide enteral feedings to maintain positive nitrogen balance (see Appendix 18-9).

C. Monitor glucose levels, preferably maintain levels below 150 mg/dL.

D. Close monitoring of fluid balance.

 Sepsis

Sepsis is a systemic inflammatory response to infection.

A. Gram-negative bacteria are most common.

B. Increased risk in clients with urinary catheters, respiratory infections, invasive procedures (arterial lines, CVP, any indwelling line).

C. At-risk clients: older adults, clients with chronic health problems, clients on immunosuppressive therapy and the clients who are malnourished.

D. Exaggerated body response to an antigen, resulting in release of endotoxins that affect platelets and cause vasodilatation, increased capillary permeability, and development of MODS.

E. Clinical manifestations.

1. Compromised respiratory function.

a. Initially, hyperventilation occurs as a compensating mechanism.

b. Hypoventilation and respiratory acidosis occur when compensation fails.

c. Respiratory failure and development of ARDS (Chapter 15).

2. Compromised cardiac function.

a. Initially increased cardiac output with decreased systemic vascular resistance (SVR) secondary to hypermetabolic state.

b. Cardiac decompensation with development of severe hypotension and MODS.

3. Development of severe hypotension progressing to septic shock despite adequate fluid resuscitation.

4. Development of (SIRS) progressing to MODS.

Treatment

A. Prevention of infection.

B. Aggressive treatment of infections.

C. Aggressive pulmonary support.

D. Fluid resuscitation.

Nursing Interventions

See care of a client in shock (Chapter 16).

Antibiotic-Resistant Infections

A. Strains of bacteria that have developed a resistance to common antibiotics (multiple drug-resistant organisms (MDROs).

1. Methicillin-resistant *Staphylococcus aureus:* wound, skin and soft tissue, pneumonia.

2. Vancomycin-resistant *Enterococcus faecalis:* urinary tract infections.

3. Penicillin resistant *Streptococcus pneumoniae:* pneumonia.

4. Cephalosporin resistant *Klebsiella pneumoniae:* pneumonia.

B. Transmission.

1. Most common mode of transmission is from person to person, including from health care workers to hospitalized clients.

2. Healthcare-associated infections (HAIs).

C. Clients at increased risk.
   1. Treatment with multiple antibiotics.
   2. Multiple hospitalizations.
   3. Older adults with chronic conditions.
   4. Clients with compromised immune function.

Treatment
Cultures, followed by administration of antibiotics sensitive to bacteria.

Nursing Interventions
Goal: To decrease spread of infection.
A. Routine cultures of health care workers.
B. Identification of clients at increased risk.

C. Add contact precautions to the standard precautions:
   1. Private room.
   2. Gown and gloves.
   3. Masks are not necessary unless the client has a respiratory tract infection.
   4. Teach family the importance of gloves and gowns.
D. Notify nurse epidemiologist when client is diagnosed with an antibiotic-resistant infection.
E. A common mode of transmission is via the hands of health care workers; handwashing is critical, even before and after removal of gloves.

Appendix 6-1 ELECTROLYTE IMBALANCES: POTASSIUM

Normal Serum Potassium (K⁺) Levels: 3.5-5.0 mEq/L

Hypokalemia: Serum K^+ below 3.5 mEq/L

CAUSES	SYMPTOMS	NURSING IMPLICATIONS

Decreased intake of K^+
GI loss:
  Vomiting
  Diarrhea
  Fistulas
  Nasogastric suction without replacement
Skin loss: diaphoresis
Excessive renal excretion:
  Diuretics
  Increasing aldosterone
Alkalosis
Steroid therapy
Diabetics: Insulin and glucose moves K^+ into cell
	Fatigue, muscle weakness, hyporeflexia
	Decreased muscle tone and reflexes
	Confusion, drowsiness, fatigue bradycardia, weak irregular pulse
	ECG changes: flat T wave, S-T depression, U waves, PVCs
	GI: Decreased bowel sounds, development of ileus, nausea, vomiting
		1. Identify source of depletion.
		2. Monitor K^+ levels.
		3. Encourage foods high in K^+.
		4. Replace K^+ (oral potassium supplements and IV).
		5. Maintain accurate I&O records.
		6. Evaluate for digitalis toxicity (low serum K^+ potentiates digitalis).
		7. Evaluate for alkalosis.
		8. Provide client education regarding diuretics.

Hyperkalemia: Serum K^+ above 5.0 mEq/L

CAUSES	SYMPTOMS	NURSING IMPLICATIONS

Decreased urinary excretion:
  Renal failure
  Decreased aldosterone
  Decreased secretion
Potassium sparing diuretics
Massive tissue injury:
  Burns
  Trauma
  Fever; sepsis
Excessive administration of IV K^+
Salt substitutes containing potassium
Acidosis
	Drowsiness
	Muscle weakness and twitching paresthesia of hands and feet and around the mouth
	GI-Diarrhea with hyperactive bowel sounds
	ECG changes:
	  Peaked T waves
	  Prolonged P-R interval
	  Widened QRS complex
	Dysrhythmias:
	  Bradycardia with ventricular ectopic beats (irregular pulse)
	  Ventricular fibrillation
	  Cardiac arrest (Figure 6-5)
		1. Identify origin of increase.
		2. Monitor K^+ levels.
		3. Administer diuretics and fluids, if renal function is adequate.
		4. Administer hypertonic glucose and insulin to initiate K^+ transfer into cell.
		5. Utilize exchange resins: **Kayexalate.**
		6. Be prepared for a cardiac emergency.
		7. Maintain accurate I&O records.

ECG, Electrocardiogram; *GI*, gastrointestinal; *I&O*, intake and output; *IV*, intravenous; *PVCs*, premature ventricular contractions.

FIGURE 6-5 Hyperkalemia. (From Zerwekh J, Claborn J, Gaglione T: *Mosby's fluid and electrolyte memory notecards: visual, mnemonic, and memory aids for nurses*, ed 2, St. Louis, 2010, Mosby.)

Appendix 6-2	MEDICATIONS TO CORRECT POTASSIUM IMBALANCE

MEDICATIONS | **NURSING IMPLICATIONS**

Potassium Supplements

Oral:
  Potassium chloride (KCl)
  Sustained release:
  K-Dur, Micro-K, Slow-K
  Potassium gluconate **(Kaon)**
IV:
  Potassium acetate
▲ High-Alert Medication (Box 5-1, p. 86)

1. Sustained-release preparations are better tolerated and more convenient.
2. Oral preparations generally have unpleasant taste and are irritating to GI system; they should be administered with a full glass of water or juice.
3. Pediatric implications: make sure child/infant is urinating adequately before beginning supplementation.
4. Potassium acetate is the only IV preparation.
5. IV K+ *must* be diluted and administered by IV drip. Do not give K+ IM or by IV push; may cause cardiac arrest. Administer no more than 10 mEq of K+ intravenously per 1 hour.
6. IV K+ solutions are irritating to the vein. If pain occurs, either slow the infusion rate or dilute solution in larger volume of fluid.
7. Administer with caution to clients with heart disease and those taking digitalis preparations.

Exchange Resin

Sodium polystyrene sulfonate **(Kayexalate):**
  PO or rectal retention enema
  (Medication is not absorbed systemically.)

1. Laxatives are given to facilitate excretion of the resin.
2. Cleansing enema precedes the Kayexalate retention enema to enhance effectiveness.
3. Carefully evaluate the client with CHF and/or hypertension.
4. Monitor serum electrolytes.
5. Use with caution in clients requiring sodium restriction.

CHF, Congestive heart failure; *GI,* gastrointestinal; *IM,* intramuscularly; *IV,* intravenous; *PO,* by mouth (orally).

Appendix 6-3 ELECTROLYTE IMBALANCES: SODIUM

CAUSES	SYMPTOMS	NURSING IMPLICATIONS

Normal Serum Sodium (Na⁺) Levels: 135-145 mEq/L

Hyponatremia: Serum Na⁺ below 135 mEq/L (loss of sodium or water excess)

CAUSES	SYMPTOMS	NURSING IMPLICATIONS
Inadequate Na⁺ intake (rare)	***Solution deficit (Na⁺ loss):***	1. Identify source of depletion.
Loss of sodium-rich fluids	CNS problems: changes in level	2. Maintain accurate I&O records, and
Cystic fibrosis	of consciousness, confusion seizures	determine weight daily (best measurement
Fluid gain, over hydration (dilutional)	Weakness, restlessness	of fluid status).
Decreased renal excretion:	Oliguria	3. Irrigate nasogastric tubes with normal
Diuretics	Abdominal cramps	saline solution.
Adrenal insufficiency	Postural hypotension	4. 0.9% NaCl (normal saline) IV or
Increased ADH	Cold and clammy skin	half-strength 0.45% NaCl if client has
Edema	***Dilutional hyponatremia (water excess):***	sodium deficit.
Excessive administration of D₅W	CNS problems: confusion, headache,	5. If seizures are present, may administer IV
Gastrointestinal losses	seizures	hypertonic solution containing 3% NaCl.
Massive tissue injury:	Hypertension	6. Monitor blood pressure.
Burns	Muscle twitching, cramping	7. Restrict fluid intake if client has fluid
Trauma	Increased urine	excess.
	Weight gain	8. Occurs in clients who are NPO, taking
		diuretics, perspiring, vomiting, having
		diarrhea; clients with burns or excessive
		administration of D₅W.
		9. Occurs in renal disease, Addison's disease,
		and diabetic acidosis.

> **⏸ NURSING PRIORITY:** Older adult clients and infants are at higher risk because of variations in total body water; carefully monitor clients receiving fluid replacement with D₅W

Hypernatremia: Serum Na⁺ above 145 mEq/L (sodium retention or water loss)

CAUSES	SYMPTOMS	NURSING IMPLICATIONS
Decreased fluid intake	***Fluid excess (Na⁺ retention):***	1. Identify origin of increase.
Excessive salt intake	Pitting edema	2. Maintain accurate I&O records, and
Excessive water loss:	Weight gain	determine weight daily.
Diarrhea	Flushed skin	3. Administer D₅W IV if fluid is normal or
Febrile state	Lethargic	there is a fluid deficit.
Diuretics	Hypertension	4. Administer diuretics to remove excess Na⁺.
Increased renal retention	Decreased hematocrit	5. Restrict fluid intake if client has fluid
Cushing's syndrome	***Fluid deficit (hemoconcentration of Na+,***	excess.
	water loss):	6. Assess for cerebral edema—lethargy,
	Concentrated urine	headache, nausea, vomiting, increased BP.
	Dry mucous membranes	
	Flushed skin, tachycardia increased	
	temperature weight loss,	
	decreased CVP	

ADH, Antidiuretic hormone; *BP*, blood pressure; *CNS*, central nervous system; *CVP*, central venous pressure; *D₅W*, 5% dextrose in water; *I&O*, intake and output; *IV*, intravenously; *NPO*, nothing by mouth.

Appendix 6-4 MEDICATIONS TO CORRECT SODIUM IMBALANCE

MEDICATION	NURSING IMPLICATIONS
Sodium supplements	
Sodium chloride (NaCl, table salt)	1. Administer with caution in clients with CHF, renal problems, edema, or hypertension.
Saline solutions: 0.9% and 0.45% saline	2. Determine weight daily; maintain accurate I&O records to evaluate fluid retention.
solution for infusion	3. Evaluate serum Na⁺ levels.
▲ High-Alert Medication	4. Do not store containers of sodium chloride above a concentration of 0.9% (normal saline)
	on the nursing unit.

CHF, Congestive heart failure; *I&O*, intake and output.

Appendix 6-5   ELECTROLYTE IMBALANCES: CALCIUM

CAUSES

SYMPTOMS

NURSING IMPLICATIONS

Normal Serum Calcium (Ca⁺⁺) Levels: 9-11 mg/dl or 4-5 mEq/L
Hypocalcemia: Serum Ca⁺⁺ below 8.6 mg/dl or below 4 mEq/L, or below 3.5 mEq/L in infants

CAUSES	SYMPTOMS	NURSING IMPLICATIONS
Acute pancreatitis Laxative abuse Dietary lack of Ca⁺⁺ and vitamin D Hypoparathyroidism Hyperphosphatemia Excessive blood transfusions Excessive IV fluids Alkalosis	Tetany: + Chvostek's sign; + Trousseau's sign (Chapter 13) Neuromuscular irritability Numbness and tingling in extremities or around mouth Laryngeal stridor Seizures Abdominal cramping and distention Hyperreflexia Dysrhythmias	1. Identify origin of deficiency. 2. Keep Ca⁺⁺ replacement medications easily accessible for clients who have had thyroid or parathyroid surgically removed. 3. Assess for tetany. 4. Reduce environmental stimuli for both adults and infants. 5. Institute seizure precautions. 6. Provide client education regarding Ca⁺⁺ intake.

Infants:

Early onset—decreased activity of parathyroid; infants of diabetic mothers; premature infants; exchange transfusion *Late onset*—decreased dietary intake, infants who are fed evaporated milk formulas containing phosphorus, intestinal malabsorption	*Early onset in infant*: restlessness, edema, apnea, intermittent cyanosis, vomiting, abdominal distention, high-pitched cry *Late onset in infant:* increasing CNS excitability	1. Teach parents to use infant formulas and or oral supplements until the child is 1 year old. 2. Do not give a child whole cow's milk until 1 year old.

Hypercalcemia: Serum Ca⁺⁺ above 10.5 mg/dl or above 5 mEq/L

Metastatic malignancy Hyperparathyroidism Thiazide diuretics Prolonged immobilization Vitamin D overdose	Anorexia, nausea, constipation CNS depression Decreasing muscle tone, coordination Pathological fractures Dysrhythmias—increases sensitivity to digitalis preparations.	1. Identify origin of increase. 2. Administer loop diuretics to facilitate removal of serum Ca⁺⁺, normal saline fluid replacement. 3. Increase client's fluid intake 3000 to 4000 mL/24 hours. 4. Decrease Ca⁺⁺ intake. 5. Encourage client mobility. 6. Provide client education regarding supplemental vitamins. 7. Increase fiber intake. 8. Assess client taking digitalis for symptoms of toxicity.

CNS, Central nervous system; *IV*, intravenous.

Appendix 6-6   MEDICATIONS TO CORRECT CALCIUM IMBALANCE

MEDICATION

ACTION

NURSING IMPLICATIONS

Calcium Salts

MEDICATION	ACTION	NURSING IMPLICATIONS
Calcium citrate **(Citracal):** PO Calcium gluconate: IV, PO Calcium carbonate **(TUMS, Rolaids):** PO Loop diuretics may be used to enhance excretion of calcium in treatment of hypercalcemia.	Activator for coagulation enzyme factors Necessary for cardiac muscle function IV infusion for treatment of hypocalcemic tetany Adjunctive therapy to prevent hypocalcemia during exchange transfusion	1. May be given in conjunction with vitamin D to enhance absorption. 2. PO supplements are more effective if taken ½-1 hr after meals. 3. Prevent IV infiltration; Ca⁺⁺ solutions cause tissue hypoxia and sloughing. 4. Do not add Ca⁺⁺ preparations to solutions containing carbonates or phosphates. 5. Use with caution for client receiving digitalis. 6. Monitor infusion rate carefully; sudden increase in serum Ca⁺⁺ level may precipitate severe cardiac dysrhythmias. 7. Corticosteroids decrease Ca⁺⁺ absorption. Administer several hours apart.

IV, Intravenous; *PO*, by mouth.

Appendix 6-7 ANTIINFLAMMATORY MEDICATIONS

General Nursing Implications

— Give oral medications with or after meals to decrease GI irritation and side effects.
— Following therapy, withdrawal from steroids *must be done* gradually.
— For clients on long-term therapy, increased amounts of corticosteroids will be required during periods of stress such as surgery.
— Decreases client's ability to respond to and fight infection.
— Closely evaluate the client on digitalis preparations and thiazide diuretics for the development of hypokalemia.
— Use with NSAIDs increases risk for intestinal irritation and perforation (Appendix 3-3).
— Uses: Inflammatory conditions—respiratory, gastrointestinal, joint inflammation, and skin conditions. Adrenocortical hormone replacement if adrenal glands are insufficient or have been removed. Suppress rejection of transplanted organs.

MEDICATIONS	SIDE EFFECTS	NURSING IMPLICATIONS

Adrenocortical Hormones (Corticosteroids, Glucocorticoids):

Antiinflammatory action: Inhibit synthesis of chemical mediators (histamine, prostaglandins), thereby suppressing inflammatory response. Suppress infiltration of area by phagocytes and suppress production of lymphocytes, further reducing the immune response and inflammation. During stress, an increase release of corticosteroids occurs to maintain blood pressure and plasma levels of glucose. Used as immunosuppressant for delaying organ rejection. Long-term use will suppress the function of the adrenal glands.

Hydrocortisone base **(Cortef)**: PO Hydrocortisone sodium succinate **(Solu-Cortef)**: IV, IM Dexamethasone **(Decadron)**: PO, IV, IM, topical Prednisone **(Deltasone, Meticorten)**: PO Methylprednisolone **(Medrol)**: PO, IM, IV Methylprednisolone sodium succinate **(Solu-Medrol)**: IV	Increased susceptibility to infections (bodywide) GI upset, gastric irritation Osteoporosis Psychologic disturbances (depression, euphoria) Hypokalemia Hyperglycemia Hypertension (caused by sodium and water retention) Cushing's syndrome: moon face, buffalo hump, distended abdomen, thin arms and legs, excessive hair growth Cataracts	1. Administer medication before 9:00 a.m. to decrease adrenal cortical suppression. 2. Monitor for psychologic changes. 3. Decrease salt intake in diet; encourage high-protein and high-potassium diet. 4. Determine weight daily; evaluate weight gain and blood pressure. 5. Topical steroids usually do not provoke physical evidence of absorption. *Teaching:* Take medication in the morning with food. Diet should include adequate K⁺ intake and decreased Na⁺ intake. Do not stop taking the medication or change the dosing without a doctor's order. Report to health care provider: any early signs of infection; or a weight gain of 5 lb or more in a week. Do not take a live virus vaccine (MMR, varicella). Do not take with aspirin products.

> ⚠ **NURSING PRIORITY:** It is critical that clients on corticosteroids do not stop taking the medications abruptly. This can result in a significant drop in blood pressure and hypoglycemia. Clients should advise all their health care providers if they are on steroids.

GI, Gastrointestinal; *IM,* intramuscular; *IV,* intravenous; *PO,* by mouth (orally).

Appendix 6-8 INFECTION CONTROL PROCEDURES

General Information

— Many clients with disease-specific isolation precautions require only standard precautions.

— The specific substances covered by standard precautions include blood and all other body fluids, body secretions, and body excretions, even if blood is not visible. Moisture from perspiration (sweat) is an exception.

— Transmission-based precautions are followed, in addition to standard precautions, whenever a client is known or suspected to be infected with contagious pathogens.

Standard Precautions

1. Wash hands before and after client care and after removing gloves. Wash hands immediately with soap and water if visibly contaminated with blood or body fluids.
2. Wear gloves if there is a possibility you might come in contact with any body fluid or contaminated surfaces or objects.
3. Change gloves between tasks and procedures on the same client if moving from a contaminated body area (perineal area) to a clean body area. Do not wash gloves for reuse.
4. Wear gloves, gown, eye protection (goggles, glasses) or face shield and a mask during procedures likely to generate droplets of blood or body fluids.
5. Wear a gown when there is risk clothing will come in contact with body fluids. Perform hand hygiene after removing the gown. Do not reuse gowns, even if they are not soiled.
6. Have used client care equipment properly cleaned; discard any single-use items after use.
7. Ensure that hospital procedures for routine care, cleaning, and disinfection of environmental surfaces, beds, bedrails, and bedside equipment are followed.
8. Place contaminated linens in a leak-proof bag; handle contaminated linens in a manner that prevents contamination and transfer of microorganisms.
9. Discard all sharps in puncture resistant container. Do not bend, break, reinsert them into their original sheaths, or handle them unnecessarily. Discard them intact immediately after use.
10. Place clients who pose a risk for transmission to others in a private room. This includes clients who cannot contain secretions/excretions or wound drainage, infants with respiratory or intestinal infections.
11. Practice good hand hygiene.

Respiratory Hygiene and Cough Etiquette

• Educate health care personnel regarding measures to contain their own respiratory secretions.
• Post signs in strategic places regarding covering the mouth and nose when coughing or sneezing; provide non-touch receptacles for disposal of tissue.

Safe Injection Practices

• Use single-dose vials for parenteral administration when possible.
• If multidose vials must be used, the needle or cannula and the syringe used to access the vial must be sterile.
• Do not use the same syringe to administer medications to multiple clients, even if the needle is changed.
• Do not keep multidose vials in the immediate client treatment area.

Infection Control for Lumbar Punctures

• Wear a surgical mask when placing a catheter or injecting material into the spinal column or subdural space (myelogram, lumbar puncture, spinal or epidural anesthesia).

Airborne Precautions (droplet smaller than 5 mcg)

1. Place client in airborne isolation infection room (AIIR) as soon as possible.
2. Personal protection equipment (PPE):
   • Wear respiratory protection (N95 respirator mask approved by the National Institute for Occupational Safety and Health [NIOSH]) when entering the room.
   • Wear gloves, and gown when entering the room, remove prior to leaving room.
3. Limit client transport and client movement out of the room. Health care personnel who are not immune are restricted from entering the client's room.
4. Conditions requiring use of airborne precautions – pulmonary or laryngeal tuberculosis, varicella, rubella and smallpox.

Droplet Precautions (droplets larger than 5 mcg)

1. Applicable to clients known to be, or suspected of being, infected with pathogens that are transmitted via respiratory droplets (sneezing, coughing, talking).
2. Place the client in a private room whenever possible; may place two clients in the same room if they are infected with the same pathogen.
3. PPE:
   • Wear a mask when entering the client room or examination area.
   • No recommendation regarding routine use of eye protection.
4. Place a mask on the client if transporting in the health care setting.
5. Instruct client and family regarding respiratory hygiene/cough etiquette.
6. Limit movement of the client from the room; if the client must leave the room, have him or her wear a surgical mask.

Contact Precautions

1. Applicable to clients with diseases easily transmitted by direct contact such as gastrointestinal, respiratory tract, skin, or wound infections and clients colonized with multidrug-resistant bacteria.
2. Place the client in a private room if condition may facilitate transmission—uncontrolled drainage, incontinence. May place two clients infected with same pathogen in the same room.
3. PPE:
   • Wear a gown when entering the client's room; remove gown prior to leaving the room.
   • Wear gloves when entering the client's room. Always change gloves after contact with infected material. Remove gloves before leaving the client's room and perform hand hygiene; do not touch anything in the room as you are leaving.
   • Wear gloves when touching the client's intact skin and surfaces and articles in close proximity to the client.
4. Dedicate use of noncritical client care equipment to the single client; if common equipment use is unavoidable, the equipment must be disinfected before use on another client.

Appendix 6-8   INFECTION CONTROL PROCEDURES—cont'd

5. Limit the transport or movement of the client outside the room; if necessary to move client, ensure that infected or colonized areas of the client's body are contained and covered.
6. Evidence shows that multiple drug-resistant organisms (MDROs) are carried from one person to another via the hands of health care personnel.

Protective Environment Precautions

1. May be used for clients who are severely immunosuppressed—clients with stem cell transplants, clients with organ transplant, AIDS clients.

2. Place the client in a private room that has positive-pressure air flow and high-efficiency particulate air (HEPA) filtration for incoming air.
3. Wear respiratory protection (N95 respirator mask), gloves, and gown when entering the room.
4. Limit client transport and client movement out of the room.
5. No fresh flowers, fruits, or potted plants allowed in room.

> **ALERT** Use critical thinking to ensure standard transmission-based precautions are implemented; prevent environmental spread of infectious diseases.

Center for Disease Control and Prevention: Standard precautions. In *Guidelines for isolation precautions: preventing transmission of infectious agents in health care settings,* 2009. Available at www.cdc.gov/ncidod/dhqp/gl_isolation_standard.html.

Appendix 6-9   ANTIBIOTIC MEDICATIONS   ℞

General Nursing Implications

— Always assess for antibiotic allergies, especially penicillin allergy, before administration.
— If cultures are ordered, they should be obtained before the administration of the first dose.
— Teach the client to finish the entire prescribed course of medication even though he or she may feel well.
— Schedule IM and IV administration at evenly spaced intervals around the clock.
— Give most oral antibiotic drugs on an empty stomach (1 hour before or 2 hours after meals).
— Take medications with a full glass of water.
— Observe for hypersensitivity:
  • Anaphylaxis—hypotension, respiratory distress, urticaria, angioedema, vomiting, diarrhea
  • Serum sickness—fever, vasculitis, generalized lymphadenopathy, edema of joints, bronchospasm
— Observe for superinfection:
  • Stomatitis—sore mouth, white patches on oral mucosa, black furry tongue, diarrhea
  • Monilial vaginitis—rash in perineal area, itching, vaginal discharge
  • New localized signs and symptoms—redness, heat, edema, pain, drainage, cough
  • Recurrence of systemic signs and symptoms—fever, malaise

MEDICATIONS	SIDE EFFECTS	NURSING IMPLICATIONS
Penicillin: *Bactericidal:* Interferes with the formation of the bacterial cell wall		
Natural penicillins Penicillin V **(PEN VEE K, Veetids):** PO, IV Aminopenicillins Amoxicillin **(Amoxil):** PO Ampicillin **(Principen, Totacillin):** PO, IM, IV *Penicillinase-resistant penicillins* Cloxacillin **(Tegopen):** PO Nafcillin: IV *Extended-spectrum penicillin* Ticarcillin disodium **(Ticar):** IM, IV Penicillin with beta-lactamase inhibitor Amoxicillin with clavulanic acid **(Augmentin):** PO	Parenteral injection—more hazardous than oral administration Diarrhea, especially in children Allergic reactions: skin rashes, joint pain, dermatitis, kidney damage Anaphylactic reaction (hypersensitivity): decreased BP, increased pulse, respiratory distress, diaphoresis Ticarcillin—hypernatremia	1. Observe for allergic reactions and have emergency equipment available. 2. Amoxicillin can be scheduled without regard to meals. 3. Observe client for 30 minutes after IM or IV administration for symptoms of allergic reactions. 4. Clients with beta-hemolytic strep infections should receive penicillin for a minimum of 10 days to prevent development of rheumatic fever or glomerulonephritis. 5. Discard liquid forms of penicillin after 7 days at room temperature and 14 days when refrigerated. 6. For IV administration, dilute reconstituted penicillin in 50 to 100 mL of 5% dextrose or 0.9% sodium chloride injection and infuse over 30 to 60 minutes.

Continued

Appendix 6-9   ANTIBIOTIC MEDICATIONS—cont'd

MEDICATIONS	SIDE EFFECTS	NURSING IMPLICATIONS

Aminoglycoside: *Bactericidal:* Interferes with protein synthesis

Gentamicin **(Garamycin):** IM, IV Amikacin **(Amikin):** IM, IV Tobramycin **(Nebcin):** IV, nebulizer Neomycin sulfate **(Mycitradin):** PO, IM, topical, ophthalmic	Ototoxicity—hearing loss is irreversible Nephrotoxicity—albuminuria, casts, oliguria Skin rash, headache, hypotension, pain, and tenderness at injection site Oral Neomycin is not absorbed systemically	1. Monitor serum peak and trough levels to determine toxic levels. 2. Neurotoxicity may be increased if given soon after surgery. 3. Assess for ototoxicity (change in hearing, ringing in the ears, dizziness, or unsteady gait) and nephrotoxicity (monitor BUN and creatinine). 4. Not commonly used for long-term therapy. 5. Encourage PO fluids of 2000-3000 mL of fluid daily. 6. For IV piggyback medications, administer over 30-60 minutes. 7. Neomycin PO may be used to suppress intestinal flora before surgery and to suppress ammonia formation in clients with cirrhosis.

Cephalosporins: *Bactericidal:* Broad-spectrum; interfere with the formation of the bacterial cell wall

First generation Cefadroxil **(Duricef, Ultracef):** PO Cephalexin **(Keflex):** PO Cefazolin **(Kefzol, Ancef):** IM, IV *Second generation* Cefuroxime **(Ceftin, Zinacef):** PO, IM, IV Loracarbef **(Lorabid):** PO Cefoxitin **(Mefoxin):** IM, IV *Third generation* Cefixime **(Suprax):** PO Ceftriaxone **(Rocephin):** IM, IV *Fourth generation* Cefepime **(Maxipime):** IM, IV	Hypersensitivity—rash, superinfection GI upset, neutropenia (decreased WBCs), pain at injection site, renal damage seizures	1. Give oral cephalosporins with food or milk. 2. Administer IM medications deep into the muscle. 3. Should not be given to clients with a known allergy to penicillin. 4. Decrease phlebitis at IV site by diluting solution and administering it slowly. 5. Antibacterial activity increases from first generation to fourth generation: treatment usually begins with first generation to prevent development of increased resistance.

Tetracyclines: *Bacteriostatic:* Broad-spectrum; interfere with protein synthesis of infectious organism and thus diminish its growth and reproduction

Tetracycline **(Sumycin):** PO, IV, IM Doxycycline **(Vibramycin):** PO, IV Demeclocycline **(Declomycin):** PO Minocycline **(Minocin):** PO, IV	PO may cause GI irritation (loose stools, diarrhea), sore throat, photosensitivity Diarrhea may indicate severe suprainfection in bowel Discoloration of teeth in children up to 8 years old Can cause staining of developing teeth in the fetus if taken after fourth month of gestation	1. Administer on empty stomach; withhold antacids, dairy foods, and foods high in calcium at least 2 hours after PO administration; do not administer with milk. 2. Can give doxycycline and minocycline with food. 3. Do not give at the same time as iron preparations. Give them as far apart as possible (e.g., 2-3 hours). 4. Advise client to avoid direct or artificial sunlight. 5. If diarrhea occurs, important to determine cause. 6. Observe for development of superinfections.

Appendix 6-9 ANTIBIOTIC MEDICATIONS—cont'd

MEDICATIONS	SIDE EFFECTS	NURSING IMPLICATIONS
Sulfonamides: *Bacteriostatic:* Suppress bacterial growth by inhibiting synthesis of folic acid		
Sulfamethoxazole: PO (available only in combination with trimethoprim) Sulfisoxazole **(Gantrisin):** PO, IV, IM Trimethoprim sulfamethoxazole **(TMP-SMZ, Bactrim, Septra):** PO, IV	Blood dyscrasias—hemolytic anemia Hypersensitivity—rash, "drug fever," photosensitivity Renal dysfunction—crystalluria (irritation and obstruction) (Stevens-Johnson syndrome)	1. Encourage 8-10 glasses of water per day to prevent crystalluria. 2. Contraindicated during pregnancy and for nursing mothers and infants under 2 months of age. 3. Avoid prolonged exposure to sun.
Sulfasalzine **(Azulfidine):** PO	Nausea, vomiting, diarrhea Hepatitis, bone marrow suppression	1. Antiinflammatory properties used to treat irritable bowel (IBS), rheumatoid arthritis. 2. Monitor CBC. 3. Maintain adequate hydration. 4. Urine may turn orange.
Macrolides: *Bacteriostatic:* Inhibit protein synthesis		
Erythromycin base **(Erythrocin):** PO, Azithromycin **(Zithromax):** PO, IV Clarithromycin **(Biaxin):** PO	Nausea, vomiting, abdominal distress, diarrhea Cholestatic hepatitis: abnormal liver function studies, jaundice, fever	1. Administer with a full glass of water.
Fluoroquinolones: *Bactericidal:* Inhibit bacterial DNA		
Ciprofloxacin **(Cipro):** PO, IV Levofloxacin **(Levaquin):** PO, IV	GI: Nausea, vomiting, abdominal distress, diarrhea CNS: dizziness, headache, confusion Superinfections, hypersensitivity	1. Absorption is reduced by milk products, antacids. 2. Administer IV infusions over 60 minutes.
Other Antibiotics		
Metronidazole **(Flagyl):** PO, IV	Nausea, dry mouth, headache Disulfiram reaction when taken with alcohol: nausea, copious vomiting, flushing, palpitations, headache; may last 30 minutes to an hour	1. Classified as an antiprotozoal antibiotic; is effective against anaerobic microorganisms. 2. Avoid concurrent use with alcohol or products containing alcohol. Will cause a disulfiram reaction.
Vancomycin **(Vancocin):** PO, IV	Ototoxicity, thrombophlebitis at site Red man syndrome: flushing, rash, pruritus, tachycardia, and hypotension	1. Acts by inhibiting cell wall synthesis; used only for serious infections. 2. IV infusions over at least 60 minutes to prevent adverse effects. 3. Serum peak and trough levels are monitored.
Linezolid **(Zyvox):** PO, IV	GI: diarrhea, nausea Myelosuppression—anemia, leukopenia, thrombocytopenia	1. New class of antibiotics—oxazolidinones. 2. Monitor for blood dyscrasias. 3. Reserved for treatment of infections from MDROs.
Antifungal		
Nystatin **(Mycostatin):** PO, topical		1. Used for treatment of candidiasis (mouth, esophagus, vagina). 2. Oral treatment encourage client to hold medication in their mouth and "swish" around to provide good contact with all affected areas.

BUN, Blood urea nitrogen; *GI,* gastrointestinal; *IM,* intramuscular; *IV,* intravenous; *PO,* by mouth; *MDRO,* multiple drug resistant organisms.

Appendix 6-10 VASCULAR ACCESS LINES

Central Line: A single or multilumen catheter inserted into the venous system and progressed into the thoracic cavity with the end of the line in the superior vena cava or the right atrium

Nursing Implications for Central Line

— Most common insertion is percutaneous into the subclavian or jugular vein.
  - A central line is necessary for a central venous pressure (CVP) reading and for total parenteral nutrition solutions.
  - Obtain a chest x-ray to evaluate for a possible pneumothorax after insertion of catheter into subclavian vein.
— Pulmonary artery catheters have a port at the level of the right atrium for central venous pressure measurement.
— When changing the tubing on straight central lines, position the client flat (if tolerated) and have client hold his or her breath and bear down when the line is opened. Immediately connect the new line and have the client breathe normally. Because the catheter goes into the thoracic cavity, it is subjected to changes in pressure, which increase the risk for air embolus.
— Maintain sterile technique when changing the dressing on the puncture site.

ALERT Assist with invasive procedures (e.g., central line placement). Obtain blood specimens peripherally or through a central line. Access implanted venous access devices.

Vascular Access Devices: Long-term vascular lines for clients receiving intravenous (IV) therapy for 3 months or longer.

- **Implanted ports (MediPort, Port-A-Cath):** MediPort vascular access line port is implanted under the skin; activities are not restricted (Figure 6-6).
- **Tunneled ports (Hickman, Broviac):** Hickman line requires surgical placement; has an external port. The distal tips of both catheters lie in the superior vena cava just above the right atrium. Not used to obtain CVP readings.
- **PICC:** A peripherally inserted central catheter (PICC) line is inserted into a large peripheral vein of the upper arm and threaded into the subclavian vein and has an external port; area requires a sterile occlusive dressing; may be used to obtain blood samples.
- **Triple- or double-lumen lines:** A venous catheter that contains two or three separate ports and lines that are encased and inserted as one line; may be part of the vascular access device (VAD). Because each line is separate, the infusing solutions do not mix.

Nursing Implications for Vascular Access Devices

- **Flushing:** Routine flushing may be required unless there is a continuous IV infusion. This may be done with normal saline solution, heparin, or fibrinolytics. Type of solution, frequency, and volume depend on IV therapy and whether blood was drawn from the line, as well as institution policy. Excessive force should never be used to irrigate the line. Syringes smaller than 10 mL should not be used because the smaller the syringe, the greater the pressure exerted. The push-pause technique is an important flushing method used for prevention of deposits in ports or catheter lumens.

⚠ NURSING PRIORITY: Do not flush a PICC catheter if there is resistance or if catheter is occluded; increased pressure may cause catheter to rupture and or produce a catheter emboli.

- **Accessing:** Gloves are worn and appropriate skin preparation is done for implanted ports; external injection ports and connectors are cleansed before accessing.
- **Dressing changes:** Implanted sites require cleansing after exit but do not require a dressing. External sites (PICCs and ports) require dressings, either gauze or transparent. Gauze dressings are changed if they are contaminated or if observation of the site is required; dressing is routinely changed every 48 hours. Transparent dressings may not be changed for 5-7 days.
- **Changing lines:** Clamping may be necessary during a tubing change to prevent air emboli; always use a flat or padded clamp to prevent damaging the line. If the line cannot be clamped, have the client hold his or her breath and bear down (Valsalva maneuver) during the line change.

Arterial Lines: Used to obtain arterial blood sample for ABGs and for blood pressure monitoring.

- **Measurements:** Arterial lines are used to evaluate blood pressure measurements. Measurement should be obtained at the end of respiration to avoid effect of respiratory cycle on arterial pressure.
- **Arterial blood sample:** Blood is withdrawn to evaluate ABGs.

Nursing Implications for Arterial Line

- **Complications:** hemorrhage, infection, thrombus formation, neurologic damage.
  - Maintain Leur Lok connection to prevent problem with accidental disconnection and bleeding from site.
  - Prevent thrombus formation and maintain line patency by maintaining pressure on line at 300 mm Hg to provide continuous flush at 3-6 mL per hour.

FIGURE 6-6 Implantable vascular access port. (From Potter PA, Perry AG: *Fundamentals of nursing,* ed 7, St. Louis, 2009, Mosby.)

Appendix 6-10   VASCULAR ACCESS LINES—cont'd

- Perform Allen's test (see Arterial Blood Gas Studies in Appendix 15-1) to determine adequate circulation to hand before placing line in radial artery.
- Assess for infection at insertion site; if present, remove catheter and change all tubing and equipment for new site.

- Prevent infection by changing pressure tubing, fluid bag, and transducer every 96 hours.
- Assess vascular status distal to arterial line by checking capillary refill, as well as color of extremity.
- Assess neurologic status distal to arterial line by checking for presence of tingling, pain, or paresthesia.

Study Questions Homeostasis

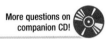
More questions on companion CD!

1. The nurse would identify which set of blood gas values as consistent with a diagnosis of respiratory acidosis in a client?
   1 pH 7.0; PCO_2 42.
   2 pH 7.46; PCO_2 38.
   3 pH 7.35; PCO_2 44.
   4 pH 7.32; PCO_2 48.

2. An older adult client is experiencing difficulty with edema and fluid overload. What nursing intervention would be the most accurate in evaluating the client's fluid balance?
   1 Measure the intake and output.
   2 Check for thirst and tissue turgor.
   3 Evaluate changes in daily weight.
   4 Evaluate vital signs every 3 hours.

3. The nurse is admitting a client from the postoperative recovery area. Postoperative orders are D_5 ½ NS with 40 mEq/L of KCl. The current liter of lactated Ringer's solution has 450 mL left to infuse. What should the nurse do?
   1 Finish the current liter of fluid.
   2 Ask the client if he needs to void.
   3 Hang the ordered IV.
   4 Assess the IV site.

4. The nurse is reviewing the health care provider's orders for a new client. The client has just returned from the surgical recovery area. The client is NPO, he has a nasogastric tube, and his vital signs are stable. Which order would the nurse question?
   1 20 mEq potassium IV push.
   2 1000 mL D_5 ½ NaCl to infuse at 125 mL per hour.
   3 Assist client to dangle at bedside in AM.
   4 Cefoxitin (Mefoxin) 1g IV in 50 mL D_5W over 30 minutes.

5. The nurse is assisting a client to ambulate. Upon standing at the bedside, the client becomes weak and sits back down on the bed. The nurse should assess the client for what problem?
   1 Sodium imbalance.
   2 Altered renal function.
   3 Fluid deficit.
   4 Hyperkalemia.

6. What information is most important to teach a client who is receiving steroid therapy?
   1 Record daily weights to determine weight gain.
   2 Increase dose of medication as needed.
   3 Do not discontinue medication abruptly.
   4 Increase fluid intake.

7. Which of the following clients would most likely experience a problem with maintaining a normal electrolyte balance?
   1 A client with peripheral edema and heart failure.
   2 A client with a history of alcohol intake and liver damage.
   3 A child with an acute episode of nephrotic syndrome.
   4 A client with obstructive lung disease.

8. The nurse is admitting a 5-month-old infant. The physician has ordered an IV solution of normal saline. There is also an order for potassium chloride (KCl) to be added to the solution. The infant's temperature is 101° F rectally, and the pulse is 120 beats/min; the infant is irritable and has not voided. What would be the next best nursing action?
   1 Wait for 1 hour from admission time and then begin the infusion of normal saline with the KCl.
   2 Feed the infant before adding the KCl to the infusing solution.
   3 Consider the order a stat order and begin the infusion immediately.
   4 Start the normal saline infusion and hold the KCl until adequate urinary output has been documented.

9. A client's condition has put him at an increased risk for development of a problem with excess fluid volume. What nursing intervention would provide the most accurate information for evaluating the clients' fluid status?
   1 Obtaining the client's daily weight before breakfast each day.
   2 Measuring fluid intake and output and comparing with values from the previous day.
   3 Assessing the blood pressure and comparing it with previous readings.
   4 Auscultating the lungs for the presence of adventitious breath sounds.

10. A older adult client has an order for continuous fluid replacement at 75 mL per hour. The nurse is preparing to start the IV. What site would be appropriate, and what is the equipment of choice?
    1 A 22-gauge butterfly, right arm antecubital area.
    2 An 18-gauge, 3-inch IV cannula (intercath), inserted in the left hand.
    3 An 18-gauge, 1-inch IV cannula (intercath), in the antecubital area of left arm.
    4 A 22-gauge, 1-inch intercath, top of the left hand.

11. A client has just received 250 mL of packed cells and is now receiving 1000 mL of D_5W at 150 mL/hour. The client tells the nurse that he feels dizzy and has a headache. The nurse observes the distended jugular veins with the client in a semi-Fowler's position. What would be the nurse's initial response?
    1 Notify the physician with the client's vital signs and complaints.
    2 Check vital signs and place the client in semi-Fowler's position.
    3 Reduce the D_5W infusion to keep vein open rate.
    4 Increase the rate of the IV because of the obvious signs of dehydration.

12. The nurse is performing a dressing change on a client who has a *Staphylococcus* infection in an abdominal incision. What infection control precautions will the nurse implement? Select all that apply:
    _____ 1 Wear clean gloves to remove the old dressing.
    _____ 2 Put on a gown when entering the room.
    _____ 3 Wear a face shield.
    _____ 4 Dispose of the gown and mask in container outside the client's door.
    _____ 5 Leave all extra dressing supplies in the room.
    _____ 6 Carefully cleanse the stethoscope and scissors that came in contact with the client.

13. The client is receiving an IV of 0.9% NaCl at 125 mL per hour. The client had a colon resection this morning. He has a nasogastric tube to suction and an ileostomy, and he is becoming increasingly restless. The nurse reviews the serum laboratory values. Which value would cause the nurse the most concern?
    1 Blood urea nitrogen 32 mg/dL.
    2 Serum glucose 190 mg/dL.
    3 Hemoglobin 13.5, hematocrit 41%.
    4 Sodium 155 mEq/L.

14. A client has returned to the room from the postoperative recovery area. He is lethargic but responsive. He has O_2 via nasal cannula at 4 L/min and an IV infusing at 125 mL/hr. On the initial nursing assessment, the nurse notes that the O_2 saturation on the pulse oximetry is 82%. What is the priority nursing action?
    1 Perform a complete neurologic check.
    2 Increase the O_2 flow and recheck the pulse oximetry.
    3 Suction the client and recheck the vital signs.
    4 Stimulate the client to cough and deep-breathe.

15. The nurse is admitting a 15-year-old client with type 1 diabetes for control of his diabetes. What values on the arterial blood gases would indicate the client is developing a complication as a result of his poorly controlled diabetes?
    1 $Paco_2$ 48 mm Hg, pH 7.37, Po_2 98 mm Hg, HCO_3^- 24 mEq/L.
    2 $Paco_2$ 33 mm Hg, pH 7.48, Po_2 88 mm Hg, HCO_3^- 26 mEq/L.
    3 $Paco_2$ 40 mm Hg, pH 7.45, HCO_3^- 32 mEq/L, O_2 saturation 90%.
    4 $Paco_2$ 38 mm Hg, pH 7.31, HCO_3^- 22 mEq/L, base excess −2.

16. A client is complaining of pain at the peripheral IV site. The nurse determines the IV is not infusing, assesses the site, and finds the area swollen, pale, and cool to touch. What is the best nursing action?
    1 Discontinue the IV and apply warm, moist packs to the involved area.
    2 Slow the IV infusion and see whether the swollen area decreases.
    3 Notify the health care provider regarding the status of the IV.
    4 Discontinue the IV and start another IV in the same vein, distal to the current site.

17. A client is being seen in the emergency department after an accident. He has no obvious physical injuries, and his blood pressure is 158/90 mm Hg. He is crying loudly, wringing his hands, and pacing the floor. His respiratory rate is 32 breaths/min, and he complains of being lightheaded. What is the best nursing response?
    1 Have him lie down and begin O_2 per nasal cannula at 4 L/min.
    2 Put him on a stretcher and begin a head-to-toe assessment.
    3 Perform a quick neurologic exam to determine his level of orientation.
    4 Have him sit down and help him breathe into a paper sack.

18. The nurse is documenting information regarding an IV insertion. What information is important to include? Select all that apply:
    _____ 1 Time and date of insertion.
    _____ 2 Type of catheter and size.
    _____ 3 Name of vein used.
    _____ 4 Status of fluid infusing.
    _____ 5 Protective measures used.
    _____ 6 Who ordered the IV and at what time.

Answers and rationales to these questions are in the section at the end of the book titled Chapter Study Questions: Answers and Rationales.

CHAPTER SEVEN

Immune System

PHYSIOLOGY OF THE IMMUNE SYSTEM

A. The lymphoid system is composed of organs and cells that participate in the immune response.
1. Primary lymphoid organs.
   a. Thymus.
      (1) Production of T cells.
      (2) Maturation and differentiation of the T cells (lymphocytes). T cells become either T cytotoxic (CD8), or T helper (CD4) cells.
      (3) Provide for long-term immunity.
   b. Bone marrow.
      (1) Production of B cells.
      (2) Differentiate into plasma cells that produce antibodies (immunoglobulins).
2. Peripheral lymphoid organs.
   a. Lymph nodes: filter out foreign material and circulate the lymphocytes.
   b. Spleen: produces lymphocytes and plasma cells; filters the blood.
   c. Mucosal-associated lymphoid tissue: the gastrointestinal tract, the bronchi in the respiratory tract, the genital tract and the skin all contain associated lymphoid tissue.
   d. Tonsils: trap and remove invading organisms.
B. Body recognizes foreign proteins, called *antigens*, which will elicit a response from the immune system—the production of antibodies, which attack and destroy the invading antigens.
C. Antigens are foreign to the body and are frequently associated with bacteria, viruses, or other pathogens; antigens react with antibodies or antigen receptors on B and T cells.
D. Allergens are antigens that produce an allergic response.
E. Inflammatory response—an innate resistance or natural barrier that responds to the site of tissue injury; examples include infection, mechanical injury, ischemia, temperature extremes.
1. Redness, heat, swelling, and pain occur secondary to vasodilatation, increased vascular permeability, and white blood cell migration to site of injury.
2. Complement system consists of plasma proteins that directly destroy pathogens, activated by the formation of an antigen-antibody complex (immune complex).
3. Complement cells are found in the innate as well as the acquired immune response.

Immunologic Responses

A. Humoral response.
1. Antibodies, produced by the plasma cells, circulate through the blood and bind to and inactivate antigens or infectious agents.
2. B lymphocytes (plasma cells) recognize the antigen and become activated, differentiated plasma cells, which produce immunoglobulins.
   a. Immunoglobulin M (IgM): provides the initial antibody response; a large molecule that is primarily confined to the intravascular space.
   b. Immunoglobulin G (IgG): main serum antibody; assumes a major role in bloodborne and tissue infections; the longest-acting immunoglobulin; crosses placenta and provides natural passive immunity in the newborn.
   c. Immunoglobulin A (IgA): appears in body fluids; prevents absorption of antigens from food; plays an important role against infection in respiratory passages.
   d. Immunoglobulin E (IgE): appears in serum and interstitial fluids; is associated with immediate hypersensitivity reactions (anaphylactic and atopic reactions); assists in the defense against parasitic infections.
B. Cell-mediated response—stem cells originate in the bone marrow and travel to the thymus, where they mature into functional T cells.
1. A response is initiated through recognition of antigens by T cells (T lymphocytes, macrophages, and natural killer cells).
2. Differentiation of the T cells into specific cells that react directly with the antigen.
   a. T cytotoxic (CD8) cells—antigen-specific; sensitized by exposure to the antigen; a second exposure will result in a more intense and rapid cell-mediated response.
   b. T helper (CD4) cells—differentiate into cytokines, which give directions to cells; changes the proliferation of the cell, as well as the activity or the secretion of the cell.
   c. Natural killer (NK) cells—large lymphocytes that recognize and kill cells from viruses, tumors or transplanted tissue; cells do not require a previous sensitization to the antigen.

119

3. Provides cellular immunity, delayed hypersensitivity reactions; recognizes tumor cells and inhibits tumor growth; rejects foreign tissue (organ transplants) and produces autoimmune disorders.

C. Humoral and cellular responses are not independent—but *inter*dependent—and an effective immune response is based on the interactions of both responses.

D. Properties of the immunologic response.
  1. *Specificity:* the formation of a specific antibody for each antigen; antibodies produced against one pathogen will not protect the body from other pathogens.
  2. *Memory:* both responses are capable of "remembering" the antigen and responding more rapidly if exposed to same antigen again.
  3. *Self-recognition:* the immune system has the ability to distinguish self or self-antigens from nonself or foreign antigens; the self-antigens do not illicit the immune response.

E. Inflammatory response.
  1. Early inflammatory response is self-limiting. It destroys injurious agents and removes them from the site. Also confines agents to the area, stimulates the immune response, and promotes healing.
  2. Chronic inflammation lasts 2 weeks or longer, frequently preceded by an unsuccessful acute response. Infiltration of lymphocytes and macrophages occur in an attempt to protect the body; the area may be walled off to form a granuloma (e.g., the granuloma associated with tuberculosis).

F. Types of specific immunity (Table 7-1).
  1. Natural immunity: no prior contact with an antigen.
  2. Acquired immunity: develops either actively or passively.

G. Effects of aging on immune response.
  1. Infants are protected at birth by maternal antibodies that cross the placenta; an infant's antibody system begins to function around 6 months of age.
  2. Newborns have a transiently depressed inflammatory response and immune function; they are prone

to infections associated with staphylococci and *Candida*.

3. Aging decreases the size and activity of the thymus, which results in a diminished response of the cell-mediated immunity. A decline in efficiency of humoral immunity also occurs because of a decrease in antibody production in response to antigens.

4. Older clients are at increased risk for impaired inflammation and wound healing secondary to chronic diseases (cardiovascular, diabetes), as well as medications that impair the inflammatory response (steroids).

> **■ NURSING PRIORITY** Clients who have a compromised immune system, from either disease or medications, should not take any immunizations until they have checked with their doctor.

DISORDERS OF THE IMMUNE SYSTEM

Hypersensitivity

A. Type I (IgE-mediated reaction; IgE antibodies involved).
  1. Occurs when a person has been previously sensitized to a specific antigen.
  2. When same antigen reappears, it interacts with the IgE; this activates the release of chemical mediators, primarily histamine.
  3. Histamine: major chemical mediator.
    a. Smooth muscle contraction (spasms of bronchial muscles and airway obstruction).
    b. Capillary vasodilatation and increased capillary permeability, leading to vascular collapse (decreased blood pressure).
    c. Increased nasal stuffiness and bronchial secretions.
    d. Reaction usually begins within minutes after exposure.

Table 7-1	**ACQUIRED IMMUNITY**	
Type	**Characteristics**	**Examples**
Active: Antibodies synthesized by body in response to antigen stimulation.	***Natural:*** Contact with an antigen through exposure; develops slowly, often lifetime protection.	Recovery from childhood diseases (e.g., chicken pox, measles, mumps).
	Artificial: Immunization with an antigen develops slowly; may provide protection for several years, but "boosters" may be required.	Immunization with live or attenuated vaccines (varicella, IPV, MMR). Toxoid immunization (tetanus toxoid, diphtheria toxoid).
Passive: Antibodies produced in one individual and transferred to another.	***Natural:*** Immunity from placenta and colostrum transferred from mother to child; provides immediate temporary protection.	Maternal immunoglobulin in the neonate.
	Artificial: Injection of serum from immune human or animal; short-lived but immediate immunity.	Gamma globulin; injection of animal hyperimmune serum (diphtheria antitoxin, tetanus antitoxin).

IPV, Inactivated polio vaccine; *MMR,* measles-mumps-rubella vaccine.

4. Conditions associated with type I.
   a. Anaphylaxis (most severe).
   b. Atopic reactions (most common).
      (1) Allergic rhinitis (hay fever).
      (2) Urticaria (hives).
      (3) Bronchial asthma.
B. Type II (cytotoxic; direct binding of IgG and IgM antibodies to an antigen).
   1. Antibodies destroy cell on which antigen is bound, causing tissue injury.
   2. The normal process of phagocytosis is accelerated and begins to damage healthy body tissue.
   3. Conditions associated with type II.
      a. Hemolytic disease of the newborn (Rh factor).
      b. Leukopenia and thrombocytopenia.
      c. ABO blood incompatibility (hemolytic reaction).
      d. Goodpasture syndrome (an antibody-mediated reaction involving the lungs and kidneys).
C. Type III (immune complex; IgG and IgM antibodies involved).
   1. Circulating immune complexes (antibody-antigen complex) are too small to be effectively removed and are deposited in the body tissue.
   2. When the immune complex is deposited in the body tissue (kidneys, skin, joints, blood vessels, and lungs), local tissue inflammation and cell wall damage occur.
   3. Symptoms depend on number of complexes present as well as the area of the body involved (autoimmune conditions).
      a. Persistent infections (streptococcal infections) combined with a poor antibody response may lead to the formation of immune complex that is eventually deposited in an affected organ.
         (1) Endocarditis (Chapter 17).
         (2) Acute glomerulonephritis (Chapter 23).
      b. Rheumatoid arthritis (Chapter 21).
      c. Systemic lupus erythematosus.
D. Type IV (cell-mediated; delayed hypersensitivity).
   1. The T cells are sensitized to an antigen from a previous exposure; occurs 24 to 48 hours after exposure, may take 72 hours to reach maximum intensity.
   2. The sensitized T cells initiate the inflammatory response, leading to cellular damage as well as damage to the surrounding tissue.
   3. Conditions associated with type IV.
      a. Tuberculosis, skin testing.
      b. Contact dermatitis (poison ivy).
      c. Transplant rejection.

Anaphylactic Reaction

Type I occurs in clients who are highly sensitized to a specific allergen—medications, blood products, insect stings. The antigen-antibody response precipitates the release of histamine, causing vasodilatation and increased capillary permeability (Figure 7-1).

Assessment

A. Risk factors.
   1. History of exposure to allergen.
      a. Amount of allergen.
      b. Absorption of ingested allergen.
      c. Antibody levels from previous exposure.
      d. Occupational, social, and environmental factors.
   2. The more rapid the onset of symptoms after exposure, the more severe the reaction.
B. Clinical manifestations—depend on the level of prior sensitivity and the amount of allergen.
   1. Mild to moderate: peripheral tingling/itching (pruritus, urticaria), sensation of warmth, edema of the lips and tongue, nasal congestion, flushing, anxiety.
   2. May rapidly progress to acute anxiety, difficulty breathing (bronchospasm, laryngeal edema), GI cramping, cyanosis, and hypotension; can be fatal.

Diagnostics

According to symptoms and exposure to allergen.

Treatment

A. Mild to moderate reactions—antihistamines and/or epinephrine 0.2 to 0.5 mL (1:1000 solution), administered subcutaneously or intramuscularly (Appendix 7-2).

> **⚠ NURSING PRIORITY** When administering epinephrine, make sure you have the correct concentration of solution. It is administered in concentrations of 0.1% or 1:1,000 subcutaneously or IM, and 0.01% or 1:10,000 IV or intracardiac. Intravenous solutions are more dilute due to potential fatal reactions.

B. Severe reactions—epinephrine 0.5 mL (concentration of 1:10,000), administered intravenously at 5- to 10-minute intervals (1 mg over at least 1 minute).
C. Oxygen in high concentrations.

ANAPHYLACTIC REACTION

Causes:
- Insect Stings (bee, wasp, ant)
- Medication Reaction
- Food Allergy (peanuts, eggs, shellfish)

Iodine

- Rapid Onset
- Dyspnea
  - Tight Throat
  - Bronchospasm
  - Laryngeal Edema
- Feelings of Apprehension
- Tingling and Swelling in Mouth, Face, Throat and Tongue
- Itching
- ↓ BP
- Tachycardia
- Loss Of Consciousness

©2007 Nursing Education Consultants, Inc.

FIGURE 7-1 Anaphylaxis. (From Zerwekh J, Claborn J: *Memory notebook of nursing,* vol 2, ed 3, Ingram, Texas, 2007, Nursing Education Consultants.)

D. IV fluids (Lactated Ringer's or 0.9% saline), vasopressor agents, and volume expanders to maintain circulatory status.

E. Maintain patent airway—intubation or tracheostomy may be necessary.

F. Corticosteroids to reduce inflammatory response (see Appendix 6-7).

ALERT Manage a medical emergency. Anaphylaxis is an immediate response, and symptoms progress very rapidly. Emergency treatment should be initiated immediately if anaphylaxis is suspected. Death from an anaphylactic reaction is most often caused by bronchospasm and edema of the airway.

Nursing Interventions

Goal: To assess clients for predisposition to hypersensitivity reactions.

ALERT Check for client allergies.

A. Evaluate client history regarding reactions to:
1. Medications, especially penicillin.
2. Foods (e.g., seafood or iodine, eggs, peanuts).
3. Insect bites.
4. Vaccines, especially egg-cultured types.
5. Blood products (transfusion reaction).
6. Diagnostic agents (e.g., iodine-based contrast media).

B. If hypersensitivity is suspected, a localized skin test may be done before the administration of substance.

C. Prevention is the priority.

Goal: To maintain adequate ventilation.

! NURSING PRIORITY Airway positioning and mouth-to-mouth resuscitation will not provide adequate ventilation when client has airway edema. An emergency tracheotomy or intubation may be indicated.

A. Maintain bed rest; place client in low Fowler's position with the legs elevated.

B. High oxygen concentrations if airway is compromised.

C. Anticipate use of airway adjuncts (tracheostomy, endotracheal intubation).

D. Administration of medications to reverse bronchospasm (albuterol, corticosteroid, epinephrine).

Goal: To restore adequate circulation.

A. Administer IV fluids (normal saline or lactated Ringer's solution) to correct loss of fluid to third-space shifts and vasodilation.

B. Carefully titrate fluid replacement with vital signs.

! NURSING PRIORITY Monitor the client's fluid status closely; as fluid begins to shift back into the vascular compartment, it is very easy to cause fluid overload.

C. Vasopressors and volume expanders may be used to increase blood pressure if fluid replacement is not effective.

Goal: Client teaching to prevent recurrence.

A. Once causative agent is identified, instruct client accordingly.

B. Advise client to wear identification tag or bracelet.

C. Explain to client that if he or she had any level of allergic reaction previously, the next exposure could be worse (penicillin, insect stings, etc.).

Autoimmune Conditions

A. Conditions in which body tolerance has been disrupted and the body tissue or cells cannot recognize their own cells (self-recognition). A critical aspect of the immune response is the ability of the body to recognize normal tissue and to not invade or destroy it.

B. An autoimmune condition occurs when the immune system can no longer recognize the normal tissue; reacts against self-antigens and begins to destroy the host tissue.

C. Some autoimmune responses are very tissue specific and invade only that specific tissue, whereas others response may have body-wide effects.

D. Autoimmune response and disease occurrence.
1. The direct action of the autoantibody on the cell surface. This causes destruction of the cell (cytotoxic); may activate the inflammatory response.
2. An alteration of both B cells and or T cells can produce auto-sensitized T cells and cause tissue damage.

E. Autoimmune response may be systemic or organ-specific.
1. Systemic diseases (rheumatic disorders: autoimmune and inflammatory).
   a. Chronic pain and progressive immobility are characteristics.
   b. Connective tissue disorders: systemic lupus erythematosus (SLE).
   c. Rheumatic disorders: rheumatoid arthritis.
2. Organ-specific diseases.
   a. Myasthenia gravis, multiple sclerosis.
   b. Hyperthyroid (Graves' disease).
   c. Addison's disease.
   d. Type 1 diabetes mellitus.

Systemic Lupus Erythematosus (SLE)

SLE is a multisystem inflammatory autoimmune disorder; the disease affects multiple organs. SLE is characterized by a diffuse production of autoantibodies that attack and cause damage to body organs and tissue.

A. Tissue injury in SLE results from deposition of the immune complexes throughout the body (kidneys, heart, skin, brain, and joints); this activates the inflammatory response.

B. The severity of symptoms varies greatly throughout the course of the disease; periods of exacerbation and remission occur.

Assessment

A. Risk factors.
1. More common in women, 20 to 40 years of age.
2. Familial tendencies.
3. May be triggered by environmental stimulus, infections, and medications; sun exposure most common.

B. Clinical manifestations (Figure 7-2).
1. Initially may be nonspecific: weight loss, fatigue, and fever.
2. Integumentary: characteristic "butterfly" rash over face in about 50% of clients; erythematous rash on areas of the body exposed to sunlight (photosensitivity); alopecia; dry scaly scalp; palmer erythema.
3. Musculoskeletal: arthritis, diffuse swelling with joint and muscle pain.
4. Renal system involvement: lupus nephritis, proteinuria, and glomerulonephritis.
5. Cardiovascular system.
   a. Raynaud's phenomenon: caused by peripheral vasospasm.
   b. Pericarditis: may progress to endocarditis.
   c. Vascular inflammation of the small vessels. Most commonly affects the small vessels of the fingers and the gastrointestinal tract.
6. Neurologic disorders: seizures, cognitive dysfunction.
7. Hematologic disorders: anemia, leukopenia, thrombocytopenia.
8. Emotional lability: severe depression and anxiety.
9. Respiratory system: dyspnea and pleurisy.
10. Gastrointestinal system: ulcers in the oral mucosa or nasopharyngeal membranes.

Diagnostics

A. No specific test is diagnostic; assess configuration of symptoms.
B. Presence of antinuclear antibody (ANA), high levels of anti-DNA, and presence of anti-Smith (Sm) are most suggestive of a diagnosis of SLE.
C. C-reactive protein (CRP), erythrocyte sedimentation rate (ESR)—monitor progress of inflammation.

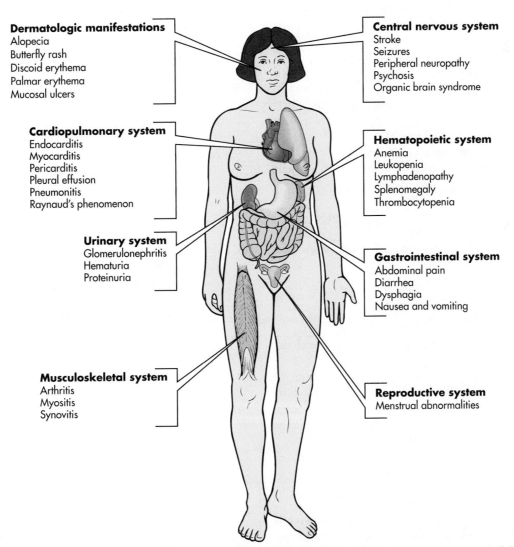

Dermatologic manifestations
Alopecia
Butterfly rash
Discoid erythema
Palmar erythema
Mucosal ulcers

Central nervous system
Stroke
Seizures
Peripheral neuropathy
Psychosis
Organic brain syndrome

Cardiopulmonary system
Endocarditis
Myocarditis
Pericarditis
Pleural effusion
Pneumonitis
Raynaud's phenomenon

Hematopoietic system
Anemia
Leukopenia
Lymphadenopathy
Splenomegaly
Thrombocytopenia

Urinary system
Glomerulonephritis
Hematuria
Proteinuria

Gastrointestinal system
Abdominal pain
Diarrhea
Dysphagia
Nausea and vomiting

Musculoskeletal system
Arthritis
Myositis
Synovitis

Reproductive system
Menstrual abnormalities

FIGURE 7-2 Systemic lupus erythematosus. (From Lewis SL et al: *Medical-surgical nursing: assessment and management of clinical problems,* ed 7, St. Louis, 2007, Mosby.)

Treatment

SLE has no known cure.

A. Nonsteroidal antiinflammatory medications (see Appendix 3-3).
B. Corticosteroids for exacerbations polyarthritis (see Appendix 6-7).
C. Immunosuppressants (see Appendix 23-3).
D. Antimalarial agents (e.g., hydroxychloroquine [Plaquenil]).

Nursing Interventions

Goal: To prevent exacerbations.

A. Maintain good nutritional status; eat a low-cholesterol diet.
B. Avoid exposure to infections.
C. Teach client about skin problems: discoid lesions, loss of hair, dry scaly scalp.
D. Teach client personal hygiene to prevent urinary tract infections.
E. Make sure client understands how to take medications.
F. Avoid exposure to sunlight; use a sunscreen with a high SPF when exposure is unavoidable.
G. Contact physician before participating in any immunization procedures.
H. Counseling regarding pregnancy.

Goal: To maintain adequate tissue perfusion.

A. Assess for indications of impaired peripheral perfusion—numbness, tingling, and weakness of hands and feet.
B. Prevent injury to extremities—especially fingers.
C. Carefully evaluate fluid status with regard to cardiac status, fluid retention, and weight gain.

Goal: To promote effective pain control.

A. Establish schedule to conserve energy, but still maintain physical activity.
B. NSAIDs to control arthritic pain.
C. Nonpharmacologic therapies to supplement analgesics (Chapter 3).
D. Evaluate response of pain to decrease inflammation from corticosteroids.

Goal: To maintain renal function.

A. Monitor for peripheral edema, hypertension, hematuria, decreased output.
B. Monitor blood urea nitrogen and creatinine levels.
C. Monitor for urinary tract infections (glomerulonephritis).
D. Assess for peripheral edema and excess fluid volume.

Goal: To assist client to maintain psychologic equilibrium.

A. Observe for behavioral changes that may indicate central nervous system involvement: headaches, inappropriate speech, difficulty concentrating.
B. Encourage client to participate in support groups and to seek counseling to deal with stress.

Acquired Immunodeficiency Syndrome

Acquired immunodeficiency syndrome (AIDS) is a condition resulting from severe impairment of the immune system's ability to respond to invading pathogens; AIDS ultimately affects all body systems.

A. Occurs as a result of being infected with the human immunodeficiency virus (HIV).
B. Once a client is infected, he or she will harbor the virus for the rest of his life.
C. The disease progression is highly individualized; the average time between the HIV infection and the development of AIDS is about 11 years, during which the symptoms are frequently vague and nonspecific.

Transmission of Human Immunodeficiency Virus

A. Blood transmission.
   1. Needle-sticks that occur when the client has a high viral load carry a higher risk than those that occur when client is at a low viral load.
   2. Exposure to an infected client's blood via open wounds or mucous membranes carries a lower risk than does a needle-stick.
   3. Transmission via blood transfusions has been greatly reduced with the screening of donated blood.
      a. A risk remains when the blood is donated within the first few months of infection and the screening blood test does not identify the donor as being HIV-positive.
      b. Clotting factors for hemophilia clients are treated with chemicals and/or heat to decrease the risk for transmission.
B. Sexual transmission—most common mode of transmission.
   1. Sexual practices, not preferences, place people at increased risk.
   2. Risk for infection is greater for the partner who receives the semen during oral, vaginal, or anal sex.
   3. Any sexual activity that involves direct contact with vaginal secretions and semen may transmit HIV.
C. Perinatal transmission.
   1. Exposure can occur during pregnancy, at the time of delivery, or during the postpartum period through breast milk.
   2. 25% of infants born to HIV-positive mothers are infected.
   3. Prophylactic antiviral medications during pregnancy can reduce rate of transmission.
   4. Decreased incidence occurs with cesarean delivery of HIV-positive mothers.
D. HIV *cannot* be transmitted by:
   1. Hugging, kissing, holding hands, or other nonsexual contact.
   2. Inanimate objects (money, doorknobs, bathtubs, toilet seats, etc).
   3. Dishes, silverware, or food handled by an infected person.
   4. Animals or insects.
E. CD4+ T helper cells are the regulating cells in the immune system; the level of CD4+ T cells is used to monitor the stages and progression of the virus;

normal CD4+ T cell count is at least 800 cells/mm³ of blood.

F. The viral load in the semen, blood, vaginal secretions, or breast milk is an important variable in the transmission.

Clinical Manifestations

A. Acute HIV infection.
1. Intense viral replication and dissemination of HIV throughout the body.
2. Symptoms are mild, ranging from no symptoms to flu-like symptoms (fever, night sweats, chills, headache).
3. Window of seroconversion: time period from when the person is infected with the virus until HIV antibodies can be detected.
4. Average time for seroconversion to occur is 1 to 3 weeks.
5. A client may have vague, nonspecific symptoms for years.
6. During this period, there is a high viral load and the CD4+ T cell count falls, but only temporarily.
B. Early chronic infection—CD4+ T cell count greater than 500 cells/mm³ and low viral load.
1. Viral replication has reached a steady state.
2. Considered asymptomatic phase; however, chronic vague symptoms persist.
3. Persistent generalized lymphadenopathy.
C. Intermediate chronic infection—CD4+ T cell count between 200 and 500 cells/mm³ and increased viral load.
1. Exacerbation of symptoms.
2. Client begins to experience localized infections, increased lymphadenopathy, and neurologic manifestations.
   a. *Candida* is a common problem—persistent oropharyngeal or vulvovaginal candidiasis.
   b. Hairy oral leukoplakia, which may also be indication of progression of disease.
   c. Shingles, oral or genital herpes lesions.
   d. Kaposi's sarcoma.
      (1) A cutaneous skin lesion that looks like a bruise; later will turn dark violet or black.
      (2) Invades body organs, extremities, skin, and torso.
      (3) May become very painful.
D. Late chronic infection, or AIDS (acquired immunodeficiency syndrome)—CD4+ T cell count less than 200 cells/mm³ and viral load increases. Diagnosis of AIDS is made when the HIV-positive client develops at least one of the following disease processes.
1. CD4+ T cell count below 200 cells/mm³.
2. AIDS dementia complex.
3. Wasting syndrome caused by HIV.
4. At least one opportunistic cancer—invasive cervical cancer, Kaposi's sarcoma, primary lymphoma of the brain.
5. At least one opportunistic infection—fungal, bacterial, or protozoal infection.

Opportunistic Diseases

A. Diseases and infections that occur in clients with AIDS are called *opportunistic* because they take advantage of the suppressed immune system.
1. The type of infection and its extent varies with each client, depending on the extent of immunosuppression.
2. Single opportunistic infections are rare; a client usually has multiple infections.
B. Infections may be delayed or prevented by antiretroviral therapy, vaccines (hepatitis B, influenza, and pneumococcal), and disease-specific prevention.
C. *Coccidioides jiroveci* pneumonia, *Pneumocystis jirovecii* pneumonia (previously called *Pneumocystis carinii* PCP).
1. May be caused by a pathogen in the body that is dormant.
2. Is not common in healthy individuals; immune system must be compromised for the infection to occur.
3. Symptoms: fever, night sweats, nonproductive cough, progressive dyspnea.
D. Tuberculosis (see Chapter 15).
E. Fungal infections: histoplasmosis (pneumonia, meningitis), coccidioidomycosis (pneumonia).
F. Kaposi's sarcoma: a bruised, dry-appearing skin lesion; may be present internally as well.
G. Candidiasis of the esophagus, mouth, vagina.

Diagnostics

A. HIV-antibody testing.
1. Enzyme immunoassay testing (EIA): detects the serum antibodies that bind to the HIV antigens. After the acute HIV invasion, an increase in the viral load and a decrease in CD4+ count occur; the client begins to develop antibodies to the HIV. If client has history of recent exposure, retesting is recommended at 3 weeks, 6 weeks, and 3 months.
2. If the EIA test result is positive, then it is repeated; if it remains positive, the Western blot (WB) and immunofluorescence assay (IFA) tests are done to confirm the HIV-positive results.
3. If the EIA is consistently positive and the WB and IFA results are positive, the client is considered to be HIV-antibody positive.

B. Rapid HIV tests—ready in minutes, but results are preliminary and must be confirmed; client needs to return for an antibody-based test (Western blot) 2-4 months later.
1. The OraQuick Rapid HIV-1 Antibody Test and the Reveal Rapid HIV-1 Antibody Test measure HIV antibodies in the blood.
2. OraQuick ADVANCE Rapid HIV-1/2 Antibody Test measures HIV antibodies in the saliva.
C. CD4+ T cell (receptor cell on the T4 helper cell) count: below 200 cells/mm^3 in an HIV-positive client indicates progression to acute HIV infection (T4, T4 helper, and CD4+ are synonymous terms).
D. Serum monitoring after diagnosis.
1. CD4+ T cell counts and plasma assays (HIV RNA viral load).
2. Evaluation for drug resistance.

Treatment

A. Medications: antiretroviral therapy (ART) (Appendix 7-1).
1. Prescribed according to the viral load and the CD4+ T cell counts.
2. Combination of at least two different drug classes.
3. Women should begin ART even if they are pregnant.
4. Combination drug therapy attacks virus at different stages of replication.
B. Medications do not cure the client, but decrease the viral replication and slow disease process.
C. Adherence to drug schedules is critical—nonadherence to drug regimen can lead to mutations of the virus and increased virus resistance.

> **! NURSING PRIORITY** Frequently, the treatment for the client with AIDS causes problems in other areas: the high-dose antibiotics may increase the level of leukopenia, and the chemotherapy medications will further decrease the bone marrow functions. The client with AIDS receiving chemotherapy will be even further immunosuppressed.

Nursing Interventions

See Nursing Interventions for immunocompromised clients.
Goal: To provide and promote client and public education regarding transmission of HIV.

> **! NURSING PRIORITY** Public and client teaching regarding the transmission of the HIV is vital in the control of this disease. The period of time from when the client is infected until the condition is diagnosed is when the majority of new infections are transmitted.

A. Safe sex.
1. Maintain monogamous relationships.
2. Sex with female or male prostitutes is a high-risk activity.
3. Avoid all direct contact with a partner's mouth, penis, vagina, or rectum if the HIV status of the partner is not known.

4. Avoid all sexual activities that cause cuts or tears in the vagina, on the penis, or in the rectum.
5. Males should wear a condom if multiple partners are involved.
6. If the HIV status of a sexual partner is not known, a condom should always be used during intercourse.
7. Anyone who has been involved in any high-risk sexual activities or who has injected IV recreational drugs should have a blood test to determine presence of the HIV.
B. Needles should not be recapped or shared. Dispose of them in an impenetrable sealed container.

 Home Care

A. An employee in a health care setting should advise employer of HIV-positive status.
B. Kitchen and bathroom facilities may be shared, provided that normal sanitary practices are observed.
C. Clean up spills of body fluids or waste immediately with a solution of 1 part bleach to 10 parts water. A bleach solution can be used to disinfect kitchen and bathroom floors, showers, sinks, and toilet bowls.
D. Towels and washcloths should not be shared without laundering.
E. Sanitary napkins, tampons, and any bloody dressings should be wrapped in a plastic bag and placed in a trash container.
F. Needles should not be recapped. Dispose of them in an impenetrable sealed container.
G. Do not donate blood or plasma, body organs, or semen.

Pediatric Acquired Immunodeficiency Syndrome

The majority of children with AIDS were infected in the perinatal period. Cases related to blood transfusions are relatively rare.

> **! NURSING PRIORITY** HIV-positive mothers should not breastfeed their infants.

Assessment

A. Risk factors.
1. Pediatric infection from transfused blood is virtually nonexistent.
2. Sexual activity and IV drug use are the major causes of HIV infection in adolescents.
3. Infants born to mothers who are HIV-positive account for the majority of children with HIV infection; ART therapy during pregnancy reduces risk for transmission to fetus.
4. Children rarely have Kaposi's sarcoma; PCP is most common opportunistic infection.
B. Clinical manifestations.
1. Infants affected during the prenatal period have rapid disease progression.
2. HIV-positive infants usually have symptoms by 18 to 24 months of age.

3. Infants diagnosed within the first year of life have a poor prognosis, as do those who develop *Pneumocystis jirovecii pneumonia* (PCP), and progressive encephalopathy.
4. Symptoms include lymphadenopathy, hepatosplenomegaly, oral candidiasis, chronic diarrhea, and failure to thrive.
5. Severe symptoms include the AIDS-defining illnesses such as PCP, wasting syndrome, HIV encephalopathy, *Candida* esophagitis, and cryptosporidiosis.
6. Immune categories are based on CD4+ counts; these are age-adjusted.

Diagnostics

A. EIA and WB for children 18 months or older.
B. Newborn: polymerase chain reaction (PCR); p24 antigen detection; majority of infants who are HIV-positive can be identified by 3 months of age.
C. Maternal antibodies to the HIV may persist for up to 18 months.
D. Positive results on two separate occasions and from separate blood specimens for p24 antigen detection, polymerase chain reaction, and virus culture are required to confirm diagnosis of HIV infection.

Treatment

Treatment for children is essentially the same as that for an adult.

Nursing Interventions Specific to Children

Goal: To maintain homeostasis.
A. Infants and children should receive the standard immunizations against childhood diseases. Measles-mumps-rubella (MMR) and varicella (chicken pox) vaccines may be given if the child is not severely immunocompromised.
B. Pneumococcal and influenza vaccines are recommended.
C. Nutritional support; high-calorie, high-protein diet.
D. Antifungal medications to prevent fungal infections.
E. Educate adolescents regarding safe sex.

Home Care

A. Teach parent(s) how to care for the child.
1. How to administer medications and importance of administering medications as scheduled.
2. Symptoms of complications: PCP, *Candida*, failure to thrive.
3. Teach parents standard precautions, including proper handling of diapers and avoidance of contact with blood and body fluids.
4. Prevent biting behaviors in young children.
5. Help parents deal with child's pain—multiple procedures, infections (abscessed tooth, otitis media).
   a. Aggressive management of pain with NSAIDs, opioids, muscle relaxants.
   b. Ongoing assessment of pain in nonverbal children—irritability, lack of interaction, lack of play.

B. Teach parents how to prevent transmission of disease.
C. Course of disease in infants and children is very unpredictable.
D. Work with school personnel to maintain privacy/confidentiality.
E. Promote normal growth and development.

Nursing Interventions for Immunocompromised Clients

Goal: To monitor for and/or prevent opportunistic infections.
A. The type, location, and severity of the infection depend on the disease progress and the client's immunosuppressive state.
B. Antimicrobial medications are given in high doses for an extended period. Medications may cause neutropenia.
C. Protect from iatrogenic infections or hospital-associated infections.
D. Observe hospitalized client and/or teach client symptoms of opportunistic infections.
   1. Persistent unexplained fever, night sweats.
   2. Thrush (white spots in the mouth).
   3. Persistent diarrhea and weight loss.

Goal: To maintain ventilation and prevent pulmonary involvement.
A. PCP prophylaxis may be maintained with trimethoprim-sulfamethoxazole.
B. Rifabutin is used for *Mycobacterium avium* prophylaxis.
C. Frequent assessments for pulmonary changes and hypoxemia.
D. Activities may be unlimited, or bed rest may be prescribed.
E. Supplemental oxygen.
F. Coughing and deep-breathing exercises.
G. Carefully evaluate respiratory function if narcotic analgesics are used.
H. Assess activity tolerance.

Goal: To assist client to minimize the effects of neurologic changes.
A. Frequent assessment of neurologic status.
B. Assess for visual changes.
C. Observe for neurologic infections, specifically meningitis.
D. If client is confused, provide care directed to reorientation.
E. Provide a safe and supportive environment, according to the neurologic deficits.

Goal: To maintain adequate nutritional intake.
A. Teach client regarding nutrition and caloric intake (high-calorie, high-protein diet; nutrition to correct deficiencies).
B. Encourage high-calorie snacks throughout the day.
C. Encourage client to eat several small meals throughout the day.
D. May need to include dietary supplements.
E. Assess client for lactose intolerance.
F. Avoid foods or beverages that may cause oral, esophageal, or gastric irritation.

G. Tube feedings or parenteral nutrition may be necessary.

Goal: To maintain fluid and electrolyte status.
A. Evaluate weight gain and loss.
B. Assess for chronic diarrhea.
C. Encourage fluids that assist in maintaining electrolyte balance.

Goal: To prevent formation of pressure ulcers and excoriation of the skin.
A. Wash perineal and anal areas; allow areas to dry thoroughly.
B. Observe bony prominence for adequacy of circulation and development of a pressure ulcer.
C. Do not put any lotions on reddened areas or open lesions.
D. Teach client the importance of frequent changes in position.
E. Use gel pads, foam mattress pads, and other devices to prevent skin breakdown in pressure prone areas (heels and sacrum).

Goal: To assist client to maintain psychologic equilibrium.
A. Encourage client to express feelings and concerns.
B. Assess for altered self-esteem, family stress, and economic pressures; provide referrals and assistance.

C. Encourage client to maintain as much independence as possible.
D. Help client take advantage of community services available.
E. Do not be judgmental regarding client's lifestyle.
F. Maintain frequent contact with the client.

Home Care for the Immunocompromised Client

A. Maintain personal hygiene and practice standard precautions; wash hands frequently.
B. Do not share personal items such as toothbrushes, razors, and enema equipment.
C. Teach client how to prevent infection.
  1. Cook all vegetables and meats, and peel fruit before eating; this eliminates many sources of microorganisms.
  2. Avoid contact with animal waste (e.g., litter boxes, bird cages, or fish); this further decreases contact with microorganisms.
  3. Avoid crowds and people with respiratory tract infections.
D. Do not get pregnant.

Appendix 7-1   ANTIRETROVIRAL THERAPY (ART)

General Nursing Implications
— Highly active antiretroviral therapy (HAART) used for treatment of clients with HIV and AIDS.
— Report any sore throat, fever, or other signs of infection to health care provider.
— Very important to administer the medication at the same time each day to maintain consistent blood levels and to decrease drug resistance.
— No vaccines or immunity-conferring agents while client is immunosuppressed.
— Maintain standard precautions, use contact, droplet, and airborne precautions as indicated.
— Medications do not cure AIDS or reduce the risk for transmission.

MEDICATIONS	SIDE EFFECTS	NURSING IMPLICATIONS
Nonnucleoside Reverse Transcriptase Inhibitors (NNRTIs): All bind directly to the HIV transcriptase and inhibit the enzyme.		
Nevirapine **(Viramune, NVP):** PO	Rash (may be severe—blistering, joint pain, oral lesions), hepatotoxic, hepatitis	Viramune: Monitor LFTs; rash may be so severe that drug is discontinued.
Delavirdine **(Rescriptor, DLV):** PO	Rash (may be severe), hepatotoxic, GI symptoms	Rescriptor: Monitor LFTs; rash may be so severe that drug is discontinued.
Efavirenz **(Sustiva, EFV):** PO	Rash, hepatotoxic, teratogenic, CNS symptoms	Sustiva: Monitor LFTs; avoid pregnancy, avoid taking with St John's wort.

Appendix 7-1 ANTIRETROVIRAL THERAPY (ART)—cont'd

Nucleoside/Nucleotide Reverse Transcriptase Inhibitors (NRTIs): All NTRIs suppress the synthesis of viral DNA by reverse transcriptase. Medications are given with other antiretroviral agents; they are not used alone due to rapid development of resistance.

MEDICATIONS	SIDE EFFECTS	NURSING IMPLICATIONS
Didanosine **(Videx):** PO	Nausea, diarrhea, peripheral neuropathy, liver damage, pancreatitis.	Food decreases absorption; give on empty stomach 30 min before eating or 2 hr after.
Stavudine **(Zerit):** PO	Pancreatitis, lactic acidosis, diarrhea, peripheral neuropathy	Report peripheral neuropathy; do not use in pregnancy.
Zidovudine **(ZDV, Retrovir, AZT, azidothymidine):** PO, IV	Bone marrow suppression, anemia, neutropenia	Maintain upright position to decrease esophageal irritation; monitor levels of anemia and neutropenia.
Lamivudine **(Epivir):** PO	Headache, nausea, malaise/fatigue, diarrhea	St. John's wort may decrease concentration.
Abacavir **(Ziagen):** PO	Hypersensitivity, pulmonary problems.	ETOH increases risk for hypersensitivity reactions; report respiratory changes.

Protease Inhibitors (PIs): Bind to the active site of the HIV and render the virus immature and noninfectious; are not given alone due to development of increased resistance.
Adverse effects of all PIs: Fat maldistribution, hyperlipidemia, hyperglycemia, bone loss, hepatotoxic.
Shared interactions: St John's wort, decreases the effectiveness of PIs.

MEDICATIONS	SIDE EFFECTS	NURSING IMPLICATIONS
Saquinavir **(Fortovase, Invirase):** PO	GI affects, headache	Do not give with grapefruit juice; take with food; check for drug interactions.
Ritonavir **(Norvir):** PO	GI discomfort, perioral paresthesia	Food increases levels; take with food for tolerance.
Indinavir **(Crixivan):** PO	GI discomfort, renal damage	Take 1 hr before or 2 hours after meals.
Nelfinavir **(Viracept):** PO	Diarrhea, rash	Take with food.
Amprenavir **(Agenerase):** PO	N/V, diarrhea, rash,	Contraindicated in pregnancy, renal or hepatic failure; high-fat meals decrease absorption.
Lopinavir/ritonavir **(Kaletra):** PO	N/V, diarrhea, increased fatigue	Moderate fat meal increases absorption; take with food.

HIV Fusion Inhibitor: Blocks entry of HIV into CD4 T cells.

MEDICATIONS	SIDE EFFECTS	NURSING IMPLICATIONS
Enfuvirtide **(Fuzeon, T-20):** subQ	Injection site reaction, bacterial pneumonia, hypersensitivity reactions	Use small-gauge needle to decrease skin reaction; monitor respiratory status.

AIDS, Acquired immunodeficiency syndrome; *GI,* gastrointestinal; *HIV,* human immunodeficiency virus; *IV,* intravenous; *PO,* by mouth (orally); *subQ,* subcutaneous.

Appendix 7-2   MEDICATIONS FOR ALLERGIC REACTIONS

MEDICATIONS | **SIDE EFFECTS** | **NURSING IMPLICATIONS**

Antihistamines: Selectively block histamine receptor sites.

H₁—First Generation

Diphenhydramine (**Benadryl**): PO, IM, IV
Clemastine (**Tavist Allergy**): PO
Promethazine (**Phenergan**): PO, IV, IM

	Side	Nursing

Dry mouth, dizziness, blurred vision, urinary retention, constipation, and sedation
Children: paradoxic reactions

1. Advise client not to engage in activity that requires mental alertness for safety.
2. Should not take medication with alcohol.
3. Should not be used in clients with asthma.

H₁—Second Generation

Cetirizine (**Zyrtec**): PO
Fexofenadine (**Allegra**): PO
Loratadine (**Claritin**): PO

Dry mouth and throat
Paradoxic reaction in children

1. Second generation is nonsedating.
2. Do not have anticholinergic properties of first generation.
3. Should not be taken with alcohol.
4. Are much more expensive than first generation.

Nasal Sprays

Fluticasone (**Flonase, Flovent**)
Triamcinolone (**Nasacort**)

Nasopharyngeal irritation

1. Teach client to clear nasal passages before using.
2. Hold spray bottle upright and insert tip into nostril.
3. Used to treat allergic rhinitis.

Adrenergic Agonist: Stimulates alpha₁, alpha₂, beta₁, and beta₂ adrenergic receptors.
Action: Relaxes smooth muscle of bronchial tree (decreases respiratory distress), cardiac stimulant (increases cardiac rate), produces vasoconstriction (increases blood pressure), drug of choice for anaphylactic reactions.

Epinephrine (**Adrenalin, EpiPen**): subQ, IV
1%—1:100—oral inhalation
0.1%—1:1,000—subQ, IM
0.01%—1:10,000—IV, intracardiac.

Hypertension, dysrhythmias, angina, hyperglycemia
Necrosis at IV site if extravasation occurs

1. Clients at risk for anaphylaxis should carry emergency epinephrine (EpiPen).
2. EpiPen—sensitive to extreme heat and light; discard if it is brown in color, has a precipitate, or has passed its expiration date.
3. Advise clients to obtain medical assistance immediately if epinephrine is used.
4. 0.1 to 0.5 mL of 1:1000 dilution subQ or IM is used for mild to moderate reaction.
5. 0.5 mL of 1:10,000 dilution subcutaneously or IV is used for severe reactions and advanced cardiac life support.
6. Drug of choice for severe anaphylactic reactions.
7. Closely monitor pulse rate and blood pressure.

Study Questions Immune System

More questions on companion CD!
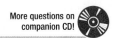

1. To evaluate the progress of the client's systemic lupus erythematosus (SLE), the nurse evaluates which data?
   1 Increased serum complement fixation, which correlates with reduction of "butterfly" rash
   2 Increasing levels of C-reactive protein (CRP) and erythrocyte sedimentation rate (ESR)
   3 Overall bone marrow proliferation, which correlates with symptoms of inflammation
   4 Presence of antinuclear antibodies (ANA), which correlates with a diminishing immune process

2. The mother of a 15-month-old child who is immunosuppressed asks about continuation of the childhood vaccines. Which immunizations are not recommended to be given to the child during immunosuppression?
   1 Diphtheria, tetanus, and pertussis (DTaP); hepatitis B
   2 *Haemophilus influenzae* B
   3 Varicella; measles, mumps, and rubella (MMR)
   4 Inactivated polio; diphtheria, tetanus, and pertussis (DTaP)

3. A client returns to the clinic to receive evaluation of his routine purified protein derivative (PPD) test for tuberculosis screening. The test result is positive. What is the best nursing interpretation of this information?
   1 This is a serious type II reaction and could indicate that he has active tuberculosis; he will need further evaluation immediately.
   2 The positive results indicate the client has been exposed to the tuberculosis bacilli and has had a delayed type IV response.
   3 The client's immune system has been compromised, which allows the immune system to build up antibodies against the pathogen.
   4 An autoimmune response has occurred and the client will need further evaluation to determine appropriate treatment.

4. A nurse is caring for a client who received a penicillin injection about 15 minutes earlier. The client complains of tingling around the mouth, and this rapidly progresses to severe dyspnea and respiratory distress. What are the priority nursing actions?
   1 Anticipate need for possibility of endotracheal intubation, begin oxygen, call for assistance, and obtain emergency cart.
   2 Place the client in supine position and assess for patent airway and presence of breath sounds.
   3 Start oxygen at 6 L/min via nasal cannula; review chart for history of a penicillin allergy.
   4 Place the client in semi-Fowler's position, perform a chin-lift to open the airway, and assess for air movement.

5. The nurse is administering medications to a client who has no allergy band on his arm. The nurse tells the client she has his penicillin medication. The client states that the last time he had penicillin, it made his mouth tingle and his hands itch. What would be the best nursing action?
   1 Administer the medication since there is no indication that the client is allergic to penicillin.
   2 Hold the medication and contact the physician regarding the client's statement about his previous experience with penicillin.
   3 Hold the medication and review the clients chart to determine whether there is a penicillin allergy noted.
   4 Notify the nursing supervisor regarding the client's statement and request further evaluation of the client.

6. A client has systemic lupus erythematosus (SLE). What statement best describes this client's immune response?
   1 A delayed hypersensitivity that is cell-mediated
   2 An immediate reaction to prior exposure
   3 An immune complex that forms with antibody production
   4 An immune response that no longer recognizes normal body tissue

7. A client is diagnosed with an immunodeficiency disease. The nurse would understand what as characteristic of this condition?
   1 Occurs when a client's body is unable to defend itself from an invading microorganism
   2 Creates a severe, sudden problem that is characterized by increased vascular permeability
   3 Is precipitated by the destruction of the normal lymphocytes in the attempt to reduce the serum level of the antigen
   4 Is a condition in which the normal immune response is interrupted and the body cells do not recognize healthy tissue

8. An infant has an acquired active immunity. Which statement best explains this type of immunity?
   1 The infant has received immunizations.
   2 Immunity was transferred from the mother to the infant.
   3 The infant is recovering from a childhood disease that conferred immunity.
   4 The infant has received gamma globulin after exposure to hepatitis.

9. The nurse is preparing discharge teaching for a woman newly diagnosed with SLE. What will be important for the nurse to include in the teaching plan? Select all that apply.
   ____ 1 Wear sunscreen and protective clothing when in direct sunlight.
   ____ 2 Avoid nonsteroidal antiinflammatory drugs to prevent bleeding episodes.
   ____ 3 Plan activities that encourage range of motion in extremities.
   ____ 4 Advise the client that pregnancy is contraindicated.

____ 5 Observe fingertips for changes in circulation.

____ 6 Help the client prioritize self-care activity.

10. A client with a diagnosis of AIDS has developed *Pneumocystis jirovecii* pneumonia (PCP). What will be important for the nurse to include in the nursing care plan?
    1 Put a mask on the client whenever he has visitors in his room.
    2 Explain to the client why he cannot go outside his room.
    3 Wear a mask and gown when providing direct care to the client.
    4 Wear a gown and gloves when assisting the client with personal hygiene.

11. A client is worried he may have been exposed to AIDS. What will be important for the nurse to explain to this client?
    1 Symptoms of AIDS will develop immediately in sexually active individuals.
    2 Clients may remain asymptomatic for an indefinite period of time.
    3 Symptoms of AIDS are usually seen before the client is found to be HIV-positive.
    4 After exposure to the virus, symptoms may develop within 6 to 12 weeks or as late as 6 months.

12. The nurse is caring for a client who is categorized as HIV-positive, acute infection. What would the nurse anticipate finding on the nursing assessment?
    1 Fatigue, weight loss, night sweats
    2 Confusion, disorientation, loss of coordination
    3 Dyspnea, tachycardia on exertion, fever
    4 Red, raised lesions on neck and face, fever

13. A woman explains to the nurse that she thinks she has been exposed to the HIV. However, she had a test 1 week after the exposure and the result was negative. What is most important for the nurse to explain to this client?
    1 Make sure she understands the importance of safe sex practices, especially the use of condoms and contraceptive practices to prevent pregnancy.
    2 Even though the client tested negative, she needs to have a series of follow-up blood tests because of the possibility of seroconversion.
    3 It is important that she obtain counseling regarding the transmission of the virus and how she may protect herself and her partner.
    4 The client should abstain from sexual activity for the next 3 months until the blood test confirms that she is negative for HIV.

14. A client is experiencing difficulty breathing, periorbital swelling, flushing, and itching. He had a diagnostic test in which an iodine-based dye was used about an hour earlier. What medication will the nurse anticipate administering immediately?
    1 A bronchodilator such as aminophylline (Theophylline)
    2 A corticosteroid such as dexamethasone (Decadron)

3 An antihistamine such as diphenhydramine (Benadryl)
4 An adrenergic agonist such as epinephrine (Adrenalin)

15. The nurse is reviewing with a certified nursing assistant (CNA) the care for a child who is diagnosed with acquired immunodeficiency syndrome (AIDS) and has developed *Pneumocystis* pneumonia. Which of the following precautions would the nurse review with the CNA?
    1 Strict handwashing
    2 Airborne precautions
    3 Contact precautions
    4 Standard precautions

16. The nurse is assisting a client with his antiretroviral therapy. What can the nurse do to help the client take his medications as prescribed?
    1 Assess the client's activities of daily living and his lifestyle routine to determine when he can most easily remember to take his medications.
    2 Provide the client with brochures that explain the side effects of the medications and why it is so important for him to adhere to his medication schedule.
    3 Plan for him to visit with other clients who use the same antiretroviral therapy and have them explain to the client how they handle their medications.
    4 Emphasize to the client how important it is to take the medications on the schedule prescribed so that the virus will not get stronger.

17. The nurse is caring for a client who is experiencing a severe anaphylactic reaction caused by an allergy to peanuts. After administering subcutaneous epinephrine and beginning oxygen administration, what would be the next most important nursing action?
    1 Administer analgesics to relieve the pain.
    2 Start an IV for fluid administration.
    3 Insert a catheter to determine urinary output.
    4 Obtain a history of possible reactions to penicillin.

18. A client with AIDS has several cutaneous lesions identified as Kaposi's sarcoma. How will the nurse care for these areas?
    1 Gently cleanse the areas, keeping them dry and free of abrasions.
    2 Place sterile, saline-soaked gauze over the areas.
    3 Apply a topical corticosteroid cream.
    4 Decrease infection by applying an antibiotic ointment.

Answers and rationales to these questions are in the section at the end of the book titled Chapter Study Questions: Answers and Rationales.

CHAPTER EIGHT

Abnormal Cell Growth

CHARACTERISTICS OF CANCER

Cancer must be regarded as a group of disease entities with different causes, manifestations, treatments, and prognoses. The basic disease process begins when normal cells undergo change and begin to proliferate in an abnormal manner.

Major Dysfunction in the Cell

A. Cellular proliferation: cancer cells divide in an indiscriminate, unregulated manner and exhibit significant variations in structure and size.

B. Loss of contact inhibition: cells have no regard for cellular boundaries; normal cells respect boundaries and do not invade adjacent areas or organs.

C. Cancer can arise from any cell in the body that can evade the normal regulatory controls of proliferation or growth and cellular differentiation.

D. Cell biology.
  1. *Predetermined* means that the stem cell of specific tissue will differentiate and mature for only that tissue.
  2. A state of equilibrium is constantly being maintained between cellular proliferation and cellular degeneration.
  3. Cancer cells divide indiscriminately.

E. Tumors (neoplasms).
  1. Benign: encapsulated neoplasm that remains localized in the tissue of origin and is typically not harmful.
     a. Exerts pressure on surrounding organs.
     b. Will decrease blood supply to the normal tissue.
  2. Malignant: nonencapsulated neoplasm that invades surrounding tissue. Depends on the stage of the neoplasm as to whether metastasis (spreading to distant body parts) occurs. Four primary mechanisms by which the neoplasm spreads (Figure 8-1).
     a. Vascular system: cancer cells penetrate vessels and circulate until trapped. The cancer cells may penetrate the vessel wall and invade adjacent organs and tissues.
     b. Lymphatic system: cancer cells penetrate the lymphatic system and are distributed along lymphatic channels.
     c. Implantation: cancer cells implant into a body organ. Certain cells have an affinity for particular organs and body areas.
     d. Seeding: a primary tumor sloughs off tumor cells into a body cavity, such as the peritoneal cavity.
  3. Common sites for metastasis: brain, liver, lungs, spinal cord, and bone.

Etiology

A. Viruses: incorporate into the genetic structure of the cell causing mutations (e.g., Kaposi's sarcoma from HIV; hepatitis B virus and hepatocellular cancer; human papilloma virus and cervical cancer).

B. Radiation: exposure to sunlight and radiation (bone cancer in radiologists; increased incidence of cancer in children who were exposed to radiation during fetal development).

C. Chemical agents: produce toxic effects by altering DNA structure in body cells (e.g., dyes, asbestos, tars, tobacco use, chronic irritation or inflammation); there may be an extended latency period from time of exposure to development of the cancer.

D. Genetic and familial factors: DNA damage occurs in cells where chromosomal patterns are abnormal, which increases the individual's susceptibility to cancer.

E. Hormonal agents: tumor growth is promoted by disturbances in hormonal balance of the body's own (endogenous) hormones or administration of exogenous hormones (e.g., prolonged estrogen replacement, oral contraceptives).

F. Idiopathic: many cancers—e.g., breast, colon, rectal, lymphatic, bone marrow, and pancreatic cancers—arise spontaneously from unknown causes.

Prevention

A. Cancer prevention.
  1. Eat a balanced diet that includes fresh fruits and vegetables, adequate amount of fiber, and decreased fats and preservatives; avoid smoked and salt-cured foods containing increased nitrates (see Figure 2-4).
  2. Avoid exposure to known carcinogens—e.g., cigarette smoking and sun exposure.

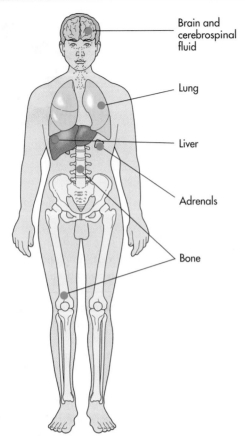

FIGURE 8-1 Pathogenesis of blood-borne metastasis. (From Lewis SL et al: *Medical-surgical nursing: assessment and management of clinical problems,* ed 7, St. Louis, 2007, Mosby.)

3. Keep weight in normal range: obesity is associated with cancer of uterus, gallbladder, breast, and colon.
4. Get enough rest and sleep—at least 6 to 8 hours per night.
5. Decreased stress, or perception of stress, improves ability to effectively manage stress.
6. Engage in at least 30 minutes of moderate to vigorous exercise 5 days a week.
7. Limit alcohol use.

B. Screening guidelines—early detection.
1. Pap test: screening should begin within 3 years of becoming sexually active or at age 21; thereafter should be done annually or every 2 years. Age 30, after 3 normal Pap tests, then Pap screening every 3-4 years.
2. Digital rectal examination (DRE): DRE with prostate-specific antigen blood test should be offered to men annually beginning at age 50. African-American males and those men with strong family history should begin at age 45.
3. Colon: beginning at age 50, all clients should have either a yearly fecal occult blood test or a flexible sigmoidoscopy every 5 years and/or both, depending on the client's risk factors.
4. Breast: annual mammogram and clinical breast exam (CBE) for women over 40. Women ages 20-39 should have a CBE every 3 years. Monthly breast self-

examination is an option for women in their 20s, but *does not replace* need for CBE or mammogram (see Chapter 22).
5. Testicular self-examination: monthly from age 20 to 40 (see Chapter 22).

Classification of Malignant Tumors

A. Cellular origin or anatomic classification: tumor is identified by the tissue of origin.
1. Epithelial tissue (*-carcinoma*): surface epithelium—carcinoma; glandular epithelium—adenocarcinoma.
2. Connective tissue (*-sarcoma*): cartilage—chondrosarcoma; striated muscle bone—rhabdomyosarcoma; fibrous tissue—fibrosarcoma; bone—osteosarcoma.
3. Nervous system tissue (*-oma*): meninges—meningeal sarcoma; nerve cells—neuroblastoma.
4. Hematopoietic tissue (*-oma*): lymphoid tumors—Hodgkin's lymphoma; plasma cells—multiple myeloma; bone marrow—lymphocytic and myelogenous leukemia.

B. TNM classification (staging) (Box 8-1).

TREATMENT OF CANCER

Diagnostics

A. Common cancer diagnostic studies.
1. Chest x-ray.
2. Tissue biopsy.
3. Radiologic studies: mammography, ultrasonography.

Box 8-1 TNM STAGING CLASSIFICATION

T: Tumor size
N: Degree of involvement of lymph nodes
M: Absence or presence of metastasis

T: Primary Tumor
TX: Tumor can't be measured or found
T0: No evidence of primary tumor
Tis: Cancer is in situ (tumor has not started growing into the surrounding structures)
T1-T4: Describe the size and/or level of invasion into nearby structures—the higher the T number, the larger the tumor and/or the further it may have grown into nearby structures

N: Regional Lymph Nodes
NX: Nearby lymph nodes can't be measured or found
N0: Nearby lymph nodes do not contain cancer
N1-N3: Describe the size, location, and/or the number of lymph nodes involved—the higher the N number, the more lymph nodes are involved

M: Distant Metastasis
MX: Metastasis can't be measured or found
M0: No known distant metastases
M1: Distant metastases present
Example: Tis, NX, M0-cancer in situ; unable to clinically assess distant lymph nodes; no evidence of distant metastasis

Adapted from American Joint Committee on Cancer: *What is cancer staging?* Available at www.cancerstaging.org/whatis.html. Accessed October 2008.

4. Radioisotopic scans: bone, liver, lung, brain.
5. Spiral computed tomography (CT).
6. Cytology studies (bone marrow aspiration, urine and cerebrospinal fluid analysis, cell washings, Pap smears and bronchial washings).
7. Position emission tomography (PET) scan.
8. Tumor markers.
9. Sigmoidoscopy or colonoscopy examinations—including stool for occult blood.
10. CBC, chemistry profile, liver function tests.
11. Bone marrow examination (if hematolymphoid malignancy is suspected).

ALERT Assist client in maintaining an optimum level of health; evaluate incorporation of healthy behaviors into lifestyle (screening, immunizations); instruct client on ways to promote health.

B. Biopsy.
1. Used for definitive diagnosis.
2. Needle: tissue samples are obtained by aspiration or with a large-bore needle.
3. Incisional: a scalpel or dermal punch is used to obtain a tissue sample.
4. Excisional: involves removal of the entire tumor.
5. Endoscopic biopsy: direct biopsy through an endoscopy of the area (gastrointestinal, respiratory, genitourinary tracts).

Goals of Cancer Therapy

A. Prophylaxis: to provide treatment when no tumor is detectable but when client is known to be at risk for tumor development, spread, or recurrence.
B. Control: client's cancer is not cured but controlled by therapy over long periods of time.
C. Cure: client will be disease-free and live to normal life expectancy.
D. Palliative: to maintain as high a quality of life for the client as possible when cure and control are not possible.

Modalities of Cancer Treatment

NURSING PRIORITY Therapy generally involves using two or more modalities of treatment.

A. Surgery.
1. Diagnostic surgery: obtains tissue samples (biopsies) for diagnostic purposes and to determine methods of treatment.
2. Clinical staging surgery: determines the extent of the cancer; presence and location of metastatic lesions.
3. Curative and/or control surgery: removal of cancers that are localized to the area of origin; extent of resection determined by the type and spread of tumor.
4. Palliative surgery: does not impair the growth or spread of the cancer but improves the client's quality of life. May be done to relieve pain, decrease obstruction, relieve pressure, and/or to prevent hemorrhage.
5. Supportive care: surgeries to support cancer treatment (e.g. suprapubic cystostomy for prostate cancer, feeding tubes).
6. Reconstructive surgery: restoration of the client's form, function, and appearance after radical surgery for cancer.
7. Preventive surgery: for clients who are in a high-risk category, certain surgical procedures may prevent the future development of cancer (e.g. prophylactic mastectomy).

B. Chemotherapy: overall goal of chemotherapy is to destroy the cancer cells without excessively damaging the normal cells (Appendix 8-1).

NURSING PRIORITY The therapeutic ratio is the guiding principle of chemotherapy. The aim is to administer an antineoplastic agent dose large enough to eradicate cancer cells but small enough to limit adverse effects to safe and tolerable levels.

1. Medications are highly toxic and destroy healthy cells, as well as cancer cells.
2. Combination chemotherapy is more effective than single-dose therapy.
3. Adjuvant therapy: after the initial therapy (surgical or radiation), medications are used to eliminate or slow replication of any remaining cancer cells. For example, tamoxifen may be given in the early stages of breast cancer to block the effects of estrogen, thereby helping to prevent the development of cancer in the other breast.
4. Myelosuppressive effects usually peak in 7 to 10 days after chemotherapy, causing low platelet counts as well as critically low white blood cell counts (leukopenia/neutropenia). The period of time when client is at the lowest level of neutrophil count is called the nadir; this represents the point at which the client is at the highest risk for infection.

ALERT Follow procedures for handling biohazardous materials (e.g., chemotherapeutic agents, radiation sources).

5. Vascular access methods of administration (Appendix 6-10).
   a. Peripherally inserted central catheters (PICC): external access central lines.
   b. Tunneled venous access port: catheter is tunneled from exit site to the venous insertion site (Port-A-Cath, Hickman catheter, or Groshong catheter).
   c. Implanted infusion venous access port: a single or double subcutaneous injection port is connected to a central venous catheter. The catheter is placed in a vein, and the other end is connected to a port that is sutured or implanted into the chest wall.

C. Regional chemotherapy.
1. Intrathecal or intraventricular: a surgically implanted device positioned under the scalp; used to deliver

chemotherapy to the cerebrospinal fluid (e.g. Ommaya reservoir).

2. Intraperitoneal: delivery of chemotherapy into the peritoneal cavity.
3. Intraarterial: catheter placed into an artery and then connected to an infusion pump.

D. Nursing interventions in chemotherapy (Table 8-1).
   1. Assess client for symptoms of bone marrow depression (increased bruising and bleeding, sore throat, fever, increased fatigue).
   2. Prevent exposure of client to people with communicable diseases or infections.
   3. Before therapy, establish a baseline regarding intake and output, bowel habits, oral hygiene, psychologic status, and family relationships.
   4. Monitor intake and output; maintain adequate hydration to prevent urinary complications.
   5. Inform client that alopecia, if it occurs, is usually transient.
   6. Some chemotherapeutic medications are highly irritant (vesicant) and must be administered intravenously into an area of high blood flow (central venous access lines) to provide rapid dilution.

E. Radiation therapy: radiation destroys the cell's ability to reproduce by damaging the cellular DNA. Cells that are rapidly reproducing are vulnerable to the effects of radiation. Radiation treats select regions of the body to achieve a focused control of the disease.
   1. Types of radiation therapy.
      a. External beam therapy (teletherapy): radiation source is outside the body and directed toward the area of the tumor.
         (1) Decreases the incidence of skin surface damage.
         (2) Client should not wash off the markers for the radiation sites.

> **! NURSING PRIORITY** Clients who receive radiation therapy should not be bathed with soap over the radiation site and should avoid use of lotions and powders.

      b. Internal radiation (brachytherapy, closed therapy, sealed source therapy): the sealed source of radiation is implanted directly into the tumor or into a body cavity around a tumor.
         (1) *Brachy-* means "short distance"—radiation given very close to the tumor, where it can be focused precisely on abnormal cells.
         (2) May be used to treat gynecologic malignancies, as well as lung or head and neck malignancies.
         (3) Sealed sources of radiation are temporarily implanted into the tumor area (Box 8-2).
      c. Unsealed source (radiopharmaceutic or isotope): Radioisotopes may be given intravenously or orally. Body fluids become contaminated.
   2. Adverse effects of radiation therapy.

> **! NURSING PRIORITY** Adverse effects are related to radiation dose delivered within a specified time, method of delivery, and client's overall health status.

      a. Skin reactions.
         (1) Skin erythema, followed by dry desquamation of the skin in the treatment field.
         (2) Wet desquamation, particularly in areas of skinfolds (breast, perineum, axillary); skin may be blistered.
         (3) Loss of hair on the skin in the treatment field.
         (4) Skin pigmentation and discoloration.
      b. Gastrointestinal disturbances are more pronounced when radiation is delivered to area closely associated with the GI tract.
      c. Cystitis when radiation source is near to urinary tract.
      d. Radiation pneumonitis.
      e. Pericarditis may occur when chest wall receives radiation.
   3. Safety precautions to prevent excessive exposure for health care providers (Figure 8-2; also see Box 8-2).
      a. Time: coordinate client care to minimize caregiver's exposure to the client.
      b. Distance: maintain the maximum distance possible to provide client care. Attempt to maintain distance of 6 feet from the source of radiation.
      c. Shielding: in practice, lead shielding is difficult to work with and is generally not necessary if time and distance principles are observed.

> **ALERT** Follow protocol when handling biohazardous materials (e.g., radiation therapy implants, chemotherapeutic agents). Time, distance, and shielding are critical concepts in caring for a client with a radiation implant.

Box 8-2 NURSING CARE FOR CLIENTS WITH SEALED RADIOACTIVE IMPLANTS

- Plan care so minimal time is spent in the room.
- When close care or prolonged care is required, use a lead shield or wear a lead apron.
- Wear a film badge to measure exposure; do not share film badges.
- Mark on the room and the client care record that pregnant women (including nurses), infants, and children under 16 years should not come in contact with the client during treatment.
- Limit visitors to 30 minutes per day and advise them to stay about 6 feet from the client.
- Save all dressings and bed linens until radioactive source is removed; follow guidelines from radiation safety officer.
- Keep long-handled forceps and lead container in the room in case of dislodgment of a radioactive source.

Table 8-1	**NURSING IMPLICATIONS AND CHEMOTHERAPY**

Problem	*Nursing Implications*
Bone marrow suppression: Thrombocytopenia (decreased platelets)	1. Initiate bleeding precautions and observe for bleeding tendency (bruising, hematuria, bleeding gums, etc). 2. Decrease invasive procedures; minimize injections.
Anemia (decreased hemoglobin)	1. Fatigue is normal with chemotherapy; client should report any significant increase in fatigue. 2. Encourage diet high in protein, calories, and iron; administer iron supplements.
Leukopenia (decreased white cells)	1. Advise health care provider regarding any unexplained temperature elevation above 100° F. 2. Monitor neutrophil levels. 3. Protect client from exposure to infections: frequent hand hygiene, location of room, screen visitors, etc. 4. See Goals for Self-Care.
Pulmonary toxicity	1. Monitor for persistent nonproductive cough, fever, exertional dyspnea, and tachypnea. 2. Most cases are cumulative dose related and can be fatal.
Hyperuricemia (increased serum levels of uric acid)	1. Encourage fluid intake up to 3000 mL daily, if allowed. 2. Assess for involvement of the kidney, ureters, and bladder. 3. Allopurinol (Zyloprim) may be used as prevention or as treatment.
Alopecia	1. Encourage client to wear something to cover the scalp (e.g., wig, scarf, turban, hat). 2. Avoid exposure of scalp to sunlight. 3. Do not rub scalp; do not use hair rollers, hair dryers, curlers, or curling irons. 4. Hair usually grows back in 3-4 weeks after chemotherapy; is usually a different texture and color.

Stomatitis (mucositis)	1. Encourage good oral hygiene and frequent oral checks.
	  a. Encourage frequent mouth rinses of saline solution to keep mucous membranes moist.
	  b. Brush teeth with a small, soft toothbrush after every meal and at bedtime.
	  c. Remove dentures to prevent further irritation.
	2. Avoid alcohol, spicy or hot foods; mechanical soft, bland diet may be ordered.
	3. Rinse mouth with antacid solutions or viscous lidocaine for pain control.

GI: anorexia, nausea and vomiting, diarrhea, and constipation	1. Assist client to maintain good nutrition.
	  a. Discuss food preferences with client and dietitian; encourage small, frequent meals.
	  b. Correlate meals with antiemetic medications.
	  c. Encourage family to provide client with favorite foods.
	  d. Increase calories, protein, and iron; encourage supplemental vitamins.
	2. Monitor hydration status and electrolyte imbalances.
	3. Evaluate skin around anal area in the client with diarrhea; prevent excoriation.
	4. May be prone to constipation—maintain high fluid and high fiber intake.
	5. Monitor weight.

Tissue irritation, necrosis, ulceration from infusion therapy	1. Vesicant medications should be administered via a central line to promote dilution of medication. Monitor site for infection. 2. If multiple drugs are administered, flush between each administration.

⚠ NURSING PRIORITY Observe client for side effects of a chemotherapeutic agent. If extravasation occurs with a vesicant medication in a peripheral site:
(a) Stop the infusion: remove any remaining drug in the tubing or needle.
(b) Contact physician and consult hospital policy and precautions for specific medication.
(c) Antidote medication may be instilled directly into the infiltrated area.
(d) Ice or heat may be applied to site, depending on the medication; the extremity may be elevated for the first 24 to 48 hours after extravasation.

GI, Gastrointestinal; *IV*, intravenous.

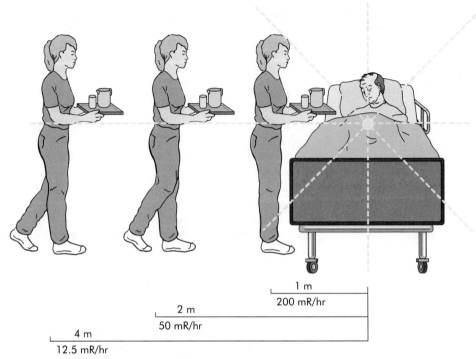

FIGURE 8-2 Radiation safety. The nurse nearest the source of radioactivity (the client) is more exposed. Radiation is subject to the inverse-square law. If a person stands 2 meters away from the source of radiation, he or she will receive one-fourth as much exposure as when standing only 1 meter away. At 4 meters, only one-sixteenth of the exposure is received. (From Monahan FD et al: *Phipps' medical-surgical nursing: health and illness perspectives,* ed 8, St. Louis, 2007, Mosby.)

4. Nursing implications for client receiving external radiation.
   a. Explain that skin reactions after radiation therapy may not develop for 10 to 14 days and may not subside until 2 to 4 weeks after treatment.
   b. Gently cleanse skin with a mild soap; do not remove skin markings.
   c. Avoid tight-fitting clothing; encourage loose-fitting cotton clothes.
   d. Avoid direct sunlight on radiation area.
   e. Avoid exposure of treatment area to all heat and/or cold sources (hot baths, hot water bottles, ice packs).
   f. Do not apply any perfumed or medicated lotions or creams.
   g. Advise client to avoid swimming during treatment period; chemicals can irritate the skin.
   h. Do not use tape, adhesive bandages, cosmetics, lotions, perfumes, powders, or deodorants on the skin in the treatment field.
   i. Closely monitor skin condition on area where x-ray treatment is directed.
5. Nursing implications for a client with an internal radiation source (sealed source) (see Box 8-2).
   a. Observe time, distance, and shield precautions for health care workers as well as all visitors; private room for client.
   b. Use badges or radiation monitors for caregivers having direct client contact.
   c. List on the chart.
      (1) Type of radiation.
      (2) Time inserted.
      (3) Anticipated removal time.
      (4) Specific precautions for the type of radiation used.
   d. Determine specific nursing care related to implant.
      (1) Uterine implant: prevent dislodgement—maintain bed rest; do not elevate head of bed past 20 degrees; low-residue diet; urinary retention catheter; prevent complications of immobility.
      (2) Head and neck implant: closely observe for minor oozing or bleeding from area; radiation may invade the carotid artery. If massive bleeding occurs, apply direct digital pressure to the site and call for assistance.
6. Nursing implications for the client receiving systemic (intravenous) radiation therapy.
   a. Systemically administered radionuclides—radioisotopes (e.g., I^{131} for thyroid cancer)—will initially cause radioactive body secretions.
   b. Keep linens, dressings, and trash in client's room until radiation safety office determines how and when they can be removed.
   c. Be aware of the type of radiation administered and the half-life of the isotope; this will determine how long the body secretions are radioactive.

F. Hematopoietic stem cell transplantation: transplanted cells engraft or bond tightly to existing bone marrow cells.

G. Pediatrics: long-term effects of treatment on the child.
   1. Impaired growth and development, especially from radiation to growth centers of the bone during early childhood and adolescence.
   2. Damage to the central nervous system.
   3. Gonadal aberrations, including reproductive, hormonal, genetic, and teratogenic effects.
   4. Disturbances to other organs, including pneumonitis, pericarditis, pleurisy, hypothyroidism, and cystitis.

Oncologic Emergencies

A. Life-threatening problems arising from tumor progression, response to chemotherapy or radiation therapy, extensive surgical resection.

B. Obstructive emergencies: caused by tumor growth and obstruction of an organ or blood vessel.
   1. Superior venal caval syndrome: may be associated with Hodgkin's disease or lung cancer.
      a. Symptoms: periorbital and facial edema; distention of the veins in the head, neck and chest; headache and possible seizures.
      b. Treatment: radiation or chemotherapy.
   2. Tracheobronchial compromise: may occur in the upper or lower airway; most commonly occurs secondary to a lung tumor.
      a. Symptoms: strider and hypoxia.
      b. Treatment: bronchodilators, steroids, and possible intubation.
   3. Spinal cord compression: caused by a tumor growth into the epidural space of the spinal cord.
      a. Symptoms: intense, severe back pain; motor weakness and dysfunction; sensory paresthesia; changes in bowel and bladder.
      b. Treatment: radiation and corticosteroids.
   4. Intestinal obstruction from tumor growth: see Chapter 18.

C. Third-space syndrome: fluid shifts from the vascular space to the interstitial space; may be associated with extensive surgical resection.
   1. Symptoms: hypovolemia with hypotension, tachycardia, low CVP, decreased urine output.
   2. Treatment: fluid replacement; however, hypervolemia can occur very easily.

D. Metabolic emergencies.
   1. Syndrome of inappropriate antidiuretic hormone (SIADH): results from production of ADH by the cancer cells or by stimulation of ADH production by the chemotherapy.
      a. Symptoms: sustained production of antidiuretic hormone (ADH) leading to water retention, hyponatremia (dilutional), weight gain, weakness, GI disturbances.
      b. Treatment: correct sodium balance-water balance; treat underlying malignancy.

   2. Hypercalcemia: results from metastatic disease of the bone or secretion of parathyroid-like hormone by the cancer cells (see Chapter 6).
      a. Symptoms: apathy, fatigue, muscle weakness, polyuria, GI disturbances, electrocardiogram changes. Immobility and dehydration also contribute to development of hypercalcemia.
      b. Treatment: long-term treatment aimed at primary malignancy; hydration, diuretics, and bisphosphonates
   3. Tumor lysis syndrome: often triggered by chemotherapy when a large number of cancer cells die and a host of intracellular components are released into the blood.
      a. Symptoms: four hallmark signs—hyperuricemia, hyperphosphatemia, hyperkalemia, and hypocalcemia—may occur within the first 24-48 hours after initiation of treatment.
      b. Treatment: increase fluids to support renal function, correct electrolyte imbalances, adequate hydration to decrease uric acid concentrations.

E. Infiltrative emergencies.
   1. Cardiac tamponade (Chapter 17).
   2. Carotid artery rupture: associated with head and neck cancer and neck radiation therapy; treatment involves ligation of the carotid artery.

Nursing Interventions

Goal: To maintain client at optimum psychosocial level.

A. Encourage verbalization.

B. Assist client to understand disease process and therapeutic regimen.

C. Include family in the care.

D. Assist client to cope with changes in body image caused by alopecia (see Table 8-1).

E. Assess client's coping skills and support systems. Encourage communication and be an active listener.

F. Recognize client's emotional outbursts and anger as part of the coping process.

G. Encourage measures to maintain client's ego.
   1. Allow client to participate in his or her own care and make decisions.
   2. Maintain active listening.
   3. Encourage personal lifestyle choices (clothing, makeup, hobbies, etc).
   4. Discuss body image issues.

Goal: To maintain nutrition (see Table 8-1).

A. Diet: appropriate to age level.

B. Hyperalimentation (see Chapter 18) to maintain adequate intake.

C. Prevent and/or decrease complications associated with nutrition.

Goal: To maintain normal elimination pattern (see Table 8-1).

A. Prevent and/or decrease complications of diarrhea.

B. Prevent constipation.

C. Prevent urinary tract infections, primarily cystitis.

1. Maintain adequate fluid intake (at least 3000 mL per day).
2. Frequently assess for symptoms of cystitis (see Chapter 23).
3. Avoid bladder catheterization if possible.
4. Check urine for presence of hematuria.
5. Encourage frequent voiding.
D. Assess for the development of vesicovaginal or rectovaginal fistulas.

Goal: To prevent and/or decrease infectious process (see Table 8-1).

A. Monitor white cell counts, be aware of onset and point of nadir.
B. Meticulous personal hygiene including frequent handwashing.
C. Child should be isolated from others with communicable diseases.
D. Frequently assess for potential infectious processes.
E. Fresh fruits and vegetables should be eaten only after they have been cooked, peeled, or washed thoroughly.
F. See goals for self-care.

Goal: To decrease hematologic complications.

A. Evaluate for decreasing platelet levels and thrombocytopenia.

> **! NURSING PRIORITY** Institute bleeding precautions if platelet count is less than 50,000/mm³.

B. Administer platelets and whole blood transfusions as indicated.
C. Evaluate areas of potential bleeding.
1. Mucous membranes, nosebleed (epistaxis).
2. Urinary tract (hematuria), stool (melena).
3. GI bleeding (hematemesis).
4. Implement bleeding precautions (see Box 14-1).

> **! NURSING PRIORITY** Advise client to use electric razor and a soft-bristle toothbrush.

D. Anemia (see Table 8-1).
1. Maintain adequate rest; encourage client to pace activities to avoid fatigue.
2. Maintain adequate oxygenation.
3. Assess for problems with erythropoiesis.
4. Evaluate respiratory and cardiac systems for mechanisms of compensation.

Goal: To relieve pain (see Chapter 3).

A. Evaluate client and family responses to pain.
B. Evaluate characteristics of pain: determine whether pain control is to be palliative.
C. Administer medications for pain relief.
D. Utilize nonpharmacologic approaches to pain relief (positioning, imagery, hypnosis, etc.).

Goal: To recognize complications specific to radiation and chemotherapy.

A. Alopecia.
B. Hemorrhagic problems.

C. Gastrointestinal distress (anorexia, ulcerations, nausea, vomiting).
D. Bone marrow depression (myelosuppression).
1. Thrombocytopenia.
2. Anemia.
3. Neutropenia.
E. Skin reactions.
F. Decreased immune response.

> **! NURSING PRIORITY** It is important for the nurse to be able to differentiate between toxic effects of medication or radiation therapy and the progression of the disease process.

Home Care

Goal: To effectively manage pain to provide client optimal rest and pain relief.

A. Assess quality, intensity, timing, and location of pain to establish baseline.
B. Identify provoking and alleviating factors and adjust environment accordingly.
C. Assess other psychologic factors affecting pain tolerance (fear, anxiety, agitation, and past experiences with pain).
D. Discuss questions regarding addiction to narcotic analgesics.
E. Assist client with nonpharmacologic pain therapies (Chapter 3).
F. Layer pain management strategies as needed; medicate with narcotic and non-narcotic analgesics as necessary.
G. Advocate for patient-controlled analgesia when appropriate.
H. Assess effectiveness of therapies and medications and modify as necessary.
I. Provide a calm, healthy environment with appropriate lighting and personal belongings as warranted by disease progression.
J. When appropriate, suggest hospice care, which can provide compassion, concern, and support for the terminally ill client.

Goal: To decrease or limit exposure to infection.

A. Limit number of people having direct contact with the client.
B. Good oral hygiene: regular flossing if there is no bleeding problem and no tissue irritation; soft toothbrush; avoid irritating foods.
C. Client should avoid coming in direct contact with animal excreta (cat litter boxes, bird cages, etc).
D. Teach client to take his or her temperature daily and report temperature over 100° F (38° C).
E. Use antipyretics cautiously because they tend to mask infection.
F. Teach client that peak of neutropenia (nadir), or highest risk for infection, occurs within 7 to 14 days after the administration of chemotherapy.
G. Teach client about radiation-induced skin reactions and provide nursing care for these skin reactions.
1. Moisturize skin 3 to 4 times a day with nonperfumed, nonmedicated cream or lotion.

2. If moist desquamation occurs, cleanse gently with normal saline solution; area should be gently patted dry or air-dried; expose areas to air for 10 to 15 minutes three times a day.
3. Avoid use of perfumes, deodorants, powders, and cosmetics to affected area.
4. Wear loose-fitting cotton clothing; avoid swimming.
5. If dry desquamation is present, apply lotion that is not perfumed, not medicated, and does not contain alcohol.

H. Teach client importance of frequent handwashing.

Goal: To maintain optimum psychosocial function.
A. Assess coping mechanisms.
B. Assess family/significant other resources.
C. Provide opportunities for client to express feelings, concerns, and fears.
D. Encourage activity; one of the best activities is walking for about 30 minutes at a rate that is comfortable.

Appendix 8-1 CANCER CHEMOTHERAPY

General Nursing Implications
— Observe for adverse effects (see Table 8-1).
— Dosage is usually based on client's body weight.
— Monitor client and laboratory values for evidence of bone marrow suppression: infection from loss of neutrophils, bleeding from loss of thrombocytes, and anemia from loss of erythrocytes.
— Avoid contact with skin when preparing chemotherapy medications that are vesicants.
— Do not administer a vesicant through a hand or wrist intravenous site; most are administered via a CVAD.
— General side effects of antineoplastic agents: nausea, vomiting, diarrhea, anorexia, alopecia, hyperuricemia, nephrotoxicity.
— Monitor renal and hepatic function to evaluate ability of client to break down and excrete chemotherapeutic agents.

MEDICATION	SIDE EFFECTS	NURSING IMPLICATIONS
ALERT Follow procedure for handling biohazardous materials (e.g., chemotherapeutic agents.)		
Alkylating Agents Kills cells by alkylation of the DNA; all are dose limiting by bone marrow suppression.		
Cyclophosphamide (**Cytoxan, Neosar**)	Renal, hepatotoxic	1. Monitor for hemorrhagic cystitis; encourage high fluid intake
Mechlorethamine (nitrogen mustard) (**Mustargen**)	Blood dycrasias	1. Strong vesicant; prevent extravasation and direct contact with the skin
Chlorambucil (**Leukeran**)	Pulmonary infiltrates and pulmonary fibrosis, hepatotoxic	1. Monitor respiratory status and maintain good respiratory hygiene
Busulfan (**Myleran**)	Pulmonary infiltrates and pulmonary fibrosis, sterility	1. Monitor respiratory status and maintain good respiratory hygiene
Ifosfamide (**Mitoxana**)	Hemorrhagic cystitis	1. High risk for cystitis; urinalysis done before each dose
Carmustine (**BCNU**)	Crosses the blood-brain barrier May have delayed bone marrow suppression	1. Nadir occurs at 4-6 weeks after beginning treatment 2. May have severe nausea and vomiting
Platinum Compounds Cisplatin (**Platinol**) Carboplatin (**Paraplatin**)	Renal damage is dose-limiting factor Neurotoxicity, ototoxicity Dose limited by bone marrow suppression	1. Produces nausea and vomiting within an hour of administration 2. Assess for tinnitus and hearing loss 3. Encourage high fluid intake; may be coupled with diuretics

Continued

Appendix 8-1   CANCER CHEMOTHERAPY—cont'd

MEDICATION	SIDE EFFECTS	NURSING IMPLICATIONS
Antimetabolites Disrupt critical cellular metabolism; cell-cycle specific. Dose limited by bone marrow suppression.		

Folic Acid Analogs

MEDICATION	SIDE EFFECTS	NURSING IMPLICATIONS
Methotrexate sodium (**Folex, Mexate**)	Pulmonary infiltrates and fibrosis; oral and GI ulceration High doses can damage kidney Teratogenic	1. Leucovorin may be administered to increase uptake; can be potentially dangerous 2. Monitor GI status; potential of intestinal perforation; nausea and vomiting occur early 3. Encourage high fluid intake to promote drug excretion 4. Avoid pregnancy for at least 6 months 5. Do not take folic acid.
Premetrexed (**Alimta**)	Teratogenic GI toxicity—stomatitis and diarrhea may be dose limiting	1. Vitamin B_{12} and folic acid to decrease bone marrow and GI toxicity 2. Avoid in pregnancy

Pyrimidine Analogs

MEDICATION	SIDE EFFECTS	NURSING IMPLICATIONS
Cytarabine (**ARA-C**)	High doses may cause pulmonary edema and neurotoxicity	1. Nausea and vomiting after bolus administration 2. Monitor pulmonary status and fluid balance
Fluorouracil (**Adrucil**)	Stomatitis, GI ulceration	1. Monitor and report early GI symptoms; may be discontinued

Purine Analogs

MEDICATION	SIDE EFFECTS	NURSING IMPLICATIONS
Mercaptopurine (**Purinethol**)	Hepatic dysfunction, GI ulceration Mutagenic	1. Monitor for jaundice 2. Allopurinol increases risk for toxicity
Thioguanine (**Tabloid**)	Hepatic dysfunction; GI ulceration	1. Monitor for jaundice

MEDICATION	SIDE EFFECTS	NURSING IMPLICATIONS
Antitumor Antibiotics Interfere with DNA synthesis; are not used to treat infections. Poor GI absorption, given IV.		

Anthracyclines

MEDICATION	SIDE EFFECTS	NURSING IMPLICATIONS
	Cause bone marrow suppression and cardiac damage	
Doxorubicin (**Adriamycin**) Daunorubicin (**DaunoXome**)	Acute dysrhythmias, delayed cardiotoxicity; heart failure	1. Dysrhythmias may occur minutes after administration 2. Monitor cardiac status and rhythm 3. Encourage follow-up after therapy to evaluate cardiac status

Nonanthracyclines

MEDICATION	SIDE EFFECTS	NURSING IMPLICATIONS
Dactinomycin (**Actinomycin-D, Cosmegen**)	Bone marrow suppression and GI mucositis are dose limiting	1. Strong vesicant 2. Monitor mouth for ulcerations
Bleomycin (**Blenoxane**)	Pulmonary injury is dose limiting	1. Monitor pulmonary functions and report any adverse changes
Mitomycin (**Mutamycin**)	Bone marrow suppression is dose limiting	1. Nadir occurs in about 3-4 weeks 2. Monitor for anemia and renal damage

Appendix 8-1   CANCER CHEMOTHERAPY—cont'd

MEDICATION	SIDE EFFECTS	NURSING IMPLICATIONS
Mitotic Inhibitors Prevent cell division.		
Vinca Alkaloids		
Vincristine **(Oncovin, Vincasar)**	Peripheral neuropathy is dose limiting Autonomic nerve system damage	1. Assess reflexes, weakness, paresthesias, sensory loss 2. Autonomic nervous system: constipation and urinary hesitancy 3. Severe vesicant
Vinblastine **(Velban)**	Dose limiting by bone marrow suppression	1. Severe vesicant
Taxanes Paclitaxel **(Taxol, Onxol)**	Severe hypersensitivity reactions Dose limiting by bone marrow suppression, peripheral neuropathy, and cardiac problems Severe neutropenia	1. Administered by 24-hour infusion 2. Assess for bradycardia and heart blocks 3. Assess reflexes, weakness, paresthesias, sensory loss
Docetaxel **(Taxotere)**	Hepatotoxic	1. Monitor LFS
Hormonal Agents Mimic or block the action of hormones.		
Androgen Antagonist Leuprolide **(Eligard, Lupron)**	Used to treat prostate cancer Impotence Increased risk for fractures	1. Encourage activity to minimize bone loss; increase intake of calcium and vitamin D; increase weight-bearing activities
Flutamide **(Eulexin)**	Gynecomastia	
Antiestrogens Tamoxifen **(Nolvadex)**	Used to treat breast cancer Increases incidence of endometrial cancer and thromboembolic problems	1. Dosage for prevention of breast cancer continues for 5 years 2. Teach activities to prevent venous stasis
Raloxifene **(Evista)** Fulvestrant **(Faslodex)** Anastrozole **(Arimidex)**	Do not increase incidence of endometrial cancer Increases risk for osteoporosis	1. Used to treat breast cancer in postmenopausal women 2. Encourage activity to minimize bone loss: increase intake of calcium and vitamin D; increase weight-bearing activities.
Immunostimulants Biologic response modifiers alter the host response to cancer cells.		
Interferon 2a **(Roferon-A)**	Flu-like symptoms (fever, chills, fatigue, myalgia) Profound fatigue may be dose limiting	1. Symptoms tend to diminish with continued therapy
Aldesleukin **(Interleukin 2)**	Flu-like symptoms (fever, chills, fatigue), nausea, vomiting, diarrhea Hypotension, anemia Hepatotoxicity, nephrotoxicity Capillary leak syndrome (CLS): hypotension, reduced organ perfusion, pulmonary edema	1. Toxicity is common in most clients, may be administered in an intensive care setting, toxicity occurs soon after administration 2. CLS: observe for adequate renal perfusion, hypotension 3. Monitor urine output and liver and renal function studies

BP, Blood pressure; *ECG*, electrocardiogram; *GI*, gastrointestinal; *IV*, intravenous; *CVAD*, central venous access device.

Study Questions Abnormal Cell Growth

More questions on companion CD!

1. The nurse receives report on assigned clients. One client is reported to be at the nadir for his cancer chemotherapy. How will this affect the nursing care plan?
   1 Implement bleeding precautions.
   2 Reinforce measures and teaching regarding preventing infections.
   3 Anticipate nutritional problems caused by nausea and vomiting.
   4 Assess for problems with fluid balance.

2. The nurse is assessing a client after beginning external radiation. What is a nursing observation that confirms the presence of early side effects of the radiation?
   1 A gradual weight loss and GI disturbances
   2 Skin erythema followed by dry desquamation
   3 Vertigo when sitting up quickly
   4 Excoriation and blisters on the affected skin

3. What are the nursing interventions regarding the care of a client with a vaginal radium implant?
   1 Clamp and drain the urinary retention catheter.
   2 Provide a high-residue diet.
   3 Place the client in a semiprivate room.
   4 Raise the head of the bed no more than 20 degrees.

4. What is an important aspect of client teaching regarding external radiation therapy?
   1 Remain isolated after treatments.
   2 Fast before the treatment.
   3 Schedule treatments monthly.
   4 Leave skin markings between treatments.

5. A client is receiving chemotherapy with several antineoplastic agents. Which nursing observation is considered a common side effect of chemotherapy?
   1 Slow, slurred speech
   2 Increased leukocytes on complete blood count
   3 Gingivitis and oral ulcers
   4 Sinus dysrhythmias with bradycardia

6. A client is going to begin external radiation therapy for his lung cancer. Which comment by the client would indicate to the nurse the need for additional teaching?
   1. "I will shower with a mild soap and check my skin for areas of redness."
   2. "I am looking forward to swimming laps again for my exercise."
   3. "I am going to eat small meals and increase the protein and fiber in my diet."
   4. "I will use only unscented emollient creams to the dry skin areas on my chest."

7. The nurse is evaluating a central venous line before administering the client's chemotherapy. What observation would cause the nurse the most concern?
   1 Nurse is unable to withdraw blood into line.
   2 Dressing was changed 24 hours ago.
   3 Inflammation and exudate are present at the insertion site.
   4 Fluid infusing is D_5W and 0.45% normal saline.

8. The nurse understands that the following are general adverse effects of antineoplastic drugs. Select all that apply.
   _____ 1. Urinary retention
   _____ 2. Infertility
   _____ 3. Stomatitis
   _____ 4. Bone marrow depression
   _____ 5. Extravasation
   _____ 6. Nausea

9. The nurse is updating a teaching plan for a client who has cancer and has been taking doxorubicin (Adriamycin) for the past several months. What is important to review with the client?
   1 Report symptoms of hematuria.
   2 Increase intake of oral fluids.
   3 Avoid folic acid intake.
   4 Report symptoms of dyspnea.

10. A client is receiving busulfan (Myleran). The nurse would notify the physician regarding which assessment finding?
    1 Persistent nonproductive, dry cough
    2 Hemoglobin 13 g/dL, hematocrit 38%
    3 Nausea and vomiting
    4 Low serum uric acid

11. A client asks the nurse why he has to take several chemotherapy agents at the same time. The nurse's response would be based on which principle?
    1 The more medications that can be given together, the shorter the treatment period.
    2 The cost is decreased because the medications are administered at the same time.
    3 Multiple medications given together will attack the cancer cells at different levels.
    4 One medication will interact with another to reduce incidence of side effects.

12. A client has developed stomatitis while receiving chemotherapy. What would be an appropriate intervention to suggest for the pain associated with the stomatitis?
    1 Use lemon-flavored glycerin swabs.
    2 Apply antacid coating solutions and viscous lidocaine.
    3 Brush oral plaques off with a soft toothbrush.
    4 Have client swish mouth with a weak hydrogen peroxide solution.

13. What is a common side effect of radiation therapy that is not associated with the effect of radiation in the treatment field?
    1 Reddened skin
    2 Bone marrow suppression
    3 Fatigue
    4 GI disturbances

Answers and rationales to these questions are in the section at the end of the book titled Chapter Study Questions: Answers and Rationales.

CHAPTER NINE

Psychiatric Nursing Concepts

SELF-CONCEPT

A. *Self-concept:* all beliefs, convictions, and ideas that constitute an individual's knowledge of himself or herself and influence the individual's relationships with others.

B. *Self-esteem:* an individual's personal judgment of his or her own worth obtained by analyzing how well his or her behavior conforms to his or her self-ideal.

C. *Self-ideal:* an individual's perception of how he or she should behave based on certain personal standards.

> **! NURSING PRIORITY** A healthy self-concept, (i.e., positive self-esteem) is essential to psychologic well-being; it is universal, (i.e., something everyone wants and needs).

Assessment

A. Factors affecting self-esteem.
1. Parental rejection in early childhood experiences.
2. Lack of recognition and appreciation by parents as child grows older.
3. Overpossessiveness, overpermissiveness, and control by one or both parents.
4. Unrealistic self-ideals or goals.

> **! OLDER ADULT PRIORITY** The use of wheelchairs, canes, walkers, hearing aids, or any combination of these will have an impact on the self-esteem of the older client.

B. Behaviors associated with low self-esteem.
1. Self-derision and criticism: describes self as stupid, no good, or a loser.
2. Self-diminution: minimizes one's ability.
3. Guilt and worrying.
4. Postponing decisions and denying pleasure.
5. Disturbed interpersonal relationships.
6. Self-destructiveness and boredom.
7. Polarizing view of life.

> **ALERT** Promoting a positive self-concept is basic to all psychotherapeutic interventions. Look for options that focus on this concept; acknowledging the client as a person is an example.

Nursing Interventions

A. Expand self-awareness.
1. Promote an open, trusting relationship.
2. Work and expand on whatever ego strength the client possesses.
3. Maximize the client's participation in the therapeutic relationship.

B. Self-exploration.
1. Encourage the client to accept his or her own feelings and thoughts.
2. Help the client clarify his or her concept of self and relationship with others through appropriate self-disclosure.
3. Explore with the client maladaptive thinking patterns such as:
   a. Catastrophizing: thinking that the worst will happen.
   b. Minimizing and maximizing: tendency to minimize the positive and maximize the negative.
   c. Black-and-white thinking: tendency to look at situations in extremes; no middle ground.
   d. Overgeneralization: thinking that if something happens once, it will happen again.
   e. Self-reference: tendency to believe that other people are particularly aware of the client's own mistakes.
   f. Filtering: selectively taking certain details out of context while neglecting to look at more positive facts.
4. Communicate empathically, not sympathetically, and remind the client that he or she has the power to change himself or herself.

C. Self-evaluation.
1. Encourage client to define and identify problem.
2. Identify irrational beliefs such as:
   a. "I must be loved by everyone."
   b. "I must be competent and never make mistakes."
   c. "My whole life is a disaster if it doesn't turn out exactly as planned."
3. Identify areas of strength by exploring the client's hobbies, skills, work, school, character traits, personal abilities, etc.

! **PEDIATRIC PRIORITY** If parents help children identify and accomplish goals that are important to them, children begin to develop a sense of personal competence and independence.

4. Explore client's adaptive and maladaptive coping responses.
   a. Determine "pay-offs" for maintaining self-defeating behaviors such as:
      (1) Procrastination.
      (2) Avoiding risks and commitments.
      (3) Retreating from the present situation.
      (4) Not accepting responsibility for one's actions.
   b. Identify the disadvantages of the maladaptive coping responses.

! **NURSING PRIORITY** An individual's functional level of overall self-esteem may change markedly from day to day and moment to moment.

D. Realistic planning.
   1. Help client identify alternative solutions.
   2. Encourage creative visualization to enhance self-esteem through goal setting.
   3. Help client set realistic goals by encouraging him or her to participate in new experiences.
E. Commitment to action.
   1. Providing an opportunity for client to experience success is essential.
   2. Reinforce strengths, abilities, and skills.

BODY IMAGE

Evaluation of Body Image Alteration
A. Types of body image disturbances.
   1. Changes in body size, shape, or appearance (rapid weight gain or loss, plastic surgery, pregnancy).
   2. Pathologic processes causing changes in structure or function of one's body (e.g., Parkinson's disease, cancer, heart disease).
   3. Failure of a body part to function properly (paraplegia or stroke).
   4. Physical changes associated with normal growth and development (puberty, aging process).
   5. Threatening medical or nursing procedures (catheterization, radiation therapy, organ transplantation).
B. Principles.
   1. Body characteristics that have been present from birth or acquired early in life seem to have less emotional significance than those arising later.
   2. Body image changes, handicaps, or changes in body function that occur abruptly are far more traumatic than ones that develop gradually.
   3. The location of a disease or injury greatly affects the emotional response to it; internal diseases are generally less threatening than external diseases (trauma, disfigurement).

4. Changes in genitals or breasts are perceived as a great threat and reawaken fears about sexuality and virility.

Alterations of Body Image: Four Phases
A. Impact phase.
   1. Shows behaviors of despair, discouragement, and passive acceptance.
   2. Often projects guilt onto others.
   3. Senses failure in one's own body.
   4. Anger and hostility often turned inward.
B. Retreat phase.
   1. Becomes aware of the injury, illness, loss, or disfigurement.
   2. Children and older adults retreat into regressive behavior.
   3. Adolescents and adults retreat into denial.
C. Acknowledgment phase.
   1. A period of mourning the loss.
   2. Acknowledges loss, regardless of the degree involved; no longer can hide or retreat from situation.
   3. Begins to focus on strengths rather than losses.
D. Reconstruction phase.
   1. Adapts to changes in body image.
   2. Encouraged to try new approaches to life.

SPECIFIC SITUATIONS OF ALTERED BODY IMAGE AND NURSING INTERVENTIONS

ALERT Facilitate client's adjustment to changes in body image.

Obesity
Assessment
A. Body weight exceeds 20% above the normal range for age, sex, and height.
B. Feeding behavior is gauged according to external environmental cues (i.e., odors, stress, availability of food) rather than hunger (increased gastrointestinal motility).
C. Increased incidence of diabetes, cardiovascular disease, and poor healing.
D. Obese client often has symptoms of depression, fatigue, dyspnea, tachycardia, and hypertension.

Nursing Interventions
A. Encourage behavior modification programs.
B. Promote activities and interests not related to food or eating.
C. Identify client's need to eat and relate the need to preceding events or situations.
D. Decrease guilt and anxiety related to being obese.
E. Provide long-range nutritional counseling.
F. Encourage an exercise program.
G. Assess for complications (hypertension, cardiovascular disease).

Stroke

Assessment

A. Change of body function due to loss of bowel and bladder control, speech, and cognitive skills.
B. Disordered orientations in relationship to body and position sense in space; body image boundaries disrupted.

Nursing Interventions

A. Decrease frustration related to speech problems by encouraging speech effort, speaking slowly, and clarifying statements.
B. Promote reintegration of altered body image caused by paralyzed body part by means of tactile stimulation and verbal reminders of the existing body part.

Amputation

Assessment

A. Feelings of loss, lowered self-esteem, guilt, helplessness.
B. Depression, passivity, and increased emotional vulnerability.
C. Phantom limb pain occurs in most clients: increased experience if amputation occurs after 4 years of age; almost universal experience after age 8.
D. Phantom limb pain is stronger and lasts longer in upper limbs than in lower limbs.

Nursing Interventions

A. Anticipatory guidance and therapeutic preparation of a client who is to undergo amputation.
B. Discussion of phantom limb phenomenon and exploration of client's fears regarding amputation.
C. Assist family members to work through their feelings and to accept client as a whole person.
D. Acknowledge phantom limb pain; reassure client that this is a normal process.
E. Provide pain medication as needed.

Pregnancy

Assessment

A. Produces marked changes in a woman's body, resulting in major alterations in body configuration within a short period of time.
B. Second trimester: woman becomes aware that her body is widening and requires more space.
C. Third trimester: woman is very much aware of increased size; may feel ambivalent about the changes in her body.
D. Woman perceives her body as vulnerable, yet also as a protective container for the unborn.
E. Mate experiences changed body image and sympathetic symptoms during woman's pregnancy.

Nursing Interventions

A. Explain and offer reassurance about the normal physiologic changes that are occurring.

B. Provide discussions of alterations in body image for both mates.
C. Encourage verbalization of feelings relating to changed body image.

Cancer

Assessment

A. Clients with cancer may experience many changes in body image.
B. Removal of sex organs (breasts, uterus) has a significant impact on a client's perception of sexuality.
C. Disfiguring head-and-neck surgery has a devastating impact on body image, because the face is one of the primary means by which people communicate.
D. Symptoms of depersonalization, loss of self-esteem, and depression may occur.

Nursing Interventions

A. Provide anticipatory guidance to help client cope with crisis of changed body image.
B. Set long-term goals to help client with cancer adjust to physiologic and psychologic changes.

Enterostomal Surgery

Assessment

A. Client often shocked at initial sight of ostomy.
B. Client may experience lowered self-esteem, fear of fecal or urine spillage, alteration in sexual functioning, and feelings of disfigurement and rejection.

Nursing Interventions

A. Preoperative explanation by use of drawings, models, or pictures of how stoma will appear.
B. Reassurance that reddish appearance of stoma and large size will diminish in time.
C. Encourage discussion and recognize importance of client talking with a "successful ostomate."

HUMAN SEXUALITY

Key Nursing Concepts

A. Growth and development.
  1. Observable differences in male and female behavior are seen as early as infancy.
  2. Core gender identity develops in the healthy child at about 3 or 4 years of age.
  3. Sexual problems seen in childhood are as follows: sexual misconception, gender identity disturbances, and home settings that cause sexual confusion.
  4. Rapid biologic changes seen in adolescence result in anxiety about maturation.
  5. The adolescent is faced with the following: establishing his or her identity; accepting a changed body image; coping with new energy; and resolving reappearing Oedipal conflict.

6. Sexual problems seen in adolescents include the following: guilty feelings regarding masturbation; integration of transient homosexual experiences into heterosexual relationship; resolution of conflicts related to premarital intercourse; and obtaining sex-related health services (e.g., birth control).
7. The young adult faces the task of establishing a pattern of heterosexual intimacy.
8. The middle-age adult faces the task of adjusting to physiologic changes in sexual function and the responsibilities of parenting.
9. Sexual activity and interest may continue into old age, provided the individual is healthy and has an interesting partner.

B. Principles.
1. Human sexuality is best understood when approached holistically (i.e., from psychologic, sociologic, and cultural perspectives).
2. The process of hospitalization alters one's concept of self as a sexual being.
3. Sexual role identity may be altered during the illness process.
4. Cultural variables influence one's expression of sexuality.
5. Hospitalized clients may act out sexually to test the response of others to their sexuality, to gain control of a situation, or to attract attention.
6. Sexual problems are addressed through short-term, behavior-oriented treatment; the goal is to decrease fear of performance and to facilitate communication.
7. Nursing plays a key role in sex-health education; nurses need to be aware of their own attitudes toward sex to respond helpfully to clients.

Changes in Sexuality

A. Effect of illness and injury on sexuality.
1. Depressive episodes often precipitate a decrease in libido.
2. Sexual preoccupations and overtones may be experienced by the client with psychosis.
3. Certain medications contribute to sexual dysfunction, failure to reach orgasm in women, and impotence or failure to ejaculate in men (e.g., reserpine, phenothiazine, and estrogen use in men decreases libido; androgen use in women increases libido).
4. Clients with spinal cord injuries may lose sexual functioning.
5. Trauma and disfigurement may precipitate an alteration in sexuality.

B. Effect of the aging process on sexuality.
1. Physiologic changes in women are frequently caused by decreasing estrogen supply, which results in decreased vaginal lubrication, shrinkage and loss of elasticity in vaginal canal, and decrease in breast size.
2. Physiologic changes in men include a decrease in testosterone, decrease in spermatogenesis, and a longer length of time to achieve erection, along with a decrease in the firmness of erection.

3. Prolonged abstinence from sexual activity can lead to disuse syndrome in which the physiologic changes are experienced to a greater degree.

CONCEPT OF LOSS

ALERT Evaluate coping mechanisms of client and family and provide emotional support to the client or family.

A. Definition.
1. Includes both biologic and physiologic aspects; loss of function.
2. Components of loss include death, dying, grief, and mourning.
   a. Death: represents finality, the end of one's biologic being.
   b. Dying: the social process of organizing activities that prepare for death; provides others, as well as the client, a way to prepare for the future.
   c. Grief: the sequence of subjective states that follow loss and accompany mourning.
   d. Mourning: the psychologic processes that are aroused by the loss of a loved object or person.
   e. Disenfranchised grief: loss that is not or cannot be openly expressed and acknowledged by others (e.g., miscarriage, birth of a disabled child, death of an ex-spouse, loss of hair during chemotherapy, death of a pet).

B. Nursing care of the dying client (see Chapter 3).

Coping and Reactions to Death Throughout the Life Cycle

A. Infant-toddler (ages 1-3).
1. Reactions to death and dying.
   a. No specific concept of death: thinks only in terms of living.
   b. Reacts more to pain and discomfort of illness and immobilization; separation anxiety; intrusive procedures; change in ritualistic routine.
2. Nursing interventions.
   a. Assist parents to deal with their feelings.
   b. Encourage parents' participation in child's care.
   c. Promote decreased separation anxiety by providing arrangements for parents to stay with child.

NURSING PRIORITY Parents of a dying child may have feelings of guilt and may need to talk out these feelings before being able to help each other and their child.

B. Preschooler (ages 3-5).
1. Reactions to death and dying.
   a. Death is viewed as a departure, a kind of sleep.
   b. No real understanding of the universality and inevitability of death.
   c. Life and death can change places with one another.

d. Death is viewed as gradual or temporary; the person is still alive but under a different set of conditions.

e. Often views illness and death as a punishment for his or her own thoughts or actions.

f. If a pet dies, may request a funeral, burial, or some other type of ceremony to symbolize the loss.

2. Nursing interventions.

a. Use play therapy for expression of thoughts and feelings regarding death and dying.

b. Provide a clear explanation of what death is; death is final and not sleep.

c. Permit a choice of attending a funeral; if child decides to attend, explain what will take place.

> **PEDIATRIC PRIORITY** A young child's fear of death is often a fear of aloneness, of being away from the parents. It is important for parents to interact with the nurse in the child's presence so that the nurse can be identified as a trustworthy substitute caretaker.

C. School-age child (ages 5-12).

1. Reactions to death and dying.

a. Death is personified; fantasies of a separate person or distinct personality (e.g., skeleton-man, devil, ghost, or death-man).

b. Fantasies about the unknown are often very frightening.

c. Fear of mutilation and punishment is often associated with death; anxiety is released by nightmares and superstitions.

2. Nursing interventions.

a. Respond to questions regarding funerals, burials, and memorial services.

b. Accept regressive or protest behavior.

c. Encourage verbalization of feelings and emotional reactions.

D. Adolescent (ages 12-18).

1. Reactions to death and dying.

a. Has a mature understanding of death.

b. Concerned more with the here and now (i.e., the present).

c. May have strong emotions about death (anger, frustration, despair); silent, withdrawn.

d. Often worries about physical changes in relationship to terminal illness.

e. May ask very difficult, open questions regarding death.

2. Nursing interventions.

a. Support maturational crises relating to identity.

b. Encourage verbalization of feelings.

c. Promote peer and parental emotional support.

d. Respect need for privacy and personal expressions of anger, sadness, or fear.

e. Model appropriate grieving behavior.

E. Adult.

1. Concerned about death as a disruption in lifestyle and its effect on significant others.

2. Adults tend to think about loss in terms of unmet goals and/or an impediment to future plans; often experience delayed grief and threat to emotional integrity.

F. Older adult.

1. Aware of death as inevitable; life is over.

2. Emphasis on religious belief for comfort; a time of reflection, rest, and peace.

> **ALERT** Respect differences between client's and health care provider's cultural practices.

CULTURAL DIVERSITY

Special Considerations

A. Cultures vary widely in their traditions.

B. In the United States, each particular ethnic group has its own cultural system and specific way of behaving and evaluating illness and wellness.

> **NURSING PRIORITY** Certain psychopathologic conditions may change diagnostic category entirely in different cultures. Misinterpretation and misunderstanding of clients' presenting symptoms can lead to problems in the nurse-client relationship (e.g., notion of possession [in a positive sense] by the Holy Ghost among American Pentecostal groups might be viewed by health care providers as a symptom of a mental disorder).

C. *Culture shock* occurs whenever a person leaves a familiar country, region, lifestyle, or occupation and enters a radically different environment.

Examples: Entering the hospital; moving to a new neighborhood.

Assessment of Cultural Aspects

A. Communication styles.

1. Does the client speak English fluently? If not, what language is preferred?

2. Is an interpreter needed?

> **NURSING PRIORITY** If an interpreter is needed, it is preferable to avoid using family members. Also, learning some key words from the interpreter will help the nurse in implementing care.

B. Ethnic or religious group.

1. What particular group does client identify with?

2. How closely does the client adhere to the traditional beliefs of the group?

C. Nutrition.

1. Are there certain ethnic or religious preferences about the selection or preparation of foods?

2. Are there foods to be encouraged (or avoided) when a person is ill?

D. Family relationships.
  1. Is the family matriarchal or patriarchal?
  2. What role in the family does the client hold?
E. Health beliefs.
  1. Does the client rely on folk medicine practices?
  2. Has the client been recently treated by a curandero, shaman, Voodoo doctor, medicine man, or Chinese herbalist?

PSYCHOSOCIAL ASSESSMENT

> ❗ **NURSING PRIORITY** Strong evidence suggests that factors such as genetics, environment, diet, and cultural beliefs are responsible for ethnic variations in psychotropic drug use (e.g., poor metabolism of certain psychotropic drugs because of genetic factors has been found to be responsible for drug effects in some ethnic groups).

Complete assessment includes descriptions of the intellectual functions, behavioral reactions, emotional reactions, and dynamic issues of the client relative to adaptive functioning and response to present situations.

> **ALERT** Assess client's response to illness, identify coping mechanisms of client and family, and assess the family's emotional reaction to client's illness.

Psychiatric History

Purpose: To obtain data from multiple sources (e.g., client, family, friends, police, mental health personnel) as a means of identifying patterns of functioning that are healthy, as well as patterns that create problems in the client's everyday life.

> ❗ **OLDER ADULT PRIORITY** Allow ample time to gather psychosocial data from older clients, because they are often starved for someone to listen to them.

A. General history of client.
  1. Demographic information: address, age, religious affiliation, occupation, insurance company, etc.
  2. Pertinent personal history such as birth, growth and development, illness, and marital history.
  3. Previous mental health hospitalizations or treatment.
B. Components of psychiatric history.
  1. Chief complaint: main reason client is seeking psychiatric help.
    a. Use client's own words as to why he or she is hospitalized or seeking help.
    b. Check for recent difficulties or alterations in relationships, level of functioning, behavior, perceptions, or cognitive abilities.
  2. Presenting symptoms: onset and development of symptoms or problems.
    a. Check for increased feelings of depression, anxiety, hopelessness, suspiciousness, confusion, fear.
    b. Assess for changes in bowel habits, insomnia, lethargy, weight loss or gain, anorexia, palpitations, pruritus, headaches.

  3. Family history.
    a. Have any of client's family members sought psychiatric treatment?
    b. Who was important to client in childhood? In adolescence?
    c. Was there physical, emotional, or sexual abuse?
    d. Did parents drink or use drugs?
  4. Personality profile.
    a. Assess client's interests, feelings, mood, and usual leisure activities or hobbies.
    b. How does client cope with stress?
    c. Inquire about sexual patterns: sexually active? sexual orientation? sexual difficulties?
    d. Have client describe social relationships: Who are client's friends? Who is important to client? What is a usual day like?

Mental Status Examination

The mental status examination differs from the psychiatric history in that it is used to identify an individual's present mental status.

> **ALERT** Identify changes in client's mental status.

Aspects of the Examination

> ❗ **NURSING PRIORITY** First, assess client's level of consciousness, vision, and hearing (e.g., alert, lethargic, stuporous, or comatose) and ability to comprehend the interview.

A. Mini-Mental State Examination (MMSE): developed by Folstein, Folstein, and McHugh, 1975.
  1. Widely used common mental status assessment for cognitive function.
  2. Quickly administered - questions related to orientation (person, place and time) , registration (repeating items, give client 3 common words and ask him to repeat the words), naming (point to a chair or object and ask client to name it), and reading (ask client to read and follow directions from a simple sentence).
  3. Excludes assessment of mood, abnormal psychologic experiences (hallucinations, delusions, illusions), and content and process of thinking.
B. General appearance, attitude, and behavior.
  1. Descriptors: posture, gait, activity, facial expression, mannerisms.
  2. Disturbances include deviations of activity, distortions in mobility (waxy flexibility or dyskinesia), uncooperativeness, and changes in personal hygiene.
C. Characteristics of talk and stream of thought.
  1. Descriptors: emphasis on *form*, rather than content, of client's verbal communication; loudness, flow, speed, quality, logic, level of coherence.
  2. Disturbances include the following patterns:
    a. Mutism: no verbal response.
    b. Circumstantiality: cumbersome detail in client's communication.

c. Perseveration: pattern of repeating same words or movements.

d. Flight of ideas: rapid speech, loosely connected thoughts.

e. Blocking: sudden silence, often associated with intrusion of delusional thoughts or hallucinations.

f. Echolalia: repeating the last word heard.

g. Neologism: coining of new words.

h. Verbigeration: repeating words, sentences, or phrases several times.

i. Pressured speech: an increase in the quantity of speech, usually becoming loud, rushed, and emphatic.

D. Emotional state.
1. Descriptors: client's report of subjective feelings (mood or affect) and examiner's observation of client's pervasive or dominant emotional state.
2. Disturbances include deviations such as elation, depression, apathy, incongruence, and disassociation.

E. Content of thought.
1. Descriptors: What is central theme? How does client view himself or herself (self-concept)? Is suicidal or homicidal ideation present? If so, what is potential lethality?
2. Disturbances include special preoccupations and experiences such as hallucinations, delusions, illusions, depersonalization, obsessions or compulsions, phobias, fantasies, and daydreams.

F. Sensorium and intellect.
1. Determine the degree of client's awareness and level of intellectual functioning; general ability to grasp information and calculate; abstract thinking; memory (recall of remote past experiences or recent past experiences, retention and recall of immediate impressions); reasoning and judgment.
2. Disturbances of orientation in terms of time, place, person, and self; memory, retention, attention, information, and judgment are assessed through use of standardized tests and questions.

❗ NURSING PRIORITY Because the validity and reliability of the mental status examination require the client to be reasonably oriented, begin the mental assessment examination by determining client's level of sensorium and orientation.

G. Insight evaluation—Determine whether the client can understand and appreciate the nature of his or her condition and the need for treatment.

STRESS AND ADAPTATION

Stress is a state produced by a change in the environment that is perceived as challenging, threatening, or damaging to the individual's equilibrium.

Adaptation is a constant, ongoing process that occurs along the time continuum, beginning with birth and ending with death.

Stressors

A. Physiologic stressors.
1. Chemical agents: drugs, poisons, alcohol.
2. Physical agents: heat, cold, radiation, electrical shock, trauma.
3. Infectious agents: viruses, bacteria, fungi.
4. Faulty immune mechanisms.
5. Genetic disorders.
6. Nutritional imbalance.
7. Hypoxia.

B. Psychosocial stressors.
1. Accidents and the survivors (e.g., airplane crash, hurricane, and earthquake survivors).
2. Death of a close friend; neighbor being robbed and/ or beaten.
3. Horrors of history: Auschwitz, Hiroshima, Chernobyl, etc.
4. Fear of aggression, mutilation, and destruction.
5. Events of history brought into our living rooms through various media.
6. Life crises: situational, developmental, role.
7. Inherent conflicts in all social relations.

C. Environmental stressors.
1. Noise pollution.
2. Temperature pollution.
3. Air and chemical pollution.

ALERT Implement measures to reduce environmental stressors and assist client in identifying strategies to deal with stress.

Stress Response

❗ NURSING PRIORITY Understanding of the stress response is basic to many nursing interventions.

A. Sympathetic: adrenal medullary response; fight-or-flight response (Box 9-1).
1. Increased pulse, blood glucose level, and coagulability of blood.
2. Pupils dilated.
3. Mental activity enhanced.
4. Cold, clammy skin.
5. Respirations rapid and shallow.

Box 9-1 SELYE'S GENERAL ADAPTATION SYNDROME

Stage I: Alarm Reaction
Mobilization of the body's defensive forces (antiinflammatory) and activation of the fight-or-flight mechanism.

Stage II: Stage of Resistance
Optimal adaptation to stress within a person's capabilities.

Stage III: Stage of Exhaustion
Loss of the ability to resist stress because of depletion of body resources; failure to adapt leads to death.

B. Pituitary-adrenal cortical response.
   1. Increased production of adrenocorticotropic hormone (ACTH) and mineralocorticoids (aldosterone); increased release of glucagon.
   2. The sympathetic-adrenal medullary response occurs within seconds.
   3. The pituitary-adrenal cortical response (also, called the *Selyean response*, after Hans Selye) includes the fight-or-flight response and takes minutes to hours to produce a desired effect.

Stress Reduction Methods

A. Proper nutrition.
B. Regular exercise, physical activity, and recreation.
C. Meditation, breathing exercises, creative imagery.
D. Communication, time management.
E. Biofeedback, rolfing (massage of deep connective tissue to achieve realignment of body structure), therapeutic touch, bioenergetics (decrease muscle tension by releasing feelings through physical exertion and verbal techniques).
F. Relaxation response.
   1. Quiet environment.
   2. Passive attitude.
   3. Comfortable position.
   4. A mental device or object, such as a word, sound, or phrase, to occupy the mind and keep out thoughts.
G. Group process and social support.
H. Thought-stopping, self-hypnosis, refuting irrational self-talk.

CONCEPT OF ANXIETY

An emotion, a subjective experience; a feeling state that is experienced as vague uneasiness, tension, or apprehension; occurs when the ego is threatened; provoked by the unknown; precedes all new experiences.
A. Assessment (Table 9-1).
B. Nursing management (Table 9-2).

ALERT Plan measures to help a client cope with anxiety.

Coping/Defense/Ego/Mental Mechanisms

Specific defense processes used by individuals to relieve or decrease anxieties caused by uncomfortable situations that threaten self-esteem.
A. Related principles.
   1. Primary functions are to decrease emotional conflicts, provide relief from stress, protect from feelings of inadequacy and worthlessness, prevent awareness of anxiety, and maintain an individual's self-esteem.
   2. Everyone uses defense mechanisms to a certain extent. If used to an extreme degree, defense mechanisms distort reality, interfere with interpersonal relationships, limit one's ability to work productively, and may lead to pathologic symptoms.
B. Common defense mechanisms (see Appendix 9-1).
C. Nursing management.
   1. Accept coping mechanisms.

Table 9-1	**ASSESSMENT OF ANXIETY**
Physiologic	*Psychologic*
Sympathetic Responses	**Behavioral Responses**
Tachycardia	Restlessness
Elevated blood pressure	Agitation
Increased perspiration	Tremors (fine to gross shaking of the body)
Dilated pupils	Startle reaction
Hyperventilation with difficulty breathing	Rapid speech
Cold, clammy skin	Lack of coordination
Dry mouth	Withdrawal
Constipation	
Parasympathetic Responses	**Cognitive Responses**
Urinary frequency	Impaired attention
Diarrhea	Poor concentration
	Forgetfulness
	Blocking of thought
	Decreased perceptual field
	Decreased productivity
	Confusion
Related Responses	**Affective Responses**
Headaches	Tension
Nausea or vomiting	Jittery feeling
Sleep disturbances	Worried
Muscular tension	Apprehension, nervousness
	Irritability
	Dread
	Fear
	Panic
	Fear of impending doom

   2. Discuss alternative coping mechanisms and problem-solving techniques.
   3. Assist the client in learning new or alternative coping patterns for a healthier adaptation.
   4. Use techniques to decrease anxiety.

THERAPEUTIC NURSING PROCESS

Therapeutic interpersonal relationship is the interaction between two persons: the *nurse* promotes goal-directed activities that help to alleviate the discomfort of the *client* by promoting growth and satisfying interpersonal relationships.

Characteristics

A. Goal-directed.
B. Empathetic understanding.
C. Honest, open communication.
D. Concreteness; avoids vagueness and ambiguity.
E. Acceptance; nonjudgmental attitude.
F. Involves nurse's understanding of self and personal motives and needs.

Interview Process

A. Establish rapport with the client.
B. Obtain pertinent client data.
C. Initiate client assessment.
D. Make practical arrangements for treatment.

Table 9-2	NURSING MANAGEMENT OF ANXIETY		
Level of Anxiety	*Assessment*	*Goal*	*Nursing Management*
Mild	Increased alertness, motivation, and attentiveness.	To assist client to tolerate some anxiety.	1. Help client identify and describe feelings. 2. Help client develop the capacity to tolerate mild anxiety and use it consciously and constructively.
Moderate	Perception narrowed, selective inattention, physical discomforts.	To reduce anxiety; directed toward helping client understand cause of anxiety and new ways of controlling it.	1. Provide outlet for tension, such as walking; crying; working at simple, concrete tasks.
Severe	Behavior becomes automatic; connections between details are not seen; senses are drastically reduced.	To assist in channeling anxiety.	1. Recognize own level of anxiety. 2. Link client's behavior with feelings. 3. Protect defenses and coping mechanisms. 4. Identify and modify anxiety-provoking situations.
Panic	Overwhelmed; inability to function or communicate; potential for bodily harm to self and others; loss of rational thought.	To be supportive and protective.	1. Provide nonstimulating, structured environment. 2. Avoid touching. 3. Stay with client. 4. Medicate client with tranquilizers if necessary.

Phases

A. Initial phase: Goal is to *build trust*.
   1. Explore the client's perceptions, thoughts, feelings, and actions.
   2. Identify the problem.
   3. Assess levels of anxiety of self and client.
   4. Mutually define specific goals to pursue.
B. Working phase: Goal is to *establish objectives* or a working agreement (contract).
   1. Encourage client participation.
   2. Focus on problem-solving techniques; choose between alternate courses of action and practice skills.
   3. Explore thoughts, feelings, and emotions.
   4. Develop constructive coping mechanisms.
   5. Increase independence and self-responsibility.
C. Termination phase: Goal is to *evaluate goals* set forth and terminate relationship.
   1. Plan for termination early in formation of relationship (in initial phase).
   2. Discuss client's feelings about termination.
   3. Evaluate client's progress and goal attainment.

⚠ NURSING PRIORITY To effectively interview a client, be sure to start with a broad, empathetic statement; explore normal behaviors before discussing maladaptive behaviors; phrase inquiries or questions sensitively to decrease client's anxiety; ask client to clarify vague statements; refocus on pressing problems when client begins to ramble; interrupt nonstop talking by client as tactfully as possible; express empathy toward client while he or she is expressing feelings.

Communication Theory

A. Levels of communication.
   1. Verbal communication: occurs through the medium of words—spoken or written.
   2. Nonverbal communication: includes everything that does not involve the spoken or written word; involves the five senses.
      a. Vocal cues: tone of voice, quality of voice, nervous coughing, sounds of hesitation.
      b. Action cues: body movement, posture, facial expressions, gestures, mannerisms.
      c. Object cues: dress, appearance to convey a certain "look" or message.
      d. Space: distance between two people; intimate, personal, public space.
      e. Touch: universal and basic to all nurse-client relationships; response to touch is influenced by the setting, cultural background (of client and of nurse), type of relationship, sex of communicators, and expectations.
B. Therapeutic nurse-client communication techniques.
   1. Planning and goals.
      a. Demonstrate active listening; face-to-face contact.
      b. Demonstrate unconditional positive regard, interest, congruence, respect.
      c. Develop trusting relationship; accept client's behavior and display nonjudgmental, objective attitude.
      d. Be supportive, honest, authentic, genuine.
      e. Focus on emotional needs and emotionally charged area.
      f. Focus on here-and-now behavior and expression of feelings.
      g. Attempt to understand the client's point of view.

h. Develop an awareness of the client's likes and dislikes.
i. Encourage expression of both positive and negative feelings.
j. Use broad openings and ask open-ended questions; avoid questions that can be answered by yes or no.
k. Use reflections of feelings, attitudes, and words.
l. Explore alternatives rather than answers or solutions.
m. Focus feedback on *what* is said rather than *why* it is said.
n. Paraphrase to assist in clarifying client's statements.
o. Promote sharing of feelings, information, and ideas instead of giving advice.
2. Examples of therapeutic communication responses (Table 9-3).
3. Examples of nontherapeutic communication responses (Table 9-4).

Table 9-3	THERAPEUTIC COMMUNICATION
Response	*Example*
1. Exploring	"What seems to be the problem?" "Tell me more about …"
2. Reflecting	Client: "I am really mad at my mother for grounding me." Nurse: "You sound angry."
3. Focusing	"Give an example of what you mean." "Let's look at this more closely."
4. Clarifying	"I'm not sure that I understand what you're saying." "Do you mean … ?"
5. Using general leads	"Go on …" "Talk more about …"
6. Broad opening leads	"Where would you like to begin?" "Talk more about …"
7. Validating	"Did I understand you to say …?"
8. Informing	"The time is …" "My name is …"
9. Accepting	"Yes." "Okay." Nodding, "Uh hmm."
10. Sharing observations	"You appear anxious. I noticed that you haven't been coming to lunch with the group."
11. Presenting reality	"I do not hear a noise or see the lights blinking." "I am not Cleopatra; I am your nurse."
12. Summarizing	"During the past hour we talked about …"
13. Using silence	Nurse remains silent and waits patiently for the client to begin speaking.

Table 9-4	NONTHERAPEUTIC COMMUNICATION
Response	*Example*
1. False reassurance	"Don't worry; you will be better in a few weeks." "Don't worry. I had an operation just like it; it was a snap."
2. Giving advice	"What you should do is …" "If I were you, I would do …"
3. Rejecting	"I don't like it when you …" "Please, don't ever talk about …"
4. Belittling	"Everybody feels that way." "Why, you shouldn't feel that way."
5. Probing	"Tell me more about your relationships with other men."
6. Overloading	"Hi, I am JoAnn, your student nurse. How old are you? What brought you to the hospital? How many children do you have? Do you want to fill out your menu right now?"
7. Underloading	Not giving enough information so that the meaning is clear; withholding information.
8. Clichés	"Gee, the weather is beautiful outside." "Did you watch that new TV show last night? Everybody's talking about it."

ALERT Listen to client's concerns and use therapeutic interventions to increase client's understanding of his or her behavior.

INTERVENTION MODALITIES

Crisis Intervention

A crisis is a self-limiting situation in which usual problem-solving or decision-making methods are not adequate.
A. A crisis offers opportunities for growth and renewal.
B. Crisis intervention strategy views people as capable of personal growth and able to control their own lives.
C. Types of crisis intervention strategies.
   1. Individual crisis counseling.
   2. Crisis groups.
   3. Telephone counseling.
D. Crisis intervention requires support, protection, and enhancement of the client's self-image.

ALERT Identify client in crisis; provide opportunity for client to express feelings about crisis.

Group Therapy

A structured or semistructured process in which individuals (7 to 12 members is an ideal size) are interrelated and interdependent and may share common purposes and norms.

A. Emphasis on clear communication to promote effective interaction.
B. Disturbed perceptions can be corrected through consensual validation.
C. Socially ineffective behaviors can be modified through peer pressure.
D. See Table 10-2: Group Modalities for Older Adult Clients.

> **NURSING PRIORITY** Determining a client's perception of reality is an important consideration when selecting the client to be a member of a group. For instance, a person who is psychotic would not be a good selection as a group member.

Family Therapy

> **ALERT** Provide emotional support to family, assess dynamics of family interactions, assess family's understanding of illness and emotional reaction, and help family adjust to role changes.

A treatment modality designed to bring about a change in communication and interactive patterns between and among family members.
A. A family can be viewed as a system that is dynamic. A change or movement in any part of the family system affects all other parts of the system.
B. Family seeks to maintain a balance or "homeostasis" among various forces that operate within and on it.
C. Emotional symptoms or problems of an individual may be expression of the emotional symptoms or problems in the family.
D. Therapeutic approaches involve helping family members look at themselves in the here and now and recognize the influence of past models on their behavior and expectations.

Milieu

> **ALERT** Maintain a therapeutic milieu/environment.

A scientifically planned, purposeful manipulation in the environment aimed at causing changes in the behavior and personality of the client.
A. Nurse is viewed as a facilitator and a helper to clients rather than as a therapist.
B. The *therapeutic community* is a very special kind of milieu therapy in which the total social structure of the treatment unit is involved as part of the helping process.
C. Emphasis is placed on open communication, both within and between staff and client groups.

Mind-Body-Spirit Therapies

These alternative therapies are different from traditional Western medicine; often influenced by traditional Chinese medicine, which focuses on maintaining unity with nature and balancing our energy systems.

A. Acupuncture: movement of energy through meridians of the body to restore energy balance.
B. Imagery: change reality by creating a different mental picture.
C. Therapeutic touch: manipulate and direct client's energy through the use of the practitioner's hands and direct energy from the practitioner to the client to enhance healing.
D. Massage: use of touch unblocks energy flow and connects client with practitioner.
E. Relaxation: imagery and progressive tensing and relaxing of muscle groups throughout the body.
F. Bioenergetics: removes blockages to promote the flow of bioenergy or Ch'i.
G. Transcendental meditation: quiet meditation, focusing on getting beyond the self and becoming one with the universal energy source.
H. Others: exercise, nutrition, prayer, religious practices.

> **ALERT** Assess client's use of alternative/complementary practices; evaluate client's response to alternative therapy.

Somatic Therapies

A. Restraints.
   1. Must consider client's civil liberties.
   2. Mechanical restraints include camisoles, wrist and ankle restraints, and sheet restraints.

> **NURSING PRIORITY** Legally, the nurse must have a physician's order for applying restraints and to provide for clients' biologic needs, (e.g., hygiene, elimination, nutrition, and ability to communicate).

B. Seclusion.
   1. Confinement to a room that may be locked. Often, the room is without a mattress or linens, and the client is wearing a hospital gown.
   2. There is limited opportunity for communication.

> **ALERT** Legal requirements for the nursing care of the client in seclusion vary from state to state, and specifics are usually not tested on the NCLEX-RN examination.

Psychosurgery

Surgical interruption of selected neural pathways that govern transmission of emotion between the frontal lobes of the cerebral cortex and the thalamus.
A. Recent resurgence of interest in psychosurgery as knowledge of neuroanatomy and "mapping" the cerebral cortex has become more sophisticated.
B. Area of moral and ethical debate, especially because nerve tissue, once damaged, cannot regenerate.

Electroconvulsive Therapy

See Chapter 10.

Other Therapies

A. Psychodrama: the use of structured and directed dramatization of client's emotional problems and experiences.
B. Activities therapy: a number of vital programs belong in this category, such as music therapy, occupational therapy, art therapy, recreational therapy, ROPES therapy, dance or movement therapy, etc.

COMMON BEHAVIORAL PATTERNS

ALERT Identify inappropriate behavior, use client behavior modification techniques, and use therapeutic interventions to increase client's understanding of his or her behavior.

Interpersonal Withdrawal

Behavior characterized by avoidance of interpersonal contact and a sense of unreality.
A. Physical withdrawal: client sits or stands apart from others; may hide, assume a catatonic posture, or (in extreme form) attempt suicide.
B. Verbal withdrawal: avoidance through silence or (in extreme form) mutism; silence may indicate resistance, a pensive moment, or the indication that nothing more is to be said.

Nursing Interventions

A. Avoid punishment of client.
B. Decrease isolation.
C. Invite the client to speak.
D. State the amount of time you are willing to stay with the client, whether he or she chooses to speak or not.
E. Change the context of the contact (e.g., go for a walk together).
F. Encourage the client to share responsibility for the continuance of the relationship.

Regression

A selective, defensive operation in which the individual resorts to earlier, childish, or less complex patterns of behavior that once brought the client attention or pleasure.

Nursing Interventions

A. Avoid fostering dependency and childlike attitudes.
B. Be patient and understanding.
C. Confront client directly about his or her plan.
D. Compliment client when he or she does something unusually well or assumes more responsibility.
E. Promote problem solving, reality orientation, and involvement in social activities.
F. Avoid punishment after periods of regression; instead, explore the meaning of the regressive behavior.
G. Remember that regression is a normal occurrence in young children who are hospitalized.

Anger

An unconscious process used to obtain relief from anxiety that is produced by a sense of danger; it involves a sense of powerlessness.
    Fear of expressing anger is related to fear of rejection.

Nursing Interventions

A. Have client acknowledge or name feelings.
B. Explore source of personal fear or perceived threat (e.g., illness, disability, disfigurement, or emotional crisis).
C. Encourage verbalization of anxiety.
D. Explore appropriate external expression of feelings.
E. Avoid arguing with client.
F. Acting-out behavior is often an indirect expression of anger; it attracts attention and often represents the feelings the person is experiencing.

NURSING PRIORITY Nontherapeutic responses to a client's anger include defensiveness, retaliation, condescension, and avoidance.

Hostility/Aggressiveness

An antagonistic feeling; the client wishes to hurt or humiliate others; the result may be a feeling of inadequacy or self-rejection due to a loss of self-esteem.

Nursing Interventions

ALERT Plan interventions to assist client to control aggressive behavior.

A. Prevent aggressive contact by early recognition of increased anxiety.
B. Maintain client contact rather than avoid it.
C. Encourage verbalization of feelings associated with a threat of frustration (helplessness, inadequacy, anger).
D. Reduce environmental stimuli.
E. Avoid reinforcement behavior (e.g., joking, laughing, teasing, and competitive games).
F. Use distraction, or remove the client from the immediate environment to reestablish self-control.
G. Set limits on unacceptable behavior.
H. Protect other clients.

NURSING PRIORITY When two clients are arguing, engage the dominant client first by using distraction or removing the client from the setting to allow time for deescalation and processing of the situation.

Violence

Behavior that is physically assaultive and risks injury to the self, others, and environment.

Nursing Interventions

> ❗ **NURSING PRIORITY** Immediate intervention should focus on control and safety, followed by discussion to alleviate guilt and identify alternative behaviors to help prevent future episodes of violence.

A. Establish eye contact.
  1. Conveys attention and concern.
  2. Elicits more information.
  3. Ask the person to look at you.

> ❗ **OLDER ADULT PRIORITY** Expect some older clients to have vision problems; they may not know who you are. Hearing problems occur often with older adults; don't shout or talk rapidly.

B. Avoid asking, "Why?" Instead ask, "What's bothering you?"
  1. *Why* questions are threatening and decrease self-esteem.
  2. Open-ended questions seek to identify the problem, convey concern, and elicit more information.
C. Speak to the client softly, slowly, and with assurance.
D. Give directions clearly and concisely. Tell the client what you want him or her to do.
E. Encourage client to verbalize feelings.
  1. Give the client an outlet for the physical tension—"Walk with me. Tell me what happened."
  2. Keep the conversation slow; pace yourself—"Wait, I can't follow that. Tell me what you said."
  3. Listen more than talk.
  4. Let the client walk or move around or provide something for the client to safely "pound" on to release the tension before you talk.
F. Position yourself near the door.
  1. Don't block the door.
  2. Don't box the client into a corner.
G. Self-protection and protection of other clients are primary concerns.
  1. Never remain with a potentially violent client alone; call security or other personnel.
  2. Keep a comfortable distance from client; don't intrude on his or her personal space.
    a. With a client experiencing mild or moderate anxiety: sit near, about 2 feet away.
    b. With a client experiencing severe anxiety or panic: stay 4 to 6 feet away (or farther).
  3. Be prepared to move quickly; violent clients act quickly and unpredictably.
  4. Determine that the client has no weapons before approaching him or her.
  5. Be supportive and intervene to increase client's self-esteem.
  6. Be honest; tell the client you are concerned that he or she is out of control, but you are not going to let anyone get hurt.
  7. Stay with the client, but don't touch him or her until you've asked permission and it has been given to you.
H. Once the client is in control of their behavior, review and process the situation in order to alleviate client's guilt and to discuss alternatives in case the client becomes anxious or angry in the future.

Manipulation/Acting Out

A type of controlling behavior in which an individual uses others to meet his or her own needs or to achieve specific goals; often disguises underlying feelings of inadequacy, inferiority, and unworthiness; an attempt to protect against failure or frustration and to gain power over another.

Nursing Interventions

A. Be consistent and firm in the expectations of behavior.
B. Allow some freedom within set limits.
C. Consistently enforce previously set limits.
D. Be alert to client's attempt to intimidate; allow verbal anger.
E. Avoid involvement and intellectualization.
F. Watch carefully for client's use of manipulative patterns; be alert to the many guises in which it may be manifested.
G. Keep staff united, firm, and consistent.
H. Encourage open communication about real needs and feelings.
I. Maintain a sense of authority.
J. Do not accept gifts, favors, flattery, or other forms of manipulation.

Dependence

A behavior pattern characterized by adopting a helpless, powerless stance; a reliance on other people to meet a basic need.

Nursing Interventions

A. Assess client's abilities and capacities.
B. Set firm and consistent limits on behavior.
C. Provide only help that is clearly needed.
D. Encourage problem-solving and decision-making skills; emphasize accountability.
E. Avoid making decisions for client or assuming responsibility for client's ability to make decisions.
F. Maintain an attitude of firmness and confidence in client's ability to make decisions.
G. Discourage reliance beyond actual needs.
H. Give positive reinforcements for development of independent, growth-facilitating behavior.
I. Encourage successful participation in social relationships.

Shame

The inner sense of being completely diminished or insufficient as a person (e.g., feeling "less than").

Nursing Interventions

A. Assist client to begin to *externalize* rather than internalize feelings of shame.
B. Encourage client to share feelings honestly with individuals he or she feels "safe" with.
C. Involve client in "debriefing," which is writing and talking about past experiences with shame.
D. Encourage client to make positive self-affirmations and to engage in creative visualization activities to improve self-concept.

Detachment

A behavioral process characterized by aloofness, superficiality, denial, and intellectualization during interpersonal contact.

Nursing Interventions

A. Establish awareness of the process of detachment.
B. Explore fears and fantasies inhibiting emotional expression.
C. Encourage verbalization from global generalities to specific personal comments.
D. Provide clarification of client's unclear responses.
E. Emphasize awareness and exploration of feelings.

ABUSE

Abuse is difficult to define, because the term has been politicized and is not a clinical or scientific term.

> **ALERT** Report client abuse to authorities, initiate a consultation/referral (e.g., support groups, community programs, social service, etc), and protect client from injury.

Types of Abuse

A. *Physical abuse:* nonaccidental, intentional injury inflicted on another person.
B. *Physical neglect:* willing deprivation of essential care needed to sustain basic human needs and to promote growth and development.
C. *Emotional abuse:* use of threats, verbal insults, or other acts of degradation that are intended to be injurious or damaging to another's self-esteem.
D. *Emotional neglect:* absence of a warm, interpersonal atmosphere that is necessary for psychosocial growth, development, and the promotion of positive feelings of self-worth and self-esteem.
E. *Sexual abuse:* lack of comprehension and consent on the part of the individual involved in sexual activities that are either exploitative or physically intimate in nature (e.g., rape, fondling, oral or genital contact, masturbation, unclothing, etc.).
F. *Incest:* sexual activity performed between members of a family group.

Intrafamily Abuse and Violence

Patterns of dysfunctional, violent families can frequently be traced back for several generations. Adult behavior and role models for parenting are influenced by the childhood experiences within the family system.

> **ALERT** Assess dynamics of family interactions; identify risk factors; plan interventions to assist client and family to cope.

 A. The incorporation of violence within the family teaches children that the use of violence is appropriate. When the children grow up and form their own families, they tend to recreate the same parent-child, husband-wife relationships experienced in their original family.
B. Frequently, the abuser has inappropriate expectations of family members; the abuser may expect perfection and may be obsessed with discipline and control.
C. Family members are confused regarding their roles in the family; parents may be unable to assume adult roles in the family. Adult family members who feel inadequate in their roles may use violence in an attempt to prove themselves and to maintain superiority.
D. Family is usually isolated, both physically and emotionally. The family tends to have few friends and is frequently isolated from the extended family. Family members are ashamed of what is occurring and tend to withdraw from social contacts in fear that the family activities might become known to others.
E. The *hostage response* is when victims assume responsibility for the violence inflicted on them.

Characteristics of Abuse: The Perpetrator

A. The person who abuses—the perpetrator.
 1. Perpetrator has an inability to control impulses; explosive temper; low tolerance for frustration.
 2. Possesses greater physical strength than the victim.
 3. Has low self-esteem and depression; feels he or she is a victim.
 4. Tends to project shortcomings and inadequacies onto others.
 5. Emotional immaturity; decreased capacity to delay satisfaction.
 6. Suspicious of everyone; fear of being exposed; tends to isolate self from family.
 7. High incidence of drug and alcohol abuse.
 8. Often has experienced abuse as a child; has a greater tendency to demonstrate violence in his or her adult relationships.
B. Common similarities between person who abuses and victim.
 1. Poor self-concept and feelings of insecurity.
 2. Feelings of helplessness, powerlessness, and dependence.
 3. Difficulty in handling or inability to handle anger.

Child Abuse

A. Child neglect: the failure to provide a child with the basic necessities; may be classified as physical or emotional neglect.

1. Failure to thrive: infant or child is below the normal ranges on the growth chart.
2. Infant or child does not appear to be physically cared for. Inappropriate diapering, diaper rash, strong urine smell to the body may be seen in infants who have been neglected.
3. Evidence of malnutrition.
4. Lack of adequate supervision; child is allowed to engage in dangerous play activities and sustains frequent injuries.
5. Language development may be delayed.
6. Withdrawal; inappropriate fearfulness.
7. Parents may be apathetic and unresponsive to the child's needs. The nurse is most often able to observe the parent-child interaction in school situations, in a doctor's office, or in the emergency department.

B. Physical child abuse.
 1. Symptoms.
  a. Bruises and welts from being beaten with a belt, strap, stick, or coat hanger or from being slapped repeatedly in the face.
  b. Rope burns from being tied up or beaten with a rope.
  c. Human bite marks.
  d. Burns.
   (1) Burns on the buttocks from being immersed in hot water.
   (2) Pattern of burns: round, small burns from cigarettes; patterns that suggest an object was used.
   (3) Burns are frequently on the buttocks, in genital area, or on the soles of the feet.
  e. Evidence of various fractures in different stages of healing.
  f. Internal injuries from being hit repeatedly in the abdomen.
  g. Head injuries: skull, facial fractures.
 2. Behavior symptoms.
  a. Withdrawal from physical contact with adults.
  b. Inappropriate response to pain or injury; failure to cry or seek comfort from parents.
  c. Infant may stiffen when held; child may stiffen when approached by adult or parent.
  d. Very little eye contact with adults.
  e. Child may try to protect abusing parent for fear of punishment if abuse is discovered.
 3. Parents or caretakers.
  a. Conflicting stories regarding accident or injury.
  b. Explanation of accident is inconsistent with injuries sustained (fractured skull and broken leg from "falling out of bed").
  c. Initial complaint is not associated with child's injury (child is brought to the emergency department with complaints of the "flu," and there is evidence of a skull fracture).
  d. Exaggerated concern or lack of concern related to level of child's injury.
  e. Refusal to allow further tests or additional medical care.
  f. Lack of nurturing response to injured or ill child; no cuddling, touching, or comforting child in distress.
  g. Repeated visits to various medical emergency facilities.
  h. Unrealistic expectations of the child; lack of understanding about stages of growth and development (e.g., severely spanking or beating a 1-year-old for lack of response to toilet training).

Nursing Interventions

Goal: To establish a safe environment.
A. It is important for the nurse to be knowledgeable of the legal responsibilities in regard to state practice acts and child abuse laws (Box 9-2).
B. All 50 states have a designated agency that is available on a 24-hour basis for reporting child abuse.
C. All states have mechanisms for removing the child from the immediate abusive environment.

Box 9-2   DOCUMENTATION FOR SUSPECTED ABUSE

Procedure
1. Obtain the client's or parent's permission before photographing the victim.
2. Do not make assumptions about the identity of the perpetrator.
3. Chart the exact words used by the client/child to describe the abuser.
4. Record information very objectively; do not record your feelings, assumptions, or opinions of the incident or how it occurred.

History
1. Specify the time, date, and location as described by the client.
2. Report the sequence of events before the abuse/attack.
3. Identify and explain the period of time between the abuse/attack and initiation of medical attention.
4. List other people/children in the immediate vicinity of the abuse/attack.
5. Include quotations from the client.
6. Use objective, specific documentation when recording observations of the client and the person who brought the client to the ED.
7. Observe and record the interaction of the child and the parents.

Physical Examination
1. Be very specific in describing the location, size, and shape of bruises and lacerations. If possible, photograph the client to demonstrate the extent of the injuries.
2. If possible, describe the location and extent of injuries on an anatomic diagram.
3. Identify presence of other injuries.
4. Describe the victim's reaction to pain, level of pain, and location of pain.

Goal: To educate the parents and help them to identify assistance for long-term supportive care.

A. Educate parents in regard to normal growth and development of children, the role of discipline, and the necessity for having realistic expectations.

B. Become familiar with available community resources such as crisis centers, crisis hotlines, parent effectiveness training groups, Parents Anonymous groups, etc.

 Incest

A. Assessment.
1. Victim is usually female; perpetrator of abuse is primarily male, usually between ages 30 and 50, and often the victim's father or other member of the immediate family.
2. Incest is a symptom of severe dysfunction in an individual and within the family.
3. Perpetrators of sexual exploitation.
   a. Emotionally dependent men.
   b. Feelings of inferiority and low self-esteem.
   c. Perpetrators frequently seduce their victims by being endearing and "good" to the child.
   d. Often, these men are pillars of the community and are involved in many youth activities.
   e. Frequently, the mother is unaware of the problem. If she suspects it, she may feel guilty for having such ideas.
4. Sexually exploited child.
   a. Child may fear retaliation if anyone finds out; may fear that she will not be believed if she tells anyone.
   b. Child may feel guilty for participating in the sexual activity and afraid of disruption of the family if it is revealed.
   c. Violence rarely accompanies the incest relationship.
   d. The child may be emotionally and physically dependent on the abusing parent.

Nursing Interventions

Goal: To educate children that their bodies belong to themselves and are private.

A. Instruct children to report any type of touching, fondling, or caressing that makes them feel uncomfortable.

B. Provide educational material to help parents talk about sexual assault and inappropriate fondling with their children.

Goal: To support the parents and the child and to help them identify assistance for long-term supportive care.

A. Provide support and the opportunity for the child and family members to discuss their feelings.

B. Assist the family to identify community resources; strongly encourage involvement in family counseling.

 Older Adult Abuse

A. Types of older adult abuse (Box 9-3).
B. Typical victim.

Box 9-3 OLDER ADULT CARE FOCUS

Older Adult Abuse

Types of Older Adult Abuse
- Physical: willful infliction of injury.
- Neglect: withholding goods or services (such as food or attention) to the detriment of the older adult's physical or mental health.
- Psychologic: withholding affection or imposing social isolation.
- Exploitation: dishonest or inappropriate use of the older person's property, money, or other resources.

Neglect Indicators
- Poor hygiene, nutrition, and skin integrity.
- Contractures.
- Urine burns/excoriation.
- Pressure ulcers.
- Dehydration.

---

1. Woman of advanced age with few social contacts.
2. At least one physical or mental impairment, limiting the person's ability to perform activities of daily living.

C. Assessment of elder abuse.
1. Symptoms: contusions, abrasions, sprains, burns, bruising, human bite marks, sexual molestation, untreated or previously treated conditions, erratic hair loss from hair pulling, fractures, dislocations, head and face injuries (especially orbital fractures, black eyes, and broken teeth).
2. Behavior: clinging to the abuser, extreme guardedness in the presence of the abuser, wariness of strangers, expression of ambivalence toward family/caregivers, depression, social or physical isolation, denial of abuse for fear of retaliation.

Nursing Interventions

Goal: To assess for older adult abuse.

A. Use a private, separate setting for interviewing victim and perpetrator.

B. The interview must be unbiased, accurate, and appropriately documented.

C. Avoid signs of disapproval that might evoke shame or anger in the older client; be nonjudgmental.

Goal: To establish a safe environment.

A. It is important for the nurse to be knowledgeable of the legal responsibilities in regard to state practice acts and reporting of abuse (see Box 9-2).

B. Client and family teaching in the areas of nutrition, general physical care, etc.

Spouse Abuse

A. Most often the spouse abused is the wife; frequently, the violence is a pattern in the woman's life. The violence in the family is frequently associated with alcohol; often, there is a history of the woman's parents having a violent relationship.

B. It is not uncommon for the husband or abuser to have been exposed to violent family dynamics during childhood.

C. After the violent attack, the husband is frequently remorseful, kind, and loving. He may promise that he will never do it again.

D. Women tend to stay in abuse situations. Retaliation, loss of home and children, and additional abuse are just a few of the consequences they fear if they try to escape the situation. Abuse may increase if they express a desire to become more independent.

Physical Assessment

A. Traumatic injury to the upper body, especially the face and breasts.

B. Signs of fear and an expression of helplessness.

C. May avoid friends and family for fear they will find out.

D. May exhibit feelings of shame, guilt, and embarrassment that she must seek treatment for her injuries.

Nursing Interventions

Goal: Primary prevention—education of the community regarding the risks of abuse.

Goal: Secondary prevention—screening activities that occur within the community.

Goal: Tertiary prevention—emergency treatment, counseling, and work that goes on in shelters.

> **! NURSING PRIORITY** When working with an abused woman, avoid anything that sounds like blaming her for her situation.

Rape

A. Legal definition of rape (varies from state to state): forced, violent sexual attack on an individual without his or her consent. Includes sex acts other than forced intercourse as rape; some states do not recognize rape by the husband.

B. Sexual assault is not a means of sexual gratification; it is a violent physical and emotional attack. Men attack women in an attempt to demonstrate their power and dominance; attempt to control, terrify, and degrade the woman.

C. Victims: in all age ranges; highest-risk age group is 12 to 20 years old.

D. Majority of rapes are not sudden and impulsive; they are well planned.

E. Most women know the rapist; most rape assaults occur between people of the same race.

F. Rape-trauma syndrome: variant of posttraumatic stress disorder; has two phases, an acute phase and a long-term reorganization phase.

> **! NURSING PRIORITY** Five components essential in treating rape victim: treat and document injuries, treat and evaluate for sexually transmitted diseases, evaluate and prevent pregnancy risk, arrange for follow-up counseling, and collect evidence according to protocols.

Assessment

A. Acute phase: may last a couple of weeks.
  1. Woman may experience a wide range of emotional responses: fear, shock, disbelief, anger, denial, guilt, embarrassment, etc. (there is no "normal response" to rape).
  2. Somatic reaction: physical trauma, skeletal muscle tension, GI and genitourinary symptoms/discomfort.

B. Long-term reorganization phase: occurs 2 weeks or more after rape.
  1. Intrusive thoughts (flashbacks, violent dreams, insomnia), fears, phobias.
  2. Increased motor activity (moving, taking trips, changing phone numbers) and emotional lability.

C. Advise the woman to not "clean up" after a rape, because the physical evidence may be destroyed; advise the woman to come immediately to the ED.

D. Complete physical assessment (Box 9-4).

Nursing Intervention

Goal: To assist the client through the acute phase after the rape experience.

A. Encourage the client to verbalize her feelings regarding the attack.

B. Assist her to set priorities and determine immediate needs.

C. Respond to the client in a warm, respectful, accepting manner; protect the client from becoming overwhelmed and distressed from the initial physical examination and questioning.

D. Discuss need for follow-up care and physical examination regarding possible pregnancy and sexually transmitted disease.

E. Provide information regarding physical and emotional responses to rape.

F. Provide referral information and plan for follow-up contact within the next week.

Goal: To assist the client to work through the emotional phases that commonly occur after the initial trauma.

A. Encourage mental health counseling during the first few days after the assault.

B. Assist the client to understand and recognize the period of long-term reorganization that frequently follows a sexual attack.
  1. Victim may experience sexual problems.
  2. May experience a strong urge to discuss the incident and feelings related to the attack.
  3. During the reorganization phase, client should have professional counseling to assist her to positively cope with the situation.

Box 9-4 CHECKLIST OF NURSING MANAGEMENT FOR THE RAPE VICTIM

Medical-Legal
- Valid written consent for examination, photographs, lab tests, release of information, and laboratory samples.
- Appropriate "chain of evidence" documentation: follow agency protocol.
- Protect legal rights.

Assist With Physical Examination
- Vital signs and general appearance.
- Examine for extragenital trauma: mouth, breasts, neck.
- Examine for cuts, bruises, scratches; photograph.

Pelvic Examination
- Vulvar trauma; erythema; hymen, anal, and rectal status.
- Matted hair or free hairs.
- Vaginal examination: use unlubricated speculum; look for foreign body, discharge, blood, lacerations; uterine size; adnexa, especially hematomas.

Implement Medical Treatment
- Care for injuries and emotional trauma.
- Antibiotic prophylaxis for STDs.
- Antipregnancy measures: postcoital dose of Ovral.

Document History
- Age, marital status, and parity.
- Menstrual and contraceptive history.
- Time of last coitus before assault.
- Change of clothes, bath, douche?
- Use of drugs or alcohol.
- Who, what, when, where?
- Penetration, ejaculation, condom, extragenital acts.

Obtain Laboratory Samples
- Use appropriate *evidence collection kits* and label carefully.
- Saline irrigation of vagina: 2 mL and swab; acid phosphatase, blood group antigen of semen, and precipitin test against human sperm and blood.
- Vaginal smears: Pap smear and Gram stain.
- Oral or rectal swabs and smears.
- Blood tests for serology, blood type, alcohol level.
- Cultures: cervix plus other areas, if indicated.
- Urine: pregnancy test, drugs.
- Hair: comb and clip; obtain fingernail scrapings; comb pubic hairs; clip client's pubic hair or any matted hairs.

Follow-Up and Referral
- Recommend continued follow-up and services of rape crisis center.
- Repeat serology testing for gonorrhea, chlamydia, and HIV at later date.

HIV, Human immunodeficiency virus; *STD,* sexually transmitted disease.

Appendix 9-1 UNDERSTANDING DEFENSE MECHANISMS

NAME OF DEFENSE MECHANISM	DEFINITION	EXAMPLE
Compensation	Attempting to make up for or offset deficiencies, either real or imagined, by concentrating on or developing other abilities	An adolescent who perceives herself as unattractive focuses her energies on cultivating her intellectual abilities and is on the honor roll at school.
Conversion	Symbolic expression of intrapsychic conflict expressed in physical symptoms	A man develops blindness after watching his friend get seriously injured in a race car accident.
Denial	Blocking out or disowning painful thoughts or feelings	A young mother with a newborn who has a cleft palate tells her friends everything is okay with her baby.
Displacement	Feelings are transferred, redirected, or discharged from the appropriate person or object to a less threatening person or object	A man gets reprimanded by his boss. Later, he yells at his wife when dinner is not ready.
Dissociation	Separating and detaching an idea, situation, or relationship from its emotional significance; helps the individual put aside painful feelings and often leads to a temporary alteration of consciousness or identity	A young adolescent who was the lone survivor of an airplane crash now experiences amnesia.
Identification	Attempting to pattern or resemble the personality of an admired, idealized person	A young man chooses to become a professional football player like his father.
Introjection	Acceptance of another's values and opinions as one's own	A young woman takes on the values and opinions of her peer group.

Appendix 9-1 UNDERSTANDING DEFENSE MECHANISMS—cont'd

NAME OF DEFENSE MECHANISM	DEFINITION	EXAMPLE
Projection	Attributing one's own unacceptable feelings and thoughts to others	A student who feels like a failure after getting an F on an important examination says, "It's the teacher's fault. He doesn't know how to write a test."
Rationalization	Attempting to justify or modify unacceptable needs and feelings to the ego, in an effort to maintain self-respect and prevent guilt feelings	A man drinks several alcoholic beverages each evening, saying, "I work hard, so I need to relax when I get home."
Reaction formation	Assuming attitudes and behaviors that one consciously rejects	A man is extremely polite and courteous to his mother-in-law, whom he intensely dislikes.
Regression	Retreating to an earlier, more comfortable level of adjustment	A young preschool child begins to suck his thumb and wet the bed shortly after the birth of a sibling.
Repression	An involuntary, automatic submerging of painful, unpleasant thoughts and feelings into the *unconscious*	A woman is unable to remember being sexually abused as a child.
Sublimation	Diversion of unacceptable instinctual drives into personally and socially acceptable areas to help channel forbidden impulses into constructive activities	A man who has strong competitive or aggressive drives channels his energy into building a successful business.
Suppression	Intentional exclusion of forbidden ideas and anxiety-producing situations from the *conscious* level; a voluntary forgetting and postponing mechanism	A young man is thinking so much about his date that it is interfering with his work. He decides to put it out of his mind until he leaves the office.
Undoing	Actually or symbolically attempting to erase a previous consciously intolerable experience or action; an attempt to repair feelings and actions that have created guilt and anxiety	A mother who has unjustly punished her child decides to bake the child's favorite cookies.

! NURSING PRIORITY Recognize client's use of defense mechanisms.

Study Questions Psychiatric Nursing Concepts

More questions on companion CD!

1. A 23-month-old has been admitted to the hospital. The child's mother works in a factory at night and says that if she misses any more work, she will be fired. She is worried about leaving her child in the hospital at night because he is so young. What would be an appropriate nursing response?
   1 "He is really too young to suffer any untoward consequences."
   2 "It's okay to leave; just leave a favorite toy."
   3 "It would be better if you could stay, but we will take good care of him."
   4 "You will have a lot of expenses in the future, so you better go to work."

2. A 9-year-old client with leukemia asks, "Will I die?" What is an initial therapeutic response based on the needs of the dying child?
   1 "Think about getting well instead of dying."
   2 "Tell me what you are thinking about dying."
   3 "You need to ask your doctor."
   4 "I really don't know."

3. In response to information that a 5-year-old's death is imminent, the parents express intense anger at the staff, and they are critical of the care their son is receiving. What is the purpose of therapeutic intervention on the parents' behalf?
   1 Assure them that the doctor will be told about their concerns.
   2 Determine their attitude toward the child's impending death.
   3 Inform them that their behavior will upset their child.
   4 Allow them to express their emotions about their son dying.

4. During a client care conference, there is a discussion regarding the anxiety of a 9-year-old client with leukemia. In addition to anxiety related to his death, the child might also experience anxiety about:
   1 Concerns about missing school
   2 Fear of separation from his family
   3 Concerns about being dependent on staff
   4 Knowledge of the disease process

5. An infant is scheduled for a pyloromyotomy. The mother begins to cry and says, "I'm such a bad mother." What is an appropriate response by the nurse?
   1 "Tell me what makes you think you are a bad mother."
   2 "Don't cry; your baby will be fine."
   3 "You are really having a bad time, aren't you?"
   4 The nurse says nothing and puts her arms around the mother.

6. In order for a terminally ill client to receive quality nursing care, the charge nurse needs to plan for which of the following when she assigns staff to care for the client?
   1 Assign a different staff nurse to the client every day.
   2 Assign the same full-time staff nurses every day.
   3 Use part-time nursing staff.
   4 Assign a different staff nurse every other day.

7. The nurse notes that a client is quite suspicious during an assessment interview and believes that her family is under investigation by the CIA. What would be appropriate nursing interventions with this client? Select all that apply:
   _____ 1 Use active listening skills to seek information from the client.
   _____ 2 Encourage the client to describe the problem as she sees it.
   _____ 3 Ask the client to tell you exactly what she thinks is happening.
   _____ 4 Tell the client that she is delusional and you can help her.
   _____ 5 Explain to the client that most people are not investigated by the CIA or FBI.
   _____ 6 Reassure the client that you are not with the CIA.

8. Which is an appropriate initial nursing measure in caring for a female who has been raped?
   1 Cleanse body wounds and apply cool compresses.
   2 Obtain written informed consent for examination.
   3 Determine whether the woman has bathed or douched.
   4 Obtain laboratory specimens.

9. When a child feels responsible for physical abuse inflicted upon him or her, the nurse knows the child is experiencing which of the following?
   1 Fear
   2 Hostage response
   3 Anxiety response
   4 Guilt

10. A nurse case worker suspects older adult neglect. What assessment findings would confirm this?
   1 Confusion and disorientation
   2 Recent hip fracture
   3 Poor nutrition and hygiene
   4 Dirty dishes in the sink

Answers and rationales to these questions are in the section at the end of the book titled Chapter Study Questions: Answers and Rationales.

CHAPTER TEN

Psychiatric Disorders

It is important to note that emotional disturbances must be evaluated within the context and framework of normal growth and development, since behavior that is acceptable at one age may be a symptom of disease at another age.

ALERT Modify approaches to care in accordance with client's development stages.

CHILD-RELATED DISORDERS

 Mental Retardation

A child who is mentally retarded has an IQ of 70 or below, which is associated with deficits or impairments in adaptive behavior before the age of 18 years.

Assessment
A. Causes.
  1. Down syndrome, phenylketonuria, rubella.
  2. Kernicterus (elevated bilirubin level), anoxia.
  3. Lead poisoning, meningitis, encephalitis.
  4. Neoplasms, Tay-Sachs disease.
B. Diagnostic criteria.
  1. IQ below 70.
  2. Deficit or impairment in adaptive behavior.
  3. Present before the age of 18 years.
C. Additional characteristics.
  1. Irritability, temper tantrums, stereotyped movements.
  2. Multiple neurologic abnormalities: dysfunction in vision or hearing or seizure activity.

Nursing Interventions
Goal: To promote optimum development within a family and community setting.
A. Promote feelings of self-esteem, worth, and security.
B. Educate the parents about developmental stages and tasks; deal with child's developmental, *not* chronologic, age.
Goal: To promote independence by setting realistic goals.
A. Teach basic skills in simple terms, with steps outlined.
B. Use behavior modification as a method for behavior control.
C. Use the principles of *repetition, reinforcement,* and *routine* when providing information for understanding and learning.

 Down Syndrome

Down syndrome is a common chromosomal abnormality characterized by an extra chromosome 21 (trisomy 21); incidence increases with maternal age.

Assessment
A. Physical characteristics criteria.
  1. Head: small in size; face has flat profile, sparse hair.
  2. Eyes: inner epicanthal folds; short and sparse eyelashes.
  3. Nose: small and depressed nasal bridge (saddle nose).
  4. Ears: small and sometimes low-set.
  5. Mouth: protruding tongue; high arched palate.
  6. Neck: short and broad.
  7. Abdomen: protruding.
  8. Genitalia: small penis, cryptorchidism.
  9. Hands: short, stubby fingers; simian crease (transverse palmar crease).
  10. Muscles: hypotonic.
B. Mental characteristics.
  1. Mental retardation.
  2. Slow development.

Nursing Interventions
Goal: To promote optimal development.
A. Involve child and parents in early stimulation program.
B. Promote self-care skills.
C. Help parents identify realistic goals for child.
D. Encourage parents to enroll child in special day care programs and education classes.
E. Emphasize to parents that child has same needs of play, discipline, and social interaction as all children.
Goal: To encourage early identification of Down syndrome.

It is common for pregnant women at risk (older than 35 years, family history of Down syndrome, or previous birth of a child with Down syndrome) to have an amniocentesis before the 16th week to rule out Down syndrome.

Home Care
A. Prevent respiratory tract infections by teaching parents about postural drainage and percussion.
B. Encourage use of cool mist vaporizer.

C. Stress importance of changing infant's position frequently.

D. Explain to parents about feeding difficulties; encourage small, frequent feedings; feed solid food by pushing food back inside of mouth; provide foods that will form bulk to prevent constipation.

E. Discuss with parents alternative options to home care.

F. Individuals with Down syndrome develop a clinical syndrome of dementia that has almost identical clinical and neuropathologic characteristics of Alzheimer's disease as described in individuals without Down syndrome.
  1. The main difference is the age of onset of Alzheimer's disease in individuals with Down syndrome.
  2. These clients present with clinical symptoms in their late 40s or early 50s.

 Attention-Deficit/Hyperactivity Disorder

Attention-deficit/hyperactivity disorder is a developmental disorder characterized by inappropriate inattention and impulsivity, which usually appear between ages 3 and 7 years. Names previously used: hyperkinetic syndrome, minimal brain damage, minimal brain dysfunction.

Assessment

A. Diagnostic criteria.
  1. Inattention.
    a. Fails to finish things he or she starts.
    b. Often doesn't seem to listen.
    c. Is easily distracted.
    d. Has difficulty concentrating.
    e. Has difficulty sticking to play activity.
  2. Impulsivity.
    a. Often acts before thinking.
    b. Shifts excessively from one activity to another.
    c. Has difficulty organizing work.
    d. Needs frequent supervision.
    e. Frequently calls out in class.
    f. Has difficulty waiting turn in games or group activities.
  3. Hyperactivity.
    a. Runs about or climbs on things.
    b. Has difficulty sitting still; fidgets.
    c. Has difficulty staying seated.
    d. Moves about excessively during sleep.
    e. Is always "on the go."
  4. Onset before the age of 7 years.
  5. Duration of at least 6 months.
B. Additional characteristics.
  1. Obstinacy, negativism, mood lability.
  2. Low frustration tolerance.
  3. Soft neurologic signs: motor perceptual dysfunctions (e.g., poor hand-eye coordination).

Nursing Interventions

Goal: To keep child from harming self or others.
A. Assist child to recognize when he or she feels angry.
B. Help the child to accept his or her feelings of anger.

C. Teach child appropriate expression of angry feelings.
D. Redirect violent behavior with physical outlets for child's anxiety (e.g., use of punching bag, jogging).
E. Confront child; withdraw attention when interactions with others are manipulative or exploitative.
F. Use time-out, isolation room, and restraints only when other interventions are unsuccessful.

Goal: To encourage age-appropriate, socially acceptable coping skills.
A. If child is hyperactive, make environment safe for continuous large muscle movement.
B. Provide large motor skill activities for child to participate in.
C. Provide frequent, nutritious snacks for child to "eat on the run."

Goal: To decrease anxiety and increase self-esteem.
A. Encourage child to seek out staff to discuss true feelings.
B. Offer support during times of increased anxiety; ensure physical and psychologic safety.

Goal: To administer prescribed medication.
A. Ritalin (methylphenidate) may be used; is usually discontinued when child enters adolescence.
B. Prolonged administration may produce a temporary suppression of normal weight gain. Child may be taken off medication during summer months when school is out.
C. Administer in morning (to prevent insomnia) and 30 to 45 minutes before meals.

 Autistic Disorder

The lack of responsiveness to other people (autism), lack of involvement with others, lack of verbal communication, preoccupation with inanimate objects, and ritualistic behavior are characteristic of infantile autism.

Assessment

A. Diagnostic criteria.
  1. Onset before 3 years of age.
  2. Impairment in social interactions—lack of responsiveness and involvement with others.
  3. Impairment in communication and imaginative activity.
    a. Gross deficits in language development: speech is characterized by echolalia, parrot speech (i.e., the automatic repetition of words).
    b. Pronominal reversal (the tendency to use *you* for *I*).
    c. Lack of spontaneous make-believe play.
  4. Markedly restricted, stereotypical patterns of behavior, interest, and activities.
    a. Rigid adherence to routines and rituals.
    b. Repetitive motor mannerisms—hand flapping, clapping, rocking, or rhythmic body movements.
  5. *Absence* of delusions, hallucinations, and associative looseness, which are characteristics of childhood schizophrenia.

Nursing Interventions

Goal: To increase social awareness.

A. Encourage a significant one-to-one relationship with an adult.

B. Promote and engage in peer interaction.

C. Develop play and self-care skills.

D. Do not force interactions. Begin with positive reinforcement for eye contact. Gradually introduce touch, smiling, and hugging.

Goal: To teach verbal (oral) communication.

A. Respond to verbalization by telling the child what you do not understand.

B. Respond to nonverbal cues with verbal (oral) interpretation.

C. Observe and record context in which lack of clarity of spoken word occurred.

D. Use "en face" approach (face-to-face, eye-to-eye) to convey correct nonverbal expressions by example.

Goal: To decrease unacceptable behavior.

A. Encourage child to recognize and respond to own physiologic needs and urges.

B. Encourage verbalization of body needs, but do not make an issue of it.

C. Offer fluids and encourage exercise to prevent constipation.

D. Offer the bathroom at appropriate intervals throughout the day.

E. Prevent child from hurting self or others by setting firm limits and recognizing feelings of anger, fear, and frustration.

 Separation Anxiety Disorder

Child demonstrates persistent and excessive anxiety on separation from parent or familiar surroundings.

Assessment

A. Diagnostic criteria.
1. Excessive distress when separated from home or parents.
2. Unrealistic worry about harm occurring.
3. Refusal to sleep unless near parent.
4. Refusal to attend school or other activities without parent.
5. Physical symptoms as a response to anxiety (e.g., stomachache, vomiting, headache, etc).

B. Additional characteristics.
1. Fear of the dark.
2. Excessive conformity; often demonstrates need for constant attention; may be demanding.
3. Usual age of onset any time between preschool years and 11 or 12 years.

Nursing Interventions

Goal: To reduce the level of anxiety in anxiety-provoking situations.

A. Identify factors that produce anxiety.

B. Turn night lights on to allay night fears.

C. Offer calm reassurance.

Goal: To differentiate between normal separation anxiety, which is seen in early childhood, and excessive anxiety, which is seen in separation anxiety disorders.

A. To be labeled as a separation anxiety disorder, the disturbance must have a duration of at least 2 weeks.

B. Children with this disorder tend to come from close-knit families.

 Specific Disorders With Physical Symptoms

Assessment

A. Stuttering.
1. Frequent repetitions or prolongations of sounds, syllables, or words.
2. Unusual hesitations and pauses that disrupt the flow of speech.
3. Speech may be very rapid or very slow.
4. Stuttering is often absent during singing or talking to inanimate objects.

B. Functional enuresis.
1. Repeated involuntary voiding of urine during the day or night.
2. The involuntary voiding occurs after the age at which it is expected and is not due to any physical disorder.

C. Functional encopresis (fecal incontinence).
1. Repeated voluntary or involuntary passage of feces of normal consistency in inappropriate places.
2. Smearing feces, which should be differentiated from the smearing that takes place involuntarily and in the younger child (age 1 or 2 years).

Nursing Interventions

Goal: To assess and medically evaluate for any physiologic cause related to stuttering, enuresis, or encopresis.

Goal: To promote a positive self-concept by helping child overcome feelings of shame and guilt associated with disorder.

Goal: To identify various approaches to controlling enuresis.

A. Administer imipramine (Tofranil).

B. Restrict fluids before going to bed.

C. Encourage behavioral intervention therapies (a buzzer that wakes child when he or she starts to urinate; bladder training programs).

Goal: To identify various approaches to controlling fecal incontinence.

A. If child is retaining feces, initiate a bowel-cleaning regimen.

B. If child has loose stools, he or she needs a daily bulk laxative.

C. If soiling is deliberate, help child to express feelings through other means.

D. Educate child about bodily signals (rectal pressure).

E. Teach child to sit on toilet for 10 to 15 minutes after eating to establish regular elimination pattern.

ALERT Initiate a toileting schedule.

Specific Developmental Disorders

Assessment

A. Developmental reading disorder.
1. Impairment in the development of reading skills.
2. Often referred to as *dyslexia*.
3. Slow reading speed and reduced comprehension.
B. Developmental arithmetic disorder: impairment in the development of arithmetic skills.
C. Developmental language disorder.
1. Three major types.
   a. Failure to acquire any language.
   b. Acquired language disability.
   c. Delayed language acquisition.
2. Often the result of trauma or a neurologic disorder.

Nursing Interventions

Goal: To identify specific developmental disorders in relationship to chronologic age in preschool testing.
Goal: To refer child to appropriate developmental program in school.

 Eating Disorders

This group of disorders is characterized by gross disturbances in eating behavior; it includes anorexia nervosa and bulimia nervosa.

Assessment

A. Anorexia nervosa.
1. Intense fear of becoming obese.
2. Need for control and perfectionism.
3. Disturbance of body image.
4. Occurs more often in females than males.
5. Weight loss of at least 15% of original body weight.
6. No known physical illness.
7. A life-threatening emergency: up to 15% of clients with anorexia die of malnutrition, and many are prone to suicide.
B. Bulimia nervosa.
1. Recurrent episodes of binge eating.
2. Awareness that eating pattern is abnormal.
3. Secretive binge eating and purging behaviors (diuretics, laxatives, excessive exercise).
   a. Russell's sign—bruises or calluses on the thumb or hand caused by trauma from self-induced vomiting.
   b. Erosion of tooth enamel, pharyngitis from vomiting.
4. Fear of not being able to stop eating voluntarily.
5. Depressed mood and self-induced vomiting after the eating binges.

Nursing Interventions

Goal: To exhibit no signs or symptoms of malnutrition.
A. If client is unable or unwilling to maintain adequate oral intake, a liquid diet may be administered through a nasogastric tube.
B. Consult with dietitian; determine number of calories required to provide adequate nutrition and realistic weight gain.
C. Explain to client details of behavior modification program.
D. Sit with client during mealtimes for support and to observe amount ingested. A limit (usually 30 minutes) should be imposed on time allotted for meals.
E. Observe client for at least 1 hour after meals.
F. Accompany client to bathroom, if self-induced vomiting is suspected.
G. Carefully document intake and output.
H. Weigh client immediately after he or she arises and after first voiding, usually once or twice each week, but not more often to avoid focusing on weight. Always use same scale, if possible.
I. Do not discuss food or eating with client, once protocol has been established. Do, however, offer support and positive reinforcement for obvious improvements in eating behaviors.
J. Offer support and use nonjudgmental approach with the client.
K. Administer antidepressants as ordered.
Goal: To increase self-esteem, as manifested by verbalizing positive aspects of self and exhibiting less preoccupation with own appearance, by discharge.
A. Assist client to reexamine negative perceptions of self and to recognize positive attributes.
B. Offer positive reinforcement for independently made decisions influencing client's life.
C. Offer positive reinforcement when honest feelings related to autonomy/dependence issues remain separated from maladaptive eating behaviors.
D. Help client to develop a realistic perception of body image and relationship with food.
E. Promote feelings of control within the environment through participation and independent decision making.
F. Allow client to make decisions when appropriate and realistic.
G. Help client realize that perfection is unrealistic and explore this need with the client.
H. Help client claim ownership of angry feelings and recognize that expressing them is acceptable if it is done in an appropriate manner. Be an effective role model.
Goal: To identify an eating disorder and rule out a physiologic cause.
Goal: To recognize complications.
A. Anorexia nervosa—refeeding syndrome can result if system is replenished too quickly, leading to cardiovascular collapse.
B. Bulimia nervosa—if syrup of ipecac is used to induce vomiting, and vomiting does not occur, the absorption of the ipecac can lead to cardiotoxicity and heart failure. Watch for edema and check breath sounds.

ORGANIC MENTAL DISORDERS

A. *Organic brain syndrome* is used to refer to a constellation of psychologic or behavioral signs and symptoms without reference to causes (e.g., delirium, dementia).

Box 10-1 KEY POINTS: ORGANIC MENTAL SYNDROMES

- Clients have varying degrees of awareness of the changes that are occurring, which is emotionally painful to them.
- Often, depression is mistaken for the early onset of dementia.
- Dementia disrupts the older adult couple's final stage of family development (generativity, retirement, etc.).
- Dementia interferes with family intergenerational development when adult offspring are unable to rectify past injustices, conflicts, and disappointments with parents.
- Caregiver coping is highly stressful and can be handled with a more positive approach when there is a focus on problem solving and education.
- Clients with Alzheimer's disease (AD) have loss of memory, intellectual functioning, orientation, affective regulation, motor coordination, and personality, with eventual loss of bowel and bladder control to the point of total incapacitation.

B. *Organic mental disorder* designates a particular organic brain syndrome in which the cause is known or presumed (e.g., alcohol withdrawal or delirium) (Box 10-1).

! NURSING PRIORITY The main characteristic of all these disorders is a psychologic or behavioral abnormality associated with transient or permanent dysfunction of the brain. For example, metabolic disorders, substance abuse intoxications and withdrawals, and systemic illnesses tend to cause a temporary type of brain dysfunction and may be followed by complete recovery; whereas pathologic processes can cause structural damage to the brain and are more likely to cause a permanent residual dysfunction or impairment.

Delirium

Delirium is a syndrome that usually develops over a short period of time. The constellation of symptoms typically fluctuates and is often reversible and temporary.

Assessment

A. Diagnostic criteria.
   1. A clouded sensorium or state of consciousness.
   2. Memory loss for both recent and remote events; disorientation.
   3. Signs and symptoms develop over a short period of time and tend to fluctuate during the day.
   4. Confusion, hallucinations, and delusions.
   5. Sleep disturbances.
   6. Motor activity may be increased or decreased.
   7. Speech may be incoherent.
B. Additional characteristics.
   1. Emotional disturbances: anxiety, fear, depression, anger.
   2. Age at onset: common in children and after the age of 60 years.

C. Etiologic factors.
   1. Systemic infection: meningitis, encephalitis, respiratory and urinary infection.
   2. Metabolic disorders: fluid or electrolyte imbalance.
      a. Hypoglycemia.
      b. Dehydration, vomiting.
   3. Hepatic or renal disease; thiamine deficiency.
   4. Drug intoxication and withdrawal.
   5. Circulatory problems associated with hypertension.
   6. Head trauma: seizure activity.

Nursing Interventions

Goal: To diminish effect of causative agent such as drugs, infectious organisms, or a circulatory-metabolic disorder.
A. Administer medications: antipyretics, antibiotics, or sedatives.
B. Assess for contributing factors/agents and eliminate when possible.
C. Prevent further damage by assessing for possible complications.
Goal: To provide adequate nutrition.
A. Encourage diet high in calories, protein, and vitamins, especially thiamine (vitamin B_1).
B. Encourage adequate intake and output.
Goal: To prevent complications.
A. Provide a quiet, nonstimulating environment to prevent hallucinations.
B. Ensure that safety needs are met (may fall out of bed).
C. Remove potentially harmful articles from a client's room: cigarettes, matches, lighters, sharp objects.
D. Pad side rails and headboard of bed for client with a seizure disorder.

Dementia

Dementia is a syndrome characterized by loss of intellectual abilities to such an extent that social and occupational functioning are negatively affected; involves memory, judgment, abstract thought, and changes in personality. Often, the disorders are progressive and follow an irreversible course in which the damage remains permanent (Box 10-2).
A. Diagnostic criteria.
   1. Loss of intellectual abilities that interfere with social and occupational functioning.
   2. Memory impairment.
   3. Impairment in abstract thinking, judgment, and language.

Box 10-2 ASSESSING CHANGES IN SENILE DEMENTIA

J	Judgment
A	Affect
M	Memory
C	Confusion
O	Orientation

4. Personality change demonstrated by exaggeration of previous personality traits.
5. Mini-Mental State Examination shows disorientation and lack of recall.

B. Additional characteristics.
1. Anxiety or depression may be apparent.
2. Behavior may demonstrate excessive orderliness, social withdrawal, or the tendency to relate an event in excessive detail.
3. Age at onset: found predominantly in older adults.

C. Etiologic factors.
1. Neurologic diseases: Huntington's chorea, multiple sclerosis, Parkinson's disease.
2. Cardiovascular disorders causing anoxia and brain damage: cerebral arteriosclerosis, cerebral vascular accident (stroke).
3. Central nervous system infections: tertiary neurosyphilis, tuberculosis, fungal meningitis, viral encephalitis.
4. Brain trauma: chronic subdural hematoma.
5. Toxic effects: metabolic disturbance.
   a. Pernicious anemia, hypothyroidism.
   b. Bromide intoxication.

c. Wilson's disease: hepatolenticular degeneration characterized by deficient metabolism of copper.
6. Loss of brain tissue and function in presenile conditions.

> **! OLDER ADULT PRIORITY** The cardinal rule: do not push too fast in getting information, assisting with activities of daily living, or insisting that the person socialize. Continued pressure and insistence on a task may result in combative behavior. Watch for reasons for confusion; it could be due to dehydration and electrolyte imbalance, not just "old age."

a. Alzheimer's disease (Table 10-1).
   (1) More commonly seen in older adult clients.
   (2) Irreversible—cerebral atrophy and neuritic plaques.
   (3) Recent memory loss. Client can recall events and activities of 10 years ago, but not 10 minutes ago.
   (4) Sundowner's syndrome: confused, disoriented behavior that becomes noticeable after the sun goes down and during the night.

Table 10-1	STAGES OF ALZHEIMER'S DISEASE
Stage	**Hallmarks**
Stage 1 **(Mild)** *Forgetfulness*	Shows short-term memory losses; loses things, forgets Memory aids compensate: lists, routine, organization Depression common—worsens symptoms Not diagnosable at this time
Stage 2 **(Moderate)** *Confusion*	Shows progressive memory loss; short-term memory loss impaired; memory difficulties interfere with all abilities Withdrawn from social activities Shows declines in instrumental activities of daily living (IADLs), such as money management, legal affairs, transportation, cooking, housekeeping Denial common; fears "losing his or her mind" Depression increasing common; frightened because aware of deficits; covers up for memory loss through confabulation Problems intensified when stressed, fatigued, out of own environment, ill Commonly needs day care or in-home assistance
Stage 3 **(Moderate to Severe)** *Ambulatory dementia*	Shows ADL losses (in order) willingness and ability to bathe, grooming, choosing clothing, dressing, gait and mobility, toileting, communication, reading, and writing skills Shows loss of reasoning ability, safety planning, and verbal communication Frustration common; becomes more withdrawn and self-absorbed Depression resolves as awareness of losses diminishes Has difficulty communicating; shows increasing loss of language skills Shows evidence of reduced stress threshold; institutional care usually needed
Stage 4 **(Late)** *End stage*	Family recognition disappears; does not recognize self in mirror Nonambulatory; shows little purposeful activity; often mute; may scream spontaneously Forgets how to eat, swallow, chew; commonly loses weight; emaciation common Has problems associated with immobility (e.g., pneumonia, pressure ulcers, contractures) Incontinence common; seizures may develop Most certainly institutionalized at this point Return of primitive (infantile) reflexes

From Hall, G.R. (1994). Caring for people with Alzheimer's disease using the conceptual model of progressively lowered stress threshold in the clinical setting. *Nursing Clinics of North America*, 29(1), 129-141, as cited in Varcarolis EM, Carson VB, Shoemaker NC: *Foundations of psychiatric mental health nursing*, page 435.

(5) Wandering behavior.
    (a) Restlessness and activity-seeking behavior.
    (b) The "stalking of old haunts."
(6) Disorientation and inability to sustain intentions; the person forgets what he or she set out to do.
(7) Catastrophic reactions: heightened anxiety occurring during interviewing or questioning, when a person cannot answer or perform.
(8) Combative behavior.
  b. Pick's disease or frontotemporal dementia (FTD): characterized by marked personality and behavioral changes and a decline in the ability to speak coherently.

> **❗ OLDER ADULT PRIORITY** Situations that can lead to combative behavior are threats to self-image, new things or people in environment, illusions, pressure to remember, and direct confrontation.

7. Alteration in intracranial pressure.
  a. Hydrocephalus.
  b. Brain tumor.

> **❗ NURSING PRIORITY** The 3 Rs—routine, reinforcement, and repetition—are key aspects of care, not only for the mentally retarded, but for the older adult client with dementia as well.

Nursing Interventions

Goal: To administer medication to slow the dementia disease process (see Appendix 10-1).
Goal: To provide a quiet, structured environment to increase consistency and promote feelings of security.

A. Avoid dependency.
B. Establish routine for activities of daily living.
C. Meet client's physical needs.
D. Do not isolate client from others in the unit.
E. Provide handrails, walkers, and wheelchairs.
F. Do not change schedules suddenly: *routine, reinforcement,* and *repetition* are the key aspects of care.
G. Check for hazards in the environment (e.g., rugs on floor); make sure environment is well lighted.
H. Prevent client from wandering away from care area.

> **ALERT** Orient client to reality and monitor activities of the confused client. (Knowledge about providing care for the older client, especially the client with Alzheimer's disease, is often tested).

Goal: To promote contact with reality.
A. Make brief and frequent contact.
B. Give feedback.
C. Supply stimulation to motivate client to engage in activities.
D. Use concrete ideas in communication.
E. Maintain reality orientation by encouraging client to reminisce (Table 10-2).

> **❗ NURSING PRIORITY** Reminiscence and life review help the client resume progression through the grief process associated with disappointing life events and increase self-esteem as successes are reviewed.

F. Orient client frequently to reality and surroundings.
  1. Allow client to have familiar objects around him or her.
  2. Use other items such as clocks, calendars, and daily schedules.

Table 10-2	GROUP MODALITIES FOR OLDER ADULT CLIENTS	
Remotivation Therapy	*Reminiscing Therapy*	*Psychotherapy*
Purpose of Group		
Resocialize regressed and apathetic older adult clients	Share memories	Alleviation of presenting psychiatric problems
	Increase socialization	Promote ability to interact with others in a group
	Enhance self-esteem	Increase ability to make decisions and function more independently
Format		
10-15 clients in a group	6-8 clients in a group	6-12 group members
Meet 1-2 times per week	Meet 1-2 times per week	Members share problems and problem-solving strategies with each other
Meetings highly structured in a classroom setting	Topics include holidays, travel	Group meets at regularly scheduled times
Each session has a specific topic		
Desired Outcomes		
Increases group members' sense of reality	Assists in alleviating depression	Decreases sense of isolation
Encourages a more objective self-image	Use of process of reorganization and reintegration provides an avenue for older adults to achieve a sense of identity and positive self-concept	Promotes new roles and reestablishes old roles
		Provides group support for increasing self-esteem

G. Use simple explanations and face-to-face interaction.

H. Do not shout message into client's ear.

I. Allow sufficient time for client to complete projects.

J. Reinforce reality-oriented comments and orientation to time, place, and date.

> **❗ NURSING PRIORITY** Speaking slowly and in a face-to-face position is most effective when communicating with an older adult experiencing a hearing loss. Visual cues facilitate understanding. Shouting causes distortion of high-pitched sounds, and in some instances, creates a feeling of discomfort for the client.

Goal: To provide diversion activities that enhance self-esteem.

A. Provide occupational therapy, physical therapy, and recreational therapy that client enjoys.

B. Maintain a flexible schedule; keep client from becoming bored and easily distracted.

C. Recognize specific accomplishments.

D. Encourage family involvement and provide emotional support.

E. Devise methods for assisting client with memory deficit.
  1. Name sign and picture on door identifying client's room.
  2. Identifying sign on outside of dining room door.
  3. Large clock, with oversized numbers and hands, appropriately placed.
  4. Large calendar, indicating one day at a time, with month, day, and year identified in bold print.

> **❗ NURSING PRIORITY** The 3 Ps for clients with dementia: protecting dignity, preserving function, and promoting quality of life.

📋 Anxiety Disorders

In the past, anxiety disorders were grouped together as neuroses. Anxiety can be a predominant disturbance (panic and generalized anxiety), or anxiety can be experienced as a person attempts to confront a dreaded situation (phobic disorder) or resist the obsessions and compulsions of an obsessive-compulsive disorder. In general, these are common responses to emotional problems that are very seldom treated in a psychiatric setting, because the person does not have a great defect in reality testing and does not demonstrate severe antisocial behavior. Pressures of decision making and decisions that are made in the early adult years seem to act as precipitating events in the development of anxiety disorders (Table 10-3).

> **ALERT** Identify effects of environmental stressors on client; plan measures to deal with client's anxiety; encourage client to use problem-solving skills; teach stress reduction techniques; and provide support to client who is upset or distraught.

Nursing Interventions

Goal: To promote techniques to reduce anxiety.

A. Desensitization: client is exposed serially to a specific list of anxiety-provoking situations; through techniques of progressive relaxation, the client becomes desensitized to each stimulus.

B. Reciprocal inhibition: the anxiety-provoking stimulus is paired with another stimulus that is associated with an opposite feeling to diminish the effect of the anxiety.

C. Cognitive therapy: internal dialogue or self-talk on feelings, emotions, and behavior.

D. Regular daily exercise.

E. Other therapy: hypnosis, meditation, imagery, yoga, biofeedback training.

📋 Somatoform Disorders

Somatoform disorders are disorders in which the person has physical symptoms suggesting a physiologic etiology; however, after in-depth assessment and diagnostic testing, no organic disease or physiologic abnormalities are found.

Assessment

A. Somatization disorder: recurrent, multiple complaints (from the following four areas) for which medical treatment has been sought; the client must display:
  1. Four pain symptoms (e.g., head, abdomen, back, shoulder, joints).
  2. Two gastrointestinal symptoms (e.g., nausea, bloating, diarrhea, flatulence).
  3. One sexual symptom (e.g., sexual indifference, erectile dysfunction, abnormal menses, painful menstruation, excessive bleeding).
  4. One symptom suggesting a neurologic problem (e.g., loss of sensation, blindness, double vision).

B. Conversion disorder: a loss of, or alteration in, physical functioning that suggests a physical disorder but is related to expression of a psychologic conflict or need; person appears calm while experiencing symptoms.
  1. A loss of alteration in physical function, suggesting a physical disorder.
  2. Symptoms are not under voluntary control.
  3. *La belle indifference:* an attitude toward the symptoms in which there is a lack of concern.
  4. Not a deliberate faking (malingering).
  5. "Classic conversion symptoms" usually suggest neurologic disease: paralysis, aphonia, blindness, and paresthesias.

C. Pain disorder: preoccupied with pain for which there is no physical cause.
  1. Severe and prolonged pain.
  2. Pain is nonanatomic in distribution.
  3. Evidence of a stressful life situation.
  4. Complaint excessive in relation to the observable symptoms.
  5. History of frequent visits to physician ("doctor shopping").
  6. Excessive use of analgesics without relief of pain, along with frequent requests for surgery.

Table 10-3	SELECTED ANXIETY DISORDERS	
Problem	**Description**	**Nursing Intervention**
Panic disorder (with or without agoraphobia): an extreme level of anxiety.	Agoraphobia (fear of being in places or situations; crowds, traveling). May experience shortness of breath, dizziness, diaphoresis, palpitations.	**Goal: To reduce panic level anxiety feelings by reinterpreting the feelings correctly** (see Table 9-2). 1. Anticipate administration of a tricyclic antidepressant. 2. Reduce amount of caffeine in diet.
Phobia: an intense, irrational fear of a specific object, activity, or situation.	Fear of being alone or in public places. Claustrophobia (fear of enclosed spaces). Acrophobia (fear of heights). Social phobia (fear of circumstances that may be humiliating, e.g., speaking in public, eating in restaurants).	**Goal: To reduce phobic behavior.** 1. Do not force client to come in contact with the feared object or source of anxiety. 2. Have client focus on awareness of self. 3. Distract client's attention from phobia.
Obsessive-compulsive disorder: unconscious control of anxiety by the use of rituals, thoughts, obsessions, or compulsions.	**Obsessions:** recurrent, persistent ideas, thoughts, or impulses that are not voluntarily produced. *Most common obsessions include thoughts of violence, contamination, and doubt.* **Compulsions:** repetitive, ritualistic behaviors that are performed in a certain fashion to relieve an unbearable amount of tension. *Most common compulsions include handwashing, counting, checking.*	**Goal: To assist in coping with the compulsive behavior.** 1. Accept rituals and avoid punishment or criticism; do not interrupt ritual, because this will increase anxiety. 2. Plan for extra time because of slowness and client's need for perfection. 3. Prevent physical deterioration or harm, and set limits only to prevent harmful acts (such as handwashing so excessively that it removes the skin from the hand surface). **Goal: To encourage client to develop different ways of handling anxiety.** 1. Reduce demands on the individual. 2. Convey acceptance of client, regardless of behavior. 3. Encourage alternative activity.
Post-traumatic stress disorder: involves the development of characteristic symptoms after a traumatic psychologic event in which the individual is unable to adapt or adjust (e.g., rape, military combat, airplane crashes, torture, or abuse).	Client reexperiences the traumatic event. Client withdraws, becomes isolated, and restricts emotional response. Experiences hyperalertness, insomnia, nightmares, depression, and anxiety.	**Goal: To determine precipitating stress factor in client's reaction.** 1. Reduce and prevent chronic disability. 2. Encourage verbalization of the traumatic event. **Goal: To maintain personal integrity.** 1. Provide physical, social, or occupational rehabilitation. 2. Somatic therapies are used to decrease anxiety (e.g., antianxiety agents, etc.).
Generalized anxiety disorder: unrealistic or excessive anxiety and worry about life's circumstances; differs from panic disorder in that it never remits and onset is at early age.	Physical symptoms associated with disorder are restlessness, apprehension, tension, irritability, "free-floating" anxiety.	**Goal: To reduce level of anxiety.** 1. Administer antianxiety agent. 2. Teach anxiety-reducing techniques. 3. Reduce pressure and anxiety-provoking situations around client. 4. Divert attention from symptoms.

D. Hypochondriasis: distorted interpretation of existing physical signs or bodily sensations, which leads the client to an unrealistic belief and preoccupation with the fear or belief of having a serious, debilitating disease.
  1. Preoccupied with bodily functioning: focusing on heart beat, breathing, digestion, or a minor aliment, such as a small scratch or a cough.

  2. Physical evaluation does not support the diagnosis of any physical problem.
  3. Fear or belief of having medical illness despite medical reassurance.
E. Body dysmorphic disorder: preoccupation with an imagined flaw in appearance in a normal-appearing person.

1. Excessive concern and focus on facial defect; less commonly on other parts of the body; preoccupies and dominates client's life.
2. Social isolation and depression leading to suicidal threats and repeated hospitalizations.
3. May seek plastic surgery.

Nursing Interventions

Goal: To divert attention from preoccupation with self and symptomatology.

A. Encourage purposeful activity that promotes interest and success.
B. Promote attitude that acknowledges personal integrity and self-worth.
C. Provide for client's physical needs as necessary.
D. Correct any misinformation and give correct information.
E. Encourage client to develop new interests and gain satisfaction from them.
F. Promote a good sense of humor.

Goal: To identify primary or secondary gain.

A. Primary gain: symptom has symbolic meaning to client; keeps client unaware of internal conflict and anxiety.
B. Secondary gain: a gain of attention and sympathy along with reinforcement of maladjusted behavior.

Goal: To avoid secondary gains as a source of reward and reinforcement for the disorder.

A. Focus on the individual and his or her feelings, *not* on the symptoms.
B. A calm, warm, supportive approach promotes understanding and acceptance.

Goal: To avoid reinforcing the client's symptoms.

A. Focus on feelings, *not* on symptoms.
B. Reduce pressure and anxiety-provoking situations around client.
C. Divert attention from symptoms.
D. Provide recreational activity.
E. Avoid pity and sympathetic approach to client's "illnesses" or "symptoms."

Goal: To be aware of personal response to the client.

A. Recognize and understand the client's self-perception as unable to cope.
B. Promote a nonjudgmental, understanding attitude.

Goal: To provide a supportive approach that does not focus on physical condition.

A. Help client to understand how he or she uses illness to avoid dealing with life's problems.
B. Offer empathy without sympathy.

Goal: To support alternative therapy.

A. Behavior modification.
B. Insight-oriented psychotherapy.
C. Hypnosis.
D. Acupuncture.

Psychophysiologic Disorder

A psychophysiologic disorder is a physical illness that is strongly influenced by psychologic factors. It was

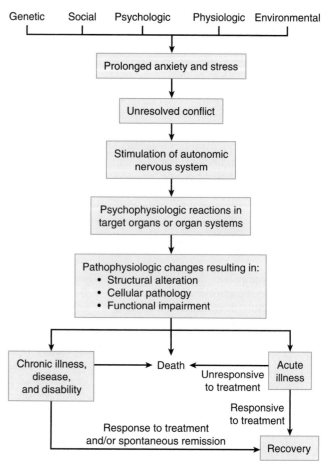

FIGURE 10-1 Concept of psychophysiologic disorder.

previously called psychosomatic disorder. It is thought that stress and anxiety arouse specific conflicts in an individual, which result in damaging effects on particular organs or organ systems that are under the control of the autonomic nervous system (Figure 10-1).

Assessment

A. Respiratory.
  1. Hyperventilation syndrome.
  2. Asthma.
B. Cardiovascular.
  1. Essential hypertension.
  2. Angina.
  3. Migraine headaches.
  4. Tachycardia.
C. Gastrointestinal.
  1. Peptic ulcer.
  2. Ulcerative colitis.
  3. Colic.
D. Integumentary.
  1. Dermatitis.
  2. Pruritus.
  3. Excessive sweating.
  4. Atopic dermatitis.
E. Musculoskeletal.
  1. Cramps.
  2. Rheumatoid arthritis.

F. Endocrine.
1. Diabetes mellitus.
2. Sexual dysfunction.
3. Hyperemesis gravidarum.
4. Hyperthyroidism.
G. Genital/urinary.
1. Amenorrhea.
2. Impotence.
3. Secondary outbreaks of herpes genitalis type 2.

Nursing Interventions

Pathophysiology of, and nursing interventions for, the psychophysiologic disorders are discussed under the appropriate body system affected.

 ## Dissociative Disorders

Dissociative disorders involve five primary symptoms: amnesia (memory loss), derealization (objects in external environment take on a quality of unreality and estrangement), depersonalization (alteration in the perception or experience of self), identity confusion (sense of conflict, puzzlement, or uncertainty in relation to one's identity), and identity alteration (organized shift in personality that occurs without the individual's awareness).

Assessment

A. Dissociative amnesia.
1. A sudden inability to recall important personal information.
2. Usually begins suddenly, after severe psychosocial stress.
3. Most often observed in the adolescent and young adult female, rarely in older adults.
B. Dissociative fugue.
1. Sudden, unexpected travel away from home with the assumption of a new identity.
2. An inability to recall one's previous identity or past.
3. No recollection of events that took place during the fugue state.
C. Dissociative identity disorder (multiple personality).
1. The existence of two or more distinct personalities, each of which determines the nature of his or her behavior and attitudes while uppermost in the person's consciousness.
2. Transition from one personality to another is sudden and often stressful.
3. Best-known examples found in literature: *Sybil* and *The Three Faces of Eve*.
D. Depersonalization disorder.
1. An alteration in the perception of the self so that the usual sense of one's own reality is temporarily lost or changed.
2. Sensations of unreality (e.g., feelings that one's extremities have changed size).
3. Onset is rapid; disappearance is gradual.

Nursing Interventions

Goal: To assist in ruling out a physical or organic disease as the cause of the dissociative disorder.
A. Many behaviors exhibited resemble postconcussion amnesia and temporal lobe epilepsy.
B. Accurate observation and description of character, duration, and frequency of the symptoms are important.
Goal: To minimize anxiety.
A. Redirect client's attention away from self.
B. Increase socialization activities.
C. Include family members in learning new ways to deal with client's behavior.
Goal: To provide insight into past traumatic experiences and learn new coping methods.
A. Long-term therapy is aimed at insight into pain of past experiences and conflicts that have been repressed.
B. Encourage awareness that dissociative behaviors are reactivated by current situations that arouse emotional pain.

PERSONALITY DISORDERS

Personality disorders create disruptive lifestyles and are characterized by inflexible and maladapted behaviors. Those with personality disorders clash with society and with cultural norms and are often placed in correctional systems, mental hospitals, and child placement facilities.

Common Characteristics

A. Problems are expressed through behavior rather than as physical symptoms of stress.
B. Disruptive lifestyle is deeply ingrained and quite difficult to change; usually related to some form of abnormal behavior or the development of a particular pattern or trait.
C. Often comes in conflict with others.
D. Pleasure principle is dominant with inadequate superego control; has difficulty with problem solving.
E. Unable to develop meaningful relationships with others and communicate effectively.
F. Rarely acknowledges that there is a problem.

Assessment

See Table 10-4 on personality disorder clusters.

> **❗ NURSING PRIORITY** Personality disorders occur when traits become rigid and manipulative.

Nursing Interventions

Goal: To promote communication and socialization in the paranoid personality.
A. Decrease social isolation.
B. Verbal and nonverbal messages should be clear and consistent.
C. To decrease anxiety, plan several brief contacts, rather than one prolonged contact.
D. Promote trust by following through on commitments.
E. Be open and honest to avoid misinterpretation.

Table 10-4	**PERSONALITY DISORDER CLUSTERS**	

Cluster A	*Cluster B*	*Cluster C*
Paranoid Personality Suspicious and mistrustful of people Secretive Questions loyalty of others Jealous Overconcerned with hidden motives and special meanings Hypersensitive and alert Exaggerates Unable to relax Takes offense quickly Impaired affect Unemotional and cold No sense of humor Absence of soft, tender, sentimental feelings Distorts reality Uses projection	**Antisocial Personality** Violates rights of others Lacks responsibility Manipulative Unable to sustain a job; frequent job changes and lengthy periods of unemployment Financial dependency Common behaviors observed—lying, stealing, truancy Aggressive sexual behavior Sexual promiscuity Excessive drinking and drug use Criminality Vagrancy Lack of remorse	**Avoidant Personality** Fear of criticism or disapproval Hypersensitive to potential rejection Views self as socially inept, personally unappealing, and inferior to others Inhibited in interpersonal relationships Reluctant to take personal risks Unwilling to get involved with people unless certain of being liked
Schizoid Personality Unable to form social relationships Cold and aloof; flat affect Indifferent to praise or criticism Has little or no desire for social involvement Appears reserved, withdrawn, and seclusive	**Borderline Personality** Unstable interpersonal relationships and moods Impulsiveness and unpredictability that may be self-damaging (e.g., spending, sex, reckless driving, drug use) Identity disturbance Recurrent suicidal behavior, gestures, or threats Self-mutilating behavior Inappropriate, intense anger; lack of anger control; shifts in mood Chronic feelings of emptiness	**Dependent Personality** Submissive; clinging behavior Fear of separation Difficulty making everyday decisions Needs others to assume responsibility Wants others to take care and nurture Feels uncomfortable or helpless when left alone Difficulty initiating projects
Schizotypal Personality Magical thinking (e.g., telepathy, superstitiousness) Ideas of reference Social isolation Recurrent illusion Oddities of thought, perception, speech, and behavior Inappropriate affect Excessive social anxiety	**Histrionic Personality** Excessive emotionality and attention-seeking behavior Uncomfortable when not center of attention Uses physical appearance to draw attention to self Self-dramatization, theatrical, and exaggerated expression of emotion Easily suggestible	**Obsessive-Compulsive Personality** Preoccupation with rules, lists, organization, schedules Perfectionistic Excessive devotion to work Overconscientious and inflexible Reluctant to delegate tasks Hoards money; frugal Rigid and stubborn in thoughts
	Narcissistic Personality Grandiose self-importance Preoccupation with fantasies of success Belief that he or she is "special or unique" Need for excessive amount of admiration Unrealistic sense of entitlement Interpersonal exploitation Lack of empathy Arrogant and haughty	

Goal: To convey to the schizoid or schizotypal client the idea that you do not perceive reality the same way as he or she does but are willing to listen, learn, and offer feedback about his or her experiences.

Goal: To promote a positive, therapeutic, interpersonal relationship.
A. Set realistic expectations.
B. Provide a model of mature behavior.
C. Use problem-solving techniques to encourage a client to make changes.
D. Anticipate and deal with depression in a client who gradually acquires enough insight to realize and accept responsibility for his or her behavior.
E. Common sources of frustration for nurses.
   1. Client's immature behavior.
   2. Poor communication skills.

Goal: To minimize manipulation and "acting out" behaviors and encourage verbal communication.
A. Set firm, consistent limits without being punitive.
B. Be aware of how client may manipulate other staff members (e.g., playing one against the other or splitting).
C. Promote expression of feelings versus acting out.
D. Promote client's acceptance of responsibility for his or her own actions and a social responsibility to others.

> **⊟ NURSING PRIORITY** A client with borderline personality disorder has a tendency to cling to one staff member, if allowed, transferring his or her maladaptive dependency to that individual. This dependency can be avoided if the client is able to establish therapeutic relationships with two or more staff members who encourage independent self-care activities.

Goal: To assist client to manage anxiety.
A. Anticipate client's needs before he or she demands attention.
B. Teach client to express his or her ideas and feelings assertively.
C. Watch for signs of defensiveness, because a client is unlikely to recognize this as a mechanism of anxiety.

Goal: To set realistic limits.
A. Break the health-attention-avoidance cycle that usually exists in relating to this type of client.
B. Support the client who is gradually making more decisions on his or her own.
C. Offer assistance only when needed.

SUBSTANCE USE DISORDERS

Substance use disorders are characterized by behavior changes, regular use of a substance (alcohol or another drug) that affects the central nervous system, and withdrawal symptoms when the substance is not taken.

Polydrug dependence involves the regular use of three or more psychoactive substances over a period of at least 6 months.

> **ALERT** Identify signs and symptoms of substance abuse/chemical dependency.

A. Substance abuse.
   1. A pattern of pathologic use.
      a. Intoxication during the day.
      b. Inability to cut down or stop drinking.
      c. Daily need of the substance in order to function.
      d. Blackouts and medical complications from use.
   2. Impairment of social or occupational functioning.
      a. Failure to meet important obligations to friends, family, and employer.
      b. Inappropriate display of erratic and impulsive behavior.
      c. Inappropriate expression of aggressive feelings.
   3. Minimum duration of at least 1 month of substance use.
B. Substance dependence: more severe than substance abuse; requires physiologic dependence as evidenced by either tolerance or withdrawal.
   1. Tolerance.
      a. Increased amounts of the substance are required to achieve the desired effect.
      b. Markedly diminished effect with regular use of the same dose.
   2. Withdrawal: a specific syndrome of symptoms, which develops when the person abruptly stops ingesting the substance.
C. Psychologic dependence.
   1. Habituation: the need to take the substance.
   2. Physiologic dependence is not necessary.
   3. No physiologic symptoms on withdrawal.
D. Common health problems.
   1. Acute problems.
      a. Poor nutritional status, loss of appetite, nausea, vomiting, and diarrhea.
      b. Central nervous system dysfunction and irritability, seizures, tremors, motor restlessness, sensitivity to light, auditory or visual disturbances, insomnia.
      c. Susceptibility to recurrent respiratory tract infections.
   2. Chronic problems.
      a. Liver dysfunction, cirrhosis, pancreatitis, hypertension.
      b. Chronic brain damage and mental deterioration, poor hygiene, dermatologic changes.
      c. Human immunodeficiency virus (HIV) seropositivity.
E. Dysfunctional behavior patterns.
   1. Manipulation.
      Examples: Legal difficulties, crime, physical assault, taking advantage of generosity.
   2. Impulsiveness.
      Examples: Inconsistent work patterns, overdose, recklessness.
   3. Dysfunctional anger.
   4. Grandiosity.
      Example: Belief that nobody has done worse things or has lost as much or taken drugs or drunk as much.

5. Denial.
6. Codependency: extreme emotional, social, or physical focus on another person, place, or thing.

F. Treatment modalities.
1. Detoxification: controlled withdrawal from alcohol or drugs by means of a medical protocol.
2. Drug treatment and rehabilitation: comprehensive program based on client outcomes; may include detoxification, family education, group counseling, and 12-step programs.
3. 12-step self-help groups: recovery built on abstinence as a daily process; requires peer support and acknowledgment that client has addiction.
4. Drug-free residential communities: therapeutic community based on a hierarchical community structure and governance, peer support, and a disciplined lifestyle.
5. Pharmacologic therapy: use of dolophine (Methadone) for opiate abuse to eliminate craving for drug.
6. Psychotherapy: may be individual, group, family, or a combination of all three; facilitates behavioral and lifestyle changes by dealing with personality issues and psychologic conflicts.

Alcohol Dependence (Alcoholism)

A chronic pattern of pathologic alcohol use is characterized by impairment in social or occupational functioning, along with tolerance or withdrawal symptoms.

General Concepts

A. Incidence.
1. An estimated 20 million Americans have alcoholism; of those who consume alcohol, 1 in 10 is an alcoholic.
2. Each year, 80 billion dollars is spent on alcohol-related illnesses, which lead to lost wages, reduced productivity, and property damage.
3. Chronic alcoholism shortens the life span by 12 years.

B. Effects of use.
1. Central nervous system depressant drug.
2. Requires no digestion; 20% is absorbed unchanged from the stomach; 80% is absorbed from the small intestine.
3. Absorbed slowly in a full stomach.
4. Measured in the bloodstream by the blood alcohol level (BAL).
5. Can be measured within 15 to 20 minutes after ingestion; reaches a peak in 60 to 90 minutes; is completely metabolized by 12 to 24 hours after the last drink.
6. Decreases inhibitions and enhances mood; slows motor reactions and subsequently prolongs reaction time.
7. In low doses, tends to increase sexual arousal; in high doses, tends to decrease it.
8. Affects critical thinking, judgment, and memory.
9. BAL of 8% to 10% (depending on the state) or more is considered intoxication.

Assessment

A. Risk factors.
1. History of alcoholism in family.
2. History of total abstinence.
3. Broken or disrupted home.
4. Last or near-last child in a large family.
5. Heavy smoking.
6. Cultural groups: Irish, Eskimo, Scandinavian, Native American.

B. Diagnostics.
1. BAL.
   a. BAL is determined by how much alcohol is consumed, how fast it is consumed, and body weight.
   b. The larger the person, the more alcohol he or she can tolerate.
   c. Usual legal guidelines for intoxication: BAL greater than 100 to 150 mg/dL.
2. Breathalyzer.
   a. About 5% to 10% of the alcohol is excreted through breathing.
   b. Used for monitoring the use of alcohol and to identify persons who are driving while intoxicated (DWI) or driving under the influence (DUI).

C. General personality characteristics of alcoholics.
1. Dependent behavior along with resentment of authority.
2. Demanding and domineering with a low tolerance for frustration.
3. Dissatisfied with life; tendency toward self-destructive acts, including suicide.
4. Low self-esteem and poor self-concept.

D. Signs and symptoms of possible alcohol abuse.
1. Sprains, bruises, and injuries of questionable origin.
2. Diarrhea and early morning vomiting.
3. Chronic cough, palpitations, and infections.
4. Frequent Monday morning illnesses; blackouts (inability to recall events or actions while intoxicated).

E. Alcohol withdrawal syndrome. Consuming one-fifth of whiskey daily for 1 month is generally considered sufficient to produce alcohol withdrawal. The withdrawal syndrome develops in heavy drinkers who have increased, decreased, or interrupted the intake of alcohol.
1. Alcohol withdrawal.
   a. Anorexia, irritability, nausea, and tremulousness.
   b. Insomnia, nightmares, irritability, hyperalertness.
   c. Tachycardia, increased blood pressure, and diaphoresis.
   d. Onset within 8 hours after cessation of drinking (usually 48 to 72 hours); clears up within 5 to 7 days.
2. Delirium tremens.
   a. Autonomic hyperactivity: tachycardia, sweating, increased blood pressure.
   b. Vivid hallucinations, delusions, confusion.
   c. Coarse, irregular tremor is almost always seen; fever may occur.

d. Onset within 24 to 72 hours after the last ingestion of alcohol; delirium tremens usually lasts 2 to 3 days.

e. Convulsions/seizures may occur ("rum fits").

f. First episode occurs after 5 to 15 years of heavy drinking.

3. Alcohol hallucinosis.

a. Auditory hallucinations.

b. Occurs within 48 hours after heavy drinking episode.

c. Often includes persecutory delusions.

d. Client may be suicidal or homicidal.

e. Spontaneous recovery within 1 week.

f. Wernicke's encephalopathy.

(1) An acute, reversible neurologic disorder.

(2) Triad of symptoms: global confusion, ataxia, and eye movement abnormality (nystagmus).

(3) Occurs primarily in clients with chronic alcoholism; may develop in illnesses that interfere with thiamine (vitamin B_1) absorption (e.g., gastric cancer, malabsorption syndrome, regional enteritis).

(4) Treatment: high doses of thiamine; 100 mg, given intramuscularly, usually reverses eye signs within 2 to 3 hours of treatment.

F. Korsakoff's syndrome (alcohol amnesiac disorder).

1. A chronic, *irreversible* disorder, often following Wernicke's encephalopathy.

2. Triad of symptoms: memory loss, learning deficit, confabulation (filling in of memory gaps with plausible stories).

G. Other disorders associated with chronic alcoholism: pneumonitis, esophageal varices, cirrhosis, pancreatitis, diabetes (these are discussed in the appropriate chapter discussing the system).

Nursing Interventions

Goal: To assess for alcoholism in a client through careful questioning.

A. Frequently used acronym—*CAGE*—suggests asking the following four questions. An answer of "yes" to any question can indicate a problem.

1. Have you ever felt the need to:
*C*ut down on your drinking?

2. Have you ever felt:
*A*nnoyed by criticism of your drinking?

3. Have you had:
*G*uilty feelings about drinking?

4. Do you ever take a morning: *E*ye-opener?

B. Identify the alcoholic client in the preoperative period.

1. Often, alcoholics are undiagnosed at the time of surgery and may go into withdrawal or delirium tremens after the NPO (nothing by mouth) period.

2. Preoperative medication doses need to be adjusted; usually, if tolerant of alcohol, clients are also tolerant of other medications, including anesthetics.

3. Client usually takes longer to be fully responsive during postoperative period; client is susceptible to severe respiratory complications; client has more difficulty with healing because of poor nutritional state.

Goal: To assist in the medical treatment of alcohol withdrawal.

A. Benzodiazepines for agitation (see Appendix 10-2).

B. Thiamine (vitamin B_1) to prevent Wernicke's encephalopathy.

C. Magnesium sulfate to increase effective of vitamin B_1. It helps reduce postwithdrawal seizures.

D. Anticonvulsant (phenobarbital), if necessary, for seizure control.

E. Encourage use of multivitamins, especially folic acid, B_{12}, and vitamin C.

F. Alpha-adrenergic blockers (clonidine) to decrease withdrawal symptoms.

G. Beta-adrenergic blockers (atenolol, propranolol) to improve vital signs and decrease cravings.

H. Encourage intake of fluids, but do not force.

Goal: To provide for the basic needs of rest, comfort, safety, and nutrition.

A. Safety measures, such as bed rest and use of bed rails, may be necessary.

B. If client is experiencing delirium tremens, stay with him or her.

C. Have room adequately lit to help reduce confusion and avoid shadows and unclear objects.

D. Monitor vital signs every 1 to 4 hours.

E. Encourage a high-carbohydrate, soft diet.

Goal: To recognize complications of alcohol use.

A. Obstetrical implications.

1. Two ounces of alcohol per day may produce a BAL, leading to fetal alcohol syndrome.

2. Chronic alcoholism can lead to maternal malnutrition, especially folic acid deficiency, bone marrow suppression, infections, and liver disease.

3. Alcohol withdrawal syndrome may occur in the intrapartal period as early as 12 to 48 hours after the last drink.

4. Delirium tremens may occur in the postpartum period.

B. Neonatal implications (fetal alcohol syndrome).

1. Teratogenic effects may be seen along with growth and developmental retardation.

2. Increased risk for anomalies of the heart, head, face, and extremities.

3. Withdrawal symptoms can occur shortly after birth and are characterized by tremors, agitation, sweating, and seizure activity.

4. Maintain seizure precautions.

C. Medical complications of alcohol abuse.

1. Trauma-related to falls, burns, hematomas.

2. Liver disease: cirrhosis, esophageal varices, hepatic coma.

3. Gastrointestinal disease: gastritis, bleeding ulcers, pancreatitis.

4. Nutritional disease: malnutrition, anemia caused by iron or vitamin B_{12} deficiency, thiamine deficiency.

5. Infections, especially pneumonia.
6. Neurologic disease: polyneuropathy and dementia.

Goal: To assist in the long-term rehabilitation of client.

A. Avoid sympathy, because clients tend to rationalize and use dependent, manipulative behavior to seek privileges.
B. Maintain a nonjudgmental attitude.
C. Set behavior limits in a firm but kind manner.
D. Place responsibility for sobriety on client; do not give advice or punish or reprimand client for failures.
E. Provide opportunities to decrease social isolation by encouraging participation in social groups and activities.
F. Encourage client to develop coping mechanisms other than alcohol to deal with stress.
G. Refer clients and family to available community resources.
   1. Alcoholics Anonymous (AA): a self-help group focusing on education, guidance, and the sharing of problems and experiences unique to the individual.
   2. Al-Anon: a self-help support group for the spouses and significant others of the alcoholic.
   3. Alateen: the support group for teenagers with an alcoholic parent.
   4. Adult Children of Alcoholics (ACOA): support group for adult children of alcoholics and dysfunctional individuals.
   5. Families Anonymous: support group for the families whose lives have been affected by the addicted client's behavior.
   6. Codependents Anonymous: support group for codependents who may be alcoholics or drug addicts and for persons who are close to an addict.
H. Promote adherence to prescribed therapeutic regimens.
   1. Disulfiram (Antabuse): a drug that produces intense side effects after ingestion of alcohol (severe nausea, vomiting, flushed face, hypotension, and blurred vision).
   2. Aversion therapy: a form of deterrent therapy attempting to induce alcohol rejection behavior by administering alcohol with an emetic.
   3. Naltrexone (Revia): opioid antagonist that decreases the craving for alcohol.
   4. Acamprosate (Campral): a drug that helps clients abstain from alcohol.

Polydrug Dependence

The regular use of three or more psychoactive substances over a period of at least 6 months.

General Concepts
A. Effects of use.
   1. Relieves anxiety.
   2. Overdose can occur.
   3. Factors affecting the degree of dependence.
      a. Physiologic and psychologic makeup of the abuser.
      b. Drug's pharmacologic action.
      c. External social and cultural factors.

B. General personality characteristics.
   1. Inability to cope with stress, frustration, or anxiety.
   2. Rebellious, immature, desire for immediate gratification.
   3. Passivity and low self-esteem.
   4. Difficulty forming warm, personal relationships.
   5. Uses defense mechanisms: denial, rationalization, intellectualization.

Assessment
A. General assessment.
   1. Determine the pattern of drug use.
      a. Which drugs are being used by the client?
      b. When was the last use?
      c. How much does client use and how often?
      d. How long has client been using drugs?
      e. What combination of drugs is being used?
   2. Determine whether there are any physical changes present (e.g., needle tracks, swollen nasal mucous membranes, reddened conjunctivae).
B. Narcotic dependence.
   Examples of narcotics: opium, heroin, morphine, meperidine (Demerol), codeine, fentanyl, methadone, OxyContin, oxycodone.
   1. Street names: horse, junk, smack (heroin); black poppy (opium); M (morphine); dollies (methadone); terp (terpin hydrate or cough syrup with codeine).
   2. Administration.
      a. Heroin: sniffed, smoked, injected intravenously (mainlining), injected subcutaneously (skin popping).
      b. Other narcotics are usually taken orally or by injection.
   3. Symptoms of use.
      a. Drowsiness and decreased blood pressure, pulse, and respiratory rate.
      b. Pinpoint pupils, needle tracks, scarring.
      c. Overdose effects: slow, shallow breathing, clammy skin, convulsions, coma, pulmonary edema, possible death.
   4. Withdrawal symptoms.
      a. Onset of symptoms approximately 8 to 12 hours after the last dose.
      b. Lacrimation, sweating, sneezing, yawning.
      c. Gooseflesh (piloerection), tremor, irritability, anorexia.
      d. Dilated pupils, abdominal cramps, vomiting, involuntary muscle spasms.
      e. Symptoms generally subside within 7 to 10 days.
C. Sedative-hypnotic dependence.
   Examples of sedative-hypnotics: barbiturates (Nembutal, Seconal) and the benzodiazepines (Librium, Valium).
   1. Street names: Peter (chloral hydrate); green and whites, roaches (Librium); red birds, red devils (secobarbital); blue birds (Amytal capsules); yellow birds (Nembutal); downers, rainbow, 7145 (barbiturates; tranquilizers).
   2. Administration: oral or injected.

3. Symptoms of use.
   a. Alterations in mood, thought, behavior.
   b. Impairment in coordination, judgment.
   c. Signs of intoxication: slurred speech, unsteady gait, decreased attention span or memory.
   d. Barbiturate use: often violent, disruptive, irresponsible behavior.
4. Withdrawal symptoms.
   a. Insomnia, anxiety, profuse sweating, weakness.
   b. Severe reactions of delirium, grand mal seizures, cardiovascular collapse.

D. Cocaine abuse.
1. Street names: coke, toot, nose candy, snow, C, powder, lady.
2. Administration: intranasal ("snorting") or by intravenous or subcutaneous injection; also smoked in pipe (free-basing).
3. Symptoms of use.
   a. Euphoria, grandiosity, and a sense of well-being.
   b. Amphetamine-like or stimulant-like effects such as increased blood pressure, racing of the heart, paranoia, anxiety.
   c. Used regularly, cocaine may disrupt eating and sleeping habits, leading to irritability and decreased concentration.

◼ NURSING PRIORITY Crack (rock) has been labeled the most addictive drug. It is a potent form of cocaine hydrochloride mixed with baking soda and water, heated (cooked), allowed to harden, and then broken or "cracked" into little pieces and smoked in cigarettes or glass water pipes. Cardiac dysrhythmias, respiratory paralysis, and seizures are some of the dangers associated with crack use.

4. Withdrawal symptoms.
   a. Severe craving.
   b. Coming down from a "high" often leads to a severe "letdown," depressed feeling.
   c. Psychologic dependence often leads to cocaine becoming a total obsession.

E. Amphetamine dependence.
   Example: dextroamphetamine (Dexedrine).
1. Street names: crank, bennies, wake-ups, uppers, speed (amphetamines).
2. Administration: oral or injected.
3. Symptoms of use.
   a. Elation, agitation, hyperactivity, irritability.
   b. Increased pulse, respiration, and blood pressure.
   c. Fine tremor, muscle twitching, and mydriasis (pupillary dilation).
   d. Large doses: convulsions, cardiovascular collapse, respiratory depression, coma, death.
4. Withdrawal symptoms.
   a. Appear within 2 to 4 days after the last dose.
   b. Depression, overwhelming fatigue, suicide attempts.

F. PCP (phencyclidine hydrochloride) abuse.
1. Street names: peace pill, hog, super pill, elephant tranquilizer, angel dust, rocket fuel, primo.
2. Administration: snorted, smoked, or orally ingested; usually smoked along with marijuana.
3. Symptoms of use.
   a. Euphoria, feeling of numbness, mood changes.
   b. Diaphoresis, eye movement changes (nystagmus), hypertension, catatonic-like stupor with eyes open.
   c. Seizures, shivering, decerebrate posturing, possible death.
   d. Synesthesia: experiencing one sense when another is actually being stimulated—e.g., seeing colors when a loud sound occurs.
4. Overdose symptoms ("bad trip"): psychosis, possible death.
   a. User may become violent, destructive, and confused.
   b. Users have been known to go berserk; users may harm themselves and others.
   c. Intoxicating symptoms lighten and worsen over a period of 48 hours.

G. Hallucinogen abuse.
   Example: LSD (lysergic acid diethylamide), psilocybin ("magic mushroom"), mescaline (peyote), DMT, MDA.
1. Street name: acid.
2. Administration: usually oral, but LSD and mescaline can be injected.
3. Symptoms of use.
   a. Pupillary dilation, tachycardia, sweating.
   b. Visual hallucinations, depersonalization, impaired judgment and mood.
   c. Flashbacks and "bad trips."
   d. Usually no signs of withdrawal symptoms after use has been discontinued.

H. Marijuana dependence.
   Example: marijuana, hashish, tetrahydrocannabinol (THC).
1. Street names: joints, reefers, pot, grass, shit, Mary Jane (marijuana), hash (hashish).
2. Administration: oral, sniffed, and smoked.
3. Symptoms of use.
   a. Euphoria, relaxation, tachycardia, and conjunctival congestion.
   b. Paranoid ideation; impaired judgment.
   c. Rarely, panic reactions and psychoses.
   d. Heavy use leads to apathy and general deterioration in all aspects of living.
   e. Overdose effects: flashbacks, bronchitis, personality changes.
4. Withdrawal symptoms.
   a. Anxiety, sleeplessness, sweating.
   b. Lack of appetite, nausea, general malaise.

I. Designer drugs.
1. Street names: Ecstasy, Adam (MDMA [methylene-dioxy-methamphetamine]), China White (MTPT).
2. Called *analog drugs* because they retain the properties of controlled drugs (e.g., MTPT is an analog of Demerol).
3. Symptoms of use and side effects are similar to those associated with the controlled substance from which they are derived.

Nursing Interventions

Goal: To assess the drug use pattern.

Goal: To assist in medical treatment during detoxification or withdrawal.

A. Narcotics.
   1. Narcotic antagonists, such as naloxone (Narcan), nalorphine (Nalline), or levallorphan (Lorfan), are administered intravenously for narcotic overdose.
   2. Withdrawal is managed with rest and nutritional therapy.
   3. Substitution therapy with propoxyphene (Darvon) may be instituted to decrease withdrawal symptoms for longer effects.
B. Depressants.
   1. Substitution therapy with a long-acting barbiturate, such as phenobarbital (Luminal), may be instituted to decrease withdrawal symptoms.
   2. Some physicians prescribe oxazepam (Serax) as needed for objective symptoms, gradually decreasing the dosage until the drug is discontinued.
C. Stimulants.
   1. Treatment of overdose is geared toward stabilization of vital signs.
   2. IV antihypertensives may be used, along with IV diazepam (Valium), to control seizures.
   3. Chlordiazepoxide (Librium) may be administered orally for the first few days while client is "crashing."
D. Hallucinogens and cannabinols.
   1. Medications are normally not prescribed for withdrawal from these substances.
   2. In the event of overdose, diazepam (Valium) or chlordiazepoxide (Librium) may be given as needed to decrease agitation.
E. Awareness that gradual withdrawal, detoxification, or dechemicalization is necessary for the client addicted to barbiturates, narcotics, and tranquilizers.
F. Abrupt withdrawal, or quitting "cold turkey," is often dangerous and can be fatal.
G. Maintain a patent airway; have oxygen available.
H. Provide a safe, quiet environment (i.e., remove harmful objects, place bed in low position).

Goal: To decrease problem behaviors of manipulation and "acting out."

A. Set firm, consistent limits.
B. Confront client with manipulative behaviors.

Goal: To promote alternative coping methods.

A. Encourage responsibility for own behavior.
B. Encourage the use of hobbies, exercise, or alternative therapies as a means to deal with frustration and anxiety.

Goal: To recognize complications of substance abuse.

A. Obstetrical implications.
   1. Narcotic addiction.
      a. Increased risk for pregnancy-induced hypertension, malpresentation, and third-trimester bleeding.
      b. Provide methadone maintenance therapy for the duration of the pregnancy—withdrawal is not advisable because of the risk to the fetus.

   2. Use of other drugs causes increased risk to mother and fetus.
B. Neonatal complications.
   1. Withdrawal symptoms depend on type of drug mother used.
   2. Restlessness, jitteriness, hyperactive reflexes, high-pitched shrill cry, feeds poorly.
   3. Maintain seizure precautions.
   4. Administer antiepileptics to treat withdrawal and prevent seizures.
   5. Swaddle infant in snug-fitting blanket.
   6. Increased risk for congenital malformations and prematurity.
C. Medical implications.
   1. Increased risk for hepatitis, malnutrition, and infections in general.

Goal: To assist in the long-term process of drug rehabilitation.

A. Refer client to drug rehabilitation programs.
B. Promote self-help residential programs that foster self-support systems and use ex-addicts as rehabilitation counselors.
C. Methadone maintenance programs.
   1. Must be 18 years old and addicted for more than 2 years, with a history of detoxification treatments.
   2. Methadone is a synthetic narcotic that appeases desire for opiates.
      a. Controlled substance; given only under urinary surveillance.
      b. Administered orally; prevents opiate withdrawal symptoms.
D. 12-step self-help groups.
   1. Narcotics Anonymous: support group for clients who are addicted to narcotics and other drugs.
   2. Nar-Anon: support group for relatives and friends of narcotic addicts.
   3. Families Anonymous.

AFFECTIVE DISORDERS

The major affective disorders are characterized by disturbances of mood.

General Concepts

A. Incidence.
   1. Approximately 1% of the adult population has had an episode of bipolar disorder.
   2. More prevalent among family members when there is a positive family history.
   3. Major depression is seen more often in women.
   4. More common in higher socioeconomic groups.
B. Causes.
   1. A variety of theories may explain affective disorders.
   2. Depressive: loss of significant others or objects; changes in levels of norepinephrine (decrease) and steroids (increase); loss of self-esteem leading to hopelessness, helplessness, and pessimism towards self and others.

3. Manic: unresolved diffuse anger and hostility; denial of depression; may develop from early childhood as a result of high parental expectations.

C. Personality characteristics associated with affective disorders.

1. Depressive: lacking in confidence, introverted, unassertive, dependent, pessimistic, feelings of inadequacy.

2. Manic: extroverted, confident, manipulative, and obsessive.

Psychodynamics

A. Manic.

1. During infancy, needs and narcissistic goals are not met, which leads to impairment in the development of self-esteem.

2. Low self-esteem and helplessness lead to need for excessive attention, affection, warmth, and appreciation.

3. Usually a massive denial of depression.

4. The air of happiness and self-confidence is a defense against dependency feelings.

B. Depressive.

1. Loss, either real or perceived, of a loved person or object.

2. Turning aggressive feelings inward and displacing them onto the self; accompanied by feelings of guilt.

3. Ambivalent feelings toward the valued/lost object.

4. Repressive guilt, which leads to feelings of helplessness and hopelessness.

Assessment

A. Bipolar disorder (Figure 10-2).

1. Manic.

a. Onset before the age of 30 years.

b. Mood: elevated, expansive, or irritable.

c. Speech: loud, rapid, difficult to interpret, punning, rhyming, and clanging (using words that sound like the meaning rather than the actual word).

d. Cognitive skills: flight of ideas, grandiose delusions, easily distracted.

e. Psychomotor activity: hyperactive, decreased need for sleep, exhibitionistic, vulgar, profane, may make inappropriate sexual advances and be obscene.

f. Course of manic episode: begins suddenly, rapidly escalates over a few days, and ends more abruptly than major depressive episodes.

2. Depressive.

a. Has had one or more manic episodes.

b. Mood: dysphoric, depressive, despairing, loss of interest or pleasure in most usual activities.

c. Cognitive process: negative view of self, world, and of the future; poverty of ideas; crying; and suicidal preoccupation.

d. Psychomotor: may have either agitation or retardation in movements, feelings of fatigue, lack of appetite, constipation, sleeping disturbances (insomnia or early morning wakefulness), and a decrease in libido.

3. Mixed.

a. Involves both manic and depressive episodes, either intermixed or alternating rapidly every few days.

b. Depressive phase symptoms are prominent and last at least a full day.

B. Major depression.

1. May occur at any age.

2. Differentiated as either a single episode or a recurring type.

3. Symptoms the same as those listed above, under "Bipolar disorder, Depressive."

4. Severity and type of depression vary with the ability to test reality.

a. Psychotic: feels worse in the morning and better as the day goes on.

b. Neurotic: wakes up feeling optimistic; mood worsens as the day passes.

C. Other disorders (not considered part of the major affective type classification).

1. Cyclothymic.

a. Chronic mood disturbance of at least 2-year duration.

b. Numerous periods of mild depression and mania.

c. Depressive mood periods: feelings of inadequacy, social withdrawal, sleeping too much, diminished work productivity.

d. Hypomanic: inflated self-esteem; uninhibited, people-seeking behavior; decreased need for sleep; increased work productivity; and sharpened or unusually creative thinking.

2. Dysthymic disorder (depressive neurosis).

a. Depressed mood with loss of interest in most usual daily activities.

BIPOLAR DISORDER

MANIC
- Onset before age 30
- Mood:
  Elevated
  Expansive
  Irritable
- Speech:
  Loud-Rapid
  Punning
  Rhyming
  Clanging
  Vulgar
- ? Wt. loss
- Grandiose delusions
- Distracted
- Hyperactive
- ↓ Need for sleep
- Inappropriate
- Flight of ideas
- Begins suddenly and escalates over several days

DEPRESSIVE
- Previous manic episodes
- Mood:
  Anxious
  Depressed
  Hopelessness
- ↓ Interest in pleasure
- Negative views
- Fatigue
- ↓ Appetite
- Constipation
- Insomnia
- ↓ Libido
- Suicidal preoccupation
- May be agitated or have movement retardation

FIGURE 10-2 Bipolar affective disorder. (From Zerwekh J, Claborn J: *Memory notebook of nursing,* vol 1, ed 4, Ingram, Texas, 2008, Nursing Education Consultants.)

b. No delusions or hallucinations.

c. Common disorder with an increased incidence in females; chronic course.

Nursing Interventions (Manic Episode)

Goal: To provide for basic human needs of safety and rest/activity.

A. Reduce outside stimuli and provide a nonstimulating environment.

B. Monitor food intake: provide a high-calorie, high-vitamin diet with finger foods, to be eaten as the client moves about.

> **❗ NURSING PRIORITY** Physiologic needs are the first priority in providing client care.

C. Encourage noncompetitive solitary activities such as walking, swimming, or painting.

D. Assist with personal hygiene.

> **❗ NURSING PRIORITY** During the manic phase, the client's physical safety is at risk because the hyperactivity may lead to exhaustion, and ultimately, cardiac failure.

Goal: To establish a therapeutic nurse-client relationship.

A. Use firm, consistent, honest approach.

B. Assess client's abilities and involve client in his or her own care planning.

C. Promote problem-solving abilities; recognize that a false sense of independence is often demonstrated by loud, boisterous behavior.

D. Do not focus on or discuss grandiose ideas.

Goal: To set limits on behavior.

A. Instructions should be clear and concise.

B. Initiate regularly scheduled contacts to demonstrate acceptance.

C. Maintain some distance between self and client to allow freedom of movement and to prevent feelings of being overpowered.

D. Maintain neutrality and objectivity: realize that client can be easily provoked by harmless remarks and may demonstrate a furious reaction but calm down very quickly.

E. Use measures to prevent overt aggression (e.g., distraction, recognition of behaviors of increased excitement).

Goal: To promote adaptive coping with constructive use of energy.

A. Do not hurry client; this leads to anxiety and hostile behavior.

> **❗ NURSING PRIORITY** In a hyperactive state, the client is extremely distractible, and responses to even the slightest stimuli are exaggerated.

B. Provide activities and constructive tasks that channel the agitated behavior (e.g., cleaning game room, going for a walk, gardening, playing catch).

Goal: To assist in the medical treatment.

A. Administer lithium (Lithane or Eskalith).

B. Teach client about lithium medication instructions (see Appendix 10-3).

C. Divalproex or valproic acid (Depakote) is used to treat lithium nonresponders.

D. Carbamazepine (Tegretol) can be used with Lithium or an antipsychotic for treatment-resistant bipolar disorder.

E. Antipsychotic drugs such as olanzapine (Zyprexa) and quetiapine (Seroquel) may be better tolerated than Lithium.

Nursing Interventions (Depressive Episode)

> **❗ NURSING PRIORITY** Depression and suicidal behaviors may be viewed as anger turned inward on the self. If this anger can be verbalized in a nonthreatening environment, the client may be able to resolve these feelings, regardless of the discomfort involved.

Goal: To assess for suicide potential.

A. Recognition of suicidal intent.

1. Self-destructive behaviors are viewed as attempts to escape unbearable life situations.

2. Anxiety and hostility are overwhelmingly present.

3. There is the presence of ambivalence; living versus self-destructive impulses.

4. Depression, low self-esteem, and feelings of hopelessness are critical to evaluate, because suicide attempts are often made when the client feels like giving up.

5. Assess for *indirect* self-destructive behavior: any activity that is detrimental to the physical well-being of the client in which the potential outcome is death.

   a. Eating disorders: anorexia nervosa, bulimia, obesity, and overeating.

   b. Noncompliance with medical treatment (e.g., diabetic who does not take insulin).

   c. Cigarette smoking, gambling, criminal and/or socially deviant activities.

   d. Alcohol and drug abuse.

   e. Participation in high-risk sports (e.g., automobile racing; skydiving).

B. Suicide danger signs (Box 10-3).

1. The presence of a suicide plan: specifics relating to method, its lethality, and likelihood for rescue.

2. Change in established patterns in routines (e.g., giving away personal items, making a will, saying good-bye).

3. Anticipation of failure: loss of a job, preoccupation with physical disease, actual or anticipated loss of a significant other.

4. Change in behavior, presence of panic, agitation, or calmness; often, as depression lifts, client has enough energy to act on suicidal feelings.

5. Hopelessness: feelings of impending doom, futility, and entrapment.

6. Withdrawal and rejection of help.

Box 10-3 SAD PERSONS SCALE

One of the most popular and easy-to-use tools available to help assess suicide risk. The more areas checked, the higher the risk.

___ **S**ex (males are more likely to successfully commit suicide)
___ **A**ge (younger than 19 or older than 45)
___ **D**epression
___ **P**revious suicide attempt
___ **E**thanol (alcohol) abuse
___ **R**ational thinking (impaired)
___ **S**ocial support lacking (including recent loss of loved one)
___ **O**rganized plan
___ **N**o spouse
___ **S**ickness (especially chronic)

Total score ranges from 0 (lowest risk) to 10 (highest risk). This scale should be used as a guideline only; use your judgment and don't neglect unspecified factors.

Box 10-4 ADOLESCENT SUICIDE

Characteristics

- History of suicide ideation
- Previous suicide attempt
- Long-term use of drugs
- Acting-out behaviors: delinquency, stealing, vandalism, academic failure, promiscuity, loss of boyfriend/girlfriend

Family Characteristics

- Unproductive, conflictual communication
- Impaired problem-solving ability
- Inconsistent positive reinforcements, plus a greater number of negative reinforcements
- Unstable home environment

C. Clients at risk (Box 10-4).
   1. Adolescents and older adults; males more likely to complete the suicide act.
   2. Clients experiencing recent stress of a maturational or situational crisis.
   3. Clients with chronic or painful illnesses.
   4. Clients with previous suicide attempts or suicidal behavior.
   5. Withdrawn, depressed, or hallucinating clients.
   6. Clients with sexual identity conflicts and those who abuse alcohol and drugs.

Goal: To provide for basic human needs of safety and protection from self-destruction.

A. Remove all potentially harmful objects (e.g., belts, sharp objects, matches, lighters, strings, etc.).
B. Maintain a one-to-one relationship and close observation.

! **NURSING PRIORITY** Be aware of special times when client might be suicidal (e.g., when suddenly cheerful, when there are fewer staff members available, upon arising in the morning, or during a busy routine day). When drug therapy is started, client may feel better and act on suicidal ideations.

C. Have client make a written contract agreeing not to harm himself or herself; provide an alternative plan of coping.
D. Administer lamotrigine (Lamictal), if ordered.

Goal: To provide for physical needs of nutrition and rest/activity.

A. Assess for changes in weight (weight loss may indicate deepening depression).
B. Encourage increased bulk and roughage in diet along with sufficient fluids if client is constipated.

! **NURSING PRIORITY** Depressed clients are particularly vulnerable to constipation as a result of psychomotor retardation.

C. Provide for adequate amount of exercise and rest; encourage client not to sleep during the day.
D. Assist with hygiene and personal appearance.

Goal: To promote expression of feelings.

A. Encourage expression of angry, guilty, or depressed feelings.
B. Convey a kind, pleasant, interested approach to promote a sense of dignity and self-worth in the client.
C. Support the client's expression of feelings by allowing the client to respond in his or her own time.
D. Seek out client; initiate frequent contact.
E. Assist with decision making when depression is severe.

Goal: To provide for meaningful socialization activities.

! **NURSING PRIORITY** The depressed client often has impaired decision-making/problem-solving ability and needs structure in his or her life. The nurse must devise a plan of therapeutic activities and provide client with a written time schedule. **Remember:** The client who is moderately depressed feels best early in the day, whereas later in the day is a better time for the severely depressed individual to participate in activities.

A. Encourage participation in activities (e.g., plan a work assignment with client to do simple tasks: straightening game room, picking up magazines).
B. Assess hobbies, sports, or activities client enjoys; encourage client's participation.
C. Encourage client to participate in small-group conversation or activity; practice social skills through role playing and psychodrama.
D. Encourage activities that promote a sense of accomplishment and enhance self-esteem.

Goal: To assist in medical treatment.

A. Administer antidepressant medication (see Appendix 10-4).
B. Assist in electroconvulsive therapy (ECT) (Box 10-5).

SCHIZOPHRENIC DISORDERS

! **NURSING PRIORITY** The schizophrenic disorders constitute the largest group of psychotic disorders in society (approximately 1% of the U.S. population).

ECT is an electric shock delivered to the brain through electrodes that are applied to both temples. The shock artificially induces a grand mal seizure.

Indications

1. Severely depressed clients who do not respond to medication.
2. High risk for suicide/starvation.
3. Overwhelming depression with delusions or hallucinations.
4. Number of treatments: usually given in a series that varies according to the client's presenting problem and response to therapy; 2 to 3 treatments per week for a period of 2 to 6 weeks.

Nursing Intervention

- To prepare client for ECT.
  1. Assess client's record for routine pretreatment checklist for information.
  2. Teach client about procedure: what to expect before, during, and after.
  3. NPO status for 6 hours before treatment.
  4. Remove dentures.
  5. Administer pretreatment medication.
- To provide support and care immediately after treatment.
  1. Provide orientation to time.
  2. Temporary memory loss is usually confusing; explain that this is a common occurrence.
  3. Assess vital signs for 30 minutes to 1 hour after treatment.
  4. Deemphasize preoccupation with ECT; promote involvement in regularly scheduled activities.
- Long-term goal: to promote and develop a positive self-concept and realistic perception of self.
  1. Encourage problem solving in social relationships; identify problem areas in relationships with others.
  2. Acknowledge and encourage statements that reflect positive attributes and/or skills.
  3. Reinforce new, alternative coping methods, especially if client uses a new method to handle sad situations and painful feelings.

Schizophrenia

Schizophrenia is a maladaptive disturbance characterized by a number of common behaviors involving disorders of thought content, mood, feeling, perception, communication, and interpersonal relationships. Onset of symptoms usually occurs in early adulthood (ages 19 to 21 years) with a duration of symptoms of at least 6 months.

General Concepts

A. Loss of ego boundaries.
B. May result from many possible factors.
  1. Organic or physiologic: genetic, biochemical (overactivity of dopamine, an insufficiency of norepinephrine, or an imbalance of both; decreased monamine oxidase activity), immunologic imbalance, a structural deviation of brain tissue, or enlarged brain ventricles.
  2. Psychosocial: individual adaptive patterns to stress, double-bind communication pattern, poor family relationships, past traumatic experiences, lack of ego strength, or a deficit in cognitive development caused by perinatal, nutritional, and maturational factors.
C. Primary mental mechanisms are repression, regression, projection, and denial.
D. Failure or inability to trust self or others.
E. Security and identity are threatened, prompting the client to withdraw from reality.

Prepsychotic Personality Characteristics

A. Aloof and indifferent.
B. Social withdrawal; peculiar behavior.
C. Relatives and friends note a change in personality.
D. Unusual perceptual experiences and disturbed communication patterns.
E. Lack of personal grooming.

Psychodynamics of Maladaptive Disturbances

A. Disturbed thought processes.
  1. Confused, chaotic, and disorganized thinking.
  2. Communicates in symbolic language in which all symbols have special meaning.
  3. Belief that one's thoughts or wishes can control other people (i.e., magical thinking).
  4. Retreats to a fantasy world, rejecting the real world of painful experience while responding to reality in a bizarre or autistic manner.
B. Disturbed affect.
  1. Difficulty expressing emotions.
  2. Absent, flat, blunted, or inappropriate affect.
  3. Inappropriate affect makes it difficult to form close relationships.
C. Disturbance in psychomotor behavior.
  1. Display of disorganized, purposeless activity.
  2. Behavior may be uninhibited and bizarre; abnormal posturing (agitated or retardation catatonia); waxy flexibility.
  3. Often appears aloof, disinterested, apathetic, and lacking motivation.
D. Disturbance in perception.
  1. Hallucinations and delusions; auditory forms are most common.
  2. Abnormal bodily sensations and hypersensitivity to sound, sight, and smell.
E. Disturbance in interpersonal relationships.
  1. Establishment of interpersonal relationships is difficult because of inability to communicate clearly and react appropriately.
  2. Difficulty relating to others.
     a. Unable to form close relationships.
     b. Has difficulty trusting others and experiences ambivalence, fear, and dependency.

c. "Need-fear dilemma": withdraws to protect self from further hurt and consequently experiences lack of warmth, trust, and intimacy.

d. "As if" phenomenon: feels rejected by others, which leads to increased isolation, perpetuating further feelings of rejection.

Types of Schizophrenia

A. Schizophrenia, disorganized.
1. Inappropriate affect; giggling and silly laughter.
2. Regressive behavior.
3. Severe thought disturbance, incoherent speech, "word salad."
4. Withdrawn, fragmentary hallucinations and delusions.

B. Schizophrenia, catatonic.
1. Stupor and excitement phases of catatonia, bizarre posturing, waxy flexibility.
2. Negativism: rigidity and mutism.

C. Schizophrenia, paranoid.
1. Delusions of persecution and grandeur.
2. Extreme suspiciousness.
3. Anger, argumentativeness, and violence.
4. Doubts about gender identity.

D. Schizophrenia, undifferentiated.
1. Mixed psychotic symptoms.
2. Unclassifiable; either does not meet the criteria of one of the subtypes or meets the criteria of more than one.

E. Schizophrenia, residual.
1. History of exhibited psychotic symptoms of schizophrenia, but not psychotic at present.
2. Continued difficulty in thinking, mood, and perception.

Assessment

A. Four A's: Eugene Bleuler's classic symptoms.
1. Associative looseness: lack of logical thought progression, resulting in disorganized and chaotic thinking.
2. Affect: emotion or feeling tone is one of indifference or is flat, blunted, exaggerated, or socially inappropriate.
3. Ambivalence: conflicting, strong feelings (e.g., love and hate) that neutralize each other, leading to psychic immobilization and difficulty in expressing other emotions.
4. Autism: extreme retreat from reality characterized by fantasies, preoccupation with daydreams, and psychotic thought processes of delusion and hallucination (Figure 10-3).
   a. Hallucinations: false sensory perceptions with no basis in reality; may be auditory, olfactory, tactile, visual, gustatory.
   b. Delusions: fixed, false beliefs not corrected by logic; develop as a defense against intolerable feelings or ideas that cause anxiety.
      (1) Delusions of grandeur: related to feelings of power, fame, splendor, magnificence.

FIGURE 10-3 Hallucinations, illusions, and delusions? (From Zerwekh J, Claborn J: *Memory notebook of nursing,* vol 1, ed 4, Ingram, Texas, 2008, Nursing Education Consultants.)

(2) Delusions of persecution: belief that others are out to harm, injure, or destroy.
   c. Ideas of reference: belief that actions and speech of others have reference to oneself; ideas symbolize feelings of guilt, insecurity, and alienation.
   d. Depersonalization: feeling alienated from oneself; difficulty distinguishing self from others; loss of boundaries between self and environment.

B. Additional characteristics.
1. Regression: extreme withdrawal and social isolation.
2. Negativism: doing the opposite of what is asked; typical behavior is to speak to no one and answer no one; used to cover feelings of unworthiness and inadequacy.
3. Religiosity: excessive religious preoccupation.
4. Lack of social awareness: crudeness and social insensitivity; neglectful of personal grooming and hygiene.

Nursing Interventions

Goal: To build trust.

ALERT Building trust is the primary goal when working with the client with schizophrenia. Maintain a therapeutic milieu; stay with client to promote safety; reducing fear and assisting client to communicate effectively are important nursing care measures.

A. Encourage free expression of feelings (either negative or positive) without fear of rejection, ridicule, or retaliation.

B. Use nonverbal level of communication to demonstrate warmth, concern, and empathy because client often distrusts words.

C. Consistency, reliability, acceptance, and persistence build trust.

D. Allow client to set pace; proceed slowly in planning social contacts.

Goal: To provide a safe and secure environment.

A. Maintain familiar routines. Make sure persons who come in contact with the client are recognizable to the client.

B. Avoid stressful situations or increasing anxiety.

Goal: To clarify and reinforce reality.

A. Involve client in reality-oriented activities.

B. Help client find satisfaction in the external environment and ways of relating to others.

C. Focus on clear communication and the immediate situation.

Goal: To promote and build self-esteem.

A. Encourage simple activities with limited concentration and *no* competition.

B. Provide successful experiences with short-range goals realistic for client's level of functioning.

C. Relieve client of decision making until he or she is ready.

D. Avoid making demands.

Goal: To encourage independent behavior.

A. Anticipate and accept negativism.

B. Avoid fostering dependency.

C. Encourage client to make his or her own decisions, using positive reinforcement.

Goal: To provide care to meet basic human needs.

A. Determine client's ability to meet responsibilities of daily living.

B. Attend to nutrition, elimination, exercise, hygiene, and signs of physical illness.

Goal: To assist in medical treatment.

A. Administer antipsychotic medications (see Appendix 10-5).

1. Assist with ECT; may be useful in some instances to modify behavior.

> **! NURSING PRIORITY** As the client's symptoms lessen, he or she will often discontinue therapy and medication, which can lead to recurrence of symptoms.

Goal: To deal effectively with withdrawn behavior.

A. Establish a therapeutic one-to-one relationship.

1. Initiate interaction by seeking out client at every opportunity.

2. Maintain a nonjudgmental, accepting manner in what is said and done.

3. Attempt to draw client into a conversation without demanding a response.

B. Promote social skills by helping client feel more secure with other people.

1. Accept one-sided conversations.

2. Accept client's negativism without comments.

C. Attend to physical needs of client as necessary.

D. Have client focus on reality.

E. Protect and restrain client from potential destructiveness to self and others.

Goal: To deal effectively with hallucinations.

A. Clarify and reinforce reality.

1. Help client recognize hallucination as a manifestation of anxiety.

2. Provide a safe, secure environment.

3. Avoid denying or arguing with client when he or she is experiencing hallucinations.

4. Acknowledge client's experience but point out that *you* do not share the same experience.

5. Do not give attention to content of hallucinations.

6. Direct client's attention to real situations, such as singing along with music.

7. Protect client from injury to self or others when he or she is prompted by "voices" or "visions."

B. Encourage social interaction to help client find satisfactory ways of relating with others.

1. Increase interaction gradually.

2. Respond verbally to anything real that client talks about.

Paranoid Disorders

Paranoid disorders are maladaptive disorders characterized by delusions, usually persecutory, and extreme suspiciousness.

General Concepts

A. Primary mental mechanism is projection.

B. Onset of paranoid behavior may be precipitated by stressful events.

1. Loss of a real or imaginary love object.

2. Experience of failure, leading to loss of self-esteem and feelings of inadequacy.

C. Delusional behavior.

1. An attempt to cope with stress and reality.

2. Associated with an extreme need to maintain self-esteem.

3. Delusions are a symbolic way to communicate with others.

4. Delusions are very real to client.

5. Delusional system usually incorporates denial of reality, followed by projection and rationalization.

Psychodynamics

A. Lack of security and trust is evident.

B. Inconsistency and failure to meet infant's basic needs lead to suspiciousness.

C. Conflicting messages and double-bind communication lead to low self-esteem.

Assessment

A. Extreme suspiciousness and withdrawal from emotional contact with others.

B. Aloof, distant, hypercritical of others.

C. Frequent complaining by letter writing or instigating legal action.

D. Resentment, anger, possible violence.

E. Delusions of grandeur and persecution and hypochondriasis.

F. Misinterpretation or distortion of reality; may refuse food and medications, insisting that he or she is being poisoned despite evidence to the contrary.

Nursing Interventions

Goal: To establish a trusting relationship.

> **ALERT** Use therapeutic interventions to increase client's understanding of behavior. The lack of trust in the paranoid client could be a test question surrounding the serving of meals or the administration of medications.

A. Maintain calm, matter-of-fact attitude.

B. Keep promises made; be honest.

C. Avoid whispering or acting secretive.

D. Allow a choice of activities and foods; involve client in treatment plan.

Goal: To increase self-esteem by providing successful experiences.

A. Allow client to set pace in closeness with others.

B. Avoid involvement in competitive, aggressive activities requiring physical contact (e.g., football, basketball).

C. Involve client in solitary activities (e.g., drawing, photography, typing) and progress to intellectual activities with others using games (e.g., chess, bridge, Scrabble).

D. Reward completion of meaningful tasks.

Goal: To help client deal effectively with delusions.

A. Clarify and focus on reality; use reality testing.

B. Avoid confirming or approving false beliefs.

C. Point out that client's beliefs are not shared.

D. Divert attention from delusions to reality; focus on here and now.

Disorders of Impulse Control

In disorders of impulse control, there is failure to resist an impulse, drive, or temptation to perform some act that may be harmful to others; the failure to resist is usually preceded by an increasing amount of tension before the act is committed but is followed by an outcome of pleasure or gratification.

Assessment

A. Pathologic gambling.
  1. Diagnostic criteria.
    a. A chronic and progressive failure to resist impulses to gamble.
    b. Disrupts, damages, or compromises family, personal, and vocational pursuits.

(1) Evidence of forgery, fraud, embezzlement.

(2) Unable to pay debts or meet other financial obligations.

(3) Borrows money, either legally or illegally.

(4) Loss of work because of frequent absenteeism.

  2. Additional characteristics.
    a. Overconfident, very energetic, "big spender."
    b. Often begins in adolescence.

B. Kleptomania (shoplifting).
  1. Recurrent impulse to steal objects.
  2. Characterized by increasing tension before stealing and a feeling of pressure or release after the act is committed.
  3. Usually done without long-term planning.

C. Pyromania (setting fires).
  1. Recurrent impulse to set fires.
  2. Usually characterized by increased amount of tension before the fire is set, with subsequent release after the act is committed.

D. Explosive disorder.
  1. A loss of control of aggressive impulses, resulting in assault or destruction of property.
  2. Behavior is usually out of proportion to the precipitating stressor.
  3. Individual usually describes "spells" or "attacks;" usually regrets the display of aggression.

Nursing Interventions

Goal: To encourage client to develop alternative ways of dealing with stress.

A. Refer client to self-help groups: Gamblers Anonymous (GAM-ANON).

B. Assist client in determining when anxiety and tension are increasing and provide a plan of action to prevent acts of stealing, setting fires, or destroying property.

Adjustment Disorders

Assessment

A. Adjustment disorders can appear at any developmental stage and are related to the developmental task at hand.

B. Usually, there is no underlying mental disorder or disease.

C. Present behavior is usually disturbed and characterized by distortions in the situation and difficulty in decision making.

Nursing Interventions

Goal: To return client to homeostasis with the fullest possible functioning level.

A. Provide empathetic understanding and support.

B. Encourage identification of specific problems and promote new problem-solving coping skills.

C. Enlist family and community support as necessary.

Appendix 10-1 ALZHEIMER'S MEDICATIONS

General Nursing Implications

— Two types: (1) *cholinesterase inhibitors*, which prevent the breakdown of acetylcholine, thus making it available at the cholinergic synapses and resulting in enhanced transmission of nerve impulses and (2) a new drug—an *NMDA receptor antagonist*—which blocks calcium influx and modulates the effects of glutamate (major excitatory transmitter in CNS).

— Drugs do not cure and do not stop disease progression, but they may slow down the progression by a few months.

MEDICATIONS	SIDE EFFECTS	NURSING IMPLICATIONS
Cholinesterase Inhibitors Donepezil **(Aricept)**: PO Galantamine **(Razadyne)**: PO Rivastigmine **(Exelon)**: PO Tacrine **(Cognex)**: PO	GI symptoms: nausea, vomiting, dyspepsia, diarrhea Dizziness and headache Tacrine: high risk for liver damage	1. Abrupt withdrawal of medication can lead to a rapid progression of symptoms. 2. Monitor for side effects since drug is typically given in high doses to produce the greatest benefit.
NMDA Receptor Antagonist Memantine **(Namenda)**: PO	Dizziness, headache, confusion, constipation	1. Used for moderate to severe cases. 2. Better tolerated than cholinesterase inhibitors.

Appendix 10-2 ANTIANXIETY AGENTS

General Nursing Implications

— Withhold or omit one or more doses if excessive drowsiness occurs.

— Assess for symptoms associated with a withdrawal syndrome in hospitalized clients: anxiety, insomnia, vomiting, tremors, palpitations, confusion, and hallucinations.

— When discontinuing, the drug dosage should be gradually decreased over a period of days, depending on the dose and length of time the client has been taking the medication.

— Schedule IV drug requires documentation.

— Promote safety with the use of side rails and assistance with ambulation as necessary.

— Teach client and family not to drink alcohol while taking an antianxiety agent and not to stop taking the medication abruptly.

MEDICATIONS	SIDE EFFECTS	NURSING IMPLICATIONS
Benzodiazepines Reduce anxiety by enhancing the action of the inhibitory neurotransmitter GABA on its receptor; also promote anticonvulsant activity and skeletal muscle relaxation.		
Chlordiazepoxide **(Librium)**: PO, IM, IV Diazepam **(Valium)**: PO, IM, IV Clonazepam **(Klonopin)**: PO Chlorazepate dipotassium **(Tranxene)**: PO Midazolam **(Versed)**: IM, IV	CNS depression, drowsiness (decreases with use), ataxia, dizziness, headaches, dry mouth *Adverse effects:* tolerance commonly develops, physical dependency	1. May cause paradoxical effects and should not be taken by mothers who are breastfeeding. 2. Assess for symptoms of leukopenia, such as sore throat, fever, and weakness. 3. Encourage client to rise slowly from a supine position and to dangle feet before standing. 4. Librium: Do not inject or add IV Librium to an existing IV infusion; inject directly into a large vein over a 1-minute period. 5. Do not mix Librium or Valium with any other drug in a syringe or add to existing IV fluids. 6. Versed is commonly used for induction of anesthesia and sedation before diagnostic tests and endoscopic exams. 7. Flumazenil **(Romazicon)** is approved for the treatment of benzodiazepine overdose; has an adverse effect of precipitating convulsions, especially in clients with a history of epilepsy. 8. *Uses:* anxiety and tension, muscle spasm, preoperative medication, acute alcohol withdrawal, and to induce sleep.

Appendix 10-2 ANTIANXIETY AGENTS—cont'd

MEDICATIONS	SIDE EFFECTS	NURSING IMPLICATIONS
Nonbenzodiazepine Agents Interact with serotonin and dopamine receptors in the brain to decrease anxiety; lack muscle-relaxant and anticonvulsant effects; do not cause sedation or physical or psychologic dependence; do not increase CNS depression caused by alcohol or other drugs.		
Buspirone **(BuSpar):** PO	Dizziness, drowsiness, headache, nausea, fatigue, insomnia	1. Not a controlled substance. 2. Some improvement can be noted in 7-10 days; however, usually takes 3-4 weeks to achieve effectiveness. 3. *Uses:* short-term relief of anxiety and anxiety disorders.

CNS, Central nervous system; *GABA,* gamma-aminobutyric acid; *IM,* intramuscularly; *IV,* intravenously; *PO,* by mouth (orally).

Appendix 10-3 ANTIMANIC MEDICATIONS

MEDICATIONS	SIDE EFFECTS	NURSING IMPLICATIONS
Lithium Carbonate Acts to lower concentrations of norepinephrine and serotonin by inhibiting their release; believed to alter sodium transport in both nerve and muscle cells. *Uses:* bipolar affective disorder (manic episode).		
Lithium **(Eskalith, Lithane):** PO	*High incidence:* increased thirst, increased urination (polyuria) *Frequent:* 1.5 mEq/L levels or less: dry mouth, lethargy, fatigue, muscle weakness, headache, GI disturbances, fine hand tremors *Adverse effects:* 1.5-2.0 mEq/L may produce vomiting, diarrhea, drowsiness, incoordination, coarse hand tremors, muscle twitching 2.0-2.5 mEq/L may result in ataxia, slurred speech, confusion, clonic movements, high output of dilute urine, blurred vision, hypotension *Acute toxicity:* seizures, oliguria, coma, peripheral vascular collapse, death	1. Monitor lithium blood levels: blood samples are obtained 12 hours after dose was given. 2. Teach client the following: a. Symptoms of lithium toxicity. b. Importance of frequent blood tests (every 2-3 days) to check lithium levels at the beginning of treatment (maintenance blood levels done every 1-3 months). c. Importance of taking dose at same time each day, preferably with meals or milk. 3. Encourage a diet containing normal amounts of salt and a fluid intake of 3 L per day; avoid caffeine because of its diuretic effect. 4. Report polyuria, prolonged vomiting, diarrhea, or fever to physician (may need to temporarily reduce dosage or discontinue use). 5. Do not crush, chew, or break the extended-release or film-coated tablets. 6. Assess clients at high risk for developing toxicity: postoperative, dehydrated, hyperthyroid, those with renal disease, or those taking diuretics. 7. Blood levels: a. Extremely narrow therapeutic range: 0.5-1.5 mEq/L. b. Toxic serum lithium level is greater than 2 mEq/L. 8. Management of lithium toxicity: possible hemodialysis. 9. Long-term use may cause goiter; may be associated with hypothyroidism.

Continued

Appendix 10-3 ANTIMANIC MEDICATIONS—cont'd

MEDICATIONS	SIDE EFFECTS	NURSING IMPLICATIONS

Other Agents Both medications listed below were originally developed and used for seizure disorders. Both have mood-stabilizing abilities.

Carbamazepine **(Tegretol):** PO	Drowsiness, dizziness, visual problems (spots before eyes, difficulty focusing, blurred vision), dry mouth *Toxic reactions*: blood dyscrasias	1. Used primarily for clients who have not responded to lithium or who cannot tolerate the side effects. 2. Avoid tasks that require alertness and motor skills until response to drug is established. 3. Monitor CBC frequently during initiation of therapy and at monthly intervals thereafter.
Valproic acid **(Depakene; Depakote):** PO	Nausea, GI upsets, drowsiness, may cause hepatotoxicity	1. Monitor liver function studies.

CBC, Complete blood count; *GI,* gastrointestinal; *PO,* by mouth (orally).

Appendix 10-4 ANTIDEPRESSANT MEDICATIONS

General Nursing Implications
— SSRIs are overtaking TCAs as drugs of choice for depression.
— Because of the potential interactions with other drugs and certain foods, MAOIs are used as second-line drugs for the treatment of depression.
— Therapeutic effect has a delayed onset of 7-21 days; however, SSRIs may take as long as 6 weeks to become effective.
— Can potentially produce cardiotoxicity, sedation, seizures, and anticholinergic effects and may induce mania in clients with bipolar disorder (SSRIs are less likely to cause these problems).
— Drugs are usually discontinued before surgery (10 days for MAOIs; 2-3 days for TCAs) because of adverse interactions with anesthetic agents.

MEDICATIONS	SIDE EFFECTS	NURSING IMPLICATIONS

Tricyclic Antidepressants (TCA) Prevent the reuptake of norepinephrine or serotonin, which results in increased concentrations of these neurotransmitters.

Imipramine hydrochloride **(Tofranil):** PO, IM Nortriptyline hydrochloride **(Aventyl):** PO Doxepin hydrochloride **(Sinequan):** PO Amitriptyline hydrochloride **(Elavil):** PO, IM	Drowsiness, dry mouth, blurred vision, constipation, weight gain, and orthostatic hypotension *Adverse reactions:* cardiac dysrhythmias, nystagmus, tremor, hypotension, restlessness	1. Should not be given at the same time as an MAOI; a time lag of 14 days is necessary when changing from one drug group to the other. 2. Because of marked sedation, client should avoid activities requiring mental alertness (driving or operating machinery). 3. Instruct client to move gradually from lying to sitting and standing positions to prevent postural hypotension. 4. **Sinequan** is tolerated better by older adults; has less effect on cardiac status; dilute the concentrate with orange juice. 5. Contraindicated in clients with epilepsy, glaucoma, and cardiovascular disease. 6. Usually given once daily at bedtime. 7. *Uses:* depression; **Tofranil** is also used to treat enuresis in children.

Appendix 10-4   ANTIDEPRESSANT MEDICATIONS—cont'd

MEDICATIONS	SIDE EFFECTS	NURSING IMPLICATIONS
Selective Serotonin Reuptake Inhibitors (SSRI) Cause selective inhibition of serotonin uptake and produce CNS excitation rather than sedation; have no effect on dopamine or norepinephrine.		
Fluoxetine (**Prozac**): PO Sertraline (**Zoloft**): PO Paroxetine (**Paxil**): PO	Nausea, headache, anxiety, nervousness, insomnia, weight gain, skin rash, sexual dysfunction	1. Medication is usually given once a day. 2. *Uses:* depression, obsessive-compulsive disorder, bulimia.
Monoamine Oxidase Inhibitors (MAOI) Inhibit the enzyme monoamine oxidase, which breaks down norepinephrine and serotonin, increasing the concentration of these neurotransmitters.		
Isocarboxazid (**Marplan**): PO Phenelzine sulfate (**Nardil**): PO Tranylcypromine (**Parnate**): PO	Drowsiness, insomnia, dry mouth, urinary retention, hypotension *Adverse reactions:* tachycardia, tachypnea, agitation, tremors, seizures, heart block, hypotension	1. Potentiate many drug actions: narcotics, barbiturates, sedatives, and atropine-like medications. 2. Have a long duration of action; therefore 2-3 weeks must go by before another drug is administered while a client is taking an MAOI. 3. Interact with specific foods and drugs (ones containing tyramine or sympathomimetic drugs). May cause a severe hypertensive crisis characterized by marked elevation of blood pressure, increased temperature, tremors, and tachycardia. Foods and drugs to avoid: coffee, tea, cola beverages, aged cheeses, beer and wine, pickled foods, avocados, and figs and many over-the-counter cold preparations, hay fever medications, and nasal decongestants. 4. Monitor for bladder distention by checking urinary output. 5. **Parnate:** most likely to cause hypertensive crisis; onset of action is more rapid. 6. *Uses:* primarily psychotic depression and depressive episode of bipolar affective disorder.
Miscellaneous Antidepressants		
Trazodone (**Desyrel**): PO	Sedation, orthostatic hypotension, nausea, vomiting, can cause priapism (prolonged, painful erection of the penis)	1. See General Nursing Implications.
Bupropion (**Wellbutrin**): PO	Weight loss, dry mouth, dizziness	1. See General Nursing Implications.

CNS, Central nervous system; *IM,* intramuscularly; *MAOIs,* monoamine oxidase inhibitors; *PO,* by mouth (orally); *SSRIs,* selective serotonin reuptake inhibitors; *TCAs,* tricyclic antidepressants.

Appendix 10-5   ANTIPSYCHOTIC (NEUROLEPTIC) MEDICATIONS

General Nursing Implications

— Use cautiously in older adult.
— Should make the client feel better and experience fewer psychotic episodes.
— Maintain a regular schedule; usually take daily dose 1-2 hours before bedtime.
— Explain to client and family the importance of compliance with medication regimen.
— Medications are not addictive.
— Discuss side effects and importance of notifying PCP if client experiences undesired or side effects.
— When mixing for parenteral use, do not mix with other drugs.
— Inject deep IM; client should stay in reclined position 30-60 minutes after dose administration.

MEDICATIONS	SIDE EFFECTS	NURSING IMPLICATIONS
Phenothiazines Block dopamine receptors and also thought to depress various portions of the reticular activating system; have peripherally exerting anticholinergic properties (atropine-like symptoms: dryness of mouth, stuffy nose, constipation, blurring of vision).		
Aliphatic types: Chlorpromazine hydrochloride **(Thorazine):** PO, IM, IV suppository Promazine hydrochloride **(Sparine):** PO, IM, IV *Piperazine types:* Prochlorperazine **(Compazine):** PO, IM, IV, suppository Fluphenazine hydrochloride **(Prolixin):** PO, IM Trifluoperazine **(Stelazine):** PO, IM *Piperidine types:* Thioridazine **(Mellaril):** PO Mesoridazine besylate **(Serentil):** PO, IM	**Extrapyramidal effects (movement disorder):** occur early in therapy and are usually managed with other drugs *Acute dystonia*—spasm of muscles of tongue, face, neck, or back; oculogyric crisis (upward deviation of the eyes); opisthotonus *Parkinsonism*—muscle tremors, rigidity, spasms, shuffling gait, stooped posture, cogwheel rigidity *Akathisia*—motor restlessness, pacing. **Tardive dyskinesia:** occurs late in therapy; symptoms are often irreversible—earliest symptom is slow, wormlike movements of the tongue; later symptoms include fine twisting, writhing movements of the tongue and face, grimacing; lip smacking; involuntary movements of the limbs, toes, fingers, and trunk **Neuroleptic malignant syndrome:** rare problem, fever (>41°C, 105°F), "leadpipe" muscle rigidity, agitation, confusion, delirium, respiratory and acute renal failure *Endocrine*—amenorrhea, increased libido in women, decreased libido in men, delayed ejaculation, increased appetite, weight gain, hypoglycemia, and edema *Dermatologic:* photosensitivity *Hypersensitivity reaction:* jaundice, agranulocytosis	1. Check blood pressure before administration; to avoid postural hypotension, encourage client to rise slowly from sitting or lying position. 2. Be aware of the antiemetic effect of the phenothiazines; may mask other pathology such as drug overdose, brain lesions, or intestinal obstruction. 3. Client teaching: protect skin from sunlight—wear long-sleeved shirts, hats, and sunscreen lotion when out in the sunlight. 4. Explain importance of reporting any signs of sore throat, fever, or symptoms of infection. 5. Encourage periodic liver function studies to be done. 6. Teach that drug may turn urine pink or reddish brown. 7. Extrapyramidal symptoms treated with anticholinergics, (e.g., **Cogentin**). 8. Long-term use of phenothiazines requires assessment of involuntary movement screening (AIMS). 9. *Uses:* severe psychoses, schizophrenia, manic phase of bipolar affective disorder, personality disorders, and severe agitation and anxiety.
Other Antipsychotic Drugs		
Haloperidol **(Haldol):** PO, IM	Significant extrapyramidal effects; low incidence of sedation, orthostatic hypotension; does not elicit photosensitivity reaction	1. May reduce prothrombin time. 2. Often used as the initial drug for treatment of psychotic disorders.

Appendix 10-5   ANTIPSYCHOTIC (NEUROLEPTIC) MEDICATIONS—cont'd

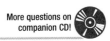

MEDICATIONS	SIDE EFFECTS	NURSING IMPLICATIONS
Risperidone **(Risperdal):** PO	Anxiety, somnolence, extrapyramidal symptoms, dizziness, constipation, GI upset, rhinitis.	1. *Uses:* tics, vocal disturbances, and psychotic schizophrenia. 2. **Risperdal** is the most frequently prescribed antipsychotic because of less serious side effects.
Clozapine **(Clozaril):** PO	Blood dyscrasias (agranulocytosis), sedation, weight gain, orthostatic hypotension, seizures, diabetes.	1. Used with caution in clients with diabetes and those with history of seizures. 2. Treatment is started slowly and gradually increased; it is important that the client not stop taking medication.

Study Questions Psychiatric Disorders

More questions on companion CD!

1. A client's feelings of despair and depression have lifted, and she tells the nurse, "I feel better now." The nurse understands that this client is:
   1. No longer a suicide risk
   2. Less of a suicide risk than when she was deeply depressed
   3. More of a suicide risk than when she was deeply depressed
   4. A suicide risk only in the evening

2. Which of the following nursing interventions should be instituted for a client experiencing a manic episode?
   1. Place the client in a quiet area, separate from others.
   2. Encourage the client to engage in some physical activity.
   3. Establish firm, set limits on behavior.
   4. Include the client in the group's activities.

3. A client demonstrates an inappropriate affect by giggling while talking about her brain being destroyed. This behavior serves what purpose for this client?
   1. Helps her to convince the staff that her problem is physical and not psychologic.
   2. Allows her to avoid the nurse's questions about the problems that resulted in her admission.
   3. Hides that she is angry with her parents for bringing her to the hospital.
   4. Protects her against the painful emotional impact of what she fears is happening to her.

4. A client experiencing severe depression is admitted to the inpatient psychiatric unit. During the initial assessment, she says, "I feel like killing myself, but I wouldn't do that because of my kids." The nurse's priority action would be to:
   1. Explore the reasons that the client might want to take her life.
   2. Determine the severity of her suicidal risk.
   3. Prevent the client from harming herself.
   4. Guide her to consider alternative ways of coping.

5. Which of the following signs and symptoms would the nurse assess for in a client with possible lithium toxicity?
   1. Hypotension, bradycardia, polyuria
   2. Tachycardia, hypertension, convulsions
   3. Diarrhea, ataxia, seizures, lethargy
   4. Urinary frequency, vomiting, fever

6. A client with schizophrenia is incontinent and urinates on the floor. The nurse's best response would be to:
   1. Ask the client to clean up after herself.
   2. Tell her that ward privileges will be withheld if it happens again.
   3. Ignore the client until her behavior improves.
   4. Clean up the urine without communicating displeasure.

7. A client's husband reports that over the past month his wife has become increasingly agitated and hyperexcitable, with a marked increase in verbal and physical activity. Based on these symptoms, the nurse concludes that the client may be experiencing which of the following?
   1. Panic attacks
   2. Paranoid behavior
   3. Free-floating anxiety
   4. Manic episode

8. When caring for a client admitted for medically monitored detoxification from alcohol, the nurse would assess for which of the following signs and symptoms of withdrawal?
   1. Anorexia, irritability, nausea, and tremulousness
   2. Bradycardia, hypotension, diaphoresis, and fever
   3. Vivid hallucinations, coarse irregular tremor
   4. Severe craving, euphoria, profuse sweating, and paranoid ideation

9. Which of the following defects is most commonly associated with Down syndrome?
   1 Deafness
   2 Congenital heart disease
   3 Hydrocephaly
   4 Muscular hypertonicity

10. When attempting to establish trust and rapport with a client experiencing schizophrenia, the priority action for the nurse would be to:
    1 Make emotional contact.
    2 Take a careful nursing history.
    3 Increase voluntary motor activity.
    4 Mutually agree to a contract.

11. Chlorpromazine (Thorazine) is ordered for a client. Which of the following signs or symptoms would the nurse include in the medication teaching about this drug?
    1 Weight loss
    2 Drowsiness
    3 Hypertension
    4 Insomnia

12. The nurse knows that which of the following is the most important factor in the successful adjustment of parents of an infant with Down syndrome?
    1 Their response to the reactions of family and friends to their infant
    2 Their ability to give physical care to their infant
    3 Their ability to talk about caring for their child and anticipated changes in their lifestyle
    4 Their understanding of the factors causing Down syndrome

13. A client is admitted to the inpatient psychiatric unit for medically monitored detoxification from alcohol. Which of the following actions would be included in the client's plan of care?
    1 Encourage increased fluid intake.
    2 Order a high-protein, high-fat diet.
    3 Provide a high-sodium, low-carbohydrate diet.
    4 Encourage ambulation and deep breathing.

14. A client with a diagnosis of schizophrenia repeatedly states, "There are flies eating my brain and making me feel weird." The client is most likely experiencing which of the following?
    1 Ideas of reference
    2 Grandiose delusions
    3 Somatic delusions
    4 Persecutory delusions

15. When preparing a client for electroconvulsive therapy (ECT), the nurse would include which of the following actions?
    1 Provide orientation to time.
    2 Assess vital signs for 30 minutes to 1 hour.
    3 Remove dentures and maintain NPO status.
    4 Encourage problem solving in social settings.

16. A client is experiencing a lack of logical thought progression, resulting in disorganized and chaotic thinking. The nurse understands this to be:
    1 Delusions of grandeur
    2 Ideas of reference
    3 Depersonalization
    4 Associative looseness

17. A client taking lithium (Eskalith) would most likely experience which of the following signs and symptoms?
    1 Increased thirst, increased urination
    2 Drowsiness, dizziness
    3 Dry mouth, blurred vision
    4 Headache, anxiety

18. A client receiving phenelzine sulfate (Nardil) must be taught to avoid which of the following foods?
    1 Chicken, eggs, and celery
    2 Aged cheeses, beer, and avocados
    3 Pasta, candy bars, and ice cream
    4 Beef, potatoes, and corn

19. A client says, "I think everyone is out to get me. I don't trust you at all." The nurse's best response would be:
    1 "I really don't think everyone is out to get you. You just think so."
    2 "I don't understand why you think everyone is out to get you. I know I am not one of those people."
    3 "How could you think everyone is out to get you when everyone is trying to help you?"
    4 "I know you think everyone is out to get you, but I don't see it that way."

20. Characteristics of borderline personality disorder include which of the following? Select all that apply:
    _____ 1 Self-mutilating behavior
    _____ 2 Impulsiveness
    _____ 3 Submissive, clinging behavior
    _____ 4 Grandiose self-importance
    _____ 5 Suspiciousness and mistrust of others
    _____ 6 Perfectionistic

Answers and rationales to these questions are in the section at the end of the book titled Chapter Study Questions: Answers and Rationales.

CHAPTER ELEVEN

Integumentary System

PHYSIOLOGY OF THE SKIN

A. Structure.
1. Epidermis—outermost layer; contains the melano-cytes and keratinocytes.
2. Dermis—connective tissue below epidermis; vascular; assists in body temperature and blood pressure regulation.

B. Glands on the skin.
1. Sebaceous glands: produce sebum, which is an oily secretion that is emptied into the hair shaft.
2. Apocrine glands: secrete an odorless fluid from the hair shaft, which, on contact with bacteria, produces a distinctive body odor.
   a. Located in the axilla, anal region, scrotum, and labia majora.
   b. Become more active at the time of puberty.
   c. Eccrine glands: sweat glands that are stimulated by elevated temperature and emotional stress.
      (1) Located all over the body, especially on the forehead, palms of the hands, and soles of the feet.
      (2) Under control of the sympathetic nervous system.

C. Functions of the skin.
1. Protection: primary function.
2. Sensory: major receptor for general sensation.
3. Water balance.
   a. 600 to 900 mL of water is lost daily through insensible perspiration.
   b. Forms a barrier that prevents loss of water and electrolytes from the internal environment.
4. Temperature regulation.
5. Involved in the activation of vitamin D.
6. Involved in wheal-and-flare reaction.
   a. Wheal: swelling.
   b. Flare: diffused redness.
   c. These responses are due to local edema caused by increased capillary permeability and dilation of the surrounding arterioles.
   d. Reaction is initiated by the release of histamine and the kinins.

System Assessment

A. Health history.
1. How long has the particular rash or lesion been present?
2. Is there any itching, burning, or discomfort associated with the problem?
3. Has the client been in contact with any irritants, sun, unusual cold, or unhygienic conditions?
4. Has anyone in the family ever had this same type of problem with his or her skin?
5. Is the client taking any medications?
6. What is the diet history? Does the client have any food allergies?

B. Physical assessment (Box 11-1).
1. Inspection.
   a. Assess the skin for color.
      (1) Jaundice.
      (2) Vitiligo: loss of melanin, resulting in white, depigmented area.
      (3) Areas to assess include the sclera, conjunctiva, nail beds, lips, and buccal mucosa.
   b. Assess for vascularity.
      (1) Determine whether there are areas of bruising, purpura, or petechiae.
      (2) Determine whether skin blanches on direct pressure.
   c. Assess lesions for type, color, size, distribution, and grouping; location and consistency.
      (1) Use metric rulers to measure the size of the lesion.
      (2) Use appropriate specific terminology to describe and report type of lesion (Table 11-1).
   d. Assess for unusual odors, especially around lesions or in the intertriginous areas (axilla, overhanging abdominal folds, and groin).
   e. Assess for chronic UV exposure and photoaging of skin—appearance of actinic (sun) keratoses (precancerous lesions), wrinkling, and telangiectasia.

(1) UVB—major factor of sunburn and nonmelanoma skin cancer.

(2) UVA—contributes to cancerous effects of UVB.

  f. Inspect hair (head and body for distribution) and nails (grooves, ridges, smoothness-thickness, detachment from nailbed).

2. Palpation.

  a. Determine temperature (use back of hand), tissue turgor (pinch under clavicle or back of hand), and mobility.

  b. Evaluate moisture and texture.

ALERT Perform a risk assessment—evaluation of skin integrity.

Box 11-1 OLDER ADULT CARE FOCUS

Differences in Skin Assessment

Skin
* Increased wrinkling and sagging, redundant flesh around eyes, slowness of skin to flatten when pinched together (tenting)
* Dry, flaking skin: excoriation from scratching
* Decreased rate of wound healing
* Evidence of bruising

Hair
* Graying; dry, scaly scalp
* Thinning, baldness

Nails
* Thick, brittle nails with diminished growth; ridging
* Prolonged return of blood with blanching

BENIND AND INFLAMMATORY DISORDERS OF THE SKIN

 Acne Vulgaris

Acne is an inflammatory disorder of the sebaceous glands and their hair follicles.

Assessment

A. More common in teenagers; may persist into adulthood.

B. Under hormonal influence during puberty; affected by presence of androgen, which stimulates the sebaceous glands to secrete sebum.

C. Inflammatory lesions or pustules; noninflammatory lesions such as open comedones (blackheads) and closed comedones (whiteheads).

D. Cysts: deep nodules that may produce scarring.

Treatment

A. Medical: topical or systemic therapy.

  1. Antibacterial and peeling agents: benzoyl peroxide and retinoic acid.

  2. Long-term antibiotic therapy.

  3. Isotretinoin (Accutane)—derivative of vitamin A, causes serious side effects; teratogenic; contraindicated during pregnancy.

Goal: To promote psychologic adjustment related to body image and appearance.

A. Counsel and assure client that problem is not related to uncleanliness, dietary intake, masturbation, or sexual activity.

B. Encourage client to talk about the problem with someone.

C. Make sure client recognizes that picking and squeezing lesions will worsen condition.

Table 11-1   COMMON DERMATOLOGIC LESIONS

Primary Lesions	*Secondary Lesions*
Macule: Flat, circumscribed area of color change in the skin without surface elevation; less than 1 cm in diameter (freckle, measles)	**Fissure:** Linear crack; may be dry or moist (athlete's foot, crack in corner of mouth)
Papule: Solid, elevated lesion, less than 1 cm in diameter (wart, elevated mole)	**Scale:** Excess epidermal cells caused by shedding (flaking of the skin)
Plaque: Circumscribed, solid lesion, greater than 1 cm in diameter (psoriasis, seborrheic keratosis)	**Scar:** Abnormal connective tissue that replaces normal skin (healed surgical incision)
Nodule: Raised, solid lesion that is larger and deeper than a papule	**Ulcer:** Loss of epidermis and dermis; crater-like; irregular shape (pressure ulcer, chancre)
Vesicle: Small elevation in skin, usually filled with serous fluid or blood; bulla: larger than a vesicle; pustule: vesicle or bulla filled with pus (chicken pox, burn, herpes zoster-shingles)	**Atrophy:** Depression in skin resulting from thinning of the layers (aged skin, striae)
Wheal: Elevation of the skin caused by edema of the dermis (insect bite, urticaria)	**Excoriation:** Area where epidermis is missing, exposing the dermis (scabies, abrasion, scratch)
Cyst: Mass of fluid-filled tissue that extends to the subcutaneous tissue or dermis	

Home Care

A. Instruct client to cleanse face twice daily but to avoid overcleansing.
B. May use a polyester sponge pad to cleanse, because it provides a mechanical removal of the epidermal layer.
C. Instruct client to keep hands away from face and to avoid any friction or trauma to the area; avoid propping hands against face, rubbing face, etc.
D. Emphasize the importance of a nutritious diet; encourage adequate food intake and use of vitamin A.
E. Avoid the use of cosmetics, shaving creams, and lotion, because they may exacerbate acne; if cosmetics are to be used, water-based makeup is preferable.
F. Instruct the client to administer medication appropriately: topical application; avoid sunlight while using medications, etc.

 Psoriasis

Psoriasis is a chronic inflammatory disorder characterized by rapid turnover of epidermal cells.

Assessment

A. Silvery scaling, plaques on the elbows, scalp, knees, palms, soles, and fingernails.
B. If scales are scraped away, a dark red base of the lesion is seen, which will produce multiple bleeding points.
C. May improve but often recurs throughout life.
D. Bilateral symmetry of symptoms is common.

Treatment

A. Medical.
  1. Topical therapy.
    a. Coal tar preparation (Anthralin).
    b. Corticosteroids.
  2. Photo chemotherapy (PUVA therapy): psoralen, ultraviolet A therapy (must wear protective eyewear during treatment and for 24 hours after therapy).
  3. Systemic therapy: antimetabolites (methotrexate); immunosuppressants.

 Home Care

A. Encourage verbalization of anxiety regarding appearance.
B. Instruct client to use a soft brush to remove scales while bathing.
C. Assess client to determine factors that may trigger skin condition (e.g., emotional stress, trauma, seasonal changes).
D. Make sure client understands treatment and implications of care related to PUVA therapy and other treatments.

 Atopic Dermatitis

Atopic dermatitis (also called eczema) is a superficial, chronic inflammatory disorder associated with allergy with a hereditary tendency (atopy); condition commonly occurs during infancy, usually between 2 and 6 months of age and often persists in adulthood.

Assessment

A. Symptoms are similar with both adults and children; reddened lesions, occur on the cheeks, arms, and legs; antecubital and popliteal space in adults; may have oozing vesicles.
B. Intense itching (worse at night).
C. As the child gets older, the lesions tend to be dry with a thickening of the skin (lichenification).
D. Infants with eczema are more likely to have allergies as children and adults and to develop asthma.

Treatment

A. Milk, eggs, wheat, and peanuts are the most commonly suspected causes in children; food allergies are not associated with adult atopic dermatitis.
B. Pruritus is treated with Benadryl, topical steroids, and immunomodulators.
C. Systemic steroids are prescribed if condition is severe.

 Home Care

A. Teach parents about dietary restrictions; provide them with written guidelines.
B. Keep fingernails and toenails cut short.
C. Feed the child when he is well rested and is not itching.
D. Assist parents to identify foods that contain eggs and other "hidden" allergenic foods.
E. Avoid overheating; decrease likelihood of perspiration (no nylon clothing).
F. Child should avoid contact with persons who have the chicken pox virus or herpes simplex.
G. Avoid immunizations with live vaccines because of the possibility of severe reactions.
H. Child should wear nonirritating clothing; wool and abrasive fabrics should be avoided.
I. Tepid bath with mild soap or an emulsifying oil followed immediately by application of an emollient; cool compresses to decrease itching.
J. Teach adults to avoid things that cause a flare-up of the condition and to treat symptoms with topical medication when they occur.

> **NURSING PRIORITY** Apply emollients (medications) immediately after bathing while skin is slightly moist to treat dry skin.

 Contact Dermatitis

Contact dermatitis **is an inflammatory skin reaction that results because the skin has come in contact with a specific irritant (***irritant contact dermatitis,* **which occurs immediately after injury to skin;** *diaper dermatitis,* **which occurs after prolonged contact with urine, feces, ointments, soaps, or friction) or an allergen (***allergic contact dermatitis,* **which is usually a symptom of delayed hypersensitivity).**

Assessment

A. Causes.
1. Poison ivy and poison oak; fabrics such as wool, polyester.
2. Cosmetics; household products such as detergents, soap, hair dye.
3. Industrial substances: paints, dyes, insecticides, rubber compounds, etc.
4. Prolonged contact with diaper wetness, fecal enzymes, increased skin pH due to urine, and friction/irritation.
B. Clinical manifestations.
1. Pruritus; hive-like papules, vesicles, and plaques (more chronic).
2. Sharply circumscribed areas (with occasional vesicle formation) that crust and ooze.

Treatment

A. Medical.
1. Topical steroids; oral steroids for severe cases.
2. Antihistamines, antipruritic agents, and antifungals (diaper dermatitis).
3. Oatmeal baths and topical soaks.
B. Skin testing to determine allergen; skin lesions usually appear within 12 to 48 hours after contact with allergen.

Home Care

A. Teach importance of washing exposed skin with cool water and soap as soon as possible after exposure (within 15 minutes is best).
B. Provide cool, tepid bath; trim fingernails, and use measures to control itching.
C. Teach about fallacy of blister fluid spreading the disease.
D. Frequent diaper changes, keep skin dry, and use protective ointment (zinc oxide or petrolatum).

 ❗ PEDIATRIC PRIORITY Talc powders may keep skin dry, but they are harmful if breathed. Plain cornstarch is safer to use.

📋 Insect Bites

Insect bites (wasp, bee, yellow jacket, hornet, fire ants, black widow spider, brown recluse spider, scorpion, tick) can range from non–life-threatening reactions to serious life-threatening reactions (due to anaphylaxis).

Assessment

A. Sharp pain, localized wheal, erythema, localized itching.
B. Non–life-threatening systemic reactions (begin several minutes to hours after bite)—urticaria, angioedema.
C. Life-threatening reactions—anaphylaxis.

Treatment

A. Medical.
1. Antihistamines, antipruritic agents, soothing baths.
2. Administration of antivenom—black widow, scorpion bite.
B. Anaphylaxis—epinephrine, corticosteroids.

Home Care

A. Teach family that hypersensitive child should wear medical alert bracelet.
B. Transfer to emergency medical care for scorpion bites in young children.

📋 Pressure Ulcer

A pressure ulcer (decubitus ulcer, bedsore) is localized injury to the skin and/or underlying tissue usually over a bony prominence, as a result of pressure, or pressure in combination with shear and/or friction.

ALERT Identify potential for skin breakdown: a pressure ulcer can be and should be prevented. Identify those clients at increased risk for ulcer development and begin preventative care as soon as possible. Do not wait for the reddened area to occur before preventative measures are initiated.

Assessment

A. Risk factors/etiology.
1. Prolonged pressure caused by immobility.
2. Malnutrition, hypoproteinemia, vitamin deficiency.
3. Infection.
4. Skin dryness, maceration, excessive skin moisture.
5. Advancing age.
6. Equipment such as casts, restraints, traction devices, etc.
B. Risk assessment instruments.
1. Braden Scale.
   a. Scores six subscales: sensory perception, moisture, activity-mobility, nutrition, friction, and shear.
   b. Total score range is 6 to 23; a lower score indicates a higher risk for pressure ulcer development.
   c. Most reliable and most often used assessment scale for pressure ulcer risk; score of 18 is cut-off for adults.
2. Pressure Ulcer Scale for Healing (PUSH Tool).
   a. Developed by the National Pressure Ulcer Advisory Panel (NPUAP) as a quick, reliable tool to monitor the change in pressure ulcer status over time.
   b. Observe and measure the pressure ulcer. Categorize the ulcer with respect to surface area (0-10), exudate (0-3), and type of wound tissue (0-4).
   c. Monitor scoring over time: 0 = healed; 17 = not healed.
C. Clinical manifestations—see Table 11-2.

Treatment

A. Medical and surgical.
1. Debridement (initial care is to remove moist, devitalized tissue).
   a. Sharp debridement: use of a scalpel or other instrument; used primarily, especially with cellulitis or sepsis.
   b. Mechanical debridement: wet-to-dry dressings, hydrotherapy, wound irrigation, and dextranomers

Table 11-2	STAGES OF PRESSURE ULCERS

Definition	Further Description	Diagram

Suspected Deep Tissue Injury

Purple or maroon localized area of discolored intact skin or blood-filled blister caused by damage of underlying soft tissue from pressure and/or shear. The area may be preceded by tissue that is painful, firm, mushy, boggy, warmer, or cooler compared with adjacent tissue.

Deep tissue injury may be difficult to detect in individuals with dark skin tones. Evolution may include a thin blister over a dark wound bed. The wound may further evolve and become covered by thin eschar. Evolution may be rapid, exposing additional layers of tissue even with optimal treatment.

SUSPECTED
DEEP TISSUE INJURY

Stage I

Intact skin with non-blanchable redness of a localized area usually over a bony prominence. Darkly pigmented skin may not have visible blanching; its color may differ from the surrounding area.

The area may be painful, firm, soft, warmer, or cooler compared with adjacent tissue. Stage I may be difficult to detect in individuals with dark skin tones. May indicate "at risk" persons (a heralding sign of risk).

STAGE 1

Stage II

Partial-thickness loss of dermis presenting as a shallow open ulcer with a red-pink wound bed, without slough. May also present as an intact or open/ruptured serum-filled blister.

Presents as a shiny or dry shallow ulcer without slough or bruising.* This stage should not be used to describe skin tears, tape burns, perineal dermatitis, maceration or excoriation.
*Bruising indicates suspected deep tissue injury.

STAGE 2

Continued

(small beads poured over secreting wounds to absorb exudate).
  c. Enzymatic and autolytic debridement: use of enzymes or synthetic dressings that cover wound and self-digest devitalized tissue by the action of enzymes that are present in wound fluids.

2. Wound cleansing (use normal saline solution for most cases).
  a. Use minimal mechanical force when cleansing to avoid trauma to the wound bed.
  b. Avoid the use of antiseptics (e.g., Dakin's solution, iodine, hydrogen peroxide).

Table 11-2	STAGES OF PRESSURE ULCERS—cont'd	

Definition	*Further Description*	*Diagram*
Stage III Full-thickness tissue loss. Subcutaneous fat may be visible, but bone, tendon, and/or muscle are not exposed. Slough may be present but does not obscure the depth of tissue loss. May include undermining and tunneling.	The depth of a stage III pressure ulcer varies by anatomic location. The bridge of the nose, ear, occiput, and malleolus do not have subcutaneous tissue, and stage III ulcers can be shallow. In contrast, areas of significant adiposity can develop extremely deep stage III pressure ulcers. Bone/tendon is not visible or directly palpable.	 STAGE 3
Stage IV Full-thickness tissue loss with exposed bone, tendon, or muscle. Slough or eschar may be present on some parts of the wound bed. Often includes undermining and tunneling.	The depth of a stage IV pressure ulcer varies by anatomic location. The bridge of the nose, ear, occiput, and malleolus do not have subcutaneous tissue, and these ulcers can be shallow. Stage IV ulcers can extend into muscle and/or supporting structures (e.g., fascia, tendon, or joint capsule), making osteomyelitis possible. Exposed bone/tendon is visible or directly palpable.	 STAGE 4
Unstageable Full-thickness tissue loss in which the base of the ulcer is covered by slough (yellow, tan, gray, green, or brown) and/or eschar (tan, brown, or black) in the wound bed.	Until enough slough and/or eschar are removed to expose the base of the wound, the true depth and stage cannot be determined. Stable (dry, adherent, intact without erythema or fluctuance) eschar on the heels serves as "the body's natural (biologic) cover" and should not be removed.	 UNSTAGEABLE

Reprinted with permission from National Pressure Ulcer Advisory Panel: Updated staging system, 2007. Available at www.npuap.org. Accessed July 31, 2008, from http://www.npuap.org/resources.htm

3. Dressings (should protect wound, be biocompatible, and hydrate).
   a. Moistened gauze.
   b. Film (transparent).
   c. Hydrocolloid (moisture and oxygen retaining).

> **! NURSING PRIORITY** Keep the ulcer tissue moist and the surrounding intact skin dry.

B. Dietary.
   1. Increased carbohydrates and protein.
   2. Increased vitamin C and zinc.

Nursing Interventions

Goal: To prevent or relieve pressure and stimulate circulation.

A. Frequent change of position; turn client every 1 to 2 hours.
B. Special beds with mattresses that provide for a continuous change in pressure across the mattress.
C. Silicone gel pads placed under the buttocks of clients in wheelchairs.
D. Sheepskin pads to provide a soft surface to protect the skin from abrasion.
E. Eggcrate-style or other foam mattress to allow circulation under the body and keep the area dry.
F. Active and passive exercises to promote circulation.

Goal: To keep skin clean and healthy and prevent the occurrence of a pressure ulcer.

A. Wash skin with mild soap and blot completely dry with soft towel.
   1. Avoid hot water and excessive rubbing.
   2. Use lotion or protective moisturizer after bathing.
B. Inspect skin frequently, especially over bony prominences.

> **! NURSING PRIORITY** Avoid massage over bony prominences. When the sidelying position is used in bed, avoid positioning client directly on the trochanter; use the 30° lateral inclined position. Do not use donut-type devices. Maintain the head of the bed at or below 30° or at the lowest degree of elevation. Teach chair-bound persons, who are able, to shift weight every 15 minutes.

C. Remove any foreign material from the bed, because it may serve as a source of irritation; keep sheets tightly stretched on bed to prevent wrinkles.

Goal: To promote healing of pressure ulcer.

A. Use methods discussed to decrease the pressure on the area in which the pressure ulcer is found.
   1. Air-fluidized beds—stage III or stage IV pressure ulcers.
   2. Static support surfaces—*not* recommended for stage III or IV.
B. Keep the ulcer area dry.
   1. Minimize skin exposure to moisture caused by incontinence, perspiration, or wound drainage.

2. Use only underpads or briefs that are made of materials that absorb moisture and provide a quick-drying surface next to the skin.
3. Position the client with the ulcer exposed to air; may use light to increase drying and promote healing.

C. Use skin barriers to decrease contamination and increase healing of a noninfected ulcer.
D. Observe the ulcer for signs of infection. Infected ulcers will have to be debrided, if healing is to occur.

SKIN INFECTIONS AND INFESTATIONS

Impetigo

Impetigo **is a bacterial skin infection caused by invasion of the epidermis by pathogenic** *Staphylococcus aureus* **and/or group A beta-hemolytic streptococci.**

Assessment

A. Pustule-like lesions with moist honey-colored crusts surrounded by redness.
B. Pruritus; spreads to surrounding areas.
C. Appears more commonly on the face, especially around the mouth.

Treatment

A. Medical.
   1. Local: topical treatment.
      a. Gentle washing two to three times a day to remove crusts.
      b. Topical mupirocin (Bactroban) antibiotic cream, if only a couple of lesions are found.
   2. Systemic antibiotic therapy is the treatment of choice with extensive lesions.

Home Care

A. Teach the client and family the importance of good handwashing and assure them that lesions heal without scarring.
B. Encourage adherence to therapeutic regimen, especially taking the full course of antibiotics.
C. Untreated impetigo may result in glomerulonephritis.

Cellulitis

Cellulitis **is an inflammation of the subcutaneous tissues often following a break in the skin caused by** *Staphylococcus aureus, Streptococcus,* **or** *Haemophilus influenzae.*

Assessment

A. Intense redness, edema with diffuse border, and tenderness.
B. Chills, malaise, and fever.

Treatment

A. Medical.
   1. Moist heat, immobilization, and elevation of part.
   2. Systemic antibiotic therapy is the treatment of choice with extensive lesions.

Home Care

A. Teach the client and family the importance of good handwashing.

B. Encourage adherence to therapeutic regimen, especially taking the full course of antibiotics.

 Fungal (Dermatophyte) Infections

Assessment

A. Types.

1. Tinea corporis (ringworm): temporary hair loss, if scalp is affected.

2. Tinea cruris (jock itch): small, red, scaly patches in the groin area.

3. Tinea pedis (athlete's foot): scaling, maceration, erythema, blistering, and pruritus; usually found between the toes.

4. Tinea unguium (onychomycosis): thickened, crumbling nails (usually toes) with yellowish discoloration.

5. Candidiasis: caused by *Candida albicans*, known as moniliasis, may affect oral mucosa, groin, and moist areas; white plaques in mouth; diffuse red rash on skin.

Treatment

A. Topical antifungal cream (see Appendix 11-2).

B. Oral antifungal medication.

C. Systemic therapy: griseofulvin; used primarily for extensive cases.

 Home Care

A. To prevent athlete's foot, client should be instructed to keep feet as dry as possible and wear socks made of absorbent cotton.

1. Talcum powder or antifungal powder may be used; **Tinactin** may be applied twice daily.

2. Encourage aeration of shoes to allow them to completely dry out.

B. Client should maintain hygienic measures to prevent the spread of fungal diseases, specifically ringworm of the scalp.

1. Family members should avoid using the same comb.

2. Scarves and hats should be washed thoroughly.

3. Examine family and household pets frequently for symptoms of the disease.

C. Client should avoid infection.

1. Any activity that allows heat, friction, and maceration to occur may lead to skin breakdown and infection.

2. Loose-fitting clothing and cotton underwear are to be encouraged.

 Parasitic Infestations

A. Pediculosis.

1. Types.

a. Pediculus humanus capitis: head lice.

b. Pediculus humanus corporis: body lice.

c. Phthirus pubis: pubic lice or crabs.

2. Clinical manifestations.

a. Intense pruritus, which may lead to secondary excoriation and infection.

b. Tiny, red, noninflammatory lesions.

c. Eggs (nits) of both head and body lice are often attached to the hair shafts.

d. Pubic lice are often spread by sexual contact.

B. Scabies: an infestation of the skin by *Sarcoptes scabiei* mites.

1. Intense itching, especially at night.

2. Burrows are seen, especially between fingers, on the surfaces of wrists, and in axillary folds.

3. Redness, swelling, and vesicular formation may be noted.

Treatment

A. Pediculosis.

1. Permethrin 1% liquid (Nix): effective against nits and lice with just one application; shampoo hair first, leave Nix on hair for 10 minutes, rinse off; may repeat in 7 days.

2. Pyrethrin compounds (e.g., Rid) for pubic and head lice.

B. Scabies: permethrin 5% cream (Elimite); cream is applied to the skin from head to soles of feet and left on for 8 to 14 hours, then washed off; only one application needed.

 Home Care

A. All family members and close contacts need to be treated for parasitic disorders; lice can survive up to 48 hours; nits can hatch in 7-10 days when shed in the environment.

B. Bedding and clothing that may have lice or nits should be washed or dry-cleaned; furniture and rugs should be vacuumed or treated.

C. Nurses should wear gloves when examining scalp to prevent spread to others.

D. When shampooing hair, use a fine-tooth comb or tweezers to remove remaining nits.

 Viral Infections

A. Herpes simplex virus (fever blister, cold sore): herpes virus type 1 (HSV-1).

1. Painful, local reaction consisting of vesicles with an erythematous base; most often appears around the mouth.

2. Contagious by direct contact; is recurrent; there is no immunity.

3. Chronic disorder that may be exacerbated by stress, trauma, menses, sunlight, fatigue, or systemic infection.

4. Recurrent episodes are characterized by appearance of lesions in the same place.

5. Not to be confused with HSV-2, which primarily occurs below the waist (genital herpes).

6. It is possible for the HSV-1 to cause genital lesions and for HSV-2 to cause oral lesions (see Sexually Transmitted Diseases in Chapter 22).

B. Herpes zoster (shingles).
1. Related to the chicken pox virus: varicella.
2. Contagious to anyone who has not had chicken pox or who may be immunosuppressed.
3. Linear patches of vesicles with an erythematous base are located along spinal and cranial nerve tracts.
4. Often unilateral and appears on the trunk; however, may also appear on the face.
5. Pain, burning, and neuralgia occur at the site before outbreak of vesicles.
6. Often precipitated by the same factors as herpes simplex infection.
C. Herpetic whitlow: occurs on fingertips and around nail cuticles; often seen in medical personnel.

Treatment

A. Usually symptomatic; application of soothing moist compresses.
B. Analgesics; gabapentin (Neurontin) for postherpetic neuralgia.
C. Antiviral agents (see Appendix 11-2).
D. Zoster vaccine is recommended for adults over 60 years regardless of whether they report a prior episode of herpes zoster.

 Home Care

A. Alleviate pain by administering analgesics.
B. Antihistamines may be administered to control the itching.
C. Usually, lesions heal without complications; herpes simplex usually heals without scarring, whereas herpes zoster may cause scarring.
D. If hospitalized, establish contact precautions for herpes zoster.

MALIGNANT SKIN NEOPLASMS

Nonmelanoma Skin Cancers

Assessment

A. Risk factors.
1. Overexposure to sunlight.
2. Fair skin type (blond or red hair and blue or green eyes).
3. Exposure to chemicals.
4. Scars from severe burns.
B. Types.
1. Actinic keratosis: premalignant type.
   a. Small macules or papules with dry, rough, adherent yellow or brown scales.
   b. Appears on face, neck, back of hand, and forearm.
   c. May slowly progress to squamous cell carcinoma.
2. Basal cell carcinoma: most common type of skin cancer.
   a. Appears as a small, waxy nodule with a translucent pearly border.
   b. Appears more frequently on the face, usually between the hairline and upper lip.

3. Squamous cell carcinoma: malignant proliferation arising from the epidermis; usually on sun-damaged skin or skin that has been irradiated or excessively scarred.
   a. May metastasize.
   b. Appears as a firm nodule with an indistinct border; may be opaque.

Malignant Melanoma

Assessment

A. Risk factors.
1. Chronic UV exposure without protection or overexposure to artificial light (tanning bed).
2. Fair skin, genetic (first-degree relative).
3. Has the highest mortality rate of any form of skin cancer (Box 11-2).
   a. Often appears in preexisting moles in the skin.
   b. Common sites include back and legs (women); trunk, head, and neck (men).
   c. Sudden or progressive change or increase in size, color, or shape of a mole.

Treatment

A. Surgical.
1. Excisional surgery; laser treatment.
2. Cryosurgery.
3. Electrodesiccation and curettage.
B. Medical.
1. Radiation therapy.
2. Chemotherapy—topical 5FU (skin cancer, except melanoma).
3. Biologic therapy (alpha-interferon, interleukin-2)—malignant melanoma.

Nursing Interventions

Goal: To assist client to understand disease process, importance of follow-up treatment, and measures to maintain health.
A. Teach the importance of avoiding unnecessary exposure to sunlight.
B. Apply protective sunscreen when outside.
C. Teach the warning signs of cancer.
D. Treat moles found in areas where there is friction or repeated irritation.
Goal: To support the client and promote psychologic homeostasis.

Box 11-2   MALIGNANT MELANOMA

Melanomas tend to have:
A Asymmetry
B Border irregularity
C Color variegation
D Diameter great than 6 mm
E Evolving or changing in some way

A. Allow for verbalization of fear and anxiety.

B. Encourage verbalization relating to altered body image when large, wide, full-thickness excisions must be made to treat malignant melanoma.

C. Point out client's resources and support effective coping mechanisms.

D. Teach the importance of examining and checking moles and any new lesions.

ELECTIVE COSMETIC PROCEDURES

A. Purpose: to improve self-image.

B. Types of elective cosmetic surgery.
1. Chemical face-lift or peel: superficial destruction of the upper layers of skin with a cauterant solution.
2. Tretinoin (Retin-A) and alpha-hydroxy acids: topical application provides reversal of photodamaged skin and normal aging by influencing epithelial cell growth and differentiation.
3. Microdermabrasion: removal of epidermis to treat acne, scars, wrinkles, etc.
4. Botulinum toxin injection: neurotoxin that causes temporary interference with neuromuscular transmission, paralyzing the affected muscle.
5. Face-lift (rhytidectomy): lifting and repositioning of facial and neck tissues.
6. Eyelid-lift (blepharoplasty): removal of redundant (excess) eyelid tissue.
7. Liposuction: technique for removing subcutaneous fat from face and body.

Nursing Interventions

Goal: To provide preoperative care.

A. Reinforce information from informed consent obtained by physician.

B. Instruct client to avoid taking vitamin E and aspirin at least 1 week before surgery to prevent bleeding.

C. Explain that wound healing and final results may not be complete until 1 year after procedure.

Goal: To provide postoperative care.

A. Administer analgesics for pain management.

B. Observe for bleeding.

C. Teach client signs and symptoms of infection.

D. Teach client who had a chemical peel to avoid the sun for 6 months to prevent hyperpigmentation, because a reduction of melanin in the skin occurs as a result of the procedure.

E. Teach client who has liposuction to wear spandex compression garments to reduce risk for bleeding and prevent fluid accumulation.

BURNS

A. Types of burns.
1. Thermal injury: most common type of burn injury; results from flames, flash (explosion), scald, or direct contact with hot object.
2. Electrical injury: intense heat is generated from electrical current and causes coagulation necrosis as current flows through the body.
3. Chemical injury: results from contact with a corrosive substance.
4. Smoke and inhalation injury: results from inhalation of air or noxious chemicals; the respiratory system frequently sustains two types of burn injuries:
   a. Smoke inhalation and topical burns on face, neck, and chest may precipitate airway edema and obstruction within 24 to 48 hours after burn injury.
   b. Inhalation of carbon monoxide combines with hemoglobin, thereby decreasing availability of oxygen to cells.

B. Fluid considerations.
1. Fluid shift and edema formation occur within first 12 hours post burn and can continue 24 to 36 hours after burn injury.
2. Fluid mobilization and diuresis occur around 48 to 72 hours post burn when the capillary integrity is restored.
3. Serum potassium levels increase and hematocrit levels increase because of hemoconcentration.
4. The increased capillary permeability and the histamine released from the injured cells precipitate a decrease in fluid volume.

Assessment

A. Respiratory—determine circumstances surrounding injury: did fire occur in an enclosed space, is there a risk for an inhalation injury?
1. Assess for burns on the face and in the mouth.
2. Examine mouth and sputum for black particles and the nasal septum for edema.
3. Assess for change in respiratory pattern indicating impending respiratory obstruction.
   a. Increased hoarseness.
   b. Drooling or difficulty swallowing.
   c. Audible wheezing, crackles, presence of stridor.
4. Assess for development of carbon monoxide poisoning.
   a. Mild: headache, decreased vision.
   b. Moderate: tinnitus, drowsiness, vertigo, altered mental state, decreased B/P, "cherry red" color from vasodilatation.

B. Evaluate cardiac output and peripheral circulation.
1. Tachycardia and hypotension may occur early.
2. Evaluate urine output to determine adequacy of tissue perfusion.
3. Evaluate peripheral circulation.

C. Identify when client ate last; check gastrointestinal function.

D. Determine hydration status.
1. Presence of hematuria.
2. Urine output (should be at least 30 mL/hr).
3. Hypotension (blood pressure below 90/60 mm Hg).

E. Presence of confusion and disorientation may occur secondary to hypoxia, low B/P, or carbon monoxide poisoning.

> **! NURSING PRIORITY** The client with burn injury is often awake, mentally alert, and cooperative at first. The level of consciousness may change as respiratory status deteriorates or as the fluid shift occurs, precipitating hypovolemia.

F. Determine the severity of the burn injury (Box 11-3 and Figure 11-1).
   1. Extent of burn surface (burn surface area).
      a. Rule of nines: generally used for adults (Figure 11-2) and estimation in children (Figure 11-3).
      b. Pediatric burns are calculated by taking into account the client's age in relation to proportion of body parts.
   2. Area of burn.
      a. Circumferential burns (burns surrounding an entire extremity) may cause severe reduction of circulation to an extremity as a result of edema

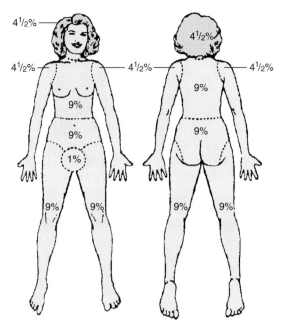

FIGURE 11-2 Rule of nines.

formation and lack of elasticity of the eschar, leading to compartmental syndrome.
      b. Location of the burn is related to the severity of the injury:
         (1) Face, neck, chest → respiratory obstruction
         (2) Hands, feet, joints, and eyes → self-care
         (3) Ears, nose → infection
   3. Age.
      a. Infants have an immature immune system and poor body defense.
      b. Older adult clients heal more slowly and are more likely to have wound infection problems and pulmonary complications.
   4. Presence of other health problems: diabetes and peripheral vascular disease delay wound healing.

Treatment

A. Respiratory status takes priority over the treatment of the burn injury.
B. If the burn area is small (less than approximately a 10% BSA), apply cold compresses or immerse injured area in cool water to decrease heat; ice should not be directly applied to the burn area.
C. Administer tetanus injection.
D. Do not put any ointment or salves on the burn area.
E. If the cause of the burn is chemical, thoroughly rinse the area with large amounts of cool water.
F. Fluid resuscitation.
   1. Used for clients with burns on 15% to 20% or more of body surface area.
   2. Placement of large bore IV catheters on admission to ED.
   3. Fluid replacement: calculation of fluid replacement begins from time of burn, not time of admission to ED.

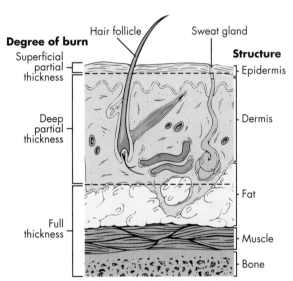

Degree of burn

Superficial partial thickness

Deep partial thickness

Full thickness

Structure

Epidermis

Dermis

Fat

Muscle

Bone

Hair follicle   Sweat gland

FIGURE 11-1 Levels of human skin involved in burns. (From Lewis SL, et al: *Medical-surgical nursing: assessment and management of clinical problems*, ed 7, St. Louis, 2007, Mosby.)

Box 11-3 DEPTH OF BURNS

- *Superficial or first-degree burn*: Area is reddened and blanches with pressure; no edema present; area is generally painful to touch.
- *Partial-thickness or second-degree burn*: Dermis and epidermis are affected; formation of large, thick-walled blisters; underlying skin is erythematous.
- *Full-thickness or third- and fourth-degree burn*: All of the skin is destroyed; may have damage to the subcutaneous tissue and muscle; usually has a dry appearance, may be white or charred; will require skin grafting to cover area; underlying structures (fascia, tendons, and bones) are severely damaged, usually blackened.

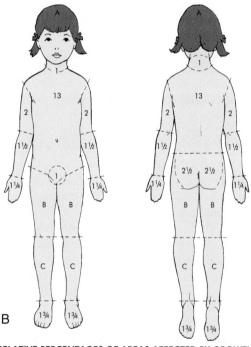

RELATIVE PERCENTAGES OF AREAS AFFECTED BY GROWTH

AREA	BIRTH	AGE 1 YR	AGE 5 YR
A = ½ of head	9½	8½	6½
B = ½ of one thigh	2¾	3¼	4
C = ½ of one leg	2½	2½	2¾

RELATIVE PERCENTAGES OF AREAS AFFECTED BY GROWTH

AREA	AGE 10 YR	AGE 15 YR	ADULT
A = ½ of head	5½	4½	3½
B = ½ of one thigh	4½	4½	4¾
C = ½ of one leg	3	3¼	3½

FIGURE 11-3 Estimation of distribution of burns in children. **A,** Children from birth to 5 years. **B,** Older children. (From Hockenberry MJ, Wilson D: *Wong's essentials of pediatric nursing,* ed 8, St. Louis, 2009, Mosby.)

a. One-half of first 24-hour fluid replacement is given during first 8 hours after burn injury.

b. One-fourth of remaining amount is given during the second and third 8-hour periods.

c. Urine output is most sensitive indicator of fluid status; fluid replacement may be titrated to keep urine output at 0.5 mL/kg or average of 30 mL/hour.

G. Maintain NPO (nothing by mouth) status; assess need for nasogastric tube.

H. Analgesics are given intravenously; do not give intramuscularly, subcutaneously, or orally because they will not be absorbed effectively.

I. Methods of wound care (area is cleaned and debrided of necrotic burned tissue).

1. Open method (exposure): burn is covered with a topical antibiotic cream and no dressing is applied.

2. Closed method of dressing: fine mesh is used to cover the burned surface; may be impregnated with antibiotic ointment, or ointment may be applied before the dressing is applied.

3. Escharotomy: procedure involves excision through the eschar to increase circulation to an extremity with circumferential burns.

4. Enzymatic debriders: collagenase, fibrinolysin, and Accuzyme may be used.

5. Wound grafting: as eschar is debrided and granulation tissue begins to form, grafts are used to protect the wound and to promote healing.

J. Nutritional support.

1. Diet is high in calories and protein.

2. In clients who have large burn surface areas, supplemental gastric tube feedings or hyperalimentation may be used.

Nursing Interventions

Goal: To maintain patent airway and prevent hypoxia.

A. Anticipate respiratory difficulty if there are any indications of inhalation injury.

1. Remain with client; frequent assessment of respiratory status.

2. Supplemental oxygen.

3. Be prepared to intubate client: airway edema can occur rapidly.

4. Assess airway as fluid resuscitation begins; may precipitate more edema.

B. Assess for carbon monoxide poisoning.

C. Anticipate transfer to burn unit if burns cover more than 15% to 20% of body surface area, depending on depth of burn, age of client, and presence of other chronic illnesses.

Goal: To evaluate fluid status and determine circulatory status and adequacy of fluid replacement.

A. Obtain client's weight on admission.

B. Assess status and time frame of fluid resuscitation; *calculation of fluid replacement begins at time of burn injury, not on arrival at hospital.*

C. Evaluate renal status and urine output: adequate output for children is 1 mL/kg/hr.

Goal: To prevent or decrease infection.

A. Implement infection control procedures to protect the client.

B. After eschar sloughs or is removed, assess wound for infection; infection is difficult to identify before the eschar sloughs.

Goal: To maintain nutrition and promote positive nitrogen balance for healing.

A. Work with dietitian to maintain nutritional intake.

B. Provide tube feedings as indicated.

C. Care of total parenteral nutrition as indicated (see Appendix 18-7).

D. Daily weight.

Goal: To prevent contractures and scarring.

A. Assist client to attempt mobilization and ambulation as soon as possible.

B. Passive and active range of motion should be initiated from the beginning of burn therapy and throughout therapy.

C. Position client to prevent flexion contractures; position of comfort for the client may increase contracture formation.

D. Use splints and exercises to prevent flexion contractures.

E. Use pressure dressings and garments to contour healing burn area to keep scars flat and prevent elevation and enlargement above the original burn injury area.

Goal: To promote acceptance and adaptation to alterations in body image.

A. Employ counselors and resource team members.

B. Maintain open communication and encourage expression of feelings.

C. Anticipate depression as a normal consequence of burn trauma; it should decrease as condition improves.

> **NURSING PRIORITY** It is important to recognize that the client's anger is not a direct attack on the care provider; it is an expression of grief and sorrow.

 Home Care

A. Physical therapy.

B. Continue high-calorie, high-protein diet.

C. Wound care management.

D. Avoid exposure of burn area to direct sunlight.

Appendix 11-1 SKIN DIAGNOSTIC STUDIES

Skin Testing

Purpose: confirm sensitivity to a specific allergen by placing antigen on or directly below skin (intradermal) to check for presence of antibodies.

1. Three methods—allergen applied to arms or back.

   Cutaneous scratch test (also known as a *tine* or *prick test*): allergen applied to a superficial scratch on skin.

   Intracutaneous injection: small amount of the allergen is injected intradermally in rows; more accurate; high risk for severe allergic reaction; used only for those who do not react to cutaneous method.

   Patch test: used to determine whether client is allergic to testing material (small amount applied on back)—returns in 48 hours for evaluation.

2. Interpreting results.

   Immediate reaction: appears within minutes after the injection; marked by erythema and a wheal; denotes a positive reaction.

   Positive reaction: indicates an antibody response to previous exposure; local wheal-and-flare response occurs.

   Negative reaction: inconclusive; may indicate that antibodies have not formed yet or that antigen was deposited too deeply in skin (not an intradermal injection); may also indicate immunosuppression.

3. Complications: range from minor itching to anaphylaxis (see Chapter 7).

> **NURSING PRIORITY** Never leave client alone during skin testing, because of the risk for anaphylaxis. If a severe reaction occurs, anticipate anti-inflammatory topical cream applied to skin site (scratch test) or a tourniquet applied to the arm (intracutaneous test) and possible epinephrine injection.

Wood's Lamp (black light)

Purpose: examination of skin with long-wave ultraviolet light that causes specific substances or areas to fluoresce (e.g., *Pseudomonas* species, fungi, patches of vitiligo).

Biopsy

Types: punch, excisional, incisional, shave

1. Verify if informed consent is needed.

2. Apply dressing and give postprocedure instructions—watch for bleeding.

Skin Culture

Purpose: identify fungal, bacterial, and viral organisms.

1. Scrap or swab affected area; label specimen and send to lab.

Microscopic Tests

Potassium hydroxide (KOH)—identifies fungal infection

Tzanck test—diagnoses of herpes infections

Mineral oil slides—diagnoses of infestations

Immunofluorescent—identifying abnormal antibody proteins (can also be a serum test)

Appendix 11-2 MEDICATIONS USED IN SKIN DISORDERS

MEDICATIONS	SIDE EFFECTS	NURSING IMPLICATIONS

General Nursing Implications
— Topical medications are used primarily for local effects when systemic absorption is undesirable.
— For topical application:
  — Apply after shower or bath for best absorption, because skin is hydrated.
  — Apply small amount of medication and rub in well.

Antifungal: Inhibits or damages fungal cell membrane, either altering permeability or disrupting cell mitosis.

MEDICATIONS	SIDE EFFECTS	NURSING IMPLICATIONS
Clotrimazole **(Lotrimin):** topical Nystatin **(Mycolog):** topical Ketoconazole **(Nizoral):** PO, topical Griseofulvin **(Fulvicin):** PO	Nausea, vomiting, abdominal pain. Hypersensitivity reaction: rash, urticaria, pruritus Hepatotoxicity Gynecomastia (ketoconazole)	1. Monitor hepatic function (when oral medication is given). 2. Avoid alcohol because of potential liver problems. 3. Check for local burning, irritation, or itching with topical application. 4. Prolonged therapy (weeks or months) is usually necessary, especially with griseofulvin (Fulvicin). 5. Take griseofulvin (Fulvicin) with foods high in fat (e.g., milk, ice cream) to decrease GI upset and assist in absorption. 6. *Uses:* tinea infections, fungal infections, candidiasis, diaper dermatitis.

Antiviral: Reduces viral shedding, pain, and time to heal.

MEDICATIONS	SIDE EFFECTS	NURSING IMPLICATIONS
Acyclovir **(Zovirax):** topical, PO, IV Penciclovir **(Denavir):** topical Vidarabine **(Ara-A, Vir-A):** IV, ophthalmic	IV: phlebitis, rash, hives PO: nausea, vomiting Topical: burning, stinging, pruritus Anorexia, nausea, vomiting Ophthalmic: burning, itching	1. Apply topically to affected area six times per day. 2. Avoid autoinoculation; wash hands frequently; apply with gloved hand. 3. Avoid sexual intercourse while genital lesions are present. 4. Drink adequate fluids. 5. Infuse IV preparations over 1 hour; use an infusion pump for accurate delivery. 6. *Uses:* herpes infections.

Antiinflammatory: Decreases the inflammatory response.

MEDICATIONS	SIDE EFFECTS	NURSING IMPLICATIONS
Triamcinolone acetonide **(Aristocort):** topical	Skin thinning, superficial dilated blood vessels (telangiectasis), acne-like eruptions, adrenal suppression	1. Triamcinolone and hydrocortisone creams come in various strengths and potency. Watch the percent strength. 2. Applied 2-3 times a day. 3. Use an occlusive dressing only if ordered. 4. Encourage client to use the least amount possible and for the shortest period of time.

Immunosuppressant: Suppresses T cells and decreases release of inflammatory mediators; alternative to glucocorticoids.

MEDICATIONS	SIDE EFFECTS	NURSING IMPLICATIONS
Pimecrolimus cream **(Elidel):** topical Tacrolimus ointment **(Protopic):** topical	Erythema, pruritus Burning sensation at application site	1. Teach clients to use sunscreen, because medication makes client sensitized to UV light. 2. Long-term effects can lead to skin cancer and lymphoma.

GI, Gastrointestinal; *IV,* intravenously; *PO,* by mouth (orally).

Appendix 11-3 TOPICAL ANTIBIOTICS FOR BURN TREATMENT

MEDICATIONS	SIDE EFFECTS	NURSING IMPLICATIONS
Topical Antibiotics: Prevent and treat infection at the burn site.		
Silver sulfadiazine **(Silvadene)**	Hypersensitivity: rash, itching, or burning sensation in unburned skin	1. Liberal amounts are spread topically with a sterile, gloved hand or on impregnated gauze rolls over the burned surface. 2. If discoloration occurs in the **Silvadene** cream, do not use. 3. A thin layer of cream is spread evenly over the entire burn surface area; reapplication is done every 12 hours. 4. Client should be bathed, "tubbed", or showered daily to aid in debridement. 5. Medication does not penetrate eschar. 6. For clients with extensive burns, monitor urine output and renal function; a significant amount of sulfa may be absorbed.
Mafenide acetate **(Sulfamylon 10%)**	Pain, burning, or stinging at application sites; excessive loss of body water; excoriation of new tissue; may be systemically absorbed and cause metabolic acidosis	1. Bacteriostatic medication diffuses rapidly through burned skin and eschar and is effective against bacteria under the eschar. 2. Dressings are not required but are frequently used. A thin layer of cream is spread evenly over the entire burn surface. 3. Monitor renal function and possible acidosis, because medication is rapidly absorbed from the burn surface and eliminated via the kidneys. 4. Pain occurs on application. 5. Watch for hyperventilation, as a compensatory mechanism when acidosis occurs.

Study Questions Integumentary System

More questions on companion CD!
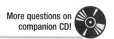

1. A client has extensive burns with eschar on the anterior trunk. What is the nurse's primary concern regarding eschar formation?
   1 It prevents fluid remobilization in the first 48 hours after burn trauma.
   2 Infection is difficult to assess before the eschar sloughs.
   3 It restricts the ability of the client to move about.
   4 Circulation to the extremities is diminished because of edema formation.

2. A client comes to the outpatient clinic with impetigo on his left arm. What information would the nurse give this client?
   1 Apply antibiotic ointment to the dried lesion.
   2 Wash the lesions with soap and water, then apply a steroid ointment.
   3 Soak the scabs off the lesion and apply an antibiotic ointment.
   4 Wash the lesions with hydrogen peroxide and apply an antifungal cream.

3. A teacher notifies the school nurse that many of the students in her third-grade class have been scratching their heads and complaining of intense itching of the scalp. The nurse notices tiny white material at the base of a student's hair shaft. What condition does this assessment reflect?
   1 Tinea capitis
   2 Pediculosis capitis
   3 Dandruff
   4 Scabies

4. In which situation would it be appropriate for the nurse to administer a patch skin test?
   1 A toddler with a possible diagnosis of cystic fibrosis
   2 A client who has a transdermal patch ordered
   3 A client scheduled for electromyography
   4 A child who is to receive ampicillin for the first time

5. What is the type of skin cancer that is most difficult to treat?
   1 Oat cell
   2 Malignant melanoma
   3 Basal cell epithelioma
   4 Squamous cell epithelioma

6. An older adult client has an open wound over the coccyx that extends through the dermis and subcutaneous tissue, exposing the deep fascia. The wound edges are distinct, and the wound bed is a pink-red color. There is no bruising or sloughing. What stage of pressure ulcer is this wound?
   1 Stage I
   2 Stage II
   3 Stage III
   4 Stage IV

7. The nurse understands that scaling around the toes, blistering, and pruritus is characteristic of what condition?
   1 Eczema
   2 Psoriasis
   3 Tinea pedis
   4 Pediculosis corporis

8. What are the physical characteristics of a client who is most susceptible to development of malignant melanoma?
   1 Light to pale skin, blond hair, blue eyes
   2 Olive complexion, oily skin, dark eyes
   3 Dark skin with freckles, dry flaky skin, hazel eyes
   4 Coarse skin, ruddy complexion, brown eyes

9. Herpes zoster has been diagnosed in an older adult client. What will the nursing management include?
   1 Apply antifungal cream to the areas daily.
   2 Maintain client on contact precautions.
   3 Administer a herpes zoster immunization.
   4 Expect to find lesions in the perineal area.

10. Which of the following nursing interventions will assist in reducing pressure points that may lead to pressure ulcers? Select all that apply:
    _____ 1 Position the client directly on the trochanter when sidelying.
    _____ 2 Avoid the use of donut-type devices.
    _____ 3 Massage bony prominences.
    _____ 4 Elevate the head of the bed as little as possible.
    _____ 5 When the client is sidelying, use the 30-degree lateral inclined position.
    _____ 6 Avoid uninterrupted sitting in any chair or wheelchair.

11. The nurse is teaching self-care to an older adult client. What would the nurse encourage the client do for his dry, itchy skin?
    1 Apply a moisturizer on all dry areas daily.
    2 Shower twice a day with a mild soap.
    3 Use a pumice stone and exfoliating sponge on areas to remove dry scaly patches.
    4 Wear protective pads on areas that show the most dryness.

12. What is the priority assessment finding for a client who has sustained burns on the face and neck?
    1 Spreading, large, clear vesicles
    2 Increased hoarseness
    3 Difficulty with vision
    4 Increased thirst

Answers and rationales to these questions are in the section at the end of the book titled Chapter Study Questions: Answers and Rationales.

CHAPTER TWELVE

Sensory System

PHYSIOLOGY OF THE EYE

A. Eyeballs.
  1. External layer.
    a. Sclera: tough, protective covering of the outside of the eye; the "white" of the eye.
    b. Cornea: transparent tissue that covers the front of the eyeball over the pupil.
    c. Conjunctiva: the thin, transparent mucous membrane that covers the outer surface of the eyeball and lines the inner surface of the eyelid.
  2. Middle layer.
    a. Choroid: pigmented layer containing large number of blood vessels that nourish the retina.
    b. Ciliary muscle: muscular body that allows the eye to focus through contraction and relaxation.
    c. Ciliary body: produces aqueous humor.
    d. Iris: controls the size of the pupil in order to regulate the amount of light that enters the eye; gives the eye its characteristic color.
    e. Pupil: the opening in the center of the *iris*; the size of the pupil determines the amount of light that enters the eye.
  3. Inner layer.
    a. Retina: thin innermost lining (or the inside back wall) of the eyeball; contains millions of light-sensitive nerve cells to coordinate and transmit signals via the optic nerve to the brain; similar to film in a camera.
    b. Macula: the part of the retina responsible for providing optimum visual focusing.
    c. Aqueous humor: fluid that fills anterior and posterior chambers; circulates through the pupil and empties into canal of Schlemm.
    d. Trabecula: mesh network through which the aqueous humor fluid drains into the canal of Schlemm.
    e. Vitreous humor: fluid that fills the cavity posterior to the lens.
    f. Crystalline lens: provides for the convergence and refraction of light rays and images onto the retina; enables vision to be focused.
    g. Optic nerve: leaves the eyeball through the retina at the location of the optic disc.
    h. Choroid: blood supply to the retina.
B. Eyelids: protective coverings of the eye.
  1. Conjunctiva: inner lining of the eyelid.
  2. Lacrimal gland: excretes lacrimal fluid (tears) to lubricate, clean, and protect the outer surface of the eye.

System Assessment

A. External assessment.
  1. Assess position and alignment of the eyes: both eyes should fixate on one visual field simultaneously.
  2. Evaluate for presence of ptosis.
  3. Inspect lids and conjunctiva for discharge or inflammation.
  4. Assess color of sclera: normally, a thin white coating; may yellow with age.
  5. Evaluate size and equality of pupils: should be equal in size and shape.
  6. Evaluate pupillary reaction to light.
    a. Direct light reflex: constriction of pupil when stimulated with light.
    b. Consensual reflex: constriction of opposite pupil when stimulated with light.
  7. Extraocular muscle function: hold finger or object about 12 inches in front of the eye and ask the client to follow the object with only the movement of the eyes; assists to evaluate for paralysis or weakness in extraocular muscle and cranial nerve function (Figure 12-1).
B. Evaluate visual acuity and check for refractive errors (see Appendix 12-1).
  1. Myopia (nearsightedness): vision for near objects is better than vision for distant objects.
  2. Hyperopia (farsightedness): vision for distant objects is better than vision for near objects.
  3. Determine any problems with double vision.
C. Assess for presence of pain and any recent change in vision.

FIGURE 12-1 Extraocular eye movements. (From: Seidel HM, et al: *Mosby's guide to physical examination,* ed 6, St. Louis, 2006, Mosby.)

ALERT Assist client to cope with sensory impairment (e.g., hearing, sight, etc.).

DISORDERS OF THE EYE

 Glaucoma

Glaucoma is a group of disorders characterized by an increase in intraocular pressure and progressive loss of peripheral vision. It is a chronic condition and a leading cause of blindness.

Types

A. Primary open-angle glaucoma (POAG chronic glaucoma): most common form. Flow of aqueous humor is slowed or stopped by obstruction, thus increasing intraocular pressure; characterized by a slow onset; chronic and progressive.
B. Primary angle-closure glaucoma (PACG—acute glaucoma): caused by rapid increase in intraocular pressure. Iris is pushed against drainage system, blocking flow of aqueous humor. Immediate treatment is required.
C. Secondary glaucoma: caused by trauma or optic neoplasm.

Assessment

A. Risk factors.
   1. Familial tendency.
   2. Aging—occurs most often in clients more than 40 years old.
   3. Chronic diseases and eye injury.
B. Diagnostics: intraocular pressure is above 22 mm Hg (see Appendix 12-1).
C. Clinical manifestations of chronic primary open-angle glaucoma (POAG)—develops slowly and frequently without symptoms.
   1. Gradual loss of peripheral vision (i.e., tunnel vision).
   2. Vague headache around lights.
   3. Blindness may eventually occur if untreated.

4. Central vision is normal, even with loss of peripheral vision.
D. Clinical manifestations of acute primary angle-closure glaucoma (PACG).
   1. Medical emergency requiring immediate treatment.
   2. Decreased central vision.
   3. Severe eye and brow pain, blurred vision.
   4. Headache.

Treatment

A. Medications (see Appendix 12-2).
   1. Topical (ophthalmic) beta blockers, carbonic anhydrase inhibitors, cholinergics (miotics), and prostaglandins may be used alone or in combination.
   2. Oral glycerin preparations promote diuresis and lower intraocular pressure.
B. Surgical intervention: most often done on outpatient basis with topical anesthetic.
   1. Argon laser trabeculoplasty: microscopic laser burns applied to the trabecula open the fluid channels facilitating outflow of aqueous humor.
   2. Trabeculectomy: creation of an artificial drain to bypass the trabecular meshwork, allowing aqueous humor to flow.

Nursing Interventions

Goal: To prevent progression of visual impairment.
A. Teaching plan.
   1. Explanation of the problem of increased intraocular pressure.
   2. Visual damage cannot be corrected, but further damage can be prevented.
   3. Correct use of prescribed medications; client must continue to take medication in order to control disease; otherwise, visual problem will progress.
   4. Importance of continued follow-up medical care.
   5. Advise all health care providers of glaucoma condition; numerous medications affect intraocular pressure; wear medical alert identification.

Goal: To decrease intraocular pressure.

A. Avoid straining at stool, lifting, or stooping.

B. Administer medications to decrease intraocular pressure.

Goal: To provide appropriate preoperative nursing measures if surgery is indicated.

A. Surgery and treatments are frequently done on an outpatient basis and with a local anesthetic. Orient the client to the surroundings and sounds that will occur during the procedure.

B. For outpatient surgery, client should wear comfortable clothes and arrange for someone to provide transportation home.

C. Postoperative instructions should be given to the client or family in writing.

Goal: To prevent client from experiencing postoperative complications (surgery frequently done under local anesthesia).

A. Administer medications: miotics, antibiotics, and steroids.

B. Be sure medication is administered in the eye for which it is ordered; the unaffected eye may be treated with a different medication.

C. Client may eat and ambulate as desired after the initial sedative effect is gone.

Home Care

A. Emphasize the importance of follow-up care.

B. Teach the client not to rub the eyes.

C. Demonstrate the correct administration of eye medication and have the client return the demonstration.

D. Advise the client to avoid activities that increase intraocular pressure.

E. Teach the client to report pain that is not relieved by prescribed analgesics.

Cataract

A cataract is a complete or partial opacity of the lens that occurs when clumps of protein compromise the sharpness of images on the retina. It may occur at birth (congenital cataract); however, it occurs most commonly in adults past middle age (senile cataracts).

Assessment

A. Risk factors.
1. Diabetes mellitus.
2. Corticosteroids: long-term systemic or topical use.
3. Age: 70% of adults over age 75 years have cataracts.

B. Clinical manifestations.
1. Painless with gradual decrease in visual acuity, blurry vision.
2. Pupil appears gray or yellowish brown to milky white.
3. Red light reflex is distorted on direct ophthalmoscopic examination.
4. Poor color perception.
5. Glare due to light scatter on lens; worse at night.

C. Diagnostics (see Appendix 12-1).

Treatment

Surgical treatment is the only method of correcting cataract; surgery is usually performed when client begins to experience problems in activities of daily living (Box 12-1). If both eyes require surgical correction, each is treated individually, about 4 to 8 weeks apart.

A. Phacoemulsification (Phaco): a small incision on the side of the cornea allowing a tiny probe to be inserted to emit ultrasound, which fragments the lens; cataract is then aspirated.

B. Intraocular lens (IOL) implant to restore visual correction.

Nursing Interventions

Goal: To provide appropriate teaching and nursing care.

A. Orient the client to the surroundings and sounds that will occur during the procedure.

Box 12-1 OLDER ADULT CARE FOCUS

Promoting Independent Activities of Daily Living for the Client With Diminished Vision

Medications
- When client is taking several medications, use containers that have different shapes (square, round, triangular).
- Obtain medication boxes with raised letters or numbers on them representing the days of the week.
- Obtain a "talking clock" that states the time.

Safety
- Remove throw rugs.
- Use unbreakable dishes, cups, and glasses.
- Keep appliance cords short and out of walkways.
- Avoid footstools in favor of a recliner with a built-in footrest.
- Label all cleansers, cleaning fluids, and caustic chemicals with large, raised lettering.
- Have hand grips installed in bathrooms.
- Put nonskid stripping on the surface of the tub floor.
- Encourage use of an electric razor.

Communication
- Teach caregivers to always introduce themselves when entering the client's room and before touching client.
- Teach the client to use telephones that have programmable automatic dialing features. Be sure to include emergency phone numbers.
- Recognize that much communication is nonverbal; therefore frequent clarification of meaning may be required.

Daily Living Considerations
- Provide information on Meals on Wheels for delivery of cooked, ready-to-eat meals.
- Encourage use of a microwave for cooking—it is safer than using a standard stove.
- Encourage the use of large-print books, newspapers, and magazines for reading. Also, many publications are available as audiotapes and CDs at local libraries and vision aid services.
- Avoid rearranging furniture and other belongings.

B. For outpatient surgery, client should wear comfortable clothes and arrange for someone to provide transportation home.

C. Before surgery, the nurse will instill mydriatic eye drops; frequently, cycloplegic drops are also used; client will be photosensitive.

D. Normal for visual acuity to be decreased immediately after surgery.

Home Care (see Box 12-1)

A. Maintain client's orientation to surroundings.

B. Eye patch may be used for about 24 hours or until the client returns to the physician for a follow-up visit.

C. Client should avoid stooping, lifting, or straining in the early postoperative period.

D. Client should avoid sleeping on the affected side.

E. Teach the client to avoid rubbing the eye; there should be minimal discomfort, and this is generally relieved by acetaminophen; report any pain that is not easily relieved.

F. Teach client how to administer eye drops (antibiotic and steroid eye drops); have client demonstrate procedure.

G. Provide written instructions; make sure the type is large enough for client to read.

Retinal Detachment

A separation of the sensory retina and the underlying epithelium, which allows fluid to collect in the space. Untreated symptomatic retinal detachment almost always results in the loss of vision in the eye.

Assessment

A. Risk factors.
  1. Severe myopia (nearsightedness).
  2. Diabetic retinopathy: sclerosed capillaries of the retina.
  3. Trauma.
  4. Degenerative changes in the retina.
  5. Previous cataract surgery.

B. Diagnostics (see Appendix 12-1).

C. Clinical manifestations.
  1. Flashes of light in the visual field.
  2. Sensation of a curtain or shadow over a portion of the visual field.
  3. Painless loss of peripheral or central vision.
  4. Area of lost vision correlates with location of retinal detachment.

Treatment

There is no medical treatment. The surgical repair may be done on an outpatient basis or may require hospitalization.

A. Laser photocoagulation: laser light beam to create inflammation and sealing of the tear or break.

B. Cryotherapy: a "supercooled" probe directed over retinal tear to produce inflammation to seal the tear.

C. Scleral buckling: extraocular surgery in which the sclera is depressed from the outside with the application of a silicone "buckle" to weld the retina in contact with the choroid (Figure 12-2).

FIGURE 12-2 Scleral buckling. (From Black JM, Hawks JH: *Medical-surgical nursing: clinical management for positive outcomes,* ed 8, Philadelphia, 2009, Saunders.)

Nursing Intervention

Goal: To enable client and significant others to discuss problems associated with detachment of the retina, the rationale for surgery, and anticipated preoperative and postoperative activities.

A. Discourage client from jerky head movements, stooping or straining; may have activity restrictions, depending on degree of detachment.

B. Local anesthesia may be used; client may be discharged within hours or may remain in hospital—depends on the degree of detachment and the type of repair.

Goal: To prevent postoperative complications.

A. Orient client to surroundings (see Box 12-1).

B. Postoperative pain may require narcotic analgesic.

C. Client may experience redness and swelling of the lids.

D. Warm or cool compresses may be used to promote comfort.

E. Postoperative medications usually include antibiotic eye drops, ophthalmic steroid drops, and dilating agents.

Goal: To help client understand and perform own eye care.

A. Activities requiring visual acuity may be restricted for several weeks (reading, driving, etc.).

B. Discourage any straining, lifting, or stooping during the postoperative recovery period.

C. Make sure client understands symptoms of detachment and importance of seeking immediate attention if it occurs again (increased incidence of reoccurrence).

Age-Related Macular Degeneration (AMD)

Most common cause of central vision loss in clients over 40 years old; related to retinal aging.

Assessment

A. Risk factors.
 1. Familial tendency: gene has been identified.
 2. Long-term exposure to UV lights and eye irritants.
B. Clinical manifestations.
 1. Blurred, darkened vision.
 2. Presence of scotomas (blind spots in visual field).
 3. Distortion of vision.
 4. Permanent loss of central vision.
 5. Wet exudative—more severe form.
  a. Development of abnormal vessels in or near macula.
  b. New vessels begin to leak and form scar tissue.
  c. Rapid onset.
 6. Dry nonexudative—less severe form.
  a. More common form.
  b. Accumulation of yellow pigment in retinal epithelium.
  c. Atrophy and degeneration of macular cells.
C. Diagnostics (see Appendix 12-1).

Treatment

Directed toward stopping progression; affected vision cannot be restored.
A. Laser treatment of abnormal vessels, macular photocoagulation of abnormal vessels.
B. Medications to inhibit growth of endothelial tissue and vessels.

Nursing Interventions

Goal: To promote prevention and/or early identification of problem and care of client with decreased visual acuity.
A. Encourage regular visual checkups.
B. Encourage diet high in leafy green vegetables and vitamins A and E, beta carotene, and zinc.
C. Promote independence in clients with decreased vision (see Box 12-1).

 Visual Impairment in Children

A. Refractory problems: same as those of an adult (see Appendix 12-1).
B. Amblyopia: reduced visual acuity in one eye; preventable if primary problem is corrected before age of 6 years.
C. Strabismus (misalignment of eyes) may result if amblyopia is not corrected.
D. Conjunctivitis: an inflammation of the conjunctiva.
 1. Characterized by redness, tearing, and exudate.
 2. Warm, moist compresses to remove crust and exudates.
 3. Always clean eye from inner canthus downward and outward to prevent contamination of other eye.
 4. May be viral, bacterial, or allergic.
 5. Treatment with antibiotic eye drops; instill after eye has been cleaned.
 6. Highly contagious; spreads easily from one eye to other.
 7. Encourage good handwashing.

E. Retinopathy of prematurity: originally known as *retrolental fibroplasia;* results in vasoconstriction of retina vessels causing retinal damage.

Nursing Interventions

A. Promote discovery of the problem as early as possible.
 1. Identify children at increased risk because of history (prematurity).
 2. Assess children for behaviors that indicate poor vision.
 3. Encourage screening for visual acuity (schools, clinics).
B. Educate parents regarding importance of therapy and continued medical follow-up.

Eye Trauma

Eye trauma may include surface injuries (e.g., burns or splash injuries), imbedded or impaled objects, or orbital trauma. History is usually congruent with eye injury.
A. Assessment and treatment are often carried out at the same time.
B. As soon as the eye injury is detected, the client should be seen by a physician (ophthalmologist).

Assessment

A. Identify eye in which trauma occurred.
B. Determine whether client has a contact lens in the affected eye.
C. Pain, inability to open the eye.
D. Decreased visual acuity: may be unable to distinguish light and images.
E. Ecchymosis, swelling.

Treatment

A. If there is visible trauma, but no penetrating object, gently apply dressing soaked with normal saline solution to prevent drying during transport.
B. Any suspected or known corneal abrasion should be examined with fluorescein, followed by ocular irrigation with normal saline solution (see Appendix 12-2, and 12-3).
C. Nonpenetrating foreign objects may be removed by irrigation with normal saline solution.
D. Penetrating foreign bodies must be removed by a physician (ophthalmologist) as soon as possible. Do not attempt to remove foreign objects from eye, but protect from movement while seeking emergency care.
E. Do not attempt to stop bleeding from the eye or the eyelid with direct pressure, do not patch the eye until type of injury is determined.
F. For chemical eye burns, before going to emergency department, irrigate the eye with copious amounts warm tap water to remove chemical. Normal saline irrigation in ED; may require short-acting ophthalmic anesthetic drops.

Nursing Interventions

Goal: To prevent further eye damage.

A. Have client "rest" the eyes: provide dimly lit room; use eye patches if necessary.

B. Irrigate eyes with normal saline solution from inner canthus to outer canthus so solution does not flow into unaffected eye.

C. Eye may remain irritated after foreign body is removed; eye patch may be necessary.

D. If penetrating eye injury is present, decrease activities that cause increased ocular pressure.

E. Keep client immobilized until evaluated by an ophthalmologist.

Goal: To care for a client with an enucleation.

A. Immediate: obtain vital signs; monitor for bleeding.

B. Instillation of topical ointments until prosthesis is fitted.

C. A clear "conformer" may be placed in the eye socket to allow the area to heal so a permanent prosthesis can be fitted.

D. Eye prosthesis.
1. Insertion: notched end of prosthesis should be closest to the client's nose; lift upper eyelid (using nondominant hand) and insert saline solution-rinsed prosthesis into socket area with top edge slipping under upper lid; gently retract lower lid until bottom edge of prosthesis slips behind it.
2. Removal: retract the lower lid and apply slight pressure just below the eye, this should release the suction holding the eye in place; assess the socket for signs of infection.
3. The prosthesis is usually cleansed with normal saline.

PHYSIOLOGY OF THE EAR

A. External ear.
1. External auditory canal: function is to transmit the collected sound waves to the tympanic membrane; outer half of canal secretes cerumen, or wax, which has a protective function.
2. Tympanic membrane: a tough membrane separating the external and middle ear; transmits vibrations from external ear to the malleus of the middle ear; normally a pearly gray color.

B. Middle ear.
1. Middle ear is filled with air at atmospheric pressure by means of the eustachian tubes; the eustachian tubes of infants and young children are shorter and wider than those of adults.
2. The external and middle ear function is to transmit and magnify sound waves by air conduction.
3. Problems in the external and middle ear cause conductive hearing loss.

C. Inner ear.
1. Bony labyrinth.
   a. Vestibule: central area contains oval window and is bathed in fluid.
   b. Semicircular canals: open into the vestibule; related to maintaining equilibrium.
   c. Cochlea: contains organ of Corti, which is the receptive end organ for hearing.
2. Disease of the inner ear or nerve pathway can result in sensorineural hearing loss.

System Assessment

A. External assessment of the ear.
1. Assess placement of the ears: low-set ears may be indicative of congenital anomalies in the newborn.
2. Movement of the auricle should not elicit pain.
3. Note presence of any discharge in the external canal.
4. With an otoscope, examine tympanic membrane for landmarks, color, and intactness.
5. Note color and consistency of cerumen.

B. Assessment of bone and air conduction (see Appendix 12-1).

C. Assess for vertigo: ask client to close eyes and stand on one foot; have client walk with eyes closed; client may fall to one side or complain of the room spinning.

DISORDERS OF THE EAR

Otitis Media

Otitis media is an infection of the middle ear caused by a viral or bacterial agent. Infants and young children are predisposed to the development of acute otitis media because of the physiologic characteristics of the ear—the eustachian tube is shorter, wider, and straighter in children than in adults.

Assessment

A. Acute otitis media (AOM).
1. May be purulent (pus-filled) or suppurative (capable of producing pus).
2. Symptoms vary with the severity of the infection.
3. Increased incidence in bottle-fed babies.

B. Repeated or persistent acute infections lead to perforation of the tympanic membrane or more severe complications such as mastoiditis.

C. Otitis media with effusion (OME): a collection of fluid in the middle ear without infection or acute symptoms that results from a blocked eustachian tube; may persist for weeks to months; most common cause of conductive hearing loss.

D. Risk factors.
1. Age: increased incidence from 6 months to 20 months; decreases with age.
2. Upper respiratory tract infection.
3. Allergies, asthma.
4. Increased incidence in infants who are exposed to passive cigarette smoke.

E. Clinical manifestations (Figure 12-3).
1. Otalgia (pain from pressure in the middle ear).
   a. Infants are irritable; may pull at their ears; sucking exacerbates pain.

FIGURE 12-3 Otitis media. (From Zerwekh J, Claborn J: *Memory notebook of nursing,* vol 2, ed 3, Ingram, Texas, 2007, Nursing Education Consultants.)

   b. Young children verbally complain of severe ear pain.
2. Fever as high as 104° F is not uncommon with AOM.
3. Otoscopic examination.
   a. AOM—tympanic membrane is immobile, bright red, and bulging, with no light reflex and purulent effusion.
   b. OME—immobile and discolored tympanic membrane.
4. Postauricular and cervical lymph node enlargement.
5. If tympanic membrane ruptures, purulent drainage or blood may be present in the outer ear; pain will decrease temporarily (AOM and OME).
6. Conductive hearing loss may occur with recurrent rupture.
7. Speech and language development may be delayed.

Treatment

A. Medications.

> ⚠ **NURSING PRIORITY** Teach the parents to administer the full course of the antibiotic.

1. Antibiotics, analgesics, antipyretics.
2. Ear drops (antibiotic and steroid combination).
3. Decongestants and antihistamines.
4. Corticosteroids for eustachian tube edema as needed.
5. OME does not require antibiotic therapy.
B. Surgical—myringotomy: drainage of the middle ear with insertion of tubes or grommets (or tympanostomy myringotomy) to relieve pressure and promote healing; used for recurrent cases that do not respond to medication; tubes also known as pressure equalizing tubes (PE tubes).

Nursing Interventions

Goal: To enable parents of clients to describe problem, handle medication schedule, and cope with home care.

A. Recurrent infections cause an increased risk for permanent hearing loss or mastoiditis with potential intracranial spread of infection.
B. Antibiotics should be continued until all prescribed medication is taken, even after all symptoms are relieved.
C. Administer acetaminophen or ibuprofen for pain and fever. There should be relief of symptoms within 24 to 72 hours; if not, the health care provider should be contacted.
D. Pain-relieving ear drops (Auralgan, Pramotic) should be used only when there is no tympanostomy tube or rupture of the tympanic membrane.

> ⚠ **NURSING PRIORITY** Aspirin should not be used for fever or pain in children 18 years or younger.

E. Control allergies and upper respiratory congestion.
F. The child should be discouraged from forcefully blowing his or her nose or holding his or her nose closed when sneezing.
G. Decrease risk for recurrence by preventing fluids from pooling around eustachian tube.
   1. Hold or elevate infant's head while feeding.
   2. Do not prop bottle or allow infant to fall asleep with a bottle.
   3. Encourage intake of water before sleeping.
H. Encourage application of a drying agent (e.g., Swim-EAR) after swimming, showering, or bathing to dry external ear canal and/or use of earplugs when child goes swimming.

Goal: Care for child after placement of tympanostomy tubes (myringotomy tubes or grommets).

A. Do not allow soapy or dirty water to get into the child's ears; use of earplugs is currently controversial.
B. Assure parents that if the ear grommet or tube falls out, it is not a significant problem.

📋 Acoustic Neuroma

A benign tumor of cranial nerve VIII, vestibulocochlear.

Assessment

A. Clinical manifestations.
   1. Sensorineural hearing loss.
   2. Tinnitus.
   3. Intermittent vertigo.
   4. Impairment of facial movement (CN VII, V).
B. Diagnostics (see Appendix 12-1 and Appendix 20-1).
C. Treatment—surgical removal of tumor.

Nursing Interventions

Goal: Promote communication and prepare client for surgery.

A. Assist hearing-impaired client with communication (Box 12-2).

Box 12-2 OLDER ADULT CARE FOCUS

Improving Communication With Hearing-Impaired Clients

- Stand in front of the client at eye level to speak. An adequate light source on your face will help with speech reading (i.e., reading lips).
- Get the client's attention by raising your hand or arm.
- Do not walk back and forth in front of the client while speaking.
- Speak clearly and in an even tone; do not shout.
- Do not chew gum, cover your mouth, or smile excessively while talking.
- Because clients rely on visual cues, watch your facial expressions.
- Encourage professional counseling in speech reading and sign language.
- Assist the client in obtaining a hearing aid; if appropriate, promote social interaction.
- Do not avoid conversation with the client; do not depend on family to interpret information.
- Investigate use of TDD (telecommunication device for the deaf).
- Use light-activated devices: door bell, smoke alarms, telephones.
- Client should avoid noisy environments where it is difficult to interpret sound.
- Provide client instruction in a quiet room with minimal distractions.

B. Determine presence of vertigo and plan for client safety.
C. Preoperative preparation (see Chapter 3).
 1. Assess level of hearing loss and communication skills.
 2. Encourage client to discuss fear regarding loss of hearing on affected side.
 3. Establish communication system for postoperative period.
Goal: To provide postoperative craniotomy care (see Chapter 20).
A. Assess for surgical interference with other cranial nerves (VII, facial; V, trigeminal; IX, glossopharyngeal).
 1. Assess for equal movement of face: smile, show teeth.
 2. Evaluate for problem swallowing.
 3. Evaluate speech.
B. Evaluate balance and hearing loss regarding ADLs and safety.

Hearing Loss

Hearing loss results from an impairment of the transmission of sound waves.
A. Conductive: results from mechanical dysfunction in transmission of sound from the outer or middle ear or both. Client will be able to benefit from a hearing aid. Example of conductive hearing loss is impacted cerumen, which often occurs in older adults.
B. Sensorineural (perceptive): results from a problem in the inner ear (cochlea) or auditory nerve pathway.

Often results from injury to cilia that transmit sound. Incoming sound cannot be analyzed correctly. Client may benefit from cochlear implant. Example of sensorineural hearing loss is presbycusis, which occurs in older adults.
C. Otosclerosis: an immobilization of the small bones in the inner ear; it occurs most often in women; an autosomal-dominant disease that is usually bilateral.
D. Congenital: rubella or nutritional deficiencies.
E. Toxicity from aminoglycosides.
F. Occupational.

Assessment

A. Risk factors.
 1. Prolonged exposure to high-intensity sound waves.

! NURSING PRIORITY Earplugs should be worn when the potential for exposure to loud noise exists.

---

 2. Repeated, chronic ear infections.
 3. Prenatal problems of rubella and eclampsia.
 4. Ototoxic medications: aminoglycosides, diuretics.
 5. Female with family history of otosclerosis.
B. Diagnostics (see Appendix 12-1).
C. Clinical manifestations.
 1. Speech problems: deterioration of present speech or delayed speech development.
 2. Fails to respond to oral communication or responds inappropriately.
 3. Excessively loud speech.
 4. General indifference to sound.
 5. Tinnitus.
 6. Responds more to facial expressions than to verbal ones.
 7. Inappropriate emotional response.

Treatment

A. Speech therapy.
B. Sign language.
C. Stapedectomy for otosclerotic lesions.
D. Cochlear implants for profound sensorineural hearing loss.

Nursing Interventions

Goal: To promote communication and socialization of the hearing-impaired client (Box 12-2).
A. Teach client how to care for hearing aid (Box 12-3).
B. Teach client how to remove ear wax if impacted cerumen is a problem; may need an ear irrigation (see Appendix 12-3).
Goal: To prevent complications after stapedectomy.
A. Assess client for dizziness, nausea, and vomiting.
B. Teach client to avoid sudden movement to prevent dizziness.
C. Maintain safety measures.
D. Instruct client that hearing may not improve until edema subsides in the operative area.

Box 12-3 OLDER ADULT CARE FOCUS

Hearing Aid Care

- Keep the hearing aid dry; do not wear it while bathing or swimming.
- Avoid using hair spray, cosmetics, or oils around the ear.
- Clean hearing aid with soft cloth and recommended cleanser; do not immerse in water.
- At night turn it off and open the battery compartment to prevent draining the battery.
- Avoid exposing it to extreme temperatures (e.g., leaving it on a window ledge in the sunlight).
- When cleaning the hearing aid, use a toothpick or pipe cleaner to remove any debris or cerumen from the hole in the middle part of the device that goes in the ear.
- If the hearing aid does not work, change the battery or check the on/off switch; check the connection between the ear mold and receiver; clean it using the steps described above, or take it to an authorized hearing aid service center.

ALERT Hearing loss is very common in older adult clients. Watch for questions about hearing loss to be incorporated into test situations pertaining to other chronic health care problems.

 Balance Disorders

The vestibular system of the inner ear maintains balance and coordination.

A. Disorders.
  1. Ménière's disease: an inner ear disorder caused by excess endolymph in the vestibular and semicircular canals; also known as endolymphatic hydrops.
  2. Labyrinthitis: an inflammation of the cochlear and/or vestibular portion of the inner ear.

Assessment

A. Diagnostics (see Appendix 12-1).
  1. Results of Weber test and auditory testing may indicate hearing loss.
  2. Romberg test (see Chapter 20 for Neurologic System Assessment).

B. Clinical manifestations.
  1. Vertigo: a sense of moving or spinning that is usually stimulated by sudden movement of the head; may occur when lying down.
  2. Sudden, severe paroxysmal episodes of vertigo (Ménière's disease).
    a. Severe nausea, vomiting.
    b. Nystagmus.
    c. Loss of balance.
    d. No pain or loss of consciousness.
  3. Fluctuating hearing loss and tinnitus (Ménière's disease).
  4. Client may have no symptoms between attacks.
  5. Manifestations become less severe with time.

Treatment

A. Medications (Ménière's disease).
  1. Atropine may stop an acute attack.
  2. Sedatives.
  3. Antihistamines, anticholinergics.
  4. Diuretics (to decrease endolymph fluid).
  5. Meclizine hydrochloride (Antivert) for prevention and treatment of "motion sickness" symptoms.
  6. Antiemetics.
B. Diet: low-sodium.

Nursing Interventions

Goal: To provide emotional and physical support during an acute attack.
A. Maintain bed rest in a quiet, dimly lit room; avoid flickering lights and television.
B. Position of comfort.
C. Avoid unnecessary nursing procedures.
D. Minimize stimulation and sudden position changes.
E. If client is severely nauseated, administer medications parenterally.
F. Maintain safety: instruct client to always call before getting out of bed.

NURSING PRIORITY As a safety precaution, instruct the client to lie down immediately if an attack feels imminent.

Appendix 12-1   OPHTHALMIC AND HEARING DIAGNOSTICS

Ophthalmic Diagnostics

Snellen chart is used in screening for visual acuity problems. Client is placed 20 feet from the chart, and visual acuity is expressed as a ratio (what the client *should* see at 20 feet compared with what he or she *can* see at 20 feet). A ratio of 20/50 means that the client can see at 20 feet what he or she should see at 50 feet.

A **noncontact tonometer** is an instrument used to measure intraocular pressure noninvasively. Normal pressure is 12 to 22 mm Hg. A puff of air is directed toward the cornea, which causes indentation and allows measurement of intraocular pressure, a screen for diagnosis of glaucoma.

Direct ophthalmoscopy is examination of the fundus or back portion of the interior of the eyeball, which provides for visual evaluation of the retina, vascular patterns, and optic disk.

Biomicroscopy (slit-lamp examination) is used to assess the anterior eye for problems of the cornea, iris, and lens and to evaluate the depth of the anterior chamber.

Refractive error evaluation determines what refractive errors have occurred because light is not correctly focused on the retina. Conditions that occur in refractive errors are:
- **Myopia** (nearsightedness)—sees near objects clearly; light ray is focused in front of the retina
- **Hyperopia** (farsightedness)—sees distant objects clearly; light ray is focused behind the retina
- **Presbyopia**—a decrease in the elasticity of the lens that causes poor accommodation for near vision (common in older adults)
- **Astigmatism**—an uneven curvature of the cornea; light rays do not focus on the retina at the same time

Hearing Diagnostics

Audiometry is used to measure a client's hearing by the use of various tones and intensities of sound produced by an audiometer.

The **Rinne test** is conducted by holding a tuning fork on the mastoid bone (bone conduction). When the client indicates that he or she no longer hears sound, the vibrating tuning fork is moved to about 2 inches from the external ear (air conduction). The client who hears normally will continue to hear the vibrations. This demonstrates that air conduction will last longer than bone conduction. When the tone is louder through air, the test result is positive and indicates normal hearing. If the bone conduction is louder than air conduction, it is indicative of a conductive loss.

The **Weber test** is conducted by placing a vibrating tuning fork on top of the client's head or in the middle of the forehead; the sound should be heard equally well in each ear. The tone is louder in an ear with unilateral conductive loss and quieter in an ear with sensorineural loss.

Otoscopy is the examination of the external ear and the tympanic membrane by the use of an otoscope.

Appendix 12-2   OPHTHALMIC MEDICATIONS

General Nursing Implications

Only use ophthalmic preparations of medications.
- To decrease systemic absorption of ophthalmic topical medications, teach client to apply gentle pressure (punctal occlusion) to the lacrimal duct (tear duct) during and immediately after instillation of drops.
- Instruct client or family in proper administration of eye drops or ointment, (i.e., maintain sterile technique and prevent dropper contamination; clearly mark each container to indicate what eye medication is for).
- Expect some blurriness from ointments; apply at bedtime, if possible, to avoid safety problems from diminished vision.
- Instruct client to report changes in vision, blurring, difficulty breathing, or flushing.
- Teach client to gently close eye and allow medication to distribute evenly over eyeball.

MEDICATIONS	SIDE EFFECTS	NURSING IMPLICATIONS
Glaucoma Medications Used to reduce production of aqueous humor and increase outflow, thereby decreasing ocular pressure.		
Alpha₂ Adrenergic Agonists Brimonidine (**Alphagan**)	Dry mouth, ocular hyperemia, local burning and stinging. Systemic absorption: hypotension	1. Can be absorbed into contact lens, wait 15 minutes after instill drops to replace contacts.
Beta Blockers **Nonselective Beta₁ and Beta₂ Blockers** Timolol maleate (**Timoptic**) Carteolol (**Ocupress**)	Eye irritation, dry eyes Bradycardia, AV block, bronchospasm	1. Assess for cardiac and respiratory changes with systemic absorption.
Selective Beta₁ Blockers Betaxolol (**Betoptic**)	Bradycardia, AV block	1. Recommended for use in clients with history of chronic pulmonary disease. Assess for systemic absorption.

MEDICATIONS	SIDE EFFECTS	NURSING IMPLICATIONS
Prostaglandin Analogs		
Latanoprost (**Xalatan**)	Increases pigmentation of eyelid and growth of eyelashes; conjunctiva hyperemia	1. Minimal systemic effects.
Travoprost (**Travatan**)		
Bimatoprost (**Lumigan**)		
Anticholinergics		
Pilocarpine hydrochloride (**IsoptoCarpine, Pilocar**): 0.25% to 10% solutions	Conjunctive irritation Provocation of asthma Headache, ciliary spasm	1. Contraindicated in clients with inflammatory eye conditions. 2. Miotic; causes constriction of pupil.

> **■ NURSING PRIORITY** Only use ophthalmic preparations of any medication for eye drops.

Cycloplegic and Mydriatics Work by blocking response of sphincter muscle of iris; produce dilation of pupil; may cause paralysis of accommodation. Used in eye examination and diagnosis.		
Atropine sulfate (**Atropisol**): 0.25% to 2% solution Cyclopentolate HCl (**Cyclogyl**): 0.5% to 1% solution Tropicamide (**Mydriacyl**)	Blurred vision, photophobia, headache, hyperemia; systemic effects: flushing, sweating, dry mouth, dizziness	1. Contraindicated in clients with glaucoma. 2. Dark glasses may be worn to decrease discomfort from photophobia. 3. Use only ophthalmic preparations.
Diagnostics Surface of eye absorbs dye, thus demonstrating corneal abrasions in eye trauma.		
Fluorescein sodium (**Fluorocyte, Fluor-L-Strip**)	Stinging, burning sensation	1. Cornea remains uncolored; abrasions and defects turn green.
Antiinfectives Used for treatment of eye infections.		
Neomycin-Polymyxin (**Neosporin**) Erythromycin (**Ilotycin**) ophthalmic ointment	Drops and ointment may cause burning or irritation.	1. Vision may be blurred. 2. Teach correct application of medication. 3. Use only eye preparations of medications.

CNS, Central nervous system; *GI*, gastrointestinal; *IV*, intravenously; *PO*, by mouth (orally).

Appendix 12-3 NURSING PROCEDURE: EAR AND EYE IRRIGATION

Ear Irrigations
Common Solutions

Warm tap water or normal saline solution.
   Hydrogen peroxide.

✓ KEY POINTS: Irrigation

- Before irrigation, visually inspect the external ear canal with otoscope to ensure that tympanic membrane is intact and that auditory canal is not obstructed by a foreign body. Do not irrigate an ear with otitis media present.
- Temperature of irrigating solution should be near body temperature (37° C, approximately 98° F). If too cold or hot, dizziness and/or nausea may occur.
- Cerumen may be softened by adding a few drops of warm mineral oil or OTC preparation.
- A rubber bulb syringe or a water pressure device may be used.
- Straighten the ear canal by either pulling the outer ear up for adults or down for children under 3 years.
- Direct water flow toward the top of the ear canal to create a circular motion.
- Do not forcefully push fluid into the ear canal, because this may rupture the eardrum. If severe pain, nausea, vomiting, or dizziness develop, stop the irrigation immediately.

Eye Irrigations
Common Solutions

Normal saline.

✓ KEY POINTS: Eye Irrigation

- Place client in position in which solution does not run into unaffected eye.
- Small amount of fluid: use a cotton ball moistened in solution.
- Moderate amount of fluid: use a plastic squeeze bottle to direct fluid along conjunctiva and over the eyeball from inner to outer canthus.
- Large amount of fluid: bags of intravenous solutions may be used to provide constant stream and adequate flushing of chemical from the eye.
- Do not allow tip of irrigating equipment to touch the eye.
- Immersion technique: place entire face in basin of lukewarm water and have client open and close eyes repeatedly.
- Avoid use of contact lenses for a period of time after eye irritation.

Study Questions Sensory System

More questions on companion CD!

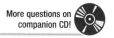

1. The nurse would question which medication order for a client with acute primary angle-closure glaucoma?
   1. Atropine (Atropisol) 1 to 2 drops in each eye now
   2. Hydrochlorothiazide (Diuril) 25 mg PO daily
   3. Propranolol (Inderal) 20 mg PO two times a day
   4. Carbamyl choline (Isopto carbachol) eye drops, 1 drop two times a day

2. A client who has glaucoma is concerned about her adult children "inheriting" the condition. What is the best nursing response?
   1. "There is no need for concern; glaucoma is not a hereditary disorder."
   2. "Your children should have an ophthalmologic examination with screening for glaucoma around age 40. After that, examinations should be done every 2 to 3 years."
   3. "There may be a genetic factor with glaucoma, and your children over 30 years old should be screened yearly."
   4. "Are your grandchildren complaining of any eye problems? Glaucoma generally skips a generation."

3. The nurse is evaluating a client recently diagnosed with chronic primary open-angle glaucoma (POAG). What will be an important nursing action?
   1. Review all medications the client is currently taking to determine whether any of them cause an increase in intraocular pressure as a side effect.
   2. Determine whether the client has experienced any sudden loss of vision accompanied by pain.
   3. Discuss with the client the importance of controlling blood pressure to decrease the potential loss of peripheral vision.
   4. Instruct the client to take analgesics as soon as any discomfort occurs in the eye and to notify clinic if pain is not relieved.

4. A child is scheduled for a myringotomy with placement of tympanostomy tubes. What is the goal of this procedure that the nurse will discuss with the parents?
   1. To decrease infection in the ear
   2. To irrigate the eustachian tube
   3. To correct a malformation in the inner ear
   4. To equalize pressure on the tympanic membrane

5. A client comes to the clinic with decreased hearing. Examination of the ear canal reveals a large amount of cerumen. What is the recommended method for removal of the cerumen?
   1. Curettage with suction and irrigation
   2. Normal saline solution irrigation
   3. D$_5$W irrigation
   4. Cotton swab applicator

6. The nurse is admitting a postoperative client after removal of an acoustic neuroma. What would be most important to include in the postoperative nursing care for this client?
   1. Determining when the client will begin chemotherapy
   2. Evaluating hearing status
   3. Assessing the client's ability to swallow
   4. Encouraging the client to discuss problems with hearing loss

7. A client's eye has been anesthetized for an ophthalmology examination. What instructions will be important for the nurse to give the client?
   1. Do not watch television for at least 1 day.
   2. Do not rub the eye for 15 to 20 minutes.
   3. Irrigate the eye every hour to prevent dryness.
   4. Wear sunglasses when in direct sunlight for the next 6 hours.

8. A child is diagnosed with conjunctivitis. Which statement indicates that the child understood the nurse's teaching?
   1. "It's okay for me to let my friends use my sunglasses while we are playing together."
   2. "It's okay for me to softly rub my eye, as long as I use the back of my hand."
   3. "I can pick the crusty stuff out of my eyelashes with my fingers when I wake up in the morning."
   4. "I will use my own washrag and towel while my eyes are sick."

9. An unknown chemical was splashed into a client's eyes. What is most important for the nurse to tell the client to do immediately?
   1. Rinse the eye with a large amount of water or saline solution.
   2. Put a pad soaked in sterile saline solution over the eye.
   3. Go to the closest emergency department.
   4. Have a co-worker visually check the eye for a foreign body.

10. Which client is at highest risk for retinal detachment?
    1. A 4-year-old with amblyopia
    2. A 17-year-old who plays physical contact sports
    3. A 33-year-old with severe ptosis and diplopia
    4. A 72-year-old with nystagmus and Bell's palsy

Answers and rationales to these questions are in the section at the end of the book titled Chapter Study Questions: Answers and Rationales.

CHAPTER THIRTEEN

Endocrine System

PHYSIOLOGY OF THE PITUITARY GLAND

A. Often referred to as the "master gland" because it secretes hormones that control hormone secretion of other endocrine glands (Figure 13-1).
B. Located in the skull beneath the hypothalamus of the brain.
C. Two lobes.
   1. Anterior pituitary: secretes hormones affecting other glands (Table 13-1).
   2. Posterior pituitary: hormones (see Table 13-1) are produced in the hypothalamus and subsequently secreted by the posterior pituitary.

System Assessment

A. Assess for growth imbalance.
   1. Evaluate overall growth pattern of child.
   2. Assess for excessive or retarded growth.
      a. In adults, assess for excessive growth of small bones and soft tissue.
      b. In children, assess for excessive or retarded growth in height.
   3. Evaluate excessive weight gain or loss.
B. Evaluate familial tendencies.
   1. Parents who displayed slower growth patterns.
   2. Compare rate of growth of siblings at age comparable to that of client.
   3. Assess for specific characteristics and/or genetic traits in the adults of the immediate family.
C. Assess for secondary sexual characteristics appropriate to age.
D. Assess intellectual development and mental changes appropriate to physical development and age.
   1. Intelligence.
   2. Increased excitability.
   3. Mental confusion, apathy.

DISORDERS OF THE PITUITARY GLAND

Hyperpituitary: Acromegaly

Acromegaly is most often the result of a benign slow-growing tumor (pituitary adenoma) that secretes growth hormones. It occurs after the closure of epiphyses of the long bones.

Assessment

A. Clinical manifestation.
   1. Enlargement of the hands and feet and hypertrophy of the skin.
   2. Changes in facial features: protruding jaw, slanting forehead, and an increase in the size of the nose.
   3. Severe enlargement of the pituitary gland may cause pressure on the optic nerve, resulting in changes in vision and headaches.
B. Diagnostics (see Appendix 13-1).
C. Complications.
   1. Headache and visual field disturbances.
   2. Diabetes mellitus/glucose intolerance.
   3. Obstructive sleep apnea.

Treatment

Surgical intervention is primary method of correcting problem; hypophysectomy may be accomplished by the transsphenoidal approach.

Nursing Interventions

Goal: To provide supportive preoperative care (see Chapter 3).
Goal: To ensure that the client will not experience complications after hypophysectomy.
A. Elevate the head 30 degrees.
B. Discourage coughing, sneezing, or straining at stool to prevent cerebrospinal fluid leak.
C. Assess for symptoms of increasing intracranial pressure (see Chapter 20).
D. Evaluate urine for excessive increase in volume (>200 mL/hr) or specific gravity <1.005 (i.e., development of diabetes insipidus).
E. Frequent oral hygiene with nonirritating solutions.
Goal: To assist client to reestablish hormone balance after hypophysectomy (adrenal insufficiency and hypothyroidism are most common complications).
A. Administer corticosteroids.
B. If output becomes excessive (because of decrease in antidiuretic hormone [ADH]), anticipate administration of ADH-regulating medications (see Appendix 13-2).

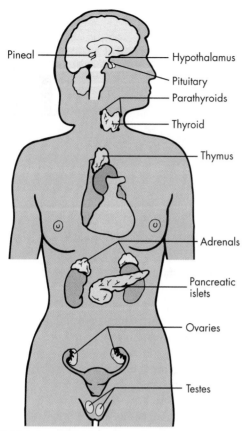

Pineal — Hypothalamus
— Pituitary
— Parathyroids
— Thyroid
— Thymus

— Adrenals

— Pancreatic islets

— Ovaries

— Testes

FIGURE 13-1 Location of the major endocrine glands. (From Lewis SL, et al: *Medical-surgical nursing: assessment and management of clinical problems,* ed 7, St. Louis, 2007, Mosby.)

C. Evaluate serum glucose levels for significant changes.
D. Monitor for problems related to hypothyroidism.
Goal: To cope with altered body image.
A. Infertility will frequently be experienced as a result of hormone changes.
B. Skeletal changes before surgery are not reversible.
C. Medication.
   1. Cortisone and thyroid hormone replacement throughout lifetime.
   2. ADH-regulating medications.
   3. Medication to support target organs involved (pancreas, thyroid, gonads).

Disorders of the Posterior Pituitary

Diabetes insipidus (DI) is characterized by a deficiency of antidiuretic hormone (ADH) or kidney's inability to respond to ADH. When it occurs, it is most often associated with neurologic conditions, surgery, tumors, head injury, or inflammatory problems.

The syndrome of inappropriate antidiuretic hormone (SIADH) is a condition in which there is continued release of ADH, regardless of the level of plasma osmolarity.
A. When there is a decrease in the serum osmolarity, the normal body response is to decrease the secretion of ADH.
B. When the normal feedback mechanism for ADH fails and the level of ADH is sustained, there is excessive water retention in the body.

Table 13-1	SUMMARY OF PITUITARY GLAND HORMONE PRODUCTION	
Hormone Produced	*Site of Action*	*Function*
Anterior Lobe		
Adrenocorticotropic hormone (ACTH)	Adrenal cortex	Growth and secretion activity of adrenal cortex (stimulates secretion of corticosteroids)
Thyroid-stimulating hormone (TSH)	Thyroid gland	Controls synthesis and secretion of thyroid hormone
Follicle-stimulating hormone (FSH)	Testes	Male: stimulates sperm production
	Ovaries	Female: stimulates development of ovarian follicles and ovulation
Luteinizing hormone (LH)	Testes	Male: stimulates spermatogenesis
	Ovaries	Female: stimulates ovulation and follicle maturation; production of estrogen and progesterone
Luteotropic hormone (LTH), Prolactin (PRL)	Mammary glands	Secretion of milk, maintenance of corpus luteum
Growth hormone (GH, somatotropin)	All body cells	Growth and maturation of bones, muscles, and other organs
Posterior Lobe		
Antidiuretic hormone (ADH)	Renal tubules	Increases reabsorption of water, thereby decreasing urinary output
Oxytocin	Smooth muscle (particularly wall of uterus and mammary glands)	Contraction of uterus at end of gestation
		Initiates let-down response of milk during lactation

NOTE: Pituitary gland secretions are controlled primarily by the hypothalamus.

C. When there is a decreased or inadequate amount of ADH, the body is unable to concentrate urine, and excessive water loss occurs.

Assessment

A. Risk factors/etiology: both conditions frequently have predisposing pathology.

B. Clinical manifestations of DI.
1. Polyuria: excretion of excessive amounts urine (greater than 200 mL/hr).
2. Polydipsia.
3. Low urine specific gravity (1.001 to 1.005).
4. Severe dehydration (tachycardia, poor skin turgor, dry mucous membranes).
5. Increase in serum sodium level (greater than 147 mEq/L).
6. Weakness.

C. Clinical manifestations of SIADH.
1. Low urinary output with weight gain and no obvious edema.
2. Decreased (dilutional) serum sodium level (less than 120 mEq/L).
3. Gastrointestinal (GI) disturbances (anorexia, nausea, abdominal cramps).
4. Cerebral edema: altered mental status, headaches, seizures.
5. High specific gravity (greater than 1.030).
6. Fatigue and muscle aches.

D. Diagnosis based on characteristic clinical manifestations.

Treatment

A. Diabetes insipidus: administration of ADH-regulating medications (see Appendix 13-2).

B. SIADH.
1. Intravenous (IV) administration of normal saline solution (if level is 126-134 mEq/L).
2. Fluid restriction (limit fluids to 500-1000 mL/24 hr).
3. Monitor sodium correction carefully. Correct deficit slowly.

Nursing Interventions

Goal: To maintain fluid and electrolyte balances (see Chapter 6).

A. Encourage intake of fluids containing electrolytes for clients with DI; restrict fluids for clients with SIADH.

B. Monitor intake and output carefully. Weigh daily.

C. Evaluate urine specific gravity for changes.

D. Assess hydration status.

E. Correlate hydration status with weight gain or loss.

F. Closely monitor sodium and potassium levels with fluid shifts (low sodium in SIADH and increased sodium in DI).

Goal: To understand the implications of the condition.

A. DI caused by other problems is usually self-limiting.

B. Correction of SIADH is based on identification and correction of the predisposing condition.

PHYSIOLOGY OF THE THYROID GLAND

A. Located in the anterior portion of the neck behind the trachea.

B. Anterior pituitary gland controls secretions of the thyroid-stimulating hormone (TSH).

C. Release of TSH is controlled by the level of thyroid hormone in the blood.

D. Primary function of thyroid hormone is to control the level of cellular metabolism by secreting thyroxin (T_4) and triiodothyronine (T_3) (Table 13-2).

E. An inadequate secretion of hormone during fetal life and neonatal development will depress metabolic activity and result in stunted physical and mental growth.

F. Disorders of the thyroid gland result in hyperfunction and hypofunction or simple enlargement of the gland.

System Assessment

A. Assess for changes in metabolism.
1. Significant increase weight or decrease in weight.
2. Diarrhea or constipation.
3. Increase or decrease in appetite.
4. Changes in vital signs.
5. Changes in texture and appearance of skin.

B. Assess for intellectual development and mental changes.
1. Intellectual level appropriate for age.
2. Increased irritability, excitability, nervousness.
3. Mental confusion, lethargy.

DISORDERS OF THE THYROID GLAND

Hyperthyroidism

Hyperthyroidism (also called Graves' disease) or thyrotoxicosis (the signs and symptoms caused by hypermetabolism) is characterized by excessive output of thyroid hormones.

Assessment

A. Risk factors.
1. More prevalent in women and older adults.
2. Peak incidence in third or fourth decade of life.
3. Probably an autoimmune condition.

Table 13-2	SUMMARY OF THYROID GLAND HORMONE PRODUCTION	
Hormone Produced	**Site of Action**	**Function**
Thyroxine (T_4)	General	Controls metabolic rate and growth and development
Triiodothyronine (T_3)		
Calcitonin (or thyrocalcitonin)	Bone	Inhibits bone resorption, lowers serum calcium levels

NOTE: Thyroid gland hormone secretion is controlled by the secretion of thyroid-stimulating hormone by the pituitary gland.

HYPERTHYROIDISM

FIGURE 13-2 Graves' disease. (From Zerwekh J, Claborn J: *Memory notebook of nursing,* vol 1, ed 4, Ingram, Texas, 2008, Nursing Education Consultants.)

B. Clinical manifestations (Figure 13-2).
   1. Increased rate of body metabolism.
      a. Intolerance to heat.
      b. Significant weight loss, despite increased appetite and food intake.
      c. Tachycardia, increase in systolic blood pressure.
      d. Increased peristalsis, leading to diarrhea.
      e. Hand tremors at rest.
   2. Visual problems.
      a. Exophthalmos (bulging eyeballs).
      b. Changes in vision.
      c. Eyelid retraction (lid lag).
   3. Changes in menstrual cycle.
   4. Enlarged, palpable thyroid gland.
   5. Labile emotional state.
C. Diagnostics (see Appendix 13-1).
   1. Increase in T_3, T_4, and free T_4 serum levels.
   2. Decrease in TSH.
   3. Radioactive iodine uptake test (I^{123}) greater than 50%.
   4. Client's physical appearance and symptoms.

Complications

A. Thyroid storm or crisis: may occur after surgery or treatment with radioactive iodine.
   1. Systolic hypertension.
   2. Tachycardia.
   3. Increased temperature (>102° F).
   4. Increased agitation and anxiety.
B. Calcium deficit may occur as a result of trauma to the parathyroid (see Hypoparathyroidism, later in this chapter).

Treatment

A. Surgical: thyroidectomy.
B. Medical.

1. Reduce thyroid tissue: irradiation of thyroid gland with radioactive iodine (I^{131}), eventually resulting in hypothyroid state.
2. Decrease thyroid synthesis and release (see Appendix 13-2).

Nursing Interventions

Goal: To decrease effects of excess thyroid hormone.
A. Decrease environmental stress (lights, visitors, noise, etc.).
B. Cool environment.
C. Sedatives, if appropriate.
D. Well-balanced meals (high in calories and high in vitamins); small meals served 4 to 6 times per day.

Goal: To protect eyes of client experiencing complications caused by eye changes.
A. Eye drops or ointment.
B. Assess for excess tearing, a sign of dry cornea.
C. Eye patches or mask may be necessary at night.

Goal: To prevent complications of thyroid storm (or crisis) (thyrotoxicosis).
A. Identify risk factors precipitating thyroid crisis.
   1. Inadequate preoperative preparation.
   2. Infection, increased emotional lability.
   3. Surgical removal of thyroid gland.
   4. After treatment of radioactive I^{131} ablation.
B. Assess for increase in hyperthyroid state.
   1. Increase in temperature, dehydration.
   2. Tachycardia (heart rate above 130 beats/min).
   3. Pulmonary edema.
   4. Nausea, vomiting, diarrhea.
   5. Increase in agitation.

Goal: To maintain homeostasis in client experiencing thyroid storm (or crisis).
A. Decrease body temperature and heart rate.
   1. Hypothermia blanket.
   2. Acetaminophen to decrease fever.
   3. Propranolol (Inderal) to treat cardiac issues.
B. Oxygen to meet increased metabolic demands.
C. IV fluids.
D. Hydrocortisone for shock and adrenal insufficiency.
E. Iodine preparations to decrease T_4 output.
F. Assess for cardiac tachydysrhythmias.
G. Propylthiouracil or methimazole (Tapazole) given to inhibit formation of thyroid hormone.

Goal: To provide preoperative nursing measures if surgery is indicated.
A. Demonstrate to client how to provide neck support after surgery.
B. Administer iodine preparations to decrease vascularity of the thyroid gland.
C. Establish baseline data for postoperative comparison.

Goal: To maintain homeostasis after thyroidectomy.
A. Maintain semi-Fowler's position to avoid tension on the suture line.
B. Administer analgesics for pain.

C. Administer IV fluids until nausea and swallowing difficulty subside.

D. Check dressings on the side and back of the neck for bleeding.

E. Assess for hematoma around the wound.

F. Apply ice collar to decrease edema.

G. Evaluate calcium levels; parathyroid may have been damaged or accidentally removed.

H. Evaluate temperature elevations; temperature increase may be early indication of thyroid storm.

> ❗ **NURSING PRIORITY** Monitor status of client who has undergone surgery (hemorrhage, airway, wound).

Goal: To prevent complication of respiratory distress after thyroidectomy.

A. Assess client frequently for noisy breathing and increased restlessness.

B. Evaluate voice changes; increasing hoarseness may be indicative of laryngeal edema.

C. Keep tracheotomy set readily available.

Goal: To decrease radiation exposure in client being treated as an in-patient with radioactive iodine (I^{131}).

A. All body secretions are contaminated because this is a systemic type of radiation.

B. Advise family members to avoid oral contact because saliva is contaminated.

C. For any body fluid spills (urine, vomitus, etc.), contact the radiation safety officer for the facility. Do not clean up the spill until directed to do so.

D. General guideline is to maintain a distance of 1 meter (a little more than 3 feet) from the client unless direct contact is necessary.

E. Infants and pregnant women should avoid contact with the client for approximately 2 days.

F. All health care personnel providing direct care to the client should wear a radiation badge.

G. Monitor client for a transient period of several days to weeks, when the symptoms of hyperthyroidism may actually worsen after radioactive iodine therapy.

> **ALERT** Observe client for side effects of chemotherapy or radiation.

 Home Care

A. Thyroid levels checked annually.

B. Lifelong thyroid replacement.

C. If excessive fatigue or tachycardia and tremors become consistent problems, notify health care provider.

 Hypothyroidism

Hypothyroidism is characterized by a slow deterioration of thyroid function. It occurs primarily in older adults and five times more frequently in women (ages 30 to 60) than in men. Myxedema coma is a life-threatening form of hypothyroidism.

Assessment

A. Early clinical manifestations.
1. Extreme fatigue, menstrual disturbances.
2. Hair loss, brittle nails, and dry skin.
3. Intolerance to cold, anorexia.
4. Constipation, apathy.

B. Late clinical manifestations.
1. Subnormal temperature.
2. Cardiac complications (bradycardia, congestive heart failure, hypotension).
3. Weight gain and edema, thickened skin.
4. Change or decrease in level of consciousness.

C. Diagnostics.
1. Decrease in serum T_3 and T_4 levels.
2. Increase in TSH level.

Treatment

A. Medical management.
1. Replacement of thyroid hormone.
2. Low-calorie diet to promote weight loss.
3. Decrease in cholesterol intake.

Complications

A. Thyroid hormone replacement will increase the workload of the heart and increase myocardial oxygen requirements.

B. Observe client for development of cardiac failure.

Nursing Interventions

Goal: To assist the client to return to hormone balance.

A. Begin thyroid replacement and evaluate client's response; advise client that it will be about 7 days before he or she begins to feel better.

B. Provide a warm environment.

> ❗ **NURSING PRIORITY** Administer sedatives and hypnotics with caution because of increased susceptibility. These medications tend to precipitate respiratory depression in the client with hypothyroidism.

C. Prevent and/or treat constipation.

D. Assess progress.
1. Decrease in body weight.
2. Intake and output balance.
3. Decrease in visible edema.
4. Energy level and mental alertness should increase in 7 to 14 days and continue to rise until normal.

E. Evaluate cardiovascular response to medication.

Goal: To assist client to understand implications of disease and requirements for health maintenance.

A. Need for lifelong drug therapy.

B. Client with diabetes needs to evaluate blood glucose levels more frequently; thyroid preparations may alter effects of hypoglycemic agents.

C. Continue to reinforce teaching as client begins to make progress; early in the disease, the client may not comprehend importance of information.

Congenital Hypothyroidism (Cretinism)

Congenital hypothyroidism is a deficiency of thyroid hormones present at birth. Symptoms depend on the amount of thyroid hormones present at birth.

Assessment

A. Condition is not generally evident in the newborn because of thyroid hormones received through the maternal circulation; may become evident at 3 to 6 months of age.
B. Early clinical manifestations.
  1. Thick, dry, mottled skin.
  2. Bradycardia.
  3. Hypotonia, hyporeflexia.
  4. Poor feeding.
  5. Hypotonic abdominal musculature.
    a. Constipation.
    b. Protruding abdomen (umbilical hernia).
C. Diagnostics.
  1. Filter-paper blood-spot thyroxine (T_4) test; if result is low, then a TSH test is done.
  2. Mandatory test in all states; should be done within 24 to 48 hours after birth.

Treatment

Medical management includes replacement of thyroid hormones. (If replacement is accomplished shortly after birth, it is possible that the child will have normal physical growth and intellectual development.)

Nursing Interventions

Goal: To identify neonates experiencing congenital hypothyroidism.
Goal: To assist parents to understand the implications of the disease and requirements for continued health maintenance.
A. Child will require lifelong medication.
B. Continue medical care to evaluate changes in thyroid replacement as the child grows.

PHYSIOLOGY OF THE PARATHYROID

Four small parathyroid glands are located near, or embedded in, the thyroid gland. The hormone secreted is parathyroid hormone (PTH), which is primarily involved in the control of serum calcium levels.

A. Function of PTH.
  1. Facilitates the mobilization of calcium and phosphorous from bone.
  2. Promotes the resorption of calcium from bone to maintain normal serum calcium levels.
  3. Promotes absorption of calcium in the GI tract (by stimulating kidneys to convert vitamin D to its active form).
  4. Renal: increases calcium reabsorption and phosphate excretion.

B. Function of calcium.
  1. Maintains normal muscle and neuromuscular responses.
  2. Necessary component of blood coagulation mechanisms.
C. Control of PTH occurs by way of the negative feedback system involving the level of serum calcium. When serum calcium levels are low, there is increased mobilization of calcium from bone, resulting in an increase in serum calcium levels.

System Assessment

A. History of problems of calcium metabolism and/or thyroid surgery.
B. Assess for changes in mental or emotional status.
C. Evaluate reflexes and neuromuscular response to stimuli.
D. Evaluate serum and urine calcium levels.

DISORDERS OF THE PARATHYROID

Hyperparathyroidism

Hyperparathyroidism is characterized by excessive secretion of PTH, resulting in hypercalcemia.

A. Normal function of PTH is to maintain serum calcium and phosphate levels.
B. Excessive PTH leads to bone damage, hypercalcemia, and kidney damage.

Assessment

A. Risk factors: more common in women after menopause.
B. Clinical manifestations.
  1. Primary hyperparathyroidism is due to adenomas, hyperplasia, or carcinomas. Bone cysts and pathologic fractures occur because of bone decalcification. Calcium is released into the blood, causing hypercalcemia.
  2. Secondary hyperparathyroidism is frequently due to chronic renal failure.
    a. Renal calculi, azotemia.
    b. Hypertension caused by renal failure.
    c. Repeated urinary tract and renal infections.
  3. Central nervous system problems of lethargy, stupor, and psychosis.
  4. GI problems.
    a. Anorexia, nausea, and vomiting.
    b. Constipation, development of peptic ulcer.
C. Diagnostics.
  1. Increased level of serum total calcium; decreased level of serum phosphorous; increased PTH.
  2. CT scan and/or x-ray film show demineralized cystic areas in bone.
  3. Increased urine calcium and phosphorous levels.

Treatment

A. Decrease level of circulating calcium.
B. Parathyroidectomy.

Nursing Interventions

Goal: To decrease the level of serum calcium.

A. High fluid intake to dilute serum calcium and urine calcium levels.

B. If IV is necessary, generally administer normal saline solution.

C. Furosemide (Lasix), a loop diuretic, may be used to increase excretion of calcium.

D. Encourage mobility, because immobility increases demineralization of bones.

E. Limit foods high in calcium.

F. Phosphate replacement.

Goal: To assess client's tolerance of and response to increased PTH level.

A. Assess for skeletal involvement.

B. Assess for renal involvement.
1. Strain urine for stones.
2. Evaluate for low back pain (renal).
3. Check for hematuria.
4. Assess intake and output carefully.

C. Assess for presence of bone pain.

D. Assess cardiac response to increased level of calcium.

Goal: To provide appropriate preoperative measures if surgery is indicated (see Chapter 3).

Goal: To prevent postoperative complications of parathyroidectomy.

A. Care of client who has undergone parathyroidectomy is same as that for client who has undergone thyroidectomy.

B. Bone pain is relieved shortly after surgery; bone lesions frequently heal; serious renal disease may not be reversible.

Hypoparathyroidism

Hypoparathyroidism is characterized by a decrease in the PTH level, resulting in hypocalcemia and elevated serum phosphate levels. Severe hypocalcemia results in tetany.

Assessment

A. Risk factors or precipitating causes.
1. Adults: inadvertent removal of parathyroid gland during thyroidectomy or radical neck dissection.
2. Children: primary cause is idiopathic (unknown).

B. Clinical manifestations.
1. Insidious onset.
   a. Muscle weakness/spasms.
   b. Loss of hair; dry skin.
2. Overt/acute tetany (potentially fatal).
   a. Bronchospasm, laryngospasm.
   b. Seizures, cardiac dysrhythmias.
   c. Circumoral paresthesia.
   d. Abdominal cramps, nausea, vomiting, diarrhea, anorexia.
   e. Positive Chvostek's sign (sign is positive when sharp tapping over the facial nerve elicits mouth, nose, and eye twitching).
   f. Trousseau's phenomenon (present when carpopedal spasm is precipitated by occluding blood flow for 3 minutes to the upper portion of the upper extremity with a blood pressure cuff).

3. Pediatrics.
   a. Carpopedal spasms, muscle cramps, twitching.
   b. Seizures: generalized or absence.
   c. Brittle hair, thin nails.

C. Diagnostics.
1. Decreased serum calcium levels.
2. Increased serum phosphate levels.
3. Low PTH levels.

Treatment

A. Vitamin D to enhance calcium absorption.

B. Increased calcium in the diet.

> **ALERT** Adjust food and fluid intake to improve fluid and electrolyte balances.

C. Acute.
1. Replace calcium through slow IV drip (calcium gluconate, calcium chloride).
2. Sedatives, anticonvulsants.

Nursing Interventions

Goal: To assist client to increase serum calcium levels.

A. Administer calcium preparations.

B. Evaluate for an increase in serum calcium levels and a decrease in serum phosphate levels.

C. Client will require lifelong medical care to maintain homeostasis.

Goal: To prevent complications of neuromuscular irritability.

A. Quiet environment.

B. Low lights.

C. Seizure precautions.

Goal: To help client avoid complications of respiratory distress.

A. Bronchodilators.

B. Tracheotomy set readily available.

C. Frequent assessment of respiratory status.

Goal: To prevent complications of cardiac problems.

A. Assess client for history of cardiac problems.

B. Assess frequently for dysrhythmias.

C. Calcium will potentiate effects of digitalis; use cautiously together.

PHYSIOLOGY OF THE PANCREAS

A. The pancreas is located in the upper left aspect of the abdominal cavity.

B. The pancreas produces the enzymes trypsin, amylase, and lipase, which are secreted into the duodenum and are necessary for the digestion and absorption of nutrients.

C. Located within the pancreas are the islets of Langerhans, which contain beta cells that are responsible for the production of insulin.

D. Insulin is necessary for maintaining normal carbohydrate metabolism and glucose utilization.

System Assessment

A. Evaluate changes in weight, particularly weight gain in an adult and weight loss in a child.
B. Evaluate alterations in fluid balance.
C. Evaluate changes in mental status.
D. Evaluate serum glucose levels.
E. Evaluate results of pancreatic enzyme studies.
F. Evaluate the abdomen for epigastric pain and abdominal discomfort.

DISORDERS OF THE PANCREAS

Diabetes Mellitus

Diabetes mellitus (DM) is a complex, multisystem disease characterized by the absence of, or a severe decrease in, the secretion or utilization of insulin.

A. Pathophysiology.
1. The primary function of insulin is to facilitate the movement of glucose from the blood into the cell, thus decreasing the blood glucose level.
   a. Necessary for the transport of glucose into the cells of the liver, muscles, and other tissues.
   b. Regulates the rate of carbohydrate metabolism and conversion to glucose, normally insulin is decreased during fasting and increased after eating (prandial).
2. Insulin is secreted by the beta cells in the islets of Langerhans in the pancreas.
3. Insulin allows the body to use carbohydrates more effectively for conversion of glucose for energy.
   a. Adequate intake of carbohydrates.
   b. Available insulin to facilitate the movement of glucose into cells.
   c. Adequate reserves of glucagon (released by pancreas; converts glycogen to glucose in the liver).
4. If carbohydrates are not available to be used for energy, cells will begin to oxidize the fats and protein stores.
   a. Breakdown of fat results in the production of ketone bodies.
   b. Protein is wasted during insulin deficiency. Protein is broken down and converted to glucose by the liver, thus contributing to the increase in circulating glucose.
   c. When fats are used as the primary energy source, the serum lipid level rises and contributes to the accelerated development of atherosclerosis.
5. When circulating glucose cannot be used for energy, the level of serum glucose will increase (hyperglycemia).
   a. Hyperglycemia will cause an increase in the osmotic gradient; water moves out of the cells into the circulating volume to decrease the osmolarity. This results in an increase in urinary output.
   b. The increase in circulating glucose exceeds the renal threshold, and glucose spills into the urine.

6. Pathophysiologic bases for symptoms.
   a. Polyuria: because of the increased serum osmolarity, there is more circulating volume; water is not reabsorbed from the renal tubules, and there is a significant increase in urine output.
   b. Polydipsia: increased loss of fluids precipitates dehydration, causing thirst.
   c. Polyphagia: tissue breakdown and wasting cause hunger.
   d. Weight loss (with type 1 DM): glucose is not available to the cells; body begins to break down fat and protein stores for energy.
B. Classification.
1. Type 1: absolute lack of insulin secretion.
   a. Absence of insulin production; client is dependent on insulin to prevent ketoacidosis and maintain life.
   b. Onset is frequently in childhood; most often diagnosed before the age of 18 years. Most common age range is 10 to 15 years.
   c. Previously called juvenile diabetes or insulin-dependent diabetes mellitus.
   d. Familial tendencies in transmission.
   e. Client will have type 1 diabetes for the rest of his or her life.
2. Type 2: combination of insulin resistance and inadequate insulin secretion to compensate.
   a. Insulin deficiency caused by defects in insulin production or by excessive demands for insulin; client is not dependent on insulin.
   b. Ketoacidosis is generally not a problem because of limited insulin production.
   c. Onset is predominately in adulthood, generally after the age of 40 years, but it may occur at any age.
   d. Previously called adult onset diabetes (AODM) or noninsulin-dependent diabetes mellitus (NIDDM).
   e. Associated with obesity; overweight people require more insulin.
   f. If not associated with obesity, there is usually a strong family history.
   g. Blood sugar often controlled by diet and oral hypoglycemics but during episodes of stress may require insulin for control.
3. Gestational diabetes.
   a. Develops during pregnancy; usually detected at 24 to 28 weeks' gestation by oral glucose tolerance test.
   b. Glucose tolerance usually returns to normal soon after delivery.
   c. Infant may be large for gestational age and may experience hypoglycemia shortly after birth.
   d. Commonly occurs again in future pregnancies; client is at increased risk for development of glucose intolerance and type 2 diabetes later in life.

Assessment

A. Clinical manifestations.
    1. Types 1 and 2.
       a. Three Ps: polyphagia, polydipsia, polyuria.
       b. Fatigue.
       c. Increased frequency of infections.
    2. Type 1.
       a. Weight loss, excessive thirst.
       b. Bed-wetting, blurred vision
       c. Complaints of abdominal pain.
       d. Rapid onset, generally over days to weeks.
    3. Type 2 (most clients asymptomatic first 5 to 10 years).
       a. Weight gain (obese), visual disturbances.
       b. Slow onset; may occur over months.
       c. Onset usually after the age of 40 years; peaks around 45 to 50 years.
       d. Fatigue and malaise.
       e. Recurrent vaginal yeast or monilia infections—frequently, this is initial symptom in women.
       f. Older adult assessment considerations (Box 13-1).

B. Diagnostics (the criteria for diagnosis are two or more abnormal test results with two or more values outside the normal range) (see Appendix 13-1).
    1. Fasting blood glucose level: above 126 mg/dL (normal glucose below 100 mg/dL).
    2. Glucose tolerance test: 2-hour glucose values are greater than 200 mg/dL.
    3. Random glucose >200 mg/dL with symptoms (three Ps, weight loss).
    4. Prediabetes: intermediate stage between normal and diabetes.
       a. Impaired glucose tolerance (IGT): 2 hours after a meal, plasma glucose is >140 mg/dL; 200 mg/dL or higher during an oral glucose tolerance test.
       b. Impaired fasting glucose (IFG): fasting blood glucose is greater than 100 mg/dL, but less than 126 mg/dL.
    5. Glycosylated hemoglobin (HbA_{1c}) is increased (less than 7% is considered good control; HbA_{1c} is not a test to diagnose diabetes.)

Box 13-1   OLDER ADULT CARE FOCUS

Diabetic Assessment Considerations and Care

- Determine mental status and manual dexterity to handle injections.
- Determine whether client can access the injection sites.
- Is client alert and mentally capable of making judgments on medications?
- Determine whether the client can pay for supplies.
- What is the client's attitude about needles and injections?
- Assess how many other medications the client is taking; problems with "polypharmacy" (too many medications).
- Determine family's or client's ability to accurately perform serum glucose testing.
- What is the client's support system?

NURSING PRIORITY The glycosylated hemoglobin level will indicate overall glucose control for approximately the past 120 days. This allows evaluation of control of the blood glucose level, regardless of increases or decreases in the blood glucose level immediately before the sample was obtained.

Treatment

A. Factors in diabetes management.
    1. Regular physical activity.
    2. Diet.
    3. Pharmacologic intervention.
▲ B. Hypoglycemic agents.
    1. Insulin: may be used in both types of diabetes. Primary function of insulin is to transport glucose into muscle and fat cells (Table 13-3).
       a. Combination premixed insulin therapy eliminates problem of mixing different types (example: NPH/regular 70/30—number refers to percentage of each type of insulin).
       b. Do not give mixtures intravenously.
       c. Response to insulin mixtures varies with individuals.
       d. Insulin will be used for glucose control during pregnancy.
    2. Oral hypoglycemic agents for noninsulin-dependent clients (see Appendix 13-2).
    3. Insulin requirement increases when:
       a. Client is seriously ill.
       b. An infection develops.
       c. Client experiences physical trauma (surgery or accidents).
       d. Growth spurts occur during adolescence and puberty.
    4. Diabetic diet.
       a. Decrease calories for weight loss.
       b. Diet to meet nutritional needs and maintain optimum glucose level. Avoid simple sugars.
       c. Decrease in cholesterol level.
       d. Meal plan.
          (1) 45% to 65% carbohydrate (low glycemic index foods and increased dietary fiber).
          (2) 25% to 30% fat (reduced saturated and trans fat foods).
          (3) 10% protein (significantly lower than for normal adult due to the stress that moderate to high protein places on the kidneys).
    5. Exercise.
       a. Planned exercise; sporadic exercise is discouraged.
       b. Glucose for exercising muscles comes from the liver.
       c. The counterregulatory hormones increase the delivery of glucose to the muscles.

ALERT Intervene to control symptoms of hypoglycemia or hyperglycemia.

Table 13-3	PROFILE OF INSULINS

▲ *Insulin*	*Nursing Implications*

Action

Rapid-acting: lispro, aspart, glulisine
Onset: 15 minutes
Peak: 60-90 minutes
Duration: 3-4 hours

Short-acting: regular
Onset: 1/2 -1 hour
Peak: 2-3 hours
Duration: 3-6 hours

Intermediate-acting:
NPH or Lente
Onset: 2-4 hours
Peak: 4-10 hours
Duration: 10-16 hours

Long-acting: glargine, detemir
Onset: 1-2 hours
Peak: no pronounced peak
Duration: 24+ hours

Rapid-Acting
Should be used in combination with longer-acting insulin.

⬛ NURSING PRIORITY Because of quick onset of action, client must eat immediately.

Short-Acting
Usually given 20-30 minutes before meals.
May be given alone or in combination with longer-acting insulins.
Given for sliding scale coverage.

⬛ NURSING PRIORITY When administering injections:

- May mix regular insulin with other insulins.
- Only regular insulin may be given IV.

Intermediate-Acting
Hypoglycemia tends to occur in mid to late afternoon.
Never give IV.
May be mixed with regular insulin.

Long-Acting
Glargine has low pH (4); CANNOT be mixed with other insulins.
Usually given once a day at bedtime, but can be administered during the day.

ALERT Intervene to control hypoglycemia/hyperglycemia. Know various insulins and nursing implications. Specifically, know when to anticipate reaction and what to teach the client about his or her insulin.

Figures from Lewis SL et al: *Medical-surgical nursing: assessment and management of clinical problems,* ed 7, St. Louis, 2007, Mosby.

⬛ NURSING PRIORITY Metabolic effects of exercise:
1. Reduces insulin needs by reducing the blood glucose level.
2. Contributes to weight loss or maintenance of normal weight.
3. Helps the body metabolize cholesterol more efficiently.
4. Promotes less extreme fluctuations in blood glucose levels.
5. Decreases blood pressure.

Complications of Insulin Therapy

A. Hypoglycemia (Table 13-4).
B. Lipoatrophy and lipohypertrophy.
   1. Associated with administration of cold insulin.
   2. May result from poor rotation of injection sites.

3. Use of human insulin greatly decreases the chance of this occurring.
C. Somogyi effect (Figure 13-3).
   1. Physiologic reflex: rebound hyperglycemia from an unrecognized hypoglycemic state.
   2. Most often occurs at night.
   3. May be treated by decreasing the evening insulin dose or by increasing the calories in the bedtime snack.
D. Dawn phenomenon (Figure 13-4).
   1. Results from nighttime release of growth hormone and cortisol.
   2. Blood glucose elevates at 5:00 to 6:00 a.m. (predawn hours).

Table 13-4	COMPARISON OF DIABETIC KETOACIDOSIS (DKA), HYPEROSMOLAR HYPERGLYCEMIA SYNDROME (HHS), AND HYPOGLYCEMIA		
	DKA	*HHS*	*Hypoglycemia*
Age	All ages, increased incidence in children.	Adult (usually seen in older adults with underlying chronic disease)	All ages
GI	Abdominal pain, anorexia, nausea, vomiting, diarrhea	Normal	Normal; may be hungry
Mental state	Dull, confusion increasing to coma	More severe neurologic symptoms due to increased osmolarity and high blood glucose level	Difficulty in concentrating, coordinating; eventually coma
Skin temperature	Warm, dry, flushed	Warm, dry, flushed	Cold, clammy
Pulse	Tachycardia, weak	Tachycardia	Tachycardia
Respirations	Initially deep and rapid; lead to Kussmaul respirations	Tachypnea	Shallow
Breath odor	Fruity, acetone	Normal	Normal
Urine output	Increased	Increased	Normal
Lab values:			
Glucose	Greater than 300 (up to 1500 mg/dL)	Greater than 600 mg/dL	Below 70 mg/dL
Ketones	High/large	Normal	Normal
pH	Acidotic (less than 7.3)	Normal	Normal
Hematocrit	High due to dehydration	High due to dehydration	Normal
Lab values: urine			
Sugar	High	High	Negative
Ketones	High	Negative	Negative
Onset	Rapid (less than 24 hr)	Slow (over many days)	Rapid
Classification of diabetes	Primarily type 1; type 2 in severe distress	Type 2	Type 1 and type 2

DKA, Diabetic ketoacidosis; *GI,* gastrointestinal; *HHNS,* hyperosmolar hyperglycemia nonketotic syndrome.

FIGURE 13-3 Somogyi effect. (From Zerwekh J, Claborn J, Gaglione T: *Mosby's pathophysiology memory notecards,* ed 1, St. Louis, 2006, Mosby.)

3. May be treated by increasing insulin for overnight period.
4. Most severe in adolescence and young adulthood with peak growth hormone.

E. Hormones that counteract insulin.
   1. Glucagon.
   2. Epinephrine.
   3. Cortisol.
   4. Growth hormone.

> **⊞ NURSING PRIORITY** Intensive control of blood glucose levels in clients with type 1 diabetes can prevent or ameliorate many of the complications.

Complications Associated with Poorly Controlled Diabetes

A. Diabetic ketoacidosis.
   1. An extreme increase in the hyperglycemic state.
   2. An increase in the mobilization of fat and protein as energy sources.
   3. Metabolism of fat results in the production of fatty acids, which are converted to ketone bodies.
   4. An increase in circulating ketone bodies precipitates the state of acidosis.
   5. Occurs predominately in type 1 diabetes.

FIGURE 13-4 Dawn phenomenon. (From Zerwekh J, Claborn J, Gaglione T: *Mosby's pathophysiology memory notecards,* ed 1, St. Louis, 2006, Mosby.)

B. Clinical manifestations of diabetic ketoacidosis (see Table 13-4).
  1. Onset.
    a. May be acute or occur over several days.
    b. May result from stress, infection, surgery, or lack of effective insulin control.
    c. Results from poorly controlled diabetes.
  2. Severe hyperglycemia (blood glucose levels of 300-800 mg/dL).
  3. Presence of metabolic acidosis (low pH [6.8-7.3] and serum bicarbonate level less than 15 mEq/L).
  4. Hyperkalemia, hypokalemia, or normal potassium level, depending on amount of water loss.
  5. Urine ketone and sugar levels are increased.
  6. Excessive weakness, increased thirst.
  7. Nausea, vomiting.
  8. Fruity (acetone) breath.
  9. Kussmaul respirations.
  10. Decreased level of consciousness.
  11. Dehydration.
  12. Increased temperature caused by dehydration.
C. Hyperglycemic-hyperosmolar state (HHS); also known as nonketotic hyperosmolar coma and/or hyperglycemic hyperosmolar nonketotic syndrome (HHNS).
  1. Occurs primarily in older adult clients with type 2 diabetes.
  2. Insulin production is adequate to prevent the breakdown of fat for cellular function, but severe hyperglycemia exists.
  3. Severe electrolyte imbalance and dehydration exist in the absence of the acidotic state.

4. Characterized by extreme hyperglycemia (values greater than 600 mg/dL).
5. Because of the ability of the body to maintain a low level of insulin production, the breakdown of fat and the production of ketone bodies do not occur. This prevents the client from developing acidosis.
6. Osmotic diuresis occurs as a result of the hyperglycemia; the client becomes dehydrated very rapidly.
D. Clinical manifestations of HHS (see Table 13-4).
  1. Warm, flushed skin, lethargy.
  2. Weakness, thirst, decreased level of consciousness.
  3. Increased temperature from dehydration.
  4. Tachycardia, decrease in blood pressure.
  5. Generally no GI problems.
  6. No acetone odor to breath or glycosuria.
  7. Severe hyperglycemia (greater than 600 mg/dL).
  8. Serum pH is normal; urine output is increased.
E. Electrolyte imbalance.
  1. As acidosis develops, potassium ions move out of cells; this leaves cellular potassium levels depleted, but the serum potassium level is usually normal because of excessive excretion.
  2. As osmotic diuresis occurs from the hyperglycemic/hyperosmolar state, serum potassium is excreted.
  3. As the client becomes more dehydrated, the serum potassium becomes concentrated and does not reflect the potassium loss.
  4. As the osmolarity and acidosis are corrected, along with the administration of insulin, the potassium will move back into the cells and result in severe hypokalemia.

Complications of Long-Term Diabetes

A. Angiopathy: premature degenerative changes in the vascular system.
  1. May affect the large vessels (macroangiopathy, early onset of atherosclerosis, and arteriosclerotic vascular problems).
  2. May affect the small vessels (microangiopathy); problems are specific to diabetes.
B. Peripheral vascular disease: combination of both types of angiopathy.
C. Hypertension.
D. Diabetic gastroparesis: delayed gastric emptying.
E. Cerebrovascular disease.
F. Coronary artery disease.
G. Ocular complications: retinopathy, cataracts, glaucoma.

PEDIATRIC PRIORITY An ophthalmologic examination should be obtained once the child is 10 years of age and has had diabetes for 3-5 years.

H. Nephropathy.
  1. Microangiopathy primarily affects the glomerular capillaries, resulting in thickening and increased permeability of the glomerular basement membrane; will progress to end-stage renal disease.

2. Recurrent pyelonephritis, particularly in women.
3. Diabetic effects on the kidneys are the single most common cause of end-stage renal failure.

I. Neuropathy: inadequate blood supply to the nerve tissue and high blood glucose levels cause metabolic changes within the neurons.
   1. Peripheral neuropathy: may be general pain and tingling; may progress to painless neuropathy.

> **⚠ NURSING PRIORITY** Painless peripheral neuropathy is a very dangerous situation for the client with diabetes. Severe injury to the lower extremities may occur, and the client will not be aware of it. Clients should be taught to daily visually inspect their feet and legs.

   2. Autonomic nerve damage: diarrhea or constipation, urinary incontinence or retention, decreased sweating, and orthostatic hypotension; impotence in men. Interferes with the client's ability to recognize episode of hypoglycemia.
   3. Approximately 60% of clients with diabetes experience neuropathy; it is the most common chronic complication.
J. Infections: An alteration in immune system response results in impairment of white cells for phagocytosis. Persistent glycosuria potentiates urinary tract infections.

Clinical Implications of Diabetes in Pregnancy

A. Effects of pregnancy on diabetes.
   1. During the first trimester of pregnancy, there is an increase in the fetal need for glucose and amino acids; this lowers the maternal blood glucose level and decreases the maternal need for additional insulin.
   2. During the second and third trimesters, the need for insulin will increase as a result of insulin resistance from major hormone changes.
   3. Oral hypoglycemic agents are not used to control diabetes in the pregnant client.
B. Effects of diabetes on pregnancy.
   1. Increase in size and number of islets of Langerhans in the client with type 2 diabetes.
   2. Increased tendency toward the development of metabolic acidosis caused by an increase in metabolic rate.
   3. Placental antagonist to insulin will decrease the effectiveness of insulin.
   4. Fetal antagonists to insulin decrease the utilization of glucose.
   5. Hormonal changes lead to decreased tolerance to glucose and increased insulin resistance (begins around 14 to 16 weeks).
C. Influence of pregnancy on diabetic control.
   1. Prone to hypoglycemia during the first trimester of pregnancy; may need to reduce insulin dosage.
   2. Increase in insulin requirements during the second and third trimesters of pregnancy may double or quadruple prepregnancy amounts.
   3. Tendency to intensify the existing complications of diabetes.

D. Monitoring fetal and maternal well-being during pregnancy, labor, and delivery.
   1. Antepartum period.
      a. Assess stability of mother's blood glucose control; insulin used rather than oral hypoglycemics.
      b. Weekly or biweekly blood glucose levels: to maintain optimum level of control.
      c. Third-trimester evaluation of fetal/placental function by determining 24-hour urinary estriol levels.
      d. Nonstress or oxytocin challenge test (stress test) done at 36 to 38 weeks' gestation to determine ability of fetus to withstand stress.
      e. Amniocentesis to obtain fluid samples to determine lecithin/sphingomyelin ratio.
   2. Intrapartum period.
      a. As long as there is evidence of adequate placental function and the infant's response to stress is appropriate, the pregnancy is allowed to progress to term, with an anticipated vaginal delivery.
      b. During labor, blood glucose levels are maintained with IV glucose and regular insulin.
      c. Fetal monitoring during labor.
   3. Postpartum period.
      a. Endocrine and metabolic changes will occur rapidly after delivery.
      b. Insulin requirements for mother will be markedly decreased and will fluctuate over next few weeks.
      c. Mother must go through a period of diabetic re-regulation.
E. Presence of diabetes predisposes the client to an increased incidence of:
   1. Pregnancy-induced hypertension.
   2. Hemorrhage.
   3. Polyhydramnios (increase in volume of amniotic fluid >2000 mL).
   4. Vaginal and urinary tract infections.
   5. Premature delivery.
   6. Intrauterine death in third trimester.
   7. Compromised newborn.
      a. Respiratory distress syndrome.
      b. Hypoglycemia.
      c. Hyperbilirubinemia.
      d. Congenital anomalies: directly associated with the degree of maternal hyperglycemia in the first trimester.

Nursing Interventions (All Types)

> **⚠ NURSING PRIORITY** Evaluating client's control of diabetes: 1. Normal fasting blood glucose 110-115 mg/dL. 2. Two hours after meals or after glucose load, blood glucose is no higher than 140 mg/dL. 3. Client is in good general health and is of normal weight. 4. Glycosylated hemoglobin is less than 7%.

Goal: To return serum glucose to normal level.

A. Initially administer regular insulin on a proportional basis according to need (Box 13-2).

▲

Box 13-2 IMPLICATIONS IN THE ADMINISTRATION OF INSULIN

1. Do not administer cold insulin; it increases pain and causes irritation at injection site.
2. An open 10-mL vial of unrefrigerated insulin should be discarded after 30 days, regardless of how much was used.
3. Do not allow insulin to freeze, and keep it away from heat and sunlight.
4. Insulin pens (NPH and 70/30) should be discarded after 1 week of storage at room temperature. Regular cartridges, which do not contain preservatives, may be left unrefrigerated for up to 1 month.
5. Extreme temperatures (less than 36° F or greater than 86° F) should be avoided.
6. Roll the vial between the palms of the hands to decrease the risk for inconsistent concentration of insulin.
7. The abdomen is the primary site for subcutaneous injections of insulin. Rotate injection sites; injection sites should be 1 inch apart.
8. Abdomen area provides most rapid insulin absorption.
9. Use only insulin syringes to administer insulin.
10. Check expiration date on insulin bottle.
11. When drawing up regular insulin with a long-acting insulin, draw up the regular (clear) insulin before the longer-acting (cloudy) insulin.
12. Regular insulin is used for administration by sliding scale and periods when blood glucose is unstable and difficult to control.
13. Using alcohol to cleanse the skin before injection is not recommended for home care. If used, hold alcohol pad in place for a few seconds but do not massage.
14. Aspirating is not recommended for self-injection.
15. Check dose with another nurse prior to administering.

B. Administer insulin 30 minutes before a meal or snack; do not administer insulin if there is no carbohydrate intake.
C. Maintain adequate fluid intake.
D. Evaluate serum electrolyte levels.
1. Do not administer potassium unless client is voiding or if urine output begins to drop.
2. Generally begin potassium replacement within 1 to 2 hours after starting insulin therapy.
3. Serum potassium levels will be misleading if the client is dehydrated or in a state of ketoacidosis.
E. Evaluate hydration status.
F. Evaluate for clinical manifestations of hypoglycemia and hyperglycemia.

ALERT Monitor hydration status and electrolyte balance.

Goal: To plan and implement a teaching regimen.
A. Assess current level of knowledge regarding diabetes.
B. Evaluate cultural and socioeconomic parameters.
C. Evaluate client's support system (family, significant others).
D. Instruct regarding sick-day guidelines (Box 13-3).

Box 13-3 DIABETIC "SICK DAY" GUIDELINES

If you do not feel well (not eating regularly or have fever, lethargy, nausea and vomiting, etc.):
1. Check your blood glucose every 3 to 4 hours and urine ketones when voiding.
2. Increase your intake of fluids that are high in carbohydrates; every hour, drink fluids that replace electrolytes: fruit drinks, sports drinks, regular soft drinks (not diet beverages).
3. If you cannot eat and you have replaced four to five meals with liquids, notify your health care provider.
4. Get plenty of rest; if possible, have someone stay with you.
5. Do not omit or skip your insulin injections or oral medications unless specifically directed to do so by your health care provider.
6. Follow your health care provider's instructions regarding blood glucose levels and insulin or oral hypoglycemic agents.
7. Stay warm, stay in bed, and do not overexert yourself.
8. Call your health care provider when:
   a. You have been ill for 1 to 2 days without getting any better.
   b. You have been vomiting or had diarrhea for more than 6 hours.
   c. Your urine self-testing shows moderate to large amounts of ketones.
   d. You are taking insulin and your blood glucose level continues to be greater than 240 mg/dL after you have taken two to three supplemental doses of regular insulin (prearranged with your provider).
   e. You are taking insulin and your blood glucose level is less than 60 mg/dL.
   f. You have type 2 diabetes, you are taking oral diabetic medications, and your premeal blood glucose levels are 240 mg/dL or greater for more than 24 hours.
   g. You have signs of severe hyperglycemia (very dry mouth or fruity odor to breath), dehydration, or confusion.
   h. You are sleepier or more tired than normal.
   i. You have stomach or chest pain or any difficulty breathing.
   j. You have any questions or concerns about what you need to do while ill.

ALERT Determine ability of family/support systems to provide care for client. Identify client's and family's strengths.

E. Administration of insulin (see Box 13-2).
1. Correct injection techniques.
2. Rotate injection site (Figure 13-5).
3. Check expiration date on the insulin.
4. Duration and peak action of prescribed insulin.
5. Allow for ample practice time.
6. Administer at the same time each day.
7. Clients following an intensive diabetes therapy program may choose to use an insulin pump or to monitor blood glucose levels four to six times a day and take injections at those times. (Figure 13-6).
   a. The insulin pump is battery-operated; insertion site is changed every 2 to 3 days; pump is refilled and reprogrammed when site is changed.

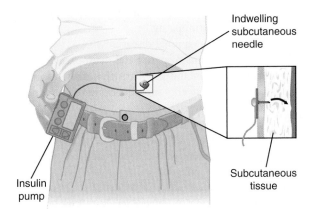

FIGURE 13-5 Sites used for insulin injection. The injection site can affect the onset, peak, and duration of action of the insulin. Insulin injected into the abdomen (area I) is absorbed fastest, followed by insulin injected into the arm (area II) and the leg (area III). (From Black JM, Hawks JH: *Medical-surgical nursing: clinical management for positive outcomes,* ed 8, Philadelphia, 2009, Saunders.)

FIGURE 13-6 Insulin pump. (From Black JM, Hawks JH: *Medical-surgical nursing: clinical management for positive outcomes,* ed 8, Philadelphia, 2009, Saunders.)

b. Delivers continuous infusion of short-acting insulin over a 24-hour period, allowing for tight glucose control.

c. Can deliver bolus of insulin based on excessive carbohydrates ingested.

d. Monitor insertion site for redness and swelling.

8. Disposable needles and syringes may be used for up to 3 days. Good handwashing is critical; needle should be recapped and stored in refrigerator to decrease bacterial growth. (Note: Reusing needles is controversial; today's needles are much thinner and

can bend to form a hook with just one injection, in which case, future use causes more tissue damage. Have client consult with his or her health care provider about this issue.)

9. Insulin pen is a compact portable device that is loaded with insulin; need to change needle with each injection.

F. Oral hypoglycemic agents.

1. Take medication as scheduled; do not skip or add doses.

2. Signs and symptoms of hypoglycemia.

3. Anticipate change in medication with pregnancy.

G. Monitoring blood glucose.

1. Self-monitoring of blood glucose (SMBG)—not necessary to use alcohol to cleanse site.

2. Use side of finger pad rather than near the center. If alternative site is used (i.e., forearm), may require different equipment.

3. Need only a large drop of blood.

H. Exercise.

1. Establish an exercise program.

2. Avoid sporadic exercise.

3. Review instructions regarding adjustment of insulin and food intake to meet requirements of increased activity.

4. Extremities involved in activity should not be used for insulin injection (e.g., arms when playing tennis).

I. Diet (Box 13-4).

1. Regularly scheduled mealtimes.

2. Understanding of food groups and balanced nutrition.

3. Incorporate family tendencies and cultural patterns into prescribed dietary regimen.

4. Provide client and family with written instructions regarding dietary needs.

J. Infection control.

1. Report infections promptly.

2. Insulin requirements may increase with severe infections.

Box 13-4 OLDER ADULT CARE FOCUS

Guidelines for Food Selection

- Avoid canned fruits that are in heavy syrup; select fruit packed in water.
- Include fresh fruits and vegetables and whole-grain cereals and breads to provide adequate dietary fiber to prevent constipation.
- Avoid casseroles, fried foods, sauces and gravies, and sweets.
- Fats (oils, margarines) that are liquid at room temperature are better than those that are solid.
- Read food labels; remember that the highest-content ingredient is listed first.
- Select foods in which the majority of calories do not come from a fat source.

3. Increased problems with vaginitis, urinary tract infections, and skin irritation.

K. Avoid injury.
1. Decreased healing capabilities, especially in lower extremities.
2. Maintain adequate blood supply to extremities; avoid tight-fitting clothing around the legs.
3. Proper foot care (see Chapter 16).

Goal: To prepare the client with diabetes for surgery.

A. Obtain base serum laboratory values for postoperative comparison.
B. Surgery should be scheduled in early morning to decrease problems with diet and insulin replacement.
C. Oral hypoglycemic agents should not be given the morning of surgery.
D. For clients with NPO (nothing by mouth) status who require insulin, an IV of 5% dextrose in water (D_5W) is frequently started.
E. Obtain a blood glucose reading about an hour before sending the client to surgery to make sure he or she is not developing hypoglycemia.

> ⚠ **NURSING PRIORITY** Evaluate intake; do not give insulin to a client on NPO status unless an IV is in place.

Goal: To maintain control of diabetic condition in the client who has had surgery.

A. IV fluids and regular insulin until client is able to take fluids orally.
B. Obtain blood glucose level four to six times a day to determine fluctuations.
C. After glucose levels stabilize, the client can usually resume taking his or her preoperative diabetic medication.
D. Observe for fluctuation of blood glucose immediately after surgery.
E. Avoid urinary bladder catheterization.
F. Evaluate peripheral circulation and prevent skin breakdown.
G. Assess for development of postoperative infections.

Goal: To identify diabetic ketoacidosis and help client return to homeostasis.

A. Establish IV access.
B. Anticipate rapid infusion of normal saline solution or plasma expanders initially, then at a maintenance rate. Administer with caution to clients with cardiac conditions.
C. Administer insulin: use IV drip (regular insulin only) during the acute phase; then administer subcutaneously as blood glucose level begins to decrease.
D. Frequent monitoring of vital signs.
E. Frequent serum glucose checks.
F. Hourly urine measurements: do not administer potassium if urine output is low or dropping.
G. Monitor blood glucose levels frequently (normally every hour).
H. Cardiac monitor to determine presence of dysrhythmias secondary to potassium levels.

I. Monitor serum electrolyte levels, particularly potassium levels.
1. Hyperkalemia may occur initially in response to the acidosis.
2. Hypokalemia occurs about 4 to 6 hours after treatment, as the acidosis is resolving.
J. Evaluate acid-base status.

Goal: To identify HHS and to help client return to homeostasis.

A. Establish IV access.
B. IV infusion to rehydrate client; normal saline solution is frequently used; closely monitor hydration status.
C. Low-dose insulin given intravenously at first to decrease blood glucose level slowly.
D. Evaluate urine output.
E. Monitor serum glucose level.
F. Evaluate acid-base status.
G. Assess client for presence of other chronic health problems.

Home Care

A. Maintain optimum weight.
B. Continue to receive long-term medical care.
C. Notify all health care providers of diagnosis of diabetes; wear medical alert identification.
D. Recognize problems of the cardiovascular system.
1. Peripheral vascular disease.
2. Decreased healing.
3. Increased risk for stroke.
4. Increased risk for myocardial infarction.
5. Presence of retinopathy.
6. Increased risk for renal disease.
E. Recognize problems of peripheral neuropathy.
F. Help client understand problems that diabetes imposes on pregnancy and the subsequent development of a high-risk pregnancy.
G. Help client understand the problem of increased susceptibility to infections.

Goal: To help the client with diabetes maintain homeostasis throughout pregnancy.

A. Prevent infection.
B. Frequent evaluation of glucose levels and monitoring of changes in insulin requirements.
C. Utilization of regular insulin rather than oral hypoglycemic agents.
D. Maintain optimum level of weight gain; labor may be induced, or cesarean delivery may be required if complications are evident.

Goal: To help the client with diabetes maintain homeostasis throughout labor and delivery.

A. IV $D_{10}W$, Ringer's lactate, or D_5 Ringer's lactate to maintain homeostasis during labor, along with continuous infusion of insulin.
B. Fetal monitoring to identify early stages of fetal distress.
C. X-ray pelvimetry to identify cephalopelvic disproportion.
D. Increased incidence of dystocia because of large infants.

E. Frequent evaluation of serum glucose levels (every 2 to 3 hours).

Goal: To help the client with diabetes return to homeostasis during the postpartum period.

A. Anticipate fluctuation in insulin requirements caused by:
   1. Loss of fetal insulin.
   2. Removal of placental influence on insulin.
   3. Changes in metabolic activity.
B. Observe for and monitor for rapid fluctuations in serum glucose levels.
C. Prevent postpartum infection.

Hypoglycemia (Insulin Reaction)

Hypoglycemia is a condition characterized by a decreased serum glucose level, which results in decreased cerebral function.

Assessment

A. Risk factors.
   1. Poorly controlled diabetes.
      a. Too little food.
      b. Increase in exercise without adequate food.
      c. Increase in insulin intake.
   2. Excessive alcohol intake with poor nutrition.
   3. Gastroenteritis or gastroparesis, which may impede absorption of food.
   4. Reflex action of insulin caused by increased carbohydrate intake (Somogyi effect).
B. Clinical manifestations.
   1. Lability of mood.
   2. Emotional changes, confusion.
   3. Headache, lightheadedness, seizures, coma.
   4. Impaired vision.
   5. Tachycardia, hypotension.
   6. Nervousness, tremors.
   7. Diaphoresis.
C. Diagnostics.
   1. Serum glucose below 70 mg/dL.
   2. Negative urine acetone test result.
   3. Normal pH.

Treatment

A. Carbohydrates by mouth if client is alert and can swallow.
   1. Milk preferred in children with a mild reaction; it provides immediate lactose, as well as protein and fat for prolonged action.
   2. Simple sugars for immediate response: orange juice, honey, candy, glucose tablets.
   3. If simple carbohydrates are taken to increase blood glucose, client should plan on eating protein or complex carbohydrates to prevent rebound hypoglycemia.
B. Glucagon can be given intravenously if client is unconscious.

Nursing Interventions

Goal: To increase serum glucose level.

A. Glucose/carbohydrate preparations as indicated.

⊞ NURSING PRIORITY When in doubt of diagnosis of hypoglycemia versus hyperglycemia, administer carbohydrates; severe hypoglycemia can rapidly result in permanent brain damage.

B. Thorough assessment of the client with diabetes for the development of hypoglycemia.

Goal: To help the client identify precipitating causes and activities to prevent the development of hypoglycemia.

A. Instruct the client with diabetes to carry simple carbohydrates.
B. Administer between-meal snacks at the peak action of insulin.
C. Between-meal snacks should limit simple carbohydrates and increase complex carbohydrates and protein.
D. Evaluate the client's understanding of insulin and control of diabetes; reaffirm teaching as appropriate.

Pancreatitis

Pancreatitis is an inflammatory condition of the pancreas.

A. Acute: characterized by an acute inflammatory process; problems range from mild edema to severe hypotension and severe hemorrhagic necrosis.
B. Chronic: characterized by progressive destruction and fibrosis of the pancreas; condition may follow acute pancreatitis but may also occur alone.

Assessment

A. Risk factors/etiology.
   1. Biliary tract obstructive disease, causing reflux of bile secretions.
   2. Alcohol intake precipitating an increase in the secretion of pancreatic enzymes.
   3. Hyperlipidemia is a common cause.
   4. Trauma.
   5. Certain drugs (thiazide diuretics, NSAIDs, estrogens, steroids, salicylates).
B. Clinical manifestations.
   1. Severe constant midepigastric pain.
      a. Radiates to the back or flank area.
      b. Exacerbated by eating.
   2. Acute.
      a. Persistent vomiting.
      b. Low-grade fever.
      c. Hypotension and tachycardia.
      d. Jaundice, if common bile duct is obstructed.
      e. Abdominal distention.
      f. Cullen's sign: periumbilical discoloration.
      g. Grey Turner's sign: flank ecchymosis.
   3. Chronic.
      a. Decrease in weight.
      b. Mild jaundice.
      c. Steatorrhea.
      d. Abdominal distention and tenderness.
      e. Hyperglycemia.

C. Diagnostics.
1. Increase in serum amylase (hallmark) and lipase levels.
2. Increase in urine amylase level.
3. Hyperglycemia.
4. Leukocytosis.
5. Elevated C reactive protein.
6. Hypocalcemia.
7. Ultrasonography.
8. Computed tomography scan.

Treatment

A. Medications.
1. Analgesics.
2. Antibiotics.
B. Decrease pancreatic stimulus.
1. NPO status; IV fluids.
2. Nasogastric suction.
3. Bed rest.
4. Diet: (if not NPO) low-fat, high-carbohydrate.
C. Surgical intervention to eliminate precipitating cause (biliary tract obstruction).

Nursing Interventions

Nursing interventions are the same for the client with acute pancreatitis and for the client with chronic pancreatitis experiencing an acute episode.
Goal: To relieve pain.
A. Administer analgesics; pain control is essential (restlessness may cause pancreatic stimulation and further secretion of enzymes).
B. Place client in side lying position with knees drawn up to chest or in semi-Fowler's position with knees flexed toward the chest.
C. Evaluate precipitating cause.
Goal: To decrease pancreatic stimulus.
A. Bed rest.
B. Maintain NPO status initially.
C. Maintain nasogastric suctioning.
D. Small frequent feedings when food is allowed.
E. Pain control.
Goal: To prevent complications.
A. Identify electrolyte imbalances, especially hypocalcemia.
B. Maintain adequate hydration.
C. Maintain respiratory status; problems occur because of pain and ascites.
D. Assess for hypoglycemia and development of diabetes.

Home Care

A. Avoid all alcohol intake.
B. Know signs of hyperglycemia and development of diabetes; understand when to return for evaluation of blood glucose level.
C. Bland diet, low in fat, high in carbohydrates (protein recommendations vary).
D. Replacement of pancreatic enzymes.

Cancer of the Pancreas

The majority of tumors occur in the head of the pancreas. As tumors grow, the bile ducts are obstructed, causing jaundice. Tumors in the body of the pancreas frequently do not cause symptoms until growth is advanced. Cancer of the pancreas has a poor prognosis.

Assessment

A. Risk factors/etiology.
1. Incidence is higher in men 45 to 65 years of age.
2. History of chronic pancreatitis is common.
3. Cigarette smoke (3 to 4 times more common among smokers)
B. Clinical manifestations.
1. Dull, aching abdominal pain.
2. Ascites.
3. Nausea, vomiting.
4. Anorexia and progressive weight loss.
5. Jaundice.
6. Clay-colored stools.
7. Dark, frothy urine.
C. Diagnostics.
1. Increased carcinoembryonic antigen (CEA) level.
2. Ultrasonography.
3. CT scan.

Treatment

A. Surgery: Whipple's procedure (radical pancreatic duodenectomy).
B. Radiation therapy.
C. Chemotherapy.

Nursing Interventions

Goal: To maintain homeostasis (see Nursing Interventions for pancreatitis).
Goal: To provide preoperative nursing measures if surgery is indicated.
A. Maintain nasogastric suctioning; assess for adequate hydration.
B. Control hyperglycemia.
C. Assess cardiac and respiratory stability.
D. Assess for development of thrombophlebitis.
Goal: To promote comfort, prevent complications, and maintain homeostasis in client who has undergone Whipple's procedure.
A. General postoperative care (see Chapter 3). Extensive surgical resection of the pancreas and surrounding tissue.
B. Evaluate for hypercoagulable state as well as bleeding tendencies.
C. Monitor for fluctuation in serum glucose levels.
D. Maintain NPO status and nasogastric suction until peristalsis returns.
E. Encourage adequate nutrition when appropriate.
1. Decrease fats and increase carbohydrates.
2. Small, frequent feedings.

F. Closely observe for development of problems from thromboemboli to coagulation problems; surgery and immobility.

 Home Care

A. Evaluate for bouts of anxiety and depression caused by severity of illness and prognosis (see Chapter 10).
B. Assist client in setting realistic goals.
C. Encourage ventilation of feelings.
D. Discuss methods for pain control.

> **❗ NURSING PRIORITY** Clients experiencing problems of the adrenal medulla have severe fluctuations in blood pressure related to the levels of catecholamines.

PHYSIOLOGY OF THE ADRENALS

The adrenal glands are located at the apex of each kidney.
A. Adrenal medulla: secretes catecholamines, epinephrine, and norepinephrine; under the influence of the sympathetic nervous system.
B. Adrenal cortex: main body of the adrenal gland; responsible for the secretion of glucocorticoids, mineralocorticoids, and adrenal sex hormones (androgens and estrogen); adrenal cortical function is essential for life (Table 13-5).
C. Function of the adrenal cortex is controlled by the negative feedback mechanisms regulating hormone release; pituitary gland secretes adrenocorticotropic hormone (ACTH), which in turn regulates hormone release of the adrenal cortex.

🦕 System Assessment

A. Adrenal medulla.
   1. Evaluate changes in blood pressure.
   2. Assess for changes in metabolic rate.
B. Adrenal cortex.
   1. Evaluate changes in weight.
   2. Evaluate changes in skin color and texture, as well as the presence and distribution of body hair.
   3. Assess cardiovascular system for instability, as evidenced by a labile blood pressure and cardiac output.
   4. Evaluate GI discomfort.
   5. Assess fluid and electrolyte changes from effects of mineralocorticoids and glucocorticoids.
   6. Assess for changes in glucose metabolism.
   7. Assess for changes in reproductive system and in sexual activity.
   8. Evaluate changes in muscle mass.

Table 13-5	**SUMMARY OF ADRENAL HORMONES**	
Hormone	*Site of Action*	*Function*
Adrenal cortex		

Mineralocorticoids* (aldosterone)	Kidney (renal tubule)	1. Increased sodium ion absorption.
		 2. Decreased potassium absorption.
		 3. Conditions causing an increase in aldosterone secretion:
		   a. Decrease in serum sodium.
		   b. Shock.

Glucocorticoids† (cortisol, hydrocortisone)	All tissues Metabolism of all food; enable individual to withstand stress	1. Increased rate of gluconeogenesis. 2. Catabolic effect on protein metabolism. 3. Antiinflammatory effect. 4. Increased secretion during times of increased body stress.
Androgens: sex hormones‡	Stimulate reproduction organs to secrete gonadal hormones	1. Responsible for secondary sexual characteristics. 2. Phases of menstrual cycle. 3. Uterine changes in pregnancy.
Females: estrogen and progesterone (ovaries)		
Males: testosterone (testes)		1. Development and maintenance of secondary sex characteristics. 2. Spermatogenesis.
Adrenal medulla§		
Epinephrine	Cardiac muscle	1. Stimulation of sympathetic nervous system. 2. Produces increase in systolic blood pressure.
Norepinephrine	Organs innervated by sympathetic nervous system	1. Increases peripheral resistance (i.e., increase in blood pressure).

*Mineralocorticoids are primarily controlled by the renin-angiotensin-aldosterone system.
†Glucocorticoids are primarily controlled by secretion of adrenocorticotropic hormone from the anterior pituitary.
‡Androgens are primarily controlled by secretions from the pituitary gland.
§Adrenal medulla hormones are primarily controlled by the sympathetic division of the autonomic nervous system.

DISORDERS OF THE ADRENALS

Pheochromocytoma

Pheochromocytoma is a rare disorder of the adrenal medulla characterized by a tumor that secretes an excess of epinephrine and norepinephrine.

A. An increase in these catecholamines produces vasoconstriction, with a precipitant increase in blood pressure, glycogenolysis, and cardiac workload.

B. Condition may become evident during pregnancy, as increasing uterine pressure precipitates problems.

Assessment

A. Clinical manifestations.
   1. Persistent or paroxysmal hypertension.
   2. Palpitations, tachycardia.
   3. Hyperglycemia.
   4. Diaphoresis.
   5. Nervousness, apprehension.
   6. Headache.

B. Diagnostics (see Appendix 13-1).
   1. Increase in urinary excretion of total free catecholamine.
   2. Increase in urinary excretion of vanillylmandelic acid and metanephrine.
   3. Serum assay of catecholamine.
   4. Magnetic resonance imaging, computed tomography scan.

C. Treatment.
   1. Medications.
      a. Antihypertensive medications (alpha-adrenergic blockers to lower blood pressure quickly).
      b. Antidysrhythmic medications.
      c. Potassium replacement.
   2. Surgery: removal of the tumor is the treatment of choice.

Nursing Interventions

Goal: To decrease client's hypertension and provide preoperative nursing measures as appropriate (see Chapter 3).

A. Decrease intake of stimulants.

B. Sedate as indicated.

C. Maintain calm, quiet environment.

D. Assess vital signs frequently.

Goal: To help client return to homeostasis after adrenalectomy.

A. Maintain normal blood pressure the first 24 to 48 hours after surgery; client is at increased risk for hemorrhage or severe hypotensive episode.
   1. Assess for blood pressure changes caused by catecholamine imbalance (both hypertension and hypotension).
   2. Administer analgesics judiciously.
   3. Administer corticosteroids as indicated.
   4. Maintain quiet, cool environment.
   5. Maintain IV fluid administration.

B. Assess for hypoglycemia.

C. Tendency toward hemorrhagic problems.

D. Monitor renal perfusion and urinary output.

E. Assess for problems of adrenal insufficiency.

Goal: To maintain health after adrenalectomy.

A. Continued medical follow-up care.

B. If both adrenals are removed, client will require lifelong replacement of adrenal hormones.

Addison's Disease (Adrenocortical Insufficiency/Adrenal Hypofunction)

Addison's disease is caused by a decrease in secretion of the adrenal cortex hormones.

A. Decreased physiologic response to stress, vascular insufficiency, and hypoglycemia.

B. Decrease in aldosterone secretions (mineralocorticoids), which normally promote concentration of sodium and water and excretion of potassium.

C. May cause an alteration in adrenal androgen secretion necessary for secondary sex characteristics.

Assessment

A. Risk factors/etiology.
   1. An autoimmunity-induced problem.
   2. Occurs after bilateral adrenalectomy.
   3. Abrupt withdrawal from long-term corticosteroid therapy.
   4. Adrenal crisis may be precipitated by client's failure to take medications.
   5. Acquired immunodeficiency syndrome (AIDS) is increasingly being identified as a cause of adrenal insufficiency.
   6. Increased emotional stress without appropriate hormone replacement.
   7. Tuberculosis.
   8. Septicemia.

B. Clinical manifestations (development of symptoms requires loss of 90% of both adrenal cortices).
   1. Onset is insidious; client may go for weeks to months before diagnosis is made.
   2. Fatigue, weakness.
   3. Weight loss.
   4. GI disturbances.
   5. Bronze pigmentation of the skin.
   6. Postural hypotension.
   7. Hyponatremia, hyperkalemia.
   8. Hypoglycemia.
   9. Adrenal crisis (Addisonian crisis).
      a. Profound fatigue.
      b. Dehydration.
      c. Vascular collapse (cyanosis and signs of shock: pallor, anxiety, weak/rapid pulse, tachypnea, and low blood pressure).

ALERT Determine whether vital signs are abnormal (e.g., hypotension, hypertension); notify others of change in the client's condition.

C. Diagnostics (see Appendix 13-1).
   1. ACTH stimulation test.
   2. Decreased serum sodium level and increased serum potassium and BUN levels.
   3. Plasma ACTH level.

Treatment

Replace adrenal hormones.

Nursing Interventions

Goal: To help client return to homeostasis.
A. Initiate and maintain IV infusion of normal saline solution.
B. Administer large doses of corticosteroids through IV bolus initially, then titrate in a diluted solution.
C. Frequent evaluation of vital signs.
D. Assess sodium and water retention.
E. Evaluate serum potassium levels.
F. Keep client immobilized and quiet.

> **! NURSING PRIORITY** If any client is experiencing difficulty with maintaining adequate blood pressure, do not move the client unless absolutely necessary. Avoid all unnecessary nursing procedures until the client's condition is stabilized.

Goal: To safely take steroid replacements (see Appendix 6-7).
A. Administer steroid preparations with food or an antacid.
B. Evaluate for edema and fluid retention.
C. Assess serum sodium and potassium levels.
D. Check daily weight.
E. Increase intake of protein and carbohydrates.
F. Evaluate for hypoglycemia.
G. Observe for cushingoid symptoms.

Home Care

A. Lifelong steroid therapy is necessary.
B. Dosage of steroids may need to be increased in times of additional stress.
C. Infection, diaphoresis, and injury will necessitate an increase in the need for steroids and may precipitate a crisis state.
D. Report gastric distress because it may be caused by steroids.
E. Carry a medical identification card.

Cushing's Syndrome (Adrenal Cortex Hypersecretion/Hypercortisolism)

Cushing's syndrome occurs as a result of excess levels of adrenal cortex hormones (primarily glucocorticoids) and, to a lesser extent, androgen and aldosterone (see Table 13-5).

> **ALERT** Evaluate client's use of medications. Implement procedures to counteract adverse effects of medication. The most common cause of Cushing's syndrome is long-term steroid therapy for chronic conditions. Many chronic conditions necessitate the use of long-term steroid therapy.

Assessment

A. Risk factors/etiology.
   1. More common in women (20 to 40 years old).
   2. Pituitary hypersecretion.
   3. A benign pituitary tumor.
   4. Iatrogenic: most often a result of long-term steroid therapy.
B. Clinical manifestations (Figure 13-7).
   1. Marked change in personality (emotional lability), irritability.
   2. Changes in appearance.
      a. Moon face.
      b. Deposit of fat on the back.
      c. Thin skin, purple striae.
      d. Truncal obesity with thin extremities.
      e. Bruises and petechiae.
   3. Persistent hyperglycemia.
   4. GI distress from increased acid production.
   5. Osteoporosis.
   6. Increased susceptibility to infection.
   7. Sodium and fluid retention; potassium depletion.
   8. Hypertension.
   9. Changes in secondary sexual characteristics.
      a. Amenorrhea (females).
      b. Hirsutism (females).
      c. Gynecomastia (males).
   10. Impotence or decreased libido.
C. Diagnostics (see Appendix 13-1).
   1. Increased serum sodium and decreased serum potassium levels.
   2. Hyperglycemia.
   3. Increased plasma cortisol levels.
   4. Loss of diurnal variation in cortisone levels.
   5. Low-dose and high-dose dexamethasone suppression test.

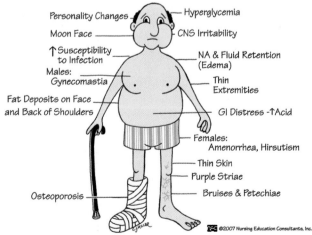

CUSHING'S SYNDROME

Personality Changes — Hyperglycemia
Moon Face — CNS Irritability
↑Susceptibility to Infection
Males: Gynecomastia — NA & Fluid Retention (Edema)
Fat Deposits on Face and Back of Shoulders — Thin Extremities
— GI Distress -↑Acid
Females: Amenorrhea, Hirsutism
— Thin Skin
— Purple Striae
Osteoporosis — Bruises & Petechiae

©2007 Nursing Education Consultants, Inc.

FIGURE 13-7 Cushing's syndrome. (From Zerwekh J, Claborn J: *Memory notebook of nursing*, vol 1, ed 4, Ingram, Texas 2008, Nursing Education Consultants.)

D. Complications.
   1. Congestive heart failure, hypertension.
   2. Pathologic fractures, psychosis.

Treatment
Treatment depends on the cause of the problem.

Nursing Interventions
Goal: To assist client to manage hormone imbalance.
A. Restrict sodium and water intake.
B. Monitor fluid and electrolyte levels.
C. Evaluate for hyperglycemia.
D. Assess for GI disturbances.
E. Prevent infection.
Goal: To prevent complications.
A. Excessive sodium and water retention: monitor for edema, hypertension, congestive heart failure.

B. Potassium depletion: monitor for cardiac arrhythmias.
C. Evaluate client's ability to cope with change in body image.
D. Evaluate for thromboembolic problems.
E. Predisposed to fractures; promote weight bearing; monitor for joint and bone pain; promote home safety.

 Home Care

A. Stress the need for continuous health care.
B. Encourage continuation of activities.
C. Have the client demonstrate an understanding of the medication regimen.
D. Help the client identify methods of coping with problems of therapy.
E. Have the client demonstrate an understanding of specific problems for which he or she needs to notify the physician.

Appendix 13-1   ENDOCRINE DIAGNOSTICS

DIAGNOSTIC TEST	NORMAL	CLINICAL/NURSING IMPLICATIONS
Thyroid		
Thyroxine (T_4)	5-12 mcg/dL Increased in hyperthyroidism, decreased in hypothyroidism	1. Stimulation of the thyroid gland by TSH will initiate the release of stored thyroid hormone.
Triiodothyronine (T_3)	70-220 ng/dL Increased in hyperthyroidism, Decreased in hypothyroidism	2. When T_3 and T_4 are low, TSH secretion increases. 3. T_3 and T_4 are used to confirm abnormal TSH.
Thyroid-stimulating hormone (TSH)	0.2-5.4 mIU/L Increased in hypothyroidism Decreased in primary hyperthyroidism	
Neonatal thyroxine (T_4)	Normal levels vary with age from 1 day to 120 days 1-3 days: 11-22 mcg/dL 1-2 wk: 10-16 mcg/dL 1-4 mo: 8-16 mcg/dL	1. Positive test result is associated with hypothyroidism. 2. Procedure is done by means of a heel puncture on infant. 3. Levels of neonatal T_4 are not interpreted in same terms as serum T_4 values; this is a completely different test.
Pancreas		
Serum glucose	Less than 100 mg/dL	1. Test is timed to rule out diabetes by determining rate of glucose absorption from serum.
Oral glucose tolerance test	1 hr: less than 200 mg/dL 2 hr: less than 140 mg/dL	2. In healthy person, insulin response to large dose of glucose is immediate. 3. Insulin and oral hypoglycemic agents should not be administered before test.

Appendix 13-1 ENDOCRINE DIAGNOSTICS—cont'd

DIAGNOSTIC TEST	NORMAL	CLINICAL/NURSING IMPLICATIONS
Glucose fasting blood sugar (FBS) Also called *fasting blood glucose (FBG)* and *fasting plasma glucose (FPG)*	Same as serum glucose (>126 mg/dL is diagnostic for diabetes)	1. Used as a screening test for problems of metabolism. 2. Maintain client in fasting state for 12 hours until blood is drawn. 3. If client is a known diabetic and experiences dizziness, weakness, or fainting, draw blood for determination of glucose level.
Glycosylated hemoglobin (HbA$_{1c}$)	Nondiabetic range is usually 4%-6% 2%-6.4% considered good diabetic control (goal is 7% or less) >8% considered poor diabetic control	1. More accurate test of diabetic control, because it measures glucose attached to hemoglobin (indicates overall control for past 90-120 days, which is the lifespan of the RBC).

ALERT Frequently, the level of the FBS is given in a question, and it is necessary to evaluate the level and determine the appropriate nursing intervention.

2-hour postprandial blood sugar	65-139 mg/dL	1. Involves measuring the serum glucose 2 hours after a meal; results are significantly increased with diabetes.
Serum amylase	30-200 U/L	1. Used to evaluate pancreatic cell damage. 2. Other intestinal conditions and inflammatory conditions cause increase.
Serum lipase	Normal values vary with method; elevated is abnormal	1. Appears in serum after damage to pancreas.
Urine sugar (Clinistix, Clinitest, Labstix)	Negative for glucose	1. Use fresh double-voided specimen. 2. A rough indicator of serum glucose levels. 3. Results may be altered by various medications.
Ketone bodies (acetone)	Negative	1. Ketone bodies occur in the urine before there is significant increase in serum ketones. 2. Use freshly voided urine.
Urinary amylase	2-hr specimen 2-34 U/hr 24-hr specimen 24-408 U/24 hr	1. In pancreatic injury, more amylase enters blood and is excreted in urine. 2. May be done on a 2-hr or a 24-hr urine specimen.
Pituitary Growth hormone (GH)	<5 ng/mL in men <18 ng/mL in women	1. NPO after midnight. 2. Maintain bed rest until serum sample is drawn.
Osmolarity urine Osmolarity serum	300 to 900 mOsm/kg of water 285 to 295 mOsm/kg of water	1. Used in evaluating ADH. 2. Do serum and urine tests at same time and compare results. 3. Normally, urine osmolarity should be higher than serum.
Adrenal Medulla Urinary vanillylmandelic acid (VMA)	<8 mg in 24 hr Increased with pheochromocytoma	1. Depending on how test is measured, there may be dietary and medication restrictions. 2. 24-hr urine collection.

Continued

Appendix 13-1 ENDOCRINE DIAGNOSTICS—cont'd

DIAGNOSTIC TEST	NORMAL	CLINICAL/NURSING IMPLICATIONS
Urine catecholamines: Epinephrine, norepinephrine	Increased in conditions that precipitate increase in catecholamine secretion	Same as for VMA.
Dopamine Metanephrine Normetanephrine		
ACTH stimulation test	Increase in plasma cortisol levels by more than 7-10 mcg/dL above baseline	1. ACTH is given as IM or IV bolus, and samples are drawn at 30 and 60 min to evaluate ability of adrenal glands to secrete steroids.
Adrenal Cortex		
ACTH suppression (dexamethasone suppression test)	Normal suppression; 50% decrease in cortisone production (cortisol level <3 mcg/dL)	1. An overnight test: a small amount of dexamethasone is administered in the evening, and serum and urine are evaluated in the morning; extensive test may cover 6 days. 2. Cushing's syndrome is ruled out if suppression is normal.
Plasma cortisol levels for diurnal variations	Secretion high in early morning, decreased in evening. 8:00 a.m.: 5-23 mcg/dL 4:00 p.m.: 3-13 mcg/dL	1. Elevation in plasma cortisol levels occurs in the morning and significant decrease in evening and night—a diurnal variation.
24-hour urine for 17-hydroxycorticosteroids and 17-ketosteroids	Male: 3-10 mg/24 hr Female: 2-8 mg/24 hr Child under 15 yr: <4.5 mg/24 hr	1. Increase in urine levels indicates hyperadrenal function.

ACTH, Adrenocorticotropic hormone; *ADH*, antidiuretic hormone; *NPO*, nothing by mouth; *RBC*, red blood cell.

Appendix 13-2 MEDICATIONS USED IN ENDOCRINE DISORDERS

MEDICATIONS	SIDE EFFECTS	NURSING IMPLICATIONS
ADH Replacement		
Desmopressin **(DDAVP):** nasal spray, PO, IV, subQ	Excessive water retention, headache, nausea, flushing	1. Monitor daily weight; correlate with intake and output.
Vasopressin **(Pitressin):** IM, subQ Lypressin **(Diapid):** nasal spray		2. Vasopressin more likely to cause adverse cardiovascular and thromboembolic problems.

Antithyroid Agents Inhibit production of thyroid hormone; do not inactivate thyroid hormone in circulating blood. They are not reliable for long-term inhibition of thyroid hormone production.

Propylthiouracil **(PTU):** PO	Agranulocytosis; abdominal discomfort; nausea, vomiting, diarrhea; crosses placenta	1. May increase anticoagulation effect of heparin and oral anticoagulants.
Methimazole **(Tapazole):** PO	Same; crosses placenta more rapidly	2. May be combined with iodine preparations. 3. Monitor CBC. 4. Store **Tapazole** in light-sensitive container. 5. May be used before surgery or treatment with radioactive iodine.
Lugol's solution: PO	Inhibits synthesis and release of thyroid hormone	1. Administer in fluid to decrease unpleasant taste. 2. May be used to decrease vascularity of thyroid gland before surgery.
Saturated solution of potassium iodide (SSKI)		

Appendix 13-2   MEDICATIONS USED IN ENDOCRINE DISORDERS—cont'd

MEDICATIONS	SIDE EFFECTS	NURSING IMPLICATIONS
Radioactive Iodine Accumulates in the thyroid gland; causes partial or total destruction of thyroid gland through radiation.		
Iodine (I^{123} or I^{131}): PO	Discomfort in thyroid area; bone marrow depression Desired effect: permanent hypothyroidism	1. Increase fluids immediately after treatment, because radioactive isotope is excreted in the urine. 2. Therapeutic dose of radioactive iodine is low; no radiation safety precautions are required. 3. Contraindicated in pregnancy.
Thyroid Replacements Replace thyroid hormone.		
Levothyroxine sodium (**Levothroid, Levoxyl, Levo-T, Novothyrox, Synthroid**): PO, IM, IV Liothyronine (**Cytomel, Triostat**)	Overdose may result in symptoms of hyperthyroidism: tachycardia, heat intolerance, nervousness	1. Be careful in reading exact name on label of medications; micrograms and milligrams are used as units of measure. 2. Generally taken once a day before breakfast. 3. Within 3-4 days, begin to see improvement; maximum effect in 4-6 weeks.
Pancreatic Enzymes Replacement enzymes to aid in digestion of starch, protein, and fat.		
Pancreatin (**Creon**): PO Pancrelipase (**Pancrease, Pangestyme, Ultrase, Viokase**): PO	GI upset and irritation of mucous membranes	1. Client is usually on a high-protein, high-carbohydrate, low-fat diet. 2. Enteric-coated tablets should not be crushed or chewed. 3. Pancreatin may be given before, during, or within 1 hr after meals. 4. Pancrelipase is given just before or with each meal or snack.
Antihypoglycemic Agent Increases plasma glucose levels and relaxes smooth muscles.		
Glucagon: IM, IV, subQ	None significant	1. Watch for symptoms of hypoglycemia and treat with food first, if conscious. 2. Client usually awakens in 5-20 min after receiving glucagon. 3. If client does not respond, anticipate IV glucose to be given.

Oral Hypoglycemic Agents Stimulate beta cells to secrete more insulin; enhance body utilization of available insulin (see Figure 13-3 for insulin).

General Nursing Implications
— Dose should be decreased for older adults.
— Use with caution in clients with renal and hepatic impairment.
— All oral hypoglycemic agents are contraindicated in pregnant clients.
— All clients should be carefully observed for symptoms of hypoglycemia and hyperglycemia.
— Medications should be taken in the morning.
— Long-term therapy may result in decreased effectiveness.

Sulfonylureas Stimulate the pancreas to make more insulin.

Chlorpropamide (**Diabinase**): PO Glipizide (**Glucotrol**): PO Glyburide (**Micronase, DiaBeta**): PO Glimepiride (**Amaryl**): PO Gliclazide (**Diamicron**): PO Tolbutamide (**Orinase**): PO Tolazamide (**Tolinase**): PO	Hypoglycemia, jaundice, GI disturbance, skin reactions (fewer side effects with second-generation agents)	1. Tolbutamide has shortest duration of action; requires multiple daily doses. 2. Glyburide has a long duration of action. 3. Interact with calcium channel blockers, oral contraceptives, glucocorticoids, phenothiazines, and thiazide diuretics.

Continued

Appendix 13-2 MEDICATIONS USED IN ENDOCRINE DISORDERS—cont'd

MEDICATIONS	SIDE EFFECTS	NURSING IMPLICATIONS
Biguanides Decrease sugar production in the liver and help the muscles use insulin to break down sugar.		
Metformin **(Glucophage):** PO	Dizziness, nausea, back pain, possible metallic taste	1. Administered with meals. 2. Is beneficial effect on lowering lipids. 3. Weight gain may occur.
Alpha-Glucosidase Inhibitors Slow down body absorption of sugar after eating; also known as *starch blockers.*		
Acarbose **(Precose):** PO Miglitol **(Glyset):** PO	Diarrhea, flatulence, abdominal pain	1. Take at beginning of meals; not effective on an empty stomach. 2. Acarbose is contraindicated in clients with inflammatory bowel disease. 3. Frequently given with sulfonylureas to increase effectiveness of both medications.
Thiazolidinediones Enhance insulin utilization at receptor sites (they do *not* increase insulin production); also referred to as *insulin sensitizers.*		
Pioglitazone **(Actos):** PO Rosiglitazone **(Avandia):** PO	Weight gain, edema	1. May affect liver function; monitor LFTs. 2. Postmenopausal women may resume ovulation; pregnancy may occur.
Meglitinides (Nonsulfonylurea Insulin Secretagogues) Stimulate release of insulin from beta cells.		
Nateglinide **(Starlix):** PO Repaglinide **(Prandin):** PO	Weight gain, hypoglycemia	1. Rapid onset and short duration. 2. Take 30 min before meals (or right at mealtime). 3. Do not take if meal is missed.
Dipeptidyl Peptidase-4 (DDP-4) Inhibitors Enhance the incretin system, stimulate release of insulin for beta cells, and decrease hepatic glucose production.		
Sitagliptin **(Januvia):** PO Vildagliptin **(Galvus):** PO	Upper respiratory tract infection, sore throat, headache, diarrhea	1. Should not be used in type 1 diabetes or for the treatment of diabetic ketoacidosis.
Injectable Drugs for Diabetes **Amylin Mimetics** Complement the effects of insulin by delaying gastric emptying and suppressing glucagon secretion.		
Pramlintide **(Symlin):** subQ	Hypoglycemia, nausea, injection site reactions	1. Teach client to take other oral medications at least 1 hour before taking or 2 hours after, because of delayed gastric emptying. 2. Injected into thigh or abdomen. 3. Cannot be mixed with insulin. **⊞ NURSING PRIORITY** Can cause severe hypoglycemia when used with insulin; usually occurs within 3 hours following injection.
Incretin Mimetics Stimulate release of insulin, decrease glucagon secretion, decrease gastric emptying, and suppress appetite.		
Exenatide **(Byetta):** subQ	Hypoglycemia, nausea, vomiting, diarrhea, headache, possible weight loss	1. Used in conjunction with metformin. 2. Monitor weight. 3. Not indicated for use with insulin.

CBC, Complete blood count; *GI,* gastrointestinal; *IM,* intramuscularly; *IV,* intravenously; *LFTs,* liver function tests; *PO,* by mouth (orally); *subQ,* subcutaneously.

Study Questions Endocrine System

More questions on companion CD!
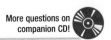

1. A client is receiving NPH insulin 20 units subcutaneously at 0700 hours daily. At 1500 hours, the nurse finds the client apparently asleep. How would the nurse know whether the client were having a hypoglycemic reaction?
   1 Feel the client and bed for dampness.
   2 Observe the client for Kussmaul respirations.
   3 Smell the client's breath for acetone odor.
   4 Check the client's pupils for dilation.

2. The nurse is caring for a client postoperative thyroidectomy. What would be an important nursing intervention?
   1 Have the client speak every 5 to 10 minutes if hoarseness is present.
   2 Provide a low-calcium diet to prevent hypercalcemia.
   3 Check the dressing at the back of the neck for bleeding.
   4 Apply a soft cervical collar to restrict neck movement.

3. The nurse is assigned to care for a new client with acute pancreatitis. What would the nurse anticipate finding during the assessment of this client?
   1 Steatorrhea, abdominal pain, fever
   2 Fever, hypoglycemia, dehydration
   3 Melena, persistent vomiting, hyperactive bowel sounds
   4 Hypoactive bowel sounds, decreased amylase and lipase levels

4. A client is found to be comatose and hypoglycemic with a blood glucose level of 50 mg/dL. What nursing action is implemented *first*?
   1 Infuse 1000 mL of D_5W over a 12-hour period.
   2 Administer 50% glucose intravenously.
   3 Check the client's urine for the presence of sugar and acetone.
   4 Encourage the client to drink orange juice with added sugar.

5. A nurse knows the clinical manifestations of a client with Addison's disease include which of the following? Select all that apply.
   _____ 1 Weight gain
   _____ 2 Hypothermia
   _____ 3 Hypertension
   _____ 4 Melanosis of skin
   _____ 5 Hypotension
   _____ 6 Hypernatremia

6. A client is prescribed levothyroxine (Synthroid) daily. What is the most important instruction to give the client for administration of this drug?
   1 Taper the dose and discontinue if mental and emotional statuses stabilize.
   2 Take it at bedtime to avoid the side effects of nausea and flatus.
   3 Call the doctor immediately at the onset of palpitations or nervousness.
   4 Decrease the intake of juices and fruits with high potassium and calcium contents.

7. What will the nurse teach the client with diabetes regarding exercise in his or her treatment program?
   1 During exercise the body will use carbohydrates for energy production, which in turn will decrease the need for insulin.
   2 With an increase in activity, the body will use more carbohydrates; therefore more insulin will be required.
   3 The increase in activity results in an increase in the use of insulin; therefore the client should decrease his or her carbohydrate intake.
   4 Exercise will improve pancreatic circulation and stimulate the islets of Langerhans to increase the production of intrinsic insulin.

8. The nurse is caring for a client who has exophthalmos associated with her thyroid disease. What is the cause of exophthalmos?
   1 Fluid and edema in the retro-orbital tissues, which increases pressure behind the eyes
   2 Impaired vision, which causes the client to squint in order to focus
   3 Increased intraocular pressure from an increase in circulating thyroid
   4 Decrease in extraocular eye movements, which results in the "thyroid stare"

9. What is a characteristic symptom of hypoglycemia that should alert the nurse to an early insulin reaction?
   1 Diaphoresis
   2 Drowsiness
   3 Severe thirst
   4 Coma

10. A client is scheduled for a routine glycosylated hemoglobin (HbA_{1c}) test. What is important for the nurse to tell the client before this test?
    1 Drink only water after midnight and come to the clinic early in the morning.
    2 Eat a normal breakfast and be at the clinic 2 hours later.
    3 Expect to be at the clinic for several hours because of the multiple blood draws.
    4 Come to the clinic at the earliest convenience to have blood drawn.

11. A client has been receiving inhalation vasopressin therapy. What will the nurse evaluate to determine the therapeutic response to this medication?
    1. Urine specific gravity
    2. Blood glucose
    3. Vital signs
    4. Oxygen saturation levels

12. A client with a diagnosis of type 2 diabetes has been ordered a course of prednisone for her severe arthritic pain. An expected change that requires close monitoring by the nurse is:
    1. Increased blood glucose level
    2. Increased platelet aggregation
    3. Increased creatinine clearance
    4. Increased ketone level in urine

13. The nurse is performing an assessment on a client who has been receiving long-term steroid therapy. What would the nurse expect to find during the assessment?
    1. Jaundice
    2. Flank pain
    3. Bulging eyes
    4. Central obesity

14. It is important for the nurse to teach the client which of the following about metformin (Glucophage)?
    1. It may cause nocturia.
    2. It should be taken at night.
    3. It should be taken with meals.
    4. It may increase the effects of aspirin.

15. A nurse assessing a client with syndrome of inappropriate antidiuretic hormone (SIADH) would expect to find which laboratory values?
    1. Serum sodium = 150 mEq/L and low urine osmolality
    2. Serum potassium = 5 mEq/L and low serum osmolality
    3. Serum sodium = 120 mEq/L and low serum osmolality
    4. Serum potassium = 3 mEq/L and high serum osmolality

16. A priority nursing diagnosis for a client admitted to the hospital with a diagnosis of diabetes insipidus is:
    1. Disturbed sleep pattern related to nocturia
    2. Activity intolerance related to muscle weakness
    3. Excess fluid volume related to intake greater than output
    4. Risk for impaired skin integrity related to generalized edema

17. A client admitted with a pheochromocytoma returns from the operating room after adrenalectomy. The nurse should carefully assess this client for:
    1. Hypokalemia
    2. Hyperglycemia
    3. Marked sodium and water retention
    4. Marked fluctuations in blood pressure

18. When caring for a client in a thyroid crisis, the nurse would question an order for:
    1. IV fluids
    2. Propranolol (Inderal)
    3. Propylthiouracil
    4. A hyperthermia blanket

19. Which medication will the nurse have available for emergency treatment of tetany in the client who has had a thyroidectomy?
    1. Calcium chloride
    2. Potassium chloride
    3. Magnesium sulfate
    4. Sodium bicarbonate

20. A client with diabetes receives a combination of regular and NPH insulin at 0700 hours. The nurse teaches the client to be alert for signs of hypoglycemia at:
    1. 12 p.m. to 1 p.m. (1200 to 1300 hours)
    2. 11 a.m. and 5 p.m. (1100 and 1700 hours)
    3. 10 a.m. and 10 p.m. (1000 and 2200 hours)
    4. 8 a.m. and 11 a.m. (0800 and 1100 hours)

Answers and rationales to these questions are in the section at the end of the book titled Chapter Study Questions: Answers and Rationales.

CHAPTER FOURTEEN

Hematologic System

PHYSIOLOGY OF THE BLOOD

A. Components.
1. Plasma: 90% water; accounts for about half of the total blood volume.
2. Formed elements (cells): account for about half of the volume.
   a. Erythrocytes (red blood cells [RBCs]).
   b. Leukocytes (white blood cells).
   c. Thrombocytes (platelets).
B. Characteristics of plasma (Figure 14-1).
1. Plasma is clear, straw-colored; it does not contain cellular elements.
2. Liquid portion of the circulating volume consists of 91% to 92% water.
3. Protein: 6% to 8% of the plasma.
   a. Albumin: most abundant protein; maintains normal colloid osmotic pressure of the plasma.
   b. Globulins.
      (1) Gamma globulins (immunoglobulins) consist primarily of antibodies produced by the plasma cells.
      (2) Alpha and beta globulins are essential factors in the clotting mechanism.
   c. Fibrinogen: necessary element in normal clot formation; produced in the liver.
   d. Prothrombin: necessary element for normal coagulation.
      (1) Produced in the liver.
      (2) Normal production is dependent on availability of adequate vitamin K.
   e. Normal body nutrients are carried by the plasma.
      (1) Carbohydrates in the form of glucose.
      (2) Proteins in the form of amino acids.
      (3) Fat in the form of lipids.
   f. Metabolic waste products are carried to organs of excretion by the plasma.
      (1) Urea, uric acid.
      (2) Lactic acid, creatinine.
C. Characteristics of erythrocytes (RBCs).
1. Formed in the red bone marrow (reticuloendothelial system); erythropoiesis is production of RBCs.
2. In early childhood, all bones contain red marrow; as child grows older, red marrow is replaced with fatty, yellow marrow.
3. In the adult, only specific bones contain red marrow (humerus, proximal end of the femur, iliac crest).
4. In conditions causing low oxygen tension, the kidneys initiate formation of erythropoietin, which then stimulates erythrocyte production.
5. Vitamin B_{12} and folic acid are necessary for the production of normal erythrocytes.
6. Erythrocytes: primary function is transportation of oxygen and carbon dioxide.
   a. Hemoglobin is the primary component of the RBC.
      (1) Serves as a buffer in the acid-base balance.
      (2) Hemoglobin combines easily with oxygen to form oxyhemoglobin.
      (3) Iron is a major component of hemoglobin and is necessary for normal oxygen transport.
      (4) Reduced hemoglobin has given up its oxygen component.
   b. Hematocrit is a fraction of the blood occupied by the erythrocytes.

> **! NURSING PRIORITY** As a general rule of thumb, the hematocrit is usually three times the hemoglobin value.

7. When RBCs are exposed to hypotonic solutions, water enters the cells, thus precipitating cellular wall rupture and destruction or hemolysis of the RBCs.
8. Hemolysis also occurs when cellular membranes are damaged, as in trauma.
9. The life span of an erythrocyte is approximately 120 days or 4 months.
10. Old erythrocytes are removed from circulation by the liver, spleen, and bone marrow; iron is salvaged and returned to the bone marrow; the remainder of each cell is converted to bile pigments, which are excreted by the liver.
D. Characteristics of the leukocytes (white blood cells).
1. Primary work of the leukocytes is accomplished when the cells leave the circulating volume and enter the body tissue.

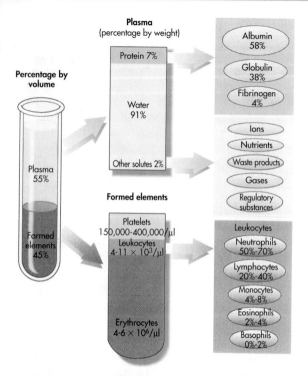

FIGURE 14-1 Approximate values for the components of blood in the adult. Normally, 45% of the blood is composed of blood cells, and 55% is composed of plasma. (From Thibodeau GA, Patton KT: *Anatomy and physiology*, ed 6, St. Louis, 2007, Mosby.)

2. Types of cells.
 a. Granulocytes (polymorphonuclear leukocytes) originate in the bone marrow.
  (1) Consist of neutrophils, eosinophils, and basophils.
  (2) Primary function is to destroy bacteria (phagocytosis).
 b. Agranular leukocytes (mononuclear) originate primarily in the lymphatic tissue.
  (1) Consist of lymphocytes and monocytes.
  (2) Assist in the removal of broken-down tissue cells.
  (3) Release substances that enhance the activity of the granulocytes.
3. Life span of the leukocyte is variable.
4. Leukocytosis refers to an overall increase in leukocytes; leukopenia refers to an overall decrease in leukocytes.
E. Characteristics of thrombocytes (platelets).
 1. Smallest of the formed cells in the circulating volume.
 2. Function: primarily involved with hemostasis; when vessel wall is damaged, platelets adhere to the area and eventually form a platelet plug to decrease bleeding.
 3. Thrombocytosis refers to a marked abnormal increase in thrombocytes; thrombocytopenia refers to a marked abnormal decrease in thrombocytes.
F. Hemostasis.
 1. Extrinsic mechanisms: clotting process initiated by tissue damage and blood loss.

2. Intrinsic mechanism: clotting mechanism within the vessel where blood loss and tissue trauma are not present.
3. Both mechanisms produce the same result: clot formation.
4. Three phases of hemostasis (coagulation).
 a. First phase: tissue injury precipitates release of platelet factor; in presence of calcium and accessory factors, thromboplastin is formed.
 b. Second phase: prothrombin is converted to thrombin; thromboplastin in phase 1 initiates the conversion of prothrombin.
 c. Third phase: thrombin converts soluble fibrinogen to insoluble fibrin (fibrin is an insoluble protein that looks like a fine network of thread or a web).
5. Erythrocytes are not part of the actual coagulation process; RBCs are essentially trapped in the fibrin mesh and give the clot its characteristic color.
6. Fibrinolysis: process by which clots, formed in tissue and small vessels, are dissolved by fibrinolysin.
G. Blood classification.
 1. Major blood groups: A, B, AB, and O.
 a. Blood compatibility and systems of classification are based on the presence or absence of specific antigens present on RBCs, as well as specific antibodies in the plasma.
 b. There are two antigens, or agglutinable substances, present on RBCs: A and B.
  (1) Neither antigen is present in O.
  (2) A is present in A.
  (3) B is present in B.
  (4) A and B are present in AB.
 c. There are two antibodies present in the plasma: anti-A and anti-B.
  (1) Both antibodies are present in O.
  (2) Anti-B is present in A.
  (3) Anti-A is present in B.
  (4) Neither is present in AB.
 d. If the antigen A on the RBCs of the donors comes in contact with the antibody A of the recipient and vice versa, agglutination and clumping will occur (e.g., type A blood transfused into type B recipient).
 e. O negative is called the *universal donor* because there are no antigens on the RBCs, and the Rh factor is not present.
 f. AB positive is called the *universal recipient* because there are no antibodies in the serum, and the Rh factor is present.
 g. In agglutination and clumping of RBCs, hemolysis occurs; hemolysis releases hemoglobin into the plasma.
 h. Problems occur with the destruction of the donor's RBCs by the plasma of the recipient's cells.
 2. Rh factor.
 a. Rh factor is present on the RBC.
 b. Rh is positive, or factor is present, in 85% to 95% of the population.

c. Rh is negative, or factor is absent, in 5% to 15% of the population.

d. Normal plasma does not contain Rh antibodies. Antibodies are formed in Rh-negative blood if transfused with Rh-positive blood; thus the recipient is sensitized to the Rh factor and subsequent Rh-positive blood might result in a severe transfusion reaction.

e. Problems of sensitization occur in the newborn when the mother is Rh negative and the infant is Rh positive (see Chapter 26).

System Assessment

A. History.
1. Disease of bone marrow and/or RBC-producing organs.
2. Treatment that depressed bone marrow activity (especially chemotherapy or radiation therapy).
3. Family history of problems (inheritance pattern).
4. Blood transfusion.

B. Bleeding problems occurring during pregnancy, labor and delivery, or immediately after delivery in both mother and infant.

C. Presence of chronic disorders or disease processes (liver, kidney, or spleen disorders).

D. Effects of aging (Table 14-1).

E. Evaluate effect hematologic disorder has on client's activities of daily living.
1. How long has client experienced symptoms?
2. What are the client's current activities and metabolic requirements?
3. Presence or absence of bleeding episodes.
4. Presence or absence of pain. If pain is present, how well is it controlled?
5. Presence of appropriate coping/defense mechanisms.

F. Assess client's current nutritional status.

G. Evaluate current blood values.

H. Evaluate status of respiratory and cardiovascular systems in maintaining homeostasis.

I. Focused examination should include the liver, spleen, skin, and lymph nodes.
1. Lymph nodes.
a. Ordinarily, lymph nodes are not palpable in adults; however, when a node is palpable, it should be small (0.5-1.0 cm).
b. Abnormal findings include nodes that are tender, hard, fixed, or enlarged. Tender nodes are often a result of the inflammatory process, whereas hard or fixed nodes are associated with malignancy.
2. Skin: abnormal findings include pallor, jaundice, purpura, petechiae, ecchymosis.
3. Liver and spleen: enlargement.

Anemias

Anemia is characterized by a low RBC count and a decrease to below normal in hemoglobin and hematocrit values.

A. Origin.
1. Defect in bone marrow production of RBCs.
2. Loss of RBCs.
a. Hemorrhage.
b. Chronic bleeding.
c. Hemolytic processes.
3. Hereditary disorders of the RBCs.
4. Inadequate nutritional intake of iron, folic acid.

B. The more rapidly an anemia occurs, the more severe the symptoms will be.

C. Healthy term infants have adequate iron storage for the first 5 to 6 months; premature infants may need iron supplementation at 2 to 3 months of age.

D. Common goal in treatment of all anemias is to identify the origin and correct the problem.
1. Assessment.
a. Pale skin, delayed wound healing, brittle thinning hair, spoon-shaped fingernails, and generalized lymphadenopathy.
b. Shortness of breath, dyspnea on exertion, tachypnea.

Table 14-1	AGE-RELATED ASSESSMENT FINDINGS FOR THE HEMATOLOGIC SYSTEM	
Assessment Area	*Hematologic System Findings*	*Older Adult Changes and Significance*
Nail beds (check for capillary refill)	Pallor, cyanosis, and decreased capillary refill are often noted in hematologic disorders.	Nails are typically thickened and discolored. Need to use another body area, such as the lips, to assess capillary refill.
Hair distribution	Thin or absent hair on trunk and extremities may indicate poor oxygenation and blood supply to area.	Older adults are losing body hair, but often in an even pattern distribution that has occurred slowly over time. Lack of hair only on lower legs and toes may indicate poor circulation.
Skin moisture and color	Skin dryness, pallor, and jaundice may occur with anemia, leukemia, etc.	Dry skin is a normal aspect of aging and thus becomes an unreliable indicator of skin moisture. Pigment loss and skin changes along with some yellowing occur with aging. Pallor that is not associated with anemia may be noted in older adults, because they tend not to go outdoors and get exposed to sunlight.

c. Tachycardia, palpitations, postural hypotension: cardiac complications can progress to cardiac decompensation.

d. Chronic fatigue, weakness, and apathy.

e. Anorexia, nausea, weight loss, constipation and diarrhea.

f. Beefy red tongue, stomatitis, hematemesis.

g. Headache, dizziness, tingling in extremities.

h. Chronic anemia may result in growth retardation in infants and children.

ALERT Identify client's ability to maintain activities of daily living.

E. Iron deficiency anemia: characterized by inadequate intake of dietary iron or excessive loss of iron.

1. Risk factors/etiology.
   a. Common in adolescents.
   b. Occurs in infants whose primary diet is milk.
   c. May occur in pregnancy.
   d. Heavy flow during menses.
2. Older adults are more prone to iron deficiency anemia because of poor dietary iron intake and decreased absorption in the small intestine.
3. Diagnostics: decreased hemoglobin and hematocrit values.
4. Clinical manifestations.
   a. May be asymptomatic in the early stages.
   b. General symptoms of anemia.
   c. Pallor, glossitis, cheilitis—three most common findings.
5. Treatment: supplemental iron intake is necessary for 6 months to replenish body storage.
   a. Supplemental iron (see Appendix 14-2).
   b. Increased dietary iron intake (see Table 2-2) .
   c. Supplemental folic acid.

ALERT Evaluate client's nutritional status; adapt a diet to meet special needs of the client; evaluate impact of condition on nutritional status.

F. Pernicious anemia: condition characterized by an inability to absorb vitamin B_{12} (cobalamin). It may be associated with loss of intrinsic factor (gastric resection), or it may be an autoimmune problem.

1. Risk factors/etiology.
   a. Generally not associated with inadequate dietary intake.
   b. More common in older adult; most common age at diagnosis is 60 years.
   c. Familial tendency.
   d. May be precipitated by gastric resection, gastritis, or chronic alcoholism.
2. Diagnostics (see Appendix 14-1).
   a. Homocysteine, cobalamin, and serum folate levels.
   b. Reduced number of RBCs and presence of abnormal RBCs.
   c. Gastric analysis for free hydrochloric acid.

3. Clinical manifestations.
   a. General symptoms of anemia, confusion.
   b. Paresthesia in the extremities, weakness, reduced vibratory sense.
   c. Loss of sense of balance, ataxia.
   d. Smooth, beefy, red tongue (glossitis).
4. Treatment.
   a. Injections of vitamin B_{12} may be required indefinitely.
   b. Maintain good nutrition with adequate iron, vitamin C, and folic acid intake.
   c. Monitor for gastric cancer—there is increased potential with pernicious anemia.

G. Aplastic anemia: characterized by depression of the bone marrow in production of all blood cell types—RBCs, WBCs, and platelets.

1. Risk factors/etiology.
   a. Examples of medications and chemicals that can precipitate aplastic anemia.
      (1) Chemotherapeutic agents, radiation.
      (2) Benzene, insecticides, arsenic.
      (3) Chloramphenicol.
      (4) Anticonvulsant medications (e.g., Dilantin).
   b. Radiation therapy.
   c. Up to 70% of cases are idiopathic in origin.
2. Diagnostics: bone marrow biopsy reveals severe decrease in all marrow elements (pancytopenia; see Appendix 14-1).
3. Clinical manifestations.
   a. General symptoms of anemia.
   b. Fever.
   c. Infections associated with neutropenia.
   d. Bleeding problems associated with thrombocytopenia.
4. Treatment.
   a. Remove causative agent.
   b. Hematopoietic stem cell transplant (see Appendix 14-4).
   c. Immunosuppression with antithymocytic globulin (ATG) and cyclosporine.

H. Folic acid deficiency anemia: associated with decreased dietary intake of folic acid.

1. Risk factors/etiology (origin very similar to that of vitamin B_{12} deficiency).
   a. Poor nutrition due to decreased folic acid intake, alcoholism, anorexia.
   b. Malabsorption syndromes.
   c. Deficiency may occur with increased demands for folic acid: infancy, adolescence, and pregnancy.
   d. Drugs: anticonvulsants and oral contraception.
   e. Hemodialysis.
2. Clinical manifestations.
   a. Slow, insidious onset.
   b. Weight loss, emaciated.
   c. May appear ill with malnourishment.
3. Diagnostics.
   a. Differentiate between folic acid deficiency and vitamin B_{12} deficiency.
   b. Serum folate levels less than 2 ng/mL.

4. Treatment: folic acid injections may be necessary initially; then oral replacement may be appropriate, 1 mg/day.

Nursing Interventions

For all clients with anemia.

Goal: To assist in establishing a diagnosis.

A. Complete nutritional evaluation.

B. History of possible causes.

Goal: To decrease body oxygen needs.

A. Assess client's tolerance to activity.

B. Provide diversional activities but also provide for adequate rest.

C. May need supplemental oxygen.

Goal: To prevent infections.

A. Decrease exposure.

B. Evaluate for temperature elevations frequently.

C. Observe for leukocytosis.

D. Maintain adequate hydration.

Goal: To assess for complications of chronic anemic state.

A. Evaluate ability of cardiovascular system to maintain adequate cardiac output.

B. Evaluate for symptoms of hypoxia (see Chapter 15).

Goal: To help client understand implications of disease and measures to maintain health.

A. Explain medical regimen.

B. Discuss importance of continuing medical follow-up.

C. Explain side effects of medications.

D. Identify foods high in iron and folic acid (see Chapter 2).

Sickle Cell Anemia

Sickle cell anemia is a problem characterized by the sickling effect of the erythrocytes, an inherited autosomal recessive disorder.

A. Basic defect of the erythrocyte is in the globulin portion of the hemoglobin.

B. Sickling problem is not apparent until around 6 months of age; the increased levels of fetal hemoglobin up to that age prevent serious sickling problems.

C. Predominantly a problem of children and adolescents. A child may be asymptomatic between crises. The problems from childhood may cause long-term complications as they become adults.

D. Pathologic changes of sickle cell disease result from:

1. Increased blood viscosity.

2. Increased RBC destruction.

3. Increased viscosity eventually precipitates ischemia and tissue necrosis caused by capillary stasis and thrombosis.

4. Cycle of occlusion, ischemia, and infarction to vascular organs.

E. Conditions precipitating sickling effect.

1. Dehydration.

2. Acidosis.

3. Hypoxia.

4. Infection with temperature elevation.

F. Pathologic effects of sickle cell disease on pregnancy.

1. Mother.

a. Increased anemia problems.

b. Increase in thromboembolic problems.

c. Increased risk for preeclampsia.

2. Infant.

a. Small for gestational age (SGA).

b. Spontaneous abortion.

c. Fetal distress caused by hypoxia.

G. Multiple body systems are involved.

Assessment

A. Risk factors/etiology.

1. Autosomal recessive disorder (see Chapter 24).

a. Normal hemoglobin (HgbA) is replaced by abnormal sickle hemoglobin (HgbS).

b. Presence of HgbS in 35% to 45% of hemoglobin indicates sickle cell trait.

2. May also occur in persons of Mediterranean, Caribbean, Arabian, East Indian, and Hispanic descent.

B. Clinical manifestations: primarily the result of obstruction caused by sickled RBCs and by increased RBC destruction.

1. Splenomegaly: caused by congestion and engorgement with sickled cells; decreases immune response.

2. Liver failure, hepatomegaly, and necrosis from severe impairment of hepatic blood flow.

3. Kidney damage caused by the congestion of glomerular capillaries and tubular arterioles.

4. Skeletal changes caused by hyperplasia and congestion of bone marrow.

C. Crisis: often precipitated by an infection or dehydration; can occur spontaneously (Figure 14-2).

1. Vaso-occlusive crisis: blood flow is impaired by sickled cells, causing ischemia and pain.

a. Extremities: occlusions in the small distal bones of the hands and the feet, characterized by pain, swelling, and decreased function (hand-foot syndrome).

b. Abdomen: severe abdominal pain.

c. Pulmonary: symptoms of pneumonia.

d. Renal: hematuria.

e. CNS: visual problems.

2. Sequestration crisis: pooling of the blood in the liver and spleen with decreased blood volume.

ALERT Recognize occurrence of a hemorrhage. Bleeding in a client with sickle cell anemia produces different symptoms than bleeding in a client who has undergone surgery; plan and implement nursing care to prevent complications; notify health care provider regarding signs of potential complications.

D. Diagnostics (see Appendix 14-1): early diagnosis, before 3 months of age, helps to minimize complications.

1. Hemoglobin electrophoresis indicates the presence and percentage of Hgb S.

2. Sickle turbidity tests (SICKLEDEX) used for screening.

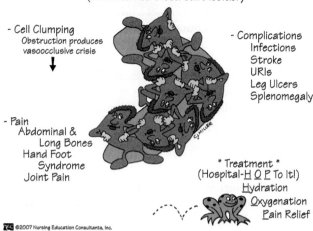

FIGURE 14-2 Sickle cell anemia crisis. (From Zerwekh J, Claborn J: *Memory notebook of nursing,* vol 2, ed 3, Ingram, Texas, 2007, Nursing Education Consultants.)

Treatment

A. Prevention of the sickling problem.
   1. Adequate hydration.
   2. Prevent infections, especially respiratory tract infections; pneumococcal vaccine is recommended.
   3. Clients generally do not require iron because of increased resorption.
   4. Daily folic acid supplement.
   5. Hydroxyurea (Droxia, Hydrea) to increase the production of Hgb F thereby reducing hemolysis and the number of sickled cells.
   6. Oxygen: assists to prevent a crisis in clients with respiratory problems, but it does not reverse a sickling crisis or reduce pain.
B. Treatment of crisis.
   1. Bed rest, hydration, antibiotics.
   2. Analgesics for pain; promote adequate oxygenation.
   3. Blood transfusions and/or exchange transfusions (see Appendix 14-3).
C. Surgery: splenectomy for severe splenic sequestration.

Nursing Interventions

Goal: To prevent sickle cell disease.
A. Participate in community screening programs and education.
B. Refer persons who are carriers (autosomal recessive trait) for genetic counseling (see Figure 24-1).
Goal: To prevent sickling crisis.
A. Maintain adequate hydration; intravenous (IV) fluids may be necessary.
B. Promote respiratory health and tissue oxygenation.
C. Prevent infection.
D. Hydroxyurea (Droxia, Hydrea): reduces sickling episodes, a long-term complication of leukemia.
Goal: To control pain.

A. Assessment of involved area.
B. Appropriate analgesics: meperidine (Demerol) is not recommended; morphine, hydromorphone, fentanyl or methadone may be used; patient-controlled analgesia (PCA) devices are frequently used to control pain.
C. Allow client to assume a position of comfort; passive range of motion may be beneficial.
D. Maintain rest if movement exacerbates pain.

> **ALERT** Determine effectiveness of pain control. Care of the child with sickle cell disease frequently centers around pain control (see Chapter 3).

Goal: To maintain adequate hydration and oxygenation.
A. Evaluate adequacy of hydration.
B. Low specific gravity may not be indicative of fluid balance if there is renal involvement.
C. Monitor IV fluid administration carefully; maintain accurate intake and output records.
D. Evaluate electrolyte balance.
E. Administer oxygen as indicated.
F. Provide good pulmonary hygiene.
G. Assess for metabolic acidosis.

> **ALERT** Monitor hydration status; evaluate client's response to parenteral administration of fluids.

Goal: To identify complication of affected organs—systematic evaluation of client to identify problems discussed in section on clinical manifestations.

Home Care

A. Increase fluids with physical activity, living in excessively hot/cold climates.
B. Seek early intervention for symptoms of infection, especially respiratory tract infection; report temperature elevations, coughing, or pain.
C. Encourage normal growth and developmental activities as tolerated by the child.
D. Client with sickle cell disease should avoid situations that may precipitate hypoxia.
   1. Traveling to high-altitude areas.
   2. Flying in an unpressurized aircraft.
   3. Participating in overly strenuous exercise.
E. Inform all significant health care personnel that child should wear medical identification.

> **ALERT** Compare physical development of client with normal development. Chronically ill children frequently are slower in growth and development; care is provided for the developmental level, not the chronologic age.

 Polycythemia Vera (Primary)

Polycythemia vera is a chronic disorder characterized by a proliferation of all red marrow cells due to a chromosomal mutation.

Assessment

A. Risk factors: usually occurs during middle age; median age is 60 years.
B. Diagnostics.
1. Increased erythrocytes, hematocrit.
2. Increased leukocytes in the bone marrow.
3. Excessive production of platelets.
4. Bone marrow biopsy demonstrates hypercellularity.
C. Clinical manifestations.
1. Early: headache, vertigo, tinnitus, pruritus.
2. Ruddy complexion (plethora).
3. Hepatosplenomegaly; peptic ulcer, dyspepsia.
4. Problems of decreased blood flow.
a. Angina, hypoxia.
b. Claudication (pain in muscles during activity).
c. Thrombophlebitis.
d. Hypertension: increased blood viscosity or peripheral resistance.
5. Complication: stroke secondary to thrombosis.

Treatment

A. Phlebotomy (2 to 3 times per week initially, then every 2 to 3 months).
B. Myelosuppressive agents (Myleran, Hydrea).
C. Symptom management: paroxetine (Paxil) for erythromelalgia (peripheral dilation of blood vessels), allopurinol (Zyloprim) for gout, interferon alpha for pruritus.

Nursing Interventions

Goal: To help client understanding dietary implications to deal with inadequate food intake due to peptic ulcer pain, dyspepsia, and symptoms of hyperuricemia (gout).

Goal: To help client understand implications of the disease and long-term health care needs (i.e., prevention of DVT).

Leukemia

Leukemia is an uncontrolled proliferation of abnormal white blood cells; eventual cellular destruction occurs as a result of the infiltration of the leukemic cells into the body tissue.

A. Highly vascular organs of the reticuloendothelial system are primarily affected; spleen, liver, and lymph nodes show marked infiltration, enlargement, and eventually fibrosis.
B. Invasion of the bone marrow by the leukemic cells can precipitate pathologic fractures.
C. Three primary consequences of leukemia.
1. Anemia from RBC destruction and bleeding.
2. Infection associated with neutropenia.
3. Bleeding tendencies caused by decreased platelets.
D. Types of leukemia.
1. Acute lymphocytic leukemia (blast or stem cell) (ALL).
a. Peak occurrences: around 4 years of age, then again around 65 years.
b. Favorable prognosis with chemotherapy.

c. Leukemic cells will infiltrate the meninges, precipitating increased intracranial pressure.
2. Acute myelogenous leukemia (AML).
a. Most common in older adults.
b. Peak incidence age 60 to 70 years.
3. Chronic myelogenous leukemia (CML).
a. Uncommon before the age of 20 years; peak incidence age 45 years.
b. Onset is generally slow.
c. Symptoms are less severe than those in acute stages of disease.
d. Presence of Philadelphia chromosome in 90% of cases.
4. Chronic lymphocytic leukemia (CLL).
a. Common malignancy of older adults; rare before age 30, and more common in men.
b. Frequently asymptomatic; often diagnosed in a chronic fatigue work-up.

Assessment

A. Clinical manifestations.
1. Anemia, infection, and bleeding tendencies occurring together.
2. Anorexia, weight loss, cough.
3. Central nervous system involvement: headache, confusion, increased irritability.
4. Fatigue, lethargy.
5. Petechiae, bruises easily, epistaxis.
6. Complaints of bone and joint pain.
7. Hepatomegaly and splenomegaly.
B. Diagnostics (see Appendix 14-1).
1. Bone marrow aspiration: increased numbers of blast (immature) cells.
2. Lumbar puncture to identify presence of leukemic cells in spinal fluid.
3. Complete blood count.
4. Studies to evaluate liver and renal function; most chemotherapy agents are detoxified in the liver and excreted by way of the renal system; these systems need to be evaluated before chemotherapy is initiated.

Treatment

A. Medications.
1. Corticosteroids.
2. Antineoplastic agents (see Appendix 8-1).
3. Xanthine-oxidase inhibitor: allopurinol (Zyloprim) decreases uric acid levels in clients receiving (see Appendix 21-2).
4. Chemotherapy usually involves an induction phase, a consolidation phase, and a maintenance phase.
5. A combination of chemotherapy agents is used initially to promote a remission.
6. Majority of children with ALL will go into remission during the induction phase.
B. Hematopoietic stem cell transplantation (see Appendix 14-4).
C. A remission is characterized by absence of leukemic cells and disappearance of all disease symptoms.

Nursing Interventions

Goal: To prevent infection.

A. Systematically assess for evidence of infection: fever, inflammation, pain.

B. Monitor temperature elevation closely; notify doctor of increase above 100.5° F (38° C).

C. Meticulous skin care, especially oral hygiene and around perianal area.

D. Protect client from exposure to infection; degree of restriction depends on immunosuppression.

E. Isolate client from persons with communicable childhood diseases, especially those with chicken pox.

F. Polio (IPV), varicella, measles-mumps-rubella, and influenza immunizations are not recommended to be given to children or adults during immunosuppression.

G. Avoid urinary catheterization if possible.

H. Encourage adequate protein and calorie intake, low-bacteria diet.

I. Maintain adequate hydration.

> **! NURSING PRIORITY** Prevention and early treatment of common infections is a priority in the care of this client.

Goal: To prevent or limit bleeding episodes (Box 14-1).

A. Use local measures to control bleeding (pressure to area; cold packs).

B. Restrict strenuous activity.

Box 14-1 BLEEDING PRECAUTIONS

Indications: Clients diagnosed with leukemia, hemophilia, or any condition that causes bleeding; clients receiving anticoagulants or thrombolytic medications.

- Limit number of venipunctures and intramuscular injections. Perform guaiac tests on stool as necessary.
- Oral hygiene:
  - Discourage flossing.
  - Use soft toothbrush or no toothbrush; may need to use cotton-tipped swabs while gums are friable.
  - Avoid harsh mouthwashes.
  - Rinse mouth frequently with mild mouthwash.
- Use electric razor for shaving.
- Assess perianal area for fissures and bleeding daily.
- Discourage client from vigorous coughing or nose blowing.
- Avoid aspirin products; evaluate NSAIDs for bleeding properties.
- Avoid catheters (urinary and suctioning) when possible.
- Avoid enemas and suppositories.
- Avoid overinflation of blood pressure cuff or leaving cuff inflated for prolonged period of time.
- Provide safe environment and prevent injury according to age (padded side rails, soft toys, house shoes, etc.).
- Monitor for bleeding episode: nosebleed, hematuria, increased bruising.

NSAIDs, Nonsteroidal antiinflammatory drugs.

C. Involve client in evaluating level of activity; decrease activity when platelet counts are low and anemia is present.

Goal: To prevent renal complications associated with chemotherapy.

A. Maintain adequate hydration to flush chemicals from the kidneys.

B. Monitor levels of uricemia.

C. Monitor renal function before and during treatment.

Goal: To provide pain relief.

A. Use acetaminophen rather than aspirin.

B. Maintain environment conducive to rest.

C. Position carefully; may coordinate positioning with administration of analgesics.

D. Evaluate effectiveness of pain relief; administer analgesic before pain becomes severe.

E. Do not exercise affected joints.

Goal: To decrease adverse effects of chemotherapy (see Chapter 8).

Goal: To prevent complications of transfusions (see Appendix 14-3).

Goal: To demonstrate an understanding of the disease and its prognosis and to display an ability to cope with the diagnosis and its consequences (physical, psychologic, social, and spiritual).

A. Assist client and family to maintain realistic expectations.

B. Be honest in discussion of the outcome and possible side effects of anticipated therapy.

C. Provide emotional support and encourage ventilation of feelings.

> **ALERT** Care of client receiving chemotherapy, blood transfusions, client and family teaching, and pain relief are all components of the exam.

Home Care

A. Do not take aspirin or medications that contain aspirin.

B. Monitor weight gain or loss.

C. Counseling to determine effect of client's or child's illness on family members.

D. Encourage family involvement in client's care.

E. Discourage pets (e.g., fish, birds, cats) because of the possibility of bacteria and virus transmission.

F. Teach family methods to stop bleeding.

G. Help parents prepare for their child's return to school.

H. Teach the importance of good handwashing and other infection prevention measures.

I. Teach family members to recognize the early signs of infection and importance of reporting these signs as soon as they are observed.

J. Provide information about community resources for the client and family—e.g., Leukemia Lymphoma Society, American Cancer Society, Meals on Wheels.

ALERT Help the family manage care of a client with long-term needs; determine the family's understanding of causes of illness; determine effectiveness of the client's support system.

Lymphomas

Characterized by malignant neoplasms originating in the bone marrow and lymphocytes. Lymphoma is the fifth most common type of cancer in the U.S.

A. Hodgkin's disease: characterized by painless enlargement of lymph nodes with progression to involve the liver and spleen. Common metastatic sites are the spleen, liver, bone marrow, and lungs. Disease is spread by extension along the lymphatic system. This is the most curable of the lymphomas.
  1. Assessment.
    a. Risk factors/etiology.
      (1) Familial tendency, more prevalent in men than in women.
      (2) May be caused by Epstein-Barr virus or exposure to occupational toxins.
      (3) Increased incidence in immunosuppressed clients.
    b. Clinical manifestations.
      (1) Initially, painless enlargement of cervical, axillary, inguinal, or mediastinal lymph nodes.
      (2) Symptoms result from pressure on adjacent organs.
      (3) Fever, malaise, night sweats.
      (4) Weight loss and fatigue are associated with a poor prognosis.
      (5) Ingestion of small amounts of alcohol cause pain at affected lymph node sites.
    c. Diagnostics: lymph node biopsy specimen showing presence of Reed-Sternberg cells.
  2. Treatment: chemotherapy and radiation.
B. Non-Hodgkin's lymphoma: a neoplastic growth (derived from B and T cells) that originates in the lymphoid tissue. It spreads malignant cells unpredictably, infiltrating the lymphoid tissue.
  1. Assessment.
    a. Risk factors/etiology.
      (1) Increased incidence in clients with immunodeficiency or autoimmune conditions who have used immunosuppressant medications.
      (2) Associated with viral infections (Epstein-Barr) and occupational exposure to carcinogens.
    b. Clinical manifestations.
      (1) Symptoms are highly variable, depending on where the disease has spread.
      (2) Lymphadenopathy that can wax and wane.
    c. Diagnostics: based on classification system of the histopathology of malignant cells.
  2. Treatment: chemotherapy and radiation.

Nursing Interventions

Goal: To maintain physiologic equilibrium (see Chapter 8).
A. Maintain hydration and nutrition.
B. Maintain good pulmonary hygiene.
C. Evaluate for shortness of breath; maintain in semi-Fowler's position.
D. Decrease body needs for oxygen.
E. Assess ability of cardiovascular system to maintain cardiac output.
F. Manage pain and effects of therapy.
Goal: To prevent infection (see "Goal: To prevent infection" in Leukemia section above).
Goal: To decrease adverse effects of chemotherapy and radiation therapy (see Chapter 8).
Goal: To help the client understand the implications of the disease and its prognosis; to have the client demonstrate the ability to cope with the diagnosis and its long-term implications (see Nursing Interventions in Chapter 8).

Multiple Myeloma (Plasma Cell Myeloma)

A malignancy of plasma cells, specifically the B lymphocytes. Infiltration occurs in the bones and soft tissues.

Assessment

A. Clinical manifestations.
  1. Back pain, bone pain (pelvis, spine and ribs most common).
  2. Pathologic fractures as a result of diffuse osteoporosis.
  3. Hypercalcemia, high serum protein levels.
  4. Renal failure.
B. Diagnostics.
  1. Serum and/or protein electrophoresis; increased Bence-Jones protein in urine.
  2. Bone marrow biopsy (see Appendix 14-1).
  3. X-ray film showing typical punched-out appearance of the bones caused by demineralization.
  4. Prognosis is based on $beta_2$-microalbuminuria and albumin.

Treatment

A. Chemotherapy (see Table 8-2) and immunomodulators (see Appendix 23-3).
B. Palliative radiation therapy.

Nursing Interventions

Goal: To maintain physiologic equilibrium.
A. Careful ambulation to decrease hypercalcemia and improve pulmonary status.
B. Adequate hydration to prevent calcium from precipitating in the kidneys; careful monitoring of hydration status.
C. Comfort measures and analgesics for pain.
D. Safety measures to prevent pathologic fractures.
  1. Do not lift anything weighing more than 10 pounds.
  2. Use proper body mechanics.

E. Braces may be necessary to support the spine.

F. Prevention of infection.

Goal: To help the client understand implications of the disease and measures to maintain health.

DISORDERS OF COAGULATION

 Hemophilia

Hemophilia is a defect in the clotting mechanism. Classically, there are two types, distinguishable only by laboratory tests. Clinically, the two types are the same, but both may occur in varying degrees of severity. The disease is most often recognized during the toddler stage.

A. Hemophilia A: factor VIII deficiency (classic hemophilia).

B. Hemophilia B: factor IX deficiency (Christmas disease).

Assessment

A. Risk factors/etiology: both types of hemophilia are sex-linked recessive disorders.

　1. Primarily affects males.

　2. Females are carriers.

B. Clinical manifestations.

　1. Persistent or prolonged bleeding that occurs from minor trauma/insults.

　2. Hemarthrosis: bleeding into joint cavities.

　3. Spontaneous hematuria.

　4. Hematoma.

　5. Intracranial hemorrhage may be fatal.

　6. Petechiae are uncommon, because platelet count is normal.

C. Diagnostics.

　1. History of bleeding episodes.

　2. Family inheritance pattern.

　3. Identification of deficient factor (factor assay).

　4. PTT, bleeding time.

Treatment

A. Factor VIII concentrate: must be reconstituted with sterile water immediately before administration; given IV push over 5-10 minutes.

B. Desmopressin (DDAVP, Stimate): synthetic vasopressin used to treat mild cases; given IV or intranasal.

C. Treatment may be carried out at home.

Nursing Interventions

Goal: To prevent spontaneous bleeding episodes (see Box 14-1).

A. Decrease risk for injury.

　1. Make environment as safe as possible without hampering motor development.

　2. Instruct client to avoid contact sports, but encourage noncontact sports (e.g., swimming).

　3. Regular exercise and physical therapy to promote muscle strength around joints and decrease bleeding episodes.

B. Preventive dental care, and prevent oral infections.

C. Maintain normal weight; increased weight causes increased strain on the joints.

D. Avoid any aspirin compounds.

E. Administer clotting factors before, during, and after invasive medical procedures.

Goal: To recognize and treat bleeding episodes.

A. Apply pressure to the area.

B. Immobilize and elevate the joints involved.

C. Do not perform passive range of motion on affected joints.

D. Apply cold pack to promote vasoconstriction.

E. Observe for signs of internal bleeding: tarry stools, slurred speech, headache.

F. Administer clotting factors in a timely manner.

Goal: To prepare client and family to administer clotting factors intravenously at home.

A. Correct technique for venipuncture.

B. Indications for use.

 C. Encourage child to learn self-administration, generally around age 9 to 12 years.

Goal: To prevent permanent joint degeneration.

A. Elevate joint and immobilize during acute bleeding episode.

B. Encourage active range of motion so child will limit movement based on pain tolerance.

C. Physical therapy after the acute phase, no weight bearing until swelling has resolved.

D. Maintain pain relief during physical therapy.

> **⚠ NURSING PRIORITY** Apply RICE to the affected joints: rest, ice, compression, elevation.

 Home Care

A. Have client and family demonstrate ability to perform IV puncture.

B. Have client and family discuss situations that call for use of IV infusion of deficient factor: endoscopy, dental work, etc.

C. Discuss with family the importance of routine prophylactic dental checkups.

D. Encourage ventilation of feelings regarding diagnosis of the disease.

E. Encourage counseling for parents regarding concern and guilt over hereditary disorder.

> **ALERT** Modify approaches in care based on child's development; determine family's understanding of the causes and/or consequences of the client's illness and ability to provide care; assist family in crisis.

 Disseminated Intravascular Coagulation

Disseminated intravascular coagulation is a secondary coagulation disorder involving widespread clotting in the

small vessels, leading to consumption of clotting factors, thereby precipitating a bleeding disorder. It is not a disease but a result of underlying conditions.

Assessment

A. Risk factors/etiology.
   1. Increase in release of coagulation factors into circulation: hemolytic processes, extensive tissue damage.
   2. Damage to the vascular endothelium (burns, transplant rejection).
   3. Shock, hemolytic processes (transfusion reactions).
   4. Infection: sepsis.
   5. Obstetrical complications: hemorrhage.
   6. Malignancies: leukemia, lymphoma, tumor lysis syndrome.
B. Clinical manifestations.
   1. Thrombocytopenia: petechiae, ecchymosis on skin and mucous membranes.
   2. Prolonged bleeding from multiple body areas.
   3. Hypotension leading to shock.
   4. Multiple organ dysfunction syndrome.
C. Diagnostics (see Appendix 14-1).
   1. Low fibrin and platelet levels.
   2. Prolonged prothrombin time (PT), partial thromboplastin time (PTT), and activated partial thromboplastin time (aPTT).
   3. Elevated fibrin split products (FSPs), and D-dimer assay.

Treatment

A. Correction of the underlying problem.
B. Platelets, fresh frozen plasma transfusions, cryoprecipitate based on precipitating cause.
C. Heparin or low-molecular-weight heparin (Lovenox)—use is controversial.
D. Recombinant human activated protein C: drotrecogin alfa (Xigris)—anticoagulant and antiinflammatory effects.
E. Treatment of shock, as indicated.

Nursing Interventions

Goal: To identify the problem early and to decrease potential adverse effects.
A. Thorough assessment of bleeding problems in clients severely compromised by other problems (shock and sepsis).
B. Nursing measures to prevent bleeding episodes (see Box 14-1).
C. Assess and support all vital systems.
Goal: To help the client's family understand the implications of the disease and demonstrate appropriate coping behaviors.
A. Provide emotional support and encourage visiting as intensive care policies and client's condition allow.

B. Encourage ventilation of feelings regarding critical illness of family member.
C. Be available to family members during visiting time.

DISORDERS OF THE SPLEEN

The spleen is affected by many disorders that can result in splenomegaly (enlarged spleen). The spleen usually contains 20 to 40 mL of blood and does not serve as a reservoir for blood volume or red blood cells.

Assessment

A. Risk factors/etiology for splenomegaly.
   1. Chronic myelogenous leukemia.
   2. Heart failure.
   3. Systemic lupus erythematosus.
B. Clinical manifestations.
   1. Hypersplenism: splenomegaly with peripheral cytopenias (anemia, leukopenia, thrombocytopenia).
   2. Pain due to splenomegaly.
   3. Splenic rupture from trauma or inadvertent tearing during other surgical procedures.
C. Diagnostics (see Appendix 14-1).
   1. Pitted or pocked RBCs or Howell-Jolly bodies.
   2. Spleen scan.

Treatment

A. Splenectomy.
B. Analgesics for pain.
C. Platelets, fresh frozen plasma transfusions.

Nursing Interventions

Goal: To identify the problem early (splenomegaly, hypersplenism, or splenic rupture) and to decrease potential adverse effects.
A. Thorough assessment of spleen problem and management to address issues of splenomegaly (pain), hypersplenism, or splenic rupture (emergency surgery).
B. Nursing measures to prevent bleeding episodes in hypersplenism (see Box 14-1).
C. Assess and support all vital systems.
D. Monitor for complications following surgery—hemorrhage, shock, fever, abdominal distention, immunologic deficiencies (IgM), infection.
Goal: To help the client's family to understand the implications of the problem and demonstrate appropriate coping behavior.
A. Provide emotional support and encourage visiting as intensive care policies and client's condition allow.
B. Encourage ventilation of feelings regarding critical illness of family member.
C. Be available to family members during visiting time.
D. Teach about lifelong risk for infection following splenectomy; encourage vaccination for pneumococcus.

Appendix 14-1   HEMATOLOGIC DIAGNOSTICS

TEST	NORMAL	CLINICAL AND NURSING IMPLICATIONS

Bone marrow aspiration or biopsy	All formed cell elements within normal range (erythrocytes, leukocytes, and platelets).	1. Evaluates presence, absence, or ratio of cells characteristic of a suspected disease (e.g., hematopoiesis pathology, chromosomal abnormalities).
		2. Preferable site is posterior iliac crest; alternate sites are sternum and anterior iliac crest.
		3. Client preparation:
		  a. Local anesthetic is used, as well as analgesics or conscious sedation.
		  b. Feeling of pressure when bone marrow is entered; pain occurs as marrow is being withdrawn.
		4. After test:
		  a. Observe for bleeding at site.
		  b. Apply pressure to site 5 to 10 minutes or longer if client is thrombocytopenic.
		  c. Bed rest for approximately 30 min afterward.
		  d. Analgesics as indicated.
		  e. Monitor for infection.

Sickle cell test (SICKLEDEX)	No hemoglobin S present.	1. Routine screening test for sickle cell trait or disorder; does not distinguish between them. 2. False-negative result in infants <3 months. 3. False-positive result can occur for up to 4 months after a transfusion of RBCs that are positive for the trait.
Hemoglobin electrophoresis	Separates various hemoglobins and allows for identification of specific problem.	1. Differentiates between trait or disorder in sickle cell anemia. 2. Diagnosis of thalassemia and hemolytic anemia.
Activated partial thromboplastin time (aPTT)	Normal 30-45 sec.	1. Sensitive in monitoring heparin; draw 1 hour before next heparin dose. 2. May be used to detect circulating anticoagulants.
Prothrombin time (PT)	12 to 15 sec or 100% (each client will have a control value).	1. Production of prothrombin depends on adequate intake and utilization of vitamin K.
International normalized ratio (INR)	Normal INR is 1.0-2.0.	2. Both tests may be used in management of Coumadin therapy. 3. INR should be maintained at 2.0-3.0 for individuals with risk for clots (atrial fibrillation, history of recent DVT) and 2.5-3.5 for individuals with mechanical heart valves.
Fibrin split products	Normal less than 10 mg/L or less than 10 mcg/mL.	1. Fibrinolysis occurs in intravascular coagulation. 2. Abnormally high levels in DIC.
Homocysteine	Normal 8-20 μmol/L.	1. An amino acid metabolized through pathways that require vitamin B_{12}. 2. Increased in B_{12} and folic acid deficiency.
D-dimer	Normal less than 250 ng/mL	1. Used to measure fibrin fragment created by fibrin degradation and clot lysis. 2. Used in management of low-molecular-weight heparin therapy.
Ferritin	Normal 10-300 ng/mL	1. Major iron storage protein reflects iron storage.

DIC, Disseminated intravascular coagulation; *DVT*, deep venous thrombosis; *RBCs*, red blood cells.

Appendix 14-2 HEMATOLOGIC MEDICATIONS

MEDICATIONS	SIDE EFFECTS	NURSING IMPLICATIONS

Iron Preparations Replacement.

Ferrous fumarate **(Feostat, Span 77, FEM Iron):** IM, PO
Ferrous gluconate **(Fergon, Ferralet):** PO
Ferrous sulfate **(Feosol, Fer-In-Sol):** PO
Iron dextran injection **(InFeD, Dexferrum):** IV, IM
	GI irritation
	Nausea
	Constipation
	Toxic reactions:
	  Fever
	  Urticaria
		1. Absorbed better on empty stomach; however, may give with meals if GI upset occurs.
		2. Liquid preparations should be diluted and given through a straw to prevent staining of the teeth.
		3. Tell client stool may be black and iron may cause constipation.
		4. Eggs, milk, cheese, and antacids inhibit oral iron absorption.
		5. Iron preparations inhibit oral tetracycline absorption. IM/IV preparations may be used if on oral tetracycline.
		  • Anaphylactic reaction can occur; test dose should be given.
		  • IM should be avoided because of pain and tissue discoloration.
		  • If given IM, use Z-track method to prevent tissue staining.
		  • IV route recommended if oral route is not acceptable.

Vitamin K Necessary for normal prothrombin activity.

Vitamin K: phytonadione **(AquaMEPHYTON):** PO, subQ, IM, IV	GI upset, rash IV not recommended because of hypersensitivity reactions	1. PO and subQ most common routes. 2. Antidote for Coumadin. 3. Observe bleeding precautions.

GI, Gastrointestinal; *IM,* intramuscularly; *IV,* intravenously; *PO,* by mouth (orally); *SQ,* subcutaneously.

Appendix 14-3 BLOOD TRANSFUSIONS

BLOOD COMPONENT FOR TRANSFUSION	PURPOSE OF ADMINISTRATION	NURSING IMPLICATIONS

Packed RBCs: 200-250 mL per unit	To increase oxygen-carrying capacity.
	To decrease risk for incompatible antibodies from the plasma.
		1. Chart:
		  Type and amount of blood product infused.
		  Time started and time completed.
		  Rate of infusion.
		  Blood unit identification number.
		2. Vital signs are taken immediately before transfusion, at 5 min and 15 min into transfusion, every hour during transfusion, and at completion of transfusion.
		3. Closely observe older adult clients for indications of fluid overload.

Platelets: 50-70 mL per unit	To treat thrombocytopenia.	1. Chart amount and type of infusion. 2. Infuse rapidly.
Fresh frozen plasma: 200-250 mL per unit	Administered for clotting factors, proteins, fluid volume.	1. Chart amount and type infused. 2. Infuse immediately after thawing. 3. Infused for 30 to 60 minutes or as client tolerates.
Whole blood: 500 mL per unit	To provide volume replacement and increase oxygen. Administered with greater than 25% blood loss.	1. Same as with packed RBCs. 2. Observations for fluid volume overload.

ALERT Administer and discontinue blood and/or blood products; check blood products according to institution policies; evaluate appropriate IV access; evaluate client's response.

Continued

Appendix 14-3   BLOOD TRANSFUSIONS—cont'd

Nursing Guidelines for Packed RBCS or Whole Blood Transfusions

1. Informed consent and alternatives should be explained to the client. Autologous (using client's own blood) and designated donor transfusions are options. If client is unable to give consent, consent should be obtained from family.
2. Obtain the type and cross-match records and the unit of blood to administer.
   Check:
   a. The ABO group on the unit against the cross-match records.
   b. The Rh type of the blood against the cross-match record.
   c. Have two RNs independently—or one RN and one physician—check the records and sign that they have checked them.
   d. Check the client's name and hospital number on the unit of blood and on the cross-match records.
   e. If any of the above do not match, DO NOT GIVE THE BLOOD.
   f. Check the expiration date on the unit of blood.
3. Administer the blood immediately after receiving it from the blood bank; blood should NEVER be stored in a unit refrigerator or allowed to sit out at room temperature. The maximum amount of time blood can be out of monitored storage is 30 min.
4. Do not add any medications to blood products.
5. Do not warm blood before transfusion, unless there are several units to be infused rapidly and client is in danger of developing a hypothermic response. If blood must be warmed, use equipment that is specifically designed for this procedure.
6. DO NOT use a microwave to warm the blood.
7. Inspect the blood bag for leaks, abnormal color, excessive air, or bubbles.
8. The average rate of transfusion in an adult is 1 unit of blood over about 3 to 4 hours, depending on the condition of the client.
9. The blood administration set should be changed after 2 units have infused to decrease risk for bacterial contamination.
10. It is not recommended to use an infusion pump; the pump increases RBC hemolysis.
11. Multiple transfusions can result in hypocalcemia.

Nursing Guidelines for Platelets and Fresh Frozen Plasma

1. Obtain type and cross-match records; check client and unit identification in same way as for packed RBCs.
2. Unit should not contain any clumps or have unusual color.
3. Fresh frozen plasma must be administered immediately.
4. Infuse each unit as fast as client will tolerate.

> ❗ **NURSING PRIORITY** The majority of major adverse transfusion reactions are due to improper identification of the blood product and the recipient.

✓ KEY POINTS: Guidelines for Performance Phase of Transfusion

- Check the doctor's order; check the labels on the blood bag against the client identification at the bedside.
- Baseline vital signs must be obtained before hanging the blood; if the client has a temperature above 101° F, advise the physician before starting the transfusion.
- Initiate the infusion with an 18-gauge or 20-gauge needle and begin infusing normal saline solution.
- Do NOT use D_5W to initiate the transfusion; it causes the blood to hemolyze and precipitate.
- Always use a standard blood administration set with a filter; DO NOT use straight IV tubing.
- Initiate infusion (rate of approximately 100 mL/hr, depending on client's condition) and remain with the client; the first 10-15 min is the most critical period of time; the majority of transfusion reactions occur during administration of the first 50 mL.
- During the transfusion, continue to monitor for circulatory overload or transfusion reaction.
- Blood deteriorates rapidly after about 2 hr or exposure to room temperature; a unit of blood should not hang longer than 4 hr.
- Components (plasma, platelets) that contain few RBCs may be administered rapidly.

TRANSFUSION REACTIONS

Hemolytic Transfusion Reaction
1. Low back pain
2. Hypotension, tachycardia, tachypnea
3. Apprehension, sense of impending doom
4. Fever, chills, flushing
5. Chest pain
6. Dyspnea
7. Onset is immediate

Allergic Reaction
1. Urticaria (hives)
2. Pruritus
3. Facial flushing
4. Severe shortness of breath, bronchospasm

NURSING MANAGEMENT

1. Stop transfusion immediately and notify physician.
2. Change the IV tubing; do not allow blood in the tubing to infuse into the client; maintain IV access.
3. Obtain first-voided urine specimen to test for blood in the urine.
4. Anticipate blood samples to be drawn by the lab.
5. With suspected renal involvement, treatment with diuretics is initiated to promote diuresis.

1. If client has a history of allergic reactions, antihistamines may be given before starting the transfusion.
2. Stop transfusion until status of reaction can be determined; if symptoms are mild and transient, the transfusion may be resumed.

Appendix 14-3   BLOOD TRANSFUSIONS—cont'd

TRANSFUSION REACTIONS

Febrile Reaction

1. Chills and fever
2. Headache, flushing
3. Muscle stiffness/pain
4. Increased anxiety

NURSING MANAGEMENT

1. Keep client covered and warm during transfusion.
2. Stop the transfusion until status of reaction can be determined.
3. Transfusion with leukocyte-poor RBCs or frozen washed packed cells may prevent this reaction in clients susceptible to fever.
4. Most common reaction.

D_5W, 5% Dextrose in water; *IV*, intravenous; *RBCs*, red blood cells; *RN*, registered nurse.

Appendix 14-4   HEMATOPOIETIC STEM CELL TRANSPLANT*

Goal: To restore hematologic and immunologic function in clients with immunologic deficiencies, leukemia, congenital or acquired anemias.

Procedure

In the adult client, approximately 400 to 800 mL of bone marrow or harvested stem cells are processed and transfused into the client. (See Appendix 14-1 for care of donor client for bone marrow aspiration.)

1. Typing:
   a. Allogenic: matching of a histocompatible donor, preferably a relative.
   b. Autologous: uses client's own bone marrow that has been collected from disease-free tissue and then frozen.
   c. Syngeneic: donor is an identical twin with perfect tissue match.
2. Immunoablative preparation pretransplant: chemotherapy and radiation to produce immunologically suppressed state before the hematopoietic transfusion; procedure takes 5 to 10 days.

Complications

1. Bacterial, viral, or fungal infection from immunosuppressed state.
2. Severe thrombocytopenia resulting in bleeding problems.
3. Graft-versus-host disease (rejection).
   a. Acute rejection generally occurs in 7 to 30 days after transplantation; chronic rejection occurs in 100 days.
   b. Erythematous rash on the palms and feet, spreading to the trunk, may be an early symptom.
   c. Altered liver enzyme profiles with liver tenderness and jaundice.
   d. Gastrointestinal disturbances: anorexia, nausea, vomiting, diarrhea.

Nursing Implications

1. Preparation of the client for immunosuppression with chemotherapy and radiation therapy.
2. Confirmation of rejection is by skin or oral mucosal biopsy.
3. Successful engraftment is indicated by formation of erythrocytes, leukocytes, and platelets, usually 2 to 5 weeks after transplantation.
4. Care of the immunosuppressed client (see Chapter 7).

---

*Includes bone marrow transplant and stem cell transplant.

Study Questions Hematologic System

More questions on companion CD!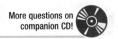

1. A client and her husband are positive for the sickle cell trait. The client asks the nurse about the chances of her children having sickle cell disease. The nurse understands that this genetic problem will reflect what pattern in the client's children?
   1 One of her children will have sickle cell disease.
   2 Only the male children will be affected.
   3 Each pregnancy carries a 25% chance of the child being affected.
   4 If she has four children, one of them will have the disease.

2. The nurse is preparing discharge teaching for a client with aplastic anemia. What will be important to include in the teaching plan? Select all that apply:
   _____ 1 Take your iron with meals every day and increase the amount of green, leafy vegetables in your diet.
   _____ 2 Establish a balance between rest and activity; avoid excessive fatigue.
   _____ 3 Rest and supplemental oxygen may be required during periods of dyspnea.
   _____ 4 Drink a glass of wine in the evening to help increase your appetite.
   _____ 5 Notify your health care provider if you begin to experience frequent bruising.
   _____ 6 Increase your intake of dairy products (milk and cheese) and protein.

3. A client is experiencing a sickle cell crisis during labor and delivery. What is the best nursing action?
   1 Maintain IV fluid infusion and assess adequacy of hydration.
   2 Administer a high concentration of oxygen.
   3 Insert a Foley catheter and monitor hourly urine output.
   4 Provide continuous sedation for pain relief.

4. The nurse is preparing a teaching plan for a family with a child who has been diagnosed with sickle cell anemia and crisis. What will the nurse include in the teaching regarding the pathophysiology of sickle cell crisis?
   1 It results from altered metabolism and dehydration.
   2 Tissue hypoxia and vascular occlusion cause the primary problems.
   3 Increased bilirubin levels will cause hypertension.
   4 There are decreased clotting factors with an increase in white blood cells.

5. A young woman comes to the clinic complaining of dizziness, weakness, and palpitations. What will be important for the nurse to evaluate initially when obtaining the health history?
   1 Activity and exercise patterns
   2 Nutritional patterns
   3 Family health status
   4 Coping and stress tolerance

6. A child with leukemia is being discharged after beginning chemotherapy. What instructions will the nurse include in the teaching plan for the parents of this child?
   1 Provide a diet low in protein and high in carbohydrates.
   2 Avoid fresh vegetables that are not cooked or peeled.
   3 Notify the doctor if the child's temperature exceeds 101° F (39° C).
   4 Increase the use of humidifiers throughout the house.

7. Which client is most likely to have iron deficiency anemia?
   1 A client with cancer receiving radiation therapy twice a week
   2 A toddler whose primary nutritional intake is milk
   3 A client with a peptic ulcer who had surgery 6 weeks ago
   4 A 15-year-old client in sickle cell crisis

8. A client with hemophilia comes to the emergency department after bumping his knee. The knee is rapidly swelling. What is the first nursing action?
   1 Initiate an IV site to begin administration of cryoprecipitate.
   2 Perform a type and cross-match for possible transfusion.
   3 Draw blood for determination of hemoglobin and hematocrit values.
   4 Apply an ice pack and compression dressings to the knee.

9. A client has an order for one unit of packed cells. What is a correct nursing action?
   1 Initiate the IV with 5% dextrose in water (D_5W) to maintain a patent access site.
   2 Initiate the transfusion within 30 minutes of receiving the blood.
   3 Monitor the client's vital signs for the first 5 minutes.
   4 Monitor the client's vital signs every 2 hours during the transfusion.

10. The nurse is caring for a client who is receiving a blood transfusion. The transfusion was started 30 minutes ago at a rate of 100 mL/hr. The client begins to complain of low back pain and headache and is increasingly restless. What is the first nursing action?
    1 Slow the infusion and evaluate the vital signs and the client's history of transfusion reactions.
    2 Stop the transfusion, disconnect the blood tubing, and begin a primary infusion of normal saline solution.
    3 Stop the infusion of blood and begin infusion of normal saline solution from the Y connector.
    4 Recheck the unit of blood for correct identification numbers and cross-match information.

Answers and rationales to these questions are in the section at the end of the book titled Chapter Study Questions: Answers and Rationales.

CHAPTER FIFTEEN

Respiratory System

The respiratory unit focuses on pathophysiologic conditions, which interfere with gas exchange. When problems of gas exchange occur, regardless of the precipitating cause, a hypoxic state is frequently the result. A thorough understanding of hypoxia and the appropriate nursing interventions for the client in a hypoxic state are a high priority.

PHYSIOLOGY OF THE RESPIRATORY SYSTEM

Organs of the Respiratory System

A. Bronchial tree.
1. Trachea divides below the carina into the right and left main stem bronchi, which extend into the lungs.
2. The right main stem bronchus is shorter, wider, and straighter than the left; therefore foreign objects are more likely to enter the right side.
3. Lobar bronchi: three in the right lung and two in the left lung; lobar bronchi subdivide several more times to form segmental and subsegmental bronchi.
4. Bronchioles: branching from the subsegmental bronchi; no cartilage in the walls. Bronchioles branch into the terminal bronchioles; no mucus glands or cilia.
B. Lungs (organs of respiration).
1. Lungs are located within the thoracic cavity (Figure 15-1)
2. Pleura: transparent serous membrane around the lung.
   a. Each lung is sealed within its own compartment by the pleura.
   b. Visceral pleura: adheres to the surface of the lung.
   c. Parietal pleura: covers the inner wall of the chest.
   d. Pleural space: potential space between the visceral and parietal pleura membrane; area between pleural layers contains a small amount of fluid to lubricate and allow for smooth motion of lung tissue during respirations.
3. Lungs.
   a. Divided into lobes.
      (1) Right lung: three lobes.
      (2) Left lung: two lobes.
   b. Each terminal bronchiole branches into respiratory bronchioles.

   c. The alveolar ducts are located at the end of the respiratory bronchioles.
   d. Alveoli: area of gas exchange; diffusion of oxygen (O_2) and carbon dioxide (CO_2) between the blood and the lungs occurs across the alveolar membrane.
   e. Surfactant is produced in the alveoli; its primary function is to reduce surface tension, which facilitates alveolar expansion and decreases the tendency of alveoli to collapse.
4. Premature infants frequently have inadequate production of surfactant.
5. Blood supply to the lungs.
   a. Pulmonary arteries to pulmonary capillaries to alveoli, where exchange of gas occurs.
   b. Bronchial arteries supply the nutrients to the lung tissue and do not participate in gas exchange.

Physiology of Respiration

External respiration is a process by which gas is exchanged between the circulating blood and the inhaled air.

A. Atmospheric pressure: pressure exerted on all body parts by surrounding air.
B. Intrathoracic pressure: pressure within the thoracic cage.
C. Gases flow from an area of high pressure to an area of low pressure; pressure below atmospheric pressure is designated as negative pressure.
D. Inspiration.
1. Stimulus to the diaphragm and the intercostal muscles by way of the central nervous system.
2. Diaphragm moves down, and intercostal muscles move outward, thereby increasing the capacity of the thoracic cavity and decreasing intrathoracic pressure to below atmospheric pressure.
3. Through the airways, the lungs are open to atmospheric pressure; air will flow into the lungs to equalize intrathoracic pressure with atmospheric pressure.
E. Expiration.
1. Diaphragm and intercostal muscles relax and return to a resting position; therefore lungs recoil and capacity is decreased.
2. Air will flow out until intrathoracic pressure is again equal to atmospheric pressure.
F. Negative pressure is greater during inspiration; therefore air flows easily into the lungs.

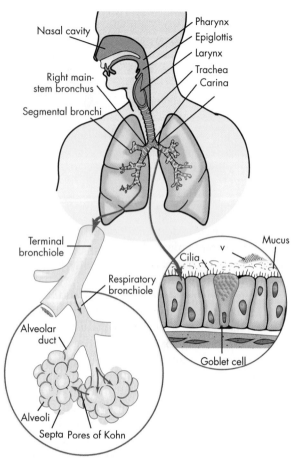

FIGURE 15-1 Respiratory system. (From Lewis SL et al: *Medical-surgical nursing: assessment and management of clinical problems*, ed 7, St. Louis, 2007, Mosby.)

G. Compliance describes how elastic the lungs are or how easily the lungs can be inflated; when compliance is decreased, the lungs are more difficult to inflate.

H. Respiratory volumes.
1. Tidal volume (VT or TV): amount of air moving in and out of the lungs in one normal breath. Normal = 500 mL (5-10 mL/kg).
2. Vital capacity (VC): amount of air forcibly exhaled in one breath after a maximum inhalation. Normal = 4500 mL.
3. Residual volume (RV): air remaining in the lungs at the end of a forced (maximum) expiration.

I. Control of respiration.
1. Movement of the diaphragm and accessory muscles of respiration is controlled by the respiratory center located in the brainstem (medulla oblongata and pons).
a. The respiratory center will control respirations by way of the spinal cord and phrenic nerve. The diaphragm is innervated by the phrenic nerve coming from the spinal cord between C-3 and C-5; the intercostal muscles are innervated by nerves from the spinal cord between T-2 and T-11.

b. Activity of the respiratory center is regulated by chemoreceptors. These receptors respond to changes in the chemical composition of the cerebrospinal fluid (CSF) and the blood (specifically, the Pao_2, $Paco_2$, and pH).
2. The medulla contains the central chemoreceptors responsive to changes in CO_2 blood levels.
a. CO_2 diffuses into cerebrospinal fluid (CSF), increasing the hydrogen ion concentration of CSF. This has a direct stimulating effect on the chemoreceptors in the medulla.
b. CO_2 saturation of the blood regulates ventilation through its effect on the pH of the CSF and the effects of the CSF on the respiratory center in the medulla.

> **⬛ NURSING PRIORITY** The primary respiratory stimulus is CO_2; when the $Paco_2$ is increased, ventilation is initiated.

3. Carotid and aortic bodies contain the peripheral chemoreceptors for arterial O_2 levels.
a. Primary function is to monitor arterial O_2 levels and stimulate the respiratory center when a decrease in Pao_2 occurs.
b. When arterial O_2 decreases to below 60 mm Hg, stimulation to breathe is initiated by the chemoreceptors.
c. In a person whose primary stimulus to breathe is hypoxia, this becomes the mechanism of ventilatory control.

J. The process of gas exchange.
1. Ventilation: the process of moving air between the atmosphere and alveoli.
2. Diffusion.
a. The process of moving O_2 and CO_2 across the alveolar capillary membrane.
b. Links the processes of ventilation and perfusion.
c. Gas diffuses across the alveolar capillary membrane from an area of high concentration to an area of low concentration.
d. Factors affecting diffusion: surface area of the lung, thickness of the alveolar capillary membrane, characteristics of the gases.

> **⬛ NURSING PRIORITY** When mucus is retained and pools in the lungs, gas diffusion is decreased; provides a medium for bacteria growth.

3. Perfusion.
a. The process of linking the venous blood flow to the alveoli.
b. Dependent on the volume of blood flowing from the right ventricle into and through the pulmonary circulation.

Oxygen and Carbon Dioxide Transport

Internal respiration is the exchange of gases between the blood and interstitial fluid. The gases are measured by an analysis of arterial blood (Table 15-1).

Table 15-1	NORMAL ARTERIAL BLOOD GAS VALUES		
Acidity index	pH	7.35-7.45
Partial pressure of dissolved oxygen	Pao_2	80 to 100 mm Hg
Percentage of hemoglobin saturated with oxygen	Sao_2	95% or above
Partial pressure of dissolved carbon dioxide	$Paco_2$	35 to 45 mm Hg
Bicarbonate	HCO_3^-	22 to 28 mEq/L

> **❗ NURSING PRIORITY** An Sao_2 below 95% indicates respiratory difficulty.

A. O_2.
   1. Transported as a dissolved gas; Pao_2 refers to the partial pressure of O_2 in arterial blood.
   2. O_2 is primarily transported chemically bound to hemoglobin; when hemoglobin leaves the pulmonary capillary bed, it is usually 95% to 100% saturated with O_2. It may be referred to as the arterial oxygen saturation (Sao_2). O_2 can also be carried (physically dissolved) in the plasma.
   3. Oxygenated hemoglobin moves through the arterial system into the cellular capillary bed, where O_2 is released from the hemoglobin and made available for cellular metabolism.
   4. Venous blood contains about 75% O_2 as it returns to the right side of the heart.
   5. O_2 delivered to the tissue is dependent on cardiac output.
B. Oxyhemoglobin dissociation curve.
   1. Curve shows the affinity of hemoglobin for O_2 at different O_2 tensions.
   2. O_2 that remains bound to hemoglobin does not contribute to cellular metabolism.
   3. Affinity of hemoglobin refers to the capacity of hemoglobin to bind to O_2.
   4. The affinity of hemoglobin for O_2 is influenced by many factors, such as hydrogen ion concentration (pH), CO_2, and body temperature.
      a. Hemoglobin binds tightly together with O_2 in an alkaline condition.
      b. Hemoglobin releases O_2 in an acid condition.
      c. As CO_2 moves into the serum at the capillary bed, it decreases the pH (acidotic), thereby enhancing O_2 release.
      d. As CO_2 moves out of the venous system into the lungs, the pH (alkalotic) is increased in the blood, thereby enhancing hemoglobin affinity for O_2.
      e. In hypothermia, blood picks up O_2 more readily from the lungs but delivers O_2 less readily to the tissues; in hyperthermia, the opposite occurs.
   5. A decrease in the arterial O_2 tension (Pao_2) and a decrease in the saturation of the hemoglobin with oxygen (Sao_2) results in a state of hypoxemia.

C. Effects of altitude on O_2 transport.
   1. At high levels (above 10,000 feet), there is reduced O_2 in the atmosphere, resulting in a lower inspired O_2 pressure and a lower Pao_2. Commercial planes are pressurized to an altitude of 8000 feet.

> **❗ NURSING PRIORITY** Clients who are on oxygen or who have a Pao_2 of less that 72 mm Hg on room air should consult with their physician before planning air travel.

   2. Body compensatory mechanisms.
      a. Increase in the number of red blood cells or hematocrit from body storage areas, thereby increasing the total hemoglobin-carrying and O_2-carrying capacity of the blood.
      b. Hyperventilation.
      c. Renal erythropoietic factor (erythropoietin) is released, thereby enhancing the production of red blood cells (secondary polycythemia). It takes approximately 4 to 5 days to actually increase red blood cell production.

> **ALERT** Apply knowledge of pathophysiology to monitoring for complications; identify client status based on pathophysiology.

   3. Extended exposure to high altitudes will result in an increased vascularization of the lungs, thus increasing the capacity of the blood to carry O_2.
   4. Problem with oxygenation at high altitudes.
      a. Decrease in O_2 supply (decrease in cardiac output or inadequate hemoglobin).
      b. Increase in body's demand.

⚷ System Assessment

A. History.
   1. Determine the frequency of upper respiratory problems and/or surgeries involving respiratory problems.
   2. Status of immunizations.
      a. Tuberculin (TB) skin test (also known as PPD or Mantoux test).
      b. Pertussis, polio, pneumococcal pneumonia vaccine (Pneumovax).
   3. Medications (including OTC, prescriptions, herbs, and vitamins).
   4. Lifestyle and occupational environments.
   5. Habits: smoking and alcohol intake.
   6. Any change in ADLs and activity secondary to respiratory problems.
B. Physical assessment.

> **ALERT** Monitor changes in the client's respiratory status. The primary indicators of respiratory disorders are sputum production, cough, dyspnea, hemoptysis, pleuritic chest pain, fatigue, change in voice, and wheezing.

1. Initially observe client's resting position.
   a. Appearance: comfortable or distressed?
   b. Assess client in the sitting position, if possible.
   c. Any dyspnea or respiratory discomfort?
2. Evaluate vital signs.
   a. Appropriate for age level?
   b. Establish database and compare with previous data.
   c. Assess client's pattern of vital signs; normal vital signs vary greatly from one individual to another (see Table 3-2).

> **ALERT** Apply knowledge of client pathophysiology when measuring vital signs; intervene when vital signs are abnormal; interpret data that need to be reported immediately.

3. Assess upper airway passages and patency of the airway.
4. Inspect the neck for symmetry; check to see whether the trachea is in midline and observe for presence of jugular vein distention.
5. Assess the lungs.
   a. Visually evaluate the chest/thorax.
      (1) Do both sides move equally?
      (2) Observe characteristics of respirations and note whether retractions are present (Figure 15-2).
      (3) Note chest wall configuration (barrel chest, kyphoscoliosis, etc.).
   b. Palpate chest for tenderness, masses, and symmetry of motion.
   c. Auscultate breath sounds; begin at lung apices and end at the bases, comparing each area side to side. Breath sounds should be present and equal bilaterally.

FIGURE 15-2 Location of retractions. (From Hockenberry MJ, Wilson D: *Wong's nursing care of infants and children,* 8th ed, St. Louis, 2007, Mosby.)

   d. Determine presence of tactile fremitus: When client says "ninety-nine," there should be equal vibrations palpated bilaterally. Over areas of consolidation, there will be an increase in the vibrations.
   e. Determine presence of adventitious breath sounds (abnormal/extra breath sounds).
      (1) Crackles: usually heard during inspiration and do not clear with cough; occur when airway contains fluid (previously also known as *rales*); sounds are not continuous (early cardiac failure, pneumonia, and atelectasis).
      (2) Wheezes: may be heard during inspiration and/or expiration; are caused by air moving through narrowed passages; sound is music-like and continuous.
      (3) Pleural friction rub: heard primarily on inspiration over an area of pleural inflammation; may be described as a grating sound.
6. Assess cough reflex and sputum production.
   a. Is cough associated with pain?
   b. What precipitates coughing episodes?
   c. Is cough productive or nonproductive?
   d. Characteristics of sputum.
      (1) Consistency.
      (2) Amount.
      (3) Color (should be clear or white).
   e. Presence of hemoptysis—duration and amount.
7. Assess for and evaluate dyspnea.
   a. Onset of dyspnea and precipitating causes.
   b. Presence of orthopnea.
   c. Presence of adventitious breath sounds.
   d. Noisy expiration.
   e. Level of tolerance of activity.
   f. Correlate vital signs with dyspnea.
   g. Cyanosis (a very late and unreliable sign of hypoxia).
      (1) For dark-skinned clients, assess the areas that are less pigmented (oral cavity, nail beds, lips, palms).
      (2) Dark-skinned clients may exhibit cyanosis in the skin as a gray hue, rather than blue.
      (3) Prolonged capillary refill time, should be less than 3 seconds.
8. Assess for and evaluate chest pain.
   a. Location of pain.
   b. Character of pain.
   c. Pain associated with cough.
   d. Pain either increased or decreased with breathing.
9. Evaluate fingers for clubbing (characteristic in clients with chronic respiratory disorders).
10. Evaluate pulmonary diagnostics (see Appendix 15-1).
    a. Hemoglobin and hematocrit (presence of polycythemia or anemia).
    b. Electrolyte imbalances.
    c. Arterial blood gases (ABGs).

RESPIRATORY DISORDERS

 Hypoxia

Hypoxia is a condition characterized by an inadequate amount of O_2 available for cellular metabolism.

ALERT Problems with respiratory status occur in all nursing disciplines. Questions may center around nursing priorities and nursing interventions in maintaining an airway and promoting ventilation in the client with respiratory difficulty. The questions may arise from any client situation (e.g., obstetrics, newborn, surgical, etc.).

A. Hypoxia occurs when signs and symptoms occur because of a decrease in Pao_2; hypoxemia occurs when the amount of O_2 in the arterial blood is less than normal.
   1. Decreased O_2 in inspired air.
   2. Disorders causing respiratory obstruction and alveolar hypoventilation.
B. Hypoxia may be caused by inadequate circulation.
   1. Shock.
   2. Cardiac failure.
C. Anemia precipitates hypoxia caused by a decrease in the O_2-carrying capacity of the blood.
   1. Inadequate red blood cell production.
   2. Deficient or abnormal hemoglobin.

Assessment

A. Risk factors/etiology.
   1. Chronic hypoxia.
      a. Chronic obstructive pulmonary disease (COPD).
      b. Cystic fibrosis.
      c. Cancer of the respiratory tract.
      d. Heart failure.
      e. Chronic anemia.
   2. Inflammatory problems affecting alveolar surface area and membrane integrity (e.g., pneumonia, bronchitis).
   3. Acute hypoxia.
      a. Acute respiratory failure.
      b. Sudden airway obstruction.
      c. Conditions affecting pulmonary expansion (e.g., respiratory paralysis).
      d. Conditions causing decreased cardiac output (heart failure, shock, cardiac arrest, etc.).
      e. Hypoventilation (brain attack or stroke, sedation, anesthesia, etc.).
B. Clinical manifestations: underlying respiratory problem, either chronic or acute (Table 15-2).
C. Diagnostics (see Appendix 15-1).
D. Compensatory mechanisms.
   1. Increase in cardiac output (tachycardia).
   2. Increase in extraction of O_2 from capillary blood.
   3. Increase in level of hemoglobin.
E. Complications.
   1. Acute.
      a. Cardiac decompensation.
      b. Progression to chronic hypoxia.
   2. Chronic.
      a. CO_2 narcosis (increase in CO_2 content of blood).
      b. Cor pulmonale.
      c. Cardiac failure.
   3. Treatment: depends on underlying problem.

NURSING PRIORITY In the client with chronic lung disease who is experiencing severe hypoxia, O_2 should never be withheld for fear of increasing the Pao_2 levels.

Nursing Interventions

Goal: To maintain good pulmonary hygiene and prevent hypoxic episode.
A. Position client to maintain patent airway.
   1. Unconscious client: position on side with the chin extended.
   2. Conscious client: elevate the head of the bed and may position on side as well.
B. Encourage coughing and deep breathing (Box 15-1).

Table 15-2	SYMPTOMS OF RESPIRATORY DISTRESS AND HYPOXIA	
Early Symptoms		**Late Symptoms**
Restlessness		Extreme restlessness to stupor
Tachycardia		Severe dyspnea
Tachypnea, exertional dyspnea		Slowing of respiratory rate
Orthopnea, tripod positioning		Bradycardia
Anxiety, difficulty speaking		Cyanosis (peripheral or
Poor judgment, confusion		central)
Disorientation		
Pediatrics		
Flaring nares (infants)		Mottling, pallor, and cyanosis
Substernal, suprasternal,		Sudden increase or sudden
supraclavicular and		decrease in agitation
intercostal retractions (see		Inaudible breath sounds
Figure 15-2)		Altered level of consciousness
Stridor—expiratory and		Inability to cry or to speak
inspiratory		
Increased agitation		

Box 15-1   EFFECTIVE COUGHING

- Increase activity before coughing: walking or turning from side to side.
- Place client in sitting position, preferably with feet on the floor.
- Client should turn his or her shoulders inward and bend head slightly forward.
- Take a gentle breath in through the nose and breathe out completely.
- Take two deep breaths through the nose and mouth and hold for 5 seconds.
- On the third deep breath, cough to clear secretions.
- Sips of warm liquids (coffee, tea, or water) may stimulate coughing.
- Demonstrate to client how to splint chest or incision during cough to decrease pain.

C. Suction client as needed and as indicated by amount of sputum and ability to cough.

D. Maintain adequate fluid intake to keep secretions liquefied.

E. Encourage exercises and ambulation as indicated by condition.

F. Administer expectorants.

G. Administer O₂ if dyspnea is present.

> ❗ **NURSING PRIORITY** Administer fluids very cautiously to a client who is having difficulty breathing. Begin with small sips of water to determine whether the client can swallow effectively—thickened liquids are easier to control. Do not begin with fluids that contain any fat (milk) or caloric value because of the increased risk for aspiration.

Goal: To implement nursing measures to decrease hypoxia. (Box 15-2).

A. Assess patency of airway (first/highest priority).
   1. Can client speak? If not, initiate emergency procedures (see Appendix 15-3).
   2. If speaking is difficult because of level of hypoxia, place in semi-Fowler's position, begin oxygen, obtain assistance, and remain with client.
   3. If client is coherent and able to speak in sentences, continue with assessment of the problem.
   4. Evaluate amount of secretions and ability to cough; suction and administer O₂ as indicated.

B. Assess use of accessory muscles, presence of retractions.

C. Maintain calm approach, because increasing anxiety will potentiate hypoxia.

> ❗ **NURSING PRIORITY** Increasing anxiety will accelerate dyspnea in a client who is experiencing severe difficulty breathing.

D. Place adult or older child in a semi-Fowler's position, if not contraindicated.

E. Place infant in an infant seat or elevate the mattress.

Box 15-2 OLDER ADULT CARE FOCUS

Respiratory Care Priorities

- Older adult client may not present with respiratory symptoms, but instead with confusion and disorientation.
- Provide adequate rest periods between activities, such as bathing, going for treatments, eating, etc.
- Increase compliance with medications by scheduling medication administration with routine activities.
- Encourage annual flu shot for individuals over age 65 and determine whether older adult has received pneumococcal vaccination.
- Evaluate client's response to changes in activity and therapy frequently.
- Administer oxygen with caution; evaluate response to increased levels of oxygen saturation.
- Maintain adequate hydration but use caution because of increased tendency for fluid volume overload.

> ❗ **NURSING PRIORITY** Position a client experiencing dyspnea with a pillow placed lengthwise behind the back and head. Do not flex the client's head forward or backward.

F. Assess color and presence of diaphoresis.

G. Evaluate vital signs: Are there significant changes from previous readings?

H. Evaluate for dysrhythmias.
   1. If the client is on a cardiac monitor, check for presence of premature atrial or ventricular contractions.
   2. Evaluate level of tachycardia.

I. Evaluate chest movements: Are they symmetrical?

J. Evaluate anterior and posterior breath sounds.

K. Assess client for chest pain with dyspnea.

L. Notify physician of significant changes in respiratory function.

M. Remain with client experiencing acute dyspnea or hypoxic episodes.

N. Assess response to O₂ therapy.

O. Monitor ABGs and pulse oximetry.

📋 Pneumothorax

Air in the pleural space results in the collapse or atelectasis of that portion of the lung. This condition is known as *pneumothorax* (Figure 15-3).

A. Tension pneumothorax: the development of a pneumothorax that allows excessive buildup of pressure (due to air that cannot escape) in the pleural space, causing a shift in the mediastinum toward the unaffected side.

> ❗ **NURSING PRIORITY** A tension pneumothorax can very rapidly become an emergency situation. It is much easier to treat the client if the pneumothorax is identified *before* it begins to exert tension on the mediastinal area.

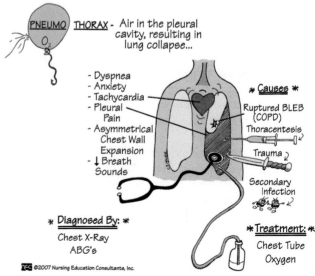

FIGURE 15-3 Pneumothorax. (From Zerwekh J, Claborn J: *Memory notebook of nursing,* vol 2, ed 3, Ingram, Texas, 2007, Nursing Education Consultants.)

Assessment

A. Risk factors/etiology.
  1. Ruptured bleb (spontaneous).
  2. Thoracentesis.
  3. Infection.
  4. Trauma (penetrating or blunt chest injury).
B. Clinical manifestations.
  1. Diminished or absent breath sounds on the affected side.
  2. Dyspnea, hypoxia.
  3. Tachycardia, tachypnea.
  4. Sudden onset of persistent chest pain, pain on affected side when breathing.
  5. Increasing anxiety.
  6. Asymmetrical chest wall expansion.
  7. Hyperresonance on percussion of affected side.
  8. Possible development of a tension pneumothorax.
    a. Decreased cardiac filling, leading to decreased cardiac output.
    b. Tracheal shift from midline toward unaffected side.
    c. Increasing problems of hypoxia.
C. Diagnostics (see Appendix 15-1).

> ⚠ **NURSING PRIORITY** When atmospheric pressure is allowed to disrupt the negative pressure in the pleural space, it will cause the lung to collapse. This requires chest tube placement to reestablish negative pressure and reinflate the lung.

Treatment

Placement of chest tubes connected to a water-sealed drainage system (see Appendix 15-4).

Nursing Interventions

Goal: To recognize the problem and prevent a severe hypoxic episode (see Hypoxia, Nursing Interventions).
A. Begin O_2 therapy.
B. Place in semi–Fowler's position.
C. Notify physician and prepare client for insertion of chest tubes.
Goal: To reinflate lung without complications.
A. Have client cough and deep-breathe every 2 hours.
B. Encourage exercise and ambulation.
C. Establish and maintain water-sealed chest drainage system (see Appendix 15-4).

📋 Pleural Effusion

Pleural effusion is caused by a collection of fluid in the pleural space. It is generally associated with other disease processes.

Assessment

A. Pathophysiology.
  1. Causes: CHF, pneumonia, TB, malignancy, pulmonary embolism, acute pancreatitis, and connective tissue disease.
  2. Transudative effusion: the result of noninflammatory conditions; caused by an increased hydrostatic pressure found in heart failure and by decreased oncotic pressure from the loss of circulating protein (chronic renal or hepatic failure).
  3. Exudative effusion: caused by an inflammatory process; occurs as a result of increased capillary permeability due to an inflammatory reaction from bacterial products or tumors.
  4. If the pleural fluid becomes purulent, the condition is referred to as empyema.
B. Clinical manifestations.
  1. Symptoms of an underlying problem.
  2. Large quantities of fluid will cause shortness of breath and dyspnea.
  3. Decreased breath sounds.
  4. Pleuritic pain on inspiration.
  5. Asymmetrical chest expansion.
C. Diagnostics (see Appendix 15-1).
  1. Malignancy may be determined by cytologic examination of the aspirated fluid.
  2. Culture and sensitivity on aspirated fluid.

Treatment

A. Thoracentesis (see Appendix 15-1) and pleurodesis (inflammation caused by a sclerosing agent, which leads to pleura sticking to chest wall).
B. If empyema develops (purulent fluid in the pleural space) area may have to be opened and allowed to drain.
C. Chest tube placement is necessary if fluid buildup is rapid, requiring removal to facilitate respirations.

Nursing Interventions

Goal: To recognize problems associated with chest tube placement and prevent an acute episode of hypoxia (see Hypoxia, Nursing Interventions).

🖐 Home Care

A. Demonstrate to client and family the prescribed method of managing wound care.
B. Client is at increased risk for respiratory tract infections.
C. The purulent fluid is localized and will not be hazardous to other family members if the basic concepts of hand hygiene and sterile technique for dressing changes are used.

📋 Open Chest Wound

An open or "sucking" chest wound is frequently caused by a penetrating injury to the chest, such as a gunshot or knife wound. If a chest tube is inadvertently pulled out of the chest, a sucking chest wound may be created.

Assessment

A. Clinical manifestations.
  1. Increase in dyspnea.
  2. A chest wound with evidence of air moving in and out via the wound.

Treatment

A. Have the client take a deep breath, hold it, and bear down against a closed glottis. Apply a light occlusive, vented dressing (taped/secured on three sides to allow air to escape) over the wound.

> **! NURSING PRIORITY** Immediately occlude the chest wound; do not leave the client to go find a dressing. If necessary, place a towel or whatever is at hand over the wound to stop the flow of air.

B. Prepare for insertion of chest tubes to water-sealed drainage system.
C. After covering the wound with a light occlusive dressing, carefully evaluate the client for development of a tension pneumothorax.

Nursing Interventions

Goal: To prevent problems of hypoxia.
Goal: To assess for development of tension pneumothorax.

Flail Chest

Flail chest is the loss of stability of the chest wall with respiratory impairment as a result of multiple rib fractures (fractures at two or more points of the ribs involved).

Assessment

A. Clinical manifestations.
 1. Paradoxical respirations: the movement of the fractured area (flailed segment) inward during inspiration and outward during expiration, or opposite to the other areas of the chest wall.
 2. Symptoms of hypoxia.
B. Diagnostics.
 1. Chest x-ray film showing multiple rib fractures.
 2. Crepitus of the ribs.

Treatment

A. Maintain patent airway.
B. Adequate pain medication to enable client to breathe deeply.
C. O_2.
D. Endotracheal intubation with mechanical ventilation for severe respiratory distress (see Appendixes 15-5 and 15-8).
E. Chest tube placement if pneumothorax occurs as a result of puncture of the lung by the fractured rib.

> **ALERT** Determine changes in client's respiratory status.

Nursing Interventions

Goal: To stabilize the chest wall and prevent complications.
A. Prepare client for endotracheal intubation and mechanical ventilation (see Appendixes 15-5 and 15-8).
B. Assess for symptoms of hypoxia.
C. Assess for symptoms of pneumothorax.

📋 Pulmonary Embolism

A pulmonary embolism (PE) is an obstruction of a pulmonary artery, most often the result of an embolism caused by a blood clot (thrombus), air, fat, amniotic fluid, bone marrow, or sepsis. The severity of the problem depends on the size of the embolus.

A. Of the clients that die from PE, the majority die because of failure to diagnose.
B. The majority of pulmonary emboli arise from thrombi in the deep veins of the legs.
C. A pulmonary embolism must originate from the venous circulation, or the right side of the heart.

Assessment

A. Common risk factors/etiology.
 1. Conditions or immobility predisposing to venous stasis and/or deep vein thrombosis: surgery within the last 3 months, stroke, spinal cord injury, and history of deep vein thrombosis (DVT).
 2. Vascular injury: intravenous (IV) catheters, thrombophlebitis, vascular disease, leg fractures.
 3. DVT: the thrombus spontaneously dislodges secondary to jarring of the area—sudden standing, changes in rate of blood flow (Valsalva maneuver, increased BP).
B. Clinical manifestations.
 1. Classic triad of symptoms: dyspnea, chest pain, and hemoptysis occurs in only 20% of clients.
 2. Most common symptoms.
  a. Increased anxiety.
  b. Sudden, unexplained dyspnea.
  c. Tachypnea.
  d. Tachycardia.
 3. Hypotension and syncope.
 4. May result in sudden death if pulmonary embolism is large.
C. Diagnostics (see Appendix 15-1).
 1. Enhanced spiral computed tomography (CT) scan (specific for PE).
 2. D-dimer test is elevated (greater than 250 mcg/L).

Treatment

A. Bed rest, semi–Fowler's position if BP permits.
B. Respiratory support: O_2, ventilator, etc.
C. Anticoagulants (heparin, low-molecular-weight heparin, or warfarin) to prevent further thrombus formation.
D. IV access for fluids and medications to maintain blood pressure.
E. Small doses of morphine sulfate may be used to decrease anxiety, alleviate chest pain, or improve tolerance to endotracheal tube.
F. Thrombolytics.

> **ALERT** Assess clients for complications caused by immobility. Immobilized clients have an increased risk for development of a pulmonary embolism. Questions require an understanding of principles for prevention of thrombophlebitis and subsequent embolism formation. It is far easier to prevent the problem than it is to treat the pulmonary embolism.

Nursing Interventions

Goal: To identify clients at increased risk and prevent and/or decrease venous stasis (see Box 16-2).

Goal: To identify problem and implement nursing measures to alleviate hypoxia (see Hypoxia, Nursing Interventions).

Goal: To monitor client's respiratory function and response to treatment.

Croup Syndromes

The term *croup* describes a group of conditions characterized by edema and inflammation of the upper respiratory tract.

A. Acute epiglottitis: a severe infection of the epiglottis, characterized by rapid inflammation and edema of the area; generally occurs in children 2 to 7 years old; may rapidly cause airway obstruction.
1. Cause: most commonly *Haemophilus influenza*.
2. Clinical manifestations: hypoxia (see Table 15-2).
   a. Rapid, abrupt onset.
   b. Sore throat, difficulty in swallowing.
   c. Inflamed epiglottis.
   d. Symptoms of increasing respiratory tract obstruction.
      (1) Characteristic position: sitting with the neck hyperextended (sniffing position) and mouth open (tripod position), drooling.
      (2) Inspiratory stridor (crowing).
      (3) Suprasternal and substernal retractions.
      (4) Increased restlessness and apprehension.
   e. High fever (above 102° F).

> ❗ **NURSING PRIORITY** The absence of spontaneous cough and the presence of drooling and agitation are cardinal signs distinctive of epiglottitis.

3. Treatment.
   a. Endotracheal intubation for obstruction (see Appendix 15-5).
   b. Humidified oxygen.
   c. Antibiotics: IV and then PO.

B. Acute laryngotracheobronchitis (croup): inflammation of the larynx and trachea, most often in children under 5 years.
1. Cause: viral agents (influenza and parainfluenza viruses, respiratory syncytial virus).
2. Slow onset, frequently preceded by upper respiratory tract infection.
3. Respiratory distress (see Table 15-2).
   a. Inspiratory stridor when disturbed, progressing to continuous stridor.
   b. Flaring of nares, use of accessory muscles of respiration.
   c. "Seal bark" cough is classic sign.
4. Low-grade fever (usually below 102° F).
5. Signs of impending obstruction.
   a. Retractions (intercostals, suprasternal, and substernal) at rest.
   b. Increased anxiety and restlessness.
   c. Tachypnea (rate may be above 60 breaths/min).
   d. Pallor and diaphoresis.
   e. Nasal flaring.

> **ALERT** Intervene when vital signs are abnormal; position client to prevent complications; interpret client data that need to be reported immediately.

6. Treatment.
   a. Maintain patent airway.
   b. Bronchodilators, racemic epinephrine (for moderate to severe croup) by inhalation.
   c. Cool mist humidification.
   d. No sedatives.
   e. Oxygen.
   f. Corticosteroids, administered intravenously, intramuscularly, or orally.

C. Acute spasmodic laryngitis: mildest form of croup; generally occurs in children 1 to 4 years old.
1. Cause: unknown.
2. Clinical manifestations.
   a. Characterized by paroxysmal attacks.
   b. Characteristically occurs at night.
   c. Mild respiratory distress (see Table 15-2).
   d. No fever.
   e. After the attack, the child appears well.
3. Treatment:
   a. Child is generally cared for at home.
   b. Usually self-limiting.
   c. Cool mist may decrease spasm.

Nursing Interventions

Goal: To maintain patent airway in hospitalized child.

A. Tracheotomy set or endotracheal intubation equipment readily available.

> ❗ **NURSING PRIORITY** For a child with epiglottitis, do not examine the throat because it may precipitate an airway spasm (laryngospasm).

B. Suction endotracheal tube or tracheotomy only as necessary.
C. Position for comfort; do not force child to lie down.
D. If child is intubated, do not leave unattended.
E. If obstruction is impending, maintain ventilation with a bag-valve mask resuscitator until child can be intubated.
F. If transport is required, allow the child to sit upright in parent's lap if possible.

Goal: To evaluate and maintain adequate ventilation.

A. Assess for increasing hypoxia.
B. Provide humidified O_2; closely evaluate because cyanosis is a late sign of hypoxia.
C. Conserve energy; prevent crying.
D. Monitor pulse oximetry for adequate oxygenation.

Goal: To maintain hydration and nutrition.

A. Do not give oral fluids until danger of aspiration is past.

ALERT Identify client potential for aspiration. In children with severe respiratory distress (rate above 60), do not give anything by mouth due to increased risk for aspiration.

B. Give IV fluids during acute episodes.
C. Provide high-calorie liquids when danger of aspiration is over.
D. Suction nares of infant before feeding.
E. Assess for adequate hydration.

 Home Care

A. Teach parents to recognize symptoms of increasing respiratory problems and when to notify physician.
B. Cool mist may assist to decrease edema and/or spasms of airway.
C. Maintain adequate fluid intake.
D. Immunization with *H. Influenza* type B vaccine.

Bronchiolitis (Respiratory Syncytial Virus)

Bronchiolitis is an inflammation of the bronchioles; alveoli are usually normal.

A. Respiratory syncytial virus (RSV) infection is most common in winter and spring (November to March), peaks in children 2-5 months old.
B. RSV is transmitted by direct contact with respiratory secretions (Appendix 6-8).
C. RSV is considered the single most important respiratory pathogen of infancy and early childhood.

Assessment

A. Cause: usually begins after an upper respiratory tract infection; incubation period of 5-8 days.
B. Reinfection is common; severity tends to decrease with age and repeated infections.
C. Clinical manifestations.
   1. Initial.
      a. Rhinorrhea and low-grade fever commonly occur first.
      b. Coughing, wheezing.
   2. Acute phase.
      a. Lethargic.
      b. Tachypnea, air hunger, retractions.
      c. Increased wheezing and coughing.
      d. Periods of apnea, poor air exchange.
D. Diagnostics: nasal secretions for RSV antigens.

Treatment

A. Rest, fluids, and high-humidity environment.
B. O₂.
C. Prevention – medication (see Appendix 15-2).

Nursing Interventions

Goal: To promote effective breathing patterns.
A. Frequent assessment for development of hypoxia (see Table 15-2); close monitoring of O_2 saturation (oximetry) levels.

B. Increase in respiratory rate and audible crackles in the lungs are indications of cardiac failure and should be reported immediately.
C. Maintain airway via position and removal of secretions.
D. Maintain adequate hydration to facilitate removal of respiratory secretions.
E. Conserve energy; avoid unnecessary procedures, but encourage parents to console and cuddle infant.

Goal: To prevent transmission of organisms.
A. If hospitalized, the child should be placed in a private room, with contact precautions in place (Appendix 6-8).
B. Decrease number of health care personnel in client's room.
C. Nurses assigned to care for these children should not be assigned the care of other children who are at high risk for respiratory tract infections.
D. Prophylaxis medication with palivizumab (Synagis) for high-risk infants.

 Home Care

A. Decreased energy level; will tire easily.
B. Small frequent feedings.
C. Teach parents how to assess for respiratory difficulty.
D. Teach parents care implications if child is receiving prophylactic medications (see Appendix 15-2).

Tonsillitis

Tonsillitis is an inflammation and infection of the palatine tonsils.

Assessment

A. Risk factors/etiology.
   1. More common in children.
   2. Increased severity in adults.
B. Clinical manifestations.
   1. Edematous, enlarged tonsils; exudate on tonsils.
   2. Difficulty swallowing and breathing.
   3. Frequently precipitates otitis media.
   4. Mouth breathing.
   5. Persistent cough, fever.
C. Diagnostics: throat culture for group A beta-hemolytic streptococci (see Appendix 15-1).

Treatment

A. Antibiotic for identified organism.
B. Surgery: tonsillectomy for severe repeated episodes of tonsillitis.

Nursing Interventions

Goal: To promote comfort and healing in home environment.
A. Nonirritating soft or liquid diet.
B. Cool mist vaporizer to maintain moisture in mucous membranes.
C. Throat lozenges, warm gargles to soothe the throat.
D. Antibiotics: important to give child all of the medication prescribed in order to prevent reoccurrence.
E. Analgesics, antipyretic (acetaminophen).

Goal: To provide preoperative nursing measures if surgery is indicated (see Chapter 3).

Goal: To maintain patent airway and evaluate for bleeding after tonsillectomy.

A. No fluids until child is fully awake; then cool, clear liquids initially. Avoid brown- or red-colored fluids and milk products.

B. Position child on side or abdomen to facilitate drainage until fully awake; when awake and alert, child may assume position of comfort but needs to remain in bed for the day.

C. Evaluate for frequent or continuous swallowing caused by bleeding; check throat with flashlight for bleeding.

D. Have nasopharyngeal suction equipment available.

E. Monitor for tachycardia, pallor, and increasing restlessness.

F. Apply ice collar to decrease edema.

G. Give oral codeine or acetaminophen for pain; aspirin is contraindicated.

H. Discourage coughing.

> **!! NURSING PRIORITY** Before the child is fully awake, position him or her on side or abdomen to prevent aspiration from bloody drainage or vomitus. Always consider the client who has had a tonsillectomy to be nauseated as a result of swallowing blood.

Home Care

A. Child will have sore throat for several days; discourage coughing and excessive activity.

B. Symptoms of bleeding are especially significant on the 5th to 10th postoperative days, when tissue sloughing may occur as a result of healing and/or infection.

C. Maintain adequate hydration; encourage intake of soft foods and nonirritating fluids.

D. A gray membrane on the sides of the throat is normal; should disappear in 1 to 2 weeks.

Pneumonia

Pneumonia is an acute inflammatory process caused by a microbial agent; it involves the lung parenchyma, including the small airways and alveoli.

Assessment

A. Predisposing conditions.
   1. Chronic upper respiratory tract infection.
   2. Prolonged immobility.
   3. Smoking.
   4. Decreased immunity (disease and/or age).
   5. Aspiration of foreign material or gastric contents.
   6. Chronic health problems: cardiac, pulmonary, diabetes, cancer, stroke.
   7. Nosocomial pneumonia: caused by tracheal intubation, intestinal/gastric tube feedings.

B. Etiology.
   1. Viral: influenza, parainfluenza, RSV (primarily infants and young children).
   2. Bacterial: *Streptococcus pneumoniae, Mycoplasma pneumoniae, Staphylococcus aureus.*
   3. Fungal (increased risk in immunocompromised clients).

C. Clinical manifestations.
   1. Fever, chills.
   2. Tachycardia.
   3. Tachypnea, dyspnea.
   4. Productive cough: thick, blood-streaked, yellow, purulent sputum.
   5. Chest pain.
   6. Malaise, altered mental status.
   7. Respiratory distress (hypoxia) (see Table 15-2).
   8. Diminished breath sounds, wheezing, crackles, tactile fremitus, dullness to percussion.
   9. Pediatrics.
      a. Feeding difficulty in infants.
      b. Cough nonproductive initially.
      c. Moderate to high fever.
      d. Adventitious breath sounds.
      e. Tachypnea.
      f. Retractions, nasal flaring

D. Diagnostics (see Appendix 15-1).

> **!! OLDER ADULT PRIORITY** An older adult client may initially present with mental confusion and volume depletion rather then respiratory symptoms and fever.

Treatment

A. Antibiotic according to organism identified (see Appendix 6-9).

> **ALERT** Administration of medications: do not start antibiotics until a good sputum specimen has been collected. An accurate culture and sensitivity test cannot be done if client has already begun receiving antibiotics.

B. Respiratory precautions: transmitted via airborne droplets (see Appendix 6-8).

C. Inhalation therapy.
   1. Cool O$_2$ mist.
   2. Postural drainage.
   3. Bronchodilators.

D. Chest physical therapy.

Nursing Interventions

Goal: To prevent occurrence.

A. Encourage mobility and ambulation if possible.

B. Good respiratory hygiene; turn, cough, and deep-breathe.

C. Identify high-risk clients.

D. Encourage pneumococcal vaccine.

Goal: To decrease infection and remove secretions to facilitate O_2 and CO_2 exchange.

A. Antibiotics.

B. Have client turn, cough, and deep-breathe.

C. Liquefy secretions.

1. Adequate hydration (administer PO fluids cautiously to prevent aspiration).

2. Cool mist inhalation.

D. Evaluate breath sounds and changes in sputum.

E. Position for comfort or place in semi-Fowler's position.

F. Nursing measures to prevent and evaluate levels of hypoxia (see Hypoxia, Nursing Interventions; also see Table 15-2).

G. Provide adequate pain control measures to facilitate coughing and deep breathing.

Goal: To teach client and family how to provide home care when appropriate.

A. Antibiotics.

B. Cool mist humidification.

C. Maintain high oral fluid intake.

D. Antipyretic: acetaminophen.

E. Frequent changes of position.

F. Understand symptoms of increasing respiratory problems and when to notify physician.

Tuberculosis

TB is a reportable communicable disease that is characterized by pulmonary manifestations.

A. Characteristics.

1. Organism is primarily transmitted through respiratory droplets; it is inhaled and implants on respiratory bronchioles or alveoli; predominately spread by repeated close contact.

2. Latent TB infection (LTBI): a client in good health is frequently able to resist the primary infection and does not have active disease; these clients will continue to harbor the TB organism.

3. The primary site or tubercle may undergo a process of degeneration or caseation; this area can erode into the bronchial tree, and TB organisms are active and present in the sputum, resulting in further spread of the disease.

4. The area may never erode but may calcify and remain dormant after the primary infection. However, the tubercle may contain living organisms that can be reactivated several years later.

5. The majority of people with a primary infection will harbor the TB bacilli in a tubercle in the lungs and will not exhibit any symptoms of an active infection.

6. May occur as an opportunistic infection in clients who are immunocompromised.

Assessment

A. Predisposing conditions.

1. Frequent close or prolonged contact with infected individual.

2. Debilitating conditions and diseases.

3. Poor nutrition and crowded living conditions.

4. Increasing age.

B. Cause: Mycobacterium tuberculosis, a gram-positive, acid-fast bacillus.

C. Clinical manifestations (up to 20% of clients may be asymptomatic).

1. Fatigue, malaise.

2. Anorexia, weight loss.

3. May have a chronic cough that progresses to more frequent and productive cough.

4. Low-grade fever and night sweats.

5. Hemoptysis is associated only with advanced condition.

6. May present with acute symptoms.

7. Clients with LTBI will have a positive skin test, but they are asymptomatic.

D. Diagnostics (see Appendix 15-1).

❗ NURSING PRIORITY A positive reaction to a TB skin test means that the person has at some time been infected with the TB bacillus and developed antibodies. It does not mean that the person has an active TB infection.

---

1. QuantiFERON-TB (QFT) rapid diagnostic: blood test to identify presence of antigens; does not take the place of sputum smears and cultures.

2. Bacteriologic studies to identify acid-fast bacilli in the sputum (see Appendix 15-1).

E. Complications.

1. Pleural effusion.

2. Pneumonia.

3. Other organ involvement.

Treatment

A. Chemotherapy (see Appendix 15-2).

1. Medical regimen involves simultaneous administration of two or more medications; this increases the therapeutic effect of medication and decreases development of resistant bacteria.

2. Sputum cultures are evaluated every 2-4 weeks initially; then monthly after sputum is negative. Sputum cultures should be negative within several weeks of beginning therapy, this depends on the medication regimen and the resistance of the bacteria.

3. Direct observed therapy (DOT): health care personnel provide the medications and observe that client swallows medication; preferred strategy for all clients.

4. Prophylaxis chemotherapy for LTBI.

a. Close contact with a client with a new diagnosis of TB.

b. Newly infected client with positive skin test reaction.

c. Client with positive skin test reaction with conditions that decrease immune response (HIV infection, steroid therapy, chemotherapy).

d. Isoniazid (INH) most often used for prophylaxis.

B. Most often treated on an outpatient basis.

Nursing Interventions

Goal: To understand implications of the disease and measures to protect others and maintain own health.

A. Evaluate client's lifestyle and identify needs regarding compliance with treatment and long-term therapy.

B. Identify community resources available for client.

> **ALERT** Identify community/home services that would facilitate a client's independent living; evaluate client's support system.

C. Understand medication schedule and importance of maintaining medication regimen.
  1. Noncompliance is a major contributor to the development of multidrug resistance and treatment failure.
  2. DOT recommended to guarantee compliance; may require client to come to public health clinic for nurse to administer medication.

> **ALERT** Evaluate client's compliance and/or ability to comply with prescribed therapy.

D. Return for sputum checks every 2 to 4 weeks during therapy.

E. Balanced diet and good nutritional status.

F. Avoid excessive fatigue; endurance will increase with treatment.

G. Identify family and close contacts who need to report to the public health department for TB screening.

H. Offer client HIV testing.

Goal: To prevent transmission of the disease.

A. When sputum is positive for the organism, implement airborne precautions for hospitalized client (see Appendix 6-8).

B. Home care: teach respiratory precautions.
  1. Cover mouth and nose when sneezing or coughing.
  2. Practice careful handwashing routine.
  3. Wear a mask when in contact with other people.
  4. Discard all secretions (nose and mouth) in plastic bags.
  5. Reevaluate periodically for active disease or secondary infection.

> **! NURSING PRIORITY** TB is most likely to be spread by clients who have active, undiagnosed TB.

Chronic Obstructive Pulmonary Disease

Also called chronic airflow limitation, chronic obstructive pulmonary disease (COPD) is a group of chronic respiratory disorders characterized by obstruction of airflow.

A. Although each of the disorders (chronic bronchitis, emphysema, and asthma) may occur individually, it is more common for two or more problems to coexist and the symptoms to overlap (most commonly bronchitis and emphysema).

FIGURE 15-4 Chronic obstructive pulmonary disease. (From Zerwekh J, Claborn J: *Memory notebook of nursing,* vol 1, ed 4, Ingram, Texas, 2008, Nursing Education Consultants.)

B. Clinical manifestations common to chronic airflow limitation (Figure 15-4).
  1. Distended neck veins, ankle edema.
  2. Orthopnea or tripod positioning, barrel chest.
  3. Prolonged expiratory time, pursed-lip breathing.
  4. Diminished breath sounds.
  5. Thorax is hyperresonant to percussion.
  6. Exertional dyspnea progressing to dyspnea at rest.
  7. Increased respiratory rate.

C. As a result of a prolonged increase in $Paco_2$ levels, the normal respiratory center in the medulla is affected; when this occurs, hypoxia will become the primary respiratory stimulus.

D. Emphysema: primarily a problem with the alveoli characterized by a loss of alveolar elasticity, overdistention, and destruction, with severe impairment of gas exchange across the alveolar membrane.
  1. Clinical manifestations of emphysema.
    a. Cough is not common.
    b. Sensation of air hunger.
    c. Use of accessory muscles of respiration.
    d. Anorexia with weight loss, thin in appearance.
    e. In general, no cardiac enlargement; cor pulmonale occurs late in disease; decreased Pao_2 with activity.
    f. ABGs are often normal until late in disease.
    g. Characteristic tripod position—leaning forward with arms braced on knees.

E. Chronic bronchitis: primarily a problem of the airway characterized by excessive mucus production and impaired ciliary function, which decreases mucus clearance. Client may develop polycythemia as a result of the low Pao_2. History of productive cough lasting 3 months for 2 consecutive years.
  1. Clinical manifestations of chronic bronchitis.
    a. Excessive, chronic sputum production (generally not discolored unless infection is present).

b. Impaired ventilation, resulting in decreased Pao_2 and symptoms of hypoxia; increased $Paco_2$ (CO_2 narcosis).

c. Respiratory symptoms: productive cough, exercise intolerance, wheezing, and shortness of breath, progressing to cyanosis.

d. Dependent edema.

e. Generally normal weight or overweight.

f. Cardiac enlargement with cor pulmonale.

Assessment

A. Risk factors/etiology.
1. Cigarette smoking (including passive smoking)—most common cause.
2. Chronic infections.
3. Inhaled irritants (from occupational exposure and air pollution).
4. Alpha$_1$-antitrypsin deficiency: enzyme deficiency leading to COPD at an early age.
5. Aging: changes in thoracic cage and respiratory muscles and loss of elastic recoil.

B. Diagnostics: see Appendix 15-1.
1. Pulmonary function studies show increased residual volume (air trapping).
2. ABGs (see Table 15-1).
   a. Changes in $Paco_2$: most often increased in bronchitis.
   b. Low Pao_2 more prominent in clients with bronchitis.
   c. Decompensated condition: decreased Pao_2, increased $Paco_2$, decreased pH—respiratory acidosis with hypoxia.

C. Complications.
1. Cor pulmonale (right-side heart failure).
2. Infections (pneumonia).
3. Peptic ulcer and gastroesophageal reflux (GERD; see Chapter 18).
4. Acute respiratory failure.

Treatment

A. Prevention or treatment of respiratory tract infections.

B. Bronchodilators (see Appendix 15-2).

C. Mucolytics and expectorants (see Appendix 15-2).

D. Chest physiotherapy (suctioning, percussion, and postural drainage).

E. Breathing exercises.

F. Exercise to maintain cardiovascular fitness; most common exercise is walking.

G. Low-flow humidified O_2.

H. Corticosteroids (see Appendix 6-7).

> **! NURSING PRIORITY** Administer low-flow O_2 for clients with emphysema. High concentrations of O_2 would decrease the client's hypoxic drive and increase respiratory distress.

Nursing Interventions

Goal: To improve ventilation.

A. Teach pursed-lip breathing: inhale through the nose and exhale against pursed lips.

B. Avoid activities increasing dyspnea.

C. Humidified O_2 (low flow via nasal cannula at a rate of 1 to 3 L/min) should be used when clients are experiencing exertional or resting hypoxemia.
1. Monitor for hypercapnia, hypoxia, and acidosis.
2. A significant increase in Pao_2 may decrease respiratory drive (O_2 toxicity).
3. Administer O_2 via nasal cannula or Venturi mask (to deliver a more precise Fio_2).
4. Assess for pressure ulcers on the top of the client's ears where the elastic holds the mask.

> **! NURSING PRIORITY** Administer O_2 therapy and evaluate results; the risk for inducing hypoventilation should not prevent the administration of O_2 at low levels to the client with COPD who is experiencing respiratory distress.

D. Assess breath sounds before and after coughing.

E. Avoid cough suppressants.

F. Place client in high-Fowler's or sitting position.

G. Maintain adequate hydration to facilitate removal of secretions.

> **! NURSING PRIORITY** The optimum amount of O_2 is the concentration that reverses the hypoxemia without causing adverse effects.

Goal: To improve activity tolerance.

A. Balance activities and dyspnea: gradually increase activities; use portable O_2 tank when walking; avoid respiratory irritants.

B. Encourage pursed-lip and diaphragmatic breathing during exercise.

C. Schedule activities after respiratory therapy.

D. Assess for negative responses to activity.

Goal: To maintain adequate nutrition.

A. Soft, high-protein, high-calorie diet—especially for underweight clients with emphysema.

B. Postural drainage completed 30 minutes before meals or 3 hours after meals.

C. Good oral hygiene after postural drainage.

D. Small frequent meals; rest before and after meals.

E. Use a bronchodilator before meals.

F. Encourage 3000 mL fluid daily unless contraindicated.

Home Care

A. Encourage client and family to verbalize feelings about condition and lifelong restriction of activities.

B. Client teaching.
1. Include client in active planning for home care.
2. Instruct client regarding community resources.
3. Instruct client regarding medication schedule and side effects of prescribed medications.

C. Recognize signs and symptoms of upper respiratory tract infection and know when to call physician.

D. Encourage activities such as walking—an increase in respiratory rate and shortness of breath will occur, but if respirations return to normal within 5 minutes of stopping activity, it is considered normal.

> **ALERT** Administer narcotics, tranquilizers, and sedatives with caution; instruct client about self-administration of prescribed medications.

Asthma

Asthma is an intermittent, reversible obstructive airway problem. It is characterized by exacerbations and remissions. Between attacks the client is generally asymptomatic. It is a common disorder of childhood but may also cause problems throughout adult life.

A. A chronic inflammatory process producing bronchial wall edema and inflammation, increased mucus secretion, and smooth muscle contraction.

B. Intermittent narrowing of the airway is caused by:
1. Constriction of the smooth muscles of the bronchi and the bronchioles (bronchospasm).
2. Excessive mucus production.
3. Mucosal edema of the respiratory tract.

C. Constriction of the smooth muscle causes significant increase in airway resistance, thereby trapping air in the lungs.

D. Emotional factors are known to play an important role in precipitating childhood asthma attacks.

E. Exercise-induced asthma: initially after exercise there is an improvement in the respiratory status, followed by a significant decline; occurs in the majority of clients; may be worse in cold, dry air and better in warm, moist air.

Assessment

A. Risk factors/etiology.
1. Hypersensitivity (allergens) and airway inflammation.
2. Exercise.
3. Air pollutants and occupational factors.
4. Pediatric implications.
   a. *Reactive airway disease* is the term used to describe asthma in children.
   b. General onset before age 3 years.
   c. Children are more likely to have airway obstruction.

B. Diagnostics (see Appendix 15-1).
1. History of hypersensitivity reactions (history of eczema in children).
2. Increased serum eosinophil count.

C. Clinical manifestations: *early-phase reactions* occur immediately and last about an hour; *late-phase reactions* do not begin until 4 to 8 hours after exposure and may last for hours or as long as 2 days, attacks may begin gradually or abruptly.

1. Episodic wheezing, chest tightness, shortness of breath, cough.
2. Use of accessory muscles in breathing, orthopnea.
3. Symptoms of hypoxia (see Table 15-2); cyanosis occurs late.
4. Increased anxiety, restlessness.
5. Difficulty speaking.
6. Thick tenacious sputum.
7. Diaphoresis.

> **PEDIATRIC PRIORITY** Children who are sweating profusely and refuse to lie down are more ill than children who lie quietly. Parents should seek immediate medical attention if a child does not respond to early treatment of an asthma attack.

D. Complications: status asthmaticus is severe asthma unresponsive to initial or conventional treatment.

Treatment

A. Medications (see Appendix 15-2).
1. Beta$_2$-adrenergic agonists (short-acting and long-acting) administered by nebulizer or metered-dose inhaler.
2. Antibiotics, if infection is present.
3. Bronchodilator.
4. Expectorants.
5. Inhaled steroids and antiinflammatory drugs to prevent and/or decrease edema.
6. Supplemental O_2 to maintain Sao$_2$ at 90%.

B. Status asthmaticus.
1. Oxygen.
2. IV fluids for hydration.
3. May require intubation and mechanical ventilation (Appendix 15-5).
4. IV bronchodilators and steroids.

C. Medications to avoid for the client with asthma.
1. Beta-adrenergic blockers.
2. Cough suppressants.

Nursing Interventions

See Hypoxia, Nursing Interventions.

Goal: To relieve asthma attacks.

A. Position for comfort: usually high-Fowler's position or tripod position.

B. Close monitoring of response to O_2 therapy: Sao$_2$ levels and changes in respiratory status.

C. Assess response to bronchodilators and aerosol therapy.

D. Carefully monitor ability to take PO fluids; risk for aspiration is increased.

E. Observe for sudden increase or decrease in restlessness, either may indicate an abrupt decrease in oxygenation.

> **NURSING PRIORITY** Determine changes in a client's respiratory status: the *inability* to hear wheezing breath sounds in the asthmatic client with acute respiratory distress may be an indication of impending respiratory obstruction.

Home Care

A. Assess emotional factors precipitating asthma attacks.
B. Educate client and family regarding identifying and avoiding allergens.
C. Implement therapeutic measures before attack becomes severe.
D. Explain purposes of prescribed medications and how to use them correctly (see Appendix 15-2).
E. Administer bronchodilators before performing postural drainage.
F. Use bronchodilators and warm up before exercise to prevent exercise-induced asthma.
G. Encourage participation in activities according to developmental level.

Cystic Fibrosis

Cystic fibrosis is a chromosomal abnormality characterized by a generalized dysfunction of the exocrine glands. The disease primarily affects the lungs, pancreas, and sweat glands.

A. The factor responsible for the multiple clinical manifestations of the disease process is the mechanical obstruction caused by thick mucus secretions.
B. Effects of disease process.
1. Pulmonary system: bronchial and bronchiolar obstruction by thick mucus, causing atelectasis and reduced area for gas exchange; the thick mucus provides an excellent medium for bacterial growth and secondary respiratory tract infections.
2. Pancreas: decreased absorption of nutrients caused by the obstruction of pancreatic ducts and lack of adequate enzymes for digestion.
3. Sweat glands: excretion of excess amounts of sodium and chloride.

Assessment

A. Risk factors/etiology.
1. Inherited as an autosomal recessive trait.
2. Most common in Caucasians.
B. Clinical manifestations.
1. Wide variation in severity and extent of manifestations, as well as period of onset.
2. Gastrointestinal tract.
a. May present with meconium ileus in the newborn.
b. Increased bulk in feces from undigested foods.
c. Increased fat in stools (steatorrhea); foul-smelling.
d. Decreased absorption of nutrients: weight loss or failure to thrive.
e. Increased appetite caused by decreased absorption of nutrients.
f. Abdominal distention.
g. Rectal prolapse related to the large bulky stools and loss of supportive tissue around rectum.
3. Genital tract.
a. In females the increased viscosity of cervical mucus may lead to decreased fertility due to blockage of sperm.

b. Males are generally sterile because of blockage or obstruction of the vas deferens.
4. Respiratory tract.
a. Evidence of respiratory tract involvement generally occurs in early childhood.
b. Increasing dyspnea, tachypnea.
c. Paroxysmal, chronic cough.
d. Pulmonary inflammation: chronic bronchiolitis and bronchitis.
e. Symptoms of chronic hypoxia: clubbing, barrel chest.
f. Mucus provides excellent medium for bacteria growth and chronic infections.
5. Excessive salt on the skin: "salty taste when kissed."
C. Diagnostics (see Appendix 15-1).
1. Sweat chloride test: normal chloride concentration range is less than 40 mEq/L, with a mean of 18 mEq/L; chloride concentration 40-60 mEq/L is suggestive of a diagnosis of cystic fibrosis.
2. Pancreatic enzymes: decrease or absence of trypsin and chymotrypsin.
3. Fat absorption in intestines is impaired.
D. Complications.
1. Frequent pulmonary infections.
2. Pneumothorax.
3. Diabetes secondary to destruction of pancreatic tissue.
4. Cor pulmonale and respiratory failure are late complications.

Treatment

Child is usually cared for at home unless complications are present.
A. Diet: high-calorie, high-protein, fats as tolerated; or decrease in fats, increased salt intake.
B. Fat-soluble vitamins A, D, E, and K in water-soluble forms.
C. Pancreatic enzyme replacement with meals (see Appendix 13-2).
D. Pulmonary therapy.
1. Physical therapy: postural drainage, breathing exercises.
2. Aerosol therapy and chest physical therapy (CPT).
3. Percussion and vibration.
4. Expectorants (see Appendix 15-2).
E. Antibiotics are given prophylactically and when there is evidence of infection.

Nursing Interventions

Goal: To promote optimum home care for child (see Chapter 3 for care of chronically ill child).
A. Identify community resources for family.
B. Assist family to identify problems and solutions congruent with their lifestyle.
C. Encourage verbalization regarding impact of child's problem on the family and the family's ability to cope with the child at home.

D. When appropriate, teach child about disease and treatment and encourage active participation in planning of care.
E. Assist parents to identify activities to promote normal growth and development.

Goal: To maintain nutrition.

A. Minimum restriction of fats; need to increase intake of pancreatic enzyme with increased fat intake.
B. Pancreatic enzymes with meals and snacks.
C. Vitamins A, D, E, and K in water-soluble form.
D. Good oral hygiene after postural drainage.
E. Postural drainage 1 to 2 hours before meals.

Goal: To prevent or minimize pulmonary complications.

A. Assist child to mobilize secretions.
   1. CPT: postural drainage, breathing exercises, nebulization treatments.
   2. Encourage active exercises appropriate to child's capacity and developmental level.
B. Prevent respiratory tract infections.
C. Prevent pneumothorax: no power lifting, intensive isometric exercises, scuba diving.

Acute Respiratory Distress Syndrome (Adult Respiratory Distress Syndrome)

Acute respiratory distress syndrome (ARDS) or noncardiogenic pulmonary edema, also referred to as shock lung and white lung, is a condition characterized by increased capillary permeability in the alveolar capillary membrane, resulting in fluid leaking into the interstitial spaces and the alveoli and a decrease in pulmonary compliance.

Assessment

A. Risk factors/etiology.
   1. Clients with multiple risk factors are more likely to develop ARDS.
   2. Risk factors.
      a. Direct lung injury: aspiration, pneumonia, chest trauma, embolism.
      b. Indirect lung injury: sepsis (most common), severe massive trauma, acute pancreatitis anaphylaxis, shock.
B. Clinical manifestations.
   1. Tachypnea and dyspnea.
   2. Increasing hypoxia not responding to increased levels of fraction of inspired O_2 (Fio_2) (see Table 15-2).
   3. Refractory hypoxemia.
   4. Tachycardia, adventitious lung sounds.
   5. Profound respiratory distress.
C. Diagnostics: see Appendix 15-1.

Treatment

Care is generally provided in an intensive care setting.

A. Maintain oxygenation.
   1. Oxygen in high levels of concentration.
   2. Endotracheal intubation and mechanical ventilation.
   3. Positive end-expiratory pressure (PEEP): used to decrease the effects of shunting and to improve pulmonary compliance.
B. Hemodynamic pressure monitoring for evidence of cardiac failure. (Appendix 17-5).
C. Treatment of underlying condition.
D. Nutritional support: requires increased calories to meet metabolic demand.

Nursing Interventions

Goal: To maintain airway patency and improve ventilation.

A. Frequent assessment for increasing respiratory difficulty; anticipate intubation or tracheotomy (see Appendix 15-5).
B. Endotracheal tube or tracheotomy suctioning.
C. Evaluate ABG reports, constant monitoring of Sao_2.
D. Sedate as necessary for client to tolerate the ventilator (see Appendix 15-8).
E. Monitor hemoglobin levels and Pao_2 saturation levels.

Goal: To maintain fluid balance.

A. Fluid balance maintained with IV hydration.
B. Evaluate serum electrolyte levels.
C. Strict intake and output, daily weights.

Goal: To assess and maintain cardiac output.

A. Assess for dysrhythmias – especially tachy dysrhythmias.
B. Correlate vital signs with other assessment changes.
C. Evaluate cardiac output in relation to fluid intake.
D. Evaluate cardiac output when PEEP is initiated because it will compromise venous return (decreased preload).

Goal: To provide emotional support to client and family.

A. Careful repeated explanation of procedures to client and to family.
B. Calm, gentle approach to decrease anxiety.
C. Be available to family at visiting times to explain procedures and equipment.
D. If endotracheal tube or tracheotomy is in place, explain to family and client that speech is only temporarily interrupted.
E. Assist client to maintain communication.

Pulmonary Edema

Pulmonary edema or acute decompensated heart failure (ADHF) is caused by an abnormal accumulation of fluid in the lung, in both the interstitial and alveolar spaces.

A. Origin is most often cardiac: pulmonary congestion occurs when the pulmonary vascular bed receives more blood from the right side of the heart (venous return) than the left side of the heart (cardiac output) can accommodate.

B. Pulmonary edema results from severe impairment in the ability of the left side of the heart to maintain cardiac output, thereby causing an engorgement of the pulmonary vascular bed.

Assessment

A. Risk factors/etiology.
   1. Alteration in capillary permeability (inhaled toxins, pneumonia, severe hypoxia).
   2. Cardiac myopathy, cardiac failure.
   3. Overhydration.
B. Clinical manifestations: hypoxia (see Table 15-2).
   1. Decreasing Pao_2.
   2. Sudden onset of dyspnea and tachypnea.
   3. Severe anxiety, restlessness, irritability.
   4. Cool, moist skin.
   5. Tachycardia (S_3, S_4 gallop)
   6. Severe coughing productive of frothy, blood-tinged sputum.
   7. Noisy, wet breath sounds that do not clear with coughing.
   8. Dependent edema.

> ! **OLDER ADULT PRIORITY** Pulmonary edema can occur very rapidly and become a medical emergency.

C. Diagnostics: BNP (B-type natriuretic peptide) levels measured to assess for heart failure (less than 100 pg/mL rules out HF).

Treatment

Condition demands immediate attention; medications are administered intravenously.

A. O_2.
   1. O_2 in high concentration.
   2. Intubation and mechanical ventilation.
   3. Use of bilevel positive airway pressure (BiPAP).
B. Sedation (morphine) or muscle paralyzing agents to allow controlled ventilation: decreases preload/vasoconstriction, as well as decreasing anxiety and pain.
C. Diuretics to reduce the cardiac preload.
D. Dopamine/dobutamine to facilitate myocardial contractility.
E. Medications to increase cardiac contractility and cardiac output (see Appendix 15-2).
F. Vasodilators to decrease afterload.

Nursing Interventions

Goal: To assess and decrease hypoxia (see Hypoxia, Nursing Interventions; also Table 15-2).

Goal: To improve ventilation (Appendixes 15-5, 15-6, 15-7, and 15-8).

A. Place in high-Fowler's position with legs dependent.
B. Administer high levels of O_2.
C. Evaluate level of hypoxia and dyspnea; may need endotracheal tube intubation and mechanical ventilation.
D. Problem may occur at night, especially in clients who are on bed rest.
E. IV sedatives/narcotics.
   1. To decrease anxiety and dyspnea and to decrease pressure in pulmonary capillary bed.
   2. Closely observe for respiratory depression.
   3. Administer a sedative to decrease anxiety if client has received a muscle paralyzing agent.
   4. May be used to assist client to tolerate ventilator.

> ! **NURSING PRIORITY** Pulmonary edema is one of the few circumstances in which a client with respiratory distress may be given a narcotic. The fear of not being able to breathe is so strong that the client cannot cooperate. When a sedative/narcotic is administered, the nurse must be ready to support ventilation if respirations become severely depressed.

F. Administer bronchodilators and evaluate client's response and common side effects.
G. Closely monitor vital signs, pulse oximetry, hemodynamic changes, and cardiac dysrhythmias.

Goal: To reduce circulating volume (preload) and cardiac workload (afterload).

A. Diuretics (see Appendix 16-6).
B. Medications to decrease afterload and increase cardiac output (see Appendix 17-2).
C. Carefully monitor all IV fluids and evaluate tolerance of hydration status.
D. Maintain client in semi- to high Fowler's position, but allow legs to remain dependent.

Goal: To provide psychologic support and decrease anxiety.

A. Approach client in a calm manner.
B. Explain procedures.
C. Administer sedatives cautiously.
D. Remain with client in acute respiratory distress.

Goal: To prevent recurrence of problem.

A. Recognize early stages.
B. Maintain client in semi-Fowler's position.
C. Decrease levels of activity.
D. Use extreme caution in administration of fluids and transfusions.

Cancer of the Upper Airway

Oral/pharyngeal cancer is uncontrollable growth of malignant cells that invade and cause damage to areas around the mouth, including the lips, cheeks, gums, tongue, soft and hard palate, the floor of the mouth, tonsils, sinuses, and even the pharynx.

Cancer of the larynx may involve the vocal cords or other areas of the larynx. The majority of lesions are squamous cell carcinomas. If detected early, this type of cancer is curable by surgical resection of the lesion (see Chapter 8).

Assessment

A. Risk factors/etiology.
  1. More common in older adult men.
  2. History of tobacco use.
B. Clinical manifestations of oral cancer.
  1. Leukoplakia: whitish or red patch on oral mucosa or tongue (premalignant lesion).
  2. Erythroplasia (erythroplakia): a red velvety patch on the mouth or tongue (premalignant lesion).
  3. A sore in the mouth that bleeds and does not heal.
  4. A lump or thickening in the cheek.
  5. Difficulty chewing or swallowing.
C. Clinical manifestations of laryngeal cancer (may be asymptomatic).
  1. Early changes.
    a. Voice changes, hoarseness.
    b. Persistent unilateral sore throat, difficulty swallowing.
    c. Feeling of foreign body in throat.
    d. Oral leukoplakia.
  2. Late changes.
    a. Pain.
    b. Dysphagia and decreased tongue mobility.
    c. Airway compromise.
D. Diagnostics: direct laryngoscopic examination with biopsy.

Treatment

Varies with the extent of the malignancy.
A. Radiation: brachytherapy—placing a radioactive source into or near the area of the tumor; may also be used with external radiation treatments (see Chapter 8).
B. Surgical intervention.
  1. Partial laryngectomy: preserves the normal airway and normal speech mechanism; if a tracheotomy is performed, it is removed after the risk for swelling and airway obstruction has subsided.
  2. Radical neck dissection or total laryngectomy, involves resection of the trachea, a permanent tracheotomy for breathing, and an alternative method of speaking (Figure 15-5).
  3. Depending on location of oral lesions, a glossectomy (removal of the tongue) and/or mandibulectomy (removal of mandible) may be performed; cancers of the oral cavity metastasize early to cervical lymph nodes.

Complications

A. Airway obstruction.
B. Hemorrhage.
C. Fistula formation.

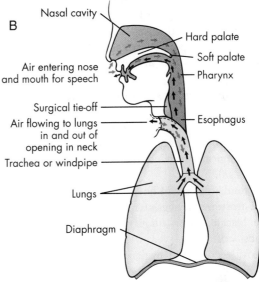

FIGURE 15-5 A, Normal airflow in and out of lungs. **B,** Airflow in and out of the lungs after total laryngectomy. Clients using esophageal speech trap air in the esophagus and release it to create sound. (From Lewis SL et al: *Medical-surgical nursing: assessment and management of clinical problems,* ed 7, St. Louis, 2007, Mosby.)

Nursing Interventions

Goal: To prevent oral and laryngeal cancer.
A. Avoid chemical, physical, or thermal trauma to the mouth.
B. Maintain good oral hygiene: regular brushing and flossing.
C. Prevent constant irritation in the mouth; repair dentures or other dental problems.
D. See a doctor for any oral lesion that does not heal in 2 to 3 weeks.

Goal: To prepare client for surgery.
A. General preoperative preparation (see Chapter 3).
B. Consult with surgeon as to the anticipated extent of the surgery, determine how airway and nutritional needs will be addressed.

C. Discuss with client the possibility of a temporary tracheotomy or, if anticipated, a permanent tracheotomy.

D. Encourage ventilation of feelings regarding a temporary or permanent loss of voice after surgery, as well as alteration in physical appearance.

E. If total laryngectomy is anticipated, schedule a visit from the speech pathologist or member of the laryngectomy club to reassure client of rehabilitation potential.

F. Establish a method of communication for immediate postoperative period.

G. Discuss nutritional considerations after surgery.

Goal: To maintain patent airway after laryngectomy.

A. If tracheotomy is not performed, evaluate for hematoma and increasing edema of the incisional area precipitating respiratory distress.

B. Place in semi-Fowler's position.

C. Administer humidified O_2 therapy.

D. Closely monitor for respiratory compromise (hypoxia).

E. Monitor vital signs for hemorrhage.

F. Avoid analgesics that depress respiration.

G. Promote good pulmonary hygiene.

H. If tracheostomy is present, suction as indicated (see Appendix 15-6).

Goal: To maintain airway; to prevent complications after tracheotomy (see Appendix 15-5).

Goal: To promote nutrition postoperatively.

A. Method of nutritional intake depends on the extent of the surgical procedure (see Appendix 18-9 for tube feedings).

B. IV fluids for first 24 hours.

C. Gastrostomy, nasogastric, or nasointestinal tubes may be placed during surgery and used until edema has subsided.

D. Provide good oral hygiene; may need to suction oral cavity if client cannot swallow.

E. Evaluate tolerance of tube feedings; treat nausea quickly to prevent vomiting (see Appendix 18-9).

F. Closely observe for swallowing difficulty with initial oral feedings.
1. Bland, nonirritating foods.
2. Thicker foods allow more control over swallowing, thin watery fluids should be avoided.

G. For a partial laryngectomy, the possibility of aspiration is a primary concern during the first few days after surgery.

ALERT Identify clients at high risk for aspiration.

Goal: To promote wound healing.

A. Assess pressure dressings and presence of edema formation.

B. Monitor wound suction devices (Hemovac, Jackson-Pratt), drainage should be serosanguineous.

C. Monitor patency of drainage tubes every 3-4 hours, fluid should gradually decrease.

D. If skin flaps were used, the wound is often left uncovered for better visualization of flap and to prevent pressure on area.

E. When drainage tubes are removed, carefully observe area for increased swelling.

F. Type of oral hygiene is indicated by the extent of the procedure.
1. Mouth irrigations.
2. Soothing mouth rinses (cool normal saline or nonirritating antiseptic solutions).
3. If dentures are present, clean mouth well before replacing.
4. Oral hygiene before and after oral intake.
5. Avoid using stiff toothbrushes and metal-tipped suction catheters.

Goal: To identify resources for speech rehabilitation after laryngectomy.

A. If a partial laryngectomy was done, client should have gradual improvement in voice; client is generally allowed to begin whispering 2 to 3 days after surgery.

B. Follow-up visit from laryngectomy club member.

C. Arrange counseling with speech pathologist.

D. Identify different methods for speech management: esophageal speech, electric/artificial larynx, or tracheoesophageal puncture (closest to normal speech).

Home Care

A. Encourage client to begin own suctioning and caring for the tracheostomy before he or she leaves the hospital.

B. Assist the family in obtaining equipment for home use.
1. System for humidification of air in home environment.
2. Suction and equipment necessary for tracheostomy care.

C. Care of stoma.
1. No swimming.
2. Wear plastic collar over stoma while showering.
3. Maintain high humidification at night to increase moisture in airway.
4. Avoid use of aerosol sprays.

D. Nutritional considerations: client cannot smell; taste will also be affected.

E. Client should carry appropriate medical identification.

F. Encourage client to put arm and shoulder on affected side through range of motion exercises to prevent functional disabilities of the shoulder and neck.

Cancer of the Lung

Cancer of the lung is a tumor arising from within the lung. It may represent the primary site or may be a metastatic site from a primary lesion elsewhere (see Chapter 8).

Assessment

A. Risk factors.
1. Smoking, including passive smoking.
2. Occupational exposure to and/or inhalation of carcinogens.

B. Clinical manifestations: nonspecific; appear late in disease.

1. Persistent chronic cough.
2. Cough initially nonproductive; then may become productive of purulent and/or blood-tinged.
3. Dyspnea and wheezing with bronchial obstruction.
4. Recurring fever.
5. Common sites of metastasis.
   a. Liver.
   b. Bones.
   c. Brain.
   d. Lymph nodes: mediastinum.
6. Pain is a late manifestation.
7. Paraneoplastic syndrome: hormone changes, skin changes, neuromuscular and vascular changes; symptoms are controlled with successful treatment of cancer.
C. Diagnostics: bronchoscopy with biopsy.

Treatment

Varies with the extent of the malignancy.
A. Radiation: may be used preoperatively to reduce tumor mass.
B. Surgery: treatment of choice early in condition.
   1. Lobectomy: removal of one lobe of the lung.
   2. Pneumonectomy: removal of the entire lung.
   3. Lung conserving resection: removal of a small area (wedge) or a segment of the lung.
C. Chemotherapy (Chapter 8).
D. Treatment may involve all three therapies.

Nursing Interventions

Goal: To prepare client for surgery.
A. General preoperative preparations (see Chapter 3).
B. Improve quality of ventilation before surgery.
   1. No smoking.
   2. Bronchodilators.
   3. Good pulmonary hygiene.
C. Discuss anticipated activities in the immediate postoperative period.
D. Encourage ventilation of feelings regarding diagnosis and impending surgery.
E. Establish baseline data for comparison after surgery.
F. Orient client to the intensive care unit, if indicated.
Goal: To maintain patent airway and promote ventilation after thoracotomy.
A. Removal of secretions from tracheobronchial tree, either by coughing or suctioning.
B. Have client cough frequently, deep-breathe, and use incentive spirometer.
C. Assess vital signs; correlate with quality of respirations.

D. Provide supplemental O_2 as indicated.
E. Control pain so that client can take deep breaths and cough.
F. Do not position the client who has undergone a wedge resection or lobe resection on the affected side for extended periods of time; this will hinder the expansion of the lung remaining on that side. If client is in stable condition, place in semi-Fowler's position to promote optimum ventilation.

NURSING PRIORITY Postoperative positioning of the client who has had thoracic surgery is important to remember, especially the client who has undergone pneumonectomy.

G. If the client who has undergone pneumonectomy experiences increased dyspnea, place him or her in semi-Fowler's position. If tolerated, positioning on the operative side is recommended to facilitate full expansion of lung on unaffected side.
H. Encourage ambulation as soon as possible.
I. Assess level of dyspnea at rest and with activity.
J. Maintain water-sealed drainage system (see Appendix 15-4). The client who has undergone pneumonectomy will not have chest tubes for lung reexpansion because there is no lung left in the pleural cavity.
Goal: To assess and support cardiac function after thoracotomy.
A. Monitor for dysrhythmias; assess adequacy of cardiac output.
B. Evaluate urine output.
C. Administer fluids and transfusions with extreme caution; client's condition is very conducive to development of fluid overload.
D. Evaluate hydration and electrolyte status.
Goal: To maintain normal range of motion and function of the affected shoulder after thoracotomy.
A. Exercises to increase abduction and mobility of the shoulders.
B. Encourage progressive exercises.
Goal: To assist client to understand measures to promote health after thoracotomy.
A. No more smoking; avoid respiratory irritants.
B. Decreased strength is common.
C. Continue activities and exercises.
D. Stop any activity that causes shortness of breath, chest pain, or undue fatigue.
E. Avoid lifting heavy objects until complete healing has occurred.
F. Return for follow-up care as indicated.

Appendix 15-1 PULMONARY DIAGNOSTICS

X-Ray Studies
Chest X-Ray Film

An x-ray film of the lungs and chest wall; no specific care is required before or after x-ray study.

Bronchoscopy

Provides for direct visualization of larynx, trachea, and bronchi; client generally receives nothing by mouth (NPO status) for 6 hours before the exam; preoperative medication is given, and the client's upper airway is anesthetized topically.

Nursing Implications
1. After the exam, evaluate the client for return of gag reflex. Maintain client's NPO status until return of gag reflex.
2. Bronchial biopsy may be done to obtain cells for cytologic exam; observe client for development of pneumothorax.

Pulmonary Angiography

Contrast material is injected into the pulmonary arteries; the angiography permits visualization of the pulmonary vasculature; definitive diagnosis for pulmonary emboli. Client should be well hydrated prior to procedure.

Contraindications: (1) dye or shellfish allergies, (2) unstable condition, (3) uncooperative client, (4) pregnancy.

Magnetic Resonance Imaging (MRI)

See Appendix 20-1.

Computerized Axial Tomography (CAT Scan)

See Appendix 20-1.

Pathology: Lab Studies
Sputum Studies

Sputum specimen should come from deep in the lungs and not be contaminated with excessive amounts of saliva. Client should be instructed to rinse mouth out with water before collection to decrease contamination.

Culture and Sensitivity Test: Performed to determine presence of pathogenic bacteria; also to determine which antibiotic the specific organism is sensitive to. Should be done before antimicrobial therapy is started.

Acid-Fast Bacilli: Sputum collection and analysis when tuberculosis (TB) is suspected; morning sputum may contain a higher concentration of organisms.

Cytologic Exam: Tumors in pulmonary system may slough cells into the sputum.

Blood Work

D-dimer: Blood test to identify degradation of fibrin; degradation products not commonly found in healthy clients. Elevated in thromboembolism and in DIC. Normal is less than 250 mcg/L.

Pulmonary Function Studies

Studies may be done: (1) to evaluate pulmonary function before surgery; (2) to evaluate response to bronchodilator therapy; (3) to differentiate diagnosis of pulmonary disease; and (4) to determine the cause of dyspnea.

Client must be alert and cooperative; client should not be sedated. Study is done in the pulmonary function laboratory; client directed to breathe into a cylinder from which a computer interprets and records data in specific values. Client should not smoke (for 12 hours) or use bronchodilating medications (for 6 hours) before the test.

Pulse Oximetry

Measurement is made by placing a sensor on the finger or earlobe; a beam of light passes through the tissue and measures the amount of oxygen-saturated hemoglobin. If probe is placed on the finger, any nail polish should be removed. Provides a method for continuously evaluating the oxygen saturation levels (Spo_2). It is noninvasive, and there are no pre- or postoximetry preparations. Readings may be incorrect if severe vasoconstriction has occurred or if Pao_2 is below 70%. Normal range is 95% or higher.

Nursing Implications
1. Pulse oximetry should be used:
   a. For the client who is on supplemental oxygen and is at increased risk for desaturation.
   b. For the chronically ill client who has a tracheotomy or is on mechanical ventilation for chronic respiratory problems.
   c. For the client who has a critical or unstable airway.
2. Pulse oximetry is not recommended to monitor oxygen satuation:
   a. For clients experiencing problems with hypovolemia or decreased blood flow to extremities.
   b. To evaluate respiratory status when ventilator changes are made.
   c. To monitor progress of client on high levels of oxygen.
   d. During cardiopulmonary resuscitation.

Arterial Blood Gas Studies

Measurement of the pH and partial pressures of dissolved gases (oxygen, carbon dioxide) of the arterial blood; requires approximately 3 mL of arterial blood, obtained through an arterial puncture. If client's oxygen concentration or ventilatory settings have been changed, or if a client has been suctioned, blood should not be drawn for at least 30 minutes (see Table 15-1). Perform Allen's test to assess collateral circulation before arterial puncture. Pressure should be maintained at the puncture site for a minimum of 5 minutes. The arterial blood sample should be tightly sealed and placed on ice.

Allen's Test: Hold client's hand, palm up. While occluding both the radial and ulnar arteries, have the client clench and unclench his or her hand several times; the hand will become pale. While continuing to apply pressure to the radial artery, release pressure on ulnar artery. Brisk color return (5-7 seconds) to the hand should occur with the radial artery still occluded. If color does not return, then ulnar artery does not provide adequate blood flow, and cannulation or puncture of radial artery should not be done.

Thoracentesis

Withdrawal of fluid from the pleural cavity; used for diagnostic and therapeutic purposes.

Nursing Implications
1. Explain procedure to client.
2. Position client.
   a. Preferably, client should sit on the side of the bed with the arms and head over the bedside table.
   b. If client is unable to assume sitting position, place on affected side with the head of the bed slightly elevated. Area containing fluid collection should be dependent.
   c. If client has a malignancy, cytotoxic drugs may be infused into the pleural space.
3. Support and reassure the client during the procedure.
4. After the procedure, position the client on his or her side with puncture side up (or in semi-Fowler's position) and monitor respiratory status and breath sounds for possible pneumothorax.

Appendix 15-1   PULMONARY DIAGNOSTICS—cont'd

Mantoux Skin Test

Mantoux test, or purified protein derivative (PPD) test, is a method of tuberculin skin testing. PPD is injected intradermally in the forearm. Results are read in 48 to 72 hours. A positive reaction means the individual has been exposed to *M. tuberculosis* recently or in the past and has developed antibodies (sensitized). It does not differentiate between active or latent infection. It may take 2 to 12 weeks after exposure for sensitivity and a positive skin test reaction to develop.

Nursing Implications

1. Intradermal injection: A small (25-gauge) needle is used to inject 0.1 mL of PPD under the skin. The needle is inserted bevel up; a raised area or "wheal" (6-10 mm) will form under the skin.
2. The most common area for injection is the inside surface of the forearm.
3. Do not aspirate; do not massage area.
4. The client should be given specific directions to return, or plans should be made to read the test in 48 to 72 hours.
5. Interpretation: The area of induration (only the part of the reaction that can be felt; induration may not be visible) is measured, not the area of erythema or inflammation.
   a. An induration of 5 mm or more is a positive reaction in immunosuppressed clients, IV drug users, and persons who have been recently exposed to active TB.
   b. An induration of 10 mm is a positive reaction for persons who are at increased risk for infection. This includes IV drug

users, clients with chronic medical conditions, children under 4 years of age, institutionalized clients, clients in long-term care facilities, and health care workers.
   c. An induration of 15 mm is a positive reaction for members of the general population who do not meet any of the other criteria.
6. A chest x-ray film, prophylactic medication, and medical follow-up are used to determine whether TB is dormant or active or whether the person was exposed and has an adequate immune response. It is also important to determine when and where the person came in contact with the TB bacillus.

Nuclear Medicine
Lung Scan: (V/Q Scan)

A procedure to determine defects in blood perfusion in the lung; particularly useful in the client believed to have a pulmonary embolus or a ventilation/perfusion problem. For the perfusion component, a radioactive dye is injected or is inhaled, and the specific uptake is recorded on x-ray film. For the ventilation component, the client breathes the tracer element through a face mask with a mouthpiece. The ventilation component requires the client's cooperation. Client is not sedated or on dietary restrictions for the exam.

ALERT Monitor laboratory values and notify primary health care provider regarding results; recognize deviations from normal; use critical thinking when evaluating client's diagnostic values.

Appendix 15-2   RESPIRATORY MEDICATIONS

Ⓡ

Bronchodilators Relax smooth muscle of the bronchi, promoting bronchodilation and reducing airway resistance; also inhibit the release of histamine.

General Nursing Implications
— Metered-dose inhalers (MDIs): Hand-held pressurized devices that deliver a measured dose of drug with each "puff." When two "puffs" are needed, 1 minute should elapse between the two "puffs." A spacer may be used to increase the delivery of the medication.
— Dry powder inhalers (DPIs) deliver more medication to lungs and do not require coordination as with an MDI; medication is delivered as a dry powder directly to the lungs; 1 minute should elapse between "puffs."
— Bronchodilators: Beta$_2$ agonists and theophylline are given with caution to the client with cardiac disease, because tachydysrhythmias and chest pain may occur.
— Aerosol delivery systems have fewer side effects and are more effective.

MEDICATIONS	SIDE EFFECTS	NURSING IMPLICATIONS
▲ Epinephrine **(Adrenaline):** subQ, IV Racemic (nebulized) epinephrine	Headache Dizziness Hypertension Tremors Dysrhythmias	1. Do not administer to clients with hypertension or dysrhythmias. 2. Primarily used to treat acute asthma attacks and anaphylactic reactions. 3. With racemic epinephrine, results should be observed in less than 2 hours.
Theophylline **(Theodur):** PO, rectal, IV Aminophylline: IV	Tachycardia Hypotension Nausea/vomiting Seizures	1. Theophylline blood levels should be determined for long-term use; therapeutic levels are between 10 and 20 mcg/mL; levels above 20 mcg/mL are toxic. 2. IV administration may cause rapid changes in vital signs. 3. Considered to be a third-line drug for use with asthma.

Continued

Appendix 15-2   RESPIRATORY MEDICATIONS—cont'd

℞

MEDICATIONS	SIDE EFFECTS	NURSING IMPLICATIONS
❗ NURSING PRIORITY Monitor blood levels of medications.		
Rapid-Acting Control		
Beta₂ Agonists		
Albuterol (**Proventil, Ventolin**): MDI, DPI, PO, aerosol Terbutaline (**Brethine**): aerosol, PO Pirbuterol (**Maxair**): MDI Levalbuterol (**Xopenex**): nebulizer Metaproterenol (**Alupent**): nebulizer, MDI	Tachycardia, tremors, and angina can occur but are rare with inhaled preparations	1. Used for short-term relief of acute reversible airway problems. 2. Not used on continuous basis in absence of symptoms. 3. Client teaching regarding proper use of MDI and/or DPI.
Anticholinergics		
Ipratropium bromide (**Atrovent**): aerosol, MDI	Nasal drying and irritation. Minimal systemic effects.	1. Nasal spray may be used for clients with allergic rhinitis and asthma. 2. MDI used to decrease bronchospasm associated with COPD. 3. Therapeutic effects begin within 30 seconds.
Long-Acting Control		
Beta₂ Agonists		
Salmeterol (**Serevent**): DPI	Headache, cough, tremors, dizziness.	1. Administered two times daily (q 12 hours). 2. Not used for short-term relief; effects begin slowly and last for up to 12 hours.
Corticosteroids		
Beclomethasone (**Beclovent, Vanceril**): MDI Triamcinolone acetonide (**Azmacort**): MDI Fluticasone (**Flovent**): MDI	Oropharyngeal candidiasis, hoarseness, throat irritation, bad taste, cough, minimal side effects.	1. Works well with seasonal and exercise-induced asthma. 2. Prophylactic use decreases number and severity of attacks. 3. May be used with beta₂ agonist. 4. Gargle after each dose and use a spacer to decrease candidiasis.
Nonsteroidal Antiinflammatory Drugs		
Cromolyn sodium (**Intal**): MDI	Inhalation: cough, dry mouth, throat irritation, and bad taste	1. Prophylactic use decreases number and severity of attacks. 2. Prevents bronchoconstriction before exposure to known precipitant (e.g., exercise). 3. Not for an acute attack.
Nedocromil sodium (**Tilade**): MDI	Unpleasant taste	1. Given to children over 6 years old. 2. Maximal effects develop within 24 hours. 3. Does not treat an acute asthmatic attack.
Leukotriene Modifiers		
Montelukast (**Singular**): PO Zafirlukast (**Accolate**): PO	Headache, GI disturbance	1. Once daily dose in the evening. 2. Administer within 1 hour before or 2 hours after eating.

Antitubercular Broad-spectrum antibiotic specific to TB bacilli.

General Nursing Implications
— Client is not contagious when sputum culture is negative for three consecutive cultures.
— Use airborne respiratory precautions when sputum is positive for bacilli.
— Treatment includes combination of medications for about 6 to 12 months.
— Monitor liver function studies for clients receiving combination therapy.
— After initial therapy, medications may be administered once daily or on a twice-weekly schedule.
— Teach clients they should not stop taking the medications when they begin to feel better.

Appendix 15-2 RESPIRATORY MEDICATIONS—cont'd

— Advise clients to return to the doctor if they notice any yellowing of the skin or eyes or begin to experience pain or swelling in joints, especially the big toe.
— Medication regimens always contain at least 2 medications to which the infection is sensitive; inadequate treatment is primary cause of increased incidence.

MEDICATIONS	SIDE EFFECTS	NURSING IMPLICATIONS
Isoniazid **(INH)**: PO, IM	Peripheral neuritis Hypersensitivity Hepatotoxicity Gastric irritation	1. Administer with (pyridoxine) vitamin B_6 to prevent peripheral neuritis. 2. Primary medication used in prophylactic treatment of TB.
Rifampin **(Rifadin)**: PO Rifapentine **(Priftin)**: PO (a derivative of rifampin)	Hepatotoxicity—hepatitis Hypersensitivity Gastric upset	1. May negate the effectiveness of birth control pills and warfarin. 2. May turn body secretions orange: urine, perspiration, tears—can stain soft contacts.
Ethambutol **(Myambutol)**: PO	Optic neuritis Allergic reactions—dermatitis, pruritus. Gastric upset	1. Give with food if GI problems occur. 2. Observe for vision changes.
Pyrazinamide **(PZA Pyrazinamide, Tebrazid)**: PO	Hepatotoxicity Increased uric acid levels	1. May take with food to reduce GI upset.
Rifabutin **(Mycobutin)**: PO	Rash, GI disturbances Hepatotoxicity	1. May turn body secretions orange: urine, perspiration, tears—can stain soft contacts. 2. Use with caution in pregnancy.

Nasal Decongestants Produce decongestion by acting on sympathetic nerve endings to produce constriction of dilated arterioles.

Phenylephrine hydrochloride **(Neosynephrine)**: intranasal Oxymetazoline **(Afrin)**: nasal spray Pseudoephedrine **(Sudafed)**: PO, nasal aerosol spray	Large dose will cause CNS stimulation, anxiety, insomnia, increased blood pressure, and tachycardia.	1. With intranasal preparations, rebound congestion may occur. 2. Not recommended for children under 6 years old. **ALERT** Evaluate client's use of home remedies and OTC medications. 3. Medications are frequently found in OTC combination decongestants. 4. Caution clients with high blood pressure to check with their health care provider before using.

Antihistamine Blocks histamine release at H_1 receptors (see Appendix 7-2).

Expectorant Stimulates removal of respiratory secretions; reduces the viscosity of the mucus.

Guaifenesin **(Robitussin, Mucinex)**: PO	Nausea GI upset	1. Increase fluid intake for effectiveness.

Antivirals used for treatment of severe respiratory syncytial virus (RSV) in hospitalized children.

Ribavirin **(Virazole)**: aerosol	Anemia, increased respiratory problems	1. Should not be used for infants receiving mechanical ventilation. 2. Carefully monitor respiratory status of infant. 3. Used on hospitalized infant. 4. Pregnant nurses should not have direct contact with medication (pregnancy category X).

Continued

Appendix 15-2 RESPIRATORY MEDICATIONS—cont'd

MEDICATIONS	SIDE EFFECTS	NURSING IMPLICATIONS
Prophylaxis: RSV		
Palivizumab **(Synagis):** IM	Hypersensitivity	1. IM injections required once a month; pain and erythema at injection site (very expensive). 2. Dosing for high-risk infants and children should begin in late fall (November) and continue through early spring (April).

CNS, Central nervous system; *GI,* gastrointestinal; *IM,* intramuscularly; *IV,* intravenously; *OTC,* over-the-counter; *PO,* by mouth (orally); *subQ,* subcutaneously; *TB,* tuberculosis; *UTI,* urinary tract infection.

Appendix 15-3 SUDDEN AIRWAY OBSTRUCTION

❗ NURSING PRIORITY The procedure to remove airway obstruction is not effective in the child with epiglottitis or sudden airway obstruction caused by inflammation of the upper airways.

Goal: To identify foreign body airway obstruction.

❗ NURSING PRIORITY If the adult client is coughing forcefully, do not interfere with attempts to cough and expel the foreign body. Do not administer any forceful blows to the back.

1. If the victim can speak or cry, there is probably adequate air exchange.
2. If the victim cannot speak or cry but is conscious, proceed to implement abdominal thrusts to clear the obstructed airway.
3. If the victim is unconscious:
   a. Call for help: dial 911/announce code blue, etc.
   b. Place client supine.
   c. Open airway using head-tilt/chin-lift method.
   d. Observe for presence of foreign body; perform finger sweep and remove if visible.
   e. Maintain open airway; if there is no evidence of breathing, deliver two effective breaths (breaths that cause visible chest rise) either mouth-to-mouth or mouth-to-nose and mouth resuscitation.
   f. If effective breaths cannot be delivered, reposition head, reopen airway, and attempt to ventilate victim again.
   g. If still unable to ventilate, initiate procedure for relieving obstructed airway.

❗ ALERT Identify and intervene in life-threatening situations; evaluate and document client's response to emergency procedures.

Goal: To clear obstructed airway—adult and child (conscious and unconscious).
1. Conscious: Perform Heimlich (abdominal thrusts) maneuver (chest thrusts if pregnant or obese) until obstruction is removed or client becomes unconscious.
   a. Stand behind client and wrap arms around waist.
   b. Make a fist and place thumb side against client's abdomen; place fist midline, just above the umbilicus, and below the xiphoid.
   c. Place other hand over fist and press into client's abdomen using quick upward thrusts.
   d. Repeat upward thrusts until foreign body is dislodged or client becomes unconscious.
   e. When client becomes unconscious, evaluate for presence of foreign body in the airway, remove if identified and attempt to ventilate.
2. Unconscious: Evaluate airway. Open airway and attempt to ventilate; if unable to ventilate, then proceed with steps for removal of foreign body.
   a. Position client supine, kneel astride the client's thighs; with the heel of the hand, apply forceful upward thrust to the abdomen well below the xiphoid and above the umbilicus.
   b. Administer five abdominal thrusts, return to the client's head, open the airway, and assess for breathing; if absent, provide two effective breaths.

Goal: To clear obstructed airway—infant (conscious and unconscious).
1. Straddle the infant over the forearm with the head dependent.
2. Deliver up to five forceful back blows between the shoulder blades.
3. Supporting the head, turn the infant back over and administer up to five chest compressions (lower one-third of the sternum, approximately one finger breadth below the nipple line).
4. Attempt to remove foreign body only if it can be visualized.
5. If infant becomes unconscious, check the mouth before giving breaths to see if foreign body can be identified.

❗ PEDIATRIC PRIORITY Do not do a blind sweep of the infant or child's mouth; the foreign body should be visualized before you attempt to sweep the mouth.

Appendix 15-4 WATER-SEALED CHEST DRAINAGE

Purposes

1. To remove air and/or fluid from the pleural cavity.
2. To restore negative pressure in the pleural cavity and promote reexpansion of the lung.

Principle of Water-Sealed Chest Drainage

The water seal (or dry seal on some equipment) serves as a one-way valve; it prevents air, under atmospheric pressure, from reentering the pleural cavity. On inspiration, air and fluid leave the pleural cavity via the chest tube; the water or dry seal keeps the air and fluid from reentering (Figure 15-6).

> **⚠ NURSING PRIORITY** There must be a seal (either water or dry seal) between the client and the atmospheric pressure.

Equipment

Three-chamber disposable chest drainage system: A molded plastic system that provides a collection chamber, a water-sealed chamber, and a suction-control chamber. When suction is applied, there should be a continuous, gentle bubbling in the water in the suction-control chamber (see Figure 15-7).

Two-chamber disposable chest drainage system: A molded plastic system that provides a water-sealed chamber where atmospheric pressure is prevented from going into client's pleural cavity via a one-way valve. The second chamber serves as a collection chamber.

Nursing Implications
Assessment

1. Evaluate for hypoxia.
2. Evaluate character of respirations.
3. Assess for symmetrical chest wall expansion.
4. Evaluate breath sounds bilaterally.
5. Palpate around insertion site for subcutaneous emphysema.

Intervention

1. Perform range of motion of the affected arm and shoulder.
2. Encourage coughing and deep breathing every 2 hours.
3. Encourage ambulation if appropriate.

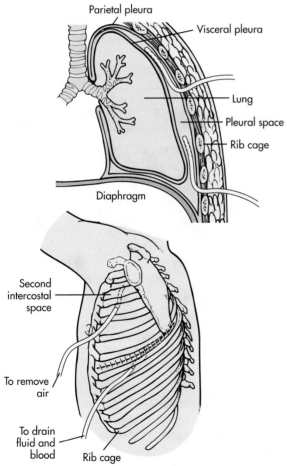

FIGURE 15-6 Placement of chest tubes. (From: Lewis SL et al: *Medical-surgical nursing: assessment and management of clinical problems,* ed 7, St. Louis, 2007, Mosby.)

FIGURE 15-7 Water-sealed chest drainage. (From Potter PA, Perry AG: *Fundamentals of nursing,* ed 7, St. Louis, 2009, Mosby.)

Continued

Appendix 15-4 WATER-SEALED CHEST DRAINAGE—cont'd

4. Administer pain medications as indicated.
5. Place in low Fowler's or semi–Fowler's position.

Observe Drainage System for Proper Functioning

1. Water level in tubing from the client should fluctuate (tidal): rise on inspiration and fall on expiration. The opposite occurs with positive-pressure mechanical ventilation.
2. Continuous bubbling should not occur in the fluid where water seal is maintained; continuous bubbling indicates an air leak; continuous bubbling should occur only in the system that maintains a third chamber for suction control.
3. Initial bubbling may occur in the water-sealed chamber with coughing or with deep respiration as air is moved out of the pleural cavity.

Maintain Water-Sealed System

1. Keep all drainage equipment below level of client's chest.
2. Evaluate for dependent loops in the tubing; this increases resistance to drainage. All extra tubing should be coiled in the bed and flow in a straight line to the system.
3. Tape all connections.
4. Note characteristics and amount of drainage. Mark level on the drainage system as needed and every 8 hours.
5. Vigorous "milking" or stripping chest tubes is controversial. Stripping should not be done routinely on clients because it increases pleural pressures.
6. Change collection chamber when it is approximately half full. Institution policy determines whether the nurse can change the collection chamber.
7. Do not clamp chest tubes during transport.

ALERT Monitor effective functioning of therapeutic devices; determine whether chest drainage is functioning properly; adjust tubes to promote drainage; identify abnormal chest tube drainage; evaluate for achievement of goal of chest tubes; assess and intervene when unexpected responses to therapy occur.

Chest Tube Removal

1. Criteria for removal of the tube:
   a. Minimum or less than 50 mL drainage per day.
   b. Fluctuations stop in the water-seal chamber.
   c. Chest x-ray film reveals expanded lung.
   d. Client had good breath sounds and is breathing comfortably.
2. Procedure.
   a. Provide pain relief about 30 minutes before procedure.
   b. Generally, the physician will want the client in a low Fowler's or semi-Fowler's position, unless contraindicated.
   c. The physician will ask the client to exhale and hold it or to exhale and bear down (a Valsalva maneuver). Either of these procedures will increase the intrathoracic pressure and prevent air from entering the pleural space.
   d. With the client holding his or her breath, the physician will quickly remove the tube and place an occlusive bandage over the area; the client can then breathe normally.
   e. Assess the client's tolerance of the procedure; a chest x-ray film should be obtained to determine that the lungs remain fully expanded.

Appendix 15-5 ARTIFICIAL AIRWAYS

Endotracheal Intubation Placement of an endotracheal (ET) tube through the mouth or nose into the trachea (Figure 15-8).

Purpose

To provide an immediate airway; to maintain a patent airway; to facilitate removal of secretions and provide method for artificial ventilation.

Nursing Interventions

1. Provide warm, humidified oxygen.
2. Establish method of communication because the client cannot speak; child is unable to cry.
3. Maintain safety measures.
   a. Prevent client from accidentally removing tube: soft hand restraints, mittens, etc.
   b. Secure ET tube to the face.
   c. Child with an ET tube requires constant attendance.
4. As soon as tube is inserted, assess symmetry of chest expansion and bilateral breath sounds. Assess for presence of bilateral breath sounds every 2 hours. If tube slips farther into the trachea, it may pass into the right main stem bronchus, obliterating the left main stem bronchus. Determine placement by checking breath sounds.
5. Cuff must remain inflated if client is on a volume ventilator. If the client has adequate spontaneous respiration and is not on a ventilator, the cuff may be left deflated.

FIGURE 15-8 Artificial airways. Position of endotracheal tube. (From Potter PA, Perry AG: *Fundamentals of nursing,* ed 7, St. Louis, 2009, Mosby.)

6. Minimal occluding volume (MOV) should be used when inflating the cuff to prevent aspiration or to maintain mechanical ventilation. This is accomplished by placing a stethoscope over the trachea or by listening to the client's breath sounds to

Appendix 15-5 ARTIFICIAL AIRWAYS—cont'd

determine when air stops moving past the cuff. A safe pressure on the cuff is 20 to 25 mm Hg.

7. Provide frequent oral hygiene; assess for pressure areas on the nose or the mouth.
8. Client's nothing-by-mouth (NPO) status is maintained as long as tube is in place.
9. Suction as indicated (see Appendix 15-6).

Tracheostomy A surgical opening in the trachea (Figure 15-9).
Purpose

To maintain airway over an extended period of time; to facilitate removal of secretions.

Nursing Interventions

Initially After Tracheostomy

1. Provide warm, humidified oxygen.
2. Small amount of bleeding around the tube is expected.
3. Observe for pulsations of the tube; it may be resting on the innominate artery; notify physician of observation.
4. Maintain frequent contact and communication with client and provide reassurance.

Maintenance of Tracheostomy

1. Provide warm, humidified oxygen.
2. Establish method of communication because client cannot speak; child is unable to cry.
3. Maintain safety measures.
    a. Secure tracheal tube to the client's neck.
    b. Use safety measures to prevent client from dislodging tube: soft restraints, trach ties, etc.
    c. Prevent clothing or bed covers from occluding area of tracheal opening.
    d. Child with a tracheostomy requires continuous attendance.
4. Assess for symmetrical expansion of chest wall and bilateral breath sounds.
5. Provide frequent oral hygiene; turn every 2 hours.
6. Inflate tracheostomy cuff during tube feedings or feedings by mouth (minimal occluding pressure).
7. Cuff must remain inflated if client is on a ventilator. If the client has adequate spontaneous respiration, the cuff may be left deflated.
8. Suction as indicated (see Appendix 15-6).

ALERT Provide tracheostomy care as necessary/appropriate.

Cuff inflation tube

Cap

Inner cannula

Fenestration

Deflated cuff

FIGURE 15-9 Artificial airways. Position of tracheostomy tube. (From Lewis SL et al: *Medical-surgical nursing: assessment and management of clinical problems,* ed 7, St. Louis, 2007, Mosby.)

9. IP tracheal tube has an obturator, it should be taped to the head of the bed. If the tracheostomy tube is accidentally removed, the obturator will be necessary for replacing the tube.
10. A fenestrated tracheostomy tube can be adapted so that air will flow throughout normal passages; frequently used when client is beginning to be weaned from the ventilator. If client has respiratory difficulty when the inner cannula is removed, immediately reinsert the cannula to provide a tracheal airway. The tube can also be plugged so that client can speak or cough through normal airway. Make sure the cuff is deflated before plugging the tracheostomy.
11. Establish means of communication; keep call light within easy reach of client.
12. If the client accidentally removes the tube, use the obturator to attempt to replace the tube in the tracheal opening. If unable to replace tracheotomy tube, hold the opening open with a hemostat until physician is available to replace the tube.

■ NURSING PRIORITY The purpose of the cuff on a tracheostomy tube or on an ET tube is to facilitate the delivery of air to the lungs, not to secure the tube position.

Appendix 15-6   SUCTIONING THROUGH ARTIFICIAL AIRWAYS

⚠ NURSING PRIORITY Suctioning the endotracheal tube or the tracheostomy is done to remove excess secretions and to maintain patent airway. Suctioning should always be done before a cuff is deflated.

1. Determine that the client needs to be suctioned.
   a. Auscultate lungs to detect presence of secretions.
   b. Observe to see whether client is experiencing immediate difficulty with removal of secretions.
2. Explain procedure if client is not familiar with it, or simply indicate you are going to assist with the removal of the secretions.
3. All equipment introduced into the trachea or the ET tube must be sterile.
4. Attach the suction catheter to the suction source while maintaining sterile technique.
5. If client is not in immediate danger of airway occlusion, hyperoxygenate with 100% O_2 for three to four hyperinflations.
6. Gently insert sterile catheter into the opening without applying suction. Insert catheter to the point of slight resistance; then pull catheter back 1 to 2 cm.
7. Apply intermittent suction as the catheter is gently rotated and withdrawn.
8. Each suctioning pass should not exceed 10 to 15 seconds in duration.
9. Reconnect client to oxygen source and evaluate whether one suctioning episode was sufficient to remove secretions.

10. Hyperoxygenate client for 1 to 5 minutes after suctioning; assess vital signs and O_2 saturation—values should return to normal or to the previous levels before suctioning.
11. Avoid suctioning client before drawing blood for determination of arterial blood gas values. Client should be allowed to stabilize for approximately 30 minutes before blood is drawn.
12. Monitor oximetry while suctioning; if oximetry does not come back to normal level immediately after suctioning, do not attempt to suction client again; replace oxygen and or ventilatory connection and continue to monitor closely.

Complications of Suctioning

1. Hypoxia: If possible, preoxygenate with high percentage of O_2 before and after suctioning.
2. Dysrhythmias: Limit suctioning to 10 to 15 seconds; monitor rhythm during suctioning; if bradycardia or tachycardia develops, discontinue suctioning immediately.
3. Bronchospasm: Try to time the suctioning with client's own cycle; insert tube during inspiration.
4. Airway trauma: Maintain suction level below 120 mm Hg.
5. Infection: Use sterile technique; assess the color and quantity of sputum suctioned.
6. Atelectasis: Use suction catheters that are approximately one-third or less of the diameter of tube.

ALERT Intervene to improve respiratory status; suction client's respiratory tract (oral, nasal, tracheostomy, and ET tube).

Appendix 15-7   OXYGEN

Goal: The goal of oxygen therapy is to maintain an optimum level of oxygenation at the lowest effective level of fraction of inspired oxygen (Fio_2).

Methods of Administration

Oxygen is measured in liters per minute flow (LPM): a range of 2 to 8 LPM is the most common order.
1. *Low-flow systems:* nasal cannula, standard mask, nonrebreather mask.
2. *High-flow systems:* Venturi mask, nebulizer mask, and ventilators. Oxygen is measured as Fio_2 in concentrations from 24% to 100%: 10 LPM oxygen flow is required to obtain accurate percentage flow.

Humidification

1. Adds water vapor to inspired gas.
2. Prevents drying and irritation of respiratory membranes.
3. Loosens thick secretions, allowing them to be more easily removed.

Indications for Oxygen Administration

1. A decrease in oxygen in the arterial blood (hypoxemia).
2. An increase in the work of breathing.
3. To decrease the cardiac workload.

ALERT Monitor client receiving oxygen therapy. Evaluate response.

Oxygen Safety in Administration

1. Properly ground all electrical equipment.
2. Do not permit any smoking by anyone in the area.
3. Use water-based, not oil-based, lubricants.
4. Use oxygen with caution in clients with chronic airway disease; most often administered via mask or nasal cannula at 2 to 4 LPM, unless client is in severe distress.
5. Oxygen supports combustion but is not explosive.

Oxygen Toxicity A medically induced condition produced by inhalation of high concentrations of oxygen over a prolonged period of time. Toxicity is directly related to concentration of oxygen, duration of therapy, and degree of lung disease present.
1. Tracheal irritation and cough.
2. Dyspnea and increasing cough.
3. Decrease in vital capacity.
4. The Pao_2 continues to decrease, even with an increasing Fio_2.
5. Atelectasis.

Appendix 15-8 VENTILATORS

ALERT Monitor and maintain clients on a ventilator.

Ventilators Deliver air at a predetermined tidal volume. The ventilator delivers the volume of air within safe ranges of pressure. A pressure limit is set, and an alarm will sound if the tidal volume cannot be delivered within the set pressure limits. The intrathoracic pressure is increased with the ventilator; this decreases the venous blood return (preload) to the right side of the heart and subsequently decreases cardiac output.

Patterns of Ventilation

1. **Assist control (AC):** The client may initiate the cycle with inspiration.
2. **Continuous mandatory ventilation (CMV):** The machine controls rate and volume of the client's ventilatory cycle.
3. **Intermittent mandatory ventilation (IMV)/synchronized intermittent mandatory ventilation (SIMV):** Delivers ventilation at inspiratory phase of client's spontaneous ventilation; may be used for weaning from ventilator.
4. **Positive end-expiratory pressure (PEEP):** Maintains positive pressure at alveolar level at end of expiration to facilitate the diffusion of oxygen. PEEP will increase the intrathoracic pressure, thus further decreasing the venous return and causing a decrease in blood pressure.
   Indications for use: Acute respiratory distress syndrome (ARDS); clients unable to maintain patent airway; neuromuscular diseases causing respiratory failure.
5. **Continuous positive airway pressure (CPAP):** Used to augment the functional residual capacity (FRC) during spontaneous breathing. Used to wean clients from ventilators and may be administered by face mask. Client or infant must have spontaneous respirations.

ALERT Identify changes in respiratory status and intervene to improve respiratory status; assess client for unexpected response to therapy.

Nursing Implications

1. All alarms should be set and checked each shift, especially low pressure and low exhaled volume.
2. A bag-valve mask resuscitator is placed in the client's room in case of mechanical failure of equipment.
3. Central venous pressure (CVP) and pulmonary artery pressure readings will be affected by the ventilator; readings should be determined in a consistent manner.

4. Ventilator setting for fraction of inspired oxygen (Fio_2), tidal volume, respiratory rate, pattern of control (AC/IMV, etc.), and PEEP should be checked and charted in the nurses' notes.
5. Assess client's tolerance of the ventilator; intravenous medications such as propofol (Diprivan) and fentanyl are frequently used. If changes, weaning, or removal of the ventilator are anticipated, do not medicate the client.
6. The client frequently experiences a high level of anxiety and fear. Explain equipment and alarms to the client and to the family. Maintain a calm, reassuring approach to the client.
7. When ventilator changes are made, carefully assess the client's response (pulse oximetry, vital signs).
8. Never allow the condensation in the tubing to flow back into fluid reservoir.

Common Ventilator Alarms

1. High pressure alarm: Sounds when tidal volume cannot be delivered at set pressure limit.
   Nursing Care: Increased secretions—suction; client biting tube—place oral airway; coughing and increased anxiety—administer sedative.
2. Low pressure alarm: Sounds when the machine cannot deliver the tidal volume because of a leak or break in the system.
   Nursing Care: Disconnection—check all connections for break in system; client stops breathing on the SIMV mode—evaluate client's tolerance; tracheostomy or endotracheal (ET) tube cuff is leaking—check for air escaping around cuff, may need to replace tracheostomy tube if cuff is ruptured.

Weaning From Ventilators

May be done via SIMV, or T-piece on ET or tracheotomy with heated mist and oxygen, or by pressure support ventilation from the ventilator. During weaning it is imperative for the nurse to maintain close observation for increasing dyspnea and hypoxia. If client experiences dyspnea, he or she should be returned to the ventilator at whatever parameters were being used, and the doctor should be notified; anticipate drawing blood for determination of arterial blood gas values.

NURSING PRIORITY Focus on the client not on the ventilator. In case of problems with the ventilator, assess the client; if adequate ventilation is not being achieved, take client off the ventilator, maintain respirations via a bag-valve mask resuscitator, and call for assistance.

Appendix 15-9   NURSING PROCEDURE: SPUTUM SPECIMEN COLLECTION

Sputum Specimen Collection This test analyzes sputum samples (material expectorated from client's lungs and bronchi during deep coughing) to diagnose respiratory disease, identify the cause of pulmonary infections, identify abnormal lung cells, and assist in managing pulmonary disease.

Nursing Implications

1. Sputum for culture and sensitivity should be collected as soon as possible to facilitate identification of bacteria and treatment.
2. Specimens for cytology and for acid-fast bacilli for TB diagnostics should be collected in the morning when bacteria and cells are most concentrated.
3. No mouthwash should be used before collection of specimen; have client rinse his mouth with water or brush his teeth with water, but do not use toothpaste.
4. Aerosol mist will assist in decreasing thickness of sputum and increasing effectiveness of coughing.
5. Maintain strict asepsis and standard precautions in collecting and transporting specimen; use sterile specimen collection container.

6. Acid-fast bacillus: Sputum collection should be done on three consecutive days.
7. Culture and sensitivity: Initial specimen should be obtained before antibiotics are administered.

Clinical Tips for Problem Solving

If client experiences pain while coughing:

- Support painful area with roll pillows to minimize pain and discomfort.
- Encourage client to take several deep breaths before beginning. This assists in triggering the cough reflex and aerates the lungs (see Box 15-1).

If client is unable to produce sputum specimen:

- Attempt procedure early in the morning, when mucus production is greatest.
- Notify physician to obtain orders for a bronchodilator or nebulization therapy.

Study Questions Respiratory System

More questions on companion CD!

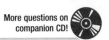

1. On the first postoperative day after a right lower lobe (RLL) lobectomy, the client deep-breathes and coughs but has difficulty raising mucus. What nursing observation would indicate the client is not adequately clearing secretions?
   1 Chest x-ray film showing right-sided pleural fluid
   2 A few scattered crackles on RLL on auscultation
   3 Increase in Paco$_2$ from 35 to 45 mm Hg
   4 Decrease in forced vital capacity

2. What nursing observation indicates the cuff on an endotracheal tube is leaking?
   1 An increase in peak pressure on the ventilator
   2 Client is able to speak.
   3 Increased swallowing efforts by client
   4 Increased crackles (rales) over left lung field

3. The client with COPD is to be discharged home while receiving continuous oxygen at a rate of 2 L/min via cannula. What information does the nurse provide to the client and his wife regarding the use of oxygen at home?
   1 Because of his need for oxygen, the client will have to limit activity at home.
   2 The use of oxygen will eliminate the client's shortness of breath.
   3 Precautions are necessary because oxygen can spontaneously ignite and explode.
   4 Use oxygen during activity to relieve the strain on the client's heart.

4. The nurse is caring for a client who is experiencing an acute asthma attack. He is dyspneic and experiencing orthopnea; his pulse rate is 120 beats/min. In what order will the nurse provide care to this client? Number the following options in the order in which they will be performed, with 1 being the first action and 4 being the last action.
   1 _____ Administer humidified oxygen.
   2 _____ Place in semi-Fowler's position.
   3 _____ Provide nebulizer treatment with bronchodilator.
   4 _____ Discuss factors that precipitate attack.

5. The wife of a client with COPD is worried about caring for her husband at home. Which statement by the nurse provides the most valid information?
   1 "You should avoid emotional situations that increase his shortness of breath."
   2 "Help your husband arrange activities so that he does as little walking as possible."
   3 "Arrange a schedule so your husband does all necessary activities before noon; then he can rest during the afternoon and evening."
   4 "Your husband will be more short of breath when he walks, but that will not hurt him."

6. Which statement correctly describes suctioning through an endotracheal tube?
   1 The catheter is inserted into the endotracheal tube; intermittent suction is applied until no further secretions are retrieved; the catheter is then withdrawn.
   2 The catheter is inserted through the nose, and the upper airway is suctioned; the catheter is then removed from the upper airway and inserted into the endotracheal tube to suction the lower airway.
   3 With suction applied, the catheter is inserted into the endotracheal tube; when resistance is met, the catheter is slowly withdrawn.
   4 The catheter is inserted into the endotracheal tube to a point of resistance, and intermittent suction is applied during withdrawal.

7. While a client's wife is visiting, she observes the client's chest drainage system and begins to nervously question the nurse regarding the amount of bloody drainage in the system. What is the best response from the nurse?
   1 "Your husband has been really sick; this must be a very difficult time. Let's sit down and talk about it."
   2 "I have checked all of the equipment and it is working fine; you do not need to worry about it."
   3 "The system is draining collected fluid from around the lungs. The drainage is expected and does not mean that he is bleeding."
   4 "The chest tube is draining the secretions from his chest; it is important for him to deep-breathe frequently."

8. The nurse is caring for an infant who is experiencing respiratory distress and being treated with continuous positive airway pressure (CPAP). The nurse knows that for this treatment to be most effective, the infant must be:
   1 Intubated with respiration maintained by controlled ventilation
   2 Able to breathe spontaneously
   3 Frequently stimulated to maintain respiratory rate
   4 Suctioned frequently to maintain alveolar ventilation

9. The nurse is assessing a client who is on a ventilator and has an endotracheal tube in place. What data confirm that the tube has migrated too far into the trachea?
   1 Decreased breath sounds are heard over the left side of the chest.
   2 Increased rhonchi are present at the lung bases bilaterally.
   3 Client is able to speak and coughs excessively.
   4 Ventilator pressure alarm continues to sound.

10. A 6-year-old client is admitted to the postoperative recovery area after a tonsillectomy. In what position will the nurse place the client?
    1 Semi-Fowler's position, with the head turned to the side
    2 Prone position, with the head of the bed slightly elevated
    3 On the back, with the head turned to the right side
    4 On the abdomen, with the head turned to the side

11. A child's mother and father are both carriers of the cystic fibrosis gene. What is the genetic basis for the possibility of this child having cystic fibrosis?
    1 One of every four offspring will have cystic fibrosis.
    2 The probability of a child having the condition is 25% with each pregnancy.
    3 Because the mother and father are both positive for the gene, all of the children will be carriers.
    4 Cystic fibrosis is inherited as an autosomal dominant trait, and all children will be carriers.

12. The nurse understands clamping a chest tube may cause what problem?
    1 Atelectasis
    2 Tension pneumothorax
    3 Bacterial infections in the pleural cavity
    4 Decrease in the rate and depth of respirations

13. On auscultation, the nurse hears wheezing in a client with asthma. Considering the pathophysiology of asthma, what would the nurse identify as the primary cause of this type of lung sound?
    1 Increased inspiratory pressure in the upper airways
    2 Dilation of the respiratory bronchioles and increased mucus
    3 Movement of air through narrowed airways
    4 Increased pulmonary compliance

14. What finding on the nursing assessment would be associated with a diagnosis of pneumonia?
    1 Diminished breath sounds
    2 Accessory use of thoracic muscles
    3 Hematemesis in the morning
    4 Dry hacking cough at night

15. The nurse is monitoring a client who is experiencing an acute asthma attack. What observations would indicate an improvement in the client's condition?
    1 Respiratory rate of 18 breaths/min
    2 Pulse oximetry of 88%
    3 Pulse rate of 110 beats/min
    4 Productive cough with rapid breathing

16. Clients with COPD usually receive low-dose oxygen via nasal cannula. The nurse understands that which problem may occur if the client receives too much oxygen?
    1 Hyperventilation
    2 Tachypnea
    3 Hypoventilation or apnea
    4 Increased snoring

17. A client has a diagnosis of right-sided empyema. Thoracentesis is to be performed in the client's room. The nurse will place the client in what position for this procedure?
    1 Prone position with feet elevated
    2 Sitting with upper torso over bedside table
    3 Lying on left side with right knee bent
    4 Semi-Fowler's position with lower torso flat

18. For a client with COPD, what is the main risk factor for pulmonary infection?
    1 Fluid imbalance with pitting edema
    2 Pooling of respiratory secretions
    3 Decreased fluid intake and loss of body weight
    4 Decreased anterior-posterior diameter of the chest

19. A client has a history of atherosclerotic heart disease with a sustained increase in his blood pressure. What side effect may occur and is important to discuss with this client before he uses an over-the-counter decongestant?
    1 Urinary frequency and diuresis
    2 Bradycardia and diarrhea
    3 Vasoconstriction and increased arterial pressure
    4 Headache and dysrhythmias

20. What symptoms would the nurse expect to observe in a 19-month-old client with a diagnosis of laryngotracheobronchitis (LTB)?
    1 Stridor on inspiration
    2 Expiratory wheezing
    3 Paroxysmal coughing
    4 Hemoptysis

Answers and rationales to these questions are in the section at the end of the book titled Chapter Study Questions: Answers and Rationales.

CHAPTER SIXTEEN

Vascular System

PHYSIOLOGY OF THE VASCULAR SYSTEM

Vessels

A. Arteries: high-pressure system that delivers oxygen and nutrients to cellular level.

B. Capillaries: capillary bed is the area of circulation where the arterioles branch into capillaries and where exchange between the circulating volume and the interstitial fluid occurs.

C. Veins: low-pressure system that returns blood and waste products from the cells to the heart; valves to prevent the backflow of blood and maintain direction of blood flow.

D. Circulatory systems.
1. Systemic circulation: flow of blood from the heart into the aorta through the arteries to the capillary bed where cellular nutrition and oxygenation occur.
2. Pulmonary circulation: flow of blood from the right ventricle through the pulmonary artery into the lungs, through the capillary beds of the lungs where the blood picks up oxygen and releases carbon dioxide and returns back into the left ventricle through the pulmonary veins.
3. Hepatic-portal circulation: flow of blood from the venous system of the stomach, intestines, spleen, and pancreas into the portal vein and through the liver for absorption of nutrients; venous blood leaves the liver through the hepatic vein and flows into the vena cava for return to the heart.

E. Lymphatic system: returns fluid and protein to circulation; maintains homeostasis of the blood proteins; assists to maintain blood volume.

Mechanics of Blood Flow

A. Blood flow is controlled by:
1. The diameter of the vessel.
2. The length of the vessel.
3. The pressure at either end of the vessel.
4. The viscosity of the blood.

B. Physiologic control.
1. Autoregulation: the ability of tissue to control its own blood flow.
   a. Lack of oxygen and accumulation of metabolic waste products initiate the autoregulatory system; enables blood supply to vital organs (brain, kidney, heart) to remain relatively constant.
   b. Collateral circulation is part of autoregulatory mechanism for long-term control of blood flow; is especially effective when obstruction to blood flow occurs gradually.
2. Nervous system control.
   a. Parasympathetic nervous system.
      (1) Regulation of the heart rate through the vagus nerve.
      (2) Baroreceptors are located in aortic arch and in carotid sinuses (carotid bodies) and are very sensitive to changes in pressure within vessel walls; an increase in pressure causes stimulation of the vagus nerve, which in turn decreases the heart rate.
   b. Sympathetic nervous system.
      (1) Primary influence is on arterioles for dilation and constriction of the vessels to maintain peripheral resistance and vasomotor tone.
      (2) Peripheral resistance is resistance of arterioles to flow of blood.
      (3) Dilation decreases peripheral resistance, thereby decreasing BP; vasoconstriction increases peripheral resistance, thereby increasing BP.
3. Normal components of serum influence BP regulation.
   a. Angiotensin and vasopressin are vasoconstrictors.
   b. Histamine is a vasodilator.
   c. Epinephrine and norepinephrine act as vasoconstrictors.

Blood Pressure

A. Systolic BP represents the ejection of blood from the heart; determined primarily by the amount of blood ejected, or the stroke volume (see Chapter 17).

B. Diastolic pressure represents the pressure remaining in the arteries at the end of systole; depends on the ability of the arteries to stretch and handle the flow of blood.

C. Pulse pressure is the difference between the systolic and diastolic pressures.

D. Autonomic nervous system influence on BP.
1. Parasympathetic system exerts control over BP through stimulation of the vagus nerve.

2. Sympathetic nervous system controls BP by:
   a. Maintaining peripheral resistance through constriction and dilation of the vessels.
   b. Increasing heart rate and force of contraction.
   c. Causing constriction of the large veins, which promotes an increase in venous return to the heart, thereby increasing cardiac output.
E. Renal influence on BP.
   1. Renin is an enzyme released by the kidneys when there is a decrease in renal blood flow.
   2. Renin breaks down to angiotensin II, a strong vasoconstrictor, thereby increasing BP.
   3. Activation of the renin-angiotensin system stimulates the adrenal cortex to increase secretion of aldosterone, thus precipitating sodium and water retention and increasing vascular volume.
F. The hypothalamus is stimulated to secrete vasopressin (antidiuretic hormone) when BP falls below normal; this increases the conservation of water, thus increasing BP.
G. System assessment: see assessment of individual system involved (Box 16-1).

DISORDERS OF THE VASCULAR SYSTEM

Atherosclerosis

A gradual thickening and narrowing of the arterial lumen; sometimes referred to as "hardening of the arteries" (Figure 16-1).

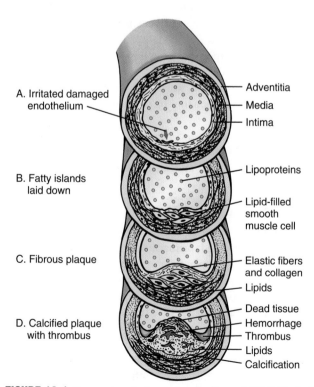

A. Irritated damaged endothelium
B. Fatty islands laid down
C. Fibrous plaque
D. Calcified plaque with thrombus

Adventitia
Media
Intima
Lipoproteins
Lipid-filled smooth muscle cell
Elastic fibers and collagen
Lipids
Dead tissue
Hemorrhage
Thrombus
Lipids
Calcification

FIGURE 16-1 Progression of atherosclerosis. (From: deWit S: Medical surgical nursing: concepts and practices, St. Louis, 2009, Saunders.)

Box 16-1 **OLDER ADULT CARE FOCUS**

Evaluation of Blood Pressure

- If a client has had hypertension for a long time, the client's "normal" BP may need to be higher to maintain adequate blood flow and allow client to perform ADLs.
- Teach client how to avoid problems with orthostatic hypotension.
- Obtain BP while client is standing, lying, and sitting. Make sure client has not had any nicotine or coffee for about an hour before BP is measured.
- Palpate for disappearance of the brachial or radial pulse when assessing BP in order to avoid the auscultatory gap.
- Compliance problems occur when client must take several medications for BP, as well as cope with other chronic health problems.

ADLs, Activities of daily living; *BP,* blood pressure.

A. Process is slow and gradually leads to a significant decrease in blood supply to the tissue.
B. Arteries commonly affected by atherosclerosis and the ensuing problems.
   1. Coronary arteries: myocardial infarction.
   2. Cerebrovascular arteries: stroke, brain accident.
   3. Aorta: aortic aneurysm, peripheral occlusive disease.
   4. Renal artery: hypertension and renal failure.
   5. Large peripheral arteries: peripheral vascular disease.

Assessment

A. Modifiable risk factors.
   1. Elevated serum cholesterol (LDL over 100 mg/dL) and triglyceride levels.
   2. Smoking.
   3. Sedentary lifestyle, obesity.
   4. Stress.
B. Nonmodifiable risk factors.
   1. Familial tendencies.
   2. Age.
   3. Gender: men at greater risk than women until age 60.
C. Conditions accelerating atherosclerotic development.
   1. Diabetes mellitus.
   2. Hypertension.
D. Clinical manifestations: depend on artery involved.
E. Diagnostics (see Appendix 16-1).

ALERT Conduct cholesterol screening sessions and adapt a diet to meet the special needs of a client.

Treatment

A. Decrease cholesterol in diet.
B. Decrease risk factors (exercise, stop smoking, decrease weight, decrease stress).
C. Antihyperlipidemic medications (see Appendix 16-2).

Table 16-1	CHOLESTEROL AND LIPOPROTEIN LEVELS
Cholesterol (total)	140-200 mg/dL
Low density lipoprotein (LDL)	Less than 130 mg/dL
High density lipoprotein (HDL)	37-70 males, 40-88 females
Triglycerides	40-190 mg/dL

D. Peripheral vasodilating medications (see Appendix 16-5).
E. Vascular surgery.

Nursing Interventions

Goal: To identify individuals at high risk.

A. Screen for and recognize modifiable and nonmodifiable risk factors.
B. Recognize significant deviations of lab values (Table 16-1).
C. Identify and control conditions that accelerate atherosclerotic development.
D. Recognize common signs and symptoms of atherosclerosis.

Hypertension

A persistent systolic BP greater than 140 mg Hg and/or diastolic BP greater than 90 mm Hg.

A. Classification.
 1. Primary hypertension (essential or idiopathic): cause unknown; accounts for approximately 90% to 95% of cases of hypertension.
 2. Secondary hypertension: sustained elevation due to a secondary underlying health problem; accounts for 10% to 15 % of cases of hypertension.
  a. Pheochromocytoma.
  b. Renal artery stenosis.
  c. Cushing's syndrome.
  d. Coarctation of the aorta (most common in children).
  e. Medications: oral contraceptives, glucocorticoids.
  f. Pregnancy-induced hypertension.
 3. Hypertensive crisis: a sudden sustained increase in the diastolic pressure above 140 mm Hg, which may be life-threatening.
  a. Medication noncompliance; undermedicating.
  b. Drug abuse (cocaine, crack).
  c. Preeclampsia or eclampsia (Chapter 24).
  d. Head injury, IICP (Chapter 20).

Assessment

A. Risk factors (Table 16-2).
B. Clinical manifestations of primary hypertension.

> **! NURSING PRIORITY** BP should be evaluated with the client lying, sitting, and standing; readings should be obtained from both arms. Legs should not be crossed.

Table 16-2	RISK FACTORS IN ESSENTIAL HYPERTENSION
Nonmodifiable Factors	
Age	Develops between 30 and 50 years of age. Poorer prognosis when developed at younger age.
Gender	More prevalent in men under 55 years; after age 55 it is more prevalent in women.
Ethnic group	The incidence of hypertension is twice as high among African Americans as among whites.
Family history	Clients with parents or siblings who have hypertension are at greater risk for high BP at a younger age.
Modifiable Factors	
Obesity	Weight gain is associated with increased frequency of hypertension. Central abdominal obesity poses greatest risk; regular exercise can reduce obesity and BP.
Stress	People exposed to repeated stress may develop hypertension more frequently.
Substance abuse	These factors are all associated with hypertension: drug abuse, drinking more than 1 oz of alcohol per day, and smoking cigarettes (nicotine).
Excess sodium intake	Can cause water retention and hypertension in some individuals; especially those who are already overweight.
Elevated serum lipids	Elevated levels of cholesterol and triglycerides are primary risk factors in atherosclerosis, which is a contributing factor to hypertension.
Sedentary lifestyle	Regular physical activity helps decrease risk.
Diabetes mellitus	Vessel disease associated with diabetes mellitus leads to high risk for hypertension.

BP, Blood pressure.

 1. Most often asymptomatic; headache, dizziness, palpitations, epistaxis may occur.
 2. Sustained (two elevated pressure readings obtained at least 1 week apart) average increase in systolic BP at 140 mm Hg or higher and increase in diastolic BP above 90 mm Hg.
 3. Cardiac effects.
  a. Coronary artery disease, heart failure.
  b. Left ventricular hypertrophy.
 4. Cerebrovascular effects.
  a. Transient ischemic attack.
  b. Stroke (cerebrovascular accident, brain attack).
 5. Progressive decrease in the function of heart, brain, kidneys, and retinas as vessel damage to these organs increases.

C. Clinical manifestations of hypertensive crisis.
   1. Diastolic pressure greater than 140 mm Hg.
   2. Classified by level of organ damage.
   3. More critical in clients with previously compromised cardiovascular system.
   4. BP is unresponsive to oral antihypertensive medications.

> **ALERT** Intervene to prevent potential neurologic complications; assess for abnormal neurologic status.

Treatment

A. Dietary management.
   1. Decrease sodium, cholesterol and saturated fats.
   2. Reduce calories (should be within 10% of ideal body weight).
   3. Limit alcohol consumption.
B. Regular exercise (walking, jogging, or swimming).
C. Stress management.
D. Avoid tobacco products.
E. Antihypertensive medications (see Appendix 16-5 and Table 16-3).
F. Diuretics to decrease circulating volume (see Appendix 16-6).

Nursing Interventions

Goal: To reduce BP in hypertensive crisis.
A. Calculate and monitor the mean arterial pressure (MAP).
   1. MAP = systolic blood pressure (SBP) + 2 × diastolic blood pressure (DBP) ÷ 3.
   2. The BP is decreased by 25% of the MAP within minutes to 1 hour.
   3. Gradual reductions over next 24-48 hours.
   4. Lowering BP too rapidly may compromise cerebral, renal, or coronary circulation.
B. BP should be monitored via an intraarterial line; titrate medication accordingly.

Table 16-3	**BLOOD PRESSURE MANAGEMENT**

1: Prehypertension—SBP 120-139, DBP 80-89: Lifestyle modifications such as weight loss, regular exercise, management of cholesterol levels, reduction of sodium intake, and alcohol and tobacco cessation.

2: Stage 1 hypertension—SBP 140-159, DBP 90-99: Begin diuretics (thiazide, loop diuretics, or potassium sparing); may consider ACE inhibitor or other antihypertensive drug for control.

3: Stage 2 hypertension—SBP greater than 160 or DBP greater than 100: Continue diuretics; add a second medication, such as a beta adrenergic blocker, an ACE inhibitor, or a calcium channel blocker, or other antihypertensive drug.

BP, Blood pressure, *SBP,* systolic blood pressure, *DBP,* diastolic blood pressure, *ACE,* angiotensin-converting enzyme.
Modified from Joint National Committee: The Seventh Report of the Joint National Committee on Prevention, Detection, Evaluation and Treatment of High Blood pressure. NIH Publication No 03-5233. Bethesda, Md, 2003.

C. Hourly urine output to monitor renal perfusion.
D. Frequent neurologic checks.
E. Maintain client on bed rest while receiving intravenous antihypertensive medications.

Goal: To identify high-risk individuals.
A. Conduct community BP screening programs.

> **ALERT** Plan and participate in the screening and education of individuals in the community (e.g., BP screenings, health fairs, school education, etc.).

B. Educate the public regarding risk factors (see Table 16-2).
C. Identify health-promoting behavior for high-risk individuals.
   1. Decrease weight.
   2. Avoid smoking; limit alcohol intake.
   3. Control diabetes.
   4. Have regular BP checkups.
   5. Engage in regular exercise: 30 to 45 minutes, three to five times a week.

> **ALERT** Identify side effects and adverse effects/contraindications; evaluate client's understanding of medications; educate client and family about medications.

Goal: To reduce BP and assist client to maintain control.
A. Assess response to medication regimen.
   1. Educate client and family member on how to take BP.
      a. Client should be seated with arm at heart level.
      b. No smoking or caffeine 30 minutes before measurement of BP.
      c. Use appropriate cuff size.
      d. Two or more readings should be averaged.
   2. BP should be monitored frequently during initial medication dosage adjustments, and at least twice a week thereafter.
   3. Instruct client regarding possible side effects (Figure 16-2).
      a. Do not stop taking medications; report side effects to health care provider.
      b. Assure client that side effects are often temporary.
      c. Sexual problems, impotence should be reported.
   4. When BP is initially decreased, evaluate client's tolerance to decrease.
      a. Postural (orthostatic) hypotension.
      b. Urinary output.
      c. Change in energy level and mental alertness.
   5. Assess factors contributing to noncompliance with medications.
      a. Cost of the medication.
      b. Failure to remember or to understand medication schedule or regimen.

> **ALERT** Compare client's current vital signs and baseline vital signs; intervene when abnormal.

FIGURE 16-2 Antihypertensives. (From Zerwekh J, Claborn J, Gaglione T: *Mosby's pharmacology memory notecards,* ed 2, St. Louis, 2008, Mosby.)

Home Care

A. Low-cholesterol, low-sodium diet.
B. Maintain optimum weight; exercise regularly.
C. Adhere to medication regimen.
1. Take medication at regular times.
2. Do not stop taking medications; call health care provider.
3. Plan with client a method to keep track of medications (e.g., using daily pill box or marking on calendar).

> **ALERT** Instruct client about self-administration of prescribed medications; evaluate client's compliance with prescribed therapy; evaluate and document client's response to therapy.

D. Avoid hot baths, steam rooms, and spas (increases vasodilation).
E. Decrease and or prevent problems of orthostatic hypotension.
1. Get up slowly, sit at the bedside to regain equilibrium, and then stand slowly.
2. Wear elastic support hose.
3. Lie or sit down when dizziness occurs.
4. Do not stand or sit for prolonged periods of time.

> **ALERT** Inform client/family/significant others of actions to maintain health and prevent disease (e.g., smoking cessation, diet, weight loss).

Aneurysm

An aneurysm is a dilation or sac formed on the wall of an arterial vessel. The aneurysm may involve only one layer or all layers of the arterial wall.
A. Types of aneurysms.
1. Berry aneurysm (see Chapter 20).
2. Abdominal aortic aneurysm: occurs primarily in the abdominal aorta below the renal arteries.
3. Thoracic aortic aneurysm: located in the aorta in the thoracic area.
4. Dissecting aneurysm: bleeding between the layers of the vessel wall; with continual bleeding, dissection of the wall of the vessel occurs. Thoracic area is the most common site for dissection.

Assessment

A. Clinical manifestations: abdominal aortic aneurysm (AAA).
1. May be asymptomatic.
2. Epigastric, back, flank or abdominal pain.
3. Pulsating abdominal mass may be palpable.
4. Signs of rupture.
a. Severe back pain.
b. Rapid hypotension and shock.
c. Abdominal distention and tenderness.
d. Hematoma formation in the flank region.
B. Clinical manifestations: thoracic aortic aneurysm.
1. Frequently asymptomatic.
2. Compression of structures in the adjacent area.
3. Dysphagia due to pressure on the esophagus.
4. Hoarseness due to pressure on the laryngeal nerve.
5. Pressure on the vena cava may cause edema of head and arms.
6. Signs of dissection and rupture.
a. Sudden constant, excruciating back and/or chest pain.
b. Rapid hypotension progressing to shock.
C. Diagnostics (see Appendix 16-1).
D. Complications: graft thrombosis, emboli, hemorrhage, paralytic ileus, and renal failure.

Treatment

A. Surgical repair of aneurysm as soon as possible.
1. Endovascular stent graft.
2. Surgical resection and graft.
B. Pain control.

Nursing Interventions

Goal: To prepare client and family for anticipated surgery.
A. Provide preoperative care (see Chapter 3).
B. Identify other chronic health problems.
C. Evaluate characteristics of pulses in the lower extremities and mark for evaluation and comparison after surgery (Figure 16-3).
D. Do not vigorously palpate the abdomen.
E. Monitor for indications of dissection or rupture.

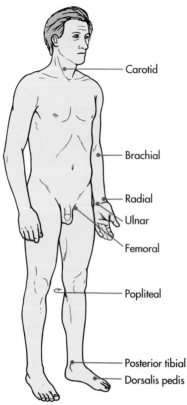

FIGURE 16-3 Common sites for palpating arteries. (From Lewis SL et al: *Medical-surgical nursing: assessment and management of clinical problems,* ed 7, St. Louis, 2007, Mosby.)

F. Maintain BP at level low enough to decrease risk for rupture, yet high enough to maintain perfusion.

Goal: To promote graft patency and circulation.

A. General postoperative care (see Chapter 3).

B. Maintain adequate BP to facilitate filling of the graft.

C. Monitor for hemorrhage.
1. Increasing abdominal girth, back pain.
2. Symptoms of hypovolemia or shock.

D. Check peripheral circulation, sensation, and movement hourly for first 24 hours.

E. If chest tubes are present, monitor function and drainage.

F. Hourly urine output; hemodynamic monitoring.

G. Evaluate blood urea nitrogen and serum creatinine levels to assess renal function.

ALERT Assess client for abnormal peripheral pulses after a procedure/surgery; determine what data need to be reported immediately.

 Home Care

A. Activity restrictions.
1. No heavy lifting for 6-12 weeks.
2. Avoid activities that involve pushing, pulling, or straining.

B. Report any signs of infection, redness, swelling, drainage, or fever.

C. Report changes in pulses, temperature, color, and sensation of extremities.

 Shock

Shock is a failure of the circulatory system to maintain adequate perfusion of vital organs.

A. Common classifications of shock (Table 16-4).
1. Hypovolemic shock: results from inadequate blood volume.
2. Cardiogenic shock: results from the heart's inability to adequately circulate blood volume.
3. Distributive shock (vasogenic): results from a change in size of the vascular space without an increase in blood volume.

Assessment

Signs and symptoms of shock are essentially the same, regardless of the precipitating cause.

A. Risk factors.
1. Increased incidence in the very young and very old.
2. Increased incidence in clients with chronic progressive disease states.
3. Trauma.
4. Postoperative hemorrhage.

B. Stages of shock.
1. Compensatory stage (initial, early, nonprogressive): the body is able to compensate (vasoconstriction, shunting); BP in low normal range but sufficient to perfuse vital organs.
2. Progressive stage (decompensated, intermediate): the body can no longer maintain an adequate supply of oxygenated blood to the tissues and vital organs; worsening of symptoms associated with decreased tissue perfusion.
3. Refractory (late, irreversible): cellular ischemia and necrosis lead to organ failure and death.

C. Clinical manifestations.
1. Compensatory stage (early).
a. Client is oriented to time, place, and date but may be restless or apprehensive with increased anxiety.
b. BP—low normal; pulse—increased or normal; respirations—increased; temperature—normal or subnormal.
c. Urine output may be slightly decreased, but within normal range.
d. MAP may decrease from 10-15 mmHg from baseline; poor perfusion of extremities with decreasing pulse pressure; vital organs are perfused.
e. Complaints of thirst and feeling cool; skin pale and cool.
f. Nausea/vomiting common as BP decreases.
2. Progressive stage (intermediate).
a. Decreasing sensory perception; decreased responsiveness to stimuli.

Table 16-4	CLASSIFICATION OF SHOCK		
Classification	*Pathophysiology*	*Conditions*	*Treatment and Clinical Implications*
Hypovolemic	Reduced venous return due to reduced blood volume; 15% to 25% reduction in volume.	Hemorrhage, burns, severe fluid loss—dehydration	1. Administer volume replacement: blood transfusion and volume expanders. 2. Administer oxygen.
Cardiogenic	Heart unable to effectively circulate the intravascular volume.	Dysrhythmias, MI, CHF	1. Monitor ECG continuously. 2. Medications to increase cardiac output. 3. Evaluate hemodynamic parameters (see Appendix 17-5). 4. Treat dysrhythmias.
Obstructive	Physical impediment to the flow of blood.	Pericardial tamponade, pulmonary embolism, vena cava compression, tension pneumothorax	1. Will have increased CVP. 2. Treatment directed toward release of obstruction.
Neurogenic	Increased venous capacity due to a loss of peripheral vasomotor tone. Cardiac function and blood volume may be normal.	Spinal cord injury (T5 or higher), drug OD, hypoglycemia, spinal anesthesia	1. Administer vasoconstrictor medications. 2. Evaluate closely for fluid overload. 3. Bradycardia may require treatment (atropine).
Systemic inflammatory response syndrome (SIRS)	Dilation of blood vessels by humoral or vasoactive substances.	Overwhelming infection; generally gram-negative organism	1. Evaluate for origin of infection. 2. IV fluids, volume expanders. 3. Cardiotonics. 4. Administer oxygen.
Anaphylactic	Antigen-antibody reaction with release of histamine, causing vasodilation and fluid shift.	Transfusion reactions, insect bites, side effect of medications, dye/food allergies	1. Maintain airway: problem with laryngeal edema. 2. Oxygen as indicated. 3. Epinephrine and Benadryl, IV.

🔲 **NURSING PRIORITY** Shock is a dynamic condition. The client's status is constantly changing, either improving or deteriorating.

CHF, Congestive heart failure; *ECG,* electrocardiogram; *IV,* intravenous; *MI,* myocardial infarction; *OD,* overdose.

b. Vital signs.
  (1) BP decrease in MAP of 20 mm Hg or more.
  (2) Pulse rate increased with weak or thready peripheral pulses.
  (3) Respirations—rate is increased with dyspnea.
c. Cold, moist skin; pallor.
d. Decrease in urine to oliguric levels.
3. Refractory (irreversible, late).
  a. Progressively decreasing level of consciousness to unresponsiveness.
  b. BP—not measurable (unable to perfuse vital organs); pulse—slow and irregular; respirations—irregular, labored.
  c. Anuria.
  d. Client becomes hypoxic and develops metabolic acidosis.
4. Diagnostics: based on the clinical manifestations and history of underlying problems.

Treatment

Depends on the underlying problem and promptness of intervention.
A. Treat underlying cause.
B. IV access and fluid resuscitation.

C. Position supine to increase venous return but not compromise pulmonary status.
D. Medication therapy (Appendix 16-7).
E. Oxygen therapy.
F. Hemodynamic monitoring (Appendix 17-9).

Nursing Interventions

Goal: To identify and correct cause of shock.
A. Rapid response to developing sign or symptoms.
  1. Maintain bed rest.
  2. Position supine; may elevate legs.
  3. Maintain airway; provide supplemental oxygen.
  4. Keep warm; no chilling.
  5. Protect from falls and injury.
B. Evaluate for progression of shock—compensating to noncompensating.
  1. Systemic inflammatory response syndrome (SIRS, Chapter 6).
  2. Multiple organ dysfunction syndrome (MODS, Chapter 6).
Goal: To maintain adequate respiratory function.
A. Administer high-flow oxygen (100%).
  1. Nonrebreather mask, bag-valve mask.
  2. Mechanical ventilation.

B. Monitor oxygenation.
   1. Pulse oximetry, ABGs.
   2. Breath sounds.
   3. Orientation, presence of confusion.
Goal: To maintain adequate circulation and/or tissue perfusion.
A. Control bleeding.
B. Maintain fluid volume.
   1. Blood and/or blood products.
   2. Intravenous (IV) fluids.
   3. Volume expanders (colloid solutions).
   4. Monitor I&O.
C. Ensure client venous access.
   1. Two large-bore (14- to 16-gauge) peripheral lines or central line for IV medications and fluid resuscitation.
   2. IM, subcutaneous, and oral meds generally not given due to inadequate and/or unpredictable perfusion.
D. Cardiogenic shock and neurogenic shock do not involve decreased circulating blood volume; monitor closely for fluid overload.
Goal: To maintain cardiac output and vascular tone.
A. Monitor hemodynamic changes.
   1. Monitor CVP, MAP, PAWP; integrate data with assessment data (see Appendix 17-9).
   2. Administer fluids to increase circulating volume.
   3. Assess adequacy of end organ perfusion (urine output, orientation, peripheral pulses).
B. Medication therapy (see Appendix 16-7).

ALERT Adjust/titrate dosage of medications based on assessment of physiologic parameters (e.g., titrating medication to maintain a specific BP). Assess client for continued decreased cardiac output; interpret data that needs to be reported immediately.

C. Monitor renal response and urinary output.
   1. Foley catheter and hourly output measurements.
   2. Maintain output greater than 30 mL/hr.
   3. Monitor BUN and creatinine.
Goal: To maintain homeostasis.
A. Ongoing neurologic evaluation.
   1. Check orientation status and LOC frequently.
   2. Reorient client as needed.
   3. Minimize sensory overload caused by hospital environment.
B. Evaluate GI status.
   1. Maintain NPO status; provide oral hygiene.
   2. Monitor bowel sounds and distention.
   3. Possible NG tube in presence of paralytic ileus and/or visceral ischemia.
C. Provide emotional support.
   1. Keep client informed of procedures and tests.
   2. Solicit support for family members (i.e. social worker, clergy, etc.).
   3. Keep family members informed of client's condition.

Peripheral Arterial Occlusive Disease

Peripheral arterial occlusive disease involves narrowing and obstruction of the arteries, especially the lower extremities. The chronic arterial obstruction progressively leads to decreased oxygen delivery to the tissues.

A. Lesions are predominantly found in the lower aorta below the renal arteries and extend through the popliteal area.
B. By the time symptoms occur, the artery is approximately 85% to 95% occluded.
C. The bifurcations at the renal, femoral, popliteal, and aortic iliac arteries are the most commonly affected sites.

Assessment

A. Risk factors: see atherosclerosis.
B. Characteristics of arterial ulcers (Table 16-5).
C. Intermittent claudication.
   1. Muscle pain and cramping with exercise; pain relieved with rest.
   2. Pain that occurs while resting or at night is indication of advanced stages.
D. Diagnostics (see Appendix 16-1).

Treatment

A. Medical.
   1. Medication therapy.
      a. Antiplatelet agents (see Appendix 16-4).
      b. Anti-platelet agents (see Appendix 16-4).
      c. Antihypertensive agents (see Appendix 16-5).
      d. Antihyperlipidemic medications (see Appendix 16-2).
   2. Stop smoking.
   3. Dietary management.
      a. Decrease cholesterol and triglyceride intake.
      b. Reduce weight if needed.
      c. Control sodium intake.
   4. Exercise program as tolerated.
   5. Control diabetes and hypertension.
B. Surgical.
   1. Peripheral atherectomy: removal of plaque within the artery.
   2. Bypass graft: bypass of an obstruction by suturing a graft proximally and distally to the obstruction.
   3. Patch graft angioplasty: artery is opened, plaque is removed, and a patch is sutured in the opening to widen the lumen.
   4. Amputation: used as a last resort when other therapies have failed and gangrene or infection is extensive.
C. Nonsurgical.
   1. Percutaneous transluminal angioplasty: use of a balloon catheter to compress the plaque against the arterial wall.
   2. Laser-assisted angioplasty: a probe is advanced through a cannula to the area of occlusion; a laser is used to vaporize the atherosclerotic plaque.
   3. Intravascular stent: placement of a stent within a narrowed vessel to maintain patency.

Table 16-5	COMPARISON OF ARTERIAL AND VENOUS LEG ULCERS	
Characteristic	**Arterial**	**Venous**
Peripheral pulses	Decreased or absent	Present; may be difficult to palpate with edema
Capillary refill	>3 sec	<3 sec
Ankle-brachial index	<0.70	>0.91
Edema	Absent unless leg constantly in dependent position	Lower leg edema
Hair	Loss of hair on legs, feet, toes	Hair may be present or absent
Ulcer location	Tips of toes, foot, or lateral malleolus	Near medial malleolus
Ulcer margin	Rounded, smooth, looks "punched out"	Irregularly shaped
Ulcer drainage	Minimal	Moderate to large amount
Ulcer tissue	Black eschar or pale pink granulation	Yellow slough or dark red, "ruddy" granulation
Pain	Intermittent claudication or rest pain in foot; ulcer may or may not be painful	Dull ache or heaviness in calf or thigh; ulcer often painful
Nails	Thickened; brittle	Normal or thickened
Skin color	Dependency rubor; elevation pallor	Bronze-brown pigmentation; varicose veins may be visible
Skin texture	Thin, shiny, friable, dry	Skin thick, hardened, and indurated
Skin temperature	Cool, temperature gradient down the leg	Warm, no temperature gradient
Dermatitis	Rarely occurs	Frequently occurs
Pruritus	Rarely occurs	Frequently occurs

From Lewis SL et al: *Medical-surgical nursing: assessment and management of clinical problems,* ed 7, St. Louis, 2007, Mosby.

Nursing Interventions

> **ALERT** Identify client with a condition that increases the risk for insufficient vascular perfusion; assess client for abnormal peripheral pulses.

Goal: To evaluate level of involvement of the extremity (Figure 16-4).
A. Assess and compare quality of peripheral pulses (see Figure 16-3).
B. Evaluate skin of the affected extremity.
 1. Color, warmth, capillary refill.
 2. Condition of the skin and nail beds.
 3. Presence of ulcers or lesions.
C. Assess tolerance to activity; determine at what point claudication occurs and whether pain at rest is present.

> **ALERT** Interpret client data that need to be reported immediately.

Goal: To prevent injury and infection.
A. Avoid vigorous rubbing of the extremity.
B. Prevent skin breakdown at pressure sites.
C. Use heel covers and bed cradle to prevent pressure on the toes and heels.
D. Visually inspect extremities for discolored areas, breaks in skin, and signs of infection.
Goal: To increase arterial blood supply.
A. Encourage moderate exercise (e.g., walking).
 1. Level of pain should be a guide to exercise; activity should be stopped when pain occurs.
 2. Goal is 30 to 60 minutes per day, 3 to 5 days a week.

B. Promote blood flow to legs.
 1. Avoid standing in one position for prolonged periods.
 2. Avoid crossing legs at the knees or ankles while in bed.
 3. Provide warmth (room temperature, extra clothing, blankets).
C. Avoid pressure in the posterior popliteal area; avoid positions, clothing, or bandages that restrict circulation to the lower extremities (hose, girdles, elastic bandages, etc.).
D. Stop smoking.
Goal: To protect the extremity with critical limb ischemia.
A. Inspection, cleansing, and lubrication of both feet.
B. Do not soak feet; keep clean and dry.
C. Cover ulcerations with dry sterile dressing.
D. Do not apply any chemicals; do not apply heat or cold.
E. Protect heels from pressure.
F. Healing is not likely to occur unless circulation is restored; protect ulcers from infection.
Goal: To evaluate and promote circulation in affected extremity after vascular surgery.
A. Frequent assessment to determine adequacy of circulation and patency of graft (see Figure 16-4).
 1. Circulation checks distal to the graft every 15 minutes × 4, then hourly × 24 hrs – notify health care provider immediately of any changes in neurocirculatory status of extremities.
 2. Monitor ankle-brachial index (ABI) measurements.
 3. Assess for compartmental syndrome (see Chapter 21) and graft thrombosis.
B. Encourage movement of the extremity as soon as client is awake; avoid flexion in the area of the graft (femoral or popliteal area).

NEUROVASCULAR ASSESSMENT

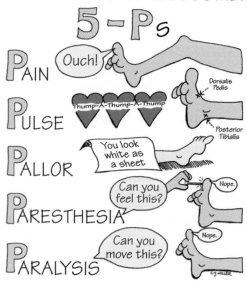

FIGURE 16-4 Neurovascular assessment (From Zerwekh J, Claborn J: *Memory notebook of nursing,* vol 1, ed 4, Ingram, Texas, 2008, Nursing Education Consultants.)

C. Assist client to ambulate as soon as possible.
D. Do not raise the knee gatch of the bed.
E. Monitor anticoagulation medications; maintain bleeding precautions.
F. Assess for development of dependent edema; may require compression dressings or diuretic.

Home Care

A. Decrease weight if appropriate.
B. Avoid standing or sitting for prolonged periods of time.
C. Teach client methods to increase circulation during normal work day (do not cross legs; use a good chair; get up and walk every hour if working at a desk).
D. Avoid tight socks, stockings, or clothing.
E. Avoid trauma to the extremities—always wear shoes.
F. Avoid tobacco products.
G. Wash and visually inspect feet daily.
H. Do not apply any type of direct heat or cold to the legs.
I. Lubricate dry skin; do not use lotions on open lesions or between the toes.
J. Seek professional care for calluses, corns, blisters, ulcers, etc.
K. File toenails straight across.
L. Wear shoes that fit well; avoid shoes that cause feet to perspire.
M. Notify health care provider of:
   1. Presence of lesions or blisters that do not heal or infections on an extremity.
   2. Increase in pain or decrease in exercise tolerance.

Chronic Venous Insufficiency and Venous Stasis Ulcers

Chronic venous insufficiency results from damage to the valves of the veins in the legs. This valvular incompetence leads to regurgitation of blood, venous pooling, and edema in the lower extremities; eventually resulting in development of venous stasis ulcers.

Assessment

A. Risk factors.
   1. Advancing age, increased venous pressure.
   2. Diabetes, obesity.
   3. Varicosities, prolonged immobility.
B. Clinical manifestations (see Table 16-5).
   1. Stasis eczema is often the first indication.
   2. "Brawny" leathery appearance to skin of lower leg.
   3. Sclerosis occurs as a result of longstanding edema; leg becomes larger at the calf.
   4. Ulcerations more commonly near the outer ankle.
   5. Ulcer appearance: irregular margins, copious exudate.
   6. Very painful.
C. Diagnostics: history and clinical manifestations.
D. Complications.
   1. Infection, cellulitis is common.
   2. Delayed or poor healing.

Treatment

A. Medical therapy.
   1. Compression therapy.
      a. Elastic compression stockings.
      b. Sequential compression devices.
      c. Unna boot (a paste bandage).
   2. Moist dressings for open wound care.
   3. Good nutritional status.
   4. Treatment of varicose veins.
B. Surgical therapy: excision of ulcer with skin grafting.

Nursing Interventions

Goal: To prevent and treat venous stasis (Box 16-2).
A. Compression devices: prevention of venous stasis is the key to healing.
   1. Compression boots/stockings: extremity may be covered with continuous compression bandage, boot, or stocking.
   2. Intermittent or sequential pneumatic compression devices: always check arterial circulation with any type of compression device.
   3. Always assess adequacy of arterial circulation prior to compression therapy.

ALERT Implement measures to promote venous return, to manage potential circulatory complications, and to monitor wounds for signs and symptoms of infection.

Box 16-2 NURSING MEASURES TO DECREASE VENOUS STASIS

- Encourage mobility; even standing at the bedside promotes venous tone.
- Elastic support stockings: Hospitalized clients should wear them all the time. Home clients generally wear them during the day. Stockings should be put on before client gets out of bed and removed when client goes to bed. Toe hole should be under the toes and heel patch over the heel. Check for constriction behind the knee and around the thigh. Do not hang feet dependently when putting stockings on; elevate the legs or put them parallel on the bed. Make sure that stockings are the correct fit by measuring the legs and ordering the appropriate size and length.
- Teach client to elevate legs for about 20 minutes every 4 or 5 hours.
- Avoid prolonged sitting; walk around every 1 to 2 hours.
- Don't cross legs when sitting or lying in bed.
- Do not wear restrictive clothing.
- Maintain adequate fluid intake; avoid dehydration.
- Use pneumatic compression devices to facilitate venous return.

Goal: To prevent infection and promote healing.
A. Keep feet clean and dry; assess for development of venous ulcers.
B. Use hydrocolloid dressings for open ulcers.
C. Maintain compression devices; monitor arterial circulation.
D. Assess for development of infections—may require debridement.

ALERT Perform or assist with dressing changes; provide wound care (e.g., central line dressing or wound dressings).

Raynaud's Phenomenon

Raynaud's phenomenon consists of intermittent episodic spasms of the arterioles, most frequently in the fingers and toes. Spasms are not necessarily correlated with other peripheral vascular problems.

Assessment

A. Clinical manifestations.
  1. Increased incidence in women age 20 to 40 years.
  2. Often associated with other systemic connective tissue diseases (e.g., lupus, scleroderma, and rheumatoid arthritis).
  3. Symptoms are precipitated by:
    a. Exposure to cold.
    b. Emotional upset.
    c. Nicotine and caffeine intake.
  4. Vasospasm in fingers, toes, ears, and/or nose leads to:
    a. Pallor and waxy appearance of the tissue.
    b. Numbness and tingling.
  5. Pulses usually remain adequate.
  6. Common findings that occur as perfusion is restored.
    a. Rubor (redness) of the tissue.
    b. Throbbing, aching, burning of the involved area.
  7. May progress to ulceration/gangrene in severe cases.
  8. Attacks are usually bilateral and intermittent; usually last only a few minutes.

Treatment

A. No cure; treatment is based on symptoms.
B. Medications: vasodilators, calcium channel blockers.

Nursing Interventions

Goal: To assist client to understand disease implications and measures to decrease episodic attacks.
A. Prevent vasospasms.
  1. Wear gloves when handling cold objects (items from the refrigerator or freezer).
  2. Protect feet, hands, nose, and ears when exposed to cold weather.
  3. Maintain warm environment.
  4. Avoid caffeine and tobacco products.
  5. Stress management.

Thromboangiitis Obliterans (Buerger's Disease)

Thromboangiitis obliterans is a condition that causes vasculitis of the small and medium-size arteries and veins of the extremities.

Assessment

A. Risk factors.
  1. Very strong relationship with tobacco use.
  2. A type of arteritis that damages arterial walls.
B. Clinical manifestations.
  1. Intermittent claudication; pain at rest in advanced stages.
  2. Usually begins distally and spreads upward.
  3. Temperature changes in affected limb.
  4. Increased sensitivity to cold in the extremity.
  5. Peripheral pulses may be diminished or absent.
C. Diagnostics.
  1. Based on clinical manifestations.
  2. Sometimes difficult to distinguish from peripheral arterial disease.
D. Complications: ulcerations and gangrene.

Treatment

A. No cure; treatment is based on symptoms; cessation of smoking early in the disease can stop symptoms and progression of the disease.
B. Medications: vasodilators, antiplatelets, calcium channel blockers.
C. Surgical therapy.
  1. Sympathectomy.
  2. Revascularization.
  3. Amputation in extreme cases.

Nursing Interventions

Goal: To evaluate level of involvement of the extremity and increase circulation to the extremity.

A. Decrease or stop smoking (also exposure to second-hand smoke).
B. Evaluate tolerance to activity.
C. Inspect feet for vascular changes.
D. Avoid extreme cold.
E. Client should not use nicotine replacement products.

> **! NURSING PRIORITY** The vascular problem has a direct relationship to cigarette smoking. For the condition to be controlled, the client must quit smoking.

Varicose Veins

Varicose veins occur when veins in the lower trunk and extremities become congested and dilated as a result of incompetent valves in the vessels and loss of elasticity of the vessel walls.

Assessment

A. Risk factors.
  1. Congenital weakness of the vessel walls.
  2. Obesity, pregnancy.
  3. Increasing age, prolonged standing.
B. Clinical manifestations.
  1. Dilated, tortuous subcutaneous veins.
  2. Cosmetic appearance of the vein is objectionable.
  3. Aching type pain after prolonged standing.
  4. Pain is generally relieved by elevating the extremity.
C. Diagnostics: positive Trendelenburg test; clinical manifestations.

Treatment

A. Medical: prevent venous stasis (see Box 16-2).
B. Surgical.
  1. Noninvasive laser therapy or high-intensity pulsed-light therapy.
  2. Sclerotherapy: injection of sclerosing agent into the affected vein.
  3. Surgical ligation of the veins; may be combined with vein stripping as well.

Nursing Interventions

Goal: To improve circulation and prevent complications.
A. Decrease venous stasis (see Box 16-2).
B. Facilitate venous return.
  1. Elastic stockings or compression wraps.
  2. Pneumatic compression devices.
  3. Range of motion and active movement of extremities to promote venous return.
C. Avoid constrictive clothing.
D. Avoid prolonged standing or sitting.

Venous Thrombosis (Thrombophlebitis)

Thrombophlebitis is the formation of a thrombus that is associated with inflammation. May be superficial or a deep vein thrombosis (DVT).

Assessment

A. Risk factors (Virchow's Triad).
  1. Venous stasis.
    a. Surgery (hip, pelvic and orthopedic surgery are associated with high risk).
    b. Pregnancy, obesity.
    c. Prolonged immobility (bed rest, long trips, prolonged sitting).
    d. Heart disease (atrial fibrillation, congestive heart failure).
  2. Hypercoagulability.
    a. Malignancies, dehydration.
    b. Blood dyscrasias.
    c. Oral contraceptives, hormone replacement therapy.
    d. Pregnancy and postpartum.
  3. Endothelial damage.
    a. IV fluids and drugs (IV catheterization, drug abuse, caustic solutions or drugs).
    b. Abdominal and pelvic surgery.
    c. Fractures and dislocations (especially of the pelvis, hip, or leg).
    d. History of DVT.

> **ALERT** Provide measures to prevent complications of immobility.

B. Clinical manifestations.
  1. Superficial thrombophlebitis.
    a. Firm, palpable, cordlike vein.
    b. Tender to touch; surrounding area warm and reddened.
  2. Deep vein thrombosis (DVT).
    a. Area around vein is tender to touch, reddened, and warm.
    b. Temperature elevation (above 100.4°F).
    c. Extremity pain and edema.
    d. Homans' sign is not considered to be an accurate indicator of thrombophlebitis (present only in about 10% of cases).
    e. May occur in deep pelvic veins.
C. Diagnostics (see Appendix 16-1).
D. Complications.
  1. DVT associated with high risk for pulmonary emboli.
  2. Chronic venous insufficiency and venous stasis ulcers.

Treatment

A. Medical.
  1. Bed rest.
  2. Elevate extremity.
  3. Anticoagulant; antiinflammatory, and fibrinolytic medications (see Appendix 16-3 and 17-5).

4. Warm moist packs.
5. Elastic support stocking if edema is present after client is ambulatory.
6. Elastic support stocking on unaffected leg only during period of bed rest.
B. Surgical (done to prevent formation of pulmonary emboli).
  1. Venous thrombectomy.
  2. Umbrella filter device in the vena cava.

Nursing Interventions

Goal: To prevent thrombophlebitis, DVT.

> ❗ **NURSING PRIORITY** The most effective way to prevent the development of a pulmonary embolus is to prevent the development of DVT.

A. Nursing measures to decrease venous stasis (see Box 16-2).
B. Prevent complications of immobilization (see Chapter 3).

C. Prophylactic anticoagulation for the high-risk client.
D. Intermittent compression devices for high-risk clients.

> **ALERT** Identify client with condition that increases risk for insufficient vascular perfusion; intervene to promote venous return.

 Home Care

A. Avoid oral contraceptives.
B. Stop smoking.
C. Use methods to decrease venous stasis (see Box 16-2).
D. Exercise regularly (especially walking).
E. Decrease weight, if appropriate.
F. Decrease sodium in diet if edema is present.
G. Follow instructions regarding anticoagulation therapy at home.
H. Understand need for follow-up health care.

Appendix 16-1   VASCULAR DIAGNOSTICS

TEST	NORMAL VALUE	THERAPEUTIC VALUE	NURSING IMPLICATIONS
Serum Studies			
Fragment D-dimer (D-dimer test)	<250 ng/mL	<250 ng/mL	1. Produced by the action of plasma on fibrin, verifies fibrinolysis has occurred. 2. Used in diagnosis of DIC and to screen for thrombosis, acute MI and PE.
PT (prothrombin time)	10-13 sec range	1.5-2.5 times normal	1. Sensitive to alterations in vitamin K. 2. Used to evaluate liver and warfarin medications.
APTT (activated partial thromboplastin time)	Activated: 24-36 sec	1.5-2.5 times normal (46-70 sec)	1. Indicator of adequacy of anticoagulation with heparin. 2. Do not draw sample from extremity with a heparin lock or infusion.
INR (international normalized ratio)		2-3 (anticoagulation)	1. Calculated level based on PT; method of standardizing values. 2. Used to evaluate warfarin (**Coumadin**).
ACT (activated coagulation time)	80-135 sec	180-240 sec or 2 times normal	1. Used to evaluate anticoagulation with heparin.
Invasive Studies			
Peripheral arteriography (angiography) Venography (phlebography)	Involves injection of a radiopaque dye into either the artery or the vein; x-ray films are obtained to identify atherosclerotic plaques, occlusions, traumatic injury, or presence of aneurysms.		1. Explain procedures to client; mild sedative may be indicated. 2. Requires informed consent. 3. After procedure: a. Perform circulatory checks distal to the puncture site. b. Observe client for allergic reactions to the dye. c. Apply pressure dressings to puncture sites, and monitor for bleeding.

Continued

Appendix 16-1 VASCULAR DIAGNOSTICS—cont'd

Noninvasive Studies

Doppler ultrasonography: Hand-held Doppler device used to detect flow of blood in peripheral arterial disease; is not sensitive to early disease changes.

Ankle-brachial index (ABI): Calculated index using a handheld Doppler; divide the ankle SBP by the highest brachial SBP; normal = 0.91 to 1.30; moderate PAD = 0.41 to 0.70.

Venous duplex scan: uses ultrasound to assess veins for flow and pressure; has become the primary diagnostic tool for DVT because it allows for visualization of the vein.

Computed tomography (CT): Allows for visualization of the arterial wall and adjacent structures; used for diagnosis of abdominal aortic aneurysm, graft occlusions.

Trendelenburg test: Client lies supine with leg elevated to promote venous drainage; a tourniquet is applied at mid-thigh, and client is asked to stand. Veins normally fill from below or distally; a varicose vein will fill from above or proximally because of the incompetent valves. Do not leave tourniquet in place longer than 1 minute.

DIC, Diffuse intravascular coagulation; *DVT,* deep vein thrombosis; *MI,* myocardial infarction; *PT,* prothrombin time; *SBP,* systolic blood pressure; *PAD,* peripheral artery disease.

Appendix 16-2 ANTIHYPERLIPIDEMIC MEDICATIONS

Antihyperlipidemics Decrease LDL cholesterol, but preferably do not decrease the HDL cholesterol. Used in combination with dietary restrictions, exercise, and smoking cessation to reduce blood lipid levels.

General Nursing Implications

— Serum liver enzymes should be monitored throughout therapy.
— Medications should be taken before meals.
— Medications should be used in conjunction with other lipid-lowering therapies (exercise, low-cholesterol diet, smoking cessation).
— Serum cholesterol and triglyceride levels should be monitored prior to and periodically throughout therapy.

MEDICATIONS	SIDE EFFECTS	NURSING IMPLICATIONS
Cholestyramine (**Questran**): PO Colestipol (**Colestid**): PO	GI disturbances Constipation	1. Supplemental fat-soluble vitamins in long-term therapy. 2. Mix powder with several ounces of fluid for administration. 3. Use with caution in presence of constipation; increase fiber and fluid intake to prevent constipation.
Nicotinic acid (**Niacin, Nicolar**): PO	Flushing GI disturbances	1. Immediately report signs of hepatotoxicity (darkening of urine, light colored stools, anorexia). 2. Flushing occurs in almost all clients; will diminish over several weeks.
Gemfibrozil (**Lopid**): PO	Diarrhea GI disturbances Abdominal pain	1. Assess for increase in muscle pain. 2. Will potentiate warfarin-derivative anticoagulants (**Coumadin**). 3. Do not confuse with hyoscyamine (**Levbid**).
Lovastatin (**Mevacor**): PO Simvastatin (**Zocor**): PO Fluvastatin (**Lescol**): PO Atorvastatin (**Lipitor**): PO Pravastatin (**Pravachol**): PO	Muscle breakdown Hepatotoxic GI disturbances	1. Give with evening meal. 2. Should not be given to clients with preexisting liver disease. 3. Assess for increase in muscle pain. 4. Monitor liver enzymes closely. 5. Do not confuse pravastatin (**Pravachol**) with lansoprazole (**Prevacid**).

GI, Gastrointestinal; *HDL,* high-density lipoprotein; *LDL,* low-density lipoprotein; *PO,* by mouth (orally).

Appendix 16-3 ANTICOAGULANTS

Anticoagulants Prolong coagulation by inactivation of clotting factors (heparin) and by decreasing synthesis of clotting factors (Coumadin ▲).

General Nursing Implications
— Increased risk for bleeding when used concurrently with other drugs, herbal remedies, or foods affecting coagulation.
— Maintain bleeding precautions.
— Second health care provider should always check order, calculation of dosage, and/or infusion pump settings when being administered intravenously (IV).
— Do not automatically discontinue according to automatic stop policies (procedures, surgery) without verifying the order; reevaluate all clients whose anticoagulants are being held for procedures and assess the need to reorder the anticoagulant therapy.

> **⚠ NURSING PRIORITY** Clarify all anticoagulant dosing for pediatric clients.

MEDICATIONS	SIDE EFFECTS	NURSING IMPLICATIONS

▲ Heparin: IV, subQ
May not be given PO
Short-term anticoagulation
	Bleeding tendencies:
	  hematuria, bleeding gums,
	  or frank hemorrhage
	Heparin-induced
	  thrombocytopenia:
	  associated with increase in
	  thrombosis
		1. Check the APTT for normal levels versus therapeutic levels.
		2. Protamine sulfate is the antidote.
		3. IV administration should be administered via infusion pump to ensure accurate dosage.
		4. Will not dissolve established clots.
		5. Check platelet levels every 2-3 days.
		6. Effective immediately after administration; anticoagulation effect has short half-life.
		7. Before starting infusion, and with each change of the container or rate of infusion, have second practitioner check drug, dosage, route, and rate.
		8. Do not store in same area as insulin; both are given by units.

Low-Molecular-Weight Heparin Enoxaparin **(Lovenox):** subQ Dalteparin sodium ▲ **(Fragmin):** subQ		1. *Use:* prophylaxis for thromboembolic problems in high-risk clients (immobility, hip or knee replacement). 2. Dosage *is not* interchangeable with heparin. 3. Leave the air lock in the prefilled syringe to prevent leakage. 4. **Lovenox** should be injected into the "love handles" of the abdomen.

Warfarin sodium
  ▲ **(Coumadin):** PO
Long-term anticoagulation
		1. Check the PT and INR to evaluate level of anticoagulation; INR greater than 3 may indicate adverse drug reaction.
		2. Vitamin K is the antidote.
		3. ***Client teaching:***
		  • Bleeding precautions (see Box 14-1).
		  • Advise all health care providers of medication.
		  • Not recommended if pregnant or lactating.
		  • Maintain routine checks on coagulation studies.
		  • Do not stop taking medication unless told to do so by health care provider.
		4. Check drug literature when administering with other medications; drug interactions are common.
		5. Oral contraceptives may decrease effectiveness.

> **ALERT** Questions about anticoagulant medications are consistently found on the examination.

▲: High-Alert Medication; *APTT,* activated prothrombin time; *INR,* international normalized ratio; *IV,* intravenously; *PO,* by mouth (orally); *PT,* prothrombin time; *subQ,* subcutaneously.

Appendix 16-4   ANTIPLATELET MEDICATIONS

MEDICATIONS	SIDE EFFECTS	NURSING IMPLICATIONS
Aspirin: PO	GI bleeding, hemorrhagic stroke	1. Given in small doses (e.g., 81 mg daily). 2. Prophylactic therapy for prevention of MI and thrombotic stroke in clients with TIAs.
Clopidogrel **(Plavix):** PO	Abdominal pain, dyspepsia, diarrhea Blood dyscrasias	1. Prophylactic treatment for prevention of MI, strokes in clients with established peripheral artery disease. 2. Expensive and slightly more effective than aspirin.
Cilostazol **(Pletal):** PO	Headache, dizziness, GI bleeding	1. Monitor for relief of intermittent claudication. 2. Grapefruit juice inhibits metabolism. 3. Administer on an empty stomach.
Ticlopidine **(Ticlid):** PO	Diarrhea, bleeding, aplastic anemia	1. Monitor coagulation studies throughout therapy. 2. Monitor cholesterol/triglyceride levels. 3. Older adult clients may have increased sensitivity to **Ticlid.**
Blood Viscosity Reducing Agent Pentoxifylline **(Trental):** PO	GI disturbances, dizziness	1. Monitor for relief of intermittent claudication in lower extremities. 2. Therapeutic effect may not be noted for 2-4 weeks. 3. Do not chew, crush or break tablets.

GI, Gastrointestinal; *MI,* myocardial infarction; *PO,* by mouth (orally); *TIA,* transient ischemic attack.

Appendix 16-5   ANTIHYPERTENSIVE MEDICATIONS

General Nursing Implications
— Advise client that postural hypotension may occur and explain how to decrease effects.
— Hypotension may be increased by hot weather, hot showers, hot tubs, and alcohol ingestion.
— Client should not abruptly discontinue medication or change dosage without consulting health care provider. Abrupt withdrawal can cause rebound hypertension.
— Encourage a low-sodium diet and weight maintenance or reduction.
— Encourage client to stop smoking.
— Have client report unpleasant side effects related to sexual dysfunction.
— Advise client not to take over-the-counter cough medications or decongestants that contain pseudoephedrine; these medications cause an increase in BP.
— Administer with meals to enhance absorption.
— Monitor BP and pulse frequently during initial dosage adjustments; and weekly during initial therapy.

MEDICATIONS	SIDE EFFECTS	NURSING IMPLICATIONS
Vasodilators Act directly on vascular smooth muscle to produce vasodilation.		
Hydralazine HCl **(Apresoline):** PO, IM, IV	Tachycardia, headache, sodium retention, drug-induced lupus syndrome	1. Advise client that postural hypotension may occur. 2. Vitamin B$_6$ may be used to prevent peripheral neuritis with long-term therapy. 3. May be used in combination with other antihypertensive medications.
▲ Nitroprusside **(Nipride):** IV	Nausea/vomiting, headache, abdominal pain, dizziness	1. Used to treat hypertensive crisis; very rapid response. 2. Solution must be prepared immediately before use and protected from light during administration; use within 24 hours. 3. Administer via infusion pump to ensure accurate flow rate. 4. Maintain continuous ECG and BP monitoring, preferably in a critical care setting.

Appendix 16-5   ANTIHYPERTENSIVE MEDICATIONS—cont'd

MEDICATIONS	SIDE EFFECTS	NURSING IMPLICATIONS

Centrally Acting Inhibitors (antiadrenergics) Decrease sympathetic effect (norepinephrine), resulting in decreased BP and peripheral resistance, decrease in heart rate, and no change in cardiac output.

Methyldopa: PO Methyldopate: IV	Hepatotoxicity, hemolytic anemia sexual dysfunction, orthostatic hypotension	1. If withdrawn abruptly, may precipitate a hypertensive crisis. 2. Do not confuse methyldopa with levodopa or L-dopa. 3. Appears on Beers list: Older adult clients may have increased sensitivity to methyldopa. Monitor for depression or altered mental status.

ACE Inhibitors Reduce peripheral vasculature resistance without increasing cardiac output, rate, or contractility; angiotension antagonists.

Captopril (**Capoten**): PO Enalapril (**Vasotec**): PO Lisinopril (**Zestril**): PO Ramipril (**Altace**): PO Moexipril (**Univasc**): PO Benazepril (**Lotensin**): PO	Postural hypotension, hyperkalemia, insomnia, nonproductive cough, loss of taste	1. Monitor closely on first dose; hypotension and first-dose syncope may occur. 2. Conserve potassium; *may not need* a potassium supplement when given with a diuretic. 3. Skipping doses or stopping drug may result in rebound hypertension.

Beta-Adrenergic Blockers See Appendix 17-2.

Calcium Channel Blockers See Appendix 17-2.

ACE, Angiotensin-converting enzyme; *BP,* blood pressure; *ECG,* electrocardiogram; *GI,* gastrointestinal; *IM,* intramuscularly; *IV,* intravenously; *PO,* by mouth (orally).

Appendix 16-6   DIURETICS (FIGURE 16-5)

General Nursing Implications

— In hospitalized clients, evaluate daily weights for fluid loss or gain.
— Maintain intake and output ratios.
— Monitor for hypokalemia, anorexia, muscle weakness, numbness, tingling, paresthesia, confusion, and excessive thirst.
— Advise client of foods that are rich in potassium.
— Administer medications in the morning.
— Teach client how to decrease effects of postural hypotension.
— Monitor BP response to medication.
— Interactions:
   — Digitalis action is increased in presence of hypokalemia.
   — Lithium levels may be increased in presence of hyponatremia.

Loop Diuretics Block sodium and chloride reabsorption, which causes water and solutes to be retained in the nephrons. Prevention of reabsorption of water back into the circulation causes an increase in excretion of the water, and thus, diuresis.

Furosemide (**Lasix**): PO, IM, IV Bumetanide (**Bumex**): PO, IM, IV Torsemide (**Demadex**): PO, IV	Dehydration, hypotension; excessive loss of potassium, sodium, chloride; hyperglycemia, hyperuricemia; muscle weakness	1. Strong diuretic that provides rapid diuresis. 2. Use with caution in older adults; CNS problems of confusion, headache. 3. Monitor closely for tinnitus/hearing loss. 4. Do not confuse **Bumex** with buprenorphine (**Buprenex**). 5. Do not confuse furosemide (**Lasix**) with torsemide (**Demadex**).

Continued

FIGURE 16-5 Diuretic water slide. (From Zerwekh J, Claborn J, Gaglione T: *Mosby's pharmacology memory notecards,* ed 2, St. Louis, 2008, Mosby.)

Thiazide Diuretics Increase renal excretion of Na Cl, K, and water. Require adequate urine output to be effective.

Chlorothiazide **(Diuril):** IV, PO
Chlorthalidone **(Hygroton):** PO
Hydrochlorothiazide
  (HydroDIURIL, Esidrix): PO
Metolazone **(Zaroxolyn):** PO
  (a thiazide-like diuretic)
	Dehydration, hypotension;
	  excessive loss of potassium,
	  hyperglycemia, hyperuricemia;
	  muscle weakness
		1. Frequently used as first-line drug to control essential hypertension.
		2. Increased risk for digitalis toxicity if taking digoxin products.
		3. If allergic to thiazides or sulfonamides, metolazone may be contraindicated.

Aldosterone Antagonist (potassium-sparing diuretics) Blocks the effect of aldosterone, inhibits the renal-angiotension-aldosterone system (RAAS); blocks receptors in the renal tubules, heart, and blood vessels. Used in treatment of heart failure, as well as hypertension.

Spironolactone **(Aldactone):** PO Triamterene **(Dyrenium):** PO	Hyperkalemia, hyponatremia, impotence, hypotension	1. May be used in combination with other diuretics to reduce potassium loss. 2. Potassium-sparing effects may result in hyperkalemia. 3. Not used for clients experiencing renal failure. 4. Avoid salt substitutes and foods containing large amounts of sodium or potassium.

Osmotic Diuretic Increases osmotic pressure of the fluid in the renal tubules, preventing reabsorption of sodium and water.

Mannitol **(Osmitrol):** IV	Pulmonary edema, CHF, tissue dehydration, nausea, vomiting	1. Stop infusion if client begins to show symptoms of CHF or pulmonary edema. 2. Use an IV filter to prevent infusion of crystals; warm vial and shake vigorously to dissolve crystals. 3. Monitor infusion site closely for infiltration and/or extravasation.

BP, Blood pressure; *CHF,* congestive heart failure; *CNS,* central nervous system; *IM,* intramuscularly; *IV,* intravenously; *PO,* by mouth (orally).

Appendix 16-7	MEDICATIONS USED FOR TREATMENT OF SHOCK

General Nursing Implications

— Most often limited to critical care settings; constant monitoring is required.
— Administered IV in diluted solution by infusion pump.
— Monitor IV infusion site closely; leakage into tissue may cause tissue sloughing.
— Administer via central line if possible.
— Carefully administered with frequent observation and evaluation of BP.
— Continuous ECG monitoring; observe client closely for cardiac dysrhythmias.
— Monitor urinary output every hour.
— Medications should not be administered to clients receiving MAOIs or tricyclic antidepressants.

MEDICATIONS	SIDE EFFECTS	NURSING IMPLICATIONS
Adrenergics Increases myocardial contractility, thereby improving cardiac output, BP, and urine output.		
▲ Dopamine **(Intropin):** IV	Dysrhythmias (tachycardia), angina, hypertension, headaches	1. Should not be given to clients with tachydysrhythmias or ventricular fibrillation. 2. Have second practitioner check drug, dosage, route, etc. 3. If extravasation occurs, stop infusion immediately; area may be infused with phentolamine mesylate **(Regitine).** 4. Closely monitor VS, cardiac rhythm, and urinary output during administration.
▲ Dobutamine **(Dobutrex):** IV	Tachycardia, dysrhythmias, hypertension	1. If extravasation occurs, stop infusion; area may be infused with phentolamine mesylate **(Regitine).**
▲ Epinephrine hydrochloride **(Adrenalin):** IV	Nervousness, restlessness, tremors, angina, dysrhythmias, tachycardia, hypertension.	1. Be sure to read label correctly and use correct strength / concentration. 2. Use in treatment of anaphylactic shock and cardiac arrest.

▲: High-Alert Medication; *ECG,* electrocardiogram; *IV,* intravenous; *MAOIs,* monoamine oxidase inhibitors; *VS,* vital signs.

Study Questions Vascular System

More questions on companion CD!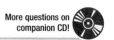

1. What is the correct reference point that the nurse would use to measure a client's central venous pressure (CVP)?
   1 Right side, midclavicular line where it intersects with the fifth intercostal space
   2 Midaxillary line at the level of the fifth intercostal space
   3 Left midsternal border at the level of the fourth intercostal space
   4 Anterior aspect of the thoracic cavity, left side at the fifth intercostal space

2. What is an important nursing action in the safe administration of heparin?
   1 Check the prothrombin time (PT) and administer the medication if it is less than 20 seconds.
   2 Use a 20-gauge, 1-inch needle and inject into the deltoid muscle and gently massage the area.
   3 Dilute in 50 mL 5% dextrose in water (D_5W) and infuse by intravenous piggyback (IVPB) over 15 minutes.
   4 Use a 25-gauge, ½-inch needle and inject the medication into the subcutaneous tissue of the abdomen.

3. While discussing her diagnosis of hypertension, a client asks the nurse how long she is going to have to take all of the medications that have been prescribed. On what principle is the nurse's response based?
   1 The client will be scheduled for an appointment in 2 months; the doctor will decrease her medications at that time.
   2 As soon as her blood pressure (BP) returns to normal levels, the client will be able to stop taking her medications.
   3 To maintain stable control of her BP, the client will have to take the medications indefinitely.
   4 The nurse cannot discuss the medications with the client; the client will need to talk with the doctor.

4. The nurse is teaching a client about home care and treatment of venous stasis ulcers on his leg. What should be included in the nurse's instructions? Select all that apply:
   _____ 1 Dressings do not need to be changed frequently because there is minimal drainage.
   _____ 2 Healing will be facilitated by wearing leg compression devices.
   _____ 3 When the client is in the sitting position, he should keep his legs elevated.
   _____ 4 Avoid standing for prolonged periods of time.
   _____ 5 Cool packs can be applied to the ulcers to decrease inflammation.
   _____ 6 Soak the affected extremity in warm water every evening

5. The nurse is caring for a client who is 6 hours postpartum. What nursing actions are directed toward the prevention of postpartum thrombophlebitis?
   1 Encourage early ambulation and increased fluid intake.
   2 Allow bathroom privileges only and elevate the lower extremities.
   3 Administer anticoagulants and evaluate the clotting factors.
   4 Encourage the client to breastfeed the infant as soon as possible.

6. The nurse is preparing to administer spironolactone (Aldactone) to a client. After assessing the client, what data indicate the need to withhold the medication?
   1 Potassium level of 5.8 mEq/L
   2 Apical pulse rate of 58 beats/min
   3 BP of 130/90 mm Hg
   4 Urine output of 30 mL/hr

7. Which nursing action would be most effective in preventing venous stasis in the postoperative surgical client?
   1 Raise the foot of the bed for 1 hour; then lower it to stimulate blood flow.
   2 Massage the lower extremities every 6 hours.
   3 Facilitate active range of motion of the upper body to stimulate cardiac output.
   4 Help the client walk as soon as and as often as possible.

8. A client has had her blood pressure evaluated weekly for 1 month. At the end of the month, the nurse averages out the weekly blood pressures at 150/96 mm Hg. The client is 20 pounds overweight, and her cholesterol is 240 mg/dL. What is important information for the nurse to include in the teaching plan for this client?
   1 Refer her to the doctor for further follow-up and medications.
   2 Increase the fiber in her diet and begin a daily 30-minute workout.
   3 Reduce her sodium intake and decrease the dietary calories that come from fat.
   4 Reduce her cholesterol intake for 1 month and check her BP three times a week.

9. Four hours after aortic-femoral bypass graft surgery, the nurse assesses the client and is unable to palpate pulses in the operative leg. The client complains of pain in the leg. What is the first nursing action?
   1 Massage the leg and apply warm towels.
   2 Elevate the leg and recheck the pulse.
   3 Call the physician immediately.
   4 Help the client ambulate.

Answers and rationales to these questions are in the section at the end of the book titled Chapter Study Questions: Answers and Rationales.

CHAPTER SEVENTEEN

Cardiac System

PHYSIOLOGY OF THE CARDIAC SYSTEM

Structure of the Heart

A. The heart is located in the mediastinal space of the thoracic cavity.

B. The apex of the heart points downward and to the left; the apex comes in contact with the chest wall at about the fifth to sixth intercostal space. In the healthy individual, the point of maximum impulse (PMI) may be palpated here; this is also the area to auscultate when evaluating the apical heart rate.

C. The heart is contained in a loose sac called the pericardium.
1. Fibrous pericardium: the outer surface.
2. Parietal layer: lines the fibrous pericardium.
3. Epicardial (visceral layer): vascular and adherent to the heart.
4. There is a potential space between the visceral and parietal layers of the pericardium. This area contains about 5 to 20 mL of pericardial fluid to lubricate the sac and prevent friction from cardiac movement.

D. Myocardial wall.
1. Epicardium: the outer surface.
2. Myocardium: the middle layer of cardiac muscle.
3. Endocardium: the lining of the inner surface of the cardiac chambers.

E. Cardiac chambers (Figure 17-1).
1. Four chambers are located within the heart; these chambers represent two pumps.
2. Both atria are the receiving chambers; both ventricles are the ejecting chambers.
3. The right side of the heart has a thinner myocardium than the left side and is a low-pressure system.
4. The left ventricle is composed of a thicker muscle, is a high-pressure system, and is capable of generating enough force to eject blood through the aortic valve and through the systemic circulation.

F. Cardiac valves: maintain the directional flow of blood through the heart chambers.
1. Atrioventricular valves are controlled and supported by papillary muscle connected to the ventricular muscle and chordae tendineae extending from papillary muscle to valve leaflets.

a. The tricuspid valve lies between the right atrium and the right ventricle.
b. The mitral valve lies between the left atrium and the left ventricle.
c. Both valves prevent backflow of blood from the ventricles into the atria during systole.
2. Semilunar valves (cusp valves) are controlled by the backward pressure of blood flow at the end of systole.
a. Pulmonic valve: the outflow valve of the right ventricle into the pulmonary circulation.
b. Aortic valve: the outflow valve of the left ventricle into the aorta.
c. Both valves prevent the backflow of blood from the pulmonary artery and the aortic arch into the ventricle during diastole.

G. Direction of blood flow through the heart structure (see Figure 17-1).
1. From the venous system, the blood enters the right atrium via the superior and inferior vena cavae; it flows through the tricuspid valve into the right ventricle; it is ejected through the pulmonic valve into the pulmonary artery; and it flows to the lungs for oxygenation.
2. Oxygenated blood returns to the left atrium via the pulmonary veins; it flows through the mitral valve into the left ventricle; it is ejected through the aortic valve into the aortic arch; and it flows into the systemic circulation.
3. The pulmonary artery is the only artery in the circulatory system to carry deoxygenated blood; the pulmonary vein is the only vein in the circulatory system to carry oxygenated blood.

Cardiac Function

A. One complete cardiac cycle consists of contraction of the myocardium (systole) and subsequent relaxation of the myocardium (diastole).

B. The amount of blood ejected with ventricular contraction is the stroke volume.

C. Starling's law of the heart: the greater the cardiac muscles are stretched, the more forceful the contraction. If an increased amount of blood flows into the heart, the heart will increase the force of contraction and eject a larger amount of blood.

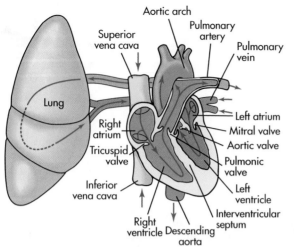

FIGURE 17-1 Blood flow through the heart. (From Lewis SL et al: *Medical-surgical nursing: assessment and management of clinical problems,* ed 7, St. Louis, 2007, Mosby.)

FIGURE 17-2 Preload and afterload. (From Zerwekh J, Claborn J: *Memory notebook of nursing,* vol 1, ed 4, Ingram, Texas, 2008, Nursing Education Consultants.)

D. Cardiac output (CO = SV × HR).
1. The cardiac output can be determined by multiplying the stroke volume (SV) by the heart rate (HR) in beats per minute (CO = SV × HR).
2. The heart pumps approximately 5 L of blood every minute.
3. The heart rate increases with exercise; therefore, cardiac output increases.
4. The cardiac output will vary according to the amount of venous return (preload).
5. Factors regulating stroke volume.
   a. Degree of stretch of the cardiac muscle before contraction (Starling's law): determined by the volume of blood in the ventricle at the end of diastole or diastolic filling.
   b. Contractility: ability of the myocardium to contract; contractility is increased by circulating catecholamines and medications such as digitalis.
   c. Preload: the filling of the ventricles at the end of diastole. The more the ventricles fill, the more the cardiac muscles are stretched, and the greater the force of the contraction during systole (Starling's law). If there is a decrease in the preload, there is also a decrease in contractility and in cardiac output.
   d. Afterload: the pressure in the aorta that the ventricles must overcome to pump blood into the systemic circulation. A decrease in the afterload causes a decrease in the workload of the ventricles; this in turn helps increase the stroke volume and the cardiac output (Figure 17-2).
E. Innervation of the myocardium (autonomic nervous system).
1. Parasympathetic (vagus nerve) stimulation.
   a. Slows rate of impulse generation at the sinoatrial (SA) node.

   b. Slows transmission of the impulse through the atrioventricular (AV) node.
   c. Atropine blocks vagal stimulation to the heart.
2. Sympathetic stimulation.
   a. Increases heart rate.
   b. Increases force of contraction.
F. Factors that increase myocardial oxygen demands.
1. Increased heart rate.
2. Increased force of contractions.
3. Increased afterload.
G. Cardiac compensatory mechanisms: when the normal compensatory mechanisms cannot maintain cardiac output to meet body needs, the client is in a state of cardiac decompensation.
1. Acute.
   a. Sympathetic nervous system receptors initiate an increase in the release of epinephrine and norepinephrine to increase the cardiac rate and myocardial contractility.
   b. Increased diastolic filling (preload) increases cardiac output by increasing the stretch of the myocardial muscle fibers, thus increasing the contractility (Starling's law). In a healthy heart, this is the mechanism that functions when there is a need for increased cardiac output, as in exercise. The increase in the stretch of the myocardial fibers and the increase in the contractile force also require an increase in oxygen consumption. If the myocardial fibers have a decreased oxygen supply and/or the demand on the myocardial muscle is increased for a prolonged period, decompensation will occur.
2. Chronic: ventricular hypertrophy increases cardiac output by increasing the size of the myocardial muscle. This also increases the myocardial need for

oxygen, and in the diseased myocardium, the hypertrophy will eventually lead to a decompensated state.

Myocardial Blood Supply

A. Coronary arteries.
1. Originate at the coronary sinus, just outside the aortic valve.
2. Provide the only source of oxygenated blood for the myocardium.
3. Arteries fill during diastole; a diastolic pressure of 60 mm Hg is required to adequately perfuse the coronary arteries.
B. Collateral circulation.
1. There are no direct connections between the large coronary arteries.
2. When gradual occlusion of large coronary vessels occurs as a result of arteriosclerotic heart disease (ASHD), the smaller vessels increase in size and provide alternative blood flow.
3. Because of the development of collateral circulation, coronary artery disease may be well advanced before the client experiences symptoms.

Conduction System

A. Controls the rate and rhythm of the heart.
B. Located in the myocardium are pathways for conduction of an electrical impulse that initiates contraction of the heart muscle.
C. Characteristics of cells in the conduction system.
1. Automaticity: the ability of certain conductive pathway cells to initiate an impulse spontaneously and consistently.
2. Excitability: the ability of a cell to respond to an impulse.
3. Conductivity: the ability of a cell to conduct an electrical impulse.
4. Refractoriness: the inability of a cell to respond to incoming stimuli.
D. Impulse generation.
1. Resting state: cell is ready to receive an impulse.
2. Depolarization: flow of electrical current along cardiac membrane, initiating muscle contraction.
3. Repolarization: cells regain the electrical charge and are returned to a resting state.
E. Relationship of conducting pathways to the electrocardiogram (ECG) (Figure 17-3).
1. P wave: indicative of the impulse generated from the sinoatrial node; initiates atrial depolarization.
2. PR interval: delay of the impulse at the atrioventricular node and bundle of His to promote ventricular filling.
3. QRS complex: passage of the impulse through the bundle of His, down the bundle branches, through the Purkinje fibers; depolarization of the ventricle occurs.
4. T wave: ventricular repolarization and return to the resting state.
5. S-T segment: above the baseline in cardiac injury and below the baseline with ischemia.

FIGURE 17-3 Normal electrocardiogram (ECG). (From Hockenberry MJ, Wilson D: *Wong's nursing care of infants and children,* ed 8, St. Louis, 2007, Mosby.)

System Assessment

A. Health history.
1. Identify presence of risk factors for the development of arteriosclerotic disease.
2. Coping strategies.
3. Respiratory.
a. History of difficulty breathing.
b. Medications taken for respiratory problems.
c. Determine normal activity level.
4. Circulation.
a. History of chest discomfort (Table 17-1).
b. History of edema, weight gain.
c. History of syncope.
d. Medications taken for the heart or for high blood pressure.
B. Physical assessment.
1. What is the general appearance of the client: Is there any evidence of distress? What is the client's level of orientation and ability to think clearly?
2. Evaluate blood pressure.
a. Pulse pressure: the difference between systolic and diastolic pressure.
b. Assess for postural hypotension (decrease in blood pressure when client stands).
c. Take blood pressure sitting, standing, and lying if client is having problems with pressure changes (see Chapter 16 for accurate blood pressure measurement).
d. Paradoxical blood pressure (paradoxical pulse): a decrease in systolic blood pressure of at least 10 mm Hg that occurs during inspiration.
3. Evaluate quality and rate of pulse; assess for dysrhythmias (see Appendix 17-7 for determining dysrhythmias).
a. Pulse deficit: the radial pulse rate is less than the apical pulse rate; occurs in atrial fibrillation.

b. Pulsus alternans: regular rhythm but quality of pulse alternates with strong beats and weak beats.

c. Thready pulse: weak and rapid; difficult to count.

4. Assess quality and pattern of respirations and evidence of respiratory difficulty.

5. Auscultation of the heart (Figure 17-4).

a. Heart sounds heard during the cardiac cycle.

(1) S_1: closure of the mitral and tricuspid valves.

(2) S_2: closure of the aortic and pulmonic valves.

(3) S_3: represents rapid ventricular filling; normal in children and young adults; in adults older than 30 years, it may be an indication of volume overload, ventricular dysfunction secondary to hypertension.

(4) S_4: extra sounds heard during atrial contraction are abnormal; may indicate a forceful atrial contraction due to increased resistance.

b. Presence of murmurs created by turbulent blood flow: graded on a scale of loudness.

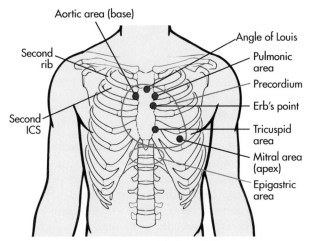

FIGURE 17-4 Cardiac auscultatory sites. (From Lewis SL et al: *Medical-surgical nursing: assessment and management of clinical problems*, ed 7, St. Louis, 2007, Mosby.)

(1) Abnormal flow through diseased valves: stenosis and insufficiency.

(2) Abnormal flow of blood between cardiac chambers (congenital heart disease).

c. Presence of a friction rub: usually heard over the apex during S_1 and S_2; can be heard best with client sitting and leaning forward.

> **ALERT** Identify common abnormal heart sounds (e.g., S_3, S_4).

6. Evaluate adequacy of peripheral vascular circulation and check for presence of peripheral edema.

7. Evaluate for presence of chest discomfort (see Table 17-1).

a. Location.

b. Intensity of pain.

c. Precipitating causes.

> **ALERT** Perform focused assessment or reassessment; interpret data that need to be reported immediately (see Box 17-1).

DISORDERS OF THE CARDIAC SYSTEM

Angina Pectoris

Arteriosclerotic heart disease (ASHD), also called coronary artery disease (CAD), occurs as a result of the atherosclerotic process (see Chapter 16) in the coronary arteries. Angina pectoris is caused by myocardial ischemia due to narrowed or blocked coronary arteries. The buildup of plaque or fatty material in the coronary artery causes a narrowing of the lumen of the artery and precipitates myocardial ischemia that causes chest pain.

A. Pain (angina) occurs when the oxygen demands of the heart muscle exceed the ability of the coronary arteries to deliver it.

Table 17-1	ASSESSING CHEST PAIN (PQRST)			
P—Precipitating Factors	*Q—Quality*	*R—Region and Radiation*	*S—Symptoms and Signs (associated with chest pain)*	*T—Timing and Response to Treatment*
May occur without precipitators	Pressure	Substernal or retrosternal	Diaphoresis, cold clammy skin	Sudden onset
Physical exertion	Squeezing	Spreads across the chest	Nausea, vomiting	Constant
Emotional stress	Heaviness	Radiates to the inside	Dyspnea	Duration >30 min
Eating a large meal	Smothering	of either or both	Orthopnea	Not relieved with
	Burning	arms, the neck, jaw,	Syncope	nitrates or rest
	Severe pain	back, upper	Apprehension	Relief with narcotics
	Increases with movement	abdomen	Dysrhythmias	
			Palpitations	
			Auscultation of extra heart sounds	
			Auscultation of crackles	
			Weakness	

B. Temporary ischemia does not cause permanent damage to the myocardium. Pain frequently subsides when the precipitating factor is removed.
C. Types of angina.
  1. Chronic stable angina: predictable with level of stress or exertion; consistently responds well to medication; pain rarely occurs at rest.
  2. Unstable angina (acute coronary syndrome).
    a. Unstable angina pain occurs spontaneously at rest (usually between midnight and 8 a.m.); progressive in frequency of attacks; unpredictable, not relieved with sublingual nitroglycerin.
    b. Variant angina (Prinzmetal angina) pain that tends to be cyclic caused by coronary spasms.
  3. New onset angina: first symptoms of angina that most frequently occur after exertion.

Assessment

A. Risk factors/etiology.
  1. ASHD (Box 17-1).
  2. Cardiac ischemia.
  3. Aortic valve disease (impedes filling of the coronary arteries).
  4. Increased cardiac demands.
    a. Exercise, emotional stress.
    b. Heavy meals, thyrotoxicosis.
    c. Exposure to cold temperature.
B. Clinical manifestations—chronic stable angina.
  1. Pain in varying levels of severity (see Table 17-1).
  2. Pain most often is located behind or just to the left of the sternum.
  3. Pain may radiate to neck, jaw, and shoulders.

  4. Client may describe pain as squeezing, choking, or constricting or as a vague feeling of pressure and indigestion.
  5. Client will frequently deny seriousness of the pain.
  6. Most clients correlate pain with activity and increased cardiac demands.
  7. Pain is of short duration, generally lasting about 5 minutes; may be longer if associated with anger or heavy meals.
  8. Accompanying symptoms may include diaphoresis, increased anxiety, pallor, and dyspnea.
C. Diagnostics—chronic stable angina (see Appendix 17-1).

Treatment—Chronic Stable Angina

A. Primary goal of treatment is to relieve pain and prevent future attacks.
B. Medication.
  1. Vasodilators: nitroglycerin (Appendix 17-2).
  2. Beta-adrenergic blockers (Appendix 17-3).
  3. Calcium-channel blockers (Appendix 17-3).
  4. Antiplatelet medications (see Appendix 16-4).
C. Procedures/surgical intervention.
  1. Percutaneous coronary intervention (PCI): a balloon is threaded from an artery in the groin to the affected coronary artery. The balloon is then inflated in an effort to compress the plaque and dilate the narrowed artery reestablishing blood flow to the myocardium.
  2. Laser angioplasty: a special catheter with a laser tip is inserted into coronary artery. When confronted with a blockage, the laser emits pulsating beams of light that vaporize the plaque.
  3. Atherectomy: technique in which the catheter has a rotating shaver on the tip that cuts away the plaque.
  4. An intracoronary stent is an expandable wire mesh that can be inserted during any of the above procedures. A stent serves as a scaffold to maintain patency of the coronary artery.
  5. Cardiac revascularization: coronary artery bypass graft (CABG) surgery, open heart surgery.
D. Restricted activity.
E. Supplemental oxygen.
F. Control of the modifiable risk factors (see Box 17-1).

Acute Coronary Syndrome: Unstable Angina Pectoris

According to the American Heart Association, acute coronary syndrome (ACS) includes the various degrees of coronary artery occlusion that can develop in individuals with coronary atherosclerosis.

A. Includes unstable angina, non-ST-segment elevation myocardial infarction (MI), and ST-segment elevation MI, all of which can lead to sudden cardiac death.
B. Unstable angina pectoris occurs when a thrombus partially occludes a coronary artery causing prolonged symptoms of ischemia which can occur at rest.

Assessment

A. Risk factors/etiology.
1. Family history of coronary artery disease.
2. Hypertension, hypercholesterolemia.
3. Diabetes, smoking.
4. Average age for 1st MI - men over 64.5 years, women over 70.5 years.
5. Women are at increased risk after menopause.
B. Clinical manifestations.
1. Two or more anginal events within the past 24 hours.
2. Prolonged chest pain (greater than 20 minutes).
3. Presenting symptoms in women: indigestion, pain between the shoulders, shortness of breath, and anxiety.
4. Hypotension, bradycardia, or tachycardia.
5. New onset S_3.
C. Diagnostics (Appendix 17-1).
1. 12-lead ECG.
   a. ST segment elevation (STEMI), traditional.
   b. Non-ST elevation MI (NSTEMI), common in women.
2. Elevated cardiac troponin 1.
3. Elevated CK-MB.
4. Presence of unstable angina.
D. Treatment (initial).
1. Bed rest.
2. Monitor vital signs, including oxygen saturation level.
3. Supplemental oxygen at 4 L/min via nasal cannula (maintain O_2 sat above 90%).
4. Reduce coronary reocclusion with antiplatelet medications (Appendix 16-4).
5. Reduce and control ischemic pain: vasodilators (nitroglycerin, sublingual, spray or IV, see Appendix 17-2), narcotics (morphine sulfate IV—if pain not relieved by the nitroglycerin).
6. Beta-adrenergic receptor blockers (Appendix 17-3) to decrease cardiac demand for oxygen; anticoagulants (Appendix 16-3) to prevent emboli.
7. Complete fibrinolytic checklist and, if appropriate, initiate fibrinolytic therapy (Appendix 17-5).
8. Transmyocardial laser revascularization (TMR): laser probe is inserted into the wall of the left ventricle; channels are created to promote the development of revascularization.

Complications

A. Dysrhythmias (see Appendix 17-7).
B. Myocardial infarction (MI).

Nursing Interventions for Angina and Acute Coronary Syndrome

ALERT Intervene to improve client's cardiovascular status; assess client for decreased cardiac output; meet client's pain management needs; use critical thinking when addressing pain management.

Goal: To decrease pain and increase myocardial oxygenation.

A. Begin supplemental oxygen.
B. Position client in reclining position with head elevated.
C. Assess characteristics of pain: administer morphine for pain control.
D. Administer medications.
1. Administer nitroglycerin (sublingually, IV, or spray; see Appendix 17-2): evaluate client's response; pain from chronic angina is usually relieved; pain from acute angina may not be relieved.
2. Narcotic analgesics (IV morphine in small increments until pain subsides).
3. Antiplatelet agent (see Appendix 16-4).
E. Maintain calm, reassuring atmosphere.
F. Establish venous access for fluids and IV medications.
G. Notify physician if pain does not respond to medication or if vital signs deteriorate.

! NURSING PRIORITY To relieve chest pain and to decrease cardiac damage resulting from an inadequate blood and oxygen supply to the myocardium, there must be an immediate reduction in the workload of the heart that results in a decrease in oxygen consumption: rest, nitroglycerin, oxygen therapy.

Goal: To evaluate characteristics of anginal pain and client's overall response.

A. Does pain increase with breathing? (Anginal pain is generally not affected by breathing or changes of position.)
B. Assess activity tolerance or precipitating factor.
C. Assess changes in characteristics of pain (see Table 17-1).
D. Evaluate response of pain to treatment or progression to more severe level.
E. Obtain a 12-lead ECG.
F. Evaluate vital signs.
1. Presence of S_3 gallop, which may indicate heart failure.
2. Presence of jugular vein distention; peripheral edema.
3. Presence of dyspnea or wet breath sounds.
4. Adequacy of cardiac output: peripheral pulses, urinary output, level of consciousness.
G. Continuous ECG monitoring: assess for presence of dysrhythmia and impact on cardiac output.
H. Monitor troponin levels (Appendix 17-1).
I. Assess client's psychosocial response: denial is common; anger, fear and depression occur in both client and family.

ALERT Intervene to improve client's cardiovascular status; provide client with strategies to manage decreased cardiac output.

Goal: To provide care after percutaneous coronary intervention (with or without stent).

A. Monitor for chest pain and hypotension; reocclusion is a primary complication.
B. Assess for bleeding or hematoma formation.

C. Frequently assess status of circulation distal to area of cannulation.

D. A sheath may be left in place; monitor area for bleeding; if bleeding occurs, put manual pressure on the area and notify the physician.

E. Prevent flexion of affected extremity and maintain bed rest for 6 to 8 hours.

F. Client is to avoid heavy lifting; may return to work in 1 to 2 weeks.

G. Notify the doctor of any chest pain, syncope, or bleeding at the site.

H. Assess ECG for evidence of ST-segment changes.

Home Care

A. Education regarding ASHD.
   1. Client will be able to identify personal risk factors and appropriate health practices to decrease risk factors.
   2. Client will be able to identify factors precipitating pain.

B. Determine that client understands his or her medication regimen (Box 17-2).

C. Assess understanding of diet and exercise regimen.

D. Assess understanding of seeking medical assistance if pain persists and is not relieved by medication.

E. Help client identify resources for counseling to decrease stress.

F. Advise client not to take erectile dysfunction drugs (Appendix 22-1) if on nitrates for chest pain.

Box 17-2 CLIENT EDUCATION FOR NITROGLYCERIN ADMINISTRATION

1. Keep in a tightly closed, dark glass container.
2. Carry supply at all times—either sublingual (SL) tablets or translingual spray; do not swallow sublingual tablets.
3. Fresh tablets should cause a slight burning under the tongue.
4. Date all opened containers and discard all medication that is 24 months old.
5. Take nitroglycerin prophylactically to avoid pain—before sexual intercourse, exercise, walking, etc.
6. Take nitroglycerin when pain begins; stop all activity.
7. If pain is not relieved in 5 minutes, call 911 and activate EMS.
8. While waiting for EMS response, if chest pain remains unrelieved, take another SL pill or 1 metered spray.
9. Remain lying down; orthostatic hypotension can be a problem.
10. Long-acting preparations should not be abruptly discontinued; this may precipitate vasospasm.
11. To decrease development of tolerance in long-acting preparations, schedule an 8-hour nitro-free period each day, preferable at night.
12. Do not take erectile dysfunction drugs with nitroglycerine.

ALERT Instruct clients about self-administration of medications.

 Acute Coronary Syndrome: Myocardial Infarction

A myocardial infarction (MI), also called coronary occlusion or heart attack, is a total occlusion of a portion of a coronary artery. After the occlusion, myocardial ischemia, injury, or death occurs.

A. Infarction most often occurs in the area of the left ventricle.

B. The severity of the situation depends on the area of the heart involved, as well as the size of the infarction.

C. Healing process.
   1. In the first 24 hours, the inflammatory process is well established; leukocytes invade the area, and cardiac enzymes are released from the damaged cells.
   2. In 4 to 10 days: necrotic zone is well defined.
   3. In 10 to 14 days: the formation of scar tissue foundation begins.

D. The presence of pre-established collateral circulation will assist in decreasing the size of the necrotic area.

NURSING PRIORITY Danger of death from an MI is greatest during the first 2 hours.

Assessment

A. Risk factors/etiology (see unstable angina).

B. Clinical manifestations.
   1. Typical pain is severe, substernal, crushing, and unrelieved by nitroglycerin.
   2. Denial of the seriousness of the pain; clients with MI frequently wait more than 2 hours to seek assistance.
   3. Dyspnea, nausea, vomiting, indigestion.
   4. Pale, dusky skin.
   5. Pain may radiate down arm or up the jaw.
   6. Onset is usually sudden.
   7. Diaphoresis; extreme weakness.
   8. Decrease in blood pressure, tachycardia, syncope.

C. Diagnostics: see acute angina (see Appendix 17-1).

Treatment (Figure 17-5)

A. Bed rest.

B. Monitor vital signs, oxygen saturation, and ECG.

C. Supplemental oxygen at 4 L/min via nasal cannula (maintain O_2 sat above 90%).

D. Pain relief (morphine sulfate IV).

E. Beta-adrenergic receptor blockers (Appendix 17-3); antiplatelets (Appendix 16-4); anticoagulants (Appendix 16-3).

F. Antidysrhythmic agents (Appendix 17-4).

G. Reperfusion (fibrinolytic) therapy (Appendix 17-5).

H. Percutaneous coronary intervention (PCI): "door-to-balloon" goal of 90 minutes for optimum response.

I. Cardiac surgery if appropriate.

Complications

A. Dysrhythmias (see Appendix 17-7).

B. Cardiogenic shock.

C. Heart failure (congestive heart failure).

IMMEDIATE TREATMENT OF AN M.I.

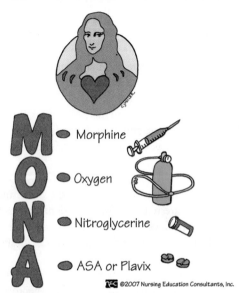

- M • Morphine
- O • Oxygen
- N • Nitroglycerine
- A • ASA or Plavix

©2007 Nursing Education Consultants, Inc.

FIGURE 17-5 MONA: Immediate treatment of an MI. (From Zerwekh J, Claborn J: *Memory notebook of nursing,* vol 2, ed 3, Ingram, Texas, 2007, Nursing Education Consultants.)

Nursing Interventions

Goal: To decrease pain and increase myocardial oxygenation (see Nursing Interventions for Angina and Acute Coronary Syndrome).

> **! NURSING PRIORITY** As long as chest pain persists, cardiac ischemia continues. If client experiences tachycardia, decrease activity whether client has chest pain or not.

Goal: To evaluate characteristics of cardiac pain and client's overall response (also see Nursing Interventions for Angina and Acute Coronary Syndrome).

A. Continuous cardiac monitoring to identify and treat dysrhythmias affecting cardiac output.
B. Frequent assessment for dysrhythmias, murmurs, and presence of S_3, S_4.
C. Maintain IV access.
D. Maintain bed rest for the first 24 hours.

> **ALERT** Meet client's pain management needs; provide medication for pain relief; use clinical decision making when administering medications; monitor for effects of pain medication.

E. Frequent assessment of chest pain.
F. Evaluate urinary output and renal response.
G. Assess respiratory system for pulmonary congestion.
H. Evaluate peripheral circulation; assess for dependent edema.
I. Maintain NPO (nothing by mouth) status initially; then allow clear liquids; progress to light meals that are low in sodium and cholesterol.

J. Promote normal bowel pattern.
1. Stool softeners.
2. Bedside commode.
3. Caution against stimulation of the vagus nerve (Valsalva maneuver).
4. Increase fiber in diet.

> **ALERT** Identify potential/actual stressors for the client; implement measures to reduce environmental stress; promote methods to reduce stress.

K. Decrease anxiety.
1. Keep client informed regarding progress and immediate plan of care.
2. Decrease sensory overload.
3. Encourage verbalization of concerns and fears.
L. Monitor for changes in neurologic status: confusion, disorientation, etc.
M. Monitor progressive activity.
1. Encourage progressive activity: walking in hallway 3 to 4 times a day with gradual increasing increments.
2. Decrease in 20 mm Hg in systolic B/P, changes in heart rate greater than 20 bpm, shortness of breath, and or chest pain indicate poor tolerance to activity.
3. Assess heart rhythm, fatigue, and blood pressure after each activity.
4. Resting tachycardia is a contraindication to activity.

> **ALERT** Determine changes in client's cardiovascular system. Monitor progress of client with cardiac disease and evaluate tolerance to changes in activity.

Home Care

A. Participate in organized cardiac rehabilitation program.
1. Progressive monitored exercise.
2. Dietary modifications.
3. Stress management.
4. Continued education regarding ASHD and decreasing personal risk factors.
B. Understand medication regimen.
C. Teach client how to take his or her pulse and check for rate and regularity.
D. Teach client how to evaluate response to exercise (dyspnea, tachycardia, chest pain, etc.).
1. Remain close to home to begin walking program.
2. Client should always carry nitroglycerine when walking or exercising.
3. Client should check pulse rate before, halfway through, and at the end of activity.
4. Stop activity for pulse increase of more than 20 bpm, shortness of breath, chest pain, or dizziness.
E. Call the doctor for pain not controlled by nitroglycerin, significant changes in pulse rate, decreased tolerance to activity, syncope, or an increase in dyspnea.

F. Sexual intercourse can generally be resumed in 4 to 6 weeks after MI or when the client can walk one block or climb two flights of stairs without difficulty.
   1. Do not drink any alcohol before sexual activity.
   2. Take nitroglycerin before sexual activity.
   3. Do not have sex after a heavy meal.
   4. Position for intercourse does not influence cardiac workload.
   5. Do not take erectile dysfunction medications (Appendix 22-1) if taking nitrates.

> **ALERT** Assess client's ability to perform self-care. Determine whether the client with cardiac disease understands the illness and whether he or she can demonstrate knowledge of care.

Heart Failure (HF)

Heart failure (also referred to as congestive heart failure [CHF] and chronic heart failure) includes cardiac decompensation, cardiac insufficiency, ventricular failure, and ultimately results in the inability of the heart to pump adequate amounts of blood into the systemic circulation to meet tissue metabolic demands.

Physiology of Heart Failure

A. Left-sided heart failure.
   1. Results from failure of the left ventricle to maintain adequate cardiac output.
   2. Blood backs up into the left atrium and into the pulmonary veins.
   3. Increasing pressure in the pulmonary capillary bed causes lungs to become congested, resulting in impaired gas exchange.
   4. Precipitating factors.
      a. MI (left ventricular infarct).
      b. Hypertension.
      c. Aortic and mitral value disease.
B. Right-sided heart failure.
   1. The right ventricle is unable to maintain adequate output.
   2. Blood backs up into the systemic circulation and causes peripheral edema.
   3. Precipitating factors.
      a. Left-sided heart failure.
      b. Chronic pulmonary disease.
C. Each side of the heart is dependent on the other for adequate function.
   1. Left-sided failure results in pulmonary congestion; this causes an increase in pulmonary pressure, which further increases the workload and pressure in the right side of the heart and precipitates failure.
   2. The majority of clinical situations involve failure of both sides of the heart.
D. High-output versus low-output failure.
   1. High-output failure occurs when the body's needs for oxygen are excessively increased; the heart increases output but is still unable to meet the body's needs (hyperthyroid and anemia).
   2. Low-output failure occurs when the myocardium is so damaged that it cannot maintain adequate cardiac output; it is the failure of the heart as a pump.
E. Cardiac compensatory mechanisms will attempt to maintain the body requirements for cardiac output; when these mechanisms become ineffective, cardiac decompensation or failure will occur.
F. Edema development in heart failure.
   1. Decreased cardiac output leads to decrease in renal perfusion, the kidneys respond by stimulating the adrenal cortex to increase the secretion of aldosterone, thus increasing the retention of sodium and water.
   2. With an increase in the venous pressure from the increased circulating volume, there is an increase in the capillary pressure; and dependent, pitting edema occurs.
G. In children, HF occurs most often as the result of a structural problem of the heart. Ventricular function may not be impaired, but symptoms occur because of increased pulmonary artery pressure and pulmonary venous congestion.

> **ALERT** If a test question states that a client is in heart failure, assume that both sides are in failure unless indicated otherwise.

Assessment

A. Risk factors/etiology.
   1. Myocardial disease, valvular disease.
   2. Hypertension.
   3. Congenital heart disease.
   4. Fluid overload.
B. Clinical manifestations (Box 17-3).
   1. Impaired cardiac function.
      a. Tachycardia evaluated according to age level (see Table 15-2).
      b. Cardiomegaly from dilation and hypertrophy; PMI is displaced.
      c. S_3 or S_4 (heart gallop) caused by impaired ventricular function.

> **ALERT** Reevaluate the client with abnormal heart sounds.

      d. In infants, failure to thrive and failure to gain adequate weight.
      e. Poor perfusion: cool extremities, weak pulses, poor capillary refill.
   2. Pulmonary congestion.
      a. Dyspnea, dyspnea on exertion, tachypnea.
      b. Orthopnea: infants and adults.
      c. Paroxysmal nocturnal dyspnea occurs while client is asleep.
      d. Symptoms of respiratory distress and hypoxia (see Table 15-2).
      e. Congested breath sounds, cough.
      f. Feeding difficulties in infants, caused by dyspnea.
      g. Increase in pulmonary artery pressure (PAP) and pulmonary arterial wedge pressure (PAWP) (see Appendix 17-9).

Box 17-3   ASSESSMENT FINDINGS OF HEART FAILURE

Right-Sided (Systemic Symptoms)
Neck vein distention
Generalized edema (anasarca)
Dependent pitting edema
Nausea, vomiting
Anorexia
Altered GI function
Weight gain
Ascites
Decreased urinary output
Liver engorgement
Electrolyte imbalances
Dysrhythmias
Elevated CVP

Left-Sided (Pulmonary Symptoms)
Dusky skin and nail beds
Chest pain
Tachycardia
Decreased systolic BP
Ventricular ectopic beats
Presence of S_3 and S_4
Shift of the PMI to the left
Irritability, restlessness
Decreased cardiac output
Increased PAWP
Wheezing crackles
Dyspnea
Productive cough

BP, Blood pressure; *CVP,* central venous pressure; *GI,* gastrointestinal; *PMI,* point of maximum impulse; *PAWP,* pulmonary arterial wedge pressure.

3. Systemic congestion.
   a. Hepatomegaly: may be an early sign in children.
   b. Dependent edema generalized in infants; evaluate by weight gain.
   c. Peripheral pitting edema.
   d. Ascites.
   e. Increase in central venous pressure (CVP) (see Appendix 17-9).

> **ALERT** Determine changes in client's cardiovascular status as related to the client's HF; interpret what data need to be reported immediately.

C. Diagnostics (see Appendix 17-1).

Treatment

A. Treatment of the underlying problem.
B. Prevention.
   1. Administration of prophylactic antibiotics to clients with rheumatic heart disease before medical procedures to prevent mitral valve damage.
   2. Effective early treatment of hypertension.
   3. Early treatment of dysrhythmia.
C. Oxygen.

D. Activity limitations.
E. Medications: treatment for HF includes reduction of the preload and afterload, as well as improvement of the contractility of the myocardium.
   1. Cardiac glycosides (Appendix 17-6).
   2. Diuretics (see Appendix 16-6).
   3. Aldosterone antagonists (see Appendix 16-6).
   4. Vasodilators (see Appendix 16-5).
   5. Angiotension-converting enzyme (ACE) inhibitors (see Appendix 16-5).
   6. Beta blockers (adrenergic receptor antagonists) (Appendix 17-3).
   7. Electrolyte replacement, carefully monitor serum potassium levels.
F. Decreased sodium diet, as well as fluid restrictions, for adults and older children.
G. Sodium and fluids may not be restricted for infants and children; infants seldom need fluid restriction because of difficulty feeding.

Complications

A. Pulmonary edema (Chapter 15).
B. Cardiogenic shock.
C. Dysrhythmias.

> **⚠ NURSING PRIORITY** The goals for therapeutic intervention in clients with CHF are to:
> - Improve cardiac output: digitalis and oxygen.
> - Decrease cardiac afterload: decrease activity, administer vasodilator.
> - Decrease cardiac preload: diuretics; decrease sodium and fluid intake; place client in semi-Fowler's position.

Nursing Interventions

Goal: To decrease cardiac demands and improve cardiac output.
A. Assess vital signs and compare with other physical assessment data.
B. Conserve energy.
   1. Encourage rest alternated with activity.
   2. Monitor pulse, respiratory rate, and dysrhythmias during periods of activity.
C. Avoid chilling; it increases oxygen consumption, especially in infants.
D. Supplemental oxygen, especially when needed with increased activity.
E. Provide uninterrupted sleep, when possible.
F. Minimize crying in children and infants.
G. Decrease stress and anxiety; encourage parents to remain with child.

> **ALERT** Check for interactions among client's drugs, foods, and fluids. For clients receiving digitalis and diuretics, it is very important to monitor the serum potassium level. A significant decrease in the serum potassium level may affect cardiac rhythm and can precipitate digitalis toxicity.

Goal: To decrease circulating volume.
A. Assess breath sounds; check for distended neck veins and peripheral edema.

B. Low-sodium diet and fluid restriction in adults and older children.

C. Evaluate fluid retention by determining accurate daily weight (1 kg or 2.2 lb weight gain = 1 L of fluid loss or retention).

D. Accurate intake and output; monitor electrolyte balance and therapeutic effect of fluid loss.

Goal: To reduce respiratory distress.

A. Position.
   1. Adult may be placed in Fowler's or semi-Fowler's position or may sit in an armchair.
   2. When in semi-Fowler's position, do not elevate client's legs; this increases venous return (preload).
   3. An infant or small child may breathe better in a side-lying position with the knees drawn up to the chest.
   4. An infant may be placed in an infant seat.
   5. Make sure diapers are loosely pinned and safety restraints do not hinder maximum expansion of the chest.
   6. Hold infant upright over the shoulder with knees flexed (knee-chest position).

B. Administer oxygen: use oxygen hood for infants and nasal cannula for adults and older children; supplemental oxygen to keep saturation levels at or above 90%.

C. Evaluate breath sounds, evaluate adventitious breath sounds and presence of congestion.

D. Do not allow infants to cry for extend periods.

> **! PEDIATRIC NURSING PRIORITY** Infants: if cyanosis decreases with crying, the problem is usually pulmonary; if cyanosis increases with crying, the problem is usually cardiac.

Goal: To monitor for development of hypoxia (see Chapter 15).

Goal: To maintain nutrition.

A. Provide small, frequent meals of easily digestible foods; allow client adequate time to eat.

B. Assist client with cultural implications in dietary management.

C. An infant will require increased calories due to increased metabolic rate.
   1. May require tube feedings.
   2. An infant does not generally require fluid restriction, because of decreased fluid intake secondary to the dyspnea.
   3. Do not prop the bottle; burp the infant frequently.
   4. Decreased calorie intake will result in decreased strength, decreased weight gain, and failure to meet developmental motor skills.

Home Care

A. Client should begin walking short distances, 250 to 300 feet, at least three to four times per week; distance can be increased as tolerated (no shortness of breath, dizziness, chest pain, or tachycardia).

B. Teach client how to count his or her pulse.

C. Teach client to do daily weights every morning, before breakfast and with similar clothes on (nightgown, pajamas, etc.).

D. Discuss use of and safety factors for home oxygen.

E. Contact health care provider for:
   1. Weight gain of 3 to 5 pounds over a week or 1 to 2 pounds overnight.
   2. Increase in dyspnea or angina, especially with decreased activity or at rest.
   3. Decrease in activity tolerance that exceeds 3 or 4 days.
   4. Increased urination at night; presence or increase in peripheral edema.
   5. Cough or respiratory congestion that lasts longer than 3 or 4 days.

F. Provide written instructions for medications, especially if they are on digitalis.

G. Assess client's home situation and ability of caregivers.

Rheumatic Heart Disease

Rheumatic heart disease is an inflammatory disease that is usually self-limiting. The primary concern is the development of rheumatic heart disease involving the endocardium and cardiac valves.

A. Usually preceded by a group A beta-hemolytic streptococcal infection.

> **! NURSING PRIORITY** Prevention and adequate treatment of streptococcal infections prevent the development of rheumatic heart disease.

B. Myocardial involvement is characterized by the development of valvulitis, pericarditis, and myocarditis.
   1. Valvulitis produces scarring of the cardiac valves.
   2. Rheumatic carditis is the only symptom that produces permanent damage, most often involves damage to the endocardium and primarily to the mitral valve.
   3. Rheumatic fever usually occurs during childhood, but manifestations of cardiac damage may not be evident for years.

Assessment

A. Risk factors/etiology: previous infection by group A beta-hemolytic streptococcus.

B. Clinical manifestations: symptoms vary; no specific symptom or lab test is diagnostic of rheumatic fever. Criteria for the diagnosis require a combination of symptoms to be present.
   1. Carditis.
      a. Tachycardia out of proportion to fever.
      b. Long high-pitched apical systolic murmur beginning with S_1 and continuing throughout cycle.
      c. Pericarditis, pericardial friction rub, and complaints of chest pain.
   2. Migratory polyarthritis.
   3. Chorea.
   4. Erythema marginatum.
   5. Subcutaneous nodules over bony prominences.
   6. History of a recent streptococcal infection.

Treatment

A. Adequate treatment of initial streptococcal infection.

B. Rest and decreased activity until tachycardia subsides.

C. Salicylates to control inflammatory process.
D. Prophylactic treatment: client is susceptible to reoccurrence of rheumatic fever.
1. Begin after immediate therapy is complete.
2. Monthly administration of penicillin over extended period of time, depending on extent of cardiac involvement.
3. Administration of additional prophylactic antibiotics when invasive procedures are necessary (genitourinary procedures, dental work, etc.).

Complications

Severe valvular damage precipitates the development of HF and may require open heart surgery for replacement of diseased valve.

Nursing Interventions

Child is generally cared for in the home environment.

Goal: To assist parents and family to provide home environment conducive to healing and recovery.
A. Decrease activity if pulse rate is increased or if child is febrile.
B. Friends may visit for short periods; child is not contagious.
C. Maintain adequate nutrition.
1. May be anorexic during the febrile phase.
2. Provide soft or liquid foods as tolerated.
3. Assist child with feeding if choreic movements are severe.
4. Maintain adequate hydration.
D. Salicylates to control inflammatory process and as analgesics for arthralgia.
E. Reassure child that chorea and joint involvement are only temporary and there will be no residual damage.

Goal: To help parents understand need for long-term prophylactic antibiotic therapy.
A. Importance of preventing recurring infections.
B. Include child in planning, especially when numerous injections are involved.
C. Importance of prophylactic therapy before invasive procedures.
D. Continued medical follow-up for the development of valvular problems as child grows.
E. Follow-up required with females; cardiac problems may not be manifested until woman is pregnant.

Endocarditis (Bacterial, Infective)

Endocarditis is an infection of the valves and inner lining or endocardium of the heart.
A. Organisms tend to grow on the endocardium in an area of increased turbulence of blood flow or in areas of previous cardiac damage (rheumatic heart disease, congenital malformations).
B. Bacteria may enter from any site of localized infection.
C. Organisms grow on the endocardium and produce a characteristic vegetation consisting of fibrin deposits, leukocytes, and microbes; the vegetation may then invade adjacent valves.
D. Vegetation is fragile and may break off, resulting in emboli.

Assessment

A. Risk factors/etiology.
1. Most often bacterial, but may be fungal or viral.
2. History of endocarditis, prosthetic valves, or acquired valvular disease.
3. IV drug abuse.
4. History of recent invasive procedures.
B. Clinical manifestations.
1. Symptoms of systemic infection: low-grade fever, chills, weakness, malaise.
2. Murmur develops; or changes in previous murmurs occur.
3. Symptoms associated with heart failure.
4. Vascular symptoms.
a. Petechiae in conjunctiva, lips, buccal mucosa, on the ankle, and in the antecubital and popliteal areas.
b. Osler's nodes on fingertips.
c. Janeway lesions: small, flat, painless red spots on the palm and soles.
5. Symptoms associated with emboli.
a. Spleen: splenomegaly, upper left quadrant pain.
b. Kidney: flank pain, hematuria.
c. Brain: hemiplegia, decreased level of consciousness, visual changes.
C. Diagnostics.
1. Echocardiography.
2. Blood cultures, drawn 30 minutes apart.

Treatment

A. IV antibiotic therapy for 4 to 6 weeks (see Appendix 6-9).
B. Bed rest if high fever or evidence of heart failure is present.
C. Prophylactic antibiotics for 3 to 5 years in children with history of rheumatic carditis.
D. Surgical intervention for severe valvular damage.

Complications

A. HF secondary to valve damage.
B. General systemic emboli.

Nursing Interventions

Goal: To help parents understand the need for long-term prophylactic therapy (see Nursing Interventions under Rheumatic Heart Disease).

Goal: To maintain homeostasis and prevent complications.
A. IV antibiotic medications.
B. Assess activity tolerance; activities may be restricted until:
1. Temperature is normal.
2. Resting pulse is below 100 beats/min.
3. ECG is stable.
C. Evaluate for occurrence of emboli and heart failure.

Home Care

A. Good oral hygiene: daily care and regular dental visits.
B. Avoid excessive fatigue; plan rest periods and activity.
C. Client and family must understand the need for continued antibiotics.
D. Report temperature elevations, fever, chills, anorexia, weight loss, and increased fatigue.
E. Advise all health care providers of history of endocarditis.

Pericarditis

Pericarditis is an inflammation of the pericardium. The pericardial space is a cavity between the inner and the outer layers of the pericardium.

A. Acute pericarditis: may be dry or may cause excessive fluid accumulation in the pericardial space.
B. Chronic constrictive pericarditis: results from scarring and causes a loss of elasticity; the scarring and thickening of the pericardium prevent adequate cardiac filling during diastole.

Assessment

A. Risk factors/etiology.
   1. Acute pericarditis.
      a. Infection.
      b. Myocardial infarction.
         (1) Acute pericarditis may occur within 48-72 hours after an MI.
         (2) Dressler's syndrome occurs about 4-6 weeks after an MI.
   2. Chronic constrictive pericarditis: usually begins with acute episode; fluid is gradually absorbed with scarring and thickening.
B. Clinical manifestations.
   1. Acute.
      a. Pericardial friction rub caused by myocardium rubbing against inflamed pericardium.
      b. Pain increases with deep inspiration and lying supine; sitting may relieve pain; pain may radiate, making it difficult to differentiate from angina.
   2. Chronic: symptoms are characteristic of gradually occurring HF and decreased cardiac output; chest pain is not a prominent symptom.
C. Diagnostics: acute and chronic (see Appendix 17-1).
   1. Increased leukocytes.
   2. Inflammation: increased C-reactive protein (CRP), increased erythrocyte sedimentation rate (ESR).

Complications

A. Pericardial effusion (fluid in pericardial space) can result in cardiac tamponade.

Treatment

A. Acute episode.
   1. Treat underlying problem.
   2. Bed rest.
   3. Antiinflammatory medications (NSAIDs).
   4. If pleural effusion and tamponade occur, pericardiocentesis (aspiration of fluid from the pericardial sac) is performed.

Nursing Interventions

Goal: To maintain homeostasis and promote comfort.
A. Assess characteristics of pain; administer appropriate analgesics.
B. Upright position, with client leaning forward, may relieve the pain.
C. Decrease anxiety, because client often associates problem with an MI; help client distinguish the difference.
D. Observe for symptoms of cardiac tamponade.
   1. Paradoxical blood pressure: precipitous decrease in systolic blood pressure on inspiration.
   2. CVP increased; presence of jugular venous distension.
   3. Heart sounds are muffled or distant.
   4. Narrowing pulse pressure.
   5. Tachypnea, tachycardia, decrease in cardiac output.
E. In a client with chronic pericarditis, evaluate for symptoms of HF and initiate appropriate nursing intervention.

Cardiac Valve Disorders

A. Causes of valve disease.
   1. Congenital heart disease.
   2. Rheumatic heart disease.
   3. Bacterial endocarditis.
   4. Ischemia caused by ASHD.
B. Mitral valve is the most common area of involvement, followed by the aortic valve (see Figure 17-1).
C. Valvular stenosis: a narrowing of the valve opening and progressive obstruction to blood flow; increase in workload of the cardiac chamber pumping through the stenosed valve.
D. Valvular insufficiency (incompetency, regurgitation): impaired closure of the valve allows blood to flow back into the cardiac chamber, thereby increasing the workload of the heart.
E. Mitral valve.
   1. Stenosis: increases workload on the left atrium as it attempts to force blood through the narrowed valve.
   2. Mitral insufficiency (regurgitation): with each cardiac contraction, the left ventricle forces blood back into the left atrium.
   3. With both conditions, the left atrium dilates and hypertrophies because of an increase in workload. This causes an increase in pulmonary pressure and the subsequent development of HF.
F. Aortic valve.
   1. Aortic stenosis: increased (afterload) work of the left ventricle as it attempts to propel blood through the narrowed valve.

2. Aortic insufficiency: increased (afterload) work of the left ventricle as blood leaks back into the left ventricle after contraction.
3. With both conditions, the left ventricle dilates and hypertrophies as a result of increased pressure; this precipitates left ventricular failure.

Assessment

A. Risk factors: associated with history of rheumatic fever, endocarditis, cardiovascular disease.
B. Clinical manifestations—mitral valve disorders.
   1. Exertional dyspnea progressing to orthopnea.
   2. Progressive fatigue caused by decrease in cardiac output.
   3. Cardiac murmur (diastolic), palpitations.
   4. Systemic embolization.
   5. Atrial fibrillation.
C. Clinical manifestations—aortic valve disorders.
   1. Syncope and vertigo.
   2. Angina (condition interferes with coronary artery filling).
   3. Dysrhythmia, systolic murmur in stenosis.
   4. Dyspnea and increasing fatigue, heart failure.
D. Diagnostics (see Appendix 17-1).

Treatment

A. Prevention of heart failure (HF, CHF), pulmonary edema, thromboembolism, and endocarditis.
   1. Digitalis (see Appendix 17-6).
   2. Diuretics.
   3. Beta-blockers to decrease cardiac rate.
B. Prophylactic anticoagulation to prevent thrombus formation.
C. Prophylactic antibiotics.
D. Open heart surgery for valve replacement when there is evidence of progressive cardiac failure.
E. Percutaneous transluminal balloon valvuloplasty (PTBV): performed in cardiac catheterization lab; balloon is threaded through the affected valve in an attempt to separate the valve leaflets.

Nursing Interventions

Goal: To prevent development of rheumatic heart disease and provide prophylactic treatment to individuals with history of rheumatic heart disease.
Goal: To prevent and/or to identify early development of HF (see Heart Failure, Nursing Interventions).

> **! NURSING PRIORITY** Primary care for the client with cardiac valve disease consists of maintaining homeostasis and preventing the development of HF. The client should be advised to avoid excessive fatigue and should be assessed according to the level of activity tolerance.

Cardiovascular Disease in Pregnancy

Rheumatic heart disease (mitral valve problems) and congenital heart defects account for the greatest incidence of cardiac disease in pregnancy.

A. Normal physiologic alterations of pregnancy that increase cardiovascular stress.
   1. Increase in oxygen requirements.
   2. 30% to 50% increase in cardiac output; peaks at 20 to 26 weeks' gestation.
   3. Increase in plasma volume.
   4. Weight gain.
   5. Hemodynamic changes during delivery.
B. As normal pregnancy advances, the cardiovascular system is unable to maintain adequate output to meet increasing demands. Classification of the severity of cardiac disease in pregnancy (including relation to prescription of physical activity) is presented in Table 17-2.

Assessment

Clinical manifestations indicative of cardiac decompensation are those of impending CHF.
A. Frequent cough, progressive dyspnea.
B. Progressive general edema, jugular venous distension (JVD).
C. Palpitations.
D. Excessive fatigue for level of activity.
E. Dysrhythmia, atrial fibrillation, and tachycardia.
F. Congested breath sounds.
G. Cardiac decompensation increases with length of gestation; highest incidence of HF is observed at 28 to 32 weeks' gestation.

Treatment

A. Management of the pregnant client.
   1. Balanced nutritional intake; iron supplements.
   2. Limited physical activity; stop any activity that increases shortness of breath.

Table 17-2	CLASSIFICATION OF CARDIOVASCULAR DISEASE

Class	Description
I	Clients with no limitations on activities; they suffer no symptoms from ordinary activities
II	Clients with slight, mild limitation of activity; they are comfortable at rest or with mild exertion
III	Clients with marked limitation of activity; they are comfortable only at rest
IV	Clients who should be at complete rest, confined to a bed or chair; any physical activity brings on discomfort, and symptoms occur even at rest

> **! NURSING PRIORITY** The functional classification of the disease is determined at 3 months' gestation and again at 7 to 8 months' gestation. Pregnant women may progress from class I or II to III or IV during pregnancy. Women with cyanotic congenital heart disease do not fit into the New York Heart Association (NYHA) classifications because the causes of their exercise-induced symptoms are not related to heart failure.

Adapted from the Criteria Committee, New York Heart Association (NYHA), Boston, 2005.

3. Diuretics, digitalis, anticoagulants, and antidysrhythmics may be given.
4. May be hospitalized at 28 to 32 weeks' gestation because of impending HF.
5. If coagulation problems occur, heparin is usually used because it does not cross the placenta.

B. Management of the client during labor and delivery.
1. Supplemental oxygen.
2. Epidural regional anesthesia is generally used for delivery.

C. Management of the client during the postpartum period: treated symptomatically according to status of cardiovascular system; the first 24 to 48 hours postpartum is period of highest risk for HF in the mother.

Nursing Interventions

Goal: To assist client to maintain homeostasis during pregnancy.

A. Written information regarding nutritional needs.
B. Nursing assessment and client education regarding early symptoms of HF.
C. Frequent rest periods; activity may be severely restricted during the last trimester.

> **■ NURSING PRIORITY** One of the most effective means of decreasing the cardiac workload is to decrease activity; therefore the pregnant client needs to avoid excessive fatigue to prevent or decrease cardiac decompensation.

D. Decrease stress by keeping client informed of progress.

Goal: To help client maintain homeostasis during labor and delivery.

A. Position client on side with head and shoulders elevated.
B. Observe for increasing dyspnea, cough, or adventitious breath sounds during labor.
C. Evaluate information from continuous fetal and maternal monitoring.
D. Encourage open glottis pushing during labor; prevent Valsalva maneuver.
E. Prepare for vaginal delivery.
F. Provide pain relief as indicated.
1. Pain increases cardiac work.
2. Evaluate effects of analgesia on fetus.

> **ALERT** Interpret what data from a client need to be reported immediately.

Goal: To maintain homeostasis in the postpartum period.

A. Assessment of cardiac adaptation to changes in hemodynamics.
1. Increased blood flow due to decreased abdominal pressure may precipitate reflux bradycardia.
2. Assess for chest pain and adequacy of cardiac output.

B. Maintain semi-Fowler's position or side lying position with the head elevated.

C. Gradual progression of activities (depending on cardiac status) as indicated by:
1. Pulse rate.
2. Respiratory status.
3. Activity tolerance.

D. Progressive ambulation as soon as tolerated to prevent venous thrombosis.
E. Assist mother and family to prepare for discharge.

Congenital Heart Disease

A. Clinical manifestations depend on the severity of the defect and the adequacy of pulmonary blood flow.
B. Normal pressure in the right side of the heart is lower than pressure in the left side; there is an increased blood flow from an area of high pressure to an area of low pressure.
1. When there is an opening between the right and left side of the heart, oxygenated blood will shunt from the left side of the heart to the right side (right-to-left shunt).
2. When the pressures on the right side of the heart exceed the pressure on the left side of the heart, unoxygenated blood from the right side will flow into the left side and unoxygenated blood will flow into the systemic circulation (left-to-right shunt).

C. Physical consequences of congenital heart defects.
1. Delayed physical development.
   a. Failure to gain weight, caused by inability to maintain adequate caloric intake to meet increased metabolic demands.
   b. Tachycardia and tachypnea precipitate increase in caloric requirements.
2. Excessive fatigue, especially during feedings.
3. Frequent upper respiratory tract infections.
4. Dyspnea, tachycardia, tachypnea.
5. Hypercyanotic spells (called "blue" spells or "tet" spells): infant suddenly becomes acutely cyanotic and hyperpneic; occur most often in children 2 months to 1 year of age.

D. Diagnostics (see Appendix 17-1).

Defects With Increased Pulmonary Artery Blood Flow

Increased blood volume on the right side of the heart increases the flow of blood through the pulmonary artery. This may decrease the systemic blood flow.

A. Atrial septal defect (ASD): opening in the septum between the atrium; blood shunts from left to the right; often caused by failure of foramen ovale to close (Figure 17-6).
B. Ventricular septal defect (VSD): opening in the septum between the ventricles; blood shunts from left side to right side (Figure 17-7).
C. Patent ductus arteriosis (PDA): failure of the fetal ductus arteriosus to close after birth; blood is shunted from the left side to the right side; may be treated with indomethacin or ibuprofen (Advil), nonsteroidal antiinflammatory drugs that change the oxygen concentration of

FIGURE 17-6 Atrial septal defect. (From Hockenberry MJ, Wilson D: *Wong's nursing care of infants and children,* ed 8, St. Louis, 2007, Mosby.)

FIGURE 17-8 Patent ductus arteriosus. (From Hockenberry MJ, Wilson D: *Wong's nursing care of infants and children,* ed 8, St. Louis, 2007, Mosby.)

FIGURE 17-7 Ventricular septal defect. (From Hockenberry MJ, Wilson D: *Wong's nursing care of infants and children,* ed 8, St. Louis, 2007, Mosby.)

FIGURE 17-9 Coarctation of the aorta. (From Hockenberry MJ, Wilson D: *Wong's nursing care of infants and children,* ed 8, St. Louis, 2007, Mosby.)

the tissue and enhance tissue changes that close the defect (Figure 17-8).

D. Clinical manifestations.
1. May be asymptomatic.
2. Signs of CHF are common.
3. Characteristics murmurs.

Obstructive Defects With Decreased Pulmonary Artery Blood Flow

Problems occur when the normal blood flow through the heart meets an obstruction. The pressure in the ventricle and in the artery prior to the obstruction is increased; pressure beyond the obstruction is decreased.

A. Coarctation of the aorta: a narrowing of the aorta; specific symptoms depend on the location of the coarcta-

tion in relation to arteries coming off the aortic arch (Figure 17-9).
1. Clinical manifestations.
   a. Marked differences in blood pressure in the upper and lower extremities; area proximal to the defect has a high pressure and a bounding pulse.
      (1) Epistaxis.
      (2) Headaches.
      (3) Bounding radial and temporal pulses.
      (4) Dizziness and fainting.
   b. Area distal to defect has decreased blood pressure and weaker pulse.
      (1) Lower extremities are cooler; mottling is present.
      (2) Weak peripheral and femoral pulses.
   c. May develop CHF.

2. Increased risk for hypertension, ruptured aorta, aortic aneurysm, and stroke.
B. Aortic stenosis: a narrowing or constriction of the aortic valve that increases resistance to blood flow from the left ventricle into systemic circulation; increases pulmonary vascular congestion.
   1. Clinical manifestations.
      a. Decreased cardiac output, faint pulses, hypotension, tachycardia.
      b. Children have exercise intolerance and may have chest pain.
      c. Characteristic murmur.
   2. At risk for bacterial endocarditis and coronary insufficiency.

Defects With Decreased Pulmonary Blood Flow

An anatomic defect is present between the right and left sides of the heart (ASD or VSD). There is increased pulmonary artery resistance to blood flow; therefore pressure increases in the right side of the heart. As the resistance in the pulmonary circulation increases, pressure in the right ventricle increases. This pressure increases until it is greater than pressure on the left side of the heart and unoxygenated (unsaturated) blood moves into the left side of the heart (right-to-left shunt).
A. Tetralogy of Fallot: consists of four defects—ventricular septal defect (VSD), pulmonic stenosis, overriding aorta, and right ventricular hypertrophy (Figure 17-10).
   1. Clinical manifestations depend on the size of the VSD and the pressures in the heart.
      a. May be acutely cyanotic at birth or may have minimal cyanosis due to patent ductus arteriosus.
      b. Child may have mild cyanosis that progresses.
      c. Infant may experience acute episodes of hypoxia (blue spells, tet spells), may occur during agitation or crying.

d. Posturing or squatting in the older child.
e. CHF does not develop, because overload of right ventricle flows into the aorta and the left ventricle; therefore pulmonary congestion does not occur.
   2. At risk for emboli, seizures, changes in level of consciousness, or sudden death from anoxia.
B. Tricuspid atresia: tricuspid valve does not develop, and there is no opening from the right atrium to the right ventricle; an ASD, or patent foramen ovale, is present and provides mixing of oxygenated and unoxygenated blood.
   1. Clinical manifestations.
      a. Cyanosis usually occurs during newborn period.
      b. Tachycardia, dyspnea.
      c. Older children have chronic hypoxemia and clubbing.
   2. Continuous infusion of prostaglandin E_1 may be used to maintain a patent ductus arteriosus.

Mixed Defects

Mixed defects are present when the survival of the infant depends on the mixing of oxygenated and unoxygenated blood for survival. Pulmonary congestion occurs as a result of the increased flow of blood into pulmonary vasculature.
A. Transposition of great vessels: the pulmonary artery receives blood from the left ventricle, and the aorta receives blood from the right ventricle. A communicated defect—ASD, VSD, or patent ductus arteriosus—must be present to provide for mixing of oxygenated and unoxygenated blood (Figure 17-11).
   1. Clinical manifestations depend on size of associated defects and mixing of blood.
      a. Newborns with minimal communication defects are cyanotic at birth.

FIGURE 17-10 Tetralogy of Fallot. (From Hockenberry MJ, Wilson D: *Wong's nursing care of infants and children,* ed 8, St. Louis, 2007, Mosby.)

FIGURE 17-11 Transposition of the great vessels. (From Hockenberry MJ, Wilson D: *Wong's nursing care of infants and children,* ed 8, St. Louis, 2007, Mosby.)

FIGURE 17-12 Truncus arteriosus. (From Hockenberry MJ, Wilson D: *Wong's nursing care of infants and children*, ed 8, St. Louis, 2007, Mosby.)

    b. Symptoms of CHF.
    c. Cardiomegaly develops shortly after birth.
  2. Prostaglandins may be given to maintain patency of ductus arteriosus to promote mixing of blood.
B. Truncus arteriosus: the pulmonary artery and aorta fail to separate; results in a single vessel that receives blood from both ventricles (Figure 17-12).
  1. Clinical manifestations.
    a. Cyanosis and CHF develop in infancy.
    b. Characteristic murmur.
  2. Multiple surgical repairs are necessary to replace conduits as child grows.

Nursing Interventions

Goal: To evaluate infant's response to cardiac defect.
A. Evaluate infant's Apgar scores at birth.
B. Evaluate adequacy of weight gain in first few months.
C. Assess feeding problems.
  1. Poor sucking reflex.
  2. Poor coordination of sucking, swallowing, and breathing.
  3. Fatigues easily during feeding.
D. Frequency of upper respiratory tract infections.
E. Determine whether cyanosis occurs at rest or is precipitated by activity.
F. Presence and quality of pulses in extremities.
G. Bacterial endocarditis is a primary concern before and after correction of a congenital defect; all fevers should be reported.
Goal: To promote oxygenation.
A. Effectively cope with hypercyanotic spells (blue spells, tet spells).
  1. Occurs suddenly, often when the infant is agitated.
  2. Hold the infant upright in a knee chest position; this reduces the venous return and increases systemic vascular resistance, which increases pressure on the right

side of the heart and diverts more blood flow through the pulmonary artery.
  3. Administer 100% O_2 via a face mask until respirations are improved.
  4. Maintain good hydration and carefully monitor hemoglobin levels.
  5. Older child may assume squatting position to increase peripheral resistance and decrease right-to-left shunting.
B. Supplemental oxygen, good pulmonary hygiene, and chest physiotherapy to maintain oxygen saturation levels.
C. Prevent overexertion, decrease excessive crying, and promote rest in order to conserve energy and caloric expenditure.
D. Maintain hydration for pulmonary hygiene and to prevent embolic problems and stroke.
E. Infants may require gavage feeding if respiratory distress limits oral feeding.
Goal: To assist parents in adjusting to diagnosis.
A. Allow family to grieve over loss of perfect infant.
B. Evaluate parents' level of understanding of the child's problem.
C. Foster early parent-infant attachment; encourage touching, holding, feeding, and general physical contact.
D. Help the family develop a relationship that fosters optimum growth and development of all family members. (See Chapter 3 for psychosocial aspects of caring for chronically ill children.)

> **ALERT** Provide emotional support to family; assist family members in managing care of a child with a chronic illness.

Goal: To detect, prevent, and treat CHF.
Goal: To provide appropriate nursing interventions for the client undergoing open heart surgery for repair of a defect.

Cardiac Surgery

A. Coronary artery bypass graft (CABG), aortic and mitral valve replacements: open heart surgery is performed with the use of the cardiopulmonary bypass machine; this machine allows for full visualization of the heart while maintaining perfusion and oxygenation.
B. Closed heart surgery is performed without the use of the bypass machine.
  1. Minimally invasive direct coronary artery bypass graft (MIDCABG): one of the most common procedures are grafts to the left anterior descending artery.
  2. Aortic and mitral balloon valvuloplasty.

Nursing Interventions

For preoperative and postoperative care, see Chapter 3.
Goal: To prepare the client psychologically and physiologically for surgery.
A. Evaluate client's history for other chronic health problems.

B. Establish baseline data for postoperative comparison.

C. Provide appropriate preoperative teaching according to age level; frequently includes a visit to the intensive care unit (parents should accompany the child on the visit).

D. Discuss immediate postoperative nursing care and anticipated nursing procedures.

E. Correct metabolic and electrolyte imbalances.

F. Establish and maintain adequate hydration.

G. Anticipate adjustments in medication schedule before surgery.
  1. Digitalis dosage is usually decreased.
  2. Diuretics may be discontinued 48 hours before surgery.
  3. Long-acting insulin will be changed to regular insulin.
  4. Antihypertensive medication dosage may be modified.

H. Eliminate possible sources of infection.

Goal: To evaluate and promote cardiovascular function after surgery.

A. Maintain adequate blood pressure.

B. Evaluate for dysrhythmia; document and treat accordingly (see Appendixes 17-4 and 17-7).

C. Maintain client in semi-Fowler's position.

D. Evaluate fluid and electrolyte balances.
  1. Record daily weight and compare with previous weight.
  2. Evaluate electrolyte balance, especially potassium levels.
  3. Assess for adequate hemoglobin and hematocrit values.
  4. Evaluate hemodynamic levels for adequate volume (see Appendix 17-9).
  5. Measure urine output hourly to evaluate adequacy of renal perfusion.
  6. Administer IV fluids, as indicated.

E. Observe for hemorrhage: most often identified by increase in chest drainage.

F. Evaluate adequacy of peripheral circulation.

G. Mediastinal chest tubes are frequently placed in the pericardial sac to prevent tamponade. These tubes are cared for in the same manner as pulmonary chest tubes (Appendix 15-4).

H. Bedside hemodynamic monitoring as indicated (see Appendix 17-9).

Goal: To evaluate and promote respiratory function.

A. Mechanical ventilation via an endotracheal tube may be used for approximately 12 to 24 hours after surgery. Generally, children are extubated sooner than adults.

B. Maintain water-sealed drainage for mediastinal/chest tubes (see Appendix 15-4).

C. Pulmonary hygiene via endotracheal tube; carefully assess pulse oximetry during suctioning.

D. Promote good respiratory hygiene after extubation (fluids, incentive spirometry, activity).

E. Evaluate arterial blood gases for adequate oxygenation, as well as acid-base balance.

F. Encourage activity as soon as possible; client should be out of bed on the first postoperative day.

G. Monitor pulse oximetry levels.

Goal: To evaluate neurologic status for complications after surgery.

A. Recovery from anesthesia within appropriate time frame.

B. Able to move all extremities equally.

C. Appropriate response to verbal command.

D. Assess for changes in neurologic status.

Goal: To prevent complications of immobility (see Chapter 3) after surgery.

Goal: To decrease anxiety and promote comfort after surgery.

A. Frequent orientation to surroundings.

B. Careful explanation of all procedures.

C. Prevent sensory overload.

D. Promote uninterrupted sleep.

E. Administer pain medications as appropriate.

Common Complications After Cardiac Surgery

A. Dysrhythmia (see Appendix 17-7).
  1. Premature ventricular contractions.
  2. Ventricular tachycardia.
  3. Atrial dysrhythmias are common with mitral valve replacement.
  4. Conduction blocks.

B. Hypovolemia.
  1. Low cardiac output may be due to hypovolemia.
  2. Frequently, vasoconstriction is present immediately after surgery. Vasodilation occurs as client's body temperature increases and precipitates hypovolemia.
  3. Evaluate hemodynamic parameters for adequacy of cardiac output.
  4. Observe client closely for response to fluid replacement, because fluid overload occurs very rapidly, especially in children.

C. Emboli.
  1. Pulmonary emboli.
  2. Arterial emboli.
    a. Occur most frequently after valvular surgery.
    b. Client may be receiving prophylactic anticoagulants.
    c. Evaluate neurologic system for evidence of cerebral emboli.

D. Cardiac tamponade.
  1. Pressure on the heart caused by a collection of fluid in pericardial sac.
  2. May be caused by fluid collecting postoperatively or from pericarditis.
  3. Pressure prevents adequate filling of ventricles, thereby decreasing cardiac output.
  4. Paradoxical blood pressure: precipitous decrease in systolic blood pressure on inspiration; diagnostic for tamponade.
  5. CVP is frequently increased; blood pressure is decreased.
  6. Heart sounds are described as distant.

7. A decrease in drainage may occur in the mediastinal tubes.
8. Treatment involves reestablishing patency of mediastinal tube, surgical exploration of bleeding areas or pericardiocentesis with pericarditis.

E. Psychosis (most common in adults).
1. Characteristics.
    a. Inappropriate verbal response.
    b. Disorientation to time and place.
    c. Visual and auditory hallucinations.
    d. Paranoid delusions.
2. Prevention of psychosis.
    a. Maintain orientation to time and place.
    b. Maintain continuity in nursing staff.
    c. Carefully explain all procedures.
    d. Encourage ventilation of feelings.

Appendix 17-1 CARDIAC DIAGNOSTICS

Serum Laboratory Studies
Cardiac Enzymes

Creatinine kinase (CK): CK isoenzyme MB (CK-MB). Increases greater than 5% of total creatine kinase are highly indicative of MI. Increases occur within 4 to 6 hours after an MI, peak in 12 to 24 hours, and return to normal in 24-36 hours.

Cardiac troponin T and cardiac troponin I: Normal level is <0.2 ng/mL (for T) and <0.03 ng/dL (for I). Levels are elevated within 4 to 6 hours after an MI and peak within 10 to 24 hours. Elevated levels are highly indicative of myocardial damage.

Nursing Implications

1. Enzymes must be drawn on admission and obtained in a serial manner thereafter. There is a characteristic pattern to the increases and decreases of enzyme levels in a client with an MI.
2. The larger the infarction, the larger the enzyme response.
3. Evaluate serial levels of the enzymes; increased levels of troponin are the most significant and diagnostic of myocardial damage.
4. Cardiac-specific troponin helps discriminate from other tissue injury.

❗ NURSING PRIORITY For a client with an increase in CK-MB$_2$ and an increase in cardiac troponin levels, it is important to monitor closely for symptoms of acute coronary syndrome (ACS or MI). In a client with ACS serum levels may be checked every 6 to 8 hours during the acute phase.

C-Reactive Protein (CRP), Highly Sensitive C-Reactive Protein (hs-CRP)

Identification of the protein that is synthesized by the liver and is not normally present in the blood except when there is tissue trauma. The response to the test assists in evaluating the severity and course of inflammatory conditions. Highly sensitive CRP (hs-CRP) may be used to identify risk for developing an MI.

Normal: Less than 1 mg/L or 8 mg/dL; increasing level is significant and may indicate some degree of inflammatory response caused by plaque formation.

Serum Electrolytes
ECG changes with potassium levels.
Hyperkalemia
1. Tall, peaked T wave.
2. Widening of the QRS.
3. Cardiac arrest.

Hypokalemia
1. Premature ventricular contractions (PVCs).
2. Ventricular tachycardia.
3. Ventricular fibrillation.

Erythrocyte Sedimentation Rate

Used as a gauge for evaluating progression of inflammatory conditions; inflammatory process precipitates a rapid settling of the red blood cells.

Normal values vary greatly, depending on the laboratory method used.

B-Type Natriuretic Peptide (BNP)

First whole blood marker for identifying and treating heart failure. Serial BNP values may be determined to evaluate left ventricular function; assists to identify heart failure versus respiratory failure as cause of dyspnea. Normal is less than 100 pg/mL.

Noninvasive Diagnostics
Electrocardiogram (ECG)

A graphic representation of the electrical activity of the heart, generally conducted by using a 12-lead format. Test to identify conduction in rhythm disorders and the occurrence of ischemia, injury, or death of myocardial tissue.

Holter Monitor

Client is connected to a small portable ECG unit with recorder that records the client's heart activity for approximately 24 to 48 hours. The client keeps a log of activity, pain, and palpitations. Client should not remove leads but is encouraged to maintain normal activity; client should not shower or bathe while the monitor is in place. The recording is analyzed and compared with the client's activity log.

Event Monitor (Transtelephonic Event Recorder)

Client is connected to portable ECG unit with a recorder. The client can activate the recorder whenever he or she feels any type of dizziness or palpitations. Monitor may be worn for extended periods of time. Monitor leads and battery are removed for showering but should be reconnected immediately. Recordings are transmitted over the phone.

Exercise Stress Test

This test involves the client exercising, usually on a treadmill, which increases speed and incline to increase the heart rate. ECG leads are attached to the client, and the response of the heart to exercise is evaluated.

Appendix 17-1 CARDIAC DIAGNOSTICS—cont'd

Nursing Implications

1. Provide appropriate pretest preparation; establish baseline vital signs and cardiac rhythm.
2. Client should:
   a. Avoid smoking, eating, or drinking any caffeine beverages for 3 hours before the test.
   b. Avoid stimulants, eating, and extreme temperature changes immediately after the test.
3. Cardiac monitoring is done constantly during test.
4. Reasons for terminating an exercise stress test: chest pain, significant increase or decrease in blood pressure, or significant ECG changes.
5. If any of the above changes occur, the test is terminated and the stress test result is said to be positive.

Echocardiogram

An ultrasound procedure to evaluate valvular function, cardiac chamber size, ventricular muscle, and septal motion. The ultrasound waves are displayed on a graph and interpreted.

Transesophageal Echocardiography

Provides a higher-quality picture than regular echocardiogram. The throat is anesthetized, and a flexible endoscope is passed into the esophagus to the level of the heart. Sedation is used during the procedure.

Nursing Implications

1. Maintain NPO for 4 to 8 hours before test.
2. Check for gag and swallow reflex before client resumes oral intake of fluids.

Invasive Diagnostics
Cardiac Catheterization

An invasive procedure in which a catheter is passed through the brachial or femoral artery for left-side cardiac catheterization; the brachial or femoral vein for right-side cardiac catheterization. Cardiac catheterization will provide data regarding status of the coronary arteries, as well as cardiac muscle function, valvular functions, and left ventricular function (ejection fraction).

Nursing Implications

1. Pretest preparation.
   a. Maintain NPO status for 6 hours before test.
   b. Check for dye allergy, especially allergy to iodine and contrast media.
   c. Record quality of distal pulses for comparison after test.
   d. Determine whether any medications need to be withheld.
   e. Appropriate client education (feeling of warmth when dye is injected; will be awake during procedure; report any chest pain; need to lie still).
2. After the test.
   a. Evaluate catheterization entry site (most often femoral) for hematoma formation. Notify physician immediately for excessive bleeding at the site, dramatic changes in blood pressure.
   b. Evaluate circulatory status (pulses distal to catheterization site, color, sensation of the extremity). Notify physician immediately for a decrease in peripheral circulation or neurovascular changes in affected extremity.
   c. Assess for dysrhythmias.
   d. Maintain bed rest; avoid flexion; keep extremity straight for 3 to 6 hours.
   e. Keep head of bed elevated at 30° or less.
   f. Encourage oral intake of fluids; IV access may be maintained.

Positron Emission Tomography (PET)

Very sensitive in identifying viable and nonviable cardiac tissue. The procedure takes about 2 to 3 hours, and a radioactive dye is injected intravenously, followed by glucose. A client's glucose must be between 60-140 mg/dL before the test.

Appendix 17-2 NITRATES

Nitrates Increase blood supply to the heart by dilating the coronary arteries; cardiac workload is reduced due to decrease in venous return because of peripheral vasodilation.

MEDICATIONS	SIDE EFFECTS	NURSING IMPLICATIONS
Nitroglycerin **(NTG, Nitrostat):** sublingual Nitroglycerin **(Nitro-BID, Nitrol):** topical (patch) Nitroglycerin ointment **(Nitropaste):** topical, by the inch Nitroglycerin translingual spray Isosorbide dinitrate **(Isordil, Sorbitrate):** PO	Headaches (will diminish with therapy), postural hypotension, syncope, blurred vision, dry mouth, reflex tachycardia	1. Advise client that alcohol will potentiate postural hypotension. 2. Educate client regarding self-medication (see Box 17-2). 3. Do not take with erectile dysfunction drugs. 4. Topical or transdermal application is used for sustained protection against anginal attacks. 5. Avoid skin contact with topical form; remove all previous applications when applying topical form. 6. Sublingual tablets and translingual spray given for an immediate response.

MEDICATIONS	SIDE EFFECTS	NURSING IMPLICATIONS

Calcium Channel Blockers Blockade of calcium channel receptors in the heart causes decreased cardiac contractility and a decreased rate of sinus and AV node conduction. Used to treat chronic stable angina, hypertension, and supraventricular dysrhythmias.

Diltiazem (**Cardizem**): PO, IV Nifedipine (**Procardia**): PO Verapamil (**Calan, Isoptin**): IV, PO	Constipation, exacerbation of CHF, hypotension, bradycardia, peripheral edema	1. Nifedipine is less likely to exacerbate preexisting cardiac conditions; is not effective in treating dysrhythmias. 2. Intensifies cardiosuppressant effects of beta-blocker medications.

Beta-Adrenergic Blocking Agents (adrenergic antagonists) Blockade of beta$_1$ receptors in the heart causes decreased heart rate, and decreased rate of AV conduction. Used to treat hypertension as well as angina. Beta blockers should be administered to all clients experiencing unstable angina or having an MI unless contraindicated. Give with caution to clients with history of bronchospasm.

▲ Labetalol (**Trandate**): PO, IV Metoprolol (**Lopressor, Toprol XL**): PO, IV Propranolol (**Inderal**): PO, IV Atenolol (**Tenormin**): PO, IV ▲ High-Alert Medications: all IV preparations. Carvedilol (**Coreg**): PO Note: Carvedilol, bisoprolol, and metoprolol sustained release are used to treat HF.	Bradycardia, hypotension, depression, lethargy and fatigue	1. High-alert medications. 2. Closely monitor cardiac client—may precipitate heart failure, but is also used to treat heart failure. 3. Teach client how to decrease effects of postural hypotension. 4. Teach client not to stop taking medication when he or she feels better. 5. Bradycardia is common adverse effect. 6. If client has diabetes, blood glucose control may be impaired.

Antidysrhythmics Decrease cardiac excitability; delay cardiac conduction in either the atrium or ventricle. Atropine is cardiac stimulant for bradycardia.

General Nursing Implications
— Assess client for changes in cardiac rhythm and impact on cardiac output.
— Evaluate effect of medication on dysrhythmia and resulting effects on cardiac output.
— Client should be on bedrest and have a cardiac monitor attached during IV administration.
— Have atropine available for cardiac depression resulting in symptomatic bradycardia.
— All cardiac depressant medications are contraindicated in clients with sinus node or AV node blocks.
— Digitalis will enhance cardiac depressant effects.
— Closely monitor for dysrhythmias that are precipitated by the treatment.
— See Appendix 17-7: Cardiac Dysrhythmias.

MEDICATIONS	SIDE EFFECTS	NURSING IMPLICATIONS
Quinidine sulfate (**Quinidine Sulfate, Quinidex**): PO	Hypotension Diarrhea, nausea, vomiting	1. Administer with food. 2. Monitor for ECG changes for toxicity—widened QRS and prolonged QT. 3. *Uses:* supraventricular tachycardia and ventricular dysrhythmias.
Atropine: subQ, IV	Tachycardia Dry mouth, blurred vision, dilated pupils	1. *Use:* block cardiac stimulation, primarily for bradycardias that are hemodynamically significant or for PVCs related to slow heart rate. 2. Assess client's cardiac output in response to the bradycardic episode.
Adenosine (**Adenocard, Adenoscan**): IV	Significant hypotension AV heart block	1. *Use:* first drug for stable, narrow-complex supraventricular tachycardia (SVT). 2. Has a rapid half-life; therefore must be given rapidly undiluted over 1 to 3 sec followed by 20 mL of normal saline.

MEDICATIONS	SIDE EFFECTS	NURSING IMPLICATIONS
Amiodarone hydrochloride **(Cordarone):** PO, IV ▲ High-Alert Medication: IV route	AV heart block, hypotension Toxicity—lung and visual problems	1. *Use:* life-threatening ventricular arrhythmias, atrial fibrillation. 2. Do not administer with other drugs that prolong the QT interval. 3. Continually monitor ECG during IV infusion.
Lidocaine hydrochloride **(Xylocaine):** IV ▲ High-Alert Medication: IV route	Drowsiness, confusion, seizures, severe depression of cardiac conduction	1. *Use:* ventricular dysrhythmias. 2. Must use IV preparatioin of **Lidocaine** for IV infusion.
Mexiletine **(Mexitil):** PO	GI disturbances—nausea/ vomiting, diarrhea; CNS disturbances— tremor, dizziness	1. *Use:* prevent/control ventricular dysrhythmias.
Procainamide **(Pronestyl):** PO, IV	Abdominal pain, cramping, hypotension, prolonged QT interval Long-term use: systemic lupus erythematosus- like syndrome (pain and inflammation of joints) Blood dyscrasias	1. *Use:* short- and long-term control of ventricular and supraventricular dysrhythmias. 2. Client should report any joint pain and inflammation. 3. Closely monitor for bradycardia and hypotension. 4. Do not take OTC cold preparations.
Propranolol hydrochloride **(Inderal):** PO, IV ▲ High-Alert Medication: IV route	See previous discussion of beta-adrenergic blockers	1. *Use:* long- and short-term treatment and prevention of tachycardia.

Appendix 17-5   FIBRINOLYTIC MEDICATIONS

▲ **Fibrinolytics** work by different actions to initiate fibrinolysis of a clot. Medications are not clot specific; they will break up a clot on a surgical incision as well as a clot from an MI (see Fibrinolytic Therapy below).

General Nursing Implications

— Therapy should begin as soon as the MI is diagnosed or when there is a history of prolonged angina. For best results, from admission in the ED until medication is administered is 30 min (door-to-needle), or within 60 min of onset of symptoms.
— Bleeding precautions (see Table 9-1).

▲ MEDICATIONS	SIDE EFFECTS	NURSING IMPLICATIONS
Alteplase **(tPA, Activase):** IV Reteplase **(Retavase):** IV Streptokinase **(Streptase, Kabikinase):** IV	Bleeding and hypotension	1. Obtain base vital signs and coagulation studies. 2. Monitor for allergic reactions with streptokinase. 3. Avoid venipunctures during and after infusion. 4. *Use:* MI, PE, DVT; contraindicated in clients with active bleeding.

Fibrinolytic Therapy

"Door-to-needle goal" of 30 min for most optimum results
If a client has any of the following, fibrinolytic therapy may be contraindicated:
• Systolic BP >180 mm Hg or diastolic BP >110 mm Hg
• Significant closed head or facial trauma within the past 3 months
• History of intracranial hemorrhage
• Currently on anticoagulants
• CPR >10 min
• Pregnancy
• Serious systemic disease (liver, kidney)

Appendix 17-6   CARDIAC GLYCOSIDES

▲ **Cardiac Glycosides (e.g., digitalis)** Increase myocardial contractility, thereby increasing cardiac output. Decrease heart rate by slowing conduction of impulses through the AV node. Enhance diuresis by increasing renal perfusion.

General Nursing Implications

— Take the apical pulse for a full minute; if the rate is below 60 beats/min in an adult or below 90 to 110 beats/min in infants and young children, or below 70 in a child, hold the medication and notify the physician.

— Evaluate for tachycardia, bradycardia, and irregular pulse. If there is significant change in rate and rhythm, hold the medication and notify the physician.

— Evaluate serum potassium levels and response to diuretics; hypokalemia potentiates action of digitalis.

— Gastrointestinal symptoms are frequently the first indication of digitalis toxicity.

— Teach client not to increase or double a dose in the case of a missed dose; if client vomits, do not give an additional dose.

— Quinidine, verapamil, and ACE inhibitors increase plasma levels of digitalis.

— To achieve maximum results rapidly, an initial loading dose is administered; then dose is reduced to a maintenance dose.

— Digibind is a digitalis antagonist and may be used for digitalis toxicity; watch for decreased potassium levels and client's response to decreased digitalis levels.

MEDICATION	SIDE EFFECTS	NURSING IMPLICATIONS
▲ Digoxin **(Lanoxin):** PO, IV	Most common: anorexia, nausea, vomiting Most serious: drug-induced dysrhythmias Visual disturbances, fatigue Children/infants: frequent vomiting, poor feeding, or slow heart rate may indicate toxicity	1. Therapeutic plasma levels of digoxin are 0.5-2.0 ng/mL. 2. First sign of toxicity is usually GI symptoms. 3. *Uses:* supraventricular tachycardia, CHF.

⊞ OLDER ADULT PRIORITY Older adults are more sensitive to digitalis and are more likely to experience toxicity.

Appendix 17-7   CARDIAC DYSRHYTHMIAS

A *dysrhythmia* is defined as an interruption in the normal conduction of the heart, either in the rate or the rhythm.

ALERT Initiate, maintain, and/or evaluate telemetry monitoring; identify abnormal cardiac rhythms; and initiate protocols to manage cardiac arrhythmias.

Characteristics of Normal Sinus Rhythm

Rate: 60 to 100 beats/min
Rhythm: regular
P waves: present, precede each QRS complex
P-R interval: 0.12 to 0.20 sec
QRS complex: present and under 0.10 sec
Dysrhythmias may be classified according to rate—either bradycardia or tachycardia. They are also classified according to their origin—atrial or ventricular. Ventricular dysrhythmias are more life-threatening than atrial dysrhythmias. (See Common Dysrhythmias below.)

Nursing Implications

1. Identify dysrhythmia and evaluate client's tolerance.
2. Monitor adequacy of cardiac output, keep on bed rest, and oxygen.

3. Convert abnormal rhythm to normal sinus rhythm—medications or cardioversion.
4. Prevent complications.

Interpretation of Electrocardiogram

1. Determine heart rate. Count the P waves in a 6-sec strip to determine the atrial rate and count the R or Q waves to determine the ventricular rate.
2. Are the QRS complexes occurring at regular intervals?
3. Are P waves present for each QRS complex?
4. Measure the P-R interval.
5. Measure the QRS interval.
6. Identify the T wave and S-T segment.
7. Analyze any abnormalities.
8. Correlate findings with characteristics of normal sinus rhythm.

ALERT Identify cardiac rhythm strip abnormalities (sinus tachycardia, premature ventricular contractions, V-tach, atrial and ventricular fibrillation); initiate, maintain, and/or evaluate telemetry monitoring; intervene to improve client cardiovascular status; initiate protocol to manage cardiac dysrhythmias (see Appendix 17-4).

Appendix 17-7   CARDIAC DYSRHYTHMIAS—cont'd

Common Dysrhythmias

RHYTHM	CHARACTERISTICS	INTERVENTIONS/IMPLICATIONS
Sinus bradycardia	Sinus rhythm below a rate of 60 beats/min	Assess client for tolerance of the rate. If hypotension or decreasing LOC occurs, the rhythm is treated. *Treatment:* atropine.
Sinus tachycardia	Regular rhythm; P waves present Rate: 100 to 150 beats/min	Assess client for tolerance of the rate. Most often caused by caffeine, alcohol, or physiologic response to stimuli. Treatment based on underlying cause. *Treatment:* adenosine, beta-blockers, pain control.
Paroxysmal atrial (supraventricular) tachycardia	Rhythm is intermittent and is initiated suddenly; terminates suddenly with or without treatment	
Atrial fibrillation	Grossly irregular rate; cannot identify P waves or P-R interval on ECG Controlled rate: 60 to 100 beats/min Uncontrolled rate: 140 to 180 beats/min	Assess client for tolerance to rapid cardiac rate. Most common dysrhythmia. Evaluate client for systemic emboli (pulmonary emboli or an embolic stroke) from clots that tend to form in fibrillating atrium; a decrease in cardiac output will occur with tachycardia; maintain bed rest until rate is controlled. Pulse deficit will occur with rapid rate. Anticoagulation before cardioversion if client is in AF for longer than 48 hours. *Treatment:* digitalis, calcium channel blockers, beta blockers, cardioversion.

AV Block

First-degree block PRI 0.32	Prolonged P-R interval; all P waves are followed by a QRS complex May result from digitalis toxicity, electrolyte imbalance, or myocardial ischemia	Identify and treat the underlying cause. Must have an ECG tracing to identify.

Continued

Appendix 17-7 CARDIAC DYSRHYTHMIAS—cont'd

RHYTHM	CHARACTERISTICS	INTERVENTIONS/IMPLICATIONS
Third-degree or complete block 	No correlation between atrial impulses and ventricular response Rate: atrial rate 80 to 90 beats/min, with ventricular rate around 30 beats/min PR interval (PRI) is variable	May occur after an MI; symptoms depend on client's tolerance to rhythm; very unstable and may lead to asystole. *Treatment:* atropine, isoproterenol, dopamine until pacing can be established with a pacemaker.
Premature ventricular contractions or beats (PVCs, PVBs) 	Premature ectopic beats; occur within a basic rhythm; are of ventricular origin; no P waves; wide, bizarre QRS complex	Indicative of ventricular irritability; considered to be significant and should be treated if they: 1. Occur in excess of 6 beats/min. 2. Occur in a consecutive manner or in pairs. 3. Occur on a T wave of a preceding complex. 4. Cause a pulse deficit. *Treatment:* oxygen, electrolyte replacement, lidocaine, procainamide; PVCs frequently precede ventricular tachycardia.
Ventricular tachycardia 	Looks like a row of PVCs in configuration, wide and bizarre; very rapid rate of 125 to 200 beats/min	Severe decrease in cardiac output; potentially life-threatening situation. May have a pulse or be pulseless. If pulseless initiate CPR. *Treatment:* lidocaine, amiodarone, procainamide, cardioversion.
Ventricular fibrillation 	Very rapid, disorganized rate; cannot identify QRS complexes; erratic conduction	Client is unresponsive, with no pulse; initiate a code and begin CPR. *Treatment:* defibrillation, lidocaine.
Asystole	No electrical activity "Straight line"	No cardiac output. Initiate CPR. *Treatment:* external pacemaker, epinephrine, atropine.

Illustrations from Phipps W et al: *Medical-surgical nursing: health and illness perspectives,* ed 8, St. Louis, 2007, Mosby.
AV, Atrioventricular; *CPR,* cardiopulmonary resuscitation; *ECG,* electrocardiogram; *LOC,* level of consciousness; *MI,* myocardial infarction; *PVCs,* premature ventricular contractions.

Appendix 17-8 PACEMAKERS

Temporary Pacing

Noninvasive: application of two large external electrodes attached to an external pulse generator.

Invasive: wire electrodes are in contact with the heart and are attached to a battery operated pulse generator. Wires may be placed on the epicardium during heart surgery; leads are passed through the chest wall. Wires may also be placed via a catheter inserted in the antecubital vein and lodged in the right atrium and/or ventricle. Used in emergency situations and in severe cases of bradycardia. Anticipate placement of permanent pacemaker.

Permanent: An internal generator is inserted into soft tissue of upper chest or abdomen, and electrodes are positioned in the atrium and ventricles. PM may synchronize pacing between atrium and ventricle. (Figure 17-13). Procedure is planned and conducted under optimal conditions; used in persistent chronic heart block, dysrhythmias, and/or severe bradycardia.

Pacing Modes

Synchronous demand: The heart is stimulated to beat when the client's pulse rate falls below a set value or rate (majority of pacemakers have a set rate between 60 and 72 beats/min; if client's pulse rate falls below the set value, the pacemaker initiates a heartbeat). The pacemaker "senses" the normal heartbeat and the following conduction. If a normal cardiac beat is initiated and conducted, the pacemaker does not initiate an impulse.

Atrioventricular: The ventricle is sensed, and the atrium is paced. If the ventricle does not depolarize, then it is also paced.

Universal atrioventricular: Both the atrial and ventricular circuits sense and pace in the respective chambers. This most closely resembles the normal conduction system.

Pacemaker Failure A cardiac monitor or an electrocardiogram (ECG) must be available to verify pacemaker failure.

Failure to sense: The pacemaker fails to recognize spontaneous heart beats and will fire inappropriately. This is dangerous because the pacer impulse may be discharged during a critical time in the cardiac cycle.

Failure to pace: A malfunction in the pacemaker generator; it may also be due to dislodgment of the leads.

Failure to capture: May occur with a low battery or poor connection. The pacemaker is discharging the impulse; however, there is no responding cardiac contraction.

Nursing Implications

1. Assess for dysrhythmias; rate should not fall below preset level.
2. Maintain bed rest if pulse rate drops below preset level.
3. Hypotension, syncope, and bradycardia should not occur.

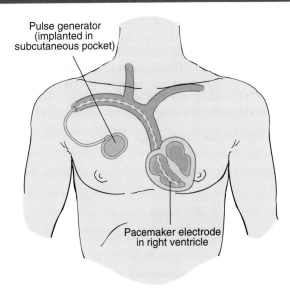

FIGURE 17-13 Permanent pacemaker placement. (From Monahan FD et al: *Phipps' medical-surgical nursing: health and illness perspectives,* ed 8, St. Louis, 2007, Mosby.)

Client Education

1. Notify all health care providers of pacemaker placement and parameters; wear a medical alert identification.
2. Avoid constrictive clothing that puts pressure on or irritates the site; report any signs of infection.
3. Safe environment: Avoid areas of high voltage, magnetic force fields (MRIs).
4. Avoid activity that requires vigorous movement of arms and shoulders or any direct blows to PM site.
5. Teach client to check his pulse and report if pulse rate is below 60 and client is experiencing symptoms; if this occurs, the pacemaker is not functioning properly, and this needs to be reported immediately.
6. Advise client to immediately report episodes of syncope.
7. Follow-up care and monitoring of pacemaker are important.
8. Client may travel without restrictions.

ALERT Connect and maintain pacing devices; monitor pacemaker and implantable cardioverter defibrillator functions.

Appendix 17-9   BEDSIDE HEMODYNAMIC MONITORING

Central Venous Pressure Monitoring

Central venous pressure (CVP) is an indication of the pressure within the right atrium or within the large veins in the thoracic cavity. An intravenous (IV) catheter is placed in the superior vena cava or in the right atrium via the subclavian vein or jugular vein. A CVP reading may also be obtained from the proximal lumen of the pulmonary artery catheter. (Figure 17-14)

Interpretation of Pressure Readings

Normal response may range from 4 to 10 mm of H_2O pressure. CVP is a dynamic measurement; it must be correlated with client's overall clinical status for correct interpretation.

Factors That Affect CVP Reading

1. Venous return to the heart (venous tone and vascular volume)
2. Intrathoracic pressure
3. Function of the left side of the heart
4. Coughing or straining (increase CVP)

> **! NURSING PRIORITY**   The CVP is an index of the ability of the right side of the heart to handle venous return. Rising CVP may indicate hypervolemia or poor cardiac contractility. Decreasing CVP may indicate a state of hypovolemia or vasodilation.

Nursing Considerations

1. Each CVP reading should be measured from the same zero level point (level of the right atrium or the phlebostatic axis).

The zero level on the manometer or the transducer should be placed at this level to obtain the reading. Client should be supine when the measurements are obtained; head may be slightly elevated, but the position should be consistent for all measurements.
2. If the CVP catheter is patent within the thoracic cavity, the fluid in the manometer or the digital readout will fluctuate with respirations or changes in thoracic pressure when the reading is obtained.
3. Patency of the CVP line is maintained via IV infusion drip.
4. Catheter should be stabilized on the skin at the insertion site, and an occlusive sterile dressing should be applied.

Complications

Air emboli and infections

> **! NURSING PRIORITY**   To obtain hemodynamic measurements, the zero point of the transducer must be at the level of the right atrium, which is the midaxillary line at the fourth or fifth intercostal space.

Pulmonary Artery Pressure Monitoring (Swan-Ganz Catheter)

A multilumen catheter (Figure 17-15) is inserted and advanced through the right atrium and right ventricle into the pulmonary artery. The flow of blood carries the catheter into the pulmonary artery. Heparinized saline solution is infused under pressure to maintain the patency of the line.

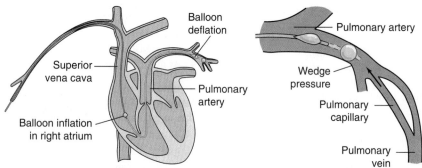

FIGURE 17-14   Pulmonary artery catheter. (From Monahan FD et al: *Phipps' medical-surgical nursing: health and illness perspectives,* ed 8, St. Louis, 2007, Mosby.)

FIGURE 17-15   Four-lumen thermodilution pulmonary artery catheter. (From Monahan FD et al: *Phipps' medical-surgical nursing: health and illness perspectives,* ed 8, St. Louis, 2007, Mosby.)

Appendix 17-9 BEDSIDE HEMODYNAMIC MONITORING—cont'd

Interpretation of Pressure Readings

Pressure readings are obtained via a transducer; for readings to be accurate, the zero level of the transducer must be at the level of the right atrium or the phlebostatic axis (see CVP).

Right atrial (RA) pressure: Normal is 1-8 mm Hg; a direct measurement of the pressure in the right atrium.

Pulmonary artery pressure (PAP): Normal is 15-25 mm Hg systolic and 5-15 mm Hg diastolic, with a mean pressure around 12-15 mm Hg. Mean PAP is increased in clients with chronic pulmonary diseases and those with CHF.

Pulmonary capillary wedge pressure (PAWP or PCWP): Normal is 4-12 mm Hg. It is determined as a mean pressure and is obtained by inflating or wedging a small balloon on the catheter tip in a distal branch of the pulmonary artery. The wedge pressure is indicative of pressure in the left cardiac chambers and reflects the function of the left atrium and ventricle. An upward trend is indicative of increases in pressure and/or fluid, whereas a downward trend indicates fluid, dehydration, or severe vasodilation.

Nursing Implications

1. Maintain patency of line via a heparinized flush solution administered under pressure.
2. The transducer should be at the level of the right atrium to ensure accurate measurements. Catheter should be secured to the skin and covered with an occlusive dressing. Each time the PCWP is evaluated, it is imperative that the balloon or the wedge be deflated to prevent pulmonary infarction, which is validated on the pressure monitor.

ALERT Evaluate invasive monitoring data obtained with a pulmonary artery pressure.

Complications

Infections, sepsis, ventricular dysrhythmias, pulmonary infarction, air emboli

---

Appendix 17-10 CARDIOPULMONARY RESUSCITATION (CPR) FOR HEALTH CARE PROVIDERS

The **American Heart Association (AHA) has established standards for cardiopulmonary resuscitation for the health care provider. For further delineation of the procedure, consult the American Heart Association Cardiopulmonary Resuscitation Guidelines. For health care providers, the American Heart Association uses the term** *infant* **to refer to individuals between birth and 1 year of age;** *child* **is used to refer to those who are between 1 year of age and the onset of puberty.**

1. **Airway.**
   - Identify that the victim is unconscious.
   - Activate the emergency medical services (EMS) system.
   - Obtain automated external defibrillator (AED). Use AED as soon as it is available for all adults and children for sudden, witnessed collapse and for in-hospital clients.
   - Place victim in position to open airway.
   - Open the airway: head-tilt/chin-lift maneuver.
   - Check for adequate breathing (look, listen, and feel for breaths).
   - If victim is breathing, place in recovery position.
   - If victim is not breathing, give 2 rescue breaths using mouth to mouth, or a pocket mask or bag mask.
2. **Breathing.**
   - Maintain the open airway.
   - Pinch nostrils closed.
   - Give two breaths that make the chest rise, at 1 sec per breath, using mouth-to-mouth technique (mouth–to–nose and mouth technique may be used for small children and infants).
   - Do not give "extra" breaths; do not give large, forceful breaths.
   - When an advanced airway is present, ventilate at the rate of 8-10/min; do not pause for compressions.
3. **Check the pulse** for no more than 10 sec.
   - Adult and child: Check the carotid pulse.
   - Infant: Check the brachial or femoral pulse.
   - If the pulse is absent, begin chest compressions—cycles of 30 compressions and 2 breaths until ACLS or PALS standards are initiated.

- If the pulse is present, continue rescue breathing, and recheck pulse every 2 min. If, despite adequate ventilation, the heart rate of an infant or child remains under 60 bpm, chest compressions should be started.
- Adult: 1 breath every 5-6 sec, 10-12 per min.
- Child and infant: 1 breath every 3-5 sec, 12-20 breaths per min.
- Advanced airway present (laryngeal mask airway, endotracheal tube): 1 breath every 6-8 sec without trying to synchronize breaths with compressions.

PEDIATRIC PRIORITY Be careful not to hyperextend the infant's head; this may block the airway. Don't pinch the infant's nose shut—cover the nose with your mouth instead. Breathe slowly, just enough to make the chest rise.

4. **External cardiac compression.**
   - Place the victim on a firm surface. If the client is in a bed, put a cardiac board behind him or her. DO NOT attempt to remove the victim from the bed.
   - Locate the lower half of the sternum in the adult. For the adult, place one hand over the lower sternum; place the other hand on top of the previous hand. For a child (age 1 year to puberty), use the heel of one hand, or two hands based on the size of the child, and press on the center of the chest at the nipple line. For an infant, locate the nipple line; the area for compression is one finger's width below the line.
   - Depress the sternum 1½ to 2 inches in the adult; in children and infants depress approximately one-third to one-half of depth of chest.
   - Push hard and fast; allow the chest to recoil completely between compressions and as few interruptions as possible.
   Adult and child:
   One rescuer and two rescuers: 30 compressions (rate of 100 per min) to 2 ventilations.

Continued

Appendix 17-10   CARDIOPULMONARY RESUSCITATION (CPR) FOR HEALTH CARE PROVIDERS—cont'd

Infant:

One rescuer: 30 compressions (rate of 100 per min) to 2 ventilations.

Two rescuers: 15 compressions to 2 ventilations.

Defibrillation: Use automatic electronic defibrillator (AED) as soon as available for sudden collapse and for in-hospital clients.

Steps for using an automated external defibrillator (AED):

1. Provide CPR until the AED arrives.
2. On arrival, open the case and turn the power on.
3. Select the correct pads for the size and age of the victim (only use the child pads/system for children less than 8 years old).
4. Attach the adhesive electrodes—one on the upper-right side of the chest directly below the clavicle, the other below the left nipple below the left armpit.
5. Attach the connecting cable to the AED.
6. Compressions will need to be discontinued while the rhythm is analyzed.
7. If shock is indicated, loudly state "Clear!" and visually check to ensure that no one is touching the client.

8. Press the SHOCK button.
9. Resume CPR immediately with cycles of 30 compressions to 2 breaths.

After 2 min, the AED will prompt you to repeat steps 6 through 9.

5. **Termination of CPR.** A rescuer who is not a physician should continue resuscitation efforts until one of the following occurs:
   - Spontaneous circulation and ventilation have been restored.
   - Resuscitation efforts are transferred to another equally responsible person who continues the resuscitation procedure.
   - A physician, or physician-directed person, assumes responsibility for resuscitation procedure.
   - The victim is transferred to an emergency medical service (e.g., paramedics and ambulance).
   - The rescuer is exhausted and unable to continue resuscitation.

ALERT Identify and intervene in life-threatening client situations. Notify primary health care provider about unexpected response/emergency situation of client.

Appendix 17-11   NONDRUG TREATMENT OF DYSRHYTHMIAS

Defibrillation is depolarization of the electrical impulses in the heart to allow the heart's own intrinsic pacemaker to regain control of cardiac rhythm.

Defibrillation (Unsynchronized)

Depolarization of cardiac cells in an emergency situation with a life-threatening dysrhythmia:

1. Always begin cardiopulmonary resuscitation (CPR) if client has no pulse and is unconscious; do not wait for a defibrillator.
2. Make sure everyone is clear of the bed and the client is not lying in fluids.
3. Make sure everyone is clear from touching the bed or client.
4. Synchronization is turned off.
5. Defibrillation is started at 200 J and progresses to a higher energy level (300-360 J).
6. Document rhythm after defibrillation.
7. Remain with client and closely assess for adequacy and stability of cardiac output and cardiac rhythm.

Synchronized Cardioversion

Depolarization of cardiac cells to allow the sinus node to regain control of cardiac rhythm:

1. An elective, planned procedure or used when client has a tachycardic rhythm with a pulse rate greater than 150.
2. Requires client teaching and informed consent when it is an elective procedure.
3. Document rhythm before synchronized cardioversion and immediately afterward.
4. The defibrillator is set (synchronized) to deliver the electrical discharge during the QRS complex; this prevents the discharge from occurring on the T wave. Look for the sync markers on the R wave.

5. Verbalize "Clear!" loudly and validate that no one is touching the client or bed before administering the shock.
6. Cardioversion is started at 50 J to 100 J.
7. Remain with client and closely assess for adequacy and stability of cardiac output and cardiac rhythm.

Implantable Cardioverter Defibrillators (ICD)

1. Used in clients who have survived one or more episodes of sudden death from ventricular dysrhythmias or from refractory ventricular dysrhythmias not associated with a myocardial infarction.
2. Implantable device can also be used as a pacemaker.
3. Inserted in a subcutaneous pocket in the subclavicular or abdominal area.
4. Client should avoid contact sports, increase activity gradually, and carry ICD identification information.
5. Client should avoid working over large motors and should move away from devices if dizziness occurs; client should avoid magnets directly over area of ICD.
6. Common response to device is anxiety and fear.
7. Assess for fluid hazards; intravenous fluids and urine may conduct voltage.
8. Client should sit or lie down if they become dizzy or if they feel the ICD discharge.

Radiofrequency Catheter Ablation

1. Used in clients who experience atrial tachycardia or AV nodal reentrant tachycardia. Electrophysiologic testing identifies the small region of the myocardium generating the dysrhythmia. A radiofrequency catheter is placed at the site, and the catheter is activated to generate RF energy. This energy destroys the tissue eliminating the dysrhythmia.
2. Complications are minimal but can include AV blocks and myocardial perforation.

Study Questions Cardiac System

More questions on companion CD!
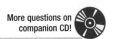

1. A client with a diagnosis of acute coronary syndrome is on a cardiac monitor. The nurse interprets the monitor rhythm to be ventricular tachycardia at a rate of 160 beats/min. The client is awake and coherent, and oxygen is being administered at a rate of 6 L/min via a nasal cannula. What is the first nursing action?
   1 Immediately defibrillate.
   2 Administer lidocaine IV push.
   3 Initiate transvenous pacing.
   4 Administer adenosine IV push.

2. The nurse is caring for a client with cor pulmonale, or right-side heart failure. What nursing assessment information correlates with an increase in venous pressure?
   1 Jugular vein distention with client sitting at a 45-degree angle
   2 Crackling sounds over the lower lobes with client in an upright position
   3 Bradycardia, restlessness, and an increase in respiratory rate
   4 Decreased pulsations at the point of maximum impulse

3. The nurse is administering nitroglycerin intravenously to relieve chest pain. What is the therapeutic action of this medication?
   1 Increases glomerular filtration, which results in decreased venous return
   2 Enhances contractility of the myocardium, which increases oxygen delivery
   3 Produces an immediate analgesic effect and relieves chest pain
   4 Increases the coronary blood supply and decreases the afterload

4. In discharge planning for the client with heart failure, the nurse discusses the importance of adequate rest. What information is most important?
   1 A warm, quiet room is necessary.
   2 Bed rest promotes venous return.
   3 A hospital bed is necessary.
   4 Adequate rest decreases cardiac workload.

5. The nurse is assessing a client whose condition is being stabilized after experiencing an acute coronary syndrome (myocardial infarction). What finding on the nursing assessment would indicate *inadequate* renal perfusion?
   1 Decreasing serum blood urea nitrogen (BUN) level
   2 Urine specific gravity of less than 1.010
   3 Urine output of less than 30 mL/hr
   4 Low urine osmolarity and creatinine clearance

6. The nurse applies a Nitro-Dur patch on a client who has undergone cardiac surgery. What nursing observation indicates that a Nitro-Dur patch is achieving the desired effect?
   1 Chest pain is completely relieved.
   2 Client performs activities of daily living without chest pain.
   3 Pain is controlled with frequent changes of patch.
   4 Client tolerates increased activity without pain.

7. The nurse has been assigned a group of cardiac clients. What would be the most important information for the nurse to check on the initial evaluation of each client? Select all that apply:
   _____ 1 Presence of cardiac pain
   _____ 2 Medications taken prior to hospitalization
   _____ 3 Presence of jugular vein distention
   _____ 4 Heart sounds and apical rate
   _____ 5 Presence of diaphoresis
   _____ 6 History of difficulty breathing

8. During the night, a client with a diagnosis of acute coronary syndrome (myocardial infraction) is found to be restless and diaphoretic. What is the best nursing action?
   1 Check his temperature and determine his serum blood glucose level.
   2 Turn the alarms low and promote sleep by decreasing the number of interruptions.
   3 Check the monitor to determine his cardiac rhythm and evaluate vital signs.
   4 Call the physician to obtain an order for sedation.

9. The nurse is caring for a client who begins to exhibit the cardiac rhythm shown in the illustration below. As the nurse observes, the rhythm remains the same. What is the best nursing action?
   1 Call an emergency code and begin resuscitation.
   2 Turn client on his left side and take his blood pressure.
   3 Prepare to administer lidocaine IV push.
   4 Take the apical pulse for a full minute.

10. The nurse is providing preoperative care for client who is scheduled for cardiac surgery. During the preoperative preparation, what is an important nursing action?
    1. Perform a thorough nursing assessment to provide an accurate baseline for evaluation after surgery.
    2. Discuss with the client the steps of myocardial cellular metabolism and the anticipated surgical response.
    3. Provide preoperative education regarding the mechanics of the cardiopulmonary bypass machine.
    4. Discuss with the client and family the anticipated amount of postoperative chest tube drainage.

11. An older adult client is taking digitalis, 0.025 mg twice a day, and Lasix (furosemide), 40 mg daily, for CHF. She has complained of increasing lethargy and nausea over the past 2 days; however, she is still able to take her medication. Her blood pressure is 150/98 mm Hg; pulse is 110 beats/min and irregular; respiratory rate is 18 breaths/min. What laboratory information is most important for the nurse to evaluate?
    1. Hemoglobin, hematocrit, and white blood cell count
    2. Arterial blood gases and acid-base balance
    3. Blood urea nitrogen (BUN) and serum creatinine levels
    4. Serum electrolyte levels, particularly potassium

12. During the shift hand-off report, the nurse learns that one of the assigned clients is in first-degree heart block. What is a nursing measure to assess the status of this dysrhythmia?
    1. Count the radial pulse for 1 full minute.
    2. Determine the cardiac rate at the PMI.
    3. Evaluate an ECG or monitor strip.
    4. Hourly pulse checks and correlate with blood pressure.

13. The nurse is preparing a client for a cardiac catheterization. What is the best explanation regarding the purpose of a cardiac catheterization with coronary angiography?
    1. Evaluate the exercise tolerance.
    2. Study the conduction system.
    3. Evaluate coronary artery blood flow.
    4. Measure the myocardial contractility.

14. A client is admitted for evaluation of his permanent pacemaker. What data would confirm that the pacemaker is *not* working correctly?
    1. Pulse rate of 96 beats/min with regular rate and rhythm
    2. Irregular pulse rate with premature ventricular beats
    3. Atrial premature beats shown on the monitor
    4. Pulse rate of 48 beats/min with premature ventricular beats

15. The nurse is assessing the pulse of a client in atrial fibrillation. Based on the graphic below, where should the stethoscope be placed to correctly auscultate this client's pulse?

16. The vital signs of a client with cardiac disease are as follows: blood pressure of 100/78 mm Hg, pulse of 46 beats/min, and respiratory rate of 18 breaths/min. Atropine (atropine sulfate) is administered IV push. What nursing assessment indicates a therapeutic response to the medication?
    1. Pulse rate has increased to 70 beats/min.
    2. Systolic blood pressure has increased by 20 mm Hg.
    3. Pupils are dilated.
    4. Oral secretions have decreased.

17. The nurse is taking the history of a client with heart failure (congestive heart failure) caused by chronic hypertension. The nurse identifies what data as supportive of the client's medical diagnosis?
    1. Dyspnea after walking about half a block
    2. Weight loss of 15 pounds over last 3 months
    3. Lower extremity edema in the evenings
    4. Dizziness and fainting when rising too quickly

18. A client is admitted with mitral valve disease and left ventricular dysfunction. What is the most reliable test to determine cardiac status?
    1. Electrocardiogram
    2. Stress test
    3. Cardiac angiogram
    4. Echocardiogram

19. What would be an important home care goal for a client who has bacterial endocarditis?
    1. To begin an exercise regimen as soon as possible
    2. To monitor urinary output
    3. To continue antibiotic therapy
    4. To decrease activity until pulse stabilizes

Answers and rationales to these questions are in the section at the end of the book titled Chapter Study Questions: Answers and Rationales.

CHAPTER EIGHTEEN

Gastrointestinal System

PHYSIOLOGY OF THE GASTROINTESTINAL SYSTEM

Digestion, Absorption, and Elimination Process

A. Digestion: physical and chemical breakdown of food.
   1. Length of time food remains in stomach depends on type of food, gastric motility, and psychologic factors; average time is 3 to 4 hours.
   2. The pH of the stomach is acidic, which promotes production of pepsin to begin the initial breakdown of proteins.
   3. Chyme (food mixed with gastric secretions) moves through the pylorus into the small intestine.
   4. Intestinal digestive enzymes are released from the villi in the small intestine.
B. Absorption: transfer of food products into circulation.
   1. Occurs in small intestine, where villi provide absorptive surface area; minimal amount of nutrients are absorbed in the stomach.
   2. Carbohydrates are broken down into monosaccharides, fats to glycerol and fatty acids, and proteins to amino acids; all are absorbed through the villi of the small intestine.
   3. Intrinsic factor is secreted in the stomach and promotes absorption of vitamin B_{12} (cobalamin) in the small intestine.
   4. Presence of chyme in small intestine stimulates contraction of the gallbladder and relaxation of the sphincter of Oddi; this process releases bile for digestion of fats.
C. Elimination: excretion of waste products.
   1. Large intestine absorbs water and electrolytes and forms feces.
   2. Serves as a reservoir for fecal mass until defecation occurs.

System Assessment

A. Evaluate client's history.
   1. Dietary and bowel habits.
   2. Nausea, vomiting, diarrhea, indigestion, constipation, flatulence: precipitating and alleviating factors.
   3. Pain related to gastrointestinal (GI) tract.
   4. Previous problems associated with GI tract, including gastritis, hepatitis, colitis, gallbladder disease, peptic or duodenal ulcer, hernia, and hemorrhoids.
   5. Unexplained or unplanned weight gain or loss.
   6. Medication history, including over-the-counter (OTC) and prescription drugs.
   7. Previous surgeries related to GI system.
B. Assess vital signs for client's overall status.
C. Assess for presence and characteristics of abdominal pain.
D. Assess client's mouth.
   1. Presence of adequate saliva, condition of teeth and tongue.
   2. Presence of the gag reflex.
   3. Presence of oral lesions.
E. Evaluate the abdomen (client should be lying flat).
   1. Inspect: divide the abdomen into four quadrants and perform visual inspection for contour, scars, masses, and movement (aortic pulsation may be visible). Figure 18-1 shows anatomic divisions of the abdomen.
   2. Auscultate: each quadrant should be auscultated for bowel sounds.
      a. Bowel sounds are considered absent if no sound is heard for 5 minutes in any one quadrant.
      b. Normally, soft gurgles should be heard every 5 to 20 seconds.
      c. Borborygmi: loud, gurgling bowel sounds; may precede diarrhea.

ALERT To determine characteristics of bowel sounds, note presence in each quadrant, as well as frequency and pitch.

   3. Percussion: purpose is to determine presence of fluid, distention and/or masses.
      a. Tympany is a high-pitched hollow sound commonly heard over areas distended with air.
      b. Dullness is a short high-pitched sound with little resonance; heard over fluid or solid masses.
   4. Palpation: purpose is to determine areas of tenderness, resistance, and swelling; deep palpation is used to identify organs and possible masses.
      a. Begin with light palpation of each quadrant; observe facial expression for any area of discomfort and/or guarding.

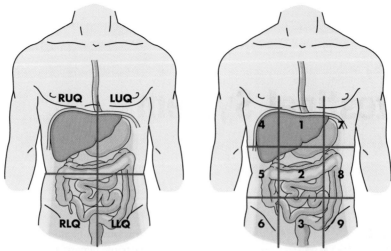

FIGURE 18-1 Anatomic Divisions of the Abdomen. **Left,** Abdomen divided into four quadrants. **Right,** Abdomen divided into nine topographic regions: *1,* epigastrium; *2,* umbilical; *3,* suprapubic; *4,* right hypochondrium; *5,* right lumbar or flank; *6,* right inguinal or iliac; *7,* left hypochondrium; *8,* left lumbar or flank; *9,* left inguinal or mac. (From Monahan FD et al: *Phipps' medical-surgical nursing: health and illness perspectives,* ed 8, St. Louis, 2007, Mosby.)

   b. Begin in area of least discomfort; if there is a problem area, palpate it last.

   c. Check for rebound tenderness by pressing two fingers firmly over painful site and withdraw them rapidly; pain occurs on release of pressure.

F. Assess rectal area for lesions, hemorrhoids, or ulcerations.

G. Evaluate elimination patterns and effects of aging on GI tract (Box 18-1).

H. Evaluate dietary pattern and fluid intake.

I. Assess stool specimen.
   1. Color, consistency, odor.
   2. Presence of blood or mucus.

DISORDERS OF THE GASTROINTESTINAL (GI) SYSTEM

Nausea and Vomiting

Nausea is an unpleasant feeling that vomiting is imminent. Vomiting is an involuntary act in which the stomach contracts and forcefully expels gastric contents.

 A. Loss of fluid and electrolytes is the primary consequence of repeated vomiting; the very young and the older adult are more susceptible to complications of fluid imbalances.

B. Prolonged vomiting will precipitate a metabolic problem.
   1. Metabolic alkalosis is associated with prolonged vomiting and loss of hydrochloric acid.
   2. Metabolic acidosis occurs with *severe* prolonged vomiting of contents of the small intestine, resulting in loss of bicarbonate.

Assessment

A. Precipitating causes.
   1. Pathogenic: related to a disease process (GI obstruction, toxic substances, etc.).

Box 18-1 **OLDER ADULT CARE FOCUS**

Changes in Gastrointestinal System Related to Aging

• Decreased hydrochloric acid and decreased absorption of vitamins; encourage frequent small feedings that are high in vitamins.

• Decreased peristalsis and decreased sensation to defecate; encourage diet high in fiber and minimum of 2000 mL of fluid daily; encourage physical activity.

• Decreased lipase from pancreas to aid in fat digestion; encourage smaller meals because diarrhea may be caused by increased fat intake.

• Decreased liver activity with decreased production of enzymes for drug metabolism, tendency toward accumulation of medications; instruct clients not to double up on their medications, especially cardiac medications.

   2. Iatrogenic: resulting from a disease treatment.
      a. Chemotherapy/radiation.
      b. Medications.
      c. Surgery (postoperative complication).
   3. Pregnancy: vomiting most often occurs in the morning.
   4. Vomiting in children is common.
   5. Further investigation and intervention is needed for progressively severe vomiting, persistent vomiting over 24 hours, and/or symptoms of dehydration.

ALERT Monitor client's hydration status; modify client's care based on results of diagnostic tests.

B. Assessment.
   1. Identify precipitating cause.
   2. Assess frequency of vomiting, amount of vomiting, and contents of vomitus.

3. Hematemesis: presence of blood in vomitus.
   a. Bright red blood is indicative of bleeding.
   b. Coffee-ground material is indicative of blood retained in the stomach; the digestive process has broken down the hemoglobin.
4. Projectile vomiting: vomiting not preceded by nausea in which vomitus is expelled with excessive force.
5. Presence of fecal odor and bile in vomitus indicates a backflow of intestinal contents into stomach.
6. Vomiting in children is usually self-limiting; assess for fever, diarrhea, and abdominal pain accompanying nausea and vomiting.

C. Diagnostics: clinical manifestations.

Treatment

A. Eliminate the precipitating cause.
B. Antiemetics (see Appendix 18-2).
C. Parenteral replacement of fluid if loss is excessive (Chapter 6).

Nursing Interventions

Goal: To prevent recurrence of nausea and vomiting and ensuing complications.

A. Prophylactic antiemetics for the client with a tendency to vomit.
B. Prompt removal of unpleasant odors, used emesis container, and soiled linens.
C. Good oral hygiene.
D. Place conscious client on side or in semi-Fowler's position; place unconscious client on side with head of bed slightly elevated to promote drainage of oral cavity.
E. Withhold food and beverages initially after vomiting; begin oral intake slowly—for adults, begin with tea, water, or oral rehydrating solutions at room temperature; for infants and children, begin with oral rehydrating solutions.
F. Assess surgical client for presence of bowel sounds and distention; do not begin oral administration of fluids if abdomen is tender or distended or no bowel sounds are present.
G. Support abdominal and thoracic incisions during vomiting.

ALERT Identify client potential for aspiration; intervene to prevent aspiration.

Goal: To relieve nausea and vomiting.
A. Administer antiemetics.
B. Evaluate precipitating causes; relieve if possible.
C. Gastric decompression with a nasogastric tube may be used for prolonged vomiting.

Goal: To assess client's response to prolonged vomiting.
A. Monitor fluid and electrolyte status (Chapter 6).
B. Assess for continued presence of gastric distention.
C. Assess for adequate hydration.
D. Assess for presence of other symptoms.

 Constipation

Constipation exists when there is a decrease in frequency of bowel movements; stool is hard and difficult to pass, and there is less than one bowel movement every 3 days.

Assessment

A. Precipitating causes.
   1. Decreased fiber and fluid intake.
   2. Immobility, inadequate exercise.
   3. Medications: narcotics, antidepressants, iron supplements, anticonvulsants.
   4. Older adult client.
   5. Overuse of laxatives.
   6. Ignoring the urge to defecate.
   7. Diverticulosis, tumors, intestinal obstructions.

ALERT Evaluate client's use of home remedies and OTC drugs. Assess what the client is using to treat constipation; frequently, the older adult client is using harsh laxatives.

B. Clinical manifestations.
   1. Abdominal distention.
   2. Decrease in the amount of stool.
   3. Dry, hard stool; straining to pass stool.
   4. Impaction.
      a. Constipation, rectal discomfort.
      b. Anorexia, nausea, vomiting.
      c. Diarrhea around impacted stool.

C. Diagnostics: clinical manifestations.

Treatment

A. Change dietary intake: increase intake of high-fiber foods and fluids.
B. Bulk laxatives, stool softeners, or enemas for occasional constipation problem (see Appendix 18-3).
C. Instruct client to maintain normal bowel schedule and not to ignore urge to defecate.
D. Discourage long-term use of laxatives and enemas.
E. Encourage regular exercise.

Nursing Interventions

ALERT Assess and intervene when client has a problem with elimination.

Goal: To identify client at risk for developing constipation and institute preventive measures (Box 18-2).

Goal: To implement treatment measures for fecal impaction removal.
A. An impaction may be present if client has had no bowel movement for 3 days or has passed only small amounts of semisoft or liquid stool.
B. Steps in removing impaction:
   1. Manually check for presence of impaction with non-sterile, lubricated gloved finger.

Box 18-2 OLDER ADULT CARE FOCUS

Preventing Fecal Impaction

- Increase intake of high-fiber foods: raw vegetables, whole-grain breads and cereals, fresh fruits.
- Increase fluid intake.
- Maintain regular activity: daily walking, swimming, or biking. If confined to wheelchair, change position frequently, perform leg raises and abdominal muscle contractions.
- Discourage use of laxatives and enemas: client may become dependent on them. If absolutely necessary, warm mineral oil enemas may soften and lubricate stool.
- Encourage use of bulk-forming products to provide increased fiber (methylcellulose, psyllium).
- Encourage bowel movement at same time each day.
- Try to position client on bedside commode rather than on a bedpan.
- If client is experiencing diarrhea, check to see if stool is oozing around an impaction.

2. Gently attempt to break up impaction using a scissor motion with the fingers.
3. Emphasis is on *prevention* of impaction (see Box 18-2).

> ⚠ **NURSING PRIORITY** Monitor client's heart rate during and after digital removal of feces; vagal stimulation can precipitate bradycardia.

Diarrhea

Diarrhea is the rapid movement of intestinal contents through the small bowel.

A. Significant increase in number of stools, along with an increase in looseness of stool.
B. Infants and older adults are most susceptible to complications of dehydration and hypovolemia.
C. Acute diarrhea is most often caused by an infection and is self-limiting when all causative agents or irritants have been evacuated.
D. Rotavirus is the most common pathogen in young children hospitalized for treatment of diarrhea.
   1. Affects all age groups and is most common in cool weather.
   2. Incubation period is 48 hours.
   3. Important source of nosocomial infections in hospital.
   4. Children 6 to 24 months old are at increased risk for complications.

Assessment

A. Precipitating causes.
   1. Bacteria (*Escherichia coli*, *Salmonella*), viruses (rotavirus), and parasites (*Giardia lamblia*).
   2. Food poisoning (frequently, infection by bacteria).
   3. Medications (antibiotics and antacids).
   4. Food intolerance (lactose intolerance) or allergies to certain foods.
   5. Malabsorption problems: celiac disease and cystic fibrosis.
B. Clinical manifestations.
   1. Frequent, loose, watery bowel movements; sense of urgency.
   2. Stools may contain undigested food, mucus, pus, or blood; frequently are foul smelling.
   3. Abdominal bloating, cramping, distention, and vomiting frequently occur with diarrhea.
   4. Hyperactive bowel sounds.
   5. May precipitate dehydration, hypokalemia, and hypovolemia, progressing to shock.
C. Diagnostics: stool examination; enzyme immunoassay (EIA) for rotavirus.

Treatment

A. Identify and treat the underlying problem.
B. Decrease activity and irritation of the GI tract by decreasing intake.
C. Parenteral replacement of fluids and electrolytes, if diarrhea is severe.
D. Do not administer antidiarrheal medications if causative agent is bacterial or parasitic. Antidiarrheals prevent client from purging the bacteria or parasite and traps the causative organism(s) in the intestines and prolongs the problem (Appendix 18-4).
E. Viral infections are either treated with medication or left to run their course, depending on the severity and type of virus.
F. Rotavirus vaccine (RotaTeq) should not be given to severely immunocompromised infants.

Nursing Interventions

Goal: To decrease diarrhea and prevent complications.
A. Identify precipitating causes and eliminate, if possible.
B. Offer soft, easily digestible food; does not have to be clear liquids.
C. Fluid and electrolyte replacement.
   1. Administer oral rehydrating solutions (ORSs); progress fluids and diet as tolerated.
   2. Frequently offer ORSs in small amounts at room temperature; do not offer high-carbohydrate fluids (juices), carbonated fluids, broth, or sports drinks.
   3. Nausea and vomiting are not contraindications to offering ORSs.
D. Maintain good hygiene in the rectal area to prevent skin excoriation.

Goal: To evaluate client's response to diarrhea.
A. Evaluate changes in vital signs correlating with fluid loss and hydration status (Chapter 6).
B. Evaluate electrolyte changes and urine specific gravity.
C. Record intake and output and daily weight if diarrhea is progressive.
D. Inspect abdomen for distention, auscultate for bowel sounds, and palpate for areas of tenderness.

Goal: To prevent spread of diarrhea.

A. Good hand hygiene.

B. Initiate contact precautions (Appendix 6-8).

1. Proper disposal of diapers and soiled linens close to bedside.

2. Instruct family regarding hand hygiene techniques.

3. Maintain separate clean and dirty areas in the room; keep bedpans, soiled linens, and soiled diapers away from clean areas.

C. Instruct parents regarding importance of hand hygiene and how to care for infant or child at home.

> ❗ **NURSING PRIORITY** Consider acute onset diarrhea as infectious until the cause is determined.

📋 Gastroesophageal Reflux Disease

Gastroesophageal reflux disease (GERD) is caused by the backward flow or reflux of gastric contents into the esophagus (esophageal reflux). Amount of damage depends on the amount and composition of gastric contents, as well as the ability of the esophagus to remove the acidic fluids.

A. Gastric contents are able to move from area of increased pressure (stomach) to area of lower pressure (esophagus) through the malfunctioning lower esophageal sphincter (LES), reflux occurs, and the esophagus is exposed to acid (Figure 18-2).

B. The acid breaks down the esophageal mucosa, and an inflammatory response is initiated.

C. Hiatal hernia: a herniation of a portion of the stomach into the esophagus; frequently presents with same symptoms as GERD; clinical course and management are the same.

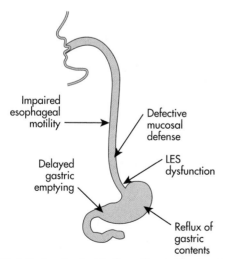

FIGURE 18-2 Factors involved in the pathogenesis of gastroesophageal reflux disease (GERD) (From Lewis SL et al: *Medical-surgical nursing: assessment and management of clinical problems,* ed 7, St. Louis, 2007, Mosby.)

Assessment

A. Risk factors.

1. Lifestyle factors: obesity; smoking; excess alcohol intake; consumption of high-fat or acidic foods; eating large meals; consumption of caffeine and carbonated beverages; stress.

2. Pathologic predisposing factors: PUD, asthma, cystic fibrosis, cancer.

3. Medications decreasing LES pressure: calcium channel blockers, nitrates, anticholinergics.

4. Anatomic factors: eating heavy meal before lying down, strenuous exercise after eating, scoliosis, poor esophageal sphincter tone, consuming an excessive amount of food and beverage.

5. Clients with prolonged chronic GERD are at increased risk for cancer.

B. Clinical manifestations.

1. Reflux esophagitis (heartburn, dyspepsia).

2. Increased pain after meals; may be relieved by antacids.

3. Activities that increase intraabdominal pressure increase esophageal discomfort.

4. Pain may radiate to back and neck.

5. Regurgitation not associated with belching or nausea.

C. Complications.

1. Aspiration of gastric contents: pneumonia, chronic bronchitis.

2. Dental erosion.

D. Diagnostics: 24-hour pH monitoring, esophageal manometry, esophagoscopy (Appendix 18-1).

Treatment

A. Medical.

1. Diet therapy: avoid intake of fatty foods; eat small, frequent meals; try chewing gum after and between meals.

2. Avoid wine and other alcoholic beverages, caffeinated drinks, chocolate.

3. Medications: histamine-2 receptor antagonists (H$_2$R blockers), proton pump inhibitors (PPIs) (Appendix 18-5), and GI stimulants or promotility drugs (Appendix 18-2).

B. Surgical: fundoplication or antireflux surgery.

C. Endoscopic intervention at lower esophagus and gastroesophageal sphincter (fundoplication, radiofrequency, sclerosing agents).

Nursing Interventions

Goal: To decrease esophageal reflux.

A. Avoid drinking beverages during meals, including alcohol and carbonated beverages.

B. Avoid temperature extremes in foods.

C. Avoid drinking fluids 3 hours before bedtime.

D. Elevate the head of the bed on 6- to 8-inch blocks.

E. If overweight, lose weight to decrease abdominal pressure gradient.

F. Avoid tobacco, NSAIDs, and salicylates.

G. Decrease intake of highly seasoned foods and tomato products.

H. Eat small, frequent meals (up to 5 per day at 3-hour intervals) to prevent gastric dilation.

I. Avoid any food that precipitates discomfort (fats, caffeine, chocolate, nicotine will decrease esophageal sphincter tone).

J. Do not lie down for 2 to 3 hours after eating.

Gastritis

Gastritis is an inflammation and breakdown of the normal gastric mucosa barrier.

A. Acute gastritis is generally self-limiting with no residual damage.

B. May be chronic or acute, diffuse or localized.

Assessment

A. Risk factors/etiology.
1. Often caused by dietary indiscretion (gastric irritants: coffee, aspirin, alcohol).
2. Smoking or exposure to radiation, psychologic stress.
3. Microorganisms: *Helicobacter pylori*, contaminated foods (*Staphylococcus* or *Salmonella* organisms).
4. Medications causing gastric irritation (aspirin, corticosteroids, chemotherapy).
5. Prolonged alcohol abuse, binge drinking.
6. Acute gastritis is a common problem in intensive care units because of stress. Clients with burns, uremia, sepsis, shock, mechanical ventilation, or multiorgan dysfunction who are not receiving enteral feeding are at significantly increased risk.

> **! NURSING PRIORITY** Best practice for the prevention of gastritis in clients who are ventilator dependent is the routine administration of antiulcerative medication (Appendix 18-5).

B. Clinical manifestations (may be asymptomatic).
1. Epigastric tenderness.
2. Anorexia, nausea, vomiting.
3. Chronic gastritis: frequently caused by the *Helicobacter pylori*.
   a. May precipitate pernicious anemia.
   b. Associated with peptic ulcer disease.

C. Diagnostics (Appendix 18-1).
1. Endoscopy with biopsy to rule out gastric carcinoma.
2. Stool examination for occult blood.
3. Gastric analysis for decreased acid production (achlorhydria).
4. Serum, stool, and gastric biopsy for *H. pylori*.

D. Complications.
1. Ulceration and hemorrhaging (Figure 18-3).
2. Cancer of the stomach.

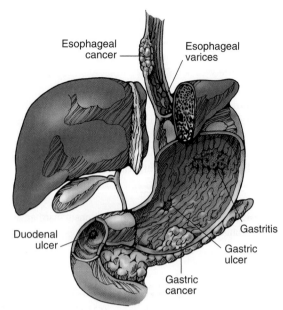

FIGURE 18-3 Common causes of gastrointestinal bleeding. (From Ignatavicius DD, Workman ML: *Medical-surgical nursing: patient-centered collaborative care,* ed 6, Philadelphia, 2010, Saunders.)

Treatment

A. Eliminate cause.

B. Medical management.
1. Antiemetics, antacids, PPIs and H_2R blockers (Appendix 18-5).
2. Treatment for *H. pylori* with antibiotics and PPIs.

C. Surgical intervention, if medical treatment fails or hemorrhage occurs.

Nursing Interventions

Goal: To decrease gastric irritation.

A. Nothing by mouth (NPO status) initially, with IV fluid and electrolyte replacement.

B. Plan of care for nausea and vomiting.

C. Begin ORSs as client tolerates them.

Goal: To monitor fluid status and prevent dehydration (Chapter 6).

Goal: To assist client to identify and avoid precipitating causes.

Gastroenteritis

Gastroenteritis is the irritation and inflammation of the mucosa of the stomach and small bowel.

Assessment

A. Risk factors/etiology.
1. Equal incidence in men and women but more severe in infants and older adults.
2. Salmonella: fecal oral transmission by direct contact or via contaminated food.
3. Staphylococcal: transmission via foods that were handled by contaminated carrier.
4. Dysentery: E. coli and Shigella.

B. Clinical manifestations.
1. Abdominal cramping, distention, and pain.
2. Nausea, vomiting, and diarrhea.
3. Anorexia, fever and chills.
C. Diagnostics: stool culture.

Treatment

A. Nothing by mouth until nausea subsides.
B. Rehydrate with water and ORSs.
C. Client resumes eating with bland, easily digestible foods.
D. Appropriate medication for causative agents.

Nursing Interventions

See Nursing Interventions section under Nausea and Vomiting.

Obesity

An imbalance between energy expenditure and caloric intake that results in an abnormal increase in fat cells.
A. According to the CDC, 65% of people in the United States over age 20 are obese.
B. Children are considered overweight if their weight is in the 95th percentile or higher for their age, gender, and height on the growth chart.
C. Classified according to the body mass index (BMI); see Chapter 2.

Assessment

A. Risk factors.
1. Genetic predisposition.
2. Sedentary lifestyle: energy intake (food) exceeds energy expenditure.
3. Sociocultural: environment conducive to excessive caloric intake.
4. Obesity puts client at increased risk for cardiovascular, respiratory, and musculoskeletal problems, as well as increased risk for development of diabetes.
B. Clinical manifestations.
1. A BMI of 25 to 29.9 kg/m^2 is considered overweight.
2. A BMI of over 30 kg/m^2 is considered obese.
3. Android obesity: fat is distributed over the abdomen and upper body (apple-shaped).
4. Gynecoid obesity: fat is distributed over the upper legs (pear-shaped).
5. Android obesity is considered to be a higher risk for obesity-related problems, especially elevated triglyceride and lipid levels as well as the development of type 2 diabetes.

Treatment

A. Lifestyle changes and modification of dietary intake.
B. Bariatric surgery.
1. Laproscopic adjustable-banded gastroplasty (LABG) involves placing a band around the fundus of the stomach; band may or may not be inflatable.
2. Malabsorptive: Roux-en-Y bypass (REG) or gastric bypass involves bypassing segments of small intestine so less food is absorbed.

3. Combination of restrictive and malabsorptive surgery: the stomach is decreased in size with formation of a gastric pouch that empties directly into the jejunum; greatest loss of weight is usually achieved over the first year.

Nursing Interventions

Goal: To prepare client for surgery (Chapter 3).
A. Discuss the importance of early ambulation to reduce complications.
B. Length of time in hospital depends on procedure.
C. Dietary changes.
Goal: To maintain homeostasis postoperatively (Chapter 3).
A. Immediately postoperative airway may be a problem; maintain good pulmonary hygiene; positive end expiratory pressure (PEEP) and or ventilator support may be necessary.
B. Increased risks for thromboembolic problems: sequential compression stockings, encourage early ambulation and administer thromboprophylaxis with low-molecular-weight heparin.
C. Do not adjust an NG tube, and do not insert NG tube even if there is protocol to do so for nausea and vomiting; notify surgeon.
D. Observe client for development of anastomotic leaks: increasing back, shoulder and or abdominal pain, unexplained tachycardia or decrease urine output; notify surgeon of these findings.
E. May use abdominal binder to protect incision.
F. In client with diabetes, assess for fluctuations in serum blood glucose; may require less antihypoglycemics.
G. Client with malabsorption surgery may experience dumping syndrome (Box 18-3).

Home Care

A. Diet.
1. Eat at least 3 meals a day; chew food completely.
2. Drink fluids throughout the day, but do not drink fluids with meals.
3. Avoid high-calorie, high-sugar, and high-fat foods.
4. Stop eating when you feel full.
5. Try to get 50 to 60 g of protein daily; may need to take a protein supplement.
6. Learn how to avoid dumping syndrome (see Box 18-3).
B. Take a chewable or liquid multivitamin with iron.
C. Can expect to lose 50% to 70% of excess body weight over 5 years.
D. For women, do not try to get pregnant for about 18 months after surgery.
E. Join a support group for long-term psychosocial implications.

Peptic Ulcer Disease

Peptic ulcer disease (PUD) is an erosion of the GI mucosa by hydrochloric acid and pepsin. Any location in the GI tract that comes in contact with gastric secretions is susceptible to ulcer development.

Box 18-3 DUMPING SYNDROME

Condition occurs when a large bolus of gastric chyme and hypertonic fluid enter the intestine.

Goal: To assess for symptoms of condition.

- Weakness, dizziness, tachycardia.
- Epigastric fullness, abdominal cramping, hyperactive bowel sounds.
- Diaphoresis.
- Generally occurs within 15 to 30 minutes after eating.
- Usually self-limiting and resolves in about 6 to 12 months.

Goal: To prevent dumping syndrome.

- Decrease amount of food eaten at one meal; eat small meals at 3-hour intervals.
- Decrease simple carbohydrates; increase proteins and high-fiber foods as tolerated.
- No added fluid with meal; fluids can be taken 30 to 45 minutes before meals or 1 hour after meals.
- Decrease concentrated sweets; add fruits high in pectin to diet (peaches, plums, apples) to slow carbohydrate absorption in small intestine.
- Position client in semi-recumbent position during meals; client may lie down on the left side for 20 to 30 minutes after meals to delay stomach emptying.
- Hypoglycemia may occur 2 to 3 hours after eating, caused by rapid entry of carbohydrates into jejunum.

ALERT Implement measures to improve client's nutritional intake. Prevent dumping syndrome and/or care for client experiencing dumping syndrome.

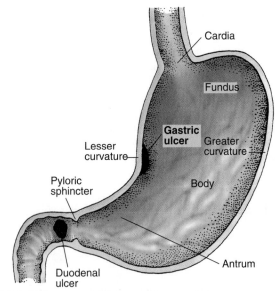

FIGURE 18-4 The most common sites for peptic ulcers. (From Ignata-vicius DD, Workman ML: *Medical-surgical nursing: patient-centered collaborative care,* ed 6, Philadelphia, 2010, Saunders.)

A. Types of peptic ulcers (Figure 18-4).
1. Duodenal (most common).
2. Gastric.
3. Physiologic stress ulcers.
B. Histamine release occurs with the erosion of the gastric mucosa in both duodenal and gastric ulcers. This results in vasodilation and increased capillary permeability, which further stimulates the secretion of gastric acid and pepsin. The continued erosion will eventually damage the blood vessels, leading to hemorrhage or erosion through gastric mucosa.
C. Characteristics.
1. Risk factors.
a. *Helicobacter pylori:* most common factor in both types of ulcers.
b. Medications: aspirin, NSAIDs, corticosteroids, reserpine.
c. Alcohol abuse, smoking.
d. Chronic gastritis.
e. Hot, rough, or spicy foods are not a factor.
f. Duodenal ulcers are associated with high secretion of HCL acid.
g. Physiologic stress ulcers are associated with physical stress: burns, sepsis, and trauma.
2. Clinical manifestations.
a. Burning pain lasting minutes to hours; the pain associated with ulcers may be confusing, and

symptoms may overlap from one type of ulcer to another.
(1) Gastric ulcers: pain is high in epigastric area; occurs 1 to 2 hours after eating.
(2) Duodenal ulcers: pain is in midepigastric area, just below the xiphoid process, or in the back; occurs 2 to 4 hours after eating and is relieved by antacids or eating.

! NURSING PRIORITY Be careful to avoid confusing ulcer pain and indigestion with angina; do not administer antacids to cardiac clients complaining of midepigastric distress or "heartburn."

Diagnostics

A. *Helicobacter pylori:* breath test; serum and stool analysis; differentiation is made between colonization and infection.
B. Gastric analysis with possible biopsy.

Treatment

A. Medications (see Appendix 18-5).
1. Medications to eliminate *H. pylori* bacteria.
a. Metronidazole (Flagyl).
b. Omeprazole (Prilosec).
c. Clarithromycin (Biaxin), amoxicillin, tetracycline.
2. Antacids.
3. Histamine-2 receptor (H_2R) antagonists.
4. Prostaglandin analogs and proton pump inhibitors (PPIs).
B. Lifestyle modifications.
1. Eat a nonirritating or bland diet; avoid foods that cause discomfort.

2. Decrease or stop smoking.
3. Minimize use of NSAIDs and antiinflammatory medications.
4. Decrease or eliminate alcohol consumption.

Complications

A. Frequently result in an emergency situation—initially treated conservatively; however, surgery may be necessary.
B. Hemorrhage: bleeding when ulcer erodes through a vessel (see Figure 18-3).
   1. Clinical manifestations.
      a. Pain, nausea, vomiting.
      b. Hematemesis, melena, or both.
      c. More common in duodenal ulcers.
      d. Vital signs may reveal symptoms of shock (Chapter 16).
   2. Treatment.
      a. Fluid volume replacement: blood, normal saline, Ringer's lactate.
      b. Medications to decrease acid production (Appendix 18-5).
      c. NPO, nasogastric tube; saline lavage may be done.
      d. Surgery if unresponsive to conservative therapy.

> **❗ NURSING PRIORITY** Recognize and implement measures to manage potential circulatory complications (e.g., occurrence of a hemorrhage); carefully evaluate the client's blood pressure. Orthostatic hypotension (a blood pressure decrease of 10 mm Hg or more) may be indicative of hypovolemia.

C. Perforation.
   1. Clinical manifestations.
      a. Sudden, severe, unrelenting abdominal pain.
      b. Rigid, "board-like" abdomen.
      c. Hyperactive to absent bowel sounds.
      d. Severity of peritonitis is proportional to size of perforation and amount of gastric spillage (see Figure 18-6).
   2. Treatment.
      a. Antibiotics.
      b. Perforation may seal, if not, laparoscopic or surgical closure.
      c. Fluid volume replacement.
D. Gastric outlet obstruction: more common in duodenal ulcers in the area of the pyloric valve.
   1. Clinical manifestations.
      a. Gradual onset of symptoms.
      b. History of PUD.
      c. Swelling, dilation of stomach.
      d. Vomiting: foul-smelling and frequently projectile.
      e. Relief may be obtained by vomiting.
   2. Treatment.
      a. Decompress the stomach with NG suctioning; maintain continuous decompression to allow for healing.

b. Fluid volume replacement.
c. Antiulcer medications.
d. Pyloroplasty to enlarge opening of pyloric valve.
E. Surgical interventions for intractable ulcers and/or complications.
   1. Partial gastrectomy: removal of majority of stomach (antrum and pylorus) with anastomosis to either the duodenum or the jejunum.
   2. Vagotomy: severing of the vagus nerve to decrease acid-secreting stimulus to gastric cells.
   3. Pyloroplasty (pyloric stenosis repair): enlargement of pyloric valve to facilitate passage of gastric contents into the small intestine; may be done in combination with vagotomy.
F. Postoperative complications.
   1. Dumping syndrome: affects up to half of clients who have undergone gastrectomy (see Box 18-3).
   2. Postprandial hypoglycemia: results from dumping syndrome; concentrated carbohydrates cause hyperglycemia, and excessive insulin is released, causing hypoglycemia about 2 hours after meals.

> **ALERT** Teach client methods to prevent and/or manage complications associated with diagnosis.

Nursing Interventions

Goal: To promote health and prevent reoccurrence of PUD.
A. Identify factors in lifestyle contributing to development of ulcer.
B. Identify factors that precipitate pain and discomfort.
C. Avoid aspirin compounds and NSAIDs.
D. Identify presence of *H. pylori* and follow therapy; ulcers tend to reoccur, so discontinuation or interruption of therapy can be detrimental.
E. Client should not take any other medications or OTC drugs that are not prescribed.

> **ALERT** Evaluate use of home remedies and OTC drugs. The client with PUD may have been using antacids for a prolonged time.

Goal: To relieve acute pain and promote healing.
A. Dietary modifications.
   1. May be NPO with NG suctioning for acute episode of gastric pain with nausea and vomiting (Appendix 18-8).
   2. Nonirritating, bland foods are generally tolerated better during healing of acute episodes.
   3. Encourage small, frequent meals.
   4. Help client identify specific dietary habits that exacerbate or precipitate pain.
B. Identify characteristics of pain and activities that increase or decrease pain.
Goal: To promote homeostasis for client with gastric obstruction.

A. Nasogastric suctioning and careful assessment of hydration status; IV fluid replacement.

B. Reposition client from side to side to maintain good gastric suctioning.

C. After several days of decompression, NG tube may be clamped for short periods and gastric residual measured; less than 200 mL residual is within normal range.

D. When gastric residual is within normal amount, oral feedings may begin at 30 mL per hour and gradually increased; closely monitor for signs of obstruction.

Goal: To promote homeostasis when client is hemorrhaging.

A. Assess client response to hemorrhage.
   1. Evaluate hemoglobin and hematocrit levels.
   2. Assess for distention, increase in pain, and tenderness.
   3. Correlate vital signs with changes in client's overall condition.
   4. Assess stools and nasogastric drainage for presence of blood.

B. Maintain nasogastric decompression and suctioning (Appendix 18-8).
   1. Insert nasogastric tube for removal of gastric contents and maintain gastric suction.
   2. May implement saline solution lavage.

C. Monitor for hypovolemia and maintain hydration status (Chapter 6).
   1. Establish peripheral infusion line, preferably with large-gauge needle for blood infusion.
   2. Insert indwelling urinary catheter to monitor urinary output; evaluate urine specific gravity.
   3. Prepare to administer whole blood transfusion (see Appendix 14-3) and IV fluids.

D. Hemodynamic monitoring (Appendix 17-9).

E. Maintain NPO status, begin oxygen administration, maintain bed rest, and position client supine with legs slightly elevated.

Goal: To assess for complications of perforation and peritonitis (see Acute Abdomen section).

Goal: To assist client to return to homeostasis after gastric resection.

A. Provide general postoperative care as indicated (see Chapter 3).

B. Maintain nasogastric suction until peristalsis returns (see Appendix 18-8).

ALERT Monitor and maintain GI drainage. Distention and obstruction of the nasogastric tube is a common problem for this client.

C. Assess continuously for:
   1. Increasing abdominal distention.
   2. Nausea, vomiting.
   3. Changes in bowel sounds.

D. No oral fluids until client tolerates clamping and/or removal of nasogastric tube.

E. Begin oral fluids slowly: clear liquids first; then progress to bland, soft diet.

F. Based on client's condition, total parenteral nutrition may be necessary to maintain adequate nutrition (Appendix 18-7).

G. Encourage ambulation to promote peristalsis.

Goal: To identify dumping syndrome (see Box 18-3).

Goal: To prevent the development of pernicious anemia after total gastric resection (see discussion of vitamin B_{12} deficiency, Chapter 14).

 Appendicitis

Appendicitis is the inflammation and obstruction of the appendix, leading to bacterial infection. If appendicitis is not treated, the appendix can become gangrenous and burst, causing peritonitis and septicemia, which could progress to death. It is the most common reason for emergency abdominal surgery in children.

A. Obstruction of the blind sac of the appendix precipitates inflammation, ulceration, and necrosis.

B. If the necrotic area ruptures, intestinal contents spill into the peritoneal cavity, causing peritonitis.

Assessment

A. Risk factors/etiology.
   1. Age: peak at 10 to 12 years of age; uncommon in children younger than 2 years.
   2. Diet: risk associated with a diet low in fiber and high in refined sugars and carbohydrates.
   3. Obstruction to opening of appendix: hardened fecal matter, foreign bodies, or microorganisms.

B. Clinical manifestations (Figure 18-5).
   1. Abdominal cramping and pain, beginning near the navel and then migrating toward McBurney's point (right lower quadrant); pain worsens with time.
   2. Rovsing sign: pain in right lower quadrant when palpating or percussing other quadrants.
   3. Anorexia, nausea, vomiting, diarrhea.
   4. Low-grade fever.

APPENDICITIS

- Peak incidence 10-12 years
- Begins as dull, steady pain in periumbilical area...
Progresses over 4-6 hours & localizes to right lower quadrant

- Low grade fever
- Nausea
- Anorexia

- Sudden pain relief may indicate rupture of appendix (Leads to peritonitis)

Diagnosis
• Clinical signs and symptoms
• ↑ WBC
• Abdominal Sonogram
• Exploratory Lap

- Rebound Pain or Tenderness (RLQ) at McBurney's Point

CJ.MILLER ©2007 Nursing Education Consultants, Inc.

FIGURE 18-5 Appendicitis. (From Zerwekh J, Claborn J: *Memory notebook of nursing,* vol 2, ed 3, Ingram, Texas, 2007, Nursing Education Consultants)

5. Side-lying position with knees flexed.
6. Client complains of pain when asked to cough; asking client to cough is better assessment method than palpating for rebound tenderness.
7. Sudden relief from pain may indicate rupture of appendix.

C. Diagnostics: no specific diagnostic tool; diagnosis made from compilation of findings.
   1. Clinical manifestations.
   2. Urinalysis to rule out urinary tract infection.
   3. Abdominal ultrasonography and CT to differentiate from other abdominal problems.
   4. CBC reveals elevated white blood cell count.
   5. Pregnancy test for adolescent females to rule out ectopic pregnancy.

D. Complications: rupture and peritonitis.

Treatment

A. Presurgery: fluid resuscitation, prophylactic antibiotic therapy; after diagnosis of appendicitis has been established, pain management with analgesics.
B. Open appendectomy or laparoscopic appendectomy.
C. Abdominal laparotomy and peritoneal lavage if appendix has ruptured.

Nursing Interventions

Goal: To assess clinical manifestations and to prepare for surgery.
A. Careful nursing assessment for clinical manifestations (Box 18-4).
B. Maintain NPO status until otherwise indicated.
C. Maintain bed rest in position of comfort.

> **ALERT** Determine need for administration of pain medications. Do not give narcotics for pain control before a diagnosis of appendicitis is confirmed, because this could mask signs if the appendix ruptures.

D. Do not apply heat to the abdomen; cold applications may provide some relief or comfort.

Box 18-4 UNDIAGNOSED ABDOMINAL PAIN

DO NOT
Give anything by mouth.
Put any heat on the abdomen.
Give an enema.
Give strong narcotics.
Give a laxative.

DO
Maintain bed rest.
Place in a position of comfort.
Assess hydration.
Assess abdominal status: distention, bowel sounds, passage of stool or flatus, generalized or local pain.
Keep client NPO until notified otherwise.

E. Do not administer enemas.
F. Avoid unnecessary palpation of abdomen.

> **ALERT** Determine whether client is prepared for surgery or procedures. Appendicitis is a very common problem; know how to care for client during diagnostic phase.

Goal: To maintain homeostasis and healing after appendectomy (see Chapter 3).
Goal: To prevent abdominal distention and to assess bowel function after abdominal laparotomy.
A. Maintain NPO status; then begin clear liquid diet, progressing to soft diet as tolerated.
B. Gastric decompression by nasogastric tube; maintain patency and suction (Appendix 18-8).
C. Monitor abdomen for distention and increased pain.
D. Assess peristaltic activity.
E. Evaluate and record character of bowel movements.
Goal: To decrease infection and promote healing after abdominal laparotomy.
A. Place client in semi-Fowler's position to localize and prevent spread of infection and reduce abdominal tension.
B. Antibiotics are usually administered via IV infusion; monitor response to antibiotics and status of IV infusion site.
C. Monitor vital signs frequently (every 2 to 4 hours) and evaluate for escalation of infectious process.
D. Provide appropriate wound care; evaluate drainage from abdominal Penrose drains and incisional area.
Goal: To maintain adequate hydration and nutrition and to promote comfort after abdominal laparotomy.
A. Maintain adequate hydration via IV infusion.
B. Evaluate tolerance of oral liquids when nasogastric tube is removed.
C. Begin oral administration of clear liquids when peristalsis returns.
D. Progress diet as tolerated.
E. Administer analgesics as indicated.

> **ALERT** Identify infection; peritonitis is common after surgery for a ruptured appendix.

Acute Abdomen

Acute abdomen encompasses a broad spectrum of urgent pathologies frequently requiring emergent surgical intervention. Also called *peritonitis*, this condition is characterized by a generalized inflammation of the peritoneal cavity, resulting in an intraabdominal infection.

A. Intestinal motility is decreased, and fluid accumulates as a result of the inability of the intestine to reabsorb fluid.
B. Fluid leaks into the peritoneal cavity, precipitating fluid, electrolyte, and protein losses, as well as fluid depletion.

Assessment

A. Risk factors/etiology.
1. Chemical peritonitis may result from an infection, the perforation of peptic ulcer, or a ruptured ectopic pregnancy.
2. Bacterial peritonitis results from traumatic injury (abdominal trauma, ruptured appendix).
3. Chemical peritonitis is rapidly followed by bacterial peritonitis.
4. Pancreatic necrosis, pyelonephritis, ectopic pregnancy, malignancy, bile duct obstruction, and duodenal ulcer may cause acute abdomen.

ALERT Monitor status of client who has undergone surgery; identify infection. Peritonitis is a potential complication any time the abdomen is entered, either through trauma or for surgery.

B. Clinical manifestations (Figure 18-6).
1. Presence of precipitating cause.
2. Sharp or knife-like pain and/or dull and deep-seated pain over involved area; rebound tenderness; pain may radiate to back, shoulder, or scapula.
3. Sudden, excruciating pain suggests the possibility of rupture.
4. Abdominal mass or distention: note color and contour of abdomen.
5. Abdominal muscle rigidity ("board-like" abdomen), guarding.
6. Unexplained persistent or labile fever.
7. Anorexia, nausea, vomiting.
8. Tachycardia, hypotension, shallow respirations: signs of impending or actual shock.
9. Decreased or absent bowel sounds.
10. Hypovolemia, dehydration.
11. Shallow respirations in attempt to avoid pain.
C. Diagnostics.
1. CBC for elevated white blood cell count and hemoconcentration of fluid shifts (Chapter 6).

2. Abdominal CT and ultrasonography.
3. Peritoneal lavage (aspiration) to evaluate abdominal fluid.

Treatment

A. Identify and treat precipitating cause; frequently requires surgical intervention.
B. Narcotic analgesic may be administered during diagnostic phase to ensure client cooperation.
C. Antibiotics.
D. IV fluids and electrolyte replacement.
E. Decrease abdominal distention: NPO, NG tube.

Nursing Interventions

Goal: To provide pain control, wound care, prevent complications of immobility, and monitor postoperative progress (Chapter 3).
Goal: To maintain fluid and electrolyte balances and reduce gastric distention.
A. Maintain nasogastric suction (Appendix 18-8).
B. Maintain IV fluid replacement: normal saline or lactated Ringer's solution to maintain hydration and urine output of 30 mL/hr; assess urine specific gravity.
C. Administer potassium supplements with caution because of possible renal complications.
D. Assess level of distention and return of peristalsis and bowel function.
E. Maintain intake and output records.
F. Assess for problems of dehydration and hypovolemia (Chapter 6).
G. Encourage activities to facilitate return of bowel function.
1. Encourage ambulation.
2. Attempt to decrease analgesics and maintain adequate pain control.
3. Maintain adequate hydration.

FIGURE 18-6 Peritonitis. (From Zerwekh J, Claborn J: *Memory notebook of nursing,* vol 2, ed 3, Ingram, Texas, 2007, Nursing Education Consultants.)

Goal: To reduce infectious process.

A. Administer antibiotics via IV infusion; assess client's tolerance of antibiotics and status of infusion site.

B. Evaluate vital signs and correlate with progress of infectious process.

C. Maintain in semi-Fowler's position to enhance respirations, as well as to localize drainage and prevent formation of subdiaphragmatic abscess.

Diverticular Disease

When a diverticulum (a pouch-like herniation of superficial layers of the colon through weakened muscle of the bowel wall) becomes inflamed, it is known as diverticulitis. Multiple diverticula are known as diverticulosis. Meckel's diverticulum is diverticular disease of the ileum in children. It is the most common congenital anomaly of the GI tract in children.

Assessment

A. Risk factors/etiology.
1. Diet.
   a. Low-fiber diet; high intake of processed foods.
   b. Constipation.
   c. Indigestible fibers (corn, seeds, etc.) may precipitate diverticulitis, but they do not contribute to the development of diverticula.
2. Age: 50% of adults are affected by age 80 years.
3. As diverticula form, the colon wall becomes thickened; diverticulitis results from retention of stool and bacteria in the diverticulum.
4. Inactivity and constipation.

B. Clinical manifestations.
1. Diverticular disease is frequently asymptomatic; symptoms vary with degree of inflammation.
2. Diverticulitis occurs when undigested food and bacteria are trapped in the diverticula.
   a. Fever.
   b. Left lower quadrant pain; may be accompanied by nausea and vomiting.
   c. Abdominal distention and increased pain on palpation.
   d. May progress to abscess, intestinal obstruction, and/or perforation.

C. Diagnostics (Appendix 18-1).
1. Computed tomography and/or ultrasound.
2. Barium enema or colonoscopy are contraindicated in acute diverticulitis.

Treatment

A. Management of uncomplicated diverticulum.
1. High-fiber diet.
2. Decreased intake of fat and red meat.
3. Stool softeners, bulk laxatives.
4. Increased activity: walking, exercise.

B. Diverticulitis.
1. Oral antibiotics when symptoms are mild.
2. Antispasmodic medications.
3. Liquid or low-fiber diet.

C. Severe diverticulitis.
1. Broad-spectrum antibiotics.
2. Bowel rest: NPO; may have an NG tube; hydration with IV fluids.
3. Pain management with opioids; avoid morphine (decreases peristalsis).
4. Surgery for obstruction, abscess, hemorrhage, or perforation.

Goal: To help client understand dietary implications and maintain prescribed therapy to prevent exacerbations.

A. Teach client about eating a high-fiber diet when asymptomatic.

B. Maintain high fluid intake.

ALERT Adapt the diet to the special needs of the client; determine client's ability to perform self-care.

C. Weight reduction, if indicated.

D. Avoid activities that increase intraabdominal pressure (e.g., straining at stool, bending, lifting); avoid wearing tight restrictive clothing.

E. Use bulk laxatives, avoid enemas and harsh laxatives.

Goal: To decrease colon activity in client with diverticulitis.

A. Maintain clear liquids or NPO status.

B. Bed rest.

C. Adequate hydration via parenteral fluids.

D. As attack subsides, gradually introduce food and fluids.

Home Care

A. High-fiber diet to prevent diverticulitis.

B. If client has any abdominal distress, all fiber should be avoided until tenderness resolves.

C. Report fevers, constant abdominal pain, and dark, tarry stools.

Inflammatory Bowel Disease (IBD)

IBD is characterized by chronic inflammation of the intestine with periods of remission and exacerbation. It is considered an autoimmune disease; tissue damage is due to overactive sustained inflammatory response.

A. **Crohn's disease** (ileitis or enteritis) is inflammation occurring anywhere along the GI tract; patches of inflammation occur next to healthy bowel tissue; most frequent site is the terminal ileum.

B. **Ulcerative colitis** is an inflammation and ulceration that most commonly occurs in the sigmoid colon and rectum; inflammation frequently begins in the rectum and spreads in a continuous manner up the colon; seldom is the small intestine involved.

C. Clients frequently experience periods of complete remission that alternate with exacerbations.

D. Even though the two conditions have different criteria for diagnosis, a clear differentiation cannot be made between them in about one-third of the cases.

Assessment

A. Risk factors/etiology.
   1. Familial tendency.
   2. Commonly occur in the teenage years, with a second peak in occurrence in clients 60 years old and older.
   3. Altered inflammatory response.
B. Clinical manifestations—Crohn's disease.
   1. Steatorrhea, multiple diarrhea stools per day.
   2. Weight loss; nutritional deficiencies; impaired absorption of vitamin B_{12} (cobalamin).
   3. Intermittent fever.
   4. Entire thickness of bowel wall is involved; fistulas are not uncommon.
   5. Nausea, cramping, flatulence.
C. Clinical manifestations—ulcerative colitis.
   1. Rectal bleeding.
   2. Diarrhea, one to two diarrhea stools per day; may contain small amounts of blood.
   3. Number of stools increases with exacerbation of condition; 10-20 stools per day in acute exacerbation.
   4. Increased in systemic symptoms (fever, malaise, anorexia) with exacerbation.
   5. Tenesmus (uncontrollable straining).
   6. Minimal small bowel involvement.
D. Diagnostics (see Appendix 18-1).

Complications

A. Crohn's disease.
   1. Perirectal and intraabdominal fistulas; fissures and rectal abscesses.
   2. Perforation and peritonitis.
   3. Nutritional deficiencies, especially of fat-soluble vitamins.
B. Ulcerative colitis.
   1. Perforation and peritonitis with toxic megacolon.
   2. Increased risk for cancer after 10 years.

Treatment

A. Dietary modifications: increased calories, protein, and fluids. Encourage client to eat small servings several times a day.
B. Medications for Crohn's disease.
   1. Antiinflammatory: aminosalicylates (sulfasalazine; see Appendix 6-9) and corticosteroids (see Appendix 6-7).
   2. Antimicrobials: prevent or treat infection.
   3. Immunosuppressants to decrease or suppress the immune response (see Appendix 23-3).
   4. Antidiarrheals.
C. Medications for ulcerative colitis: aminosalicylates and corticosteroids to decrease inflammation.
D. Surgical intervention may be necessary if client fails to respond to medical management and if fistulas, perforation, bleeding, or intestinal obstruction occur.
   1. Total removal of colon, rectum, and anus with formation of permanent ileostomy (Appendix 18-12).
   2. Total removal of colon, rectum, and anus with formation of continent ileostomy (Kock's pouch).
   3. Minimally invasive surgery (MIS) involves a laparoscopy to remove small areas of diseased tissue in the ileum and ileocecal areas.

Nursing Interventions

Goal: To promote hemodynamic stability and hydration.
A. Evaluate and maintain adequate hydration status.
B. Encourage good fluid intake (3000 mL/day).
C. Evaluate electrolyte status; monitor potassium level if on corticosteroids.
D. Assess characteristics in patterns of stool.

Goal: To promote nutrition.
A. Balanced diet with increased protein and calories.
B. Assess for iron deficiency anemia due to blood loss and reduced intake of iron.
C. Assess for anemia due to lack of absorption of vitamin B_{12} (cobalamin); monthly injections or daily oral or nasal spray may be necessary.
D. Help client identify and avoid foods that precipitate diarrhea.
E. Parenteral nutrition or enteral feeding may be necessary because of malabsorption (Appendix 18-7, Appendix 18-9).
F. Supplemental folic acid for clients on long-term sulfasalazine treatment.
G. Supplemental liquid nutrition.

Goal: To promote emotional and psychosocial stability.
A. Frequent bowel movements, rectal discomfort, and uncontrollable disease result in anxiety, frustration, and depression—promote comfort by keeping anal area clean and keeping room clear of offensive odors.
B. Establish trust, encourage self-care strategies, explain all procedures and treatments.
C. Encourage rest to prevent fatigue.
D. Symptoms of reoccurrence of the problem—call the physician if these occur.
   1. Continued diarrhea and weight loss.
   2. Chills, fever, malaise.

Home Care

A. Dietary modifications, avoidance of foods that cause diarrhea.
B. Medication regimen: precautions regarding steroids or immunosuppressive medications.
C. Dressings and wound care if fistula is present.
D. Identify appropriate measures to decrease stress in lifestyle.
E. Acute symptoms may be exacerbated or, as disease progresses, may become chronic.

Intestinal Obstruction

Interference with normal peristalsis and impairment to forward flow of intestinal contents is known as intestinal obstruction.

FIGURE 18-7 Bowel obstructions. (From Lewis SL et al: *Medical-surgical nursing: assessment and management of clinical problems,* ed 7, St. Louis, 2007, Mosby.)

A. Types of obstruction (Figure 18-7).
  1. Mechanical obstruction.
    a. Strangulated hernia.
    b. Intussusception: the telescoping of one portion of the intestine into another (occurs most often in infants and small children).
    c. Volvulus: twisting of the bowel.
    d. Tumors: cancer (most frequent cause of obstruction in older adults).
    e. Adhesions.
  2. Neurogenic: interference with nerve supply in the intestine.
    a. Paralytic ileus or adynamic ileus occurring as a result of abdominal surgery or inflammatory process.
    b. Potential sequelae from spinal cord injury.
  3. Vascular obstruction: interference with the blood supply to the bowel.
    a. Infarction of superior mesenteric artery.
    b. Bowel obstructions related to intestinal ischemia may occur very rapidly and may be life-threatening.
B. Regardless of the precipitating cause, the ensuing problems are a result of the obstructive process.
C. The higher the obstruction in the intestine, the more rapidly symptoms will occur.
D. Fluid, gas, and intestinal contents accumulate proximal to the obstruction. This causes distention proximal to the obstruction and bowel collapse distal to the obstruction.
E. As fluid accumulation increases, so does pressure against the bowel. This precipitates extravasation of fluids and electrolytes into the peritoneal cavity. Increased pressure may cause the bowel to rupture.

F. Increased pressure causes an increase in capillary permeability and leakage of fluids and electrolytes into peritoneal fluid; this leads to a severe reduction in circulating volume.
G. Intussusception is the most common cause of intestinal obstruction in children from ages 3 months to 6 years.
H. The location of the obstruction determines the extent of fluid and electrolyte imbalance and acid-base imbalance.
  1. Dehydration and electrolyte imbalance do not occur rapidly if obstruction is in the large intestine.
  2. If the obstruction is located high in the intestine, dehydration occurs rapidly because of the inability of the intestine to reabsorb fluids; metabolic alkalosis develops from loss of gastric acid due to vomiting or NG suctioning.

Assessment

A. Risk factors/etiology: identify type of obstruction and precipitating cause.
B. Clinical manifestations.
  1. Vomiting.
    a. Occurs early and is more severe if the obstruction is high.
    b. Higher obstruction may contain bile, and vomiting may be projectile.
    c. Vomiting caused by lower obstructions occurs more slowly and may be foul smelling due to the presence of bacteria and fecal material.
  2. Abdominal distention.
  3. Bowel sounds initially may be hyperactive proximal to the obstruction and decreased or absent distal to the obstruction; eventually, all bowel sounds will be absent.

4. Colicky-type abdominal pain.
5. Fluid and electrolyte imbalances, dehydration.
6. Intussusception.
   a. Child is healthy with sudden occurrence of acute abdominal pain.
   b. Child may pass one normal stool; then as condition deteriorates, the child may pass a stool described as "currant jelly" (a mixture of blood and mucus).
   c. A "sausage-shaped" mass may be palpated in the abdomen.

ALERT Determine characteristics of bowel sounds. This is particularly important for the client with intestinal problems.

C. Diagnostics (Appendix 18-1).
   a. Abdominal x-ray to differentiate obstruction from perforation.
   b. Barium enema to identify area of obstruction; only done after a bowel perforation has been ruled out.

Complications

A. Infection/septicemia.
B. Gangrene of the bowel.
C. Perforation of the bowel.
D. Severe dehydration and electrolyte imbalances.

Treatment

A. Mechanical and vascular intestinal obstructions are generally treated surgically; ileostomy or colostomy may be necessary.
B. Conservative treatment includes nasogastric suctioning and decompression (Appendix 18-8).
C. Fluid and electrolyte replacement.
D. Intussusception: hydrostatic reduction by water-soluble contrast, air, or barium enema.

Nursing Interventions

Goal: To prepare client for diagnostic evaluation and to maintain ongoing nursing assessment for pertinent data (see Appendix 18-1).
A. Monitor all stools; passage of normal stool may indicate reduction of the obstruction, especially an intussusception.
B. Classic signs and symptoms of intussusception may not be present; observe child for diarrhea, anorexia, vomiting, and episodic abdominal pain.
Goal: To decrease gastric distention and to maintain hydration and electrolyte balance.
A. Maintain NPO status.
B. Maintain nasogastric suction (Appendix 18-8).
C. Monitor IV fluid replacement: most often normal saline or lactated Ringer's solution.
D. Administer potassium supplements with caution because of complications of decreased renal function.
E. Evaluate peristalsis, presence of any bowel function.
F. Maintain accurate intake and output records.
G. Assess for dehydration, hypovolemia, and electrolyte imbalance (Chapter 6).

H. Measure abdominal girth to determine whether distention is increasing.
I. Encourage activities to facilitate return of bowel function.
   1. Encourage physical activity, as tolerated.
   2. Attempt to decrease amount of medication required for effective pain control.
   3. Maintain hydration.
J. Frequently, the position of comfort is side-lying with knees flexed.
Goal: To provide appropriate preoperative preparation when surgery is indicated (see Chapter 3).
Goal: To maintain homeostasis and promote healing after abdominal laparotomy (see Chapter 3).
Goal: To decrease infection and promote healing after surgery.
A. Monitor client's response to antibiotics.
B. Monitor vital signs frequently and evaluate for presence or escalation of infectious process.
C. Provide wound care. Evaluate drainage and healing from abdominal Penrose or Jackson-Pratt drains, as well as from abdominal incisional area.

ALERT Empty and reestablish negative pressure of portable wound suction devices (Hemovac and Jackson-Pratt drains).

Goal: To reestablish normal nutrition and promote comfort after abdominal laparotomy.
A. Evaluate tolerance of liquids when nasogastric tube is removed.
B. Begin administration of clear liquids initially and continue to evaluate for peristalsis and/or distention, nausea, and vomiting.
C. Progress diet as tolerated.
D. Administer analgesics as indicated.
E. Promote psychologic comfort.
   1. Respond promptly to requests.
   2. Carefully explain procedures.
   3. Encourage questions and ventilation of feelings regarding status of illness.
   4. Encourage parents to ask questions and to room-in with infant or child; rapidity of the onset of child's condition challenges parents' ability to cope.

Hernia

A hernia is a protrusion of the intestine through an abnormal opening or weakened area of the abdominal wall.
A. Types.
   1. Inguinal: a weakness in which the spermatic cord in men and the round ligament in women passes through the abdominal wall in the groin area; more common in men; most common type of hernia in children.
   2. Femoral: protrusion of the intestine through the femoral ring; more common in women.
   3. Umbilical: occurs most often in children when the umbilical opening fails to close adequately; most

common hernia in infants; may occur in adults when the rectus muscle is weak from surgical incision.

4. Incisional or ventral: weakness in the abdominal wall caused by a previous incision.

5. Classification.
   a. Reducible: hernia may be replaced into the abdominal cavity by manual manipulation.
   b. Incarcerated or irreducible: hernia cannot be pushed back into place.
   c. Strangulated: blood supply and intestinal flow in the herniated area are obstructed; strangulated hernia leads to intestinal obstruction.

B. Risk factors.
   1. Chronic cough, such as smoker's cough or cough associated with cystic fibrosis.
   2. Obesity or weakened abdominal musculature.
   3. Straining during bowel movement or lifting heavy objects.
   4. Pregnancy.

Assessment

A. Clinical manifestations.
   1. Hernia protrudes over the involved area when the client stands or strains, or when the infant cries.
   2. Severe pain occurs if hernia becomes strangulated.
   3. Strangulated hernia produces symptoms of intestinal obstruction.

B. Diagnostics (Appendix 18-1).

Treatment

A. Preferably elective surgery through abdominal incision.
B. Laparoscopic hernia repair.
C. Emergency surgery for strangulated hernias producing intestinal obstruction.

Nursing Interventions

Goal: To prepare client for surgery, if indicated (see Chapter 3).

Goal: To maintain homeostasis and promote healing after herniorrhaphy.

A. General postoperative nursing care (see Chapter 3).
B. Repair of an indirect inguinal hernia: assess male clients for development of scrotal edema.
C. Encourage deep breathing and activity.
D. If coughing occurs, teach client how to splint the incision.
E. Refrain from heavy lifting for approximately 6 to 8 weeks after surgery.
F. Wound care.
   a. Keep wound clean and dry: use occlusive dressing or leave open to air.
   b. Change diapers frequently and/or prevent irritation and contamination in incisional area.

Pyloric Stenosis

Pyloric stenosis is the obstruction of the pyloric sphincter by hypertrophy and hyperplasia of the circular muscle of the pylorus.

Assessment

A. Risk factors/etiology.
   1. Occurs most often in first-born, full-term male infants (infantile hypertrophic pyloric stenosis).
   2. Seen more frequently in Caucasian infants.
   3. First-born male infant of a mother who was affected is at increased risk.

B. Clinical manifestations.
   1. Onset of vomiting may be gradual, usually occurs at 3 weeks or as late as 5 months; is progressive and may be projectile.
   2. Emesis is not bile stained but may be curdled from length of time in stomach.
   3. Vomiting occurs shortly after feeding.
   4. Infant is hungry and irritable.
   5. Infant does not appear to be in pain or acute distress.
   6. Weight loss occurs, if untreated.
   7. Stools decrease in number and in size.
   8. Dehydration occurs as condition progresses; hypochloremia and hypokalemia occur as vomiting continues.
   9. Upper abdomen is distended, and an "olive-shaped" mass may be palpated in the right epigastric area.

C. Diagnostics (Appendix 18-1).

D. Treatment: surgical release of the pyloric muscle (pyloromyotomy).

Nursing Interventions

Goal: To maintain hydration and gastric decompression; to initiate appropriate preoperative nursing activities (Appendix 18-8).

A. Maintain nasogastric decompression if NG tube is in place and record type and amount of drainage.
B. Assess hydration status and electrolyte balance—especially serum calcium, sodium, and potassium levels.
C. NPO status with continuous IV infusion (most often saline solutions) may be required.
D. Accurate intake and output records: complete description of all vomitus and stools.
E. Monitor vital signs and check for signs of peritonitis.
F. Preoperative teaching for parents.

Goal: To maintain adequate hydration and promote healing after pyloromyotomy.

A. Postoperative vomiting in the first 24 to 48 hours is not uncommon; maintain IV fluids until infant tolerates adequate oral intake.
B. Continue to monitor infant in the same manner as in the preoperative period.
C. Feedings are initiated early; bottle-fed infant may begin with clear liquids containing glucose and electrolytes, small amounts offered frequently.
D. Breastfed infants: mother can express breast milk and offer small amounts in a bottle or initially limit nursing time.

Goal: To help parents provide appropriate home care after pyloromyotomy.

A. No residual problems are anticipated after surgery.
B. Instruct parents regarding care of the incisional area.

Cancer of the Stomach

Tumors in the cardia and fundus of the stomach are associated with a poor prognosis.

A. Cancer (adenocarcinoma) occurs in the wall of the stomach.

B. Metastasis generally occurs by direct extension of the malignant growth into adjacent organs and structures (esophagus, spleen, pancreas, etc.).

C. Because of the ability of the stomach to accommodate the growing tumor, symptoms may not be evident until metastasis has occurred.

Assessment

A. Risk factors/etiology.
   1. Increased incidence in men.
   2. Peak incidence in seventh decade.
   3. Presence of *H. pylori* is considered an increased risk factor
   4. Increased incidence in presence of other chronic gastric problems.

B. Clinical manifestations.
   1. Early symptoms.
      a. Loss of appetite, persistent indigestion.
      b. Early satiety, dyspepsia.
      c. Nausea, vomiting.
      d. Blood in stool.
   2. Later symptoms.
      a. Pain often exacerbated by eating.
      b. Weight loss, anemia.
      c. Nausea and vomiting due to impending GI obstruction.
      d. Presence of a palpable mass in the stomach; ascites from involvement of peritoneal cavity.

C. Diagnostics (Appendix 18-1).
   1. Gastroscopy and biopsy.
   2. Full-body imaging for metastasis.

Treatment

Gastrectomy is the preferred method of treatment.

Nursing Interventions

See Nursing Interventions for gastric resection under Peptic Ulcer Disease.

Cancer of the Colon and Rectum (Colorectal Cancer)

Colorectal cancer (cancer of the colon and/or the rectum) is the third most common cancer in the United States and the second leading cause of cancer-related deaths.

A. 85% of colorectal cancers arise from adenomatous polyps that can be detected and removed by sigmoidoscopy or colonoscopy.

B. Symptoms frequently do not appear until condition is advanced with metastatic sites.

C. Most common areas of metastasis include regional lymph nodes, liver, lungs, and peritoneum.

Assessment

A. Risk factors/etiology.
   1. Family history (first-degree relative) of colorectal cancer.
   2. Incidence increases significantly after the age of 50.
   3. History of inflammatory bowel disease.
   4. High-fat, high-calorie, low-residue diet with high intake of red meat increases anaerobic bacteria in bowel, which convert bile acids into carcinogens.
   5. Alcohol, tobacco use, and obesity are also associated with increased risk.

B. Clinical manifestations.
   1. Symptoms are vague early in disease state and may take years to present.
   2. Bloody stools, melena (dark tarry) stools.
   3. Change in bowel habits: constipation and diarrhea.
   4. Change in shape of stool (pencil- or ribbon-shaped in sigmoid or rectal cancer).
   5. Weakness and fatigue from iron deficiency anemia and chronic blood loss.
   6. Pain, anorexia, and unexpected weight loss are late symptoms.
   7. Bowel obstruction may lead to perforation and peritonitis.

C. Diagnostics (Appendix 18-1).
   1. Sigmoidoscopy and colonoscopy with biopsies.
   2. Carcinoembryonic antigen (CEA) tumor marker detected in blood.

Treatment

A. Colon resection: may have resection with or without a colostomy or may have an abdominal-perineal resection that includes resection of the sigmoid colon, rectum, and anus.

B. Laser photocoagulation: destroys small tumors and palliative for large tumors obstructing bowel.

C. Endoscopic excision or electrocoagulation for small, localized tumors or for clients who are poor surgical candidates.

D. Radiation therapy: external, intracavity, or implanted; may be used preoperatively to shrink tumor size.

E. Chemotherapy: reduces recurrence and prolongs survival in stage II and III rectal tumors.

Nursing Interventions

Goal: To provide information to high-risk clients.

A. Diet: high-fiber, low-fat diet with a decreased intake of red meat.

B. Digital rectal exams yearly after age 40.

C. Annual fecal occult blood testing after age 50.

D. Flexible sigmoidoscopy or colonoscopy every 3 or 5 years after age 50 for high risk; otherwise every 10 years for average risk.

Goal: To provide preoperative care.

A. Determine extent of surgery anticipated; colostomy is not always done.

B. Bowel preparation: low-residue diet, cathartics 24 hours before surgery; enemas may or may not be used the evening before surgery.

C. Oral neomycin to decrease bacteria in the bowel.

D. If colostomy is to be done, discuss implications and identify appropriate area for stoma on abdomen (see Appendix 18-12).

E. Prepare client for change in body image if colostomy is indicated.

Goal: To provide appropriate wound care after abdominal-perineal resection.

A. Client will have three incisional areas.
  1. Abdominal incision.
  2. Incisional area for colostomy.
  3. Perineal incision.

> **ALERT** Identify factors interfering with wound healing and/or symptoms of infection.

B. Perineal wound.
  1. Wound may be left open to heal by secondary intention: provide warm sitz baths (100.4° to 100.6° F) for 10 to 20 minutes to promote debridement, increase circulation to the area, and promote comfort.
  2. Wound may be partially closed with drains (Jackson-Pratt and/or Hemovac) in place: assess the wound for integrity of suture line and presence of infection; drainage should be serosanguineous; drains remain in place until drainage is less than 50 mL/24 hour (Chapter 3).
  3. Wound may be open and packed: drainage is profuse first several hours after surgery; may require frequent reinforcement and dressing change; drainage is serosanguineous.

C. Position client with a perineal wound on his or her side; do not allow client to sit for prolonged period until wound is healed.

D. Assess status of stoma and healing of abdominal incision (see Appendix 18-12).

Goal: To maintain homeostasis and promote healing after abdominal-perineal resection or colon resection (see Chapter 3).

A. Infections, hemorrhage, wound disruption, thrombophlebitis, and stoma problems are the most common complications.

B. Help client begin to become independent with colostomy care early in recovery period (see Appendix 18-12).

Goal: To provide psychosocial support.

A. Emotional support is essential with cancer diagnosis; recovery is long and frequently painful.

B. Sexual dysfunction may occur; determine from physician if nerve paths for erection and ejaculation were in area of resection; provide opportunity for questions.

C. Keep room clean and free of offensive smells; client may be very self-conscious regarding open wound and/or stoma; provide opportunity for questions and discussion.

 Home Care

A. Recovery period is long; help client and family identify community resources.

B. Help client and family identify resources and obtain equipment for colostomy care (see Appendix 18-12).

C. Instruct client in care of perineal wound if it is not healed.
  1. Sitz baths: always check temperature of water; wound tissue can be easily damaged.
  2. Presence of continuous drainage may indicate a fistula.

D. Identify community resources for client: home health visits, social services, etc.

E. Assess client's ability to care for stoma; help client begin self-care before discharge (Appendix 18-12).

 Celiac Disease (Malabsorption Syndrome)

Celiac disease is also known as *sprue, gluten enteropathy,* and *malabsorption syndrome.* This disease is an immune reaction to rye, wheat, barley, and oat grains that leads to an inflammatory response, causing damage to the villi of the small intestines and resulting in the inability to absorb nutrients (malabsorption).

A. Previously considered a disease of childhood with symptoms beginning between the ages of 1 year and 5 years; celiac disease is now commonly seen at all ages with mean age of diagnosis being 40 years.

B. Symptoms frequently begin in early childhood, but condition may not be diagnosed until client is an adult.

C. Development of celiac disease is dependent on genetic predisposition, ingestion of gluten, and immune-mediated response.

Assessment

A. Cause: congenital defect or an autoimmune response in gluten metabolism.

B. Clinical manifestations.
  1. Symptoms may begin when child has increased intake of foods containing gluten: cereals, crackers, breads, cookies, pastas, etc.
  2. Foul-smelling diarrhea with abdominal distention and anorexia in infants and toddlers.
  3. Poor weight gain in children, failure to thrive.
  4. Constipation, vomiting, and abdominal pain may be the initial presenting symptoms in adults.
  5. Vitamin deficiency leads to central nervous system impairment and bone malformation.
  6. May be associated with other autoimmune conditions (rheumatoid arthritis, type 1 diabetes, thyroid disease).

C. Diagnostics: biopsy of duodenum and small intestine.

Treatment

Primarily dietary management: gluten-free diet.

Nursing Interventions

Goal: To help client and family understand diet therapy and promote optimal nutrition intake.

A. Written information regarding a gluten-free diet; corn, rice, potato, and soy products may be substituted for wheat in diet.

B. Diet should be well balanced and high in protein.

C. Teach client and/or family how to read food labels for gluten content; thickenings, soups, instant foods may contain hidden sources of gluten.

D. Important to discuss the necessity of maintaining a life-long gluten-restricted diet; problems may occur in clients who relax their diet and experience an exacerbation of the disease state.

E. Lack of adherence to dietary restrictions may precipitate growth retardation, anemia, and bone deformities.

ALERT Adapt the diet to meet client's specific needs.

Hirschsprung's Disease

Hirschsprung's disease (congenital aganglionic megacolon) is characterized by a congenital absence of ganglionic cells that innervate a segment of the colon wall.

A. Clinical symptoms vary depending on the age when symptoms are recognized, the length of the affected bowel, and presence of inflammation.

B. Most common site is the rectosigmoid colon; colon proximal to the area dilates (i.e., megacolon).

Assessment

A. Risk factors/etiology: congenital anomaly.

B. Clinical manifestations.
1. May be acute and life-threatening or may be a chronic presentation.
2. Internal sphincter loses ability to relax for defecation.
3. Newborn.
   a. Failure to pass meconium within 48 hours after birth.
   b. Vomiting, abdominal distention.
   c. Reluctance to take fluids.
4. Older infant and child.
   a. Chronic constipation, impactions.
   b. Passage of ribbon-like, foul-smelling stools and diarrhea.
   c. Failure to thrive.
   d. Lack of appetite.

C. Diagnostics: rectal biopsy to confirm.

Treatment

A. Surgical correction usually involves resection of aganglionic bowel with creation of a temporary colostomy to relieve the obstruction.

B. The final repair closes the colostomy, and the bowel is reanastomosed.

Nursing Interventions

Goal: To promote normal attachment and prepare infant and parents for surgery.

A. Allow parents to ventilate feelings regarding congenital defect of infant.

B. Foster infant-parent attachment.

C. General preoperative preparation of the infant; neonate does not require any bowel preparation.

D. Careful explanation of colostomy to parents.

Goal: See Nursing Interventions for client who has undergone abdominal surgery in the Intestinal Obstruction section of this chapter.

Goal: To help parents understand and provide appropriate home care for their infant/child after colostomy (see Appendix 18-12).

A. Colostomy is most often temporary.

B. Parents should be actively involved in colostomy care before discharge.

Hemorrhoids

Dilated hemorrhoidal veins of the anus and rectum; may be internal (above the internal sphincter) or external (outside of the external sphincter).

Assessment

A. Risk factors/etiology: conditions that increase anorectal pressure.
1. Pregnancy, obesity, prolonged constipation.
2. Prolonged standing or sitting.
3. Portal hypertension.
4. Straining at bowel movement.

B. Clinical manifestations.
1. External hemorrhoids appear as protrusions at the anus.
2. Prolapsed hemorrhoids may bleed or become thrombosed.
3. Thrombosed hemorrhoid: a blood clot in a hemorrhoid that causes inflammation and pain.
4. Rectal bleeding during defecation.

C. Diagnostics: rectal examination.

Treatment

A. Conservative treatment.
1. Sitz baths, stool softeners, ointments, topical anesthetics.
2. Prevent constipation: diet high in fiber (bran) and roughage with increased water intake.
3. Avoid straining with bowel movement; keep anal area clean.

B. Aggressive treatment.
1. Ligation of prolapsed, thrombosed hemorrhoids with small rubber band.
2. Infrared coagulation for bleeding hemorrhoids.
3. Surgery for painful, large, bleeding hemorrhoids.

Nursing Interventions

Goal: To provide appropriate information to help client manage problem at home.

A. Avoid prolonged standing or sitting.
B. Take sitz baths to decrease discomfort.
C. Use OTC ointments to decrease discomfort.
D. Apply ice pack, followed by a warm sitz bath, if severe discomfort occurs.
E. Avoid constipation and straining at stool.

 Home Care

A. Encourage bulk laxatives and increased fluid intake to promote soft stool for first bowel movement.
B. Rectal pain may be severe; analgesics and local application of moist heat may be used.
C. Review preventive techniques; weight loss and avoidance of constipation.

Appendix 18-1 GASTROINTESTINAL SYSTEM DIAGNOSTICS

X-Ray
Upper Gastrointestinal Series or Barium Swallow

X-ray examination in which barium is used as a contrast material; used to diagnose structural abnormalities and problems of the esophagus and stomach. As the client swallows the barium, x-ray films are obtained to show the structures, function, position, and abnormalities of organs from mouth through jejunum.

Nursing Implications

1. Explain procedure to client (usually not done on client with acute abdomen until possibility of perforation has been ruled out).
2. Maintain client's nothing by mouth (NPO) status 8 hours before procedure.
3. Client will swallow barium to coat the GI tract for visualization of various landmarks and structures.
4. After examination, promote normal excretion of barium to prevent impaction. Barium can cause constipation, so encourage extra fluid. It may be necessary to use a stool softener or laxative to promote evacuation of barium.
5. Stool should return to normal color within 72 hours.

Lower Gastrointestinal Series or Barium Enema

X-ray examination of the colon in which barium is used as a contrast medium; barium is administered rectally.

Nursing Implications

1. Maintain client's NPO status for 8 hours before test. Client may have clear liquids the evening before the test.
2. Colon must be free of stool; laxatives and enemas are administered the evening before the test.
3. Explain to client that he or she may experience cramping and the urge to defecate during the procedure.
4. After the procedure, increase fluids and administer a laxative to assist in expelling the barium.

Endoscopy
Gastroscopy, Esophagogastroduodenoscopy (EGD), Colonoscopy, Sigmoidoscopy

Endoscopy is the direct visualization of the gastrointestinal tract (GI) via a flexible, fiberoptic, lighted scope.

Upper GI: inflammation, ulcerations, tumors; evaluation and treatment of esophageal varices.

Lower GI: evaluation of diverticular disease or irritable bowel syndrome; treatment of active bleeding or ulceration; identification of polyps, tumors, inflammation, fissures, or hemorrhoids. The endoscope is capable of obtaining biopsy specimens and clipping benign polyps.

Nursing Implications Before Procedure

1. Upper GI: NPO for up to 12 hours before procedure.
2. Lower GI: bowel prep—cathartics and/or enemas, clear liquid diet for 24 hours before test.

3. Client should avoid aspirin, NSAIDs, iron supplements, and gelatin containing red coloring for a week before procedure.
4. May give preoperative medication for relaxation and to decrease secretions.
5. For upper GI studies, a topical anesthesia will be used to anesthetize the throat before insertion of the scope.
6. Upper GI studies: assess client's mouth for dentures and removable bridges.
7. Lower GI studies: help client into the left side-lying, knee-chest position; explain the need to take a deep breath during the insertion of the scope; client may feel urge to defecate as scope is passed.
8. Conscious sedation frequently used for lower GI studies or colonoscopy.

Nursing Implications During Procedure

1. Verify informed consent and client identification.
2. For upper GI studies, confirm NPO status for past 8 hours; for lower GI studies, confirm bowel preparation.
3. Assess for presence of GI bleeding; notify physician if any bleeding is present.
4. Maintain safety: airway precautions during sedation; positioning, monitor level of sedation (Chapter 3).

Nursing Implications After Procedure

1. Upper GI: *maintain client's NPO status until the gag reflex returns;* position client on his or her side to prevent aspiration until gag or cough reflex returns; use throat lozenges or warm saline solution gargles for relief of sore throat.
2. Monitor vital signs and O_2 saturation during recovery.
3. Observe for signs of perforation: upper GI bleeding—dysphagia, substernal or epigastric pain; lower GI bleeding—rectal bleeding, increasing abdominal distention.
4. Assist client to upright position: observe for orthostatic hypotension.
5. Warm sitz bath for any anal discomfort.

Analysis of Specimens
Paracentesis; Diagnostic Peritoneal Lavage

Procedure: A catheter is inserted into the peritoneal cavity, most often just below the umbilicus.

Purposes

1. To determine effect of blunt abdominal trauma.
2. To assess for presence of ascites.
3. To identify cause of acute abdominal problems (e.g., perforation, hemorrhage).
   - To assess for intraabdominal bleeding after a blunt trauma to the abdomen. If no blood is aspirated, normal saline is infused into the peritoneal cavity. The fluid is aspirated or allowed to drain by gravity. Fluid should return clear with a slight yellow cast if there is no injury. Bloody fluids, presence

Continued

Appendix 18-1   GASTROINTESTINAL SYSTEM DIAGNOSTICS—cont'd

of bacterial or fecal material, high white or red blood cell count occur with a positive test result; immediate surgery may be required.

- If client has abdominal fluid from ascites or other abdominal pathologic conditions, a specimen of the fluid is obtained without instilling fluid.

Nursing Implications

1. A nasogastric tube may be used to maintain gastric decompression during procedure.
2. Have the client void before the procedure, if client has a full bladder at the time of insertion of the catheter, risk for bladder perforation and peritonitis is increased.
3. In clients with chronic liver problems, assess coagulation lab values before procedure.
4. Place client in semi-Fowler's position.
5. Maintain sterile field for puncture.
6. In clients with ascites, usually do not drain more than 1 L.

Complications

1. Perforation of bowel: peritonitis.
2. Introduction of air into abdominal cavity; client may complain of right referred shoulder pain (caused by air under the diaphragm).

3. Contraindicated in pregnancy and in clients with coagulation defects or possible bowel obstruction.

Stool Examination

Stool is examined for form and consistency and to determine whether it contains mucus, blood, pus, parasites, or fat. Stool will be examined for presence of occult blood.

Nursing Implications

1. Collect stool in sterile container if examining for pathologic organisms.
2. A fresh, warm stool is required for evaluation of parasites or pathogenic organisms.
3. Collect the sample from various areas of the stool.
4. The result of the guaiac test for occult blood is positive when the paper turns blue.
5. Document medications and over-the-counter drugs client is taking when sample is obtained.
6. Sample should be approximately the size of a walnut or 30 mL, if soft.

Appendix 18-2   ANTIEMETICS

MEDICATIONS	SIDE EFFECTS	NURSING IMPLICATIONS
Dopamine Antagonists Depress or blocks dopamine receptors chemoreceptor trigger zone of the brain.		
Phenothiazines—suppress emesis Chlorpromazine hydrochloride **(Thorazine):** PO, suppository, IM Promethazine **(Phenergan):** PO, IM, suppository High-Alert Medication for IV route Prochlorperazine **(Compazine):** PO, suppository, IM Thiethylperazine maleate **(Torecan):** PO, suppository, IM	Central nervous system depression, drowsiness, dizziness, blurred vision, hypotension, photosensitivity	1. Subcutaneous injection or intravenous administration may cause tissue irritation and necrosis. 2. Use with caution in children; do not administer **Thorazine** to infants less than 6 months old, **Compazine** to children weighing less than 20 lb or less than 2 years old, or **Torecan** to children less than 12 years old. 3. **Thorazine** should be used only in situations of severe nausea or vomiting. Can also be used for intractable hiccups. 4. **Torecan:** cautious use in clients with liver and kidney diseases.
Prokinetics—stimulate motility Metoclopramide **(Reglan):** PO, IM, IV	Restlessness, drowsiness, fatigue, anxiety, headache	1. Used to decrease problems with esophageal reflux and nausea and vomiting associated with chemotherapy. 2. Use with caution in clients when increase in peristalsis may be detrimental (perforation, obstruction).
Antihistamines Depress the chemoreceptor trigger zone, block histamine receptors.		
Hydroxyzine **(Atarax, Vistaril):** PO, IM Dimenhydrinate **(Dramamine, Marmine):** PO, suppository, IM	Sedation; anticholinergic effects—blurred vision, dry mouth, difficulty in urination and constipation; paradoxical excitation may occur in children	1. Caution client regarding sedation: should avoid activities that require mental alertness. 2. Administer early to prevent vomiting. 3. Use with caution in clients with glaucoma and asthma. 4. Subcutaneous injection may cause tissue irritation and necrosis; use Z-track injection technique.

GI, Gastrointestinal; *IM,* intramuscular; *IV,* intravenous; *PO,* by mouth (oral).

Appendix 18-3 LAXATIVES

General Nursing Implications

— Laxatives should be avoided in clients who have nausea, vomiting, undiagnosed abdominal pain and cramping, and/or any indications of appendicitis.
— Dietary fiber should be taken for prevention of, and as first-line treatment for, constipation.
— Daily intake of fluids should be increased.
— Constipation is determined by stool firmness and frequency.
— Increasing activity will increase peristalsis and decrease constipation.
— Narcotic analgesics and anticholinergics will cause constipation.
— A laxative should be used only briefly and in the smallest amount necessary.
— Use laxatives with caution during pregnancy.

MEDICATIONS	SIDE EFFECTS	NURSING IMPLICATIONS
Bulk laxatives—stimulate peristalsis and passage of soft stool Methylcellulose **(CITRUCEL)** Psyllium **(Metamucil, Perdiem)** Fibercon Bran	Esophageal irritation, impaction, abdominal fullness, flatulence	1. Not immediately effective; 12 to 24 hours before effects are apparent. 2. Use with caution in clients with difficulty swallowing. 3. Administer with full glass of fluid to prevent problems with irritation and impaction.
Surfactants—decrease surface tension, allowing water to penetrate feces Docusate **(Colace, Surfak)**	Occasional mild abdominal cramping	1. Do not use concurrently with mineral oil. 2. Not recommended for children less than 6 years old.
Stimulants—stimulate and irritate the large intestine to promote peristalsis and defecation Bisacodyl **(Dulcolax)**: suppository, PO Senna concentrate **(Senokot, Ex-Lax)**: PO, suppository	Diarrhea, abdominal cramping	1. Use for short period of time. 2. Do not use in presence of undiagnosed abdominal pain or GI bleeding.
Bowel evacuants—nonabsorbable osmotic agents that pull fluid into the bowel Polyethylene glycol **(GoLYTELY, Colyte)**: PO, NG Magnesium citrate: PO	Nausea, bloating, abdominal fullness.	1. Primary use is in preparing the bowel for examination. 2. Clear liquids only (no gelatin with red coloring) after administration. 3. **GoLYTELY** requires the client to drink a large amount of fluid (4 L); provide 8 to 10 oz chilled at a time to increase client consumption and enhance taste. 4. Best if consumed over 3 to 4 hours. 5. Evacuants cause frequent bowel movements; advise client to plan accordingly.

Appendix 18-4 ANTIDIARRHEAL AGENTS

MEDICATIONS	SIDE EFFECTS	NURSING IMPLICATIONS
Anhydrous morphine **(Paregoric):** PO	Lightheadedness, dizziness, sedation, nausea, vomiting, paralytic ileus, abdominal cramping	1. Opioid derivatives, suppress peristalsis. 2. Not recommended during pregnancy or breastfeeding. 3. Can produce drug dependence and mild withdrawal symptoms. 4. Encourage increased fluids. 5. Avoid activities that require mental alertness.
Diphenoxylate HCl Atropine **(Lomotil):** PO Loperamide HCl **(Imodium, Kaopectate II caplets):** PO Bismuth subsalicylate **(Kaopectate, Pepto-Bismol):** PO	May precipitate constipation and an impaction	1. Absorbent, has soothing effect, and absorbs toxic substances. 2. May interfere with absorption of oral medications. 3. Should not be given to clients with fever >101°. 4. Do not give in presence of bloody diarrhea.

PO, by mouth (orally).

Appendix 18-5 ANTIULCER AGENTS

MEDICATIONS	SIDE EFFECTS	NURSING IMPLICATIONS

Antacid An alkaline substance that will neutralize gastric acid secretions; nonsystemic. Some combination antacids also relieve gas, and some work as laxatives. Several antacids form a protective coating on the stomach and upper GI tract.

MEDICATIONS	SIDE EFFECTS	NURSING IMPLICATIONS
Aluminum hydroxide **(Amphojel)** Aluminum hydroxide and magnesium salt combinations **(Gelusil, Maalox, Gaviscon)**	Constipation, phosphorus depletion with long-term use Constipation or diarrhea, hypercalcemia, renal calculi	1. Avoid administration within 1 to 2 hours of other oral medications; should be taken frequently—before and after meals and at bedtime. 2. Instruct clients to take medication even if they do not experience discomfort. 3. Clients on low-sodium diets should evaluate sodium content of various antacids. 4. Administer with caution to the client with cardiac disease, because GI symptoms may be indicative of cardiac problems.
Sodium preparations Sodium bicarbonate **(Rolaids, Tums):** PO	Rebound acid production, alkalosis	1. Discourage use of sodium bicarbonate because of occurrence of metabolic alkalosis and rebound acid production.

Histamine H$_2$ Receptor Antagonists Reduce volume and concentration of gastric acid secretion.

MEDICATIONS	SIDE EFFECTS	NURSING IMPLICATIONS
Cimetidine **(Tagamet):** PO, IV, IM	Rash, confusion, lethargy, diarrhea, dysrhythmias	1. Take 30 minutes before or after meals. 2. May be used prophylactically or for treatment of PUD. 3. Do not take with oral antacids.
Ranitidine **(Zantac):** PO, IM, IV	Headache, GI discomfort, jaundice, hepatitis	1. Use with caution in clients with liver and renal disorders. 2. Do not take with aspirin products. 3. Wait 1 hour after administration of antacids.
Nizatidine **(Axid):** PO Famotidine **(Pepcid):** PO, IV	Anemia, dizziness Headache, dizziness, constipation, diarrhea	1. Use with caution in clients with renal or hepatic problems. 2. Dosing may be done with without regard to food or to meal time. 3. Caution clients to avoid aspirin and other NSAIDs.

Appendix 18-5 ANTIULCER AGENTS—cont'd

MEDICATIONS	SIDE EFFECTS	NURSING IMPLICATIONS
Proton Pump Inhibitors Inhibit the enzyme that produces gastric acid.		
Omeprazole **(Prilosec):** PO Lansoprazole **(Prevacid):** PO	Headache, diarrhea, dizziness	1. Administer before meals. 2. Do not crush or chew; do not open capsules. 3. Sprinkle granules of **Prevacid** over food; do not chew granules. 4. The combination of omeprazole **(Prilosec)** with clarithromycin **(Biaxin)** effectively treats clients with *Helicobacter pylori* infection in duodenal ulcer.
Cytoprotective Agents Bind to diseased tissue provides a protective barrier to acid.		
Sucralfate **(Carafate):** PO	Constipation, GI discomfort	1. Avoid antacids. 2. Used for prevention and treatment of stress ulcers, gastric ulceration, and PUD. 3. May impede the absorption of medications that require an acid medium.
Prostaglandin Analogues Suppresses gastric acid secretion; increases protective mucus and mucosal blood flow.		
Misoprostol **(Cytotec)**	GI problems, headache	1. Contraindicated in pregnancy. 2. Indicated for prevention of NSAID-induced ulcers.

GI, Gastrointestinal; *IM,* intramuscular; *IV,* intravenous; *NSAID,* nonsteroidal antiinflammatory drug; *PO,* by mouth (orally); *PUD,* peptic ulcer disease.

Appendix 18-6 INTESTINAL MEDICATIONS

Intestinal Antibiotics Decrease bacteria in the GI tract; used to sterilize bowel before surgery.

MEDICATIONS	SIDE EFFECTS	NURSING IMPLICATIONS
Kanamycin sulfate **(Kantrex):** PO Neomycin sulfate **(Mycifradin sulfate):** PO	Suprainfection of the bowel	1. Do not have side effects of parenterally administered aminoglycosides.
Paromomycin **(Humatin):** PO	Vomiting and diarrhea	1. Administer with meals. 2. Administer with caution in clients with ulcerative bowel disease.

5 Aminosalicylates (5 ASA) Antiinflammatory effect in small bowel and colon; used to treat ulcerative colitis and Crohn's disease.

Sulfasalazine **(Azulfidine):** PO	Nausea, fever rash, arthalgia	1. Assess client for allergy to sulfur. 2. Should not be used with thiazide diuretics. 3. Monitor CBC; maintain adequate hydration. 4. May continue on medication to maintain remission.
Mesalamine **(Asacol):** PO, **(Pentasa):** PO enteric coated tablet **(Rowasa)** Suppository or enema	GI symptoms, headache	1. Suppository or enema has minimal systemic effects. 2. Rectal administration is usually at night.
Balsalazide **(Colazal):** PO	Abdominal pain, headache	

PO, By mouth (orally).

Appendix 18-7 PARENTERAL NUTRITION

▲ **Parenteral Nutrition (PN)** An intravenous (IV) delivery of highly concentrated nutrients and vitamins.
1. Goal is to provide adequate nutrition and to facilitate healing and growth of new body tissue.
2. Conditions that interfere with the process of nutrition: ingestion, digestion, absorption.

Goal: To maintain client in positive nitrogen balance and promote healing.

Routes of Administration

1. **Peripheral:** Partial parenteral nutrition (PPN) is administered via a large peripheral vein or peripherally inserted central catheter (PICC) when nutritional support is indicated for a short period; may use IV fat (lipid) emulsions.
2. **Central:** Total parenteral nutrition (TPN) is administered via a parenteral line (PICC, Hickman, Broviac, central line) inserted in the antecubital, jugular, or subclavian vein and threaded into the vena cava; used for nutritional support in the client who requires in excess of 2500 calories per day for an extended period. Solutions used are hypertonic with high glucose content and require rapid dilution.

Nursing Implications

1. PN may be commercially prepared and then customized in the hospital pharmacy specifically for the client's most recent blood analysis findings; *nothing should be added to solution after it has been prepared in the pharmacy.*
2. Orders are written daily, based on the current electrolyte and protein status; always check the doctor's order for correct fluid for the day.
3. Solution may be refrigerated for up to 24 hours, but solution should be taken out of refrigeration 30 minutes prior to infusion. If solution has been hanging for 24 hours, it should be discarded and a new bag of solution hung.
4. Begin PN at a slow rate (40 to 60 mL per hour) and then gradually increase rate to prescribed infusion rate. Maintain constant flow rate; if infusion of solution is behind, determine how much, divide that amount over about 24 hours, and gradually increase rate to level of previous infusion order. Do not randomly accelerate the infusion to "catch up" over an hour; *PN must be administered via an infusion pump.*
5. Monitor serum blood glucose levels on a regular basis; some institutions require glucose testing every 4 to 6 hours. May be less frequent after first week of administration.
6. Infusion is initiated and discontinued on a gradual basis to allow the pancreas to compensate for increased glucose intake. If TPN is temporarily unavailable, give $D_{10}W$ or $D_{20}W$ until PN solution is available.
7. Monitor intake and output and compare daily trends. Body weight is an indication of the adequacy of hydration. Tissue healing is an indication of adequacy of protein and positive nitrogen balance.
8. Check label on bag of solution against orders; check solution for leaks, clarity, or color changes.

Maintenance

1. A sterile occlusive dressing should be used at the catheter site; change site dressing every 48 to 72 hours or per facility protocol.
2. Change IV tubing every 24 hours or per facility protocol.
3. Do not draw blood or measure central venous pressure (CVP) from the PN line.
4. Maintain record of daily weight; desired weight gain is approximately 2 pounds per week.

ALERT Evaluate client's nutritional status: monitor client's response to TPN.

Complications

1. Hyperglycemia may be caused by too rapid infusion of solution. Blood glucose is monitored every 4 to 6 hours during initial infusion, and sliding scale insulin may be ordered.
2. Fat emulsion syndrome may occur in clients receiving IV fat (lipid) emulsion. Monitor for fever, increased triglycerides, and clotting problems.
3. Refeeding syndrome is characterized by fluid retention, electrolyte imbalances, and hyperglycemia; occurs in clients with chronic malnutrition states. Hypophosphatemia occurs and is associated with dysrhythmias and respiratory complications.
4. Site infection: Monitor site and change dressing according to policy; clients may be immunosuppressed and signs of infection may be masked. If infection is suspected (erythema, tenderness, exudates), a culture should be done and health care provider notified immediately.
   Septicemia: Strong glucose solutions provide good media for bacteria; strict aseptic techniques in dressing changes.
5. Air embolus or risk for pneumothorax (central line): Increased tendency to occur during insertion of central catheter line and during dressing changes; place client in Trendelenburg position during insertion and during dressing changes (see Appendix 6-10 for care of central line).

Appendix 18-8 NURSING PROCEDURE: NASOGASTRIC TUBES

1. **Levin tube:** Single lumen.
   a. Suctioning gastric contents.
   b. Administering tube feedings.
   c. Connect to intermittent suction.
2. **Salem sump tube:** Double lumen (smaller blue lumen vents the tube and prevents suction on the gastric mucosa, maintains intermittent suction, regardless of suction source).
   a. Suctioning gastric contents and maintaining gastric decompression.
   b. Do not clamp, irrigate, or apply suction to air vent tube.
   c. Connect to continuous low suction.

✓ KEY POINTS

ALERT Insert feeding/nasogastric tubes and determine whether characteristics of nasogastric drainage are with in normal limits.

- Before insertion, position the client in high-Fowler's position, if possible. (If client cannot tolerate high-Fowler's, place in left lateral position.)
- Use a water-soluble lubricant to facilitate insertion.
- Measure the tube from the tip of the client's nose to the earlobe and from the nose to the xiphoid process to determine the approximate amount of tube to insert to reach the stomach.
- Insert the tube through the nose into the nasopharyngeal area; flex the client's head slightly forward.
- Secure the tube to the nose; do not allow the tube to exert pressure on the upper inner portion of the nares.
- Validating placement of tube.
  a. Aspirate gastric contents.
  b. Measure pH of aspirated fluid (pH of gastric secretions is usually less than 4).
  c. It is *no longer recommended* to determine placement by injecting air and listening with a stethoscope for sound of air in the stomach.

   d. Always validate placement of a nasogastric tube prior to instilling anything into tube.
- Characteristics of nasogastric drainage.
  a. Normally is greenish yellow, with strands of mucus.
  b. Coffee-ground drainage: old blood that has been broken down in the stomach.
  c. Bright red blood: indicates bleeding in the esophagus, the stomach, or the lungs.
  d. Foul-smelling (fecal odor): occurs with reverse peristalsis in bowel obstruction; increase in amount of drainage with obstruction.
- If duodenal placement is required, have client lay in right lateral position for several hours. Provide enough excess in the tube to allow the tube to migrate down into duodenum.

Clinical Tips for Problem Solving

- **Abdominal distention:** Check for patency and adequacy of drainage, determine position of tube, assess presence of bowel sounds, and assess for respiratory compromise from distention.
- **Nausea and vomiting around tube:** Place client in semi-Fowler's position or turn to side to prevent aspiration; suction oral pharyngeal area. Attempt to aspirate gastric contents and validate placement of tube. Tube may not be far enough into stomach for adequate decompression and suction; try repositioning. If tube patency cannot be established, tube may need to be replaced.
- **Inadequate or minimal drainage:** Validate placement and patency; tube may be in too far and be past pyloric valve or not in far enough and in the upper portion of the stomach. Reassess length of tube insertion and characteristics of drainage, request x-ray for validation.

ALERT ALWAYS check the placement of a gastric tube before injecting or irrigating it; placement should be checked each shift; do not adjust or irrigate the nasogastric tube on a client after a gastric resection.

Appendix 18-9   NURSING PROCEDURE: ENTERAL FEEDING

Short-Term

1. **Nasogastric:** Provides alternative means of ingesting nutrients for clients.
2. **Nasointestinal:** A weighted tube of soft material is placed in the small intestine to decrease chance of regurgitation. A stylet or guide wire is used to progress the tube into the intestine. Do not remove stylet until tube placement has been verified via x-ray. Do not attempt to reinsert stylet while tube is in place; this could result in perforation of the tube.

Long-Term

1. **Percutaneous endoscopic gastrostomy (PEG):** A tube is inserted percutaneously into the stomach; local anesthesia and sedation are used for tube placement.
2. **Percutaneous endoscopic jejunostomy (PEJ):** A tube is inserted percutaneously into the jejunum.
3. **Gastrostomy:** A surgical opening is made into the stomach, and a gastrostomy tube is positioned with sutures.

Methods of Administering Enteral Feedings

- Continuous: Controlled with a feeding pump. Decreases nausea and diarrhea.
- Intermittent: Prescribed amount of fluid infuses via a gravity drip or feeding pump over specific time. For example, 350 mL is given over 30 minutes.
- Cyclic: Involves feeding solution infused via a pump for a part of a day, usually 12 to 16 hours. This method may be used for weaning from feedings.

Nursing Implications

- The client should be sitting or lying with the head elevated 30 to 45°. Head of bed should remain elevated for 30 to 60 minutes after feeding if intermittent or cyclic feeding is used.
- If feedings are intermittent, tube should be irrigated with water before and after feedings.

- Aspirate gastric contents to determine residual. If residual is more than 200 mL, and there are signs of intolerance (nausea, vomiting, distention), hold next feeding for 1 hour and recheck residual or, if residual is greater than half of last feeding, delay next feeding for 1 to 2 hours.
- Return aspirated contents to stomach to prevent electrolyte imbalance.
- Flush the tube with 30 to 50 mL of water:
  a. After each intermittent feeding.
  b. Every 4 to 6 hours for continuous feeding.
  c. Before and after each medication administration.
- When a PEG or PEJ tube is placed, immediately after insertion measure the length of the tube from the insertion site to the distal end and mark the tube at the skin insertion site. This tube should be routinely checked to determine whether the tube is migrating from the original insertion point.
- Prevent diarrhea:
  a. Slow, constant rate of infusion.
  b. Keep equipment clean to prevent bacterial contamination.
  c. Check for fecal impaction; diarrhea may be flowing around impaction.
  d. Identify medical conditions that would precipitate diarrhea.
- For continuous feeding, change feeding reservoir every 24 hours.

> **❗ NURSING PRIORITY** If in doubt of a tube's placement or position, stop or hold the feeding and obtain x-ray confirmation of location.

> **ALERT** Change rate and amount of tube feeding based on client's response.

Appendix 18-10   NURSING PROCEDURE: ENEMAS

Types of Enemas

Soap suds enema: Castile soap is added to tap water or normal saline. Dilute 5 mL of castile soap in 1 liter of water.

Tap water enema: Request order for specific quantity when administered to infants or children; should not be repeated because of risk for water toxicity. Use caution when administering to adults with altered cardiac and renal reserve.

Saline enemas: Are the safest enemas to administer; safe for infants and children.

Retention enema: An oil-based solution that will soften the stool. Should be retained by client 30 to 60 minutes. Typically 150 to 200 mL. May be mineral oil or similar oil; or may include antibiotics or nutritive solution.

Hypertonic enema: Used when only a small amount of fluid is tolerated (120-180 mL). Commercially prepared Fleets enema.

Carminative enema: An agent used to expel gas from the GI tract. Example is magnesium sulfate/glycerin/water (MGW).

Harris flush or return flow enema: Mild colonic irrigation of 100 to 200 mL of fluid into and out of the rectum and sigmoid colon to stimulate peristalsis. Repeated multiple times by raising and lowering container until flatus is expelled and abdominal distention is relieved.

✓ KEY POINTS: Administering an Enema

- Fill enema container with warmed solution.
- Allow solution to run through the tubing before inserting into rectum so that air is removed.
- Place client on left lateral Sims' position.
- Generously lubricate the tip of the tubing with water-soluble lubricant.
- Gently insert tubing into client's rectum (3 to 4 inches for adults, 1 inch for infants, 2 to 3 inches for children), past the external and internal sphincters.
- Raise the solution container no more than 12 to 18 inches above the client.
- Allow solution to flow slowly. If the flow is slow, the client will experience fewer cramps. The client will also be able to tolerate and retain a greater volume of solution.

Appendix 18-10   NURSING PROCEDURE: ENEMAS—cont'd

Clinical Tips for Problem Solving

If client expels solution prematurely:
- Place client in supine position with knees flexed.
- Slow the water flow and continue with the enema.

If the enema returns contain fecal material before surgery or diagnostic testing, repeat enema. If, after three enemas, returns still contain fecal material, notify physician.

If client complains of abdominal cramping during instillation of fluid:
- Slow the infusion rate by lowering the fluid bag.

ALERT Assist and intervene with client who has an alteration in elimination.

Appendix 18-11   NURSING PROCEDURE: STOOL SPECIMEN

Types of Stool

- Normal → semisoft to semisolid, brown color
- Narrow, ribbon-like stool → spastic or irritable bowel, or obstruction
- Diarrhea → spastic bowel, viral infection
- Blood and mucus, soft stool → bacterial infection
- Mixed blood or pus → colitis
- Yellow or green stool → severe, prolonged diarrhea; rapid transit through bowel
- Black stool → gastrointestinal bleeding or intake of iron supplements
- Tan, clay-colored, or white stool → liver or gallbladder problems
- Red stool → colon or rectal bleeding; some medications and foods may also cause a red coloration
- Fatty stool, pasty or greasy → intestinal malabsorption, pancreatic disease

✓ KEY POINTS: Collecting the Specimen

- Always wear gloves during procedure.
- Use clean bedpan or bedside commode to collect stool; do not use stool that has been in contact with toilet bowl water or urine.

- Collect stool specimen in a clean, dry container. If stool is to be evaluated for organisms, use a sterile container. Use a tongue blade to obtain specimens from several areas of the stool and place in the stool collection container.
- The client collecting a stool specimen for an occult blood test needs to follow directions regarding diet restrictions (no red meat, beets, or foods that may cause the stool to turn red or lead to a false-positive result).
- Stool specimen should be approximately size of a walnut. If stool is liquid, approximately 30 mL is needed.
- Take the specimen to the laboratory. Do not allow it to remain in unit.

ALERT Obtain specimen from client for laboratory tests.

Appendix 18-12   NURSING PROCEDURE: CARE OF THE CLIENT WITH AN OSTOMY

Types of Ostomies (Figure 18-8)

Colostomy: Opening of the colon through the abdominal wall; stool is generally semisoft and bowel control may be achieved.

Ileostomy: Opening of the ileum through the abdominal wall; stool drainage is liquid and excoriating; drainage is frequently continuous; therefore it is difficult to establish bowel control. Fluid and electrolyte imbalances are common complications.

Kock's ileostomy: May be referred to as a "continent" ileostomy; an internal reservoir for stool is surgically formed. Decreases problem of skin care caused by frequent irritation of stoma by drainage. Primary complications are leakage at the stoma site and peritonitis.

Goals

1. Maintain physiologic and psychologic equilibrium.
2. Assist client to maintain total care of colostomy or ileostomy before discharge.

Preoperative Care

1. Preoperative education: Actively involve family and client; encourage questions concerning the procedure.
2. Placement of stoma is evaluated, and site is selected with client standing. Select a site that is easily seen and accessible to client; select a flat area of the abdomen, avoiding skin creases and folds; select site that does not interfere with clothing.

✓ KEY POINTS: Postoperative Nursing Implications— Initial Care

- Evaluate stoma every 8 hours after surgery. It should remain pink and moist; dark blue stoma indicates ischemia.
- Measure the stoma and select an appropriately sized appliance. Mild to moderate swelling is common for the first 2 to 3 weeks after surgery, which necessitates changes in size of the appliance.
- Appliance should fit easily around the stoma and cover all healthy skin.

Continued

Appendix 18-12   NURSING PROCEDURE: CARE OF THE CLIENT WITH AN OSTOMY—cont'd

The **ascending colostomy** is done for right-sided tumors.

The **transverse (double-barreled) colostomy** is often used in such emergencies as intestinal obstruction or perforation because it can be created quickly. There are two stomas. The proximal one, closest to the small intestine, drains feces. The distal stoma drains mucus. Usually temporary.

The **transverse loop colostomy** has two openings in the transverse colon, but one stoma. Usually temporary.

Descending colostomy

Sigmoid colostomy

FIGURE 18-8 Types of colostomies. (From Monahan FD et al: *Phipps' medical-surgical nursing: health and illness perspectives*, ed 8, St. Louis, 2007, Mosby.)

- Keep the skin around the stoma clean, dry, and free of stool and intestinal secretions. Prevent contamination of the abdominal incision.
- Change the skin appliance only when it begins to leak or becomes dislodged.
- Ostomy bags should be changed when about one-third full to avoid weight of bag dislodging skin barrier.

✓ KEY POINTS: Irrigation

- Do not irrigate an ileostomy or maintain regular irrigations in child with colostomy.
- Irrigate colostomy at same time each day to assist in establishing a normal pattern of elimination.
- Involve client in care as early as possible.
- In adults, irrigate with 500 to 1000 mL of warm tap water.

> **⚠ NURSING PRIORITY** Use a cone tipped ostomy irrigator; do not use an enema tube/catheter.
> Do not irrigate more than once a day.
> Do not irrigate in the presence of diarrhea.

- Place the client in a sitting position for irrigation, preferably in the bathroom with the irrigation sleeve in the toilet.
- Elevate the solution container approximately 12 to 20 inches and allow solution to flow in gently. If cramping occurs, lower fluid or clamp the tubing.
- Allow 25 to 45 minutes for return flow. Client may want to walk around before the return starts.
- Encourage client to participate in care of his or her own colostomy. Have client perform return demonstration of colostomy irrigation before leaving the hospital.

- Assist the client to control odors: diet and odor-control tablets.
- Kock's ileostomy is drained when client experiences fullness. A nipple valve is created in surgery and drained by insertion of a catheter.

Clinical Tips for Problem Solving

If water does not flow easily into colostomy stoma:
- Check for kinks in tubing from container.
- Check height of irrigating container.
- Encourage client to change positions, relax, and take a few deep breaths.

If client experiences cramping, nausea, or dizziness during irrigation:
- Stop flow of water, leaving irrigation cone in place.
- Do not resume until cramping has passed.
- Check water temperature and height of water bag; if water is too hot or flows too rapidly, it can cause dizziness.

If client has no return of stool or water from irrigation:
- Be sure to apply drainable pouch; solution may drain as client moves around.
- Have client increase fluid intake; he or she may be dehydrated.
- Repeat irrigation next day.

If diarrhea occurs:
- Do not irrigate colostomy.
- Check client's medications; sometimes they may cause diarrhea.
- If diarrhea is excessive and/or prolonged, notify physician.

> **ALERT** Provide ostomy care.

Study Questions Gastrointestinal System

More questions on companion CD!

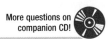

1. On the second day after gastric resection, the client's nasogastric tube is draining bile-colored liquid containing coffee-ground material. What is the best nursing action?
   1 Continue to monitor the amount of drainage and correlate it with any change in vital signs.
   2 Reposition the nasogastric tube and irrigate the tube with normal saline solution.
   3 Call the physician and discuss the possibility that the client is bleeding.
   4 Irrigate the nasogastric tube with iced saline solution and attach the tube to gravity drainage.

2. The nurse is providing preoperative care for a client who will have a gastric resection. What will the preoperative teaching include?
   1 A nasogastric tube will be in place several days after surgery.
   2 The client will be started on a low-residue, bland diet about 2 days after the surgery.
   3 Explain the anticipated prognosis and implications that the client may have a malignancy.
   4 A urinary retention catheter will be in place for 1 week after surgery.

3. The nurse is planning care for a client scheduled for gastroduodenoscopy and a barium swallow. What will the nursing care plan include?
   1 Anticipating the client will receive a low-residue diet in the evening and then receive nothing by mouth (NPO status) 6 to 12 hours before the test.
   2 Discussing with the client the nasogastric tube and the importance of gastric drainage for 24 hours after the test.
   3 Explaining to the client that he will receive nothing by mouth (NPO status) for 24 hours after the test to make sure his stomach can tolerate food.
   4 Discussing the general anesthesia and explaining to the client that he will wake up in the recovery room

4. In preparing a pediatric client for an appendectomy, the nurse would question which doctor's orders?
   1 Penicillin 600,000 units IVPB, now
   2 Obtain signed consent form from parents.
   3 Administer enemas until clear.
   4 500 mL Ringer's lactate solution at 50 mL/hr

5. What are the best nursing actions in caring for a client with appendicitis before surgery?
   Select all that apply:
   _____ 1 Maintain bed rest.
   _____ 2 Offer full liquids to maintain hydration.
   _____ 3 Position client on side, legs flexed to the abdomen with the head slightly elevated.
   _____ 4 Position client on left side; apply a warm K-Pad to the abdomen.
   _____ 5 Administer narcotic for pain and allow client to assume position of comfort.
   _____ 6 Maintain NPO and begin a peripheral IV for fluid replacement.

6. An obese client has had a combination restrictive malabsorptive bariatric surgery. What will be important for the nurse to include in discharge teaching for this client?
   1 Increase intake of foods high in iron, calcium, and vitamin B_{12} to prevent deficiencies.
   2 Do not take any added fluids with meals or immediately after meals.
   3 Elevate bed to prevent development of gastroesophageal reflux during sleep.
   4 Plan intake of three balanced meals a day with increased fluids between meals.

7. In planning discharge teaching for the client who has undergone a gastrectomy, the nurse includes what information regarding dumping syndrome?
   1 The syndrome will be a permanent problem, and the client should eat 5 to 6 small meals per day.
   2 The client should decrease the amount of fluid consumed with each meal and for 1 hour after each meal.
   3 The client should increase the amount of complex carbohydrates and fiber in the diet.
   4 Activity will decrease the problem; it should be scheduled about 1 hour after meals.

8. The nurse is assessing a child with a tentative diagnosis of appendicitis. The nursing assessment is most likely to reveal what characteristics concerning the pain?
   1 Rebound tenderness in the right lower quadrant, associated with decreased bowel sounds and vomiting
   2 Gnawing pain, radiating through to the lower back, with severe abdominal distention
   3 Sharp pain with severe gastric distention, frequently associated with hemoptysis
   4 Pain on light palpation in midepigastric area, chronic low-grade fever, and diarrhea

9. The nurse is caring for a client who has been diagnosed with a bleeding duodenal ulcer. What data identified on a nursing assessment would indicate an intestinal perforation and require immediate nursing action?
   1 Increasing abdominal distention, with increased pain and vomiting
   2 Decreasing hemoglobin and hematocrit with bloody stools
   3 Diarrhea with increased bowel sounds and hypovolemia
   4 Decreasing blood pressure with tachycardia and disorientation

10. The nurse is caring for a client who is scheduled for a gastric endoscopy. Which of the following actions must the nurse perform before the client is able to eat or drink after the endoscopy?
    1 Check oxygen saturation.
    2 Give small sips of water.
    3 Check all vital signs.
    4 Assess the client's gag reflex.

11. A client is admitted with duodenal ulcers. What will the nurse anticipate the client's history to include?
    1 Recent weight loss
    2 Increasing indigestion after meals
    3 Awakening with pain at night
    4 Episodes of vomiting

12. The nurse is preparing discharge teaching for a client with a diagnosis of gastroesophageal reflux disease (GERD). What would be important for the nurse to include in this teaching plan? Select all that apply:
    _____ 1 Elevate the head of the bed.
    _____ 2 Decrease intake of caffeine products.
    _____ 3 Take an antacid before bedtime.
    _____ 4 Increase fluid intake with meals.
    _____ 5 Take ranitidine (Zantac) at bedtime.
    _____ 6 Eat a bedtime snack of milk and protein.

13. The nurse is conducting discharge dietary teaching for a client with diverticulosis who is recovering from an acute episode of diverticulitis. Which statement by the client would indicate to the nurse that the client understood his dietary teaching?
    1 "I will need to increase my intake of protein and complex carbohydrates to increase healing."
    2 "I need to eat foods that contain a lot of fiber to prevent problems with constipation."
    3 "I will not put any added salt on my food, and I will decrease intake of foods that are high in saturated fat."
    4 "Milk and milk products can cause a lactose intolerance. If this occurs, I need to decrease my intake of these products."

14. What is the priority nursing action for the client who is complaining of nausea in the recovery room after gastric resection?
    1 Evaluate the nasogastric tube for patency.
    2 Call the physician for an antiemetic order.
    3 Place client in semi-Fowler's position so that he will not aspirate.
    4 Medicate the client with a narcotic analgesic.

15. The nurse is assisting a client immediately before a colonoscopy. The nurse will direct the client and help him move into what position?
    1 Prone
    2 Sims' lateral
    3 Slight Trendelenburg
    4 Flat with lithotomy stirrups

16. What will be important for the nurse to do when collecting a stool specimen for an occult blood (Hemoccult) test?
    1 Samples should be taken from two areas of the stool.
    2 Three separate stool samples will be required for accuracy of test.
    3 The nurse should collect about 20 mL of stool sample.
    4 Any red color on or near the specimen is considered positive.

17. A school-age child with a diagnosis of celiac disease asks the nurse, "Which foods will make me sick?" Which of the following food items would the nurse teach the child to avoid?
    1 Rice cereals, milk, and tapioca
    2 Corn cereals, milk, and fruit
    3 Corn or potato bread and peanut butter
    4 Malted milk, white bread, and spaghetti

18. The nurse practitioner orders half-strength enteral formula at a rate of 55 mL/hr. A can holds 250 mL. How many cans would the nurse need for the next 24 hours?
    Answer: _____ cans

Answers and rationales to these questions are in the section at the end of the book titled Chapter Study Questions: Answers and Rationales.

CHAPTER NINETEEN

Hepatic and Biliary System

PHYSIOLOGY OF THE HEPATIC AND BILIARY SYSTEM

Organs of the Hepatic and Biliary System

A. Liver.
1. Located in the upper right portion of the abdominal cavity just under the diaphragm; vascular organ; protected by the rib cage.
2. Blood flow into the liver is from two sources.
   a. Portal vein carries venous blood from the stomach, intestines, pancreas, and spleen into the liver. The venous blood is rich in nutrients absorbed from the gastrointestinal (GI) system.
   b. The hepatic artery provides oxygenated blood to the liver.
   c. The portal vein and hepatic artery enter the liver via a common vessel and flow through the liver tissue; blood then leaves the liver via the hepatic vein and empties into the inferior vena cava.
3. Because of pressure differences in the hepatic and portal veins, the liver may normally store 200 to 400 mL of blood.
4. The liver produces approximately 600 to 1200 mL of bile daily.
   a. Bile drains from the liver via the common bile duct.
   b. The common bile duct enters the duodenum, either close to or in conjunction with the pancreatic duct.
5. It can sustain 90% damage with loss of tissue and still remain functional.
B. Gallbladder.
1. A muscular, elastic sac located on the undersurface of the liver.
2. The cystic duct from the gallbladder joins the common bile duct from the liver.
3. The gallbladder is capable of storing 20 to 50 mL of bile. When food enters the duodenum, the gallbladder contracts; the sphincter of Oddi, which controls the release of bile, relaxes; and bile enters the intestine via the common duct.
4. When the sphincter of Oddi closes, bile flows back into the gallbladder for storage.
5. The primary function of the gallbladder is concentration and storage of bile.

Functions of the Liver

A. Synthesis of absorbed nutrients.
1. Serum glucose regulation.
   a. Glucose from carbohydrate metabolism is converted to glycogen, which is stored in the liver and released according to the body's needs.
   b. Gluconeogenesis refers to the ability of the liver to produce glucose from noncarbohydrate sources, such as amino acids and the glycerol portion of fats. This process is initiated when the body's requirements for glucose are in excess of the stored glycogen in the liver.
2. Lipid (fat) metabolism.
   a. Preliminary breakdown of fatty acids as a source of body energy.
   b. When the glucose available for metabolism is limited, fatty acids may be broken down for production of energy. This results in formation of ketone bodies.
   c. Utilization of fatty acids for production of cholesterol, lipoprotein, and phospholipid.
3. Protein metabolism.
   a. Synthesis of plasma proteins.
   b. Deaminization: breakdown of amino acids for energy or for conversion to glucose or fat.
   c. Synthesis of nonessential amino acids.
   d. Ammonia is a by-product of protein metabolism. It is converted to urea by the liver and excreted by the kidneys.
B. Synthesis of prothrombin for normal clotting mechanisms. Vitamin K is necessary for adequate prothrombin production.
C. Vitamin and mineral storage.
1. Produces and stores vitamins A and D.
2. Vitamin B_{12} and iron are stored in the liver.
D. Drug metabolism: barbiturates, amphetamines, and alcohol are metabolized by the liver.

E. Production of bile and bile salts.
   1. Bile is continuously formed in the liver.
   2. Bile salts are produced in the liver; cholesterol is a necessary constituent of bile salts.
   3. Bile and bile salts emulsify fat for digestion and absorption in the intestine.
   4. Bilirubin, a bile pigment, is excreted by the liver.
      a. The spleen removes and breaks down the hemoglobin in worn-out red blood cells. This results in the production of bilirubin.
      b. Bilirubin is carried from the spleen to the liver for excretion.
      c. Bilirubin is conjugated in the liver (made water soluble) and secreted into the bile.
         (1) A small amount of unconjugated bilirubin (indirect) is released into the circulation and is not water soluble.
         (2) Conjugated bilirubin (direct) has been processed through the liver to form a water-soluble substance.
         (3) Conjugated bilirubin is secreted into the bile and flows into the small intestine for fat digestion.
         (4) Conjugated bilirubin is converted into urobilinogen in the large intestine and is reabsorbed and returned to the liver or excreted in feces. Normally, only a small amount of urobilinogen is excreted in the urine.

System Assessment (Box 19-1)

A. History.
   1. History of liver, gallbladder, or jaundice problems.
   2. History of bleeding problems.
   3. History of reproductive problems.
   4. Medication intake.
   5. Recent association with anyone with jaundice.
   6. Alcohol consumption.
B. Physical assessment.
   1. Inspection.
      a. Skin.
         (1) Presence of vascular angiomas, skin lesions, or petechiae.
         (2) Hydration status.
         (3) Color of the skin (jaundiced).
         (4) Presence of peripheral edema.
      b. Abdomen.
         (1) Evidence of jaundice.
         (2) Contour of the abdomen.
         (3) Presence of visible abdominal wall veins.
   2. Palpation of the abdomen.
      a. Pain, tenderness, presence of distention.
      b. Hepatomegaly, splenomegaly.
C. Nutritional assessment.
   1. Weight gain or loss; dietary intake.
   2. Problems of anorexia, nausea and vomiting.

Pathophysiology of Jaundice

A. Jaundice may begin so gradually that it is not noticed immediately.
B. The increased levels of bilirubin cause a yellowish discoloration of the skin. It may be first observed as a yellow color in the sclera of the eyes. Serum bilirubin levels must exceed 2 mg/dL for jaundice to occur. The yellow discoloration is due to deposits of bilirubin in the skin and body tissue.
C. Types of jaundice.
   1. Hemolytic jaundice.
      a. Occurs with an increase in the breakdown of red blood cells, which causes an increase in the amount of unconjugated bilirubin in the blood.
      b. The liver cannot handle the increased level of unconjugated bilirubin. The bilirubin is not water soluble; therefore it cannot be excreted. Unconjugated bilirubin is lipid soluble and is capable of entering nerve cells and causing brain damage.
      c. The increased production of urobilinogen will increase the amount of bilirubin excreted in the urine and feces.
      d. Causes of hemolytic jaundice.
         (1) Blood transfusion reactions.
         (2) Sickle cell crisis.
         (3) Hemolytic anemias.
         (4) Hemolytic disease of the newborn.
   2. Hepatocellular jaundice.
      a. Results from the inability of the liver to clear normal amounts of bilirubin from the blood.
      b. Increase in serum levels of unconjugated and conjugated bilirubin.
      c. Causes of hepatocellular jaundice.
         (1) Hepatitis.
         (2) Cirrhosis.
         (3) Hepatic cancer.
   3. Obstructive jaundice.
      a. Results from an impediment to bile flow through the liver and the biliary system.
      b. The obstruction may be within the liver, or it may be outside the liver.
      c. Causes of obstructive jaundice.
         (1) Hepatitis.
         (2) Liver tumors.
         (3) Cirrhosis.
         (4) Obstruction of the common bile duct by a stone.

Box 19-1   FOCUSED ASSESSMENT: LIVER AND BILIARY

Skin color: jaundice
Changes in abdominal girth
Changes in stool: pale, frothy, fatty
History of contact with infectious individuals
Issues with indigestion and food intolerance
Type of pain
Psychosocial problems associated with alcohol use

DISORDERS OF THE HEPATIC SYSTEM

 Hepatitis

Widespread inflammation of the liver tissue is called *hepatitis*.

A. Types of hepatitis (Table 19-1).
  1. Hepatitis A virus (HAV): infectious hepatitis.
    a. Primarily a disease of children because of mode of transmission and interaction of large numbers of children in daycare centers.
    b. The mortality rate is low, but there is an increase in fatalities in the older adult population.
    c. Administration of immune serum globulin (immunoglobulin G) to exposed individuals increases the immune resistance and/or decreases the severity of the illness (passive immunization).
  2. Hepatitis B virus (HBV): serum hepatitis.
    a. Identification of HBsAg (Australian antigen).
      (1) Identification of antigen in potential blood donors has significantly decreased transmission via blood transfusions.

Table 19-1	HEPATITIS	
Hepatitis A (HAV)	**Hepatitis B (HBV)**	**Hepatitis C (HCV)**
Transmission Modes		
Predominately fecal-oral	Percutaneous inoculation with contaminated needles or instruments is the primary mode	Percutaneous (parenteral)/mucosal exposure to blood and blood products
Poor personal hygiene		High-risk sexual contact
Oral-anal sexual practices	Skin or mucous membrane break by inoculation (needle-sticks, cuts, ear piercing, tattooing, or contaminated drug paraphernalia)	Perinatal contact
Contaminated food, water, and shellfish (commonly spread by infected food handlers)		Closely associated with HBV
Carriers are most contagious just before onset of symptoms (jaundice)	Blood and blood products	
Transmission through sexual contact and percutaneous transmission are possible, but these are not primary modes of transmission	Nonpercutaneous transmission—contact with body fluids containing hepatitis B surface antigen (HBsAg) (e.g., sexual contact)—is the second most common mode	
	Infants of mothers with HBV may contract the disease in utero, at birth, or after delivery	
	Infected asymptomatic carrier	
	Hepatitis D (HDV) is very similar to HBV	
Incubation Period		
2 to 6 weeks (average: 4 weeks); also the most contagious period	6 weeks to 6 months (average: 12 weeks)	2 weeks to 6 months (average: 8 weeks)
Virus is present in feces for 7 to 10 days before a person becomes ill	Contagious as long as serum marker (surface antigen; HBsAg) appears	Most contagious 1 to 2 weeks before symptoms appear; infectivity continues during clinical course
		Large number of cases (75%-85%) develop chronic HCV
High-Risk Individuals		
Household contacts	Household contacts	Multiple blood transfusion recipients
Sexual contacts	Sexual contacts	Sexual contacts
Institutions, daycare centers, schools	Dental, laboratory, and medical personnel	IV drug users
	Multiple blood transfusion recipients	
	IV drug users	
Sources of Infection and Spread of Infection		
Crowded living conditions; poor hygiene and sanitation	Contaminated needles, syringes, and blood products	Blood and blood products, needles and syringes
Contaminated food, milk, water, and shellfish	Sexual activity with infected partners	Sexual activity with infected partners
Infected food handlers	Asymptomatic carriers	
Sexual contact	Tattoo-body piercing with contaminated needles; bites	

> **ALERT** Follow infection control guidelines; standard precautions include blood and body fluids.

IV, Intravenous.

(2) Antigen is present in blood, vaginal secretions, menstrual fluid, semen, saliva, and respiratory secretions (see Table 19-1).
- b. Administration of hepatitis B immunoglobulin will provide some temporary immunity.
- c. HBV vaccine should be administered to everyone as a standard immunization (see Table 2-1).
3. Hepatitis C (HCV).
- a. Transmission is very similar to that of HCV, with multiple causative agents; percutaneous inoculation (IV drug use), blood transfusions.
- b. Increased incidence occurs with crowded living conditions.
4. Toxic and drug-induced hepatitis.
- a. Toxic: systemic poisons: carbon tetrachloride, gold compounds.
- b. Drug-induced: isoniazid (INH), Diuril, methotrexate, methyldopa.
5. Autoimmune hepatitis.
- a. Cause is unknown; associated with other autoimmune diseases.
- b. Different treatment than viral hepatitis; treated with corticosteroids and immunosuppressants.
B. The inflammatory process causes hepatic cell degeneration and necrosis. Hepatitis A is generally self-limiting with liver regeneration and complete recovery. Hepatitis B and hepatitis C are more serious and can progress to total destruction of the liver.

ALERT Teach health promotion information; follow infection control guidelines/protocols. Prevent transmission in the hospital in addition to teaching the importance of personal hygiene.

Assessment

Regardless of the type of hepatitis, the clinical picture is similar.
A. Risk factors/etiology and sources/spread of disease (see Table 19-1).
B. Clinical manifestations: all clients experience inflammation of the liver tissue and exhibit similar symptoms.
1. Anicteric phase.
- a. Anorexia, nausea, malaise, headache.
- b. Upper right quadrant discomfort.
- c. Low-grade fever, hepatomegaly.
2. Icteric phase (jaundiced).
- a. Dark urine caused by increased excretion of bilirubin.
- b. Pruritus.
- c. Stools light and clay colored.
- d. Liver remains enlarged and tender.
3. Posticteric phase (after jaundice).
- a. Malaise, easily fatigued.
- b. Hepatomegaly remains for several weeks.
4. Anicteric hepatitis (absence of jaundice).
- a. Frequently occurs in children.
- b. Many clients with hepatitis A and hepatitis C (non-A, non-B) may not show clinical jaundice.

- c. Unexplained fever, general GI disturbances.
- d. Anorexia and malaise.

 PEDIATRIC PRIORITY Children often have diarrhea, and their symptoms are frequently attributed to gastroenteritis rather than hepatitis. Jaundice is seldom noted.

5. Onset of hepatitis A is more acute; symptoms are generally less severe.
6. Onset of hepatitis B is more insidious; symptoms are more severe.
7. Most cases of hepatitis C are asymptomatic or mild, but they tend to be persistent and lead to chronic liver disease.
C. Diagnostics (see Appendix 19-1).
1. Increased alanine aminotransferase, aspartate aminotransferase, and serum bilirubin levels.
2. Presence of HBsAg in serum of client with hepatitis B.
3. Presence of anti-HAV antibodies in blood with hepatitis A.
4. ELISA is initial screening test for hepatitis C. Recombinant immunoblot assay (RIBA) is confirmation test.

Treatment

A. No specific medications for HAV.
1. Chronic HBV and HCV: α-interferon and antivirals.
B. Encourage good nutrition; no specific dietary modifications; client will probably not tolerate a high-fat diet.
C. Decreased activity; promote rest.

Complications

A. Chronic, active hepatitis.
B. Fulminant hepatitis: severe, acute case of hepatitis.
C. Permanent destruction of liver cells, leading to cirrhosis.
D. Total destruction of the liver.

Nursing Interventions

Goal: To control and prevent hepatitis.
A. Understand characteristics of transmission and preventive measures for hepatitis A.
1. Good personal hygiene, especially handwashing.
2. Participate in community activities for health education, (e.g., environmental sanitation, food preparation, etc.).
3. Identify individuals at increased risk for exposure: those with household contact, intimate sexual contact, and/or institutional contact with those with active disease.
4. Administer immune serum globulin (immunoglobulin G) within 2 weeks of exposure, if they do not have presence of anti-HAV antibodies (antibody to HAV).
5. Preexposure prophylaxis: hepatitis A vaccine (single dose).
6. Implement standard precautions.
7. Client should abstain from sexual activity during periods of communicability.

! **OLDER ADULT PRIORITY** Older adult clients are at higher risk for liver damage and complications of hepatitis.

B. Understand characteristics of transmission and preventive measures for hepatitis B.
   1. Identify individuals at increased risk for exposure: those with oral or percutaneous contact with HBsAg-positive fluid and those who have had sexual contact with carriers within 4 weeks of the appearance of jaundice.
   2. Administration of hepatitis B vaccine.
   3. Postexposure prophylaxis: HBV vaccine series started and hepatitis B immune globulin (HBIG) given within 24 hours of exposure.
C. Understand characteristics of transmission and preventive measures for hepatitis C.
   1. No vaccine for HCV.
   2. Immunoglobulin G, antivirals, or α-interferon are not recommended.
D. Maintain strict contact-based standard precautions for hospitalized client with questionable diagnosis of hepatitis (see Appendix 6-8).

Goal: To promote healing and regeneration of liver tissue.
A. Bed rest with bathroom privileges initially; progressive activity according to liver function test results.
B. Promote psychologic and emotional rest.
   1. Strict bed rest may increase anxiety.
   2. Frequently, young adults are very concerned about body image; encourage verbalization and emphasize temporary nature of symptoms.
   3. Maintain communication and frequent contact.
C. Promote nutritional intake.
   1. Anorexia and decreased taste for food potentiate nutritional deficits.
   2. Small frequent feedings of favorite foods, good oral hygiene, and food served in a pleasant atmosphere.
D. Encourage increased fluid intake.

⫶⫶⫶ Home Care

A. Continued need for adequate rest and nutrition until liver function test results are normal.
B. Avoid alcohol and over-the-counter medications, especially those containing acetaminophen and phenothiazine.

ALERT Evaluate client's use of over-the-counter medications.

C. Clients with hepatitis B should avoid intimate and sexual contact until antibodies to the HBsAg are present and the client is no longer contagious.
D. If possible, client should have his or her own bathroom.
E. Client and family must understand importance of personal hygiene and good handwashing.
F. Client should not donate blood.

 Hepatic Cirrhosis

Hepatic cirrhosis is a chronic, progressive disease of the liver, characterized by degeneration and destruction of liver cells.
A. Liver regeneration is disorganized and results in the formation of scar tissue, which in time, will exceed the amount of normal liver tissue.
B. Types of cirrhosis.
   1. Alcoholic (previously called Laënnec's): also called portal or nutritional cirrhosis; associated with alcohol abuse; accumulation of fat in liver cells leading to widespread inflammation and destruction of liver cells, which results in widespread scar formation.
   2. Postnecrotic: can follow hepatitis or exposure to hepatotoxin.
   3. Biliary: diffuse fibrosis and scarring caused by chronic biliary obstruction and infection.
   4. Cardiac: increase in venous pressure associated with long-term right-sided heart failure.
C. Complications of cirrhosis.
   1. Portal hypertension.
      a. Structural changes in the liver result in obstruction of normal hepatic blood flow, which causes increased pressure in the portal circulation.
      b. Collateral circulation develops as the body attempts to reduce the increased portal pressure. Common areas for collateral channels are:
         (1) Lower esophagus at the area of the gastric vein.
         (2) Anterior abdominal wall.
         (3) Parietal peritoneum.
         (4) Rectum.
      c. Esophageal varices form from collateral vessels in the lower esophagus.
      d. Splenomegaly occurs from the increase of congestion in the splenic bed; may lead to leukopenia and thrombocytopenia.
      e. Caput medusae: dilated veins around the umbilical area.
   2. Peripheral edema and ascites.
      a. Edema results from:
         (1) Impaired liver synthesis of protein, resulting in decreased colloid osmotic pressure (hypoalbuminemia).
         (2) Portal hypertension, malnutrition.
      b. Ascites: accumulation of serous fluid in the peritoneal cavity.
         (1) With increased pressure in the liver, excessive protein and water leak out of the liver into the abdomen.
         (2) The presence of hypoalbuminemia results in decreased colloid osmotic pressure, which facilitates movement of fluid and protein into the abdominal cavity.
         (3) Hyperaldosteronism causes increased amounts of sodium and water to be retained.

3. Hepatic encephalopathy (coma) results from the inability of the liver to detoxify ammonia.
   a. Ammonia is a by-product of protein metabolism.
   b. Large quantities of ammonia remain in the systemic circulation and cross the blood-brain barrier, producing toxic neurologic effects.

ALERT Identify changes in mental status.

Assessment

A. Risk factors/etiology.
1. Excessive, prolonged alcohol consumption.
2. Nutritional deficiencies.
3. Frequently, a combination of alcoholism and nutritional deficiency.
4. Predisposing chronic hepatic and biliary infections.

B. Clinical manifestations.
1. GI disturbances: anorexia, indigestion, change in bowel habits, weight loss.
2. Changes in the skin.
   a. Jaundice (hepatocellular and biliary), pruritis.
   b. Spider angiomas on the face, neck, and shoulders.
   c. Palmar erythema: reddened areas on the palms that blanch with pressure.
3. Blood disorders: anemia.
4. Coagulation disorders: spontaneous bruising from thrombocytopenia.
5. Changes in sexual characteristics: gynecomastia, impotence in males; amenorrhea, vaginal bleeding in females.
6. Peripheral neuropathy: probably caused by inadequate intake of vitamin B complex.
7. Hepatomegaly, splenomegaly.
8. Portal hypertension.
   a. Esophageal varices that bleed easily.
   b. Hemorrhoids.
   c. Collateral veins visible on abdominal wall.
   d. Development of edema and ascites.
   e. Edema generally occurs in feet, ankles, and presacral area.
   f. Severe abdominal distention and weight gain with ascites.
   g. Presence of fluid waves in the abdomen.
9. Portal-systemic encephalopathy (Figure 19-1).
   a. Changes in mental responsiveness.
   b. Level of concentration: ask client to repeat a series of numbers; if client has encephalopathy, he or she will be unable to repeat a 4- to 6-digit sequence.
   c. Memory: determine client's ability to recall recent events (yesterday or past week) and remote events (last year).
   d. Apraxia: deterioration in writing and drawing; inability to construct or draw a figure.
   e. Asterixis (flapping tremors): clients with asterixis are unable to hold their hands out in front of

PORTAL SYSTEMIC ENCEPHALOPATHY (PSE)
HEPATIC ENCEPHALOPATHY (HEPATIC COMA)

FIGURE 19-1 Portal-systemic encephalopathy. (From Zerwekh J, Claborn J: *Memory notebook of nursing,* vol 1, ed 4, Ingram, Texas, 2008, Nursing Education Consultants.)

them when asked; a flapping of the hands will occur.
   f. Fetor hepaticus: musty, sweet odor to breath due to inability of liver to degrade digestive products.

C. Diagnostics (see Appendix 19-1).

Treatment

A. Cirrhosis.
1. Rest.
2. Dietary modification: increase calories and carbohydrates; protein and fat may be consumed as tolerated.
3. Vitamin supplement, especially vitamin B complex.
4. Abstinence from alcohol.

B. Ascites.
1. IV albumin or other volume replacement after a high volume paracentesis.
2. Sodium restriction in diet.
3. Fluid restriction for cases of severe ascites.
4. Diuretics.
5. Paracentesis for temporary relief.
6. Peritoneovenous shunt (LeVeen shunt): a surgical procedure for reinfusion of ascitic fluid into venous system.
7. Surgical procedures to decrease portal hypertension by shunting portal blood flow: transjugular intrahepatic portosystemic shunt (TIPS).

C. Esophageal varices.
1. Blood transfusions to restore volume from bleeding varices.
2. Administration of IV vasopressin (Pitressin) produces vasoconstriction of the splanchnic arterial bed, decreases portal blood flow, and portal hypertension.
3. Endoscopic sclerotherapy: injection of a sclerosing agent directly into esophageal varices; bleeding may recur because there has been no reduction in portal hypertension.

4. Endoscopic ligation or banding of the varices: often used in combination with sclerotherapy.
5. Balloon tamponade: mechanical compression of bleeding varices via esophageal gastric balloon tamponade (Minnesota or Sengstaken-Blakemore tube).
6. Shunting surgical procedures: decrease portal hypertension by shunting portal blood flow; usually performed after second major bleeding episode.
7. Management to prevent bleeding: beta adrenergic blockers (Inderal), repeated sclerotherapy, endoscopic ligation, and portosystemic shunts.

D. Decrease portal systemic encephalopathy.
1. Restriction of dietary protein intake.
2. Neomycin: decreases the normal flora in the intestines to reduce bacterial activity on protein.
3. Lactulose: used to reduce the amount of ammonia in the blood of clients with liver disease by drawing ammonia from the blood into the colon where it is removed from the body. May also be used to treat constipation, because it pulls water into the colon to facilitate movement of waste through the GI system.
4. Control of GI hemorrhage to decrease protein available in the intestine.

Nursing Interventions

Goal: To promote health in the client with cirrhosis.
A. Proper diet: increased protein as tolerated, adequate carbohydrates, vitamin supplements.
B. Adequate rest.

> **ALERT** Monitor client's hydration and nutritional status.

C. Avoid potential hepatotoxic over-the-counter drugs (aspirin and acetaminophen).
D. Check all body secretions for frank or occult blood.
E. Abstinence from alcohol.
F. Attention and care should be given the alcoholic client without being judgmental or moralizing.
G. Client should understand symptoms indicative of complications and when to seek medical advice.
H. Regular medical checkups.

Goal: To maintain homeostasis and promote liver function.
A. Rest and activity schedule based on clinical manifestations and lab data.
B. Measures to prevent complications of immobility (see Chapter 3).
C. Assist client to maintain self-esteem.
1. Maintain positive, accepting atmosphere in the delivery of care.
2. Encourage ventilation of feelings regarding disease.
D. Assist in activities of daily living, as necessary, to prevent undue fatigue.
E. Promote nutritional intake.
1. Good oral hygiene; between-meal nourishment.
2. Provide food preferences when possible.
3. Administer antiemetic before meals, if necessary.

4. Iron and vitamin supplements, especially vitamin B complex.
5. Nasogastric or parenteral feeding, if client is unable to maintain adequate intake.
F. Decrease discomfort of pruritus caused by jaundice: cool rather than warm baths, avoid excessive soap.
G. Good skin care to prevent breakdown.
H. Evaluate serum electrolyte levels, especially potassium and sodium levels, because of the use of diuretics to decrease ascites and edema.
I. Monitor temperature closely because of increased susceptibility to infection.
J. Assess for bleeding tendencies and prevent trauma to the mucous membranes.
K. Measure abdominal girth to determine whether it is increasing from ascitic fluid (Figure 19-2).

Goal: If esophageal varices are present, decrease risk for active bleeding.
A. Soft, nonirritating foods.
B. Discourage straining at stool.
C. Decrease esophageal reflux.
D. No salicylate compounds (aspirin).
E. Evaluate for active bleeding.
1. Monitor vital signs.
2. Assess for melena and hematemesis.

Goal: To decrease bleeding from esophageal and gastric varices.
A. Gastric lavage with iced saline solution.
B. Assess and prevent complications associated with sclerotherapy.
1. Client is sedated and the throat is anesthetized before the procedure.
2. By means of endoscopy, the physician injects the sclerosing agent into the varices.
3. Bleeding from the varices should stop within minutes.
4. Client may experience chest discomfort for 2 to 3 days; administer an analgesic.

FIGURE 19-2 Measuring abdominal girth. (From Ignatavicius DD, Workman ML: *Medical-surgical nursing: patient-centered collaborative care*, ed 6, Philadelphia, 2010, Saunders.)

5. Esophageal perforation and ulceration are complications associated with treatment; observe client for development of severe chest pain.
6. Observe for return of active bleeding.

Goal: To decrease esophageal bleeding by using an esophageal tamponade balloon.

A. Constant observation is required while the balloon is inflated.
B. The client is to receive *absolutely* nothing by mouth; provide frequent oral and nasal hygiene.
C. Constant tension/traction is applied to maintain the pressure against the esophageal sphincter by the gastric balloon. The gastric balloon is *not* to be deflated while tension is present and the esophageal balloon is inflated.
D. Keep the head of the bed elevated to decrease gastric regurgitation and nausea.
E. Keep scissors at the bedside in case the esophageal balloon moves into the oropharynx area and causes obstruction of the trachea. If this should occur, the lumen to the esophageal balloon should be cut to immediately deflate the balloon and relieve the obstruction.

Goal: To assess for and prevent complications associated with ascites.

A. Decrease sodium intake.
B. Administer diuretics, potassium supplements.
C. Daily measurements of abdominal girth.
D. Maintain semi-Fowler's position to decrease pressure on the diaphragm.
E. Assess weight daily.
F. Monitor pulse oximetry for indications of respiratory distress.

Goal: To assess for and prevent complications of hepatic encephalopathy.

A. Frequent assessment of responsiveness.
B. Assess for changes in level of orientation and motor abnormalities (asterixis).
C. Decrease production of ammonia.
  1. Increase carbohydrates and fluids.
  2. Decrease activity, because ammonia is a by-product of metabolism.
  3. GI bleeding will increase ammonia levels as a result of the breakdown of red blood cells.
  4. Lactulose to promote excretion of ammonia in the stool; diarrhea may occur.
  5. Nonabsorbable intestinal antibiotics (Appendix 6-9) will decrease protein breakdown.
D. Prompt treatment of hypokalemia.

Goal: To provide appropriate preoperative and postoperative care if surgical procedure is indicated (see Chapter 3).

A. Anastomosis of the high-pressure portal system to the low-pressure systemic venous system to create a shunt to decrease portal hypertension (portosystemic shunt), thereby decreasing problems with esophageal varices and ascites.
B. Client is at increased risk for postoperative complications.
  1. Hemorrhage, electrolyte imbalance.
  2. Seizures, delirium tremens.

C. Surgical procedures do not alter course of progressive hepatic disease.

Cancer of the Liver

Primary cancer of the liver is rare. Metastatic cancer is more common.

A. Liver is a common site for metastases because of increased rate of blood flow and capillary network.
B. Metastases are found in the liver in approximately one-half of all clients with late-stage cancer.
C. Prognosis is poor.

Assessment

A. Risk factors/etiology: malignancy elsewhere in the body.
B. Clinical manifestations.
  1. Anorexia, weight loss, fatigue, anemia.
  2. Right upper quadrant pain, ascites, jaundice.
C. Diagnostics (see Appendix 19-1).

Treatment

Treatment is primarily palliative.
A. Surgical excision of tumor, if it is localized.
B. Chemotherapy: very poor response.
C. Radiofrequency (RF) ablation uses heat to burn tumor (percutaneous approach).
D. Cryosurgery (cryoablation) uses liquid nitrogen to freeze liver tissue; not used for metastatic disease.
E. Percutaneous ethanol injection (PEI) or percutaneous acetic acid injection (PAI) used to treat unresectable liver cancer.

Nursing Interventions

Focused on maintaining comfort; nursing care is the same as that for the client with advanced cirrhosis.

Liver Transplantation

Therapeutic option for clients with end-stage liver disease; not recommended for widespread malignant disease.

Assessment

A. Rigorous prescreening process.
B. Rejection less common than with kidney transplants.

Treatment

A. Live liver transplant: portion of liver is donated.
B. Split liver transplant: donor liver is divided and given to two recipients.

Nursing Interventions

Goal: To monitor for postoperative complications.

A. Assess neuro status, monitor for hemorrhage and common respiratory problems of pneumonia, atelectasis, and pleural effusion.
B. Monitor IV fluids, nasogastric tube drainage, Jackson-Pratt drain, and T-tube drainage.

C. Administer antibiotics and analgesics.

D. Critical to monitor for infection the first 2 months after surgery; fever may be the only sign.

Goal: to provide nursing care of the immunocompromised client (see Chapter 7).

DISORDERS OF THE BILIARY TRACT

Cholelithiasis and Cholecystitis

Cholelithiasis is the presence of stones in the gallbladder; this is the most common form of biliary disease. Cholecystitis is an inflammation of the gallbladder, which is frequently associated with stones; this condition may be acute or chronic (Figure 19-3).

Assessment

A. Risk factors/etiology.

1. Cholelithiasis.
   a. Supersaturation of bile with cholesterol causes precipitate to occur.
   b. Conditions upsetting cholesterol and bile balance include infection and disturbances of cholesterol metabolism.
   c. Increased incidence in females, especially during pregnancy.
   d. Increased incidence after age 40; obesity.
2. Cholecystitis.
   a. Associated with stones.
   b. *Escherichia coli* is common bacteria involved.
   c. May also be associated with neoplasms, anesthesia, or adhesions.

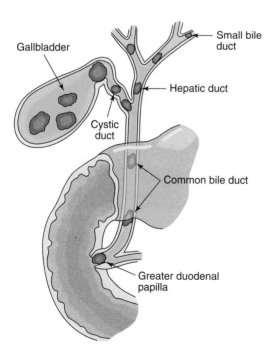

FIGURE 19-3 Common sites of gallstones. (From Monahan FD et al: *Medical-surgical nursing: health and illness perspectives,* ed 8, St. Louis, 2007, Mosby.)

> **❗ OLDER ADULT PRIORITY** Incidence of gallstone increases with age. Older adults are more likely to go from asymptomatic gallstones to serious complications of gallstones without biliary colic.

B. Clinical manifestations.

1. Cholelithiasis: severity of symptoms depends on the mobility of the stone and whether obstruction occurs.
   a. Epigastric distress, feeling of fullness.
   b. Abdominal distention.
   c. Vague pain in the right upper quadrant after consumption of meals high in fat.
2. Obstruction of cystic ducts by stones, precipitating biliary colic.
   a. Severe abdominal pain radiating to the back and shoulder.
   b. Nausea, vomiting, tachycardia, diaphoresis.
   c. Pain occurs 3-6 hours after consumption of a heavy meal, especially if high in fat.
   d. Jaundice may occur with obstruction of bile flow.
   e. Urine may become very dark, and stools may be clay colored.
3. Cholecystitis.
   a. Abdominal guarding, rigidity, rebound tenderness.
   b. Fever.
   c. Pain exacerbated by deep breathing.
   d. Onset may be sudden with severe pain.

C. Diagnostics (see Appendix 19-1).

Treatment

A. Cholecystectomy for cholelithiasis: surgical removal of the stones.

B. Cholecystitis.

1. Anticholinergics to decrease secretions and promote relaxation of the gallbladder.
2. Analgesics: hydromorphone (Dilaudid) or morphine.
3. Antibiotics.
4. Atropine and dicyclomine (Bentyl) will relieve spasms and decrease pain.
5. Ketorolac (Toradol) may be used to decrease spasms and pain in older adults.

C. Laparoscopic cholecystectomy.

1. Three small incisions are made.
2. Decreases risk to client.
3. Day surgery or overnight stay.
4. Early ambulation and decreased pain.

> **❗ NURSING PRIORITY** Common postop problem of referred pain to the shoulder due to CO_2 that was not released or absorbed by body, which can irritate the phrenic nerve and diaphragm causing difficulty breathing.

D. Decrease dietary fat intake.

Nursing Interventions

Goal: To decrease pain and inflammatory response.

A. Low-fat liquid diet during acute attack.

B. Low-fat solids added, as tolerated.

C. IV fluids and gastric decompression if nausea and vomiting are severe.

D. Antibiotics and analgesics.

E. Assess for indications of infection.

Goal: To provide appropriate preoperative nursing care if surgery is indicated (see Chapter 3).

Goal: To maintain homeostasis and prevent complications after cholecystectomy.

A. General postoperative care for clients having abdominal surgery (see Chapter 3).

B. Evaluate tolerance to diet and progress diet gradually to low-fat solids.

C. Penrose drain may be in place; client will frequently have large amounts of serosanguineous drainage; change dressing as indicated.

D. Sims' position to facilitate the movement of CO_2 gas pocket away from the diaphragm.

E. T-tube may be used to maintain patency of bile duct and to facilitate bile drainage until edema subsides (Figure 19-4).

   1. Maintain tube to gravity drainage.

   2. Observe amount and color of bile drainage.

   3. Do not irrigate or clamp tube; do not raise tube above the level of the gallbladder.

   4. Observe for bile drainage around the tube.

   5. Observe and record drainage (bloody initially, then greenish-brown).

   6. Drainage is usually around 500 mL per day for several days after surgery; drainage will gradually decrease, and the doctor will remove the tube.

   7. Typically not placed or used after a laparoscopic cholecystectomy.

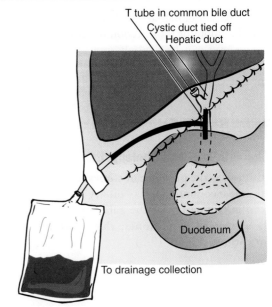

FIGURE 19-4 Placement of a T-tube. (From Black JM, Hawks JH: *Medical-surgical nursing: clinical management for positive outcomes,* ed 8, St. Louis, 2009, Mosby.)

F. Monitor urine and stool for changes in color.

Goal: To assist client to understand implications of disease process and measures to maintain health after cholecystectomy.

A. Dietary teaching regarding low-fat diet.

B. Weight reduction, if appropriate.

C. Avoid heavy lifting.

D. Understand symptoms indicating bile obstruction (i.e., stool and urine changes) and advise physician accordingly.

Appendix 19-1 DIAGNOSTICS OF THE HEPATIC AND BILIARY SYSTEM

LABORATORY TESTS	NORMAL	NURSING IMPLICATIONS
Serum Laboratory Tests		
Bilirubin		A rise in the serum level of bilirubin will occur if there is excessive destruction of red blood cells or if the liver is unable to excrete normal amounts of bilirubin.
Direct	0.1 to 0.3 mg/dL	
Indirect	0.1 to 1.0 mg/dL	
Total	0.2 to 1.3 mg/dL	
Protein studies		Proteins are responsible for maintaining the colloid oncotic pressure in the serum.
Total serum protein	6.0 to 8.0 g/dL	
Serum albumin	3.5 to 5.0 g/dL	
Serum globulin	2.0 to 3.5 g/dL	Synthesis of protein and normal serum protein levels are affected by various liver impairments.
Serum enzymes		
Lactic dehydrogenase (LDH)	50-150 units/L	Elevated in heart failure, hemolytic disorders, hepatitis, liver damage.
LDH_5		LDH_5 isoenzyme elevated in hepatitis.
Aspartate aminotransferase (AST)	10 to 26 units	Elevated in liver disease, acute hepatitis, myocardial infarction, pulmonary infarction.
Alanine aminotransferase (ALT)	10 to 35 units	Elevated in liver disease, shock.
Alkaline phosphatase (ALP)	30-120 units/L	Primary sources of ALP in body are bone and liver. Abnormally high readings may be associated with either liver or bone disease and must be correlated with presenting clinical symptoms.
Serum blood ammonia	30-70 mcg/dL	Increasing blood ammonia is indicative of the inability of the liver to convert ammonia to urea.
Hepatitis antigens and antibodies	Negative for antigens	Antigens indicate hepatitis (hepatitis B surface antigen [HBsAg] elevated in hepatitis B). Antibodies indicate exposure, current disease, or hepatitis B immunization.

Biopsy

Liver biopsy

Percutaneous needle aspiration of liver tissue

1. Informed consent procedure.
2. Client's status is NPO for 6 hours before procedure.
3. Blood coagulation study results should be available on the chart before biopsy procedure.
4. Immediately before needle insertion, have client take a deep breath, exhale completely, and hold breath. This immobilizes the chest wall and decreases the risk for penetration of the diaphragm with the needle.
5. Keep client on bed rest for 12-14 hr. Client should be positioned on the right side for 2 hr postprocedure to apply pressure and decrease risk for hemorrhage.
6. Assess for complications of pneumothorax and hemorrhage immediately after biopsy; assess for right upper abdominal pain or referred shoulder pain; observe for development of bile peritonitis.

ALERT Monitor status of client after a procedure: Position the client on right side with a pillow under the costal margin to facilitate compression of the liver.

Cholangiography

Percutaneous transhepatic cholangiography (PTC)

IV injection of radiopaque dye to visualize the biliary duct system

1. Client's status is NPO for 8 hr before the test.
2. Assess for sensitivity to iodine.
3. Evaluate for iodine reaction after the test.
4. Client should drink large amounts of fluid after test to increase excretion of dye.

Nuclear Imaging Scans (Scintigraphy)

Hepatobiliary scintigraphy (HIDA)

Shows size, shape and position of biliary system. Radionuclide (Tc-99m) injected IV; client positioned under a camera or counter to record distribution of tracer

1. Explain to client that traces of radionuclide pose minimal danger.
2. Needs to lie flat during scanning procedure.

Continued

Appendix 19-1   DIAGNOSTICS OF THE HEPATIC AND BILIARY SYSTEM—cont'd

LABORATORY TESTS	NORMAL	NURSING IMPLICATIONS
Ultrasound		
Gallbladder ultrasound		1. Client is NPO for 8-12 hours, since gas can reduce quality of images and food can cause gallbladder contraction.
Uses high-frequency sound waves to examine the gallbladder; provides information about presence of tumors and patency of vessels and detects gallstones		2. Explain to client that a conductive gel (lubricant) will be applied to the skin and a transducer placed on the area.
Hepatobiliary ultrasound		
Detects abscesses, cysts, tumors, and cirrhosis		
Endoscopy		
Endoscopic retrograde cholangiopancreatography (ERCP)		1. Client is NPO for 8 hours before procedure.
Fiberoptic endoscope and fluoroscopy inserted orally, descended into duodenum, then into common bile duct and pancreatic ducts, where contrast medium is injected for visualization of the structures.		2. Explain that sedative will be given before and during procedure.
		3. Check for allergy to contrast medium.
		4. Informed consent must be signed.
		5. Check vital signs—monitor for perforation or infection; pancreatitis is most common complication.
		6. Check for return of gag reflex before giving fluids.

ALP, Alkaline phosphatase; *ALT,* alanine aminotransferase; *AST,* aspartate aminotransferase; *INR,* international normalized ratio; *IV,* intravenous; *NPO,* nothing by mouth.

Study Questions Hepatic and Biliary System

More questions on companion CD!
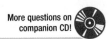

1. After administering diuretics to a client with ascites, which of the following nursing actions most ensures safe care?
   1. Monitoring serum potassium for hyperkalemia
   2. Assessing the client for hypervolemia
   3. Weighing client weekly
   4. Documenting accurate intake and output

2. A client with hepatitis B has a headache. Which analgesic(s) would be appropriate for this client? Select all that apply.
   _____ 1 Ibuprofen
   _____ 2 Naproxen
   _____ 3 Aspirin
   _____ 4 Acetaminophen
   _____ 5 Morphine
   _____ 6 Demerol

3. An obese 44-year-old woman with a history of chronic cholecystitis is to receive vitamin K before surgery. What is the purpose of this medication?
   1. To increase the digestion and utilization of fats
   2. To support the immune system and promote healing
   3. To aid in the emptying of bile from the gallbladder
   4. To facilitate coagulation activities of the blood

4. A client with cirrhosis is receiving neomycin sulfate. The nurse understands that the purpose of this medication is to
   1. Decrease gastric acidity.
   2. Acidify feces and trap ammonia in the bowel.
   3. Decrease bacterial flora.
   4. Reduce portal hypertension.

5. What statement would indicate to the nurse that the client understands the discharge teaching regarding his cirrhosis?
   1. "I will decrease vitamin B intake."
   2. "I need to continue Tylenol daily."
   3. "I will weigh myself every day in the morning."
   4. "I can eat my regular diet."

6. The nurse is caring for a client with chronic hepatitis B (HBV). What will the teaching plan for this client include?
   1. Avoid sexual activity.
   2. Report any clay-colored stools.
   3. Eat a high-protein diet.
   4. Perform daily urine bilirubin checks.

7. The client returns to his room after liver biopsy. The nurse positions the client on his left side and assesses for bleeding. What is a priority nursing assessment?
   1. Assess the vital signs.
   2. Observe for frank bleeding.
   3. Check pretest prothrombin time and partial thromboplastin time values.
   4. Determine adequacy of urinary output.

8. A client with portal hypertension and ascites has had a paracentesis to relieve respiratory compromise. What medication will the nurse anticipate the client will receive?
   1. $D_{10}W$
   2. Meperidine (Demerol)
   3. IV albumin
   4. Furosemide (Lasix)

9. The nurse is making a home visit to a client with hepatitis A (HAV). Before assessing the client, the nurse will gather the equipment and perform what action next?
   1. Wipe the bedside table with alcohol preps.
   2. Place the supplies on the bedside table.
   3. Place paper towels on the bedside table.
   4. Put on a gown and gloves.

10. While talking with a client with a diagnosis of end-stage liver disease, the nurse notices the client is unable to stay awake and seems to fall asleep in the middle of a sentence. The nurse recognizes these symptoms to be indicative of what condition?
    1. Hyperglycemia
    2. Increased bile production
    3. Increased blood ammonia levels
    4. Hypocalcemia

11. What is the primary purpose of giving lactulose (Enulose) to a client with advanced liver disease?
    1. To ensure regular bowel movements
    2. To prevent bowel obstruction
    3. To decrease ammonia levels in the blood
    4. To promote clotting

12. Which position is best for the client who has undergone a traditional abdominal cholecystectomy?
    1. Side-lying position, to prevent aspiration
    2. Semi-Fowler's position, to facilitate breathing
    3. Supine, to decrease strain on the incision line
    4. Prone, to reduce nausea

13. A client who underwent cholecystectomy 3 days ago has a T-tube that has stopped draining. What is the best nursing action?
    1. Flush the tube with 5 mL of normal saline solution.
    2. Reposition the client.
    3. Continue to monitor.
    4. Assess for tube placement.

14. The nurse is caring for a client with hepatitis A. Which type of infection precautions are appropriate for this client?
    1. Standard precautions
    2. Droplet precautions
    3. Contact precautions
    4. Bloodborne precautions

15. A new employee at a facility needs to receive the hepatitis vaccine. Which statement reflects accurate understanding of the immunization?
    1 "I need to receive six shots—one a month until I show positive antibodies to hepatitis."
    2 "Once I receive the hepatitis vaccine, I will be immune to all types of hepatitis."
    3 "I will receive three injections over a period of months, which should protect me from hepatitis B."
    4 "The hepatitis vaccine is an oral vaccine with live attenuated virus."

16. A client asks how her body can continue to function normally after a laparoscopic cholecystectomy. Which response by the nurse would be the most accurate answer to the client's question?
    1 "You should never eat a diet that is high in fat now that you do not have a gallbladder."
    2 "The primary function of the gallbladder is concentration and storage of bile."
    3 "The liver continues to secrete bile and takes over the function of the gallbladder."
    4 "The gallbladder has no known function in the human body, so removal is okay."

17. Clients with liver disease frequently develop a problem with jaundice. What would the nurse identify as the physiologic cause of jaundice?
    1 Increased levels of ammonia
    2 Increased alanine aminotransferase (ALT) level
    3 Bilirubin levels above 4 mg/dL
    4 Increased red blood cell breakdown

18. The client who has undergone a traditional cholecystectomy has a T-tube in place after surgery. What is the purpose of the T-tube in the care of this client?
    1 To remove bile leaking from the incision
    2 To provide a means of wound irrigation
    3 To drain bile from the common bile duct
    4 To prevent rupture of the inflamed gallbladder

19. What is the most important nursing intervention for the safety of a client with altered clotting mechanisms caused by hepatic cirrhosis?
    1 Promote independence in the client's activities of daily living.
    2 Administer antibiotics to decrease ammonia.
    3 Implement bleeding precautions.
    4 Increase vitamin supplements and nutritional intake.

20. A client has a diagnosis of hepatitis B. What would be the most important information for the nurse to include in a teaching plan for this client?
    1 How to sanitize all bathroom facilities
    2 Avoid sexual contact.
    3 Maintain droplet precautions.
    4 Follow up with hepatitis B vaccinations.

Answers and rationales to these questions are in the section at the end of the book titled Chapter Study Questions: Answers and Rationales.

CHAPTER TWENTY

Neurologic System

PHYSIOLOGY OF THE NERVOUS SYSTEM

A. Central nervous system (CNS) (Figure 20-1).
B. Peripheral nervous system.
 1. Twelve pairs of cranial nerves.
 2. Thirty-one pairs of spinal nerves.
 3. Autonomic nervous system (ANS).
  a. Sympathetic system: "fight or flight."
  b. Parasympathetic system.

Cells of the Nervous System

A. Neuron: the functional cell of the nervous system.
B. Function/classification.
C. Supporting cells provide support, nourishment, and protection to the neuron.
D. Myelin sheath.
 1. Dense membrane or insulator around the axon.
 2. Facilitates function of the neuron.
 3. Contributes to the blood-brain barrier to protect the CNS from harmful molecules.
E. Nerve regeneration: entire neuron is unable to undergo complete regeneration.
 1. Neuron regeneration in the CNS is very limited, possibly because of the lack of neurilemma (membrane surrounding the neuron).
 2. Scar tissue is a major deterrent to successful cellular regeneration.
F. Impulse conduction.
 1. Reflex arc.
  a. A reflex arc is the functional unit that provides pathways over which nerve impulses travel.
  b. The passage of impulses over a reflex arc is called a reflex act or a reflex and is an involuntary response to a stimulus.
  c. Reflex arc: the afferent neuron carries the stimulus to the spine, integrates it into and through the spine (CNS) to the efferent neuron, and crosses the synapse with the message from the CNS to the organ or muscle, which responds to the stimulus. This is the sequence of events evaluated when the deep tendon reflexes are tested.
 2. Synaptic transmission.
  a. A chemical synapse maintains a one-way communication link between neurons.
  b. Chemical neurotransmitters (neuromediators) facilitate the transmission of an impulse across the synapse.
   (1) Acetylcholine.
   (2) Norepinephrine.
   (3) Dopamine.
   (4) Histamine.
  c. Impulses pass in only one direction.

Central Nervous System

The brain and the spinal cord within the vertebral column make up the CNS (see Figure 20-1).

A. The brain and the spinal column are protected by the rigid bony structure of the skull and the vertebral column.
B. Meninges: protective membranes that cover the brain and are continuous with those of the spinal cord.
 1. Pia mater: a delicate vascular connective tissue layer that covers the surfaces of the brain and the spinal column; part of the blood-brain barrier.
 2. Arachnoid: a delicate nonvascular, waterproof membrane that encases the entire CNS; the subarachnoid space contains the cerebrospinal fluid (CSF).
 3. Dura mater: a tough white fibrous connective tissue, the outer layer of protection to the brain and spinal cord.
C. Cerebrospinal fluid (CSF).
 1. Serves to cushion and protect the brain and spinal cord; brain literally floats in CSF.
 2. CSF is clear, colorless, watery fluid; approximately 100 to 200 mL in total volume, with a normal fluid pressure of 60 to 100 mm H_2O.
 3. Formation and circulation of CSF (Figure 20-2).
  a. Fluid is secreted by the choroid plexus located in the ventricles of the brain.
  b. CSF flows through the lateral ventricles into the third ventricle, then flows through the aqueduct of Sylvius into the fourth ventricle, where the central canal of the spinal column opens.
  c. From the fourth ventricle, CSF flows around the spinal cord and brain.
  d. Because CSF is formed continuously, it is reabsorbed at a comparable rate by the arachnoid villi.

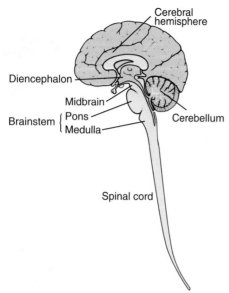

FIGURE 20-1 Major divisions of the central nervous system. (From Lewis SL et al: *Medical-surgical nursing: assessment and management of clinical problems*, ed 7, St. Louis, 2007, Mosby.)

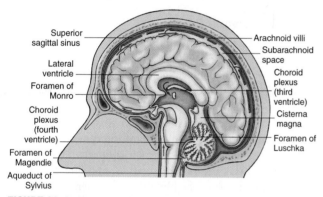

FIGURE 20-2 Circulation of the cerebrospinal fluid. (From Monahan FD et al: *Medical-surgical nursing: health and illness perspectives*, ed 8, St. Louis, 2007, Mosby.)

D. Brain.
   1. Cerebrum: the largest portion of the brain; separated into hemispheres; the cerebral cortex is the surface layer of each hemisphere.
   2. Major lobes of the central cortex.
      a. Frontal.
         (1) Responsible for intelligence and personality.
         (2) Coordination of voluntary skeletal muscle movement.
         (3) Abstract thinking, morals, judgment.
         (4) Broca's area for speech, motor-speech area, area of expressive ability (to speak and write).
      b. Parietal.
         (1) Interprets sensory nerve impulses (pain, temperature, touch).
         (2) Maintains proprioception.
         (3) Recognition of size, texture, and shape of objects.

   c. Temporal.
      (1) Auditory area: interprets meaning of certain sounds.
      (2) Wernicke's area for speech, sensory speech area, comprehension and formulation of speech (understanding spoken and written words).
   d. Occipital area: interprets vision and controls ability to understand written words.
   3. Motor areas of the cerebral cortex.
      a. Primary function is coordination and control of skeletal muscle activity.
      b. Corticospinal tracts (pyramidal tracts).
         (1) Descending tract from the motor area of the cerebral cortex to the spinal cord.
         (2) Majority of motor nerves cross in the medulla to the opposite side before descending into the spinal cord.
         (3) These corticospinal tracts do not cross over.
      c. Brain cells and the nerve fibers in the descending tracts of the CNS are called upper motor neurons.
   4. Movement is controlled by:
      a. Cerebral cortex: voluntary initiation of motor activity.
      b. Basal ganglia: assist in maintaining posture.
      c. Cerebellum: coordinates muscle movement.
   5. Cerebellum: attached to the medulla and the pons.
      a. Primarily concerned with coordination of motor movement, muscular tone, and maintenance of equilibrium.
      b. Nerve fibers spread upward to the cerebrum and downward to the pons, medulla, and spinal cord.
         (1) Visual reflexes: pupillary constriction and movement of the eye.
         (2) Auditory reflexes: turning of the head toward sound.
   6. Brainstem: consists of the pons and the medulla.
      a. Pons: contains both motor and sensory pathways relaying messages between the cerebrum and the spinal cord; also regulates respiration.
      b. Medulla oblongata: a continuation of the spinal cord as it enters into the cranial vault in the brain.
         (1) Conduction center and crossing center for the upper motor neurons.
         (2) Maintains control of cardiac rate.
         (3) Vasomotor center for constriction and dilation of vessels.
         (4) Respiratory center for changes in rate and depth of breathing.
         (5) Vomiting and swallowing reflex center.
      c. Thalamus.
         (1) Organization and distribution of incoming sensory impulses.
         (2) Activities related to consciousness.
      d. Hypothalamus.
         (1) Homeostasis: regulation of visceral activities, including body temperature, fluid and electro-

lyte regulation, motility and secretions of the gastrointestinal tract, arterial blood pressure.

(2) Nerve connections with the thalamus and the cerebral cortex make it possible for emotions to influence visceral activity (e.g., spastic colon).

(3) Regulation of endocrine glands via influence on the pituitary gland.

(4) Neurosecretion of antidiuretic hormone, which is stored in the pituitary gland.

7. Cerebral circulation.
   a. The internal carotid arteries enter the cranial vault at the temporal area.
   b. The circle of Willis is an arterial anastomosis at the base of the brain. The circle ensures continued circulation if one of the main vessels is disrupted.

E. Spinal cord.
   1. The spinal cord is continuous with the medulla and extends down the vertebral column to the level of the first or second lumbar vertebrae.
   2. Each column is divided into functional groups of nerve fibers.
      a. Ascending tracts: transmit impulses to the brain (sensory pathway).
      b. Descending tracts: transmit impulses from the brain to the various levels of the spinal cord (motor pathways).
   3. Structure.
      a. Intervertebral disks lie between the vertebrae to provide flexibility to the spinal column.

b. Nucleus pulposus is the fibrocartilaginous portion of the intravertebral disk; acts as shock absorber for the spinal cord.

4. Upper motor neurons: originate in the brain; transmit impulses from the brain to the lower motor neurons.

5. Lower motor neurons: originate in the spinal cord; transmit impulses to the muscles and organs. These neurons form the reflex arc.

6. Reflex activity.
   a. The reflex arc must be intact; the spinal cord serves as the connection between the afferent pathway (sensory) and the efferent pathway (motor).
   b. Testing of the reflex arc (deep tendon reflexes) allows evaluation of the lower motor neuron and the sensory/motor fibers from the spinal column. *For example, if the biceps reflex is normal, the lower motor neurons and the nerve fibers at C5 and C6 are intact.*

Peripheral Nervous System

The cranial and spinal nerves, which connect the CNS with the body parts, constitute the peripheral nervous system.

A. Cranial nerves (Table 20-1).
   1. Twelve pairs of cranial nerves.
   2. Originate from under the surface of the brain.

B. Spinal nerves.
   1. Each pair of nerves is numbered according to the level of the spinal cord from which it originates (e.g., C1, C2, etc.).

Table 20-1	CRANIAL NERVES	
No.	**Name**	**Function**
I	Olfactory	Sense of smell
II	Optic	Vision: conducts information from the retina
III	Oculomotor	Downward and outward movement of the eye
		Pupillary constriction and accommodation
		Muscle of the upper eyelid (ability to keep the eye open)
IV	Trochlear	Movement of the eye
V	Trigeminal:	
	Ophthalmic	Corneal reflex
	Maxillary	Sensory fibers of the face
	Mandibular	Motor nerves for chewing and swallowing
VI	Abducens	Inward movement of the eye
VII	Facial	Facial expression
		Sense of taste on anterior tongue
		Muscle of the eyelid (ability to close the eye)
VIII	Acoustic	Reception of hearing and maintenance of equilibrium
IX	Glossopharyngeal	Sense of taste on posterior tongue
		Salivation
		Swallowing or gag reflex
X	Vagus nerve	Assists in swallowing action
		Motor fibers to larynx for speech
		Innervation of organs in thorax and abdomen
		Important in respiratory, cardiac, and circulatory reflexes
XI	Accessory (spinal)	Ability to rotate the head and raise the shoulder
XII	Hypoglossal	Muscles of the tongue

2. Each spinal nerve is connected to the cord by two roots.
   a. Dorsal (posterior root): a sensory nerve carrying messages to the CNS.
   b. Ventral (anterior root): a motor nerve carrying neuron messages to glands and the peripheral areas.
C. Somatic nervous system: consists of peripheral nerve fibers sending sensory stimuli to CNS and motor nerve fibers that stimulate skeletal muscle.
D. Autonomic nervous system (ANS): regulates involuntary activity (cardiovascular, respiratory, metabolic, body temperature, etc.).
   1. Consists of two divisions that have antagonistic activity.
   2. Parasympathetic division: maintains normal body functions.
   3. Sympathetic division: prepares the body to meet a challenge or an emergency (preparation for "fight or flight") (Table 20-2).
   4. Most of the organs of the body receive innervation from both the parasympathetic and the sympathetic divisions. The divisions are usually antagonistic in effect on individual organs: one stimulates; the other relaxes.
   5. Chemical mediators: facilitate transmission of impulses in the ANS.
      a. Acetylcholine is released by the fibers in both divisions of the ANS.
      b. Norepinephrine is released primarily by the sympathetic division.

ALERT Identify pathophysiology related to an acute or chronic condition (e.g., signs and symptoms).

 System Assessment

A. History.
   1. Neurologic history.
      a. Avoid suggesting symptoms to the client.
      b. The manner in which the problems first presented and the overall course of the illness are very important.

c. Mental status must be assessed before the history data from the client can be assumed to be accurate.

NURSING PRIORITY In the older adult client, assess orientation and mental status before continuing assessment of neurologic function (Box 20-1).

2. Medical history.
   a. Assess comorbidities (Box 20-2).
   b. Complete medication profile including complementary medications.

Box 20-1   OLDER ADULT CARE FOCUS

Assessing Neurologic Function in Older Adults

Signs of Cognitive Impairment
- Significant memory loss (person, place, and time).
- Person: Does client know who he or she is, and can client give you his or her full name?
- Place: Can client identify his or her home address and where he or she is now?
- Time: What was the most recent holiday; what month, time of day, day of the week is it now?
- Does client show a lack of judgment?
- Is client agitated and/or suspicious?
- As determined from client's appearance and family's response, does client have problems with ADLs?
- Short-term memory: Can the client recall your name, name of the President, or name of his or her doctor?
- Short-term recall: Ask the client to name three or four common objects; then ask client to recall them within the next 5 minutes.
- Does the client have sensory deficits (hearing and vision) of which he or she is not aware?

Box 20-2   OLDER ADULT CARE FOCUS

Causes of Confusion in the Older Adult Client

Decreased Cardiac Output
- Myocardial infarction
- Dysrhythmias
- Congestive heart failure

Hypoxia/Respiratory Acidosis
- Pneumonia
- Infection
- Hypoventilation

Neurologic
- Vascular insufficiency
- Infections
- Cerebral edema

Metabolic—Altered Homeostasis
- Electrolyte imbalance
- Hypoglycemia/hyperglycemia
- Dehydration
- Urinary tract infections

Environmental
- Strange surroundings
- Hypothermia/hyperthermia

Table 20-2	AUTONOMIC NERVOUS SYSTEM	
Area Affected	*Sympathetic*	*Parasympathetic*
Pupil	Dilates	Constricts
Bronchi	Dilates	Constricts
Heart	Increases rate	Decreases rate
Gastrointestinal	Inhibits peristalsis	Stimulates peristalsis
	Stimulates sphincter	Inhibits sphincters
Bladder	Relaxes bladder muscle	Contracts bladder muscle
	Constricts sphincter	Relaxes sphincter
Adrenal glands	Increases secretion of epinephrine and norepinephrine	

c. Birth (or delivery) history. Was client a difficult delivery?

d. Sequence of growth and development.

3. Family history: presence of hereditary or congenital problems.

4. Personal history: activities of daily living (ADLs), any change in routine.

5. History and symptoms of current problem.

a. Paralysis or paresthesia, syncope.

b. Headache, dizziness, speech problems.

c. Visual problems, changes in personality.

d. Memory loss, nausea, vomiting.

B. Physical assessment.

1. General observation of client.

a. Posture, gait, coordination; perform Romberg test.

b. Position of rest for the infant or young child.

c. Personal hygiene, grooming.

d. Evaluate speech and ability to communicate.
   (1) Pace of speech: rapid, slow, halting.
   (2) Clarity: slurred or distinct.
   (3) Tone: high-pitched, rough.
   (4) Vocabulary: appropriate choice of words.

e. Facial features may suggest specific syndromes in children.

2. Mental status (must take into consideration the client's culture and educational background).

> ⚠ **NURSING PRIORITY** Level of consciousness and mental status are assessment data for the client with neurologic deficits.

a. Level of consciousness.
   (1) Oriented to person, place, time, and situation (in order of importance).
   (2) Appropriate response to verbal and tactile stimuli.
   (3) Memory, problem-solving abilities.

b. Mood.

c. Thought content and intellectual capacity.

d. General appearance and behavior.

3. Assess pupillary status and eye movements (Figure 20-3).

a. Size of pupils should be equal.

b. Reaction of pupils.
   (1) Accommodation: pupillary constriction to accommodate near vision.
   (2) Direct light reflex: constriction of pupil when light is shone directly into eye.
   (3) Consensual reflex: constriction of the pupil in the opposite eye when the direct light reflex is tested.

c. Evaluate ability to move eye.
   (1) Note nystagmus: fine, jerking eye movement.
   (2) Ability of eyes to move together.
   (3) Resting position of the iris should be at mid-position of the eye socket.
   (4) Assess for lid lag (ptosis).

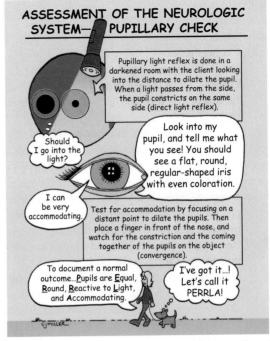

FIGURE 20-3 Assessment of the neurologic system: pupillary check. (From Zerwekh J, Gaglione T: *Mosby's assessment memory notecards: visual, mnemonic, and memory aids for nurses,* ed 1, St. Louis, 2007, Mosby.)

d. PERRLA: indicates that **P**upils are **E**qual, **R**ound, and **R**eactive to **L**ight and that **A**ccommodation is present.

> ⚠ **NURSING PRIORITY:** When assessing a client's neurologic status, always evaluate symmetry. If asymmetrical findings are detected, refine exam to determine CNS versus peripheral nervous system as origin of asymmetry.

4. Evaluate motor function.

a. Assess face and upper extremities for equality of movement and sensation.

b. Evaluate appropriateness of motor movement-spontaneous and on command.

c. Movement of extremities should always be evaluated bilaterally; tone, strength, and muscle movement of each side should be compared (e.g., bilateral hand grips of equal strength).

d. Presence of inappropriate, nonpurposeful movement (e.g., posturing).
   (1) Decerebrate: extension and adduction of the arms, hyperextension of the legs.
   (2) Decorticate: flexion, internal rotation of the arms, extension of the legs.
   (3) Presence of nonpurposeful involuntary movements such as tremors, jerking, twitching, tics, or muscle fasciculation.
   (4) Opisthotonos: extreme hyperextension of the head and dorsal arching.

e. Ability of an infant to suck and to swallow.

f. Asymmetrical contraction of facial muscles.

5. Evaluate reflexes.
   a. Gag or cough reflex.
   b. Swallow reflex.
   c. Corneal reflex.
   d. Babinski reflex: normal is negative in adults and children older than 1 year; positive sign is dorsal flexion of the foot and large toe with fanning of the other toes.
   e. Deep tendon reflexes (simple stretch reflex).
6. Assess vital signs and correlate with other data; changes often occur slowly, and the overall trend needs to be evaluated.
   a. Blood pressure and pulse: intracranial problems precipitate changes; systolic blood pressure may increase, and pulse rate may decrease.
   b. Respirations: rate, depth, and rhythm are sensitive indicators of intracranial problems.
      (1) Cheyne-Stokes respiration: periodic breathing in which hyperpnea alternates with apnea.
      (2) Neurogenic hyperventilation: regular, rapid, deep hyperpnea.
      (3) Ataxic: completely irregular pattern with random deep and shallow respirations.
   c. Temperature: evaluate changes in temperature as related to neurologic control versus infection.

DISORDERS OF THE NEUROLOGIC SYSTEM

Increased Intracranial Pressure

An increase in intracranial pressure (ICP) occurs any time there is an increase in the size or amount of intracranial contents.
A. The cranial vault is rigid, and there is minimal room for expansion of the intracranial components.
B. An increase in any one of the components necessitates a reciprocal change in other cranial contents; this frequently results in ischemia of brain tissue. An increase in ICP results from one of the following:
1. Increased intracranial blood volume (vasodilation).
2. Increased CSF.
3. Increase in the bulk of the brain tissue (edema).
C. Cerebral edema.
1. Edema occurs when there is an increase in the volume of brain tissue caused by an increase in the permeability of the walls of the cerebral vessels. Protein-rich fluid leaks into the extracellular space. Edema is most often the cause of increased ICP in adults, which reaches maximum pressure in 48 to 72 hours.
2. Cytotoxic (cellular) edema occurs as a result of hypoxia. This results in abnormal accumulation of fluid within the cells (intracellular) and a decrease in extracellular fluid.
D. Poor ventilation will precipitate respiratory acidosis, or an increase in the $Paco_2$.
1. Carbon dioxide has a vasodilating effect on the cerebral arteries, which increases cerebrovascular blood flow and increases ICP.

2. Clients should be ventilated to a normocapnic state to prevent cyclic vasodilation, which increases intracranial pressure.
E. Regardless of the cause, increased ICP will result in progressive neurologic deterioration; the specific deficiencies seen are determined by the area and extent of compression of brain tissue.
F. If the infant's cranial suture lines are open, increased ICP will cause separation of the suture lines and an increase in the circumference of the head.

! NURSING PRIORITY There is no single set of symptoms for all clients with increased ICP; symptoms depend on the cause and on how rapidly increased ICP develops.

Assessment
A. Risk factors/etiology.
1. Cerebral edema caused by some untoward event or trauma, including toxic exposure, blunt trauma, fluid and electrolyte imbalance.
2. Brain tumors.
3. Intracranial hemorrhage caused by epidural or subdural bleeding (closed head injuries or ruptured blood vessels).
4. Subarachnoid hemorrhage, hydrocephalus.
5. Cerebral embolism, resulting in necrosis and edema of areas supplied by the involved vessel.
6. Cerebral thrombosis, resulting in ischemia of the area and leading to edema and congestion of affected area.
7. Encephalitis/meningitis.
B. Clinical manifestations (bedside neurologic checks) (Figure 20-4).

ALERT Determine change in a client's neurologic status. Be able to rapidly evaluate the client and recognize incremental changes in the neurologic signs that indicate an increase in ICP (Box 20-3).

INCREASED INTRACRANIAL PRESSURE

- Changes in LOC
- Eyes
  - Papilledema
  - Pupillary Changes
  - Impaired Eye Movement
- Posturing
  - Decerebrate
  - Decorticate
  - Flaccid
- Decreased Motor Function
  - Change in Motor Ability
  - Posturing
- Headache
- Seizures
  - Impaired Sensory & Motor Function
- Changes in Vital Signs:
  - Cushing's Triad:
    - ↑ Systolic B/P
    - ↓ Pulse
    - Altered Resp Pattern
- Vomiting
- Changes in Speech
- Infants: Bulging Fontanels
  - Cranial Suture Separation
  - ↑ Head Circumference
  - High Pitched Cry

©2007 Nursing Education Consultants, Inc.

FIGURE 20-4 Increased intracranial pressure. (From Zerwekh J, Claborn J: *Memory notebook of nursing,* vol 1, ed 4, Ingram, Texas, 2008, Nursing Education Consultants.)

Box 20-3 INCREASING INTRACRANIAL PRESSURE

Adult
Early: Restless, irritable, lethargic
Intermediate: Unequal pupil response, projectile vomiting, vital signs changes
Late: Decreased level of consciousness, decreased reflexes, hypoventilation, dilated pupils, posturing

Infant/Child
Early: Poor feeding, tense fontanel, headache, nausea and vomiting, increased pitch of cry, unsteady gait
Intermediate (younger than 18 months): Increased head circumference, altered consciousness, bulging fontanel; shrill cry, severe headache, blurred vision, stiff neck
Late: Same as adult

---

1. Assess for *changes* in level of consciousness, because change is the cardinal indicator of increased intracranial pressure.
   a. Any alteration in level of consciousness (early sign for both adults and children)— irritability, restlessness, confusion, lethargy, and difficulty in arousing—may be significant.

! NURSING PRIORITY The first sign of a change in the level of ICP is a change in level of consciousness; this may progress to a decrease in level of consciousness.

   b. Inappropriate verbal and motor response; delayed or sluggish responses.
   c. As the client loses consciousness, hearing is the last sense to be lost.
2. Changes in vital signs.
   a. Increase in systolic blood pressure with increase in pulse pressure.
   b. Decrease in pulse rate.
   c. Alteration in respiratory pattern (Cheyne-Stokes respiration, hyperventilation).
   d. Assess temperature with regard to overall problems; temperature usually increases.

! NURSING PRIORITY Cushing's triad: increasing systolic pressure, with increased pulse pressure, decreased pulse rate, and Cheyne-Stokes respirations. Increased ICP is well established when this occurs.

3. Pupillary response: normal pupils should be round, midline, equal in size, and equally briskly reactive to light and should accommodate to distance. Abnormal findings include:
   a. Ipsilateral: pupillary changes occurring on the same side as a cerebral lesion.
   b. Contralateral: pupillary changes occurring on the side opposite a cerebral lesion.
   c. Unilateral dilation of pupils.
   d. Sluggish or no pupillary response to light and poor or absent accommodation.
4. Motor and sensory function: normal is indicated by the ability to move all extremities with equal strength. Abnormal findings include:
   a. Unilateral or bilateral weakness or paralysis.
   b. Failure to withdraw from painful stimuli.
   c. Posturing: decerebrate, decorticate, flaccid, or opisthotonos.
   d. Seizure activity, ataxia.
5. Headache.
   a. Constant with increasing intensity.
   b. Exacerbated by movement.
   c. Photophobia.
6. Vomiting: projectile vomiting without prior nausea.
7. Infants.
   a. Tense, bulging fontanel(s).
   b. Separated cranial sutures.
   c. Increasing frontal-occipital circumference.
   d. High-pitched cry.
C. Diagnostics (see Appendix 20-1).
   1. Direct ICP monitoring.
   2. Romberg test: measures balance. Client stands with feet together and arms at side, first with eyes open, then with eyes closed for 20 to 30 seconds.
   3. Caloric testing: test is performed at bedside by introducing cold water into the external auditory canal. If the eighth cranial nerve is stimulated, nystagmus rotates toward the irrigated ear. If no nystagmus occurs, a pathologic condition is present.
   4. Doll's eye reflex (oculocephalic reflex).
      a. Doll's eye reflex is normal when the client's head is moved from side to side and the eyes move in the direction opposite that of the turning.
      b. Doll's eye reflex is abnormal when the client's eyes remain in a fixed, midline position when the head is turned from side to side (possible brainstem involvement).
      c. Contraindicated until risk for spinal cord injury is ruled out.
   5. Papilledema: edema of the optic nerve; observed by examining retina area with an ophthalmoscope.
   6. Nuchal rigidity: herniation of brainstem may occur; an emergent crisis.
   7. Lumbar puncture is generally not performed; decrease in CSF pressure could precipitate herniation of the brainstem.

Treatment
A. Treatment of the underlying cause of increasing pressure.
B. Neurologic checks every hour or as ordered.
   1. May involve correlation of several variables including level of consciousness, vital signs, speech, facial symmetry, grasp strength, leg strength, and pupil responses.

2. Careful comparison to previous assessment is critical to detect incremental changes.

C. Intravenous (IV) and oral fluids to maintain normal fluid volume status if mean arterial pressure (MAP) is low to normal. Often, normal saline solution is fluid of choice; 5% dextrose in water potentiates cerebral edema.

D. Medications.
   1. Osmotic diuretic corticosteroids.
   2. Anticonvulsants, antihypertensives.

E. Maintain adequate ventilation by means of mechanical ventilation to lower Paco$_2$ (25 to 35 mm Hg) to prevent vasodilation of cerebral vessels.

F. Placement of ventriculoperitoneal shunt during decompression surgery.

Complications

A. CSF leaks, especially in client with basilar skull fracture, may cause meningitis.

B. Herniation: shifting of the intracranial contents from one compartment to another; involves herniation through the tentorium cerebelli; affects area for control of vital functions.

C. Permanent brain damage.

Nursing Interventions

Goal: To identify and decrease problem of increased ICP.

A. Neurologic checks, as indicated by client's status (Tables 20-3 and 20-4).

B. Maintain head of bed in semi-Fowler's position (15-30 degrees) to promote venous drainage and respiratory function.

ALERT Change client's position. If the client with increased ICP develops hypovolemic shock, do not place client in Trendelenburg position.

C. Change client's position slowly; avoid extreme hip flexion and extreme rotation or flexion of neck. Maintain the head midline.

D. Monitor urine osmolarity and specific gravity.

E. Evaluate intake and output.
   1. In response to diuretics.
   2. As correlated with changes in daily weight.
   3. For complications of diabetes insipidus (see Chapter 13).

F. Maintain intake evenly during therapeutic treatment.

Table 20-3	GLASGOW COMA SCALE (GCS)		
Category of Response	**Appropriate Stimulus**	**Response**	**Score**
Eyes open	Approach bedside	Spontaneous response	4
	Verbal command	Opening of eyes to name or command	3
	Pain	Lack of opening of eyes to previous stimuli but opening to pain	2
		Lack of opening of eyes to any stimulus	1
		Untestable	U
Best verbal response	Verbal questioning with maximum arousal	Appropriate orientation, conversant, correct identification of self, place, year, and month	5
		Confusion; conversant, but disorientated in one or more spheres	4
		Inappropriate or disorganized use of words (e.g., cursing), lack of sustained conversation	3
		Incomprehensible words, sounds (e.g., moaning)	2
		Lack of sound, even with painful stimuli	1
		Untestable	U
Best motor response	Verbal command (e.g., "raise your arm, hold up two fingers")	Obedience in response to command	6
	Pain (pressure on proximal nail bed)	Localization of pain, lack of obedience but presence of attempts to remove offending stimulus	5
		Flexion withdrawal*, flexion of arm in response to pain without abnormal flexion posture	4
		Abnormal flexion, flexing of arm at elbow and pronation, making a fist	3
		Abnormal extension, extension of arm at elbow, usually with adduction and internal rotation of arm at shoulder	2
		Lack of response	1
		Untestable	U

From Lewis SL et al: *Medical-surgical nursing: assessment and management of clinical problems,* ed 7, St. Louis, 2007, Mosby.
*Added to the original scale by many centers.

Table 20-4		MODIFIED GLASGOW COMA SCORE FOR PEDIATRIC CLIENTS	
Activity	Score	Infant's Best Response	Children (4 years or older)
Eyes opening	4	Spontaneous	Spontaneous
	3	To speech	To speech
	2	To pain	To pain
	1	No response	No response
Verbal response	5	Coos, babbles	Oriented; smiles, interacts, follows objects
	4	Irritable cry	Confused, disoriented, uncooperative
	3	Cries in response to pain	Inappropriate words, persistent cries, inconsolable, inconsistent awareness of environment
	2	Moans in response to pain	Incomprehensible sounds, agitated, restless, unaware of environment
	1	No response	No response
Motor response	6	Normal spontaneous movements	Normal spontaneous movements
	5	Withdraws from touch	Localizes pain
	4	Withdraws from pain	Withdraws from pain
	3	Abnormal flexion	Abnormal flexion
	2	Abnormal extension	Abnormal extension
	1	No response	No response

G. Minimize respiratory suctioning and ensure hyperoxygenation before suctioning.

H. Sedatives and narcotics can depress respiration; use with caution because they mask symptoms of increasing ICP.

I. Client should avoid strenuous coughing, Valsalva maneuver, and isometric muscle exercises.

J. Avoid straining with stools (increases intrathoracic pressure sporadically).

K. In infants, measure frontal-occipital circumference to evaluate increase in size of the head.

L. Control hyperthermia.

M. Maintain head and spinal column in midline position.

Goal: To maintain respiratory function.

> **❗ NURSING PRIORITY** An obstructed airway is one of the most common problems in the unconscious client; position to maintain patent airway or use airway adjuncts.

A. Prevent respiratory problems of immobility.

B. Evaluate patency of airway frequently; as level of consciousness decreases, client is at increased risk for accumulating secretions and airway obstruction by the tongue.

C. Keep Paco$_2$ levels normal.

D. Suction as necessary briefly.

E. Client may require intubation and respiratory support from a ventilator (see Appendixes 15-5 and 15-8).

Goal: To protect client from injury.

A. Maintain seizure precautions (see Appendix 20-5).

B. Restrain client only if absolutely necessary; struggling against restraints increases ICP.

C. Do not clean the ears or nasal passages of a client with a head injury or a client who has had neurosurgery. Check for evidence of a CSF leak: CSF has glucose in it; test it with a dipstick. CSF also leaves a yellow "halo" stain.

D. Aspiration is a major problem in the unconscious client; place the client in semi-Fowler's position for tube feeding after ensuring correct tube placement.

E. Maintain quiet, nonstimulating environment.

F. Inspect eyes and prevent corneal ulceration.
1. Protective closing of eyes, if eyes remain open.
2. Irrigation with normal saline solution or methylcellulose drops to restore moisture.

Goal: To maintain psychologic equilibrium.

A. Neurologic checks should be done on a continual basis to detect potential problems.

B. Encourage verbalization of fears regarding condition.

C. Give simple explanation of procedures to client and family.

D. Altered states of consciousness will cause increased anxiety and confusion; maintain reality orientation.

E. If client is unconscious, continue to talk to him or her; describe procedures and treatments; always assume that client can hear.

F. Assist parents and family to work through feelings of guilt and anger.

Goal: To prevent complications of immobility (see Chapter 3).

Goal: To maintain elimination.

A. Urinary incontinence: may use condom catheter or indwelling bladder catheter.

B. Keep perineal area clean, prevent excoriation.

C. Monitor bowel function; evaluate for fecal impaction.

> **ALERT** Notify primary health care provider when client demonstrates signs of potential complications; interpret what data for a client need to be reported immediately.

Home Care

A. Teach client and family signs of increased ICP.
B. Call the doctor if any of the following are observed:
   1. Changes in vision.
   2. Increased drainage from incision area or clear drainage in the ears.
   3. Abrupt changes in sleeping patterns or irritability.
   4. Headache that does not respond to medication.
   5. Changes in coordination, disorientation.
   6. Slurred speech, unusual behavior.
   7. Seizure activity, vomiting.
C. Review care of surgical incision, wounds, or drains.

Brain Tumors

A. Brain tumors may be benign, malignant, or metastatic; malignant brain tumors rarely metastasize outside the CNS.
B. Supratentorial: tumors occurring within the anterior two-thirds of the brain, primarily the cerebrum.
C. Infratentorial: tumors occurring in the posterior third of the brain (or below the tentorium), primarily in the cerebellum or the brainstem.
D. Regardless of the origin, site, or presence of malignancy, problems of increased ICP occur because of the limited area in the brain to accommodate an increase in the intracranial contents.

Assessment

A. Risk factors/etiology.
   1. Age: highest incidence in people older than 70 years; common in children younger than 8 years.
   2. Presence of metastatic cancer of the lung or breast.
   3. Family history: gliomas tend to occur in other family members.
   4. Occupation: people who work with high levels of radiation, formaldehyde (pathologists), vinyl chloride (plastics manufacturers), and other chemicals are at increased risk for brain tumors.
B. Clinical manifestations: symptoms correlate with the area of the brain initially involved.
   1. Headache.
      a. Recurrent. May vomit on arising and then feel better.
      b. More severe in the morning.
      c. Affected by position.
      d. Headache in infant may be identified by persistent, irritated crying and head rolling.
   2. Vomiting: initially with or without nausea; progressively becomes projectile.
   3. Papilledema (edema of the optic disc).
   4. Seizures (focal or generalized).
   5. Dizziness and vertigo.
   6. Mental status changes: lethargy and drowsiness, confusion, disorientation, and personality changes.
   7. Localized manifestations:
      a. Focal weakness: hemiparesis.
   8. Sensory disturbances.
      a. Language disturbances.
      b. Coordination disturbances.
      c. Visual disturbances.
   9. Head tilt: child may tilt the head because of damage to extraocular muscles; may be first indication of a decrease in visual acuity.
   10. Changes in vital signs indicative of increasing ICP (Cushing's triad).
   11. Cranial enlargement in the infant younger than 18 months.
C. Diagnostics (see Appendix 20-1).

Treatment

A. Medical.
   1. Dexamethasone (see Appendix 6-7).
   2. Chemotherapy.
   3. Anticonvulsants (see Appendix 20-2).
   4. Complementary and alternative medicine.
B. Radiation: x-rays, gamma knife, stereotactic radiosurgery.
C. Surgical intervention: craniotomy/craniectomy, biopsy, shunt placement, reservoir placement, laser removal.

Complications

Complications include meningitis, brainstem herniation, diabetes insipidus, and syndrome of inappropriate antidiuretic hormone secretion (see Chapter 13). Residual effects include a wide array of complications such as seizures, dysarthria, dysphasia, disequilibrium, and permanent brain damage.

Nursing Interventions

Goal: To provide appropriate preoperative nursing interventions.
A. General preoperative care with exceptions, as noted (see Chapter 3).
B. Carefully assess and discuss with surgeon the appropriateness of a preoperative enema.
C. Prepare client and family for appearance of the client after surgery, including partial or complete hair loss.
D. Encourage verbalization regarding concerns about surgery.
E. Skin preparation is usually done in the operating room.

Goal: To monitor changes in ICP after craniotomy (see Box 20-3).
A. Obtain vital signs and perform neurologic checks and cranial nerve assessments as necessary.
B. Maintain pulmonary function and hygiene.
C. Anticipate use of anticonvulsants and antiemetics.
D. Discourage coughing.
E. Carefully evaluate level of consciousness; increasing lethargy or irritability may be indicative of increasing ICP.
F. Evaluate dressing.
   1. Location and amount of drainage.
   2. Clarify with surgeon whether the nurse or the surgeon will change dressing.
   3. Evaluate for CSF leak through the incision.

G. Maintain semi-Fowler's position if there is a CSF leak from ears or nose.
H. Postoperative positioning for client who has had infratentorial surgery is as follows:
   1. Bed should be flat.
   2. Position client on either side; avoid supine position.
   3. Maintain head and neck in midline.
   4. Keep NPO for 24 hours to reduce edema around medulla and reduce vomiting.
I. Postoperative position for client who has had supratentorial surgery: semi- to low-Fowler's position.
J. Trendelenburg position is contraindicated for clients who have had either infratentorial or supratentorial surgery.
K. Maintain fluid regulation.
   1. After client is awake and the swallow and gag reflexes have returned, begin offering clear liquids by mouth.
   2. Closely monitor intake and output.
L. Evaluate neurologic status in response to fluid balance and diuretics.
M. Evaluate changes in temperature: may be due to respiratory complications or to alteration in the function of the hypothalamus.
N. Provide appropriate postoperative pain relief.
   1. Avoid narcotic analgesics.
   2. Acetaminophen is frequently used.
   3. Maintain quiet, dim atmosphere.
   4. Avoid sudden movements.
O. Prevent complications of immobility (see Chapter 3).
P. Maintain seizure precautions (see Appendix 20-5).

 Home Care

See home care for client with increasing ICP.

 Head Injury

A. Classification.
   1. Penetrating head injury: dura is pierced, as in stabbing or shooting.
   2. Closed or blunt head injury: head is either drastically accelerated (whiplash) or decelerated (collision); most common head injury in civilian life.
 B. Children and infants are more capable of absorbing direct impact because of the pliability of the skull.
C. Coup-contrecoup injury: damage to the site of impact (coup) and damage on the side opposite the site of impact (contrecoup) when brain "bounces" freely inside skull.
D. Primary injury to the brain occurs by compression and/or tearing and shearing stresses on vessels and nerves.
E. Although brain volume remains unchanged, secondary injury occurs from the cerebral edema in response to the primary injury and frequently precipitates an increase in ICP.
F. Types of head injuries (Figure 20-5).
   1. Concussion: temporary interference in brain function; may affect memory, speech, reflexes, balance, and coordination.
      a. Only small number of victims actually "black out."
      b. Usually from blunt trauma including contact sports.
      c. Usually does not cause permanent damage.
      d. Transient, self-limiting.
   2. Contusion (a bruise on the brain).
      a. Multiple areas of petechial hemorrhages.
      b. Headache, pupillary changes, dizziness, unilateral weakness.
      c. Blood supply is altered in the area of injury; swelling, ischemia, and increased ICP.
      d. May last several hours to weeks.
   3. Intracranial hemorrhage.
      a. Epidural (extradural) hematoma: a large vessel (often a meningeal artery or vein) in the dura mater is damaged; a hematoma rapidly forms between the dura and the skull, precipitating an increase in ICP.
         (1) Momentary loss of consciousness, then free of symptoms (lucid period), and then lethargy and coma-seldom evident in children.
         (2) Symptoms of increasing ICP may develop within minutes after the lucid interval.
         (3) Tentorial herniation may occur without immediate intervention.
      b. Subdural hematoma: a collection of blood between the dura and arachnoid area filling the brain vault; usually the result of serious head injury.
         (1) May be acute (manifesting in less than 24 hours) or "chronic" (developing over days to weeks).
         (2) When neurologic compromise presents, subdural hematoma becomes an emergent event.

A. Subdural hematoma   B. Epidural hematoma   C. Intracerebral hematoma

FIGURE 20-5 Formation of head injury after hematoma. (From Black JM, Hawks JH: *Medical-surgical nursing: clinical management for positive outcomes*, ed 8, Philadelphia, 2009, Saunders.)

Emergency neurosurgery may be required to relieve pressure and prevent brain herniation.

(3) Treatment may also include diuretics and anticonvulsants.

(4) Persistent neurologic complications—including dysarthria, unilateral weakness, memory loss, and seizures—may continue.

4. With presence of retinal hemorrhage, evaluate for "shaken baby syndrome."

Assessment

A. Risk factors/etiology.
1. History of trauma.
2. Epidural hematomas are rare in children younger than 4 years.
3. Subdural hematomas are common in infants and may result from birth trauma.
B. Clinical manifestations.
1. Epidural hematoma: decreased GCS, pupillary changes, unilateral weakness.
2. Subdural hematoma: headache, change in LOC, numbness, headache, slurred speech, or inability to speak.
C. Diagnostics (see Appendix 20-1).

Complications

Complications include increased ICP, meningitis, diabetes insipidus, seizures, and permanent neurologic compromise.

Treatment

! NURSING PRIORITY The primary treatment objectives for the client with a head injury are to maintain a patent airway, to prevent hypoxia and hypercapnia resulting in acidosis, and to identify the occurrence of increased ICP.

A. The majority of clients who experience concussion are treated at home.
B. A period of unconsciousness or presence of seizures is considered a serious indication of injury.
C. Surgical intervention.
1. Burr holes to evacuate the hematoma.
2. Craniotomy/craniectomy.

Nursing Interventions

Goal: To provide instruction for care of the client in the home environment (Box 20-4).
A. Problems frequently do not occur until 24 hours or more after the initial injury.
B. Observe the client for increased periods of sleep; if client is asleep, awaken every 2 to 3 hours to determine whether client can be aroused normally.
C. Maintain contact with physician for reevaluation if complications occur.
D. Health care provider should be notified when any of the following are observed:
1. Any change in level of consciousness (increased drowsiness, confusion).
2. Inability to arouse client, seizures.

Box 20-4   DISCHARGE INSTRUCTIONS FOR CLIENTS WITH HEAD INJURY

Arouse the client every 3 to 4 hours for the first 24 hours.
Anticipate complaints of dizziness, headaches.
Do not allow client to blow his nose; try to prevent sneezing.
No alcohol or sedatives for sleep.
Acetaminophen for headaches.
No exercising over next 2 to 3 days.
Call the doctor if any of the following is noted:
• Change in vision: Blurred or diplopia
• Poor coordination: Walking, grasping
• Drainage (serous or bloody) from the nose or ears
• Forceful vomiting
• Increasing sleepiness, more difficult to arouse
• Slurred speech
• Headache that does not respond to medication and continues to get worse
• Occurrence of a seizure

---

3. Bleeding or watery drainage from the ears or nose.
4. Loss of feeling or sensation in any extremity.
5. Blurred vision, slurred speech, vomiting.

ALERT Determine family's understanding of the consequences of the client's illness. Written and oral instructions should be given to the client and to the family. Increased anxiety may affect comprehension of oral directions (see Box 20-4).

Goal: To maintain homeostasis and to monitor and identify early symptoms of increased ICP.
A. Bed rest and clear liquids initially.
B. Frequent neurologic checks for increased ICP.
1. Change or decrease in level of consciousness is frequently the first indication.
2. Instruct clients with head injury not to cough, sneeze, or blow nose.
C. Evaluate drainage from nose, ears, and mouth.
1. Do not clean out the ears: place loose cotton in the auditory canal and change when soiled.
2. Check continuous clear drainage from the nose with Dextrostix; if glucose is present, it is indicative of a CSF leak; spinal fluid also dries with a yellow halo around edges of drainage.
3. If a CSF leak occurs, keep the head of the bed elevated and monitor for development of an infection (meningitis).
D. Seizure precautions (see Appendix 20-5).
E. Maintain adequate fluid intake by IV infusion or oral intake; do not overhydrate.
F. Assess for other undetected injuries; stabilize spine after head injury until spinal cord injury is ruled out.
Goal: To provide appropriate nursing interventions for the client experiencing an increase in ICP (see nursing goals for increased ICP).
Goal: To provide adequate nutritional and caloric intake for the client with a head injury.
A. Provide enteral feedings if client is unable to eat.
B. Assist client to take oral feedings once swallow reflex is normal; client is at increased risk for aspiration.

Hydrocephalus

Hydrocephalus is a condition caused by an imbalance in the production and absorption of CSF in the ventricles of the brain.

Classification: Primary

A. Noncommunicating (obstructive): circulation of CSF is blocked within the ventricular system of the brain.
B. Communicating: CSF flows freely within the ventricular system but is not adequately absorbed.

Classification: Secondary

A. Congenital.
B. Acquired—possibly from trauma, infection, or tumor.

Assessment

A. Risk factors/etiology.
  1. Neonate: usually the result of a congenital malformation.
  2. Older child, adult.
    a. Space-occupying lesion.
    b. Preexisting developmental defects.
B. Clinical manifestations: infant.
  1. Head enlargement: increasing circumference in excess of normal 2 cm per month for first 3 months.
  2. Separation of cranial suture lines.
  3. Fontanel becomes tense and bulging.
  4. Dilated scalp veins.
  5. Frontal enlargement, bulging "sunset eyes."
  6. Symptoms of increasing ICP.
C. Clinical manifestations: older child, adult.
  1. Symptoms of increasing ICP.
  2. Specific manifestations related to site of the lesion.
D. Diagnostics (see Appendix 20-1).
  1. Increasing head circumference is diagnostic in infants.

Treatment

A. Noncommunicating and communicating: ventriculo-peritoneal shunt; CSF is shunted into the peritoneum.
B. Obstructive: removal of the obstruction (cyst, hematoma, tumor).

Nursing Interventions

Goal: To monitor for the development of increasing ICP.
A. Daily measurement of the frontal-occipital circumference of the head in infants.
B. Assess for symptoms of increasing ICP (see Box 20-3).
C. Infant is often difficult to feed; administer small feedings at frequent intervals because vomiting may be a problem.
Goal: To maintain patency of the shunt and monitor ICP after shunt procedure.
A. Position supine, with head turned opposite side up to prevent pressure on the shunt valve and to prevent too-rapid depletion of CSF.
B. Position is not a problem with children who are having a shunt revision; they have not had an increase in ventricular pressure.
C. Monitor for increasing ICP and compare with previous data.

D. Monitor for infection, especially meningitis or encephalitis.

Home Care

A. Teach parents symptoms of increasing ICP.
B. Have parents participate in care of the shunt before client's discharge.
C. Encourage parents and family to ventilate feelings regarding client's condition.
D. Refer client to appropriate community agencies.

Reye's Syndrome

Reye's syndrome is a rare acute illness that occurs after a viral illness (frequently, after aspirin has been consumed) and results in fatty infiltration of the liver and subsequent liver degeneration and increased intracranial pressure.
A. Damaged liver cells no longer adequately convert ammonia to urea for excretion from the body.
B. Circulating ammonia crosses the blood-brain barrier to produce acute neurologic effects.

Assessment

A. Risk factors/etiology.
  1. Most often preceded by an acute viral infection.
  2. Primarily affects children from the age of 6 months to adolescence.
  3. Frequently, the affected child has received salicylate (aspirin) for control of fever during the preceding viral infection.
  4. With warning labels now on aspirin, problem has significantly decreased.
B. Clinical manifestations.
  1. Stage 1.
    a. Initial symptom may be severe persistent vomiting.
    b. Lethargy, listlessness.
  2. Stage 2.
    a. Irritability, disorientation.
    b. Progresses to state of increased ICP with deepening coma and posturing.
C. Diagnostics (see Appendix 19-1).
  1. Definitive diagnosis is a liver biopsy.
  2. Prolonged prothrombin time.
  3. Elevated blood ammonia levels.
  4. Elevated serum aspartate aminotransferase and alanine aminotransferase levels.

Treatment

A. Primarily supportive, based on stage of the disease; mechanical ventilation, fluid and electrolyte balance.
B. Measures to decrease ICP.
C. Early intervention critical to successful treatment.

Nursing Interventions

Goal: To monitor progress of disease state and maintain homeostasis.
A. IV fluids.
B. Monitor serum electrolytes and liver function studies.
C. Maintain respiratory status; prevent hypoxia.
D. Assess for problems of impaired coagulation.

E. Decrease stress, anxiety: child may not remember events before the critical phase.

Goal: To monitor for and implement nursing actions appropriate for increasing ICP.

Stroke (Brain Attack)

Stroke, or brain attack, is the disruption of the blood supply to an area of the brain, resulting in tissue necrosis and sudden loss of brain function. It is the leading cause of adult disability in the United States.

A. Atherosclerosis (see Chapter 16), resulting in cerebrovascular disease, frequently precedes the development of a stroke.

B. Types of stroke.
1. Ischemic stroke.
   a. Thrombotic stroke: formation of a clot that results in the narrowing of a vessel lumen and eventual occlusion; accounts for about 80% of strokes.
      (1) Associated with hypertension and diabetes (i.e., conditions that accelerate the atherosclerotic process).
      (2) Produces ischemia of the cerebral tissue distal to occlusion and edema to the surrounding areas.
   b. Embolic stroke: occlusion of a cerebral artery by an embolus.
      (1) Common site of origin is the endocardium.
      (2) May affect any age group; associated with atrial fibrillation, endocarditis, and prosthetic cardiac valves.
2. Hemorrhagic stroke.
   a. Rupture of a cerebral artery caused by hypertension, trauma, or aneurysm.
   b. Blood compresses the brain.

C. The area of edema resulting from tissue damage may precipitate more damage than the vascular damage itself.

D. TIA and RIND.
1. Transient ischemic attack (TIA, silent stroke).
   a. Brief episode, less than 24 hours, of neurologic dysfunction; usually resolves within 30 to 60 minutes.
   b. Should be considered a warning sign of an impending stroke.
   c. Neurologic dysfunction is present for minutes to hours, but no permanent neurologic deficit remains.
2. Reversible ischemic neurologic deficit (RIND).
   a. Symptoms similar to TIA.
   b. Neurologic symptoms last longer than 24 hours but less than a week.
3. Stroke: client has neurologic deficits related to mobility, sensation, and cognition.

E. Neuromuscular deficits resulting from a stroke are due to damage of motor neurons of the pyramidal tract.
1. Damage to the left side of the brain will result in paralysis of the right side of the body (Figure 20-6).

Right-brain damage (stroke on right side of the brain)	Left-brain damage (stroke on left side of the brain)
• Paralyzed left side: hemiplegia	• Paralyzed right side: hemiplegia
• Left-sided neglect	• Impaired speech/language aphasias
• Spatial-perceptual deficits	• Impaired right/left discrimination
• Tends to deny or minimize problems	• Slow performance, cautious
• Rapid performance, short attention span	• Aware of deficits: depression, anxiety
• Impulsive, safety problems	• Impaired comprehension related to language, math
• Impaired judgment	
• Impaired time concepts	

FIGURE 20-6 Manifestations of right-brain and left-brain stroke. (From Lewis SL et al: *Medical-surgical nursing: assessment and management of clinical problems,* ed 7, St. Louis, 2007, Mosby.)

2. Both upper and lower extremities of the involved side are affected.

Assessment

A. Risk factors/etiology (Box 20-5).

B. Clinical manifestations.
1. Transient ischemic attack (TIA) and reversible ischemic neurologic deficit (RIND).
   a. Visual defects: blurred vision, diplopia, blindness of one eye, tunnel vision.
   b. Transient hemiparesis, gait problems.
   c. Slurred speech, confusion.
   d. Transient numbness of an extremity.
2. Complete stroke (occurs suddenly with an embolism, more gradually with hemorrhage or thrombosis); manifestations vary according to which cerebral vessels are involved.
   a. Hemiplegia: loss of voluntary movement; damage to the right side of the brain will result in left-sided weakness and paralysis.
   b. Aphasia: defect in using and interpreting the symbols of language; may include written, printed, or spoken words.
   c. May be unaware of the affected side; neglect syndrome ensues.
   d. Cranial nerve impairment: chewing, gag reflex, dysphagia, impaired tongue movement.
   e. May be incontinent initially.
   f. Agnosia: a perceptual defect that causes a disturbance in interpreting sensory information; client

Box 20-5	RISK FACTORS ASSOCIATED WITH STROKE

Modifiable
- Smoking
- Obesity
- Increased salt intake
- Sedentary lifestyle
- Increased stress
- Oral contraceptives

Partially Modifiable
- Hypertension
- Cardiac valve disease
- Dysrhythmias
- Diabetes mellitus
- Hypercholesterolemia

Nonmodifiable
- Sex: Increased incidence in men
- Age
- Race: Increased incidence in the African-American population
- Hereditary predisposition

may not be able to recognize previously familiar objects.

   g. Cognitive impairment of memory, judgment, proprioception (awareness of one's body position).
   h. Hypotonia (flaccidity) for days to weeks, followed by hypertonia (spasticity).
   i. Visual defects.
      (1) Homonymous hemianopia: loss of same half of visual field in each eye; client has only half of normal vision.
      (2) Horner's syndrome: ptosis of the upper eyelid, constriction of the pupil, and lack of tearing in the eye.
   j. Apraxia: can move the affected limb but is unable to carry out learned movements.
   k. Increased ICP, drowsiness to coma.
   l. Pain in eye, nose, or face.
   m. Gait disturbances.
C. Diagnostics (see Appendix 20-1).

Treatment

A. Prophylactic.
   1. Aspirin, platelet inhibitors.
   2. Antihypertensives, anticoagulants.
B. Immediate treatment (differs depending on whether thrombotic or hemorrhagic stroke).
   1. Medical.
      a. Medications to decrease cerebral edema.
         (1) Osmotic diuretics.
         (2) Corticosteroids (dexamethasone).
      b. Anticoagulants for thrombotic stroke (*never* administered to a client with hemorrhagic stroke).
      c. Anticonvulsants.

   d. Thrombolytic therapy or fibrinolytic therapy (such as recombinant tissue plasminogen activator (rtPA [Retavase]) considered for nonhemorrhagic strokes within 3 hours of first manifestation of stroke signs.
   e. Antihypertensives and antidysrhythmics.
   2. Surgical.
      a. Carotid endarterectomy, especially for transient ischemic attack.
      b. Craniotomy for evacuation of hematoma.
      c. Extracranial-intracranial bypass for mild strokes.
C. Specific therapies to resolve physical, speech or occupational complications, including use of assistive devices.

Nursing Interventions

Goal: To prevent stroke through client education (see Box 20-5).
A. Identification of individuals with reversible risk factors and measures to reduce them.
B. Appropriate medical attention for control of chronic conditions conducive to the development of stroke.
C. Teach high-risk clients early signs of TIA and RIND and to seek medical attention immediately if they occur.

Goal: To maintain patent airway and adequate cerebral oxygenation.
A. Place client in side-lying position with head elevated.
B. Assess for symptoms of hypoxia; administer oxygen or assist with endotracheal intubation and mechanical ventilation as necessary (see Appendix 15-8).
C. Maintain patent airway; use oropharyngeal airway to prevent airway obstruction by the tongue.
D. Client is prone to obstructed airway and pulmonary infection; have client cough and deep-breathe every 2 hours.

Goal: To assess for and implement measures to decrease ICP (see nursing goals for increased ICP).

Goal: To maintain adequate nutritional intake.
A. Before oral feedings, evaluate need for swallow studies.
B. Administer oral feedings with caution; start after first 24 hours; check for presence of gag and swallowing reflexes before feeding.
C. Place food on the unaffected side of the mouth; begin with clear foods (gelatins).
D. Select foods that are easy to control in the mouth (thick liquids) and easy to swallow; liquids often promote coughing, because client is unable to control them.
E. Maintain high-Fowler's position for feeding.
F. Maintain privacy and unrushed atmosphere.
G. If client is unable to tolerate oral intake, enteral feedings may be initiated.

ALERT Identify potential for aspiration; assess client's ability to eat.

Goal: To preserve function of the musculoskeletal system.
A. Passive range of motion (ROM) on affected side; begin early because the exercises are more difficult if muscles begin to tighten.

B. Active ROM on unaffected side.

C. Prevent foot drop: passive exercises; rigid boots; have client out of bed as soon as possible.

D. Legs should be maintained in a neutral position; prevent external rotation of affected hip by placing a trochanter roll or rolled pillow at the thigh.

E. Reposition every 2 hours, but limit the period of time spent on the affected side.

> **❗ NURSING PRIORITY** Protect the client's affected side: do not give injections on that side, watch for pressure areas when positioning, have client spend less time on affected side than in other positions.

F. Assess for adduction and internal rotation of the affected arm; maintain arm in a neutral (slightly flexed) position with each joint slightly higher than the preceding one.

G. Restraints should be avoided because they often increase agitation.

H. Maintain joints in position of normal function to prevent flexion contractures.

I. Assist client out of bed on the unaffected side; this allows client to provide some stabilization and balance with the good side (Figure 20-7).

> **ALERT** Mobility: Assist client to ambulate, perform active and passive ROM exercises, assess for complications of immobility, prevent DVT, prevent skin breakdown and encourage independence.

Goal: To maintain homeostasis.

A. Evaluate adequacy of cardiac output.

B. Monitor hydration status: prevent fluid overload.
1. Carefully regulate IV fluid intake.
2. Evaluate response to diuretics.
3. Assess for the development of peripheral edema.
4. Restrict fluid intake, as indicated.
5. Assess respiratory parameters indicative of fluid overload.
6. Monitor daily weight.

C. Determine previous bowel patterns and promote normal elimination.
1. Avoid use of urinary catheter, if possible; if catheter is necessary, remove as soon as possible.
2. Offer bedpan or urinal every 2 hours; help establish a schedule.
3. Prevent constipation: provide increased bulk in diet, stool softeners, etc.
4. Provide privacy and decrease emotional trauma related to incontinence.

> **ALERT** Assess and manage a client with an alteration in elimination. Establish a toileting schedule; the client who has had a stroke will need assistance in reestablishing a normal bowel and bladder routine.

D. Prevent problems of skin breakdown through proper positioning and good skin hygiene.

E. Assist client to identify problems of vision.

FIGURE 20-7 Transfer from bed to wheelchair by client with hemiplegia. (From Black JM, Hawks JH: *Medical-surgical nursing: clinical management for positive outcomes,* ed 7, Philadelphia, 2005, Saunders.)

F. Maintain psychologic homeostasis.
1. Client may be very anxious because of a lack of understanding of what has happened and because of his or her inability to communicate.
2. Speak slowly and clearly and explain what has happened.
3. Assess client's communication abilities and identify methods to promote communication.

Home Care

A. Encourage independence in ADLs.
B. Provide clothing that is easy to get in and out of.
C. Active participation in ROM; have client do his or her own ROM on affected side.
D. Physical, occupational, and speech therapy for retraining of lost function.
E. Assist client to maintain sense of balance when in the sitting position; client will frequently fall to the affected side (unilateral neglect syndrome).
F. Encourage participation in carrying out daily personal hygiene.
G. Teach client safe transfer from bed to wheelchair and provide assistance as needed (see Figure 20-7).
H. Bowel and bladder training program.
1. To promote bladder tone, encourage urination (with or without assistance) every 2 hours rather than allowing the client to void when he or she feels the urge.
2. Teach client to perform Kegel exercises regularly.
3. Advise client to avoid caffeine intake.
4. Increased bulk in diet will help avoid constipation (see Table 18-2).
5. Increase fluids to 2000 mL per day as tolerated.
6. Administer stool softeners PRN.
7. Establish regular daily time for bowel movements.
I. Encourage social interaction (see Appendix 20-6).
1. Speech therapy.
2. Frequent and meaningful verbal stimuli.
3. Allow client plenty of time to respond.
4. Speak slowly and clearly; do not give too many directions at one time. Use short sentences.
5. Do not "talk down to" client or treat client as a child (elder speak).
6. Client's mental status may be normal; do not assume it is impaired.
7. Nonverbal clients do not lose their hearing ability.
J. Evaluate family support and the need for home health services.

> **ALERT** Assist family to manage care of a client with long-term care needs; determine needs of family regarding ability to provide home care after discharge.

 Cerebral Aneurysm, Subarachnoid Hemorrhage

A cerebral aneurysm occurs when a weakened saccular outpouching of the cerebral vasculature bulges from pressure on the weakened tissue. A Berry aneurysm is a cerebral aneurysm occurring in the arterial junction of the circle of Willis. A ruptured cerebral aneurysm often results in hemorrhagic stroke.

A. A subarachnoid hemorrhage is a potentially fatal condition in which blood accumulates below the arachnoid mater in the subarachnoid space; most often occurs secondary to an aneurysm.
B. An aneurysm frequently ruptures and bleeds into the subarachnoid space.
C. Symptoms occur when an aneurysm enlarges, or when it ruptures. As blood collects in the subarachnoid space, it compresses and damages the surrounding brain tissue.
D. Subarachnoid hemorrhage may lead to neurologic compromise including seizures, stroke, permanent brain damage, and even death.
E. Often, symptoms do not appear until rupture has occurred.

Assessment

A. Risk factors/etiology.
1. Age: more common in adults 30 to 60 years of age.
2. Atherosclerosis, connective tissue disease, cigarette smoking, and hypertension—causing fragility in the vessel wall.
3. Head trauma and congenital vessel weakness may increase the risk.
B. Clinical manifestations.
1. Rupture may be preceded by:
   a. Severe headache.
   b. Intermittent nausea.
2. Rupture frequently occurs without warning.
   a. Sudden severe headache, seizures.
   b. Nuchal rigidity, hemiparesis.
   c. Loss of consciousness.
   d. Symptoms of increasing ICP: nausea, vomiting, photophobia.
3. Severity of symptoms depends on the site and amount of bleeding.
C. Diagnostics (see Appendix 20-1).

Treatment

A. Aminocaproic acid: inhibits fibrinolysis in life-threatening situations.
B. Osmotic diuretics, anticonvulsants.
C. Corticosteroids: dexamethasone (Decadron).
D. Calcium channel blockers: minimize vasospasm after hemorrhage.
E. Stool softeners.
F. Analgesics for recurrent headache.
G. Fluids to maintain systolic blood pressure at 100 to 150 mm Hg (increase in volume and pressure increases blood flow through narrowed vessels).
H. Surgical intervention: ligation or "clipping" of the aneurysm to reduce the swelling and minimize the risk for re-bleeding.
I. Procedure to block abnormal arteries or veins and prevent bleeding.

Nursing Interventions

Goal: To prevent further increase in ICP and possible rupture.

A. Immediate bed rest; bathroom privileges may be permitted.

B. Prevent Valsalva maneuver.

C. Client should avoid straining, sneezing, pulling up in bed, and acute flexion of the neck.

D. Elevate head of the bed 30 degrees to 45 degrees to promote venous return.

E. Quiet, dim, nonstimulating environment: disconnect telephone; promote relaxation.

F. Constant monitoring of condition to identify occurrence of bleeding, as evidenced by symptoms of increasing ICP.

G. Administer analgesics cautiously; the client should continue to be easily aroused so that neurologic checks can be performed.

H. No hot or cold beverages or food, no caffeine, no smoking.

I. Maintain seizure precautions.

> ⚠ **NURSING PRIORITY** If the client survives the rupture of the aneurysm and re-bleeding occurs, it is most likely to occur within the next 24 to 48 hours.

Goal: To assess for and implement nursing measures to decrease ICP (see nursing goals for increased ICP).

Goal: To provide appropriate preoperative nursing interventions (see nursing goals for brain tumor).

Goal: To maintain homeostasis and monitor changes in ICP after craniotomy (see nursing goals for craniotomy).

📋 Meningitis

Meningitis is an acute viral or bacterial infection that causes inflammation of the meningeal tissue covering the brain and spinal cord.

A. Infectious process increases permeability of protective membrane and results in an increased protein concentration in the CSF.

B. Inflammatory process results in the development of cerebral edema.

C. Bacterial meningitis is less common but more severe than viral meningitis.

Assessment

A. Risk factors/etiology.
1. Pathogenic organism most often gains entry from an infection elsewhere in the body.
2. Meningococcal meningitis is the only form that is readily contagious; transmitted by direct contact with droplets from the airway of an infected person.
3. Increased mortality rate among infants.

B. Clinical manifestations: older child and adult.
1. Rash, petechiae, purpura.
2. Nuchal rigidity.
3. Chills and high fever.
4. Severe and persistent headache.
5. Increasing irritability, malaise, changes in level of consciousness.
6. Respiratory distress.
7. Generalized seizures.
8. Nausea and vomiting.
9. Positive Kernig sign: resistance or pain at the knee and the hamstring muscles when client attempts to extend the leg after thigh flexion.
10. Positive Brudzinski sign: reflex flexion of the hips when the neck is flexed.
11. Photophobia.

C. Clinical manifestations: neonate and infant.
1. Fever.
2. Apneic episodes.
3. Bulging fontanel.
4. Seizures.
5. Crying with position change.
6. Opisthotonos positioning: a dorsal arched position.
7. Changes in sleep pattern, increasing irritability.
8. Poor sucking; may refuse feedings.
9. Poor muscle tone, diminished movement.
10. Irritability.

D. Diagnostics (see Appendix 20-1).
1. Lumbar puncture reveals increasing CSF pressure; if ICP is present, then a CT scan may be done before the procedure.
2. Elevated WBCs.
3. CSF and blood cultures positive for meningococcus bacteria.

Treatment

A. Respiratory isolation until positive organism is identified.

B. IV antibiotics, steroids (see Appendixes 6-9, 6-7).

C. Optimum hydration.

D. Anticonvulsant medications (see Appendix 20-2).

E. Antivirals (see Appendix 7-1).

F. Maintain ventilation.

Complications

A. Increasing ICP resulting in permanent brain damage.

B. Visual and hearing deficits, paralysis.

C. Subdural effusion; may be aspirated or allowed to absorb when meningitis treatment is started and protein leak stops.

Nursing Interventions

Goal: To identify the causative organism, control spread, and initiate therapy.

A. Maintain respiratory droplet precautions until organism is identified; place client in a private room (Appendix 6-9).

B. Begin administration of IV antibiotics after lumbar puncture during which CSF sample was obtained.

C. Identify family members and close contacts who may require prophylactic treatment.

Goal: To monitor course of infection and prevent complications.

A. Frequent nursing assessment for increased ICP (see Box 20-3).

B. Maintain adequate hydration; cerebral edema may require limiting fluid intake.

C. Monitor infusion site for complications of IV piggyback antibiotics.

D. Assess for side effects of high dosage of antibiotics.

E. Decrease stimuli in environment: dim lights, quiet environment, no loud noises.

F. Avoid movement or positioning that increases discomfort; client generally assumes a side-lying position.

G. Seizure precautions.

H. Prevent complications of immobility.

I. Good respiratory hygiene.

J. Measures to decrease fever.

Encephalitis

Encephalitis is an inflammatory process of the CNS, or "inflammation of the brain."

Assessment

A. Risk factors/etiology.
1. Commonly occurs as a complication after a viral infection (measles, chicken pox, mumps).
2. May be transmitted by a vector such as a mosquito or tick.
3. Causative organism may be herpes simplex virus in middle-aged adults.

B. Clinical manifestations.
1. Severe headache, nuchal rigidity.
2. Sudden fever.
3. Seizures.
4. Changes in level of consciousness.
5. Motor involvement: ataxia, dysphasia, tremor, convulsions.
6. Drowsiness, confusion, disorientation.
7. Irritability.
8. Bulging fontanels in infants.

C. Diagnostics.
1. Examination of the CSF.
2. Viral studies to isolate the virus.
3. EEG for seizure activity.
4. Blood test for West Nile virus.

Treatment

A. Anticonvulsants.

B. Treatment to decrease ICP.

C. Hydration, bed rest, proper nutrition.

Nursing Interventions

Nursing interventions for encephalitis are the same as those for meningitis, with the exception of antibiotic therapy. Encephalitis is caused by a viral agent and is not responsive to antibiotic therapy; antibiotic therapy may be ordered to prevent bacterial infection.

ALERT Identify changes in client's mental status; treat client with seizures.

Spinal Cord Injury

Spinal cord injury (SCI) is damage to the spinal cord housed inside the spinal column. Most SCIs exist with the spinal cord intact yet compromised from injury or disease. SCI most often occurs as a result of direct trauma to the head or neck area.

A. Risk factors.
1. More than 80% of clients with SCIs are male.
2. More than half of SCIs occur between the ages of 16 and 35 years.
3. Also an increased risk after 60 years of age, when falls become more common.
4. Other risk factors: osteoarthritis, cancer, involvement in sports.

B. Initially after the injury, the nerve fibers swell, and circulation to the spinal cord is decreased; hemorrhage and edema occur, causing an increase in the ischemic process, which progresses to necrotic destruction of the spinal cord.

C. Consequences of SCI depend on the extent of damage, as well as the level of cord injury (Figure 20-8).
1. The higher the lesion, the more severe the sequelae.
   a. Clients with lesions at C4 or higher may require ventilatory support.
   b. Lesions between T1 and T8 often allow use of the hands.
   c. Lesions below T8 often allow upper body control.
2. Complete transection (complete cord dissolution, complete lesion): immediate loss of all sensation and

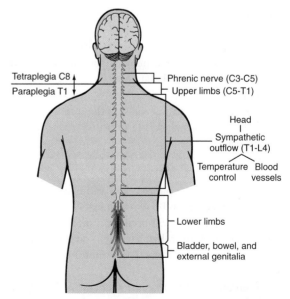

FIGURE 20-8 Spinal cord injury: areas of paralysis. (From Lewis SL et al: *Medical-surgical nursing: assessment and management of clinical problems,* ed 7, St Louis, 2007, Mosby.)

voluntary movement below the level of injury; minimal, if any, return of function.

3. Incomplete (partial).
   a. Central cord syndrome: center of cord is damaged; results primarily in impairment of upper extremities.
   b. Damage to one side of the cord (Brown-Séquard syndrome): motor function and position sense may be present on one side; temperature and sensation may be lost on the opposite side.
   c. Anterior cord damage: disruption of blood flow results in a mixed loss of sensory and motor function below the level of injury.

4. Cord edema peaks in about 2 to 3 days and subsides within about 7 days after the injury.

5. Lumbosacral injuries.
   a. Variable pattern of motor and sensory loss.
   b. Frequently result in neurogenic bowel and bladder.

D. Spinal cord shock (areflexia): temporary loss or dysfunction of spinal reflex activity; occurs predominantly in complete cord lesions; loss of communication with the higher centers of control results in flaccidity and loss of functional control below the level of injury.
   1. SCI interrupts sympathetic nerve impulse transmission; parasympathetic impulses are not counterchecked, resulting in vasodilation; loss of venous return results in hypotension, which is neurogenic shock.
   2. Hypothalamus loses control of body temperature, which assists in vasoconstriction and vasodilation.
   3. Condition may persist for several weeks and reverse spontaneously; resolution of spinal shock will be evident by return of reflexes.
   4. Hyperreflexia will occur as recovery progresses; spastic movements may be precipitated by emotion and cutaneous stimulation.

E. Autonomic dysreflexia occurs in clients with an injury at T6 or higher.
   1. A noxious stimulus below the level of injury triggers the sympathetic nervous system, which causes a release of catecholamines (epinephrine, norepinephrine).
   2. Most common stimuli causing the response are a full bladder or bowel, UTI, pressure ulcers, and skin stimulation.
   3. Severe hypertension (systolic may be greater than 300), nausea, pounding headache, bradycardia, restlessness, flushing piloerection, and blurred vision are the most common body responses.

F. Bladder dysfunction will occur as a result of the injury; normal bladder control is dependent on the sensory and motor pathways and the lower motor neurons being intact.
   1. Neurogenic bladder occurs in clients with both upper and lower motor neuron disorders.
      a. Upper motor neuron disorders produce a spastic or reflex bladder.
      b. Lower motor neuron disorders produce a flaccid bladder.
   2. Management of bladder problems depends on client's preferences and lifestyle, as well as client's functional abilities.

G. Long-term rehabilitation potential depends on the amount of damage done to the cord, which may not be evident until several weeks after the injury.

Assessment

A. Clinical manifestations: depend on level of SCI (see Figure 20-8).
   1. Injury at C3 through C5 will cause respiratory compromise.
   2. Depending on degree of injury, the degree of paralysis and amount of sensory loss below the level of injury will vary.
   3. Spinal shock.
      a. Generally occurs within 72 hours and may last for several weeks.
      b. Flaccid paralysis.
      c. Loss of sensation and absence of reflexes.
      d. Bowel and bladder dysfunction.
      e. Hypotension and bradycardia.
      f. After spinal shock, reflexes and autonomic activity return, as evidenced by development of spasticity.
   4. Autonomic dysreflexia in clients with injuries at T6 or higher.
      a. Severe hypertension, bradycardia.
      b. Complaints of headache.
      c. Flushing and diaphoresis above level of injury.

B. Diagnostics (see Appendix 20-1).

C. Complications.
   1. Respiratory stasis; pulmonary edema and emboli.
   2. Cardiovascular compromise from neurogenic shock, or autonomic dysreflexia.
   3. Skin breakdown resulting in localized and systemic infections.
   4. Immobility issues causing renal and gastrointestinal compromise.
   5. Psychologic, social, and body image issues.

Treatment

A. Emergency intervention required.

B. Corticosteroids within 8 hours of injury (methylprednisolone).

C. Immobilization of the vertebral column in cervical fracture.
   1. Cervical tongs (Crutchfield, Gardner-Wells) for cervical immobility.
   2. Halo vest/jacket traction to promote mobility.
   3. Sterno-occipital mandibular immobilizer (SOMI) brace worn with cervical fusion.

D. Spinal surgery to remove bone fragments and assure spinal alignment.

E. Respiratory support as necessary.

Nursing Interventions

Goal: To maintain stability of the vertebral column and prevent further cord damage.

A. Emergency care and treatment.
   1. Suspect SCI if there is any evidence of direct trauma to the head or neck area (contact sports, diving accidents, motor vehicle accident).
   2. Immobilize client and place on spinal board with the head and neck in a neutral position; do not allow the neck to flex.
   3. Airway, status of breathing, and circulation are the primary concerns initially after injury.
   4. Neurogenic shock may occur within the first 24 hours; observe for decreased B/P, severe bradycardia.

> **⚠ NURSING PRIORITY** Do not hyperextend the neck in a client with a suspected cervical injury. Airway should be opened by the jaw-lift method. Improper handling of the client often results in extension of the damaged area.

   5. Maintain in extended position with no twisting or turning; do not remove cervical collar or spinal board until area of injury is identified.
   6. Maintain patent airway during transportation.
B. Maintain stability of the vertebral column as indicated by the level of injury.
   1. Prescribe and maintain bed rest on firm mattress with supportive devices (sandbags, skin traction, etc.); maintain alignment in the supine position; logroll without any flexion or twisting.
   2. Maintain cervical traction: tongs are inserted into the skull with traction and weights applied; do not remove weights; logroll to maintain spinal immobility.
   3. Halo vest/jacket traction: maintains cervical immobility but allows client to be mobile.
      a. If bolts or screws come loose, keep the client immobilized and call the doctor.
      b. Clean pin sites according to facility policy, observe for infection.
      c. Roll client onto his or her side at the edge of the bed and allow client to push up from the mattress to a sitting position. *Never* use the halo vest frame to assist the client to turn or sit up.
      d. Correct size of wrench should be kept at bedside to remove the anterior bolts in case of emergency.
      e. Assist client to maintain balance when standing; the traction is heavy for a person who is weak, and the client is at increased risk for falling.
   4. Maintain extremities in neutral, functional position.

> **ALERT** Apply, maintain, or remove orthopedic devices (e.g. traction, splints, braces, casts).

C. Perform appropriate nursing intervention when surgery is indicated to stabilize the injury.

Goal: To identify level of damage and changes in neurologic status.

A. Assess respiratory function: symmetrical chest expansion, bilateral breath sounds, presence of retractions or dyspnea.
B. Motor and sensory evaluation.
   1. Ability to move extremities; strength of extremities.
   2. Sensory examination, including touch and pain.
   3. Presence of deep tendon reflexes.
C. Ongoing assessment and status of:
   1. Bladder, gastric, bowel function.
   2. Psychologic adjustment to the injury.
D. Evaluate history of how injury occurred; obtain information regarding how client was transported.
E. Determine status of pain.

Goal: To maintain respiratory function.

A. Frequent assessment of respiratory function during the first 48 hours.
   1. Changes in breathing pattern.
   2. Observe breathing pattern for use of sternocleidomastoid and intercostal muscles for respiration.
   3. Evaluate arterial blood gas values and pulse oximetry.
   4. Determine development of hypoxia.
B. Maintain adequate respiratory function, as indicated.
   1. Chest physiotherapy.
   2. Incentive spirometry.
   3. Changing position within limits of injury.
   4. Assess for complications of atelectasis, pulmonary emboli, and pneumonia.
   5. Nasopharyngeal or endotracheal suctioning based on airway and level of injury.

Goal: To maintain cardiovascular stability.

A. Spinal shock.
   1. Monitor vital signs and evaluate changes.
   2. Vagal stimulation, hypothermia, and hypoxia may precipitate spinal shock.
   3. Assess deep tendon reflexes and muscle strength as resolution of shock occurs.
B. Assess for development of autonomic dysreflexia; if it occurs:
   1. Elevate the head of the bed, and check the client's blood pressure.
   2. Assess for sources of stimuli: distended bladder (check urinary tubing), fecal impaction, constipation, tight clothing.
   3. Relieve the stimuli, and dysreflexia will subside.
   4. Maintain cardiovascular support during period of hypertension.
   5. A hypertensive crisis from dysreflexia will require immediate intervention.
C. Evaluate cardiovascular responses when turning or suctioning client.
D. Apply antiembolism stockings or elastic wraps to the legs to facilitate venous return. (Lack of muscle tone and loss of sympathetic tone in the peripheral vessels result in decreases in both venous tone and venous return, which predispose client to deep vein thrombosis.)
E. Implement measures to promote venous return.

ALERT Prevent complications of immobility; prevent venous stasis: identify symptoms of deep venous thrombosis, apply compression stockings, and change client's position.

Goal: To maintain adequate fluid and nutritional status.

A. During the first 48 hours, evaluate gastrointestinal function frequently; decrease in function may necessitate use of a nasogastric tube to decrease distention.

B. Prevent complications of nausea and vomiting.

C. Evaluate bowel sounds and client's ability to tolerate oral fluids.

D. Increase protein and calories in diet; may need to decrease calcium intake.

E. Evaluate for presence of paralytic ileus.

F. Increase roughage in diet to promote bowel function.

Goal: To prevent complications of immobility (see Chapter 3).

Goal: To promote bowel and bladder function.

A. Urine is retained as a result of the loss of autonomic and reflexive control of the bladder.

   1. Intermittent catheterization or indwelling catheter may be used initially to prevent bladder distention.

   2. Perform nursing interventions to prevent urinary tract infection; avoid urinary catheterization, if possible.

B. Determine type of bladder dysfunction based on level of injury.

C. Assess client's awareness of bladder function.

D. Initiate measures to institute bladder control.

   1. Establish a schedule for voiding; have client attempt to void every 2 hours.

   2. Use the Credé method (in adults) for manual expression of urine.

   3. May be necessary to teach client self-catheterization.

   4. Record output and evaluate for presence of residual urine.

E. Evaluate bowel functioning.

   1. Incontinence and paralytic ileus frequently occur with spinal shock.

   2. Incontinence and impaction are common later.

F. Initiate measures to promote bowel control (after spinal shock is resolved).

   1. Identify client's bowel habits before injury.

   2. Maintain sufficient fluid intake and adequate bulk in the diet.

   3. Establish specific time each day for bowel evacuation.

   4. Assess client's awareness of need to defecate.

   5. Teach client effective use of the Valsalva maneuver to induce defecation.

   6. Induce defecation by digital stimulation, suppository, or as a last resort, enema.

ALERT Assess and manage a client with alteration in elimination; initiate a toileting schedule; the client with SCI may need bowel and bladder retraining, depending on level of the injury.

Goal: To maintain psychologic equilibrium.

A. Provide simple explanations of all procedures.

B. Anticipate outbursts of anger and hostility as client begins to work through the grieving process and adjusts to changes in body image.

C. Anticipate and accept periods of depression in client.

D. Encourage independence whenever possible; allow client to participate in decisions regarding care and to gain control over environment.

ALERT Plan measures to deal with client's anxiety and promote client's adjustment to changes in body image; assist client and significant others to adjust to role changes. *Note:* These items are all part of the test plan, and the test could include questions about the client with SCI.

E. Encourage family involvement in identifying appropriate diversional activities.

F. Avoid sympathy and emphasize client's potential.

G. Initiate frank, open discussion regarding sexual functioning.

H. Assist client and family to identify community resources.

I. Assist client to set realistic short-term goals.

Myasthenia Gravis

Myasthenia gravis is a sporadic, progressive neuromuscular disease characterized by a decrease in the acetylcholine level at the receptor sites in the neuromuscular junction. This inadequate acetylcholine level results in a disturbance in nerve impulse transmission, causing progressive weakness in skeletal muscles. Myasthenia gravis literally means "grave muscle weakness."

Assessment

A. Risk factors/etiology.

   1. Autoimmune disease.

   2. More common in women younger than 40 and men older than 60 but may occur at any age.

B. Clinical manifestations.

   1. Primary problem is skeletal muscle fatigue with sustained muscle contraction; symptoms are predominantly bilateral.

     a. Muscular fatigue increases with activity.

     b. Ptosis (drooping of the eyelids) and diplopia (double vision) are frequently the first symptoms. (Ophthalmologist may be first contact regarding dysfunction.)

     c. Impairment of facial mobility and expression.

     d. Impairment of chewing and swallowing.

     e. Speech impairment (dysarthria).

     f. No sensory deficit, loss of reflexes, or muscular atrophy.

     g. Poor bowel and bladder control.

   2. Course is variable.

     a. May be progressive.

     b. May stabilize.

     c. May be characterized by short remissions and exacerbations.

3. Myasthenic crisis: an acute exacerbation of symptoms that may require intubation and mechanical ventilation to support respiratory effort; caused by major muscular weakness and inability to maintain respiratory function.
   a. Severe respiratory distress and hypoxia.
   b. Increased pulse and blood pressure.
   c. Decreased or absent cough or swallow reflex.
4. Cholinergic crisis: a toxic response to the anticholinesterase medications; anticholinesterase medications must be withheld—this response is rare with proper dosing of Mestinon.
   a. Nausea, vomiting, and diarrhea.
   b. Weakness with difficulty in swallowing, chewing, and speaking.
   c. Increased secretions and saliva.
   d. Muscle fasciculation, constricted pupils.

C. Diagnostics (see Appendix 20-1).
1. Electromyography: shows a decreasing response of muscles to stimuli.
2. Ice pack test: assess clients with ptosis; muscles improve with cold application; place pack on closed lids for 2 minutes to see whether ptosis improves.
3. Tensilon test.
   a. Used for diagnosing myasthenia gravis.
   b. Used to differentiate cholinergic crisis from myasthenic crisis.
   c. IV injection of neostigmine or edrophonium causes immediate, although short-lived, relief of muscle weakness.

Treatment

A. Anticholinesterase (cholinergic) medications (see Appendix 20-3).
1. Neostigmine (Prostigmin).
2. Pyridostigmine (Mestinon).
B. Corticosteroids (see Appendix 6-7).
C. Plasma electrophoresis (plasmapheresis): separation of plasma to remove autoantibodies from the bloodstream.
D. Immunosuppressive therapy.
E. Surgical removal of the thymus (thymectomy).

Nursing Interventions

Client may be hospitalized for acute myasthenic crisis or for respiratory tract infection.
Goal: To maintain respiratory function.
A. Assess for increasing problems of difficulty breathing. Measure forced vital capacity frequently to assess respiratory status.
B. Determine client's medication schedule. When was medication last taken?
C. Assess ability to swallow; prevent problems of aspiration.

ALERT Identify clients at high risk for aspiration; do not give the client experiencing a myasthenic crisis anything to eat or drink.

D. Evaluate effectiveness of cough reflex.
E. Be prepared to intubate or provide ventilatory assistance.
Goal: To distinguish between a myasthenic crisis and a cholinergic crisis.
A. Maintain adequate ventilatory support during crisis.
B. Assist in administration of Tensilon test to differentiate crisis.
   1. Myasthenic crisis: client's condition will improve.
   2. Cholinergic crisis: client's condition will temporarily worsen.
C. If myasthenic crisis occurs, neostigmine may be administered.
D. If cholinergic crisis occurs, atropine may be administered, and cholinergic medications may be reevaluated.
E. Avoid use of sedatives and tranquilizers, which causes respiratory depression.
F. Provide psychologic support during crisis.

Home Care

A. Teach client importance of taking medication on a regular basis; peak effect of the medication should coincide with mealtimes.
B. If ptosis becomes severe, client may need to wear an eye patch to protect cornea (alternate eye patches if problem is bilateral).
C. Emotional upset, severe fatigue, infections, and exposure to extreme temperatures may precipitate a myasthenic crisis.

Multiple Sclerosis

Multiple sclerosis (MS) is characterized by multiple areas of demyelination from inflammatory scarring of the neurons in the brain and spinal cord (CNS).
A. The progression of the disease results in total destruction of the myelin, and the nerve fibers become involved.
   1. Loss of myelin sheath causes decreased impulse conduction, destruction of the nerve axon, and a blockage of the impulse conduction.
   2. The demyelination occurs in irregular scattered patches throughout the CNS.
   3. Theories as to cause include autoimmunity and exposure to viruses.
B. Clinical course.
   1. Relapsing-remitting MS: most common course, causing sporadic attacks with exacerbations and remissions lasting days to months; client has a significant "flare-up" or exacerbation, followed by partial or complete recovery.
   2. Primary-progressive MS: after a number of years of the relapsing-remitting form, client experiences a slow steady worsening of symptoms without complete improvement between exacerbations; plateaus of severity may occur, but baseline function progressively worsens.
   3. Secondary-progressive MS: progressively worsens from onset with acute exacerbations; baseline function continues to worsen.

4. Progressive-relapsing MS: gradual progressive worsening of disease without remissions; onset in third or fourth decade of life with equal incidence in men and women.

Assessment

A. Risk factors/etiology: cause is unknown.
 1. More common in women.
 2. Problem of young adults.
 3. More common in cooler climates.
B. Clinical manifestations.
 1. Signs and symptoms vary from person to person, as well as within the same individual, depending on the area of involvement.
 2. Cerebellar dysfunction: nystagmus, ataxia, dysarthria, dysphagia.
 3. Motor dysfunction: weakness of eye muscles, weakness or spasticity of muscles in extremities.
 4. Sensory: vertigo, blurred vision, decreased hearing, tinnitus.
 5. Bowel and bladder dysfunction.
 6. Sexual dysfunction.
 7. Psychosocial.
  a. Intellectual functioning remains intact.
  b. Emotional lability: increased excitability and inappropriate euphoria.
  c. Emotional effects of the chronic illness and changes in body image.
C. Diagnostics: no definitive diagnostic test.

Treatment

A. No cure; medical treatment is directed toward slowing of the disease process and relief of symptoms.
B. Medications to decrease edema and inflammation of the nerve sites.
 1. Antiinflammatory agents.
 2. Immunosuppressive agents: interferons.
 3. Adrenocorticotropic hormone for acute exacerbations.

Nursing Interventions

Client may be hospitalized for diagnostic workup or for treatment of acute exacerbation and complications.

Goal: To maintain homeostasis and prevent complications during an acute exacerbation of disease symptoms.

A. Maintain adequate respiratory function.
 1. Prevent respiratory tract infection.
 2. Good pulmonary hygiene.
 3. Prevent aspiration; sitting position for eating.
 4. Evaluate adequacy of cough reflex.
B. Maintain urinary tract function.
 1. Prevent urinary tract infection.
 2. Increase fluid intake, at least 2000 mL/24 hr.
 3. Evaluate voiding: assess for retention and incontinence.
C. Maintain nutrition.
 1. Evaluate coughing and swallowing reflexes.
 2. Provide food that is easy to chew.

3. If client is experiencing difficulty swallowing, observe client closely during fluid intake.

Goal: To prevent complications of immobility (see Chapter 3).

Goal: To promote psychologic well-being.

A. Focus on remaining capabilities.
B. Encourage independence and assist client to gain control over environment.
C. If impotence is a problem, initiate sexual counseling.
D. Assist client to work through the grieving process.
E. Identify community resources available.

Home Care

A. Medical regimen and side effects of the medications.
B. Physical therapy to maintain muscle function and decrease spasticity.
C. Measures to maintain voiding; may need to perform self-catheterization.
D. Safety measures because of decreased sensation.
 1. Check bath water temperature.
 2. Wear protective clothing in the winter.
 3. Avoid heating pads and clothing that is constrictive.
E. Client should understand that relapses are frequently associated with an increase in physiologic and psychologic stress.

ALERT Determine client's ability to care for self; plan with family to assist client to meet self-care needs.

Guillain-Barré Syndrome

Guillain-Barré syndrome is an acute, rapidly progressing motor neuropathy involving segmental demyelination of nerve roots in the spinal cord and medulla. Demyelination causes inflammation, leading to edema, nerve root compression, decreased nerve conduction, and rapidly ascending paralysis. Both sensory and motor impairment occur. It is also called Landry's paralysis.

Assessment

A. Risk factors/etiology: cause is unknown; frequently, client has a recent history of acute illness.
B. Clinical manifestations.
 1. Progressive weakness and paralysis begin in the lower extremities and ascend bilaterally.
 2. Paralysis ascends the body symmetrically.
  a. Paralysis of respiratory muscles.
  b. Cranial nerve involvement, most often facial nerve (CN VII), produces difficulty talking and swallowing.
 3. Loss of sensation and function of bowel and bladder.
 4. Manifestations may progress rapidly over hours or may occur over 2 to 4 weeks.
 5. Muscle atrophy is minimal.
 6. Paralysis decreases as the client begins recovery; most often, there are no residual effects.

C. Diagnostics (see Appendix 20-1).
  1. Elevated protein concentration in CSF.

Treatment (Supportive)

A. Respiratory support, possibly mechanical ventilation.
B. Corticosteroids.
C. Immunosuppressives and immunoglobulins.
D. Plasmapheresis: plasma exchange.

Nursing Interventions

Goal: To evaluate progress of paralysis and initiate actions to prevent complications.

A. Evaluate rate of progress of paralysis; carefully assess changes in respiratory pattern.
B. Frequent evaluation of cough and swallow reflexes.
  1. Remain with client while client is eating; have suction equipment available.
  2. Maintain NPO (nothing by mouth) status if reflexes are involved.
C. If assent of paralysis is rapid, prepare for endotracheal intubation and respiratory assistance.
D. Prevent complications of immobility during period of paralysis (see Chapter 3).
E. Assess for involvement of the autonomic nervous system.
  1. Orthostatic hypotension.
  2. Hypertension.
  3. Cardiac dysrhythmias.
  4. Urinary retention and paralytic ileus.

Goal: To prevent complications of hypoxia if respiratory muscles become involved (see Chapter 15).

Goal: To maintain psychologic homeostasis.

A. Simple explanation of procedures.
B. Complete recovery is anticipated.
C. Provide psychologic support during period of assisted ventilation.
D. Keep client and family aware of progress of disease.

📋 Amyotrophic Lateral Sclerosis

Amyotrophic lateral sclerosis (ALS), also known as Lou Gehrig's disease, is a rapidly progressive, invariably fatal degeneration of nerves controlling voluntary muscles. Replacement of motor neurons with fibrous tissues causes hardening of anterior and lateral columns of the spinal cord, thus "lateral sclerosis."

Assessment

A. Clinical manifestations.
  1. Twitching, cramping, and muscle weakness.
  2. Dysarthria and dysphagia.
  3. Fatigue; asymmetrical muscle atrophy and weakness.

  4. Progressive muscle weakness.
    a. Begins with upper extremities and progressively involves muscles of neck and throat.
    b. Trunk and lower extremities are involved late in course of disease.
  5. Most often fatal within 2 to 5 years after onset.
  6. Intellectual functioning and all five senses are usually unaffected.
B. Diagnostics: electromyography and nerve conduction studies. Muscle biopsy may be performed to rule out other pathologies.

Treatment

A. Riluzole (Rilutek) prolongs life by a few months; protects motor neurons from degeneration and death.
B. Supportive care.

Nursing Interventions

Goal: To provide ongoing assessment in assisting client to deal with progressive symptoms.

A. Promote independence in ADLs.
  1. Conserve energy; space activities.
  2. Avoid extremes of hot and cold.
  3. Use of appliances to prolong independence in ambulation and ADLs.
B. Promote nutrition.
  1. Small frequent feedings.
  2. Have client sit upright with head slightly flexed forward while eating.
  3. Keep suction equipment easily available during meals.
C. Encourage family and client to talk about losses and the difficult choices they face.
D. Assist family and client to identify need for advanced directives and to complete them.

Muscular Dystrophy

Muscle dystrophy (MD) is a group of genetic diseases characterized by progressive weakness and skeletal muscle degeneration affecting a variety of muscle groups. The term *pseudohypertrophy* describes the characteristic muscle enlargement (caused by fatty infiltration) that occurs in muscular dystrophy.

A. Duchenne's muscular dystrophy is the most common and most severe form of MD.
B. Condition is characterized by gradual degeneration of muscle fibers and progressive symmetrical weakness and wasting of skeletal muscle.

Assessment

A. Risk factors/etiology.
  1. Genetic: sex-linked disorder primarily affecting males.
  2. Onset generally occurs between the ages of 3 and 5 years.
B. Clinical manifestations.
  1. History of delay in motor development, particularly a delay in walking.

2. Abnormal waddling gait.
   a. Child falls frequently and develops characteristic manner of rising.
   b. Gower's sign: from sitting or squatting position, the child assumes a kneeling position and pushes the torso up by "walking" his or her hands up the thighs.
3. Progressive muscle weakness, atrophy, and contractures.
   a. Ambulation is frequently impossible by the age of 9 to 11 years.
   b. Ultimately destroys essential muscles of respiration; death occurs from respiratory tract infection or cardiac failure.
C. Diagnostics.
   1. Electromyography, muscle biopsy.
   2. Serum enzymes: creatinine phosphokinase level is increased in neonate, then gradually declines.

Treatment

A. Steroids administered to boys older than 5 years of age.

Nursing Interventions

Child is frequently cared for at home and hospitalized only when complications occur.
Goal: To maintain optimal motor function as long as possible.
A. Regular physical therapy for stretching and strengthening muscles; ROM exercises.
B. Maintain child's independence in ADLs.
C. Assist family to identify resources, to adapt physiologic barriers within the home, and to promote mobility of the child in a wheelchair.
D. Assist family to identify methods of preventing respiratory tract infection; assess for respiratory problems.
E. Provide braces, splints, and assistive devices as needed.
Goal: To assist parents and child to maintain psychologic equilibrium and to adapt to chronic illness.
A. Assist parents to understand importance of independence and self-help skills; frequently, parents are overprotective of the child.
B. Counseling to assist parents and family members to identify family activities that can be modified to meet child's needs.
C. Mother may feel particularly guilty because of transmission of disease to her son.
D. Identify available community resources.
E. Counseling to assist family and child with chronic illness and child's eventual death.

 ### Cerebral Palsy

Cerebral palsy is a nonprogressive, lifelong neuromuscular genetic disorder resulting from damaged motor centers of the brain that cause nerve impulses to be incorrectly sent and/or received. The overall result is impairment of muscle control with poor muscle coordination.

Assessment

A. Risk factors/etiology.
   1. May result from existing prenatal brain abnormalities (kernicterus, hemolytic disease of newborn).
   2. Prematurity is single most important determinant of cerebral palsy; however, in about 24% of cases, cause is not identifiable.
B. Clinical manifestations.
   1. Delayed achievement of developmental milestones.
   2. Increased or decreased resistance to passive movement.
   3. Abnormal posture.
   4. Presence of infantile reflexes (tonic neck reflex, exaggerated Moro reflex).
   5. Associated disabilities.
      a. Mental retardation, seizures.
      b. Attention-deficit problems.
      c. Vision and hearing impairment.
   6. Muscle tightness and spasms.
C. Diagnostics.
   1. Diagnostic tests to rule out other neurologic dysfunction: EEG, MRI, blood tests.
   2. Frequently difficult to diagnose in early months; condition may not be evident until child attempts to sit alone or walk.
   3. Gait lab analysis: evaluates walking ability.

Treatment

A. Maintain and promote mobility with orthopedic devices and physical therapy.
B. Skeletal muscle relaxants.
C. Anticonvulsants, as indicated.

Nursing Interventions

Child is frequently cared for at home and on an outpatient basis unless complications occur.
Goal: To assist child to become as independent and self-sufficient as possible.
A. Physical therapy program designed to assist individual child to gain maximum function.
B. Assist child to progress according to developmental level and functional abilities; encourage crawling, sitting, and balancing appropriate to developmental level.
C. Assist child to carry out ADLs as age and capacities permit.
D. Speech therapy, as indicated.
E. Encourage play appropriate for age.
F. Encourage appropriate educational activities.
G. Bowel and bladder training may be difficult because of poor control.
Goal: To maintain physiologic homeostasis.
A. Maintain adequate nutrition.
   1. May experience difficulty eating because of spasticity; may drool excessively; use of manual jaw control when feeding.
   2. Encourage independence in eating and use of self-help devices.

3. Provide a balanced diet with increased caloric intake to meet extra energy demands.
B. Maintain safety precautions to prevent injury.
C. Increased susceptibility to infections, especially respiratory tract infections, because of poor control of intercostal muscles and diaphragm.
D. Increased incidence of dental problems; schedule frequent dental checkups.

Goal: To promote a positive self-image in the child and provide support to the family.
A. Use positive reinforcement frequently.
B. Assist parents to set realistic goals.
C. Encourage recreation and educational activities, especially those involving other children with cerebral palsy.
D. Encourage child to express feelings regarding the disorder.
E. Do not "talk down" to child; communicate at appropriate developmental level.
F. Assist parents in problem solving in home environment.
G. Identify available community resources.
H. Utilize principles in caring for chronically ill pediatric client (Chapter 2).

Parkinson's Disease (Paralysis Agitans)

Parkinson's disease is a progressive neurologic disorder with gradual onset that causes destruction and degeneration of nerve cells in the basal ganglia; results in damage to the extrapyramidal system, causing difficulty in control and regulation of movement.
A. Dopamine, a neurotransmitter, is responsible for normal functioning of the extrapyramidal system.
B. The condition is correlated with a depletion of or imbalance in dopamine and increased activity of acetylcholine.

Assessment
A. Risk factors/etiology.
  1. In general, onset occurs after age 60.
  2. More common in males.
B. Clinical manifestations (Figure 20-9).
  1. Tremor.
    a. Affects the arms and hands bilaterally: often, the first sign.
    b. Tremors usually occur at rest; voluntary movement may decrease tremors; tremors during voluntary movement are not as common.
    c. Described as "pill-rolling" tremor.
    d. Exacerbated by emotional stress and increased concentration.
  2. Muscle rigidity.
    a. Increased resistance to passive movement.
    b. Movement may be described as "cog-wheel rigidity" because of jerky movement of extremities.
  3. Bradykinesia: slow activity.
    a. Decreased blinking of the eyelids.
    b. Loss of ability to swallow saliva.
    c. Facial expression is blank or "mask-like."
    d. Loss of normal arm swing while walking.
    e. Difficulty initiating movement.
  4. Stooped posture, shuffling propulsive gait.
  5. May exhibit mental deterioration similar to that associated with Alzheimer's disease.
  6. Depression occurs in two-thirds of clients.
C. Diagnostics: no specific diagnostic test.

Treatment
A. Medication to enhance dopamine secretion (see Appendix 20-4).
B. Anticholinergic medications to decrease effects of acetylcholine (see Appendix 20-4).

FIGURE 20-9 Parkinson's disease. (From Zerwekh J, Claborn J: *Memory notebook of nursing*, vol 1, ed 4, Ingram, Texas, 2008, Nursing Education Consultants.)

C. Clients frequently become tolerant to medications and require adjustments in types of medications and medication schedules.

D. Surgical therapy: aim is to decrease symptoms.
1. Ablation (destruction of tissue).
2. Deep brain stimulation (DBS).

Nursing Interventions

Goal: To maintain homeostasis.

A. Encourage independence in ADLs with use of self-help devices.

B. Maintain nutrition.
1. Increase calories and protein; provide more easily chewed foods.
2. Frequent small meals.
3. Allow ample time for eating.
4. Monitor weight loss.
5. Provide pleasant atmosphere at mealtime; client frequently prefers to eat alone because of difficulty swallowing and inability to control saliva.
6. Increase fluid intake with increased bulk in the diet to decrease problem with constipation.

C. Maintain muscle function.
1. Full ROM to extremities to prevent contracture.
2. Decrease effects of tremors.
3. Exercise and stretch daily.
4. Physical therapy, as indicated.

D. Closely monitor response to or changes in response to medications.

> **ALERT** Identify situations that necessitate role changes; evaluate family involvement in health care; review necessary modifications to promote home safety.

Goal: To promote a positive self-image.

A. Encourage diversional activities.

B. Assist client to set realistic goals.

C. Explore reasons for depression; encourage client to discuss changes occurring in lifestyle.

D. Assist client in gaining control of ADLs and environment.

E. Assist client to identify and avoid activities that increase frustration levels.

F. Encourage good personal hygiene.

Headache

Headache is a very common symptom of various underlying pathologic conditions in which pain-sensitive nerve fibers respond to unacceptable levels of stress and tension, muscular contraction in the upper body, pressure from a tumor, or increased ICP.

Assessment

A. Types of headaches.
1. Tension headache (muscle contraction headache): most common of all headaches; feeling of tightness like a band around the head; onset is gradual; may be accompanied by dizziness, tinnitus, or lacrimation; associated with stress and premenstrual syndrome.
2. Migraine: constriction of intracranial vessels leading to an intense throbbing pain when vessels return to normal; prodromal or aura; crescendo quality; unilateral pain, often beginning in eye area; nausea, vomiting, photophobia—migraines are seriously debilitating and may require lifestyle and occupational changes.
3. Cluster headache: rare headache that is more common in men; occurs in numerous episodes or clusters; no aura; unilateral pain often arising in nostril and spreading to forehead and eye; often occurs at same time of day.

Treatment

A. Migraine: sumatriptan (Imitrex); dihydroergotamine mesylate (Migranal).

B. Nonsteroidal antiinflammatory drugs.

C. Relaxation, yoga, stress management.

D. Cluster headaches treated with high flow oxygen.

Nursing Interventions

A. Prevention: recognize triggers, decrease stress, adjust medications during menstrual cycle.

B. Watch for signs of ominous headache: new-onset unilateral headache in person older than 35 years; vomiting not accompanied by nausea; pain that awakens client.

C. Encourage client to keep a "headache diary" for best management and treatment.

Trigeminal Neuralgia

Trigeminal neuralgia is a fleeting unilateral sensory disturbance of cranial nerve V, causing brief, paroxysmal pain and facial spasm; also known as tic douloureux.

Assessment

A. Risk factors/etiology.
1. Onset generally occurs between 20 and 40 years of age.
2. Increased frequency with aging.

B. Clinical manifestations.
1. Abrupt onset of paroxysmal intense pain in the lower and upper jaw, cheek, and lips.
   a. Tearing of the eyes and frequent blinking.
   b. Facial twitching and grimacing.
   c. Pain is usually brief; ends as abruptly as it begins.
   d. Pain may be described as severe, stabbing, and shock-like.
2. Recurrence of pain is unpredictable.
3. Pain is initiated by cutaneous stimulation of the affected nerve area.
   a. Chewing.
   b. Washing the face.
   c. Extremes of temperature: either on the face or in food.
   d. Brushing teeth.

Treatment

A. Medical management of pain (see Appendix 20-2): carbamazepine (Tegretol) and gabapentin (Neurontin).
B. Surgical intervention.
   1. Local nerve block.
   2. Surgical intervention to interrupt nerve impulse transmission.
      a. Percutaneous stereotactic rhizotomy—destroys some of the nerve fibers; assists to manage pain.
      b. Microvascular decompression (craniotomy) to relieve pain and preserve facial sensation.

Nursing Interventions

Goal: To control pain.
A. Assess the nature of a painful attack.
B. Identify triggering factors; adjust environment to decrease factors.
   1. Keep room at an even, comfortable temperature.
   2. Avoid touching client.
   3. Avoid jarring the bed.
   4. Allow client to carry out own ADLs as necessary.
C. Administer analgesics to decrease pain.

> **⊞ NURSING PRIORITY** Because of the severe pain caused by the condition, clients are susceptible to severe depression and suicide.

Goal: To maintain nutrition.
A. Frequently, client does not eat because of reluctance to stimulate the pain.
B. Provide lukewarm food that can be easily chewed.
C. Increase protein and calories.

Home Care

A. Identify presence of corneal reflex; provide protective eye care if reflex is absent.
B. If there is loss of sensation to the side of the face, client should:
   1. Chew on the unaffected side.
   2. Avoid temperature extremes in foods.
   3. Check the mouth after eating to remove remaining particles of food.

   4. Maintain meticulous oral hygiene.
   5. Have frequent dental checkups.

Bell's Palsy

Bell's palsy is a transient cranial nerve disorder affecting the facial nerve (cranial nerve VII), characterized by a disruption of the motor branches on one side of the face, which results in muscle weakness or flaccidity on the affected side.

Assessment

A. Clinical manifestations.
   1. Lag or inability to close eyelid on affected side.
   2. Drooping of the mouth.
   3. Decreased taste sensation.
   4. Upward movement of the eyeball when the eye is being closed.
B. Diagnostics (see Appendix 20-1).

Treatment

A. Corticosteroids: administration should be started immediately after symptoms arise.
B. Antivirals.
C. Moist heat may relieve pain, if present.

Nursing Interventions

Goal: To assess nerve function and prevent complications.
A. Analgesics to decrease pain.
B. Evaluate ability of client to eat.
C. Meticulous oral hygiene.
D. Prevent drying of the cornea on the affected side.
   1. Instill methylcellulose drops frequently during the day.
   2. Ophthalmic ointment and eye patches may be required at night.
E. As function returns, active facial exercises may be performed.

Goal: To assist client to maintain a positive self-image.
A. Changes in physical appearance may be dramatic.
B. Tell client that the condition is usually self-limiting with minimal, if any, residual effects.
C. Client may require counseling, if change in facial appearance is permanent.

Appendix 20-1   NEUROLOGIC SYSTEM DIAGNOSTICS

Skull and Spine X-Ray Studies Simple x-ray films are obtained to determine fractures, calcifications, etc.

Electroencephalography (EEG) A recording of the electrical activity of the brain to physiologically assess cerebral activity; useful for diagnosing seizure disorders; used as a screening procedure for coma; also serves as an indicator for brain death. May also be used to assess sleep disorders, metabolic disorders and encephalitis.

Nursing Implications

1. Explain to client that procedure is painless and there is no danger of electrical shock.
2. Determine from physician if any medications should be withheld before test, especially tranquilizers and sedatives.
3. Frequently, coffee, tea, cola, and other stimulants are prohibited before examination.
4. Client's hair should be clean before the examination; after the exam, assist client to wash electrode paste out of hair.

Carotid Doppler Ultrasonography A noninvasive ultrasound scan to estimate blood flow in carotid and cerebral vessels to assess for stenosis. No preparation is necessary.

Magnetic Resonance Imaging (MRI) Cell nuclei have magnetic properties; the MRI machine records the signals from the cells in a manner that provides information to evaluate soft tissue structures (tumors, blood vessels).

Nursing Implications

1. Procedure will take approximately 1 hour.
2. All metal objects should be removed from the client (hearing aids, hair clips, jewelry, buckles, etc.).
3. The client will be placed in a long magnetic tunnel for the procedure.
4. Poor candidates for MRI include the following.
   a. Clients with pacemakers (the magnetic field interferes with the function of the pacemaker and interferes with the test as well).
   b. Clients with implanted insulin pumps or joint replacements.
   c. Pregnant clients.
   d. Obese clients.
   e. Any client who requires life-support equipment (the equipment will malfunction in a magnetic field).

Computerized Axial Tomography (CAT) Scan Computer-assisted x-ray examination of thin cross-sections of the brain to identify hemorrhage, tumor, edema, infarctions, and hydrocephalus. Machine is large donut-shaped tube with table through the middle.

Nursing Implications

1. Explain appearance of scanner to client and explain importance of remaining absolutely still during the procedure.
2. Remove all objects from client's hair; for 4 to 6 hours before test, client receives fluids only.
3. Dye will be injected via venipuncture; assess for iodine allergy and advise the client that he/she may experience a flushing or warm sensation when the dye is injected.
4. Contrast dye may discolor urine for about 24 hours.
5. Dye may be injected into spinal cord for assessment of intervertebral disks and bone density.

Brain Scan A scanner traces the uptake of radioactive dye in the brain tissue. The dye is concentrated in the damaged tissue; it will take approximately 2 hours after dye is injected for the scan to be completed.

Nursing Implications

1. Determine whether medications need to be withheld before procedure.
2. Client will be asked to change positions during the test in order to visualize the brain from different angles.
3. The client should not experience any pain.

Caloric Testing Test is performed at bedside by introducing cold water into the external auditory canal. It is contraindicated in the client with a ruptured tympanic membrane and is not done on the client who is awake. If the 8th cranial nerve is stimulated, nystagmus rotates toward the irrigated ear. If no nystagmus occurs, a pathologic condition is present.

Positron Emission Tomography (PET) See Appendix 17-1.

Lumbar Puncture A needle is inserted into the lumbar area at the L4-L5 level; spinal fluid is withdrawn, and spinal fluid pressure is measured; contraindicated in presence of increased intracranial pressure. Normal spinal fluid values: opening pressure, 60 to 150 mm water; specific gravity, 1.007; pH, 7.35; clear fluid; protein concentration, 15 to 45 mg/dL; glucose concentration, 45 to 75 mg/dL; no microorganisms present.

Nursing Implications

Before test

1. Have client empty bladder.
2. Explain position (lateral recumbent with knees flexed) to client (Figure 20-10).
3. Advise physician if there is a change in the client's neurologic status before the test; increased intracranial pressure is a contraindication to a lumbar puncture.

After test

1. Keep client flat at least 3 hours, and sometimes up to 12 hours, to decrease occurrence of headache.
2. Encourage high fluid intake.
3. Observe for spinal fluid leak from puncture site; if leakage occurs, it may precipitate a severe headache.

Myelogram An outpatient procedure in which dye is injected into the subarachnoid space and x-ray films of the spinal cord and vertebral column are obtained to identify spinal lesions.

FIGURE 20-10 Lumbar puncture. (From Black JM, Hawks JH: *Medical-surgical nursing: clinical management for positive outcomes,* ed 7, Philadelphia, 2005, Saunders.)

Appendix 20-1 NEUROLOGIC SYSTEM DIAGNOSTICS—cont'd

Nursing Implications
Before test
1. Same as for lumbar puncture.
2. Check whether client has any allergies to dye.

After test
1. Keep the head of the bed elevated 30 to 50 degrees to decrease dispersion of the dye in the CSF and to the brain.
2. Headache may occur as a result of irritation of the central nervous system.
3. Client should not receive any of the phenothiazines before or immediately after the examination.

Cerebral Angiogram Injection of contrast material into the cerebral circulation; series of x-ray films is taken to study the cerebral blood flow; dye is usually injected via a soft catheter that is inserted and threaded through the femoral artery.

Nursing Implications
Before test
1. Client should be well-hydrated, but should receive nothing by mouth for 6 to 8 hours before the test; client should void before procedure.
2. Determine if client has any allergies to iodine or to shell fish.
3. Inform client that he or she should remain very still during the procedure.
4. A feeling of warmth in the face and mouth and a metallic taste in the mouth are common when dye is injected.

After test
1. Evaluate client's neurologic status; complications involve occlusion of cerebral arteries.
2. Observe injection site for hematoma formation.
3. Posttest complications include continuous bleeding at injection site, rash, dizziness, and tingling in an extremity.
4. Check circulation distal to area of puncture.

Electromyography (EMG) Measures electrical discharge from a muscle. Flat electrodes or small needles are placed in the muscle. The client may be asked to move and perform simple activities; the electrical stimulus for the muscle will be recorded. Useful for diagnosis in spinal cord deformity, muscular dystrophy, myasthenia gravis or amyotrophic lateral sclerosis.

Nursing Implications
Before test
1. May determine pretest serum muscle determinations.
2. Explain to the client that small needles will be inserted into the skin.

After test
1. Client may need something for pain because of muscle stimulation.
2. Assess needle sites for areas of hematomas; apply ice pack to prevent and/or relieve.

Appendix 20-2 ANTIEPILEPTICS

MEDICATIONS	SIDE EFFECTS	NURSING IMPLICATIONS
Antiepileptics (AED) Suppress discharge of neurons within a seizure focus to reduce seizure activity.		
Phenobarbital **(Sodium Luminal):** IM, PO, rectal, IV Primidone **(Mysoline):** PO	Drowsiness, ataxia, excitation in children and the elderly	1. Client should avoid potential hazardous activities requiring mental alertness. 2. Sudden withdrawal from chronic use may precipitate symptoms. 3. Closely observe response in children and elderly. 4. Used to treat grand mal and focal seizures. 5. See Appendix 15-5 for care of client with seizures.
Phenytoin **(Dilantin):** PO, IV	Gingival hyperplasia, skin rash, hypoglycemia Bradycardia, hypotension Visual changes: nystagmus, diplopia, blurred vision	1. Administer PO preparations with meals or milk to decrease gastric irritation. 2. Frequently used with phenobarbital for control of grand mal seizures. 3. IM injection is not recommended. 4. Do not mix with any other medications when administering IV solution. 5. Promote good oral hygiene; gum hyperplasia is a problem with long-term use. 6. See Appendix 15-5 for care of client with seizures. 7. AEDs should be withdrawn slowly over 6 weeks to several months when medication therapy is discontinued.

Continued

Appendix 20-2   ANTIEPILEPTICS—cont'd

MEDICATIONS	SIDE EFFECTS	NURSING IMPLICATIONS
Divalproex sodium **(Depakote):** PO	GI disturbances, rash, weight gain, hair loss, tremor, blood dyscrasias GI, dermatologic effects, blood dyscrasias	1. Should not be given to clients with severe liver dysfunction. 2. Potentiates action of phenobarbital, phenytoin, diazepam. 3. *Uses:* seizures, bipolar disorder, migraine.
Carbamazepine **(Tegretol):** PO, suspension	Drowsiness, dizziness, headache; visual disturbances common during first few weeks of treatment	1. Wean client from medication as soon as seizures are controlled. 2. Antimanic properties as well.
Clonazepam **(Klonopin):** PO	CNS depression, ataxia	1. Antianxiety effects may assist with seizure control. 2. Monitor results of liver function tests.

CNS, Central nervous system; *GI,* gastrointestinal; *IM,* intramuscular; *IV,* intravenous; *PO,* by mouth (orally).

Appendix 20-3   CHOLINERGIC (ANTICHOLINESTERASE) MEDICATIONS

MEDICATIONS	SIDE EFFECTS	NURSING IMPLICATIONS
Cholinergic Medications Intensify transmission of impulses throughout the CNS, where acetylcholine is necessary for transmission.		
Neostigmine bromide **(Prostigmin):** PO, subQ, IM Pyridostigmine bromide **(Mestinon):** PO, IM, IV Edrophonium chloride **(Tensilon):** IV, IM	Excessive salivation, increased GI motility, urinary urgency, bradycardia, visual problems	1. Primary group of medications used for treatment of myasthenia gravis. 2. Atropine is the antidote for overdose. 3. In treatment of myasthenia gravis, medication is frequently administered 30 to 45 minutes before meals. 4. **Mestinon** is given as maintenance therapy for the client with myasthenia gravis. 5. **Tensilon** is used for diagnostic purposes; not recommended for maintenance therapy. 6. Teach client symptoms of side effects and advise client to call the doctor if they are present.

CNS, Central nervous system; *GI,* gastrointestinal; *IM,* intramuscular; *IV,* intravenous; *PO,* by mouth (orally); *subQ,* subcutaneous.

Appendix 20-4   ANTIPARKINSONISM AGENTS

MEDICATIONS	SIDE EFFECTS	NURSING IMPLICATIONS
Anticholinergics Inhibit action of acetylcholine at sites throughout the body and CNS. Decrease synaptic transmissions in the CNS.		
Benztropine mesylate **(Cogentin):** PO, IM, IV Trihexyphenidyl hydrochloride **(Artane):** PO, IM, IV Procyclidine **(Kemadrin):** PO	Paralytic ileus, urinary retention, cardiac palpitations, blurred vision, nausea and vomiting, sedation, dizziness Minor side effects such as dry mouth, jitteriness, and nausea	1. Administer PO preparations with meals to decrease gastric irritation. 2. Medications have cumulative effect. 3. Should not be used in clients with glaucoma, myasthenia gravis, GU or GI tract obstruction or in children younger than 3 years. 4. Monitor client carefully for bowel and bladder problems. 5. May be used to treat side effects of Thorazine.

Appendix 20-4 ANTIPARKINSONISM AGENTS—cont'd

MEDICATIONS	SIDE EFFECTS	NURSING IMPLICATIONS
Dopaminergics Assist to restore normal transmission of nerve impulses.		
Levodopa **(L-DOPA, Larodopa):** PO	*Early:* Anorexia, nausea and vomiting, abdominal discomfort, postural hypotension *Long-term:* Abnormal, involuntary movements, especially involving the face, mouth, and neck; behavioral disturbances involving confusion, agitation, and euphoria	1. Administer PO preparations with meals to decrease GI distress. 2. Almost all clients will experience some side effects, which are dose related; dosage gradually increased according to client's tolerance and response. 3. Onset of action is slow; therapeutic response may require several weeks to months. 4. Vitamin B_6 (pyridoxine) is antagonistic to the effects of the medication; decrease client's intake of multiple vitamins and fortified cereals.
Carbidopa/levodopa **(Sinemet):** PO	Same as for levodopa	1. Same as for levodopa. 2. Use of carbidopa significantly decreases the amount of levodopa required for therapy. 3. Prevents inhibitory effects of levodopa on vitamin B_6.
Amantadine hydrochloride **(Symmetrel):** PO	Orthostatic hypotension, dyspnea, dizziness, drowsiness, blurred vision, constipation, urinary retention (side effects are dose related)	1. Less effective than levodopa; produces a more rapid clinical response.

CNS, Central nervous system; *GI,* gastrointestinal; *GU,* genitourinary; *IM,* intramuscular; *IV,* intravenous; *PO,* by mouth (orally).

Appendix 20-5 SEIZURE DISORDERS

A seizure disorder is the interruption of normal brain functioning by uncontrolled paroxysmal discharge of electrical stimuli from the neurons.

Classification of Seizures

Simple Partial Seizures (remains conscious throughout seizure)

Rarely last longer than 1 minute; an aura may occur before the seizure.
1. Confined to a specific area (hand, arm, leg); client may experience unusual sensations.
2. One-sided movement of an extremity.
3. Autonomic changes; skin flushing, change in heart rate, epigastric discomfort.

Complex Partial Seizures (may have impairment of consciousness)

1. May loose consciousness for 1 to 3 minutes.
2. May produce automatisms (lip smacking, grimacing, repetitive hand movements).
3. Client may be unaware of environment and wonder what is happening at the beginning of the seizure.
4. In the period after the seizure, client may experience amnesia and confusion.
5. Also called temporal lobe seizures or psychomotor.

Generalized Seizures (Bilaterally Symmetric and Without Local Onset)

No warning or aura, as client loses consciousness for a few seconds to several minutes.

1. Absence (petit mal): Characterized by a short period of time when the client is in an altered level of consciousness. Staring, blinking period (followed by resumption of normal activity) is characteristic. May occur more than 100 times per day; may go unnoticed; in general, onset is in childhood between the ages of 4 and 12 years.
2. Tonic-clonic seizures: May last 2 to 5 minutes. Full recovery may take several hours; client may be confused, amnesic, and irritable during this recovery period.

Tonic phase: Loss of consciousness with stiffening and rigidity of muscles. Apnea and cyanosis are common during this period; phase generally lasts for about 1 minute.

Clonic phase: Hyperventilation, with rapid jerking movements. Tongue biting, incontinence, and heavy salivation may occur during this period (Figure 20-11).

Seizure Etiology

Acute Disorders

- Increased intracranial pressure, metabolic alterations
- Infections, febrile episodes in children (generally between 6 months and 3 years)

Continued

A

Tonic phase

B

Clonic phase

C

Postictal phase

FIGURE 20-11 Tonic-clonic seizure activity. (From Black JM, Hawks JH: *Medical-surgical nursing: clinical management for positive outcomes,* ed 8, Philadelphia, 2009, Saunders.)

Chronic (Recurrent, Epilepsy)

- Brain injury at birth, trauma, vascular disease
- Brain tumors, genetic factors, idiopathic

Nursing Assessment

1. Identify any activities that occurred immediately before the seizure.
2. Was the client aware a seizure was going to occur? If so, how did client know?
3. Describe type of movements that occurred and the body area affected (e.g., jaw clenched, tongue biting).

4. Presence of incontinence.
5. Period of apnea and cyanosis.
6. Presence of automatisms (lip smacking, grimacing, chewing).
7. Duration of seizure.
8. Changes in level of consciousness.
9. Condition of client after seizure: oriented, level of activity, any residual paralysis or muscle weakness.

> **⚠ NURSING PRIORITY** Airway management and ventilation cannot be performed on a client who is experiencing a tonic-clonic seizure. After the seizure is over, evaluate the airway and initiate ventilations as necessary.

Nursing Management

1. Remain with the client who is having a seizure; note the time the seizure began and how long it lasted.
2. Do not attempt to force anything into the client's mouth if the jaws are clenched shut.
3. If the jaws are not clenched, place an airway in the client's mouth. This protects the tongue and also provides a method of suctioning the airway, should the client vomit.
4. Protect the client from injury (risk for falling out of bed or striking self on bedrails, etc).
5. Loosen any constrictive clothing.
6. Do not restrain client during seizure activity; allow seizure movements to occur, but protect client from injury.
7. Evaluate respiratory status; if vomiting occurs, be prepared to suction the client to clear the airway and prevent aspiration.
8. Maintain calm atmosphere and provide for privacy after the seizure activity.
9. Reorient client.

> **ALERT** Report characteristics of a client's seizure; determine changes in client's neurologic status.

Client Education

1. Identify activities/events that precipitate the seizure activity.
2. Avoid alcohol intake, fatigue, and loss of sleep.
3. Take medications as directed.
4. Counseling for the family and for the client to assist them in maintaining positive coping mechanisms.
5. Wear medical alert bracelet or have identification card.

Appendix 20-6 APHASIA

Aphasia is a total loss of comprehension and use of language. Dysphasia is the difficulty related to the comprehension or use of language and is due to a partial disruption or loss; patterns of dysphasia differ because the stroke affects different parts of the brain. The condition is precipitated by a problem in the cerebral cortex. The most common cause of aphasia is a vascular problem involving the middle cerebral artery. The speech center is located in the dominant side of the cerebral hemisphere. The speech center for a right-handed person is located in the left cerebral hemisphere. Clients with aphasia are often frustrated and irritable. Emotional lability is common. Accept the behavior in a manner that prevents embarrassment for the client.

TYPES OF APHASIA

Sensory aphasia (receptive or fluent, Wernicke's area): Cannot understand oral or written communication. Client cannot interpret or comprehend speech or read.

Motor aphasia (expressive, Broca's aphasia): Inability to speak or to write. However, the client can comprehend incoming speech and can read.

Mixed: Most aphasia involves both the sensory and motor aspects of speech. Rarely is aphasia only sensory or only motor.

Global aphasia: All communication and receptive function is lost.

Dysarthria: A disturbance in the muscular control of speech. Does not affect the meaning of communication or comprehension, just the mechanics of speech—pronunciation, articulation, and phonation.

NURSING IMPLICATIONS

1. Stand in front of the client; speak clearly and slowly.
2. Do not shout or speak loudly; the client can hear.
3. Be patient; give the client time to respond; do not press him or her for immediate answers.
4. Use nonverbal communications such as touch, smiles, and gestures.
5. Assist the client with motor aphasia to practice repeating simple words such as yes, no, and please.
6. Listen carefully, try to understand, and try to communicate; this conveys to the client that you care.
7. nvolve family members in practice and assist them to identify ways they can support the client.

ALERT Assist client to communicate effectively.

Study Questions Neurologic System

More questions on companion CD!

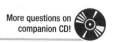

1. The nurse is obtaining a health history from a client who states he is having pain in his left arm. Which question by the nurse will elicit the most useful response from the client?
   1 "Does the pain feel like pins and needles in your arm?"
   2 "Does the pain radiate from your neck to your arms?"
   3 "Can you describe the pain you are experiencing in your arm?"
   4 "Is the numbness in your arm intermittent or constant?"

2. The nurse is assessing a client with a tentative diagnosis of a brain tumor. What would the nurse anticipate the client's primary complaint to be?
   1 Decreased appetite
   2 Frequent insomnia
   3 Recurrent headaches
   4 Peripheral edema

3. The nurse is caring for a client who has had a right-sided stroke. What would be appropriate nursing care for this client?
   1 Performing passive ROM exercises to affected side, active ROM on unaffected side
   2 Placing food on the affected side of the client's mouth
   3 Applying hot packs to the right leg to decrease muscle spasms
   4 Turning client every 2 hours and maintaining position on the right side for 2 hours

4. A client is scheduled for an electroencephalogram. What will the nurse explain to the client regarding the purpose of this test?
   1 Evaluates electrical currents of skeletal muscles
   2 Measures ultrasonic waves in the brain
   3 Determines size and location of brain activity
   4 Records brain electrical activity

5. A client who has had a stroke is aphasic; it has been a week since his stroke. He is beginning to show functional improvement and demonstrates an ability to follow verbal directions. What will rehabilitation now include?
   1 A right-leg brace
   2 Ambulation training
   3 Speech training
   4 Vocational retraining

6. The nurse is caring for a client who is doing well after his craniotomy. What will the bowel care for this client include?
   1 An enema every other day to avoid the Valsalva maneuver
   2 High-fiber diet and stool softeners to prevent constipation
   3 Low-residue diet to decrease stool formation and prevent constipation
   4 Daily checking for impaction caused by loss of bowel innervation

7. After a grand mal seizure, what nursing action is the *highest* priority?
   1 Loosen or remove constricting clothing and protect client from injuring himself or herself.
   2 Maintain a patent airway by turning the client on his side and suctioning, if necessary.
   3 Remain with the client and administer anticonvulsant medications as ordered by the physician.
   4 Describe and record events before the onset of the seizure, during the seizure, and after the seizure.

8. A client with Parkinson's disease is experiencing anorexia and vomiting. The client is taking levodopa. What will be the initial nursing activity?
   1 Assess client's food preferences.
   2 Monitor client's blood pressure.
   3 Hold client's medication and notify the physician.
   4 Administer client's medication with food.

9. An 8-year-old child is admitted after an accident where he sustained a closed head injury. The child is alert and oriented but very lethargic. There is clear fluid draining from the child's nose. What is the best nursing action?
   1 Gently suction the fluid from the nasal area.
   2 Turn from side to side only.
   3 Keep head of bed elevated.
   4 Encourage participation in games to play in bed.

10. When obtaining a health history, the nurse expects a client with a recent diagnosis of Parkinson's disease to report which sign or symptom?
    1 Weight loss
    2 Slowness of movement
    3 Continual motor tremors
    4 Depression

11. While caring for a client who has recently been diagnosed with Parkinson's disease, the nurse should understand that:
    1 Intellectual capabilities will decrease.
    2 Diversional interests may decrease.
    3 Mood fluctuations may occur.
    4 Communication skills may fluctuate.

12. Pneumonia is a common problem in children with spastic cerebral palsy. The nurse understands that this occurs because:
    1 There is an associated dysfunction of the respiratory center in the central nervous system.
    2 The immunologic system is immature and does not produce adequate antibodies to fight infection.
    3 Decreased mobility leads to stasis of secretions in the respiratory passages.
    4 There is a weakness of the voluntary muscles that control respiration.

Answers and rationales to these questions are in the section at the end of the book titled Chapter Study Questions: Answers and Rationales.

CHAPTER TWENTY-ONE

Musculoskeletal System

PHYSIOLOGY OF THE MUSCULOSKELETAL AND CONNECTIVE TISSUE

Skeletal System

A. Bone structure.
1. Periosteum: dense fibrous membrane covering the bone; periosteal vessels supply bone tissue.
2. Epiphysis: the widened area found at the end of a long bone.
3. Epiphyseal plate (growth zone): a cartilage area in children, which provides for longitudinal growth of the bone.
4. Articular cartilage: provides a smooth surface over the end of the bone to facilitate joint movement.
5. Red bone marrow: hemopoietic tissue located in the central bone cavities.

B. Bone maintenance and healing.
1. Regulatory factors determining both formation and resorption.
   a. Weight-bearing stress stimulates local bone resorption and formation; in states of immobility in which weight bearing is prevented, calcium is lost from the bone.
   b. Vitamin D promotes absorption of calcium from the gastrointestinal tract and accelerates mobilization of calcium from the bone to increase or maintain serum calcium levels.
   c. Parathyroid hormone regulates the concentration of calcium in the serum partially by promoting the transfer of calcium from the bone.
   d. Calcitonin and amino biphosphates (e.g., alendronate [Fosamax], ibandronate [Boniva]) increase the production of bone cells.
2. Bone healing.
   a. When a bone is damaged or injured, a hematoma precedes new tissue formation in the production of new bone substance.
   b. A callus is formed as minerals are deposited to organize a network for the new bone.
   c. The callus forms the initial clinical union of the bone and provides enough stability to prevent movement when bones are gently stressed.
   d. Continued bone healing provides for gradual return of the injured bone to its preinjury shape

and structural strength; this is frequently referred to as remodeling of the bone.

> **ALERT** Identify pathophysiology related to an acute or chronic condition (e.g. signs and symptoms).

Connective Tissue: Joints and Cartilage

A. Joints.
1. The action of joints permits bones to change position and facilitate body movement.
2. The diarthrodial (synovial) joint is the most common type of joint in the body.
   a. Cartilage (hyaline) covers the end of the bone.
   b. A fibrous capsule of connective tissue joins the two bones together.
      (1) Synovium (synovial membrane) lines the capsule.
      (2) Synovial fluid is secreted by the synovium and serves to decrease friction by lubricating the joint.

B. Articular cartilage is rigid, connective, avascular tissue that covers the end of each bone; nourished by capillaries in adjacent connective tissue; damaged cartilage heals slowly because of lack of direct blood supply.

C. Ligaments and tendons are tough fibrous connective tissues that provide stability while continuing to permit movement.
1. Tendons attach muscles to the bone.
2. Ligaments attach bones to joints.

Skeletal Muscle

A. Lower motor neurons control the activity of the skeletal muscles.

B. Energy is consumed when skeletal muscles contract in response to a stimulus.
1. Lactic acid, a by-product of muscle metabolism, accumulates if the amount of oxygen available to the cell is not sufficient.
2. Muscle fatigue results from:
   a. Increased work of the muscle, with inadequate oxygen supply.
   b. Depletion of glycogen and energy stores.

C. Muscle contraction.
1. Isometric: the length of the muscle remains constant; the force generated by the muscle increases—for

example, when one pushes against an immovable object.

2. Isotonic: shortening of the muscle but with no increase in muscle tension.
3. Normal activity is a combination of both types of muscle contraction.
4. Muscles accomplish movement only by contraction.
   a. Flexion: bending at a joint.
   b. Extension: straightening of a joint.
   c. Abduction: action moving away from the body.
   d. Adduction: action moving toward the body.

> **NURSING PRIORITY:** Know the terms used in referring to movement of joints.

5. Hypertrophy will occur if muscle is exercised repeatedly.
6. Atrophy will occur with muscle disuse.

System Assessment

A. History.
   1. History of musculoskeletal injuries, musculoskeletal surgeries, neuromuscular disabilities, inflammatory and metabolic conditions directly or indirectly affecting the musculoskeletal system.
   2. Familial predisposition to orthopedic problems.
   3. Level of normal activity, occupation, exercise, recreation.
   4. Existence of other chronic health problems.
B. Physical assessment.
   1. Initial inspection for gross deformities, asymmetry, and edema.
   2. Nutritional status: appropriateness of client's weight and body frame; 24-hour diet recall, dietary supplements.
   3. Joints.
      a. Movement: active and passive; examine active movement first; compare movement and range of motion (ROM) on one side of the body with movement and ROM on the opposite side.
      b. Inflammation and tenderness: with or without movement.
      c. Presence of joint deformities and dislocations.
      d. Palpate joints for crepitus.
   4. Evaluate limb length and circumference if hypertrophy or inconsistency in bone length is evident.
   5. Evaluate client's spinal alignment, posture, and gait.
   6. Evaluate skeletal muscle.
      a. Muscle strength bilaterally.
      b. Coordination of movement.
      c. Presence of atrophy or hypertrophy.
      d. Presence of involuntary muscle movement.
   7. Assess peripheral pulses and peripheral circulation.
   8. Assess for presence and characteristics of pain.
      a. Specific type of pain and exact location.
      b. Identify precipitating and/or alleviating factors (most musculoskeletal pain is relieved by rest).
      c. Ask about back pain and/or injury.

Box 21-1 BODY MECHANICS

The wider the base of support, the greater the stability.
   Position feet wide apart.
The lower the center of gravity, the greater the stability.
   Flex the knees; let the strong muscles of the legs do the work.
   Position close to client.
Face the client; keep back, pelvis, and knees aligned; avoid twisting.
Balance activity between arms and legs.
   Avoid bending to lift; this decreases strain on the back.
Encourage client to assist.
   Pivoting, turning, rolling, and leverage require less work.
Person with heaviest load should coordinate team efforts.
Obtain assistance or a lift with heavy or difficult transfers or moves.
Teach client proper body mechanics.

> **ALERT** Use ergonomic principles when providing care (assistive devices, proper lifting).

Box 21-2 OLDER ADULT CARE FOCUS

Musculoskeletal Changes

- Decreased bone density leads to more frequent fractures.
- Decrease in subcutaneous tissue results in less soft tissue over bony prominences.
- Degenerative changes in the musculoskeletal system alter posture and gait.
- Degenerative changes in cartilage and ligaments result in joint stiffness and pain.
- Range of motion of extremities decreases; older adult may need increased assistance with activities of daily living.
- Slowed movement and decreased muscle strength lead to decreased response time.
- Loss of height from disk compression, posture changes, kyphosis.

9. Sensory changes: assess for decreased sensation in extremities.
10. Body mechanics (Box 21-1, Appendix 3-1).
11. Changes in the older adult (Box 21-2).

> **ALERT** Perform a focused assessment and reassessment for changes in client condition. Recognize signs and symptoms of complications and intervene appropriately.

DISORDERS OF MUSCULOSKELETAL AND CONNECTIVE TISSUE

 Congenital Hip Dysplasia

Congenital hip dysplasia is a malformation of the hip that occurs as a result of imperfect development of the femoral head, the acetabulum, or both. The structures that support the hip joint and hold the joint together are too loose, or the joint cavity is too shallow.

Assessment

A. Risk factors/etiology.
1. Frequently associated with other congenital deformities.
2. Prenatal factors.
   a. Maternal hormone secretion.
   b. Intrauterine posture, especially frank breech position.
B. Clinical manifestations (newborn).
1. Ortolani sign: infant supine, knees flexed, hips fully abducted; a click is heard or felt as the hip is reduced by abduction.
2. Asymmetrical gluteal and thigh folds.
3. Shortening of the leg on the affected side; one knee is lower than the other (Galeazzi sign).
C. Diagnostics (see Appendix 21-1).

Treatment

A. Treatment is initiated as soon as condition is identified.
B. For the newborn, the dislocated hip is securely held in a full abduction position. This keeps the femur in the acetabulum and stabilizes the area.
1. Abduction devices.
   a. Pavlik harness: a fabric strap harness that is secured around the infant's shoulders and chest and is connected to straps around the lower leg. The harness maintains the legs in a flexed, abducted position at the hip. The harness may be removed for bathing, but the infant will wear it full time until the hip is stable.
   b. Hip spica cast: most often used when adduction contracture is present. After the removal of the cast, a protective abduction brace is fitted.
2. Closed reduction: performed in older children, 6 to 18 months old.
3. Open reduction: performed if hip is not reducible with traction or closed reduction.
C. Successful reduction becomes increasingly difficult after the age of 4 years.

Nursing Interventions

Goal: To identify hip dysplasia in the newborn before discharge.
Goal: To assist parents to understand mechanism to maintain reduction.
A. Pavlik brace: teach parents proper application of brace; undershirts should be worn beneath the brace; check skin under brace for irritation or pressure areas; no oils or lotions should be applied to skin that will be under brace.
B. Teach parents cast care if hip spica cast is applied.

> **ALERT** Apply, maintain and or remove orthopedic devices (tractions, braces, splints, casts).

Goal: To facilitate developmental progress.
A. Provide appropriate stimuli and activity for developmental level.

B. Encourage parents to hold and cuddle child.
C. Maintain normal home routine.

Clubfoot (Talipes Equinovarus)

Clubfoot is a deformity of the foot in which adduction, plantar flexion, and inversion of the foot occur in varying degrees of severity. The unilateral form occurs more commonly than the bilateral form.

Assessment

A. Risk factors/etiology (inconclusive).
1. Intrauterine compression.
2. Decreased growth of distal tibia.
B. Assessment.
1. Condition is apparent at birth.
2. In true clubfoot, there is severe limitation of ROM.
C. Diagnostics: clinical manifestations.

Treatment

Treatment is begun immediately and most often requires three stages for correction.
A. Correction of deformity: casts are applied in series for gradual stretching and straightening; massage accompanied by special bandaging may also be used.
B. Maintenance of correction: orthopedic shoes.
C. Follow-up observations to prevent recurrence of the deformity.

Nursing Interventions

Goal: To assist parents to understand mechanism of treatment to achieve correction.
A. Appropriate care of cast or brace at home.
B. Follow-up care and importance of frequent cast changes.
Goal: To facilitate developmental progress and adapt nurturing activities to meet infant's and parents' needs (same as for congenital hip dysplasia).

Herniated Lumbar Disk

The intervertebral disk forms a cushion between the vertebral bodies of the spinal column. As stress on an injured or degenerated disk occurs, the cartilage material of the disk (nucleus pulposus) herniates inward toward the spinal column, causing compression or tension on the spinal nerve root. The problem most often occurs in the lumbosacral area.

Assessment

A. Risk factors/etiology.
1. Degenerative disk disease.
2. Obesity.
3. Injury or stress to the lower back.
4. Muscle-strengthening exercises.
B. Clinical manifestations (lumbar disk).
1. Low back pain, commonly radiating down one buttock and posterior thigh.

2. Coughing, straining, sneezing, bending, twisting, and lifting exacerbate the pain.
3. Lying supine and raising the leg in an extended position will precipitate the pain.

C. Diagnostics (see Appendix 21-1).

Treatment

A. Conservative.
   1. Analgesics, muscle relaxants.
   2. Weight reduction, if appropriate.
   3. Ice may be used for first 48 hours after injury; then moist heat is a better analgesic.
   4. Activity modification, good body mechanics, back brace.
   5. Ultrasound therapy and massage.
   6. Back strengthening exercises once the pain subsides.
B. Surgical.
   1. Laminectomy: removal of the herniated portion of the disk.
   2. Microlaminectomy (diskectomy): removal of the herniated disk with use of a microscope (less trauma in the disk area, improved hemostasis, minimal nerve root involvement).
C. Alternative: acupressure or acupuncture.

Nursing Interventions

Goal: To relieve pain by means of conservative measures and prevent recurrence of problem.

A. Decrease muscle spasm/pain with analgesics, muscle relaxants, decreased activity, and cold or heat applications.
B. Begin ambulation slowly and avoid having client bend, stoop, twist, sit, or lift.
C. Instruct the client and family regarding the principles of appropriate body mechanics.
D. The client will need a firm mattress; sleeping in the prone position, especially with a pillow, should be avoided.
E. Instruct the client and family regarding lower back exercises.
F. Encourage correct posture; instruct client to avoid prolonged standing.
G. Client should sit in straight-backed chairs.
H. Semireclining position with forward flexion of lumbar spine (recliner) may be position of comfort.

Goal: To prepare client for laminectomy.

A. Perform preoperative nursing interventions, including education as appropriate.
B. Have client practice logrolling.
C. Have client practice voiding from supine position.
D. Discuss with client postoperative pain and anticipated methods to decrease pain.
E. Evaluate bowel and bladder function.
F. Identify specific characteristics of pain to be included in database for comparison with pain after surgery.
G. Establish a baseline neurologic assessment for postoperative reference.

Goal: To maintain spinal alignment after laminectomy.

A. Keep the bed in flat position.
B. Logroll client when turning.
C. Keep pillows between the legs when client is positioned on the side.
D. The client who has had microdisk surgery will have fewer limitations on mobility. Often, the client may assume a position of comfort.
E. Assist with application of back brace if ordered.

Goal: To maintain homeostasis and assess for complications after laminectomy.

A. Evaluate incision area for possible leakage of spinal fluid and bleeding – notify health care provider of clear fluid leaking from incisional area.
B. Analgesics may be given via a patient-controlled analgesia pump or epidural catheter.
C. Assess pain and determine whether there is any pain radiation.

ALERT Assess client's need for pain management and intervene as needed using non-pharmacologic comfort measures. Use pharmacological pain measures for pain management as needed.

D. Perform neurovascular checks of extremities.
E. Normal bladder function returns in 24 to 48 hours; assess current status of voiding.

⚠ NURSING PRIORITY The client who has undergone laminectomy frequently experiences difficulty voiding; this may be due to edema in the area of surgery that interferes with normal bladder sensation.

F. Ambulate as soon as indicated (frequently on first postoperative day if no fusion was done).
G. If fusion was performed, may need to apply body brace before ambulation.
H. The client who has undergone microlaminectomy experiences less pain, is frequently out of bed on the day of surgery, and has fewer complications.
I. Paralytic ileus and constipation are common complications; assess for decreased bowel sounds and abdominal distention.

ALERT Identify factors that interfere with elimination.

 ### Scoliosis

Scoliosis is a lateral curvature of the spine. If it is allowed to progress without treatment, it will severely affect the shape of the thoracic cavity and impair ventilation.

A. Idiopathic (predominant type) occurs primarily in adolescent girls.
B. Most noticeable at beginning of growth spurt, around 10 years of age.

Assessment

A. Clinical manifestations.
   1. Uneven hips and shoulders.
   2. Visible curvature of the spinal column; head and hips are not in alignment.

3. When child bends forward from the waist, there is visible asymmetry of the shoulders. The ribs and shoulder are more prominent on one side.

4. Waist line is uneven; one hip is more prominent.

B. Diagnostics.
   1. Clinical manifestations.
   2. X-ray film.

Treatment

A. Observation and monitoring for curvature less than 25 degrees.

B. Brace if curvature shows progression (used for curvatures of 25 to 40 degrees).
   1. Milwaukee brace for high thoracic curvatures.
   2. Boston brace (underarm orthosis) for thoracic-lumbar curves.

C. Surgery (used for curvatures of more than 40 degrees): spinal fusion and placement of a rod to prevent destruction of the fused segment; the rod may be left in place permanently unless it becomes displaced or causes discomfort.

Nursing Interventions

Goal: To identify defects early and promote effective conservative therapy.

A. Promote health programs in school to identify condition.

ALERT: Perform targeted screening (scoliosis, vision and hearing).

B. Assist client and parents to properly use braces.
   1. Make sure brace is properly fitted and does not inadvertently rub bony prominences.
   2. May put light T-shirt under brace for comfort.
   3. Initially, the brace is worn 20 to 23 hours per day.
   4. Brace is regularly adjusted to promote correction.
   5. If progress is good, child is weaned from the brace during the daytime and wears it only at night.
   6. Supplemental exercises.

Goal: To support normal growth and development and assist the child to develop a positive self-image.

A. Continue to encourage peer socialization.

B. Encourage independence.

C. Encourage child to participate in and be independent in scheduling of activities and other aspects of care.

D. Emphasize positive long-term outcome.

Goal: To maintain spinal alignment after surgical correction (see Care of Client After Laminectomy and Fusion).

Goal: To maintain homeostasis and assess for complications after surgical correction (see Care of Client After Laminectomy and Fusion).

Fractures

A. A fracture is a disruption or break in the continuity of the bone, which occurs most often as the result of a traumatic injury.

B. Characteristics of bones in children affecting fractures and fracture healing.
   1. Presence of epiphyseal plate; if the epiphyseal plate is damaged in the fracture, this may affect the growth of the long bone.
   2. Periosteum is thicker and stronger and has an increased blood supply; therefore healing is more rapid.
   3. Bones are more porous and allow for greater flexibility.

C. Pathologic fractures occur as a result of a disease process.

D. Classification of fractures (Figure 21-1).
   1. Type.
      a. Complete: fracture line extends through the entire bone; the periosteum is disrupted on both sides of the bone.
      b. Incomplete: fracture line extends only partially through the bone (greenstick, hairline-type fractures).
      c. Comminuted: fracture with multiple bone fragments; more common in adults.
      d. Greenstick: an incomplete fracture with bending and splintering of the bone; more common in children.
      e. Impacted: complete fracture in which bone fragments are driven into each other.
   2. Classified according to location on the bone: proximal, middle, or distal.

FIGURE 21-1 Types of Fractures. **A,** Greenstick. **B,** Transverse. **C,** Oblique. **D,** Spiral. **E,** Comminuted. **F,** Open. (Courtesy Rocky Shepheard, New London, Ohio. In Monahan FD et al: *Phipps' medical-surgical nursing: health and illness perspectives,* ed 8, St. Louis, 2007, Mosby.)

3. Stable versus unstable fracture.
   a. Stable: a portion of the periosteum usually remains intact; frequently transverse, spiral, or greenstick fractures.
   b. Unstable: bones are displaced at the time of injury, with poor approximation; frequently comminuted or impacted.
4. Simple, closed fracture: does not produce a break in the skin.
5. Complex, open, or compound fracture: involves an open wound through which the bone has protruded.

> **⚠ NURSING PRIORITY** Age, displacement of the fracture, the site of the fracture, nutritional level, medications, and blood supply to the area of injury are factors influencing time required for fracture healing to become complete. Be familiar with the terms used to describe fractures.

Assessment

A. Risk factors/etiology.
   1. Pathologic fracture.
      a. Osteoporosis.
      b. Tumors (multiple myeloma, osteogenic sarcoma).
      c. Metabolic diseases (e.g., thyroid disorders).
   2. Trauma.
B. Clinical manifestations.
   1. Edema, swelling of soft tissue around the injured site.
   2. Pain: immediate, severe.
   3. Abnormal positioning of extremity; deformity.
   4. Loss of normal function.
   5. False movement: movement occurs at the fracture site; bone should not move except at joints.
   6. Crepitus: palpable or audible crunching as the ends of the bones rub together.
   7. Discoloration of the skin around the affected area.
   8. Sensation may be impaired if there is nerve damage.
C. Diagnostics (see Appendix 21-1).

Treatment

A. Immediate immobilization of suspected fracture area.
B. Fracture reduction.
   1. Closed reduction: nonsurgical, manual realignment of the bones; then injured extremity is usually placed in a cast for continued immobilization until healing occurs.
   2. Open reduction and internal fixation (ORIF): surgical correction of alignment.
C. Traction (Figure 21-2).
   1. Purposes.
      a. Immobilization of fractures until surgical correction is done; immobilization or alignment of fracture until sufficient healing occurs to permit casting.
      b. Decrease, prevent, or correct bone or joint deformities associated with muscle diseases and bone injury.
      c. Prevent or reduce muscle spasm.

FIGURE 21-2 Traction. **A,** Balanced suspension traction with a Thomas splint and a Pearson attachment. **B,** Buck's extension traction. **C,** 90°-90° traction. (*A* from Monahan FD et al: *Phipps' medical-surgical nursing: health and illness perspectives,* ed 8, St. Louis, 2007, Mosby. *B* and *C* from Hockenberry MJ, Wilson D: *Wong's nursing care of infants and children,* ed 8, St. Louis, 2007, Mosby.)

   2. Types.
      a. Skeletal: wire or metal pin is inserted into or through the bone.
      b. Skin: force of pull is applied directly to the skin and indirectly to the bone.
D. Cast application to maintain immobility of affected area.
   1. Cast applied to immobilize joints above and below the injured area.
   2. Short or long arm or leg cast.
   3. Body jacket cast for spinal injuries.
   4. Hip spica cast for femoral fractures.
E. Fixation devices.
   1. External fixation: application of a rigid external device consisting of pins placed through the bone and held in place by a metal frame; requires meticulous care of pin insertion sites (Figure 21-3).
   2. Internal fixation: done through an open incision; hardware (pins, plates, rods, screws) is placed in the bone.
   3. Both methods may be used to treat a fracture.

Complications

A. Improper healing: delayed union, nonunion, or angulation (bone heals at a distorted angle).
B. Infection: especially in injuries resulting in an open fracture and soft tissue injury.

FIGURE 21-3 External fixation. (Courtesy Stryker, Kalamazoo, MI.)

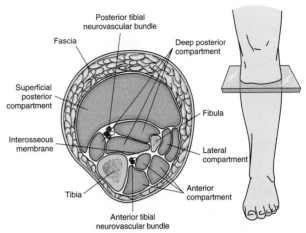

FIGURE 21-4 Compartments of the leg. (From Monahan FD et al: *Phipps' medical-surgical nursing: health and illness perspectives*, ed 8, St. Louis, 2007, Mosby.)

C. Decreased neurovascular status resulting from pressure of cast and edema formation.
1. Decreased pulses distal to injury.
2. Pain unrelieved by analgesics.
3. Edema, pallor.
4. Decreased sensory and motor function.
D. Compartment syndrome: muscle, nerves, and vessels are restricted to a confined space (myofascial compartment) within an extremity (Figure 21-4).
1. Etiology.
   a. Decreased compartment size from cast, splints, tight bandages, tight surgical closure.
   b. Increase in compartment contents caused by hemorrhage and/or edema.
2. Clinical manifestations of compartment syndrome.
   a. Muscle ischemia occurs as a result of compression of structures in the compartment.
   b. Arterial compression may not occur; pulses may still be present.

ALERT Manage a client with alteration in hemodynamics, tissue perfusion and hemostasis (cerebral, cardiac, peripheral). Recognize signs and symptoms of complications.

   c. May cause permanent damage if not relieved immediately.
   d. Clients complain of excessive pain unrelieved by analgesics.
   e. Occurrence of complication may be decreased by elevation of the extremity and application of ice packs after initial injury.
   f. Treatment is directed toward immediate release of pressure: if the client has a cast, the cast may be "bivalved"—the cast is split in half, and the halves are secured around the extremity by a wrap, such as an elastic bandage.

   g. Volkmann's ischemic contracture: compartment syndrome in the arms that compromises circulation; occurs most often as a result of short arm cast used to immobilize a fracture of the humerus.
   h. Can result in permanent damage in a short time (6-8 hours).
   i. Paresthesia is frequently the first sign; pulselessness is a late sign.
E. Venous stasis and thrombus formation are related to immobility.
F. Fat embolism.
1. Associated with fractures or surgery of long bones (especially the femur); primarily occurs in adults.
2. Clinical manifestations generally occur within 12 to 48 hours of injury.
3. Fat embolism produces symptoms of acute respiratory distress and hypoxia.
G. Blisters may be associated with twisting-type fractures or compartmental syndrome.

Nursing Interventions

Goal: To immobilize a fractured extremity and to provide emergency care before transporting victim.
A. Evaluate circulation distal to injury.

⚠ NURSING PRIORITY: Identify orthopedic situations that can cause compromised circulation and neurologic damage; intervene and obtain assistance.

B. If pulses are not present or if the extremity must be realigned to apply splint for transfer, apply just enough traction to support and immobilize the fractured extremity in a position of proper alignment. Once the traction is initiated, do not release it until the extremity has been properly splinted.

C. Splint and immobilize extremity before transfer.

> ❗ **NURSING PRIORITY** Do not apply traction to compound fractures; traction may cause more damage to tissue and vessels.

D. Elevate the affected extremity, if possible, to decrease edema.

Goal: To identify complications early, perform frequent peripheral nerve and vascular assessments distal to the area of injury or cast.

A. Impaired blood flow.
1. Pulselessness; skin pale and cool to touch.
2. Pain, swelling, edema distal to injury or cast.
3. Capillary refill greater than 3 seconds.

B. Nerve damage from excessive pressure.
1. Paresthesia, numbness distal to injury or cast.
2. Motor paralysis of previously functioning muscles.
3. Feeling of deep pain and pressure.

C. Infection: may occur within the cast.
1. Unpleasant odor, drainage (foul, purulent).
2. Generalized body temperature elevation.
3. Increased warmth over cast, "hot spot."

> **ALERT** Monitor wound for signs and symptoms of infection; identify adverse response to therapy.

D. Compartment syndrome.
1. Significant increase in pain, not responsive to analgesics.
2. Loss of movement and sensation distal to cast.
3. Skin is pale, cool to touch.
4. Edema distal to injury or cast.
5. Pulses may be present initially.

E. Notify physician immediately if any complications of compartment syndrome or compromised circulation are present.

> **ALERT** Manage care for a client with alteration in tissue perfusion (peripheral circulation). Recognize signs and symptoms of complications and intervene appropriately.

Goal: To maintain immobilization by means of a cast.

A. Plaster cast: allow cast to dry adequately before moving the client or handling the cast.
1. Encourage drying of cast by using fans and maintaining adequate circulation.
2. Avoid handling wet cast to prevent indentions in the cast, which may precipitate pressure areas inside the cast; support cast on pillows.
3. Reposition client every 2 hours to increase drying on all cast surfaces.
4. "Petaling" a cast is done to cover the rough edges and prevent crumbling of a plaster cast; edges are covered with small strips of waterproof adhesive.

5. Try not to get the cast wet; after the cast is dry and the initial edema is resolved, may use low setting on hair dryer after exposure to water.

> ❗ **NURSING PRIORITY** Teach client: DO NOT get plaster cast wet, remove any type of padding, insert any objects inside cast, bear weight on new cast for 48 hours (if weight-bearing type), or cover cast with plastic for long periods of time.

B. Synthetic casts (fiberglass, polyester cotton knit) are lighter and require a minimal amount of drying time.
1. Frequently used for upper body cast.
2. Preferable for infants and children.
3. Cast does not crumble around the edges and does not soil as easily.
4. Cast dries rapidly if it gets damp, and it does not disintegrate in water; some synthetic casts can be immersed for bathing.

C. Continue to assess for compromised circulation and compartment syndrome.

D. Body jacket cast and hip spica cast.
1. Evaluate for abdominal discomfort caused by cast compression of mesenteric artery against duodenum.
2. Relief of abdominal pressure can be achieved by means of nasogastric tube and suction or cast removal and reapplication.
3. Evaluate for pressure areas over iliac crest.

E. Elevate casted extremity, especially during the first 24 hours after application.

F. Apply ice packs over the area of injury (keeping cast dry) during the first 24 hours.

G. Encourage movement and exercise of unaffected joints.

Goal: To maintain immobilization via traction (see Figure 21-2).

A. Assume that traction is continuous unless the doctor orders otherwise.

B. Carefully assess for skin breakdown, especially under the client.

C. Do not change or remove traction weight on a client with continuous traction.

D. The traction ropes and weights should hang free from any obstructions.

E. Traction applied in one direction requires an equal countertraction to be effective.
1. Do not let the client's feet touch the end of the bed; this will cause the countertraction to be lost.
2. Do not allow the traction weights to rest on anything at the end of the bed; this negates the pull of the traction.

F. Carefully assess the pin sites in clients with skeletal traction. Osteomyelitis is a serious complication of skeletal traction.

> **ALERT** Recognize client with a condition that increases risk for insufficient vascular perfusion; monitor effective functioning of therapeutic device; prevent complications of immobility. The majority of clients with fractures will experience some level of immobility.

Goal: To prevent complications of immobility (see Chapter 3).

Goal: To prevent complications from external or internal fixation.

A. Inspect exposed skin and pin sites for infection.

B. Cleanse around pin sites.

C. Perform wound care on incisional area or area of trauma.

D. Observe carefully for development of an infection.

E. Evaluate for circulatory and neurosensory impairment.

Home Care

A. Teach client what not to do.
  1. Do not bear weight on the affected extremity until instructed to do so.
  2. Do not allow the cast to get wet (discuss alternatives to tub baths).
  3. Do not insert any objects into the cast or remove any padding.
  4. Do not move or manipulate pins on an external fixator device.

B. Client should report symptoms associated with swelling or an increase in pain, especially pain unrelieved by analgesics.

C. Assess pin sites for evidence of infection.

Specific Fractures

A. Colles' fracture.
  1. Fracture of the distal radius.
  2. Primary complication is compartment syndrome.

B. Fractured pelvis.
  1. Frequently occurs in older adults and is associated with falls.
  2. May cause serious intra-abdominal injuries (hemorrhage) and urinary tract injury.
  3. Bed rest is prescribed for clients with stable fractures.
  4. Combination of traction, cast, and surgical intervention may be used for the client with a complex fracture.
  5. Turn client only on specific orders.

C. Fractured hip: may be repaired by fixed or sliding nail plates, replacement prostheses, or hip joint replacement.
  1. Common in women older than 65 years because of loss of postural stability and loss of bone mass.
  2. Types of fractures.
    a. Intracapsular fracture (femoral neck): more difficult to heal; associated with osteoporosis; more likely to be associated with avascular necrosis due to interruption of blood supply.
    b. Extracapsular fracture: occurs outside joint capsule; usually caused by severe direct trauma or a fall.
  3. Clinical manifestations.
    a. External rotation and adduction of the affected extremity.
    b. Shortening of the length of the affected extremity.
    c. Severe pain and tenderness.

4. Treatment.
  a. Initially, Buck's traction to immobilize fracture and decrease muscle spasms (see Figure 21-2).
  b. Surgical repair as soon as client's condition allows (permits earlier mobility and prevents complications of immobility).
5. Nursing interventions after surgery (Box 21-3).
  a. Circulatory and neurologic checks distal to area of injury.
  b. Position to prevent flexion, adduction, and internal rotation, which cause dislocation of the prosthesis.

ALERT: Position client to prevent complications.

  (1) Do not adduct the affected leg past the neutral position.
  (2) Maintain the affected leg in an abducted position with an A-frame pillow or pillows between the legs.
  (3) Avoid flexion of the hip of more than 90 degrees.
  (4) Prevent internal or external rotation by using sandbags, pillows, and trochanter rolls at the thigh.
  (5) Extreme external rotation accompanied by severe pain is indicative of hip prosthesis displacement.
  c. Check physician's order regarding positioning and turning.
  d. Evaluate blood loss.
    (1) Check under the operative site for hemorrhage.
    (2) Measure the diameter of both thighs to evaluate the presence of internal bleeding in the affected extremity.

NURSING PRIORITY: The client is especially prone to complications of immobility (thromboembolism following hip fracture); use nursing interventions to minimize complications.

Box 21-3 OLDER ADULT CARE FOCUS

Musculoskeletal Nursing Implications

- Older adults have difficulty maintaining immobility after fractures; therefore fractures are frequently repaired with surgical intervention (ORIF).
- Older adults heal more slowly, so use of extremity and weight bearing are frequently delayed.
- Complications of immobility occur more frequently; mobilize hospitalized clients as early as possible.
- Do not rely on fever as the primary indication of infection; decreasing mental status is more common.
- Contractures are more common in older adults.
- Encourage older adults to use assistive devices such as canes and walkers.

D. Total hip replacement.
  1. Hip replacement may be done because of a pathologic fracture or a disease process such as arthritis.
  2. Preoperative care.
    a. Encourage client to practice using either crutches or a walker, whichever is anticipated to be used after surgery.
    b. Encourage client to practice moving from bed to a chair in the manner that will be necessary after surgery.
    c. Help the client begin practicing the postoperative exercises so that he or she will understand and be able to do them correctly after surgery.
    d. Client should discontinue use of NSAIDs and/or aspirin about a week before surgery.
  3. Postoperative care.
    a. Position supine with head slightly elevated, maintain abduction of affected leg.
    b. Quadriceps exercises.
    c. Neurologic and circulation checks.
    d. Client is mobilized on first or second postoperative day to prevent complications of immobility; may use antiembolism stockings and/or sequential compression pumps on lower extremity to prevent venous stasis.
    e. Low-molecular-weight heparin (see Appendix 16-3) may be given to prevent thrombophlebitis.
    f. Keep client's heels off the bed to prevent skin breakdown.
    g. Legs should not be crossed.

> **!** **NURSING PRIORITY** After surgery, do not allow the repaired hip to flex greater than 90 degrees; avoid adduction and internal rotation of extremity. Flexion and adduction will dislocate the hip prosthesis.

    h. Observe for signs of possible hip dislocation.
      (1) Increased hip pain.
      (2) Shortening of affected leg.
      (3) External leg rotation.
      (4) If these symptoms are observed, contact the surgeon immediately.
E. Femoral shaft fracture.
  1. Common injury in young adults and children.
  2. Treatment.
    a. Immobility is achieved by means of a spica cast in older children.
    b. 90°-90° traction (see Figure 21-2): balanced skeletal traction for fractured femur.
    c. Older child and adult.
      (1) Internal fixation (adults).
      (2) Balanced skeletal traction for 8 to 12 weeks.
      (3) Immobilization by application of a hip spica cast alone or after balanced skeletal traction.
F. Rib fractures.
  1. Usually heal in 3 to 6 weeks with no residual impairment.

  2. Painful respirations cause client's breathing to be more shallow and coughing to be restrained; this precipitates buildup of secretions and decreased ventilation, leading to atelectasis.
  3. Chest taping or strapping is not usually done because it decreases thoracic excursion.
  4. Multiple rib fractures may precipitate the development of a pneumothorax or a tension pneumothorax (see Chapter 15).
G. Mandible fracture.
  1. Wiring of jaws (intermaxillary fixation) is treatment.
  2. Postoperative problems: airway obstruction and aspiration of vomitus.
  3. Wire cutters at bedside in case of emergency (cardiac or respiratory arrest).
    a. Suction client if vomiting.
    b. Cutting wires may complicate problem.
  4. Tracheostomy set at bedside.
  5. Oral hygiene and use of pad/pencil or picture board to communicate post-op.
  6. Discharge teaching: oral care, techniques for handling secretions, diet (problems with constipation and flatus due to low-bulk, high-carbohydrate liquid supplements), how and when to use wire cutters.

Osteoporosis

Osteoporosis is a metabolic bone disease that involves an imbalance between new bone formation and bone resorption.

A. Primary osteoporosis is the most common type; occurs most often in women after menopause because low levels of estrogen are associated with an increase in bone resorption.
B. Bone loss occurs predominantly in the vertebral bodies of the spine, the femoral neck in the hip, and the distal radius of the arm. Bone mass declines, leaving the bones brittle and weak.

Assessment

A. Risk factors/etiology.
  1. Age/ethnicity: incidence increases in white and Asian women after the age of 50 years.
  2. Estrogen deficit: early menopause, estrogen-blocking medications such as tamoxifen or aromasin.
  3. Low peak bone mass: the maximum amount of bone a person achieves is peak bone mass achieved before age 20.
  4. Alcohol intake, sedentary lifestyle.
  5. Endocrine disorders of the thyroid and parathyroid glands.
  6. Nutritional deficits: insufficient intake of dietary calcium and/or vitamin D.
  7. Cigarette smoking, long-term use of corticosteroids.
B. Clinical manifestations (Figure 21-5).
  1. May be asymptomatic until x-ray films demonstrate skeletal weakening. Bone loss of 25% to 40% must

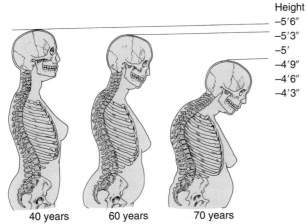

Height
—5′6″
—5′3″
—5′
—4′9″
—4′6″
—4′3″

40 years   60 years   70 years

FIGURE 21-5 Osteoporotic changes. (From Black JM, Hawks JH: *Medical-surgical nursing: clinical management for positive outcomes,* ed 8, Philadelphia, 2009, Saunders.)

occur before osteoporosis can be identified on standard x-ray films.

2. Spinal deformity and "dowager's hump."
   a. Results from repeated pathologic, spinal vertebral fractures.
   b. Gradual loss of height.
   c. Increase in spinal curvature (kyphosis).
3. Spinal fractures may occur spontaneously or as a result of minimal trauma.
4. Chronic low thoracic and midline back pain.
5. Height loss may precipitate thoracic problems, decrease in abdominal capacity, and decrease in exercise tolerance.
6. Hip fractures and vertebral collapse are the most debilitating problems.
C. Diagnostics (see Appendix 21-1).
   1. Serum laboratory values of calcium, vitamin D, phosphorus, and alkaline phosphatase may be normal or low.
   2. Computed tomography or bone density scan (DEXA) can be performed to evaluate bone loss.
      a. Bone mineral density (BMD): 2.5 standard deviations below mean of young adults is classified as osteoporosis.
      b. Osteopenia: T-score = 1.0 to 2.5, but not at level of osteoporosis.

Treatment

A. Dietary: increased intake of protein, calcium, and vitamin D.
B. Medications.
   1. Calcium supplements: daily intake of calcium should be approximately 1000 mg for men and 1500 mg for postmenopausal women.
   2. Vitamin D supplements to enhance utilization of calcium; spending 20 minutes daily in the sun will provide adequate vitamin D.
   3. Medications to facilitate increased bone density (see Appendix 21-2).

C. Exercise: activities that put moderate stress on bones by working them against gravity (walking, racquet sports, jogging).
   1. Swimming and yoga may not be as beneficial because of decreased stress on bone mass.
   2. Walking for 30 minutes 3-5 times a week is most effective exercise in preventing osteoporosis.
   3. Weight bearing exercise decreases the development of osteoporosis and possibly increases new bone formation.
D. Compression fractures of the vertebrae usually heal without surgical intervention.

Complications

Bone fractures occurring in the vertebral bodies, distal radius, or hip.

Nursing Interventions

Goal: To decrease pain and promote activities to diminish progression of disease.
A. Pain relief.
   1. Bed rest initially, firm mattress.
   2. Narcotic analgesics initially, followed by nonsteroidal antiinflammatory drugs (NSAIDs).
B. Assess bowel and bladder function; client will be prone to constipation and paralytic ileus if vertebrae are involved.
C. Regular daily exercise; encourage outdoor exercises (increases utilization of vitamin D).
D. Increased calcium intake and estrogen therapy.

Home Care

A. Decrease falls and injury by maintaining safe home environment (Box 21-4).

Box 21-4   OLDER ADULT CARE FOCUS

Protecting Joints

- If pain lasts longer than 1 hour after exercise, change the exercises that involve that joint.
- Plan activity and work that conserve energy; do important tasks first.
- Alternate activities; do not do all heavy tasks at one time.
- Minimize stress on joints; sit rather than stand, avoid prolonged repetitive movements, move around frequently, avoid stairs or prolonged grasping.
- Use largest muscles rather than smaller ones; use shoulders or arms rather than hands to push open doors; pick up items without stooping or bending; use leg muscles; women should carry purses on their shoulders rather than in their hands.
- Painful, acutely swollen inflamed joints should not be exercised beyond basic range of motion.
- Regular exercise can be done even when joints are slightly painful and stiff; swimming and bike riding maintain mobility without weight-bearing.
- Expect changes in mental status after surgery.
- There may be a role change in the family due to the client's decreased mobility.

B. The client should understand the need to continue taking medications, even if they do not make the client feel better. It is important for the client to understand that the calcium and vitamin D supplements are necessary to prevent further bone loss.

C. Do not exercise if pain occurs.

D. Avoid heavy lifting, stooping, and bending. Review and demonstrate good body mechanics with the client.

Osteomyelitis

Osteomyelitis is an infection of the bone, bone marrow, and surrounding soft tissue.

A. The most common causative organism is *Staphylococcus aureus*.

B. Inflammatory response occurs initially, with increased vascularization and edema.

C. Even though the healing process occurs, the dead bone tissue frequently forms a sequestrum, which continues to retain viable bacteria; this tissue may produce recurrent abscesses for years.

D. Classified according to acute or chronic status.

   1. Acute: sudden onset; may heal in 2 to 3 weeks or progress to chronic status.

   2. Chronic: a continuous, persistent problem or exacerbation of previous problem.

Assessment

A. Risk factors/etiology.

   1. Indirect entry of organism: hematogenous.

     a. More frequently affects growing bone.

     b. Injury and infection of adjacent soft tissue in distal femur, proximal tibia, humerus, and radius.

   2. Direct injury: can occur at any age.

     a. Trauma.

     b. Surgical procedures.

B. Clinical manifestations.

   1. Acute.

     a. Tenderness, swelling, and warmth in affected area.

     b. Drainage from infected site.

     c. Systemic symptoms: fever, chills, nausea, night sweats.

     d. Constant pain in affected area; worsens with activity.

     e. Circulatory impairment.

   2. Chronic (present longer than 1 month; failed to respond to initial course of antibiotic therapy).

     a. Drainage from wound or sinus tract.

     b. Recurrent episodes of bone pain.

     c. Diminished systemic signs: low-grade fever; local signs of infection more common.

     d. Remission and exacerbation of problem.

C. Diagnostics (see Appendix 21-1).

   1. Wound and/or blood culture.

Treatment

A. Intensive intravenous (IV) antibiotics; oral antibiotic therapy for 6 to 8 weeks.

B. Immobilization of affected area.

C. Surgical debridement may be necessary.

D. Hyperbaric oxygen therapy to stimulate circulation and healing.

Nursing Interventions

Goal: To decrease pain, promote comfort, and decrease spread of infection.

A. Administer IV piggyback antibiotics; frequently assess status of IV site.

B. Maintain correct body alignment.

   1. Move affected extremity gently and with support.

   2. Prevent contractures, especially of affected extremity.

C. If there is an open wound, maintain wound (contact) precautions (see Chapter 6).

D. Client is usually discharged with prescription for antibiotics and should keep all follow-up care appointments.

> **ALERT** Monitor wounds for signs of infection; manage wound care.

Osteogenic Sarcoma

A. Osteogenic sarcoma (osteosarcoma) is the most common primary bone cancer; it advances very rapidly with metastasis to the lungs via the blood (see Chapter 8).

B. Most commonly affects the long bones, often the distal end of the femur, proximal tibia, or proximal humerus.

Assessment

A. Risk factors/etiology.

   1. Peak incidence between 10 and 25 years of age.

   2. Increased incidence in males during adolescence.

B. Clinical manifestations.

   1. Localized pain, swelling at site of tumor usually around knee.

   2. Client may limp and be unable to function at full capacity.

C. Diagnostics (see Appendix 21-1).

   1. Computed tomography scan to determine the extent of the lesion.

   2. Radioisotope scans to evaluate for metastasis.

   3. Lung evaluation to determine whether metastatic sites are present.

   4. Results of serum laboratory studies are inconclusive; client usually has an increase in the serum alkaline phosphatase level.

   5. X-ray film will reveal the tumor location and assist in determining an appropriate biopsy site.

Treatment

A. Amputation of extremity and/or extensive surgical resection of bone and surrounding tissue. Limb salvage procedure more often done, if there is a clear margin around tumor site.

B. Chemotherapy; radiation therapy.

Nursing Interventions

Goal: To maintain homeostasis and prevent complications after surgery.

A. An extensive pressure dressing with wound drains/suction may be applied.

B. ROM is usually begun immediately; continuous passive motion may be used immediately or on first postoperative day for both upper and lower extremity surgery.

C. Muscle toning is important before weight bearing.

D. Frequent neurovascular assessment is necessary because of resection of nerves and vessels in area; extremity may also be casted or splinted for support.

Goal: To prevent complications and promote mobility after amputation (see Appendix 21-3).

Goal: To assist the client/child and family to cope with the diagnosis and build basis for rehabilitation.

A. Provide honest, straightforward information to child/client and parents regarding the situation.

B. Allow the family and client an opportunity to express their concerns and fears; surgery is extensive and may affect body image (see Chapter 9).

C. Anticipate sense of loss of control and anger over changes in body.

D. Encourage normal growth and developmental activities as appropriate; allow client to be as independent as possible.

Goal: To assist the child and the family to cope with the side effects of chemotherapy and radiation (see Chapter 8).

Amputations

Removal of part of an extremity at various anatomic locations.

Assessment

A. Indications for amputation.
   1. Peripheral vascular disease, especially vascular disease of lower extremities.
   2. Severe trauma, congenital disorders.
   3. Acute or widespread infections (e.g., gas gangrene).
   4. Malignant tumors.

B. Diagnostic tests: dependent on underlying problem.

Nursing Interventions

Goal: To prevent further loss of circulation to the extremity, promote psychologic stability, promote comfort, promote optimum level of mobility.

A. Monitor circulation before surgery.

B. Provide preoperative care regarding upper extremity exercises to promote arm strength for postoperative activities of crutch walking and gait training.

ALERT Identify and prevent complications of immobility; use positioning to prevent contractures; provide support for client with unexpected alteration in body image; assist client to ambulate and move with assistive devices; promote wound healing; assist client with use of prosthesis.

Goal: To manage pain control and residual limb wound care postoperatively.

A. Residual limb may be elevated immediate post-op; after that time, clients should avoid sitting in a chair for more than 1 hour with hips flexed or having pillow under the residual limb to prevent flexion contractions. Flexion contracture hinders use of prosthesis.

B. Client should lie on their abdomen for 30 minutes 3 to 4 times/day and position the hip in extension while prone.

C. Discuss the phenomenon of phantom limb sensation.

D. Administer analgesics; phantom limb pain is very real to the client.

E. Evaluate residual limb for bleeding and healing.

F. A rigid compression dressing (plaster molded over dressing) may be applied to prevent injury and to decrease swelling. Controlling the edema will enhance healing and promote comfort. Changes of the rigid dressing are necessary; as the residual limb heals, it also shrinks. The compression dressing may be changed three or four times before a permanent prosthesis is fitted. The compression dressing may be formed so that it can attach to a prosthesis.

G. If the client is not fitted with a rigid compression dressing, the residual limb will be shaped with a compression bandage. Ace bandage elastic wrapping is often used for compression of this type. It should be worn at all times except during physical therapy and bathing.

Goal: To assist the client to understand measures for residual limb care after the wound has healed.

A. Continually assess for skin breakdown; visually inspect the residual limb for redness, abrasions, or blistering.

B. The residual limb should be washed daily, carefully rinsed, and dried; residual soap and moisture contribute to skin breakdown.

C. Do not apply anything to the residual limb (alcohol increases skin dryness and cracking; lotions keep skin soft and hinder use of prosthesis).

Home Care

A. Client should put the prosthesis on when he or she gets up and should wear it all day. The residual limb tends to swell if the prosthesis is not applied. The more the client wears the prosthesis; the less swelling will be experienced.

B. Using a lower limb prosthesis requires 40% to 60% more energy for walking.

C. Referral to community health nurse for instruction ambulation, transfer techniques, prone positioning, and proper residual limb care.

Rheumatoid Arthritis

Rheumatoid arthritis is a chronic, systemic autoimmune disease that affects all areas of the body; inflammatory responses occur in all connective tissue. Early symptoms include inflammation of the synovial joints.

A. Joint involvement progresses in stages; if disease is diagnosed early, permanent joint deterioration may be prevented.
   1. The synovium becomes thickened and inflamed, and fluid accumulates in the joint space; this causes a pannus to form.
   2. The pannus tissue erodes the cartilage and destroys the joint.
B. Exacerbations and remissions occur; condition tends to be progressive with each exacerbation.
C. Condition is a problem of the connective tissue; inflammatory response may occur in organs throughout the body (heart, lungs, blood vessels, muscles).

Assessment

A. Risk factors/etiology.
   1. Gender: significantly increased incidence in women.
   2. May occur at any age including childhood; peak incidence occurs between 20 and 45 years of age.
   3. Genetic predisposition.
B. Clinical manifestations.
   1. Symmetrical joint involvement (hands and feet).
      a. Warm, tender, red, painful joints; primarily affects small joints, wrists, elbows, shoulders.
      b. Decrease in ROM.
      c. Decrease in strength.
      d. Stiffness and pain are worse in the morning and decrease during the day with moderate activity.
   2. Subcutaneous nodules over bony prominences.
      a. Nodules are painless; frequently occur on the elbows.
      b. May be present for weeks to months.
   3. Systemic effects.
      a. Vasculitis.
      b. Pulmonary fibrosis.
      c. Pericarditis.
      d. Sjögren's syndrome (dry eyes, etc.).
   4. Chronic deformities develop, most often in the hands.
   5. Exacerbation of symptoms may be associated with physical or emotional stress.
C. Diagnostics (see Appendix 21-1).

Treatment

A. Disease-modifying antirheumatic drugs (DMARDs) (see Appendix 21-2).
B. NSAIDs.
   1. Salicylate (aspirin).
   2. Ibuprofen, naproxen.
C. Corticosteroids (see Appendix 6-7).
D. Methotrexate (see Appendix 8-1).
E. Heat and/or cold applications.
F. Assistive devices to preserve joints and prevent deformity.
G. Physical and rehabilitative therapy.
H. Surgery: joint replacements.

Complications

A. Musculoskeletal.
   1. Severe joint deformity, flexion contracture.
   2. Diffuse skeletal demineralization.
   3. Stress fractures.
B. Systemic involvement.

Nursing Interventions

Goal: To relieve pain and preserve joint mobility and muscle strength (see Box 21-4).
A. Use warm compresses to promote relaxation and to decrease stiffness; use cold compresses to decrease inflammation.
B. If heat increases pain, cold compresses may be beneficial during an acute episode.
C. Acutely inflamed joints should be immobilized in a device that maintains a functional position.
D. Position client to maintain correct body alignment and prevent contractures, especially flexion contractures.

> **ALERT** Assess client for complications of immobility, intervene appropriately when providing care.

E. Immobility can increase the pain; ROM exercises and weight bearing may help decrease pain.
F. Antiinflammatory medications should be taken before activity and with meals or food to decrease gastric upset.
G. If client is taking steroids, he or she should wear a medical identification tag.
Goal: To assist client to prevent joint deformity, preserve joint function, and reduce inflammation and pain.
A. Regularly scheduled rest periods (excessive fatigue is a problem); balance activities with rest.
B. Protect joints (Box 21-4).
   1. Maintain functional joint alignment; avoid positions that precipitate joint contraction (sitting too long with knees bent).
   2. Warm moist or cold compresses to relieve pain and muscle spasms.
   3. Acutely inflamed joints may be splinted; splint should be removed periodically and gentle ROM exercises performed.
   4. Use large muscle groups; avoid repetitive movement of smaller joints.
C. Demonstrate ability to carry out individual exercise program.
D. Identify medications that are effective in relieving pain.
E. Chronic pain may lead to feelings of powerlessness and make the client more susceptible to false advertising regarding claims of cure and relief of chronic pain.
F. Encourage client to be independent in activities of daily living (ADLs) as long as possible.

Home Care

A. Encourage client to ventilate feelings regarding chronic progression of the disease state.
B. Evaluate family support system; help family to identify measures to assist client.

C. Modify home routine to decrease stress on joints: ADLs, dressing, etc.

D. Identify measures to assist client to maintain self-esteem: What activities can client continue to participate in? Focus on what client *can* do.

E. Assist client to set realistic goals.

F. Identify available community resources.

> **ALERT** Determine client's ability to perform self-care; assist family to manage care of client with long-term care needs.

Osteoarthritis (Degenerative Joint Disease)

Osteoarthritis is a progressive, nonsystemic, noninflammatory disease that causes a progressive degeneration of synovial joints of weight-bearing long bones.

A. Primarily associated with aging; may also be caused by musculoskeletal injury or conditions that cause repetitive damage to joints.

B. The cartilage at the ends of the long bones deteriorates and leaves the ends of the bones rubbing together; this produces a painful, swollen joint.

Assessment

A. Etiology/predisposing factors.
   1. Excessive use of a specific joint: knees in athletes, feet in dancers, etc.
   2. The hips are more commonly affected in men; in women, the hands are more commonly affected.
   3. Obesity: joints that carry excess weight are more likely to degenerate earlier.
   4. Frequently observed in older adults.

B. Clinical manifestations.
   1. Joints involved.
      a. Primarily involves weight-bearing joints; occurs as a result of mechanical stress.
      b. May also involve joints in the fingers and the vertebral column.
   2. Symptoms occurring in the joint.
      a. Pain, swelling, tenderness.
      b. Crepitation: a grating sound or feeling with movement.
      c. Instability, stiffness, and immobility.
   3. Pain occurs on motion and with weight bearing.
   4. Pain increases in severity with activity.
   5. Heberden's nodes: bony nodules on the distal finger joints.

C. Diagnostics (see Appendix 21-1).
   1. No specific lab test to confirm; diagnosis is made primarily on the basis of symptoms and history.

Treatment

A. Medications for pain relief: salicylates (aspirin), acetaminophen (Tylenol), NSAIDs (ibuprofen [Motrin]); COX-2 inhibitors (Celebrex).
   1. Intraarticular injection of corticosteroids, methotrexate, disease-modifying antirheumatic drugs, and gold compounds.

B. Activity balanced with adequate rest.

C. Weight reduction, if appropriate.

D. Physical therapy and exercise.

E. Surgical intervention with joint replacement.

Nursing Interventions

Goal: To relieve pain, prevent further stress on the joint, and maintain function.

A. Acutely inflamed joint should be immobilized with splint or brace.

B. Plan ADLs to prevent stress on involved joints and provide adequate rest periods.

C. Heat compresses can be used for relief of pain; cold compresses may be used if joint is inflamed.

D. It is very important to maintain regular exercise program; decrease activity in acutely inflamed, painful joints.

> **NURSING PRIORITY** More than 4000 mg daily of acetaminophen increase client risk for liver damage.

Goal: To help client understand measures to maintain health (see Box 21-4).

A. Identify activities requiring increased stress on involved joints.

B. Maintain regular exercise program (e.g., walking, swimming) to promote muscle strength and joint mobility.

C. Encourage independence in ADLs.

Goal: To maintain psychologic equilibrium and promote positive self-esteem.

 Juvenile Idiopathic Arthritis (Juvenile Rheumatoid Arthritis)

Juvenile idiopathic arthritis (JIA) is a new name for chronic childhood arthritis, previously called juvenile rheumatoid arthritis (JRA). It is characterized as a chronic inflammatory problem of connective tissue; it involves the synovial joints.

A. Synovium becomes thick and edematous; granulation tissue turns to scar tissue, and the joint is destroyed.

B. Reason for name change to JIA is due to the minimally applicable reference of "rheumatoid" in childhood arthritis, which is relevant only in a small number of affected children.

Assessment

A. Risk factors/etiology.
   1. Possibly autoimmune in origin.
   2. Peak onset between 1 and 3 years and 8 and 10 years of age.

B. Clinical manifestations.
   1. Morning stiffness.
   2. May have multiple joint involvement, both large and small joints.
   3. Joints may be tender and painful to touch or may be relatively free of pain.
   4. Fever, rash, and development of uveitis (inflammation of the iris and ciliary body of the eye).

C. Diagnostics: diagnosis is made by exclusion of other diseases; presence of antinuclear antibodies.

Treatment

A. Medications.
   1. NSAIDs, methotrexate.
   2. Tumor necrosis factor inhibitors.
   3. Corticosteroids in severe cases.
B. Physical therapy.
C. Moist heat is used to reduce stiffness and relieve pain.
D. Exercise, especially water exercises.

Complications

Complications include severe hip disease and loss of vision from iridocyclitis.

Nursing Interventions

Child is usually cared for at home except during severe exacerbations.

Goal: To decrease pain and promote joint mobility.
A. Moist heat to relieve joint stiffness and pain.
B. Therapeutic exercises incorporated into play activities.
C. Maintain good body alignment when child is at rest; prevent flexion contractures of affected joints.
D. Avoid overexercising painful joints.

Goal: To help child maintain normal growth and development patterns and to promote self-esteem.
A. Well-balanced diet without excessive weight gain.
B. Schedule regular exercise program appropriate to developmental level.
C. Encourage independence; allow child to participate in planning care.
D. Encourage school attendance and socialization with peers.

Gout

Gout is an arthritic condition resulting from a defect in the metabolism of uric acid (hyperuricemia).
A. Uric acid is the end product of purine metabolism.
B. Hyperuricemia may also occur in individuals receiving chemotherapy (secondary gout).

Assessment

A. Risk factors/etiology.
   1. Increased incidence in middle-aged men and with diets high in purine-rich food.
   2. Obesity, hypertension, diuretic use, excessive alcohol consumption.
B. Clinical manifestations.
   1. Intense pain and inflammation of one or more small joints, especially those in the large toe.
   2. Characterized by remissions and exacerbations of acute joint pain.
   3. Onset is generally rapid with swollen, inflamed, painful joints.
   4. Presence of tophi or uric acid crystals in the area around the large toe and the outer ear.
   5. Tophi may be present in subcutaneous tissue.
C. Diagnostics: persistent hyperuricemia: level greater than 6 mg/dL.

Treatment

A. Medications.
   1. Antigout (see Appendix 21-2).
   2. NSAIDs for pain and also to assist in preventing attacks.
B. Decrease amount of purine in diet (see Chapter 2).

Complications

A. Uric acid kidney stones.
B. Secondary osteoarthritis.

Nursing Interventions

Goal: To prevent acute attack, promote comfort, and maintain joint mobility.
A. Medications should be given early in the attack to decrease the severity of the attack.
B. Protect affected joint: immobilize, no weight bearing.
C. Cold packs may decrease pain.
D. Decreased amount of purine in diet.
E. Encourage high fluid intake to increase excretion of uric acid and to prevent the development of uric acid stones.
F. Assist client to identify activities and aspects of lifestyle that precipitate attacks.
   1. Dietary habits (decrease purine intake).
   2. Decrease alcohol consumption.

Appendix 21-1 DIAGNOSTIC STUDIES

Serum Diagnostics

Rheumatoid factor (RF): Used to determine presence of autoantibodies (rheumatoid factor) found in clients with connective tissue disease; if antibody is present, it is suggestive of rheumatoid arthritis; the higher the antibody titer, the greater the degree of inflammation.

Antinuclear antibody (ANA): Measures the presence of antibodies that destroy the nucleus of body tissue cells (i.e., those seen in connective tissue diseases); a positive test result is associated with systemic lupus erythematosus.

Complement: Essential body protein to measure immune and inflammatory reactions; usually depleted in rheumatoid arthritis.

Alkaline phosphatase: Enzyme produced by osteoblasts; elevated levels found in osteoporosis, healing fractures, bone cancer, osteomalacia.

Aldolase: Elevated levels in muscular dystrophy.

Creatine kinase (CK): Elevated levels found in muscular dystrophy and traumatic skeletal muscle injury.

Invasive Diagnostics

Arthroscopy: Involves the use of an arthroscope inserted into a joint for visualization of the joint structure; preferably, procedure is conducted in the operating room with strict asepsis and performed with either local or general anesthesia; frequently used to diagnose structural abnormalities of the knee.

Nursing Implications
1. Perform preoperative nursing interventions, as appropriate with the level of anesthesia to be used.
2. After procedure, wound is covered with a sterile dressing.
3. A compression bandage may be applied for 24 hours after the test.
4. Teach client symptoms of vascular compromise, mobility restrictions, and sterile dressing change procedure.
5. Walking is permitted; however, excessive exercise should be avoided for a few days.
6. Teach the client signs of infection (increased temperature, local inflammation at site).

Arthrocentesis: Incision of a joint capsule to obtain samples of synovial fluid; local anesthesia is induced, and aseptic preparation is done before fluid aspiration. Synovial fluid is examined for infection and bleeding into the joint and to confirm specific types of arthritis.

Nursing Implications
1. Explain procedure to client.
2. May be done at bedside or in an examination room.
3. Compression dressing is usually applied, and joint is rested for several hours after test.
4. Observe dressing for leakage of blood or fluid.
5. Assess the puncture site for evidence of infection.

Myelogram and CT scan: Used to determine status of vertebral disk. See Appendix 20-1.

Bone biopsy: May be performed in client's room or in a treatment room. After satisfactory local anesthesia is achieved, a long needle is inserted into the bone, or a small incision is made to obtain bone tissue.

Nursing Implications
1. Plan for analgesic to be administered before procedure.
2. If an incision was made, maintain a pressure dressing over the site.
3. Extremity is elevated to decrease edema and may be immobilized for about 12 to 24 hours.
4. Assess the puncture site or incision for evidence of infection.

Electromyelogram (EMG): Evaluates the electric potential of the muscle with muscle contraction. Small needles are inserted into the muscle and recording of electrical activity is performed.

Nursing Implications
1. Explain to client that there is discomfort with procedure.
2. No stimulants (caffeine) or sedatives 24 hours before the procedure.

Noninvasive Diagnostics

X-ray films: The most common diagnostic procedure to determine musculoskeletal problems.
1. Identify musculoskeletal problems.
2. Determine progress of disease or condition.
3. Evaluate effectiveness of treatment.

Bone scan: Radioisotopes may be injected intravenously, and bone is scanned to determine where the isotopes are "taken up." May be used to determine presence of malignancies, arthritis, and osteoporosis. No special precautions before or after test; need to encourage fluid intake to increase excretion of dye.

Computerized axial tomography (CAT scan): See Appendix 20-1.

Magnetic resonance imaging (MRI): See Appendix 20-1.

Appendix 21-2   MEDICATIONS

MEDICATIONS	SIDE EFFECTS	NURSING IMPLICATIONS
Antigout Agents Decrease the plasma uric acid levels either by inhibiting the synthesis of uric acid or increasing the excretion of uric acid.		
Colchicine: PO	Nausea, vomiting, diarrhea Toxic effects: bone marrow depression	1. Take medication at earliest indication of impending gout attack. 2. Take medication with food. 3. Promote high fluid intake to promote uric acid excretion. 4. In acute attack, administer 1 tablet every hour until symptoms subside, until GI problems occur, or until a total of 8 mg has been taken.
Allopurinol **(Zyloprim)**: PO	Rash, GI distress, fever, headache	1. Administer with food to decrease gastric upset. 2. Discontinue medication if rash occurs. 3. Use with caution in clients with renal insufficiency. 4. May be used to decrease serum uric acid levels in clients receiving chemotherapy.
Probenecid **(Benemid)**: PO	GI disturbances, headache, skin rash, fever	1. Urate tophi deposits should decrease in size with therapy. 2. Give with food.
Skeletal Muscle Relaxants Relax skeletal muscle by depressing synaptic pathways in the spinal cord.		
Methocarbamol **(Robaxin)**: PO, IM, IV Cyclobenzaprine **(Flexeril)**: PO Carisoprodol **(Soma)**: PO Baclofen **(Lioresal)**: PO	Drowsiness, dizziness, GI upset, rash, blurred vision Drowsiness, dizziness, headache, GI upset, orthostatic hypotension Drowsiness, weakness, fatigue, confusion	1. Used for muscle spasms associated with MS and spinal cord injury. 2. Caution clients to avoid activities that require mental alertness for safety (driving, using power tools, etc.). 3. Evaluate client for postural hypotension. 4. Advise client to avoid CNS depressants (e.g., alcohol, opioids, antihistamines). 5. Administer with meals to decrease GI distress.
Dantrolene **(Dantrium)**: PO, IV	Hepatotoxicity, muscle weakness, drowsiness	1. Teach clients symptoms of liver dysfunction. 2. Acts directly to relax skeletal muscle.
Calcium Medications Hormones that enhance bone density by preventing the reabsorption of calcium in bone and kidneys.		
Calcitonin-salmon **(Calcimar, Miacalcin)**: subQ, IM, nasal spray	GI upset, local inflammation at injection site, flushing	1. Monitor levels of serum calcium. 2. Treatment of established postmenopausal osteoporosis.
Bisphosphonates—alendronate **(Fosamax)**, ibandronate, **(Boniva)**: PO, nasal spray	Esophagitis, GI flushing, rash, musculoskeletal pain, fever, chills, jaw pain	1. Have client swallow tablet whole; it should not be chewed. 2. Take in morning on an empty stomach with large glass of water (6 to 8 oz) and wait at least 30 minutes before eating or lying down. 3. Make sure client has adequate intake of vitamin D. 4. Used for prevention and treatment of postmenopausal osteoporosis. 5. Client should report any signs or symptoms of gastric reflux or pain.

MEDICATIONS	SIDE EFFECTS	NURSING IMPLICATIONS
Corticosteroids See Appendix 6-7.		

Nonsteroidal Antiinflammatory Medications (NSAIDs) See Appendix 3-3.

Disease-Modifying Antirheumatic Drugs (DMARDs) Antimetabolite, antirheumatic, and antimalarial drugs that act to decrease inflammation.

MEDICATIONS	SIDE EFFECTS	NURSING IMPLICATIONS
Methotrexate **(Rheumatrex)**	Toxic effects: hepatotoxicity, bone marrow depression Nausea, vomiting, stomatitis	1. Caution women of childbearing age to avoid pregnancy. 2. Monitor CBC regularly. 3. Avoid alcohol during therapy. 4. Administer with food.
Hydroxychloroquine **(Plaquenil)**	Toxic effects: retinopathy, skeletal muscle myopathy or neuropathy Headache, anorexia, dizziness	1. Recommend eye exams every 3 months. 2. Not recommended for children. 3. Therapeutic effect may take 3 to 6 months.
Leflunomide **(Arava)**	Toxic effects: hepatotoxicity, diarrhea, teratogenesis	1. Not recommended for women who may become pregnant. 2. May slow the progression of joint damage caused by rheumatoid arthritis and improves physical function.

Biological Therapy Agents that bind TNF to decrease inflammatory and immune responses; used in cases of severe arthritis.

MEDICATIONS	SIDE EFFECTS	NURSING IMPLICATIONS
Etanercept **(Enbrel):** subQ	Increased risk for infections, injection site reactions, heart failure, headache, nausea, dizziness	1. Use cautiously in clients with heart disease. 2. Rotate injection sites at least 1 inch apart. 3. Advise clients that injection site reaction generally decreases with continued therapy. 4. Do not administer to clients with chronic or localized infections. 5. Have client report signs of infection, bruising, or bleeding.
Infliximab **(Remicade):** IV Adalimumab **(Humira):** subQ	Increased risk for opportunistic infections, abdominal pain, nausea/vomiting, headache, rash, injection site reactions	1. Avoid in clients with heart disease. 2. Assess clients for infections; administer TB skin test and chest x-ray before starting medication. 3. Rotate injection sites at least 1 inch apart. 4. Perform periodic CBCs to monitor for blood dyscrasias.

CBC, Complete blood count; *CHF,* congestive heart failure; *CNS,* central nervous system; *GI,* gastrointestinal; *IV,* intravenous; *PO,* by mouth (orally); *subQ,* subcutaneous; *TNF,* tumor necrosis factor.

Appendix 21-3 ASSISTIVE DEVICES FOR IMMOBILITY

Crutches

Measuring a Client (Figure 21-6)

- Measurement may be taken with client supine or standing.
- Supine: measure the distance from the client's axilla to a point 6 inches lateral to the heel.
- Standing: measure the distance from the client's axilla to a point 4 to 6 inches to the side and 4 to 6 inches in front of the foot.
- Adjust hand bars so that client's elbows are flexed approximately 30 degrees.

3 finger widths
(1-2 in., 2.5-5 cm)

30 degrees flexion

6 in.

6 in.

FIGURE 21-6 Crutch measurement. (From Harkreader H, Hogan MA, Thobaben M: *Fundamentals of nursing: caring and clinical judgment,* ed 3, Philadelphia, 2007, Saunders.)

- If client was measured while supine, assist client to stand with crutches. Check the distance between client's axilla and arm pieces. You should be able to put two of your fingers between client's axilla and the crutch bar.

Four-Point Alternate Gait

- The four-point alternate gait is used by clients who can bear partial weight on both feet—for example, clients with arthritis or cerebral palsy. It is a particularly safe gait, in that there are three points of support on the floor at all times.
- This gait provides a normal walking pattern and makes some use of the muscles of the lower extremities.

Three-Point Alternate Gait

- For the three-point alternate gait, the client must be able to bear the total body weight on one foot; the affected foot or leg is either partially or totally non-weight-bearing.
- In this gait both crutches are moved forward together with the affected leg while the weight is being borne by the client's hands on the crutches. The unaffected leg is then advanced forward.

Crutch Walking

- Up stairs: Unaffected leg moves up first, followed by the crutches and the affected leg.
- Down stairs: Crutches and affected leg move down first, body weight is transferred to the crutches, and the unaffected leg is moved down.

ALERT Assess client's use of assistive devices; evaluate correct use; assist client to ambulate with an assistive device.

Canes

- The cane is used on the side opposite the affected leg.
- The cane and the affected leg move together.

Walkers

- Lift the walker and place it approximately 2 feet in front.
- Gain balance before moving walker forward again; balance provides stability and equal weight bearing.

Appendix 21-4 AMPUTATIONS

* Removal of part of a body, usually an extremity at various anatomic locations.

Indications for Amputation

1. Peripheral vascular disease, especially vascular disease of lower extremities.
2. Severe trauma.
3. Acute chronic infection.
4. Malignant tumors.

Nursing Implications

1. Prevent further loss of circulation to the extremity.
2. Promote psychologic stability.
3. Promote comfort.
4. Promote optimum level of mobility.

Postoperative Care

ALERT Identify and prevent complications of immobility; use positioning to prevent contractures; provide support for client with unexpected alteration in body image; assist client to ambulate and move with assistive devices; promote wound healing; assist client with use of prosthesis.

Residual Limb Wound Care

1. The residual limb may be elevated for approximately 24 to 48 hours; after that time, keep the joint immediately above the residual limb in an extended position. Flexion contracture hinders use of prosthesis.
2. Recognize the difference between phantom limb pain (PLP) and residual limb pain (RLP). Opioid analgesics are not as effective for PLP as for RLP.
3. Phantom limb pain is very real to the client. Handle residual limb carefully when assessing site or changing dressing.
4. Evaluate residual limb for bleeding and healing.
5. A rigid compression dressing may be applied to prevent injury and to decrease swelling. Controlling the edema will enhance healing and promote comfort. Changes of the rigid dressing are necessary; as the residual limb heals, it also shrinks. Jobst air splint, a plastic inflatable device, is used and inflated to 20 mm Hg for 22 of every 24 hours.
6. If the client is not fitted with a rigid compression dressing, the residual limb will be shaped with a compression bandage. Ace bandage elastic wrapping is often used for compression of this type.
7. Discourage a semi-Fowler's position in the client with above-the-knee amputation; this position encourages flexion contraction at the hip.

Residual Limb Care after Wound Has Healed

1. Continually assess for skin breakdown; visually inspect the residual limb for redness, abrasions, or blistering.
2. The residual limb should be washed daily, carefully rinsed, and dried. Soap and moisture contribute to skin breakdown.
3. Do not apply anything to the residual limb (alcohol increases skin dryness and cracking; lotions keep skin soft and hinder use of prosthesis).
4. Client should put the prosthesis on when he or she gets up and should wear it all day. The residual limb tends to swell if the prosthesis is not applied. The more the client wears the prosthesis, the less swelling will be experienced.

Study Questions Musculoskeletal System

More questions on companion CD!
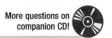

1. After a lumbar laminectomy, a client continues to complain of the same low back pain that he had before surgery. The nurse knows that this finding is caused by what problem?
   1 Failure of the surgeon to remove the client's herniated disk
   2 Swelling in the operative area that compresses adjacent structures
   3 Twisting of the client's spine when he turns from side to side
   4 Limitation of movement resulting from spinal fusion

2. The nurse is assessing a client who had a fractured femur repaired with an external fixator device. Which assessment findings would cause the nurse concern regarding the development of compartmental syndrome? Select all that apply.
   _____ 1 Decrease in pulse rate in affected leg
   _____ 2 Paresthesia distal to area of injury
   _____ 3 Toes on affected leg cool to touch and edematous
   _____ 4 Complaints that pins are hurting
   _____ 5 Complaints of leg pain unrelieved by analgesics or repositioning
   _____ 6 Client angry and calling loudly to the nurse every 10 minutes

3. In taking the health history of a client with severe painful osteoarthritis, the nurse would expect the client to report which of the following?
   1 A gradual onset of the disease, with involvement of weight-bearing joints
   2 A sudden onset of the disease, with involvement of all joints
   3 No complaints of morning stiffness
   4 Joint pain that is not affected by exercise

4. A client has a fractured hip and is currently in Buck's traction before surgery. How is the counterattraction in Buck's traction achieved?
   1 By applying a 10-pound counterweight at the knee
   2 By placing shock blocks under the head of the bed
   3 By elevating the knee gatch and elevating the head of the bed about 30 degrees
   4 By elevating the foot of the bed frame and allowing the weights to hang freely

5. The postoperative nursing care plan for a client who has had a right leg amputation includes:
   1 Applying ice packs to the residual limb for 72 hours
   2 Having the client lie on his or her abdomen for 30 minutes 3-4 times/day
   3 Wrapping the residual limb with Ace bandages from proximal to distal ends
   4 Managing client's pain with antiinflammatory medications.

6. A client has a long leg plaster cast applied. What nursing actions are implemented while the cast is still wet?
   1 Use only the fingertips when moving the cast.
   2 Keep the client and cast covered with blankets.
   3 Support the cast on plastic-covered pillows.
   4 Place a heat lamp directly over the cast.

7. A client is being treated with Buck's traction. What are important nursing interventions for this client?
   1 Remove the traction boot every 6 hours to provide skin care.
   2 Check and clean the pin sites at least three times daily.
   3 Check the area around the hip where the traction is applied.
   4 Verify that weights are in the amounts ordered and are hanging freely.

8. For a client with severe painful osteoarthritis, a regimen of heat, massage, and exercise will:
   1 Help relax muscles and relieve pain and stiffness.
   2 Restore range of motion previously lost.
   3 Prevent the inflammatory process.
   4 Help the client cope with pain effectively.

9. A client is confined to bed with a fracture of the left femur. He begins receiving subcutaneous heparin injections. What is the purpose of this medication?
   1 To prevent thrombophlebitis and pulmonary emboli associated with immobility
   2 To promote vascular perfusion by preventing formation of microemboli in the left leg
   3 To prevent venous stasis, which promotes vascular complications associated with immobility
   4 To decrease the incidence of fat emboli associated with long bone fractures

10. What is important assessment information to obtain from a client with a fractured hip?
   1 Circulation and sensation distal to the fracture
   2 Amount of swelling around the fracture site
   3 Degree of bone healing that has occurred
   4 Amount of pain that the fracture and healing are causing

11. What evaluation is important in the preoperative nursing assessment of a client with a severely herniated lumbar disk?
   1 Movement and sensation in the lower extremities
   2 Leg pain that radiates to both lower extremities
   3 Reflexes in the upper extremities
   4 Pupillary reaction to light

Answers and rationales to these questions are in the section at the end of the book titled Chapter Study Questions: Answers and Rationales.

CHAPTER TWENTY-TWO

Reproductive System

PHYSIOLOGY OF THE REPRODUCTIVE SYSTEM

Male Reproductive System

A. External genitalia.

B. Internal genitalia.
 1. Testes (gonads): spermatogenesis occurs in seminiferous tubules, and testosterone is produced by the interstitial cells.
 2. Epididymis: a tubular, coiled segment of the spermatic duct that stores spermatozoa until they are mature and then transports sperm from the testis to the vas deferens.

C. Accessory glands.
 1. Seminal vesicles: sac-like structures posterior to the prostate that secrete nearly one-third of the volume of semen; also prostaglandin.
 2. Prostate gland: produces a slightly alkalotic substance that contains high levels of acid phosphatase and serves as the vehicle for spermatozoa.

D. Semen.
 1. Male ejaculate composed of spermatozoa (2% to 5%) and seminal plasma.
 2. Alkaline pH: 7.2 to 7.4.
 3. Average volume of ejaculate: 2.5 to 4 mL; may vary from 1 to 10 mL; repeated ejaculation leads to decreased volume.
 4. Sterility: sperm count less than 20 million per milliliter (normal sperm count = 100 million per milliliter).
 5. Storage of sperm: varies from a period of several hours to 40 days, depending primarily on the frequency of ejaculation.

Female Reproductive System

A. External genitalia.
 1. Labia majora: contain an extensive venous blood supply, which leads frequently to edema and varicosities in pregnancy.
 2. Periurethral (Skene) glands: often the site of gonorrheal infection.

B. Internal genitalia.
 1. Vagina: a thin-walled, muscular membranous canal that connects the external genitalia with the center of the pelvis.
  a. The pH is acidic and is maintained by a relationship between lactic acid-producing Döderlein's bacilli (lactobacilli) and the vaginal content.
  b. Bacilli break down vaginal epithelial cells; disruption of this cycle (antibiotic therapy, douching, vaginal sprays, etc.) may destroy the normal self-cleansing action of the vagina.
 2. Cervix: protrudes into the vagina.
  a. Provides an alkaline environment to shelter sperm from the acidic vagina.
  b. Cervical mucus pH increases (alkaline) and becomes clear and more viscous at ovulation, similar to egg white consistency.
 3. Uterus: a hollow, pear-shaped, muscular pelvic organ; located between the bladder and the rectum.
  a. Uterine wall: endometrium is the inner mucosal lining; undergoes cyclic changes as a result of hormonal levels.
  b. Uterine ligaments: maintain upright position of uterus in pelvic cavity.
 4. Fallopian tubes: attached to the upper, outer section of the uterus.
  a. Distal tubules are fimbriated (fringed) and bell shaped.
  b. By their peristaltic and ciliary action, they move the ovum (egg) into the uterine cavity.
 5. Ovaries: located behind and below the fallopian tubes, produce ova, estrogen, and progesterone.

C. Breasts: divided into lobes and lobules arranged in a radial pattern, separated by fibrous tissue called Cooper's ligaments.

D. Menstrual cycle (Figure 22-1).
 1. The cyclical hormonal changes occurring from menarche to menopause.
 2. Variation in menstrual cycle length is always due to variation in the proliferation phase—once ovulation occurs, the secretory phase is 14 days in length.
 3. Fertilization: generally occurs in the outer third of the fallopian tube; a single ejaculation deposits 2.5 to 4.0 mL of semen, containing approximately 200 to 400 million spermatozoa.
 4. Implantation: The zygote (fertilized ovum) is propelled by ciliary action of the fallopian tube into the

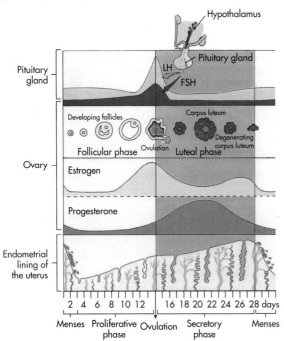

FIGURE 22-1 Female reproductive cycle. (From Lewis SL et al: *Medical-surgical nursing: assessment and management of clinical problems*, ed 7, St. Louis, 2007, Mosby.)

uterine cavity; implants in the endometrium about 7 to 10 days after fertilization.

System Assessment

A. External assessment.
   1. Assess vulvar area for discharge, erythema, swelling, or growths.
   2. Assess penis for growths, masses, erosions, ulcers, or vesicles.
   3. Inspect breasts for nipple inversion, retraction, secretions, nodules, lumps, color changes, erythema or masses.
   4. Determine whether there is any abdominal pain or tenderness on palpation.
B. Internal assessment.
   1. Pelvic examination.
      a. Collection of cells from the cervix for a Papanicolaou (Pap) smear.
      b. Bimanual examination.
   2. Digital rectal examination.
      a. To evaluate prostate for size, shape, pain, or tenderness.
      b. Useful in female pelvic exams for assessing fistulas, masses and anatomy.
C. History.
   1. Menstrual history.
      a. Age at onset.
      b. Last menstrual period.
      c. Duration of cycle, amount of flow, number of cycles per year, and use of birth control methods.
   2. Obstetrical history.

3. Urinary system.
   a. Pattern of voiding: dysuria, urgency, nocturia, frequency.
   b. Difficulty starting stream, stopping stream, or changing the force of stream; a feeling of incomplete emptying of bladder.
   c. Hematuria, incontinence, color, odor.
4. Sexual function.
   a. Ability to achieve erection and ejaculation.
   b. Problems with intercourse.
   c. Bleeding after intercourse.
   d. Exposure to sexually transmitted diseases (STDs).
   e. Change in sex drive, libido.
   f. Adequate lubrication for sexual activity.

DISORDERS OF THE REPRODUCTIVE SYSTEM

Prostate Disorders

A. Benign prostatic hypertrophy (BPH) or hyperplasia: enlargement of prostate gland tissue.
B. Cancer of the prostate: a malignancy of the prostate gland, which is a hormone-dependent adenocarcinoma; growth of the tumor is usually related to the presence of androgen hormone.

Assessment

A. Risk factors/etiology.
   1. BPH: very common in men older than 50 years.
   2. Prostatic carcinoma: rarely found in men younger than 60 years; usually found in the posterior lobe of the prostate gland.
B. Clinical manifestations.

ALERT Relate client's symptoms to adverse reactions of medication. Carefully assess the client with BPH in regard to anticholinergic medications (atropine) that cause urinary retention as a side effect.

   1. Common to both disorders.
      a. Bladder outlet obstruction.
         (1) Urinary hesitancy, frequency, urgency, and dribbling.
         (2) Nocturia, hematuria, urinary retention, and a sensation of incomplete emptying of the bladder.
         (3) Urinary retention may cause overflow urinary incontinence and dribbling after voiding.
      b. Acute retention may cause hydroureter and pressure in the kidney.
      c. Increased incidence of urinary tract infection due to residual urine.
   2. Prostatic cancer.
      a. Tumor grows slowly and is confined to capsule; therefore prostate may appear normal, thus delaying the diagnosis.
      b. On digital rectal exam, unilateral prostatic enlargement; prostate is described as "stony hard" and fixed.

c. Obstruction is rare unless BPH is also present.

d. Pain in the hip or back may be presenting symptom as a result of metastasis.

C. Diagnostics.

1. Digital rectal examination.

2. Cystoscopy and bladder scan.

3. Urinalysis with culture and sensitivity.

4. Transrectal and/or transabdominal ultrasound.

5. Rule out or diagnose cancer.

　　a. Prostate-specific antigen (normal PSA 0-4 mcg/L) for cancer.

　　b. Tumor markers for diagnosis, staging, and monitoring progress.

　　c. Needle biopsy of prostate.

Treatment

A. Medical.

1. BPH: finasteride (Proscar) and alpha adrenergic blockers to shrink prostatic tissue.

2. Radiation, hormonal therapy, and chemotherapy for malignancy.

B. Surgical: size of prostate and general health dictate the type of surgery.

1. Transurethral resection of the prostate (TURP): removal of prostatic tissue via a resectoscope, which is passed through the urethra (Figure 22-2).

2. Transurethral incision of the prostate (TUIP): making transurethral slits or incisions into prostate to relieve obstruction; effective with minimally enlarged prostate (BPH).

3. Prostatectomy: removal of the prostate via suprapubic, retropubic, or perineal approach; may be done by incision or laproscopically; most often for removal of malignancy.

4. Transurethral microwave therapy (TUMT) and transurethral needle ablation (TUNA): microwaves are delivered directly to the prostate; heat causes necrosis of tissue; both procedures are done on an outpatient basis.

5. Internal radiation therapy (brachytherapy) involves the placement of tiny radioactive "seeds" into the prostate for treatment of cancer.

6. Hormone therapy (anti-androgen medications—Lupron): depriving the cancer cells of testosterone may help slow the growth of prostatic cancer.

7. Cryotherapy (cryoablation): liquid nitrogen is applied to the prostate via a transrectal ultrasound probe; dead cells are absorbed by the body.

Complications

A. BPH.

1. Preoperative.

　　a. Urinary tract infection (UTI).

　　b. Rupture of overstretched blood vessels in the bladder and hematuria.

　　c. Hydroureter (distention of the ureter) and hydronephrosis (enlargement of kidney caused by postrenal obstruction) with resultant renal failure.

2. Postoperative.

　　a. Hemorrhage: especially in the first 24 hours.

　　b. Urinary incontinence.

　　c. Bladder spasms.

　　d. Retrograde ejaculation: semen passed into the bladder rather than out through the penis.

　　e. Infection.

B. Prostatic cancer.

1. Preoperative.

　　a. Complications are similar to BPH.

　　b. Cancer may spread via the perineal lymphatic system to the regional lymph nodes; from the veins of the prostate, it may metastasize to the pelvic bones, bladder, lungs, and liver.

2. Postoperative.

　　a. Increased problems with deep venous thrombosis caused by lithotomy position during open perineal resection.

　　b. Change in sexual functioning: impotence and failure to ejaculate.

　　c. Incontinence assessment.

Nursing Interventions

Goal: To promote elimination, to treat UTI, and to provide client education (Box 22-1).

A. Evaluate adequacy of voiding and presence of urinary retention and infection.

B. Teach client to avoid bladder distension, which results in loss of muscle tone.

1. Do not postpone the urge to void; it is important to prevent overdistention of the bladder, which further complicates the problem.

2. Avoid drinking a large amount of fluid in a short period of time.

3. Avoid alcohol because of the diuretic effect.

C. Encourage annual digital rectal examination of the prostate for all men older than 40 years.

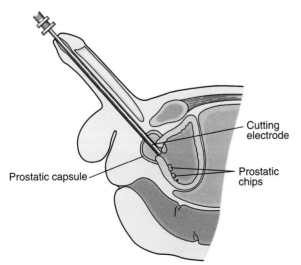

FIGURE 22-2 Transurethral resection of the prostate. (From Monahan FD et al: *Medical-surgical nursing: health and illness perspectives*, ed 8, St. Louis, 2007, Mosby.)

Cutting electrode

Prostatic capsule

Prostatic chips

D. Examination is recommended every 6 months for clients who have BPH or who have had a prostatectomy.

> **❗ NURSING PRIORITY** Assess all male clients older than 50 years for symptoms of BPH. BPH occurs in 80% of men older than 80 years.

Goal: To maintain closed irrigation after surgery in the client who has undergone TURP or suprapubic prostatectomy (Figure 22-3).

A. Continuous bladder irrigation (CBI) with sterile, antibacterial, isotonic irrigating solution (Murphy drip, closed bladder irrigation).

   1. Closed bladder irrigation is done with a triple-lumen catheter: one lumen for inflating the balloon (30 to 50 mL of water), one for maintaining outflow of urine, and one for the instillation of the continuous irrigating solution.

Box 22-1   OLDER ADULT CARE FOCUS

Benign Prostatic Hypertrophy

General

- All men over 50 years of age should be assessed for urinary retention and adequacy of bladder emptying.
- Increased problem with urinary stasis; increased straining to urinate; increased incidence of infections.

After Surgery

- Closely evaluate for presence of infection, especially UTI, respiratory.
- Assess fluid balance; confusion and agitation may be symptoms of fluid overload.
- Help the client ambulate as soon as possible—increased risk for pooling of blood in pelvic cavity and pulmonary emboli from immobility.
- Client is at increased risk for falls.
- Determine psychologic response to physical stress (confusion, disorientation); orient to surroundings frequently.

---

2. Provides continuous irrigation to prevent infection and to flush the bladder of tissue and clots after TURP.

3. If clots occur, the catheter may be irrigated, or the rate of flow may be increased until the drainage outflow clears.

4. Calculate intake and output carefully; a large amount of bladder irrigation fluid must be subtracted from total output to determine client's true urinary output.

5. Monitor/titrate CBI so the outflow is light pink without clots; notify surgeon of any increase in bleeding.

6. If catheter is occluded and does not drain properly, turn off the CBI until catheter patency is reestablished.

B. Blood clots and pieces of tissue are normal for the first 24 hours after TURP.

C. If client has excessive bleeding, the physician may increase the size of the balloon on the indwelling catheter and put traction on the catheter to compress the area of bleeding.

D. Client should void within 6 hours of removal of catheter.

> **❗ NURSING PRIORITY** Maintain continuous bladder irrigation for the client who has undergone TURP; prevent overdistention of the bladder. If client complains of pain, check the urinary drainage and make sure it is patent. Obstruction most commonly occurs in the first 24 hours as a result of clots in the bladder.

E. Bladder spasms: belladonna and opium suppositories or antispasmodics are administered as needed; spasms often occur because of the presence of clots in the catheter; check the catheter for patency.

F. The sensation of a full bladder is common while the irrigating catheter is in place; explain (repeatedly) about

---

TURP
(Transurethral Resection of the Prostate)

- Continuous or Intermittent Bladder Irrigation (C.B.I.)
  Murphy Drip
- Close observation of drainage system-
  (↑Bladder Distention causes Pain & Bleeding).
- Maintain Catheter Patency
- Bladder Spasms
- Pain Control: Analgesics & ↓ Activity first 24 hours.
- Avoid straining with BM's. ↑ Fiber diet & Laxatives.
- Complications:
  - Hemorrhage - Bleeding should gradually ↓ to light pink in 24 hrs.
  - Urinary Incontinence - Kegal Exercises
  - Infections - ↑ Fluids
  - Prevent Deep Vein Thrombosis
    - Sequential compression stockings
    - Low dose heparin
    - Discourage sitting for prolonged periods

©2007 Nursing Education Consultants, Inc.

FIGURE 22-3 Transurethral resection of the prostate. (From Zerwekh J, Claborn J: *Memory notebook of nursing,* vol 1, ed 4, Ingram, Texas, 2008, Nursing Education Consultants.)

the urinary catheter and advise the client to avoid bearing down in an attempt to void.

Goal: To provide postoperative care.

A. After client is ambulatory, encourage walking, rather than sitting for prolonged periods.

B. Teach client exercises to control urinary stream and maintain continence.
1. Have client contract perineal muscles (Kegel exercises) by squeezing buttocks together.
2. Instruct client to practice starting and stopping the stream several times while voiding.

C. Assure client that TURP does not usually cause problems relating to sexual functioning; provide an opportunity for open discussion of sexual concerns.

D. Dribbling after voiding is a common problem, which often subsides within a few weeks.

E. Teach client to avoid straining during bowel movement; encourage diet high in fiber, and administer stool softeners as needed.

F. Discuss with the client the importance of maintaining a high fluid intake to prevent UTIs.

G. Encourage client to minimize use of caffeine-containing products, which may cause bladder spasms.

Goal: To provide postoperative care for a client after radical open prostatectomy.

A. Maintain adequate pain control, frequently with patient-controlled analgesia.

B. As a result of the surgical position and postoperative immobility, client is at high risk for deep venous thrombosis.
1. Monitor sequential compression devices.
2. Apply antiembolism stockings.
3. Administer low-dose prophylactic heparin.

ALERT Identify symptoms of deep venous thrombosis.

C. Perineal prostatectomy and total prostatectomy for cancer frequently result in erectile dysfunction caused by damage to the pudendal nerves and urinary incontinence.

D. Record output from drains.

E. Emphasize importance of not straining against catheter to relieve bladder pressure.

F. Evaluate for urinary retention.

ALERT Explain procedure to client and family. It is important to clarify for the client the information the doctor gives him; however, it is the doctor's responsibility to advise the client regarding any complications he may experience with sexual functioning.

Home Care

A. If client is discharged with urinary catheter in place, teach him how to care for the catheter and how to relieve an obstruction.

B. Client should avoid use of suppositories and enemas.

C. Primary care provider should be contacted if signs of UTI are noted.

D. After removal of urinary catheter, teach client Kegel exercises to increase urinary control (see BPH).

E. Instruct client to continue high fluid intake, avoid strenuous exercise, and avoid prolonged sitting; encourage walking.

Inflammatory Disorders

A. Prostatitis: inflammation of the prostate, usually caused by bacteria (*Escherichia coli, Proteus* spp.) or by a sudden decrease in sexual activity.

B. Epididymitis: inflammation of epididymis, often associated with prostatitis or a UTI; often develops as a complication of gonorrhea; in men younger than 35 years, the primary cause is infection with *Chlamydia trachomatis*.

Assessment

A. Clinical manifestations.
1. Prostatitis.
    a. Fever and chills.
    b. Perineal, rectal, and/or back pain.
    c. Dysuria, urethral discharge.
    d. Prostate is enlarged, firm, and tender when palpated.
    e. May be acute or chronic with exacerbations.
    f. Increased risk with catheterizations, bladder infection, or alternative sexual activity.
2. Epididymitis.
    a. Pain and tenderness in the inguinal canal.
    b. Painful swelling in the scrotum and groin.
    c. Fever and chills.
    d. Pyuria and bacteriuria.
    e. Feeling of "heaviness" in the testicle(s).

B. Diagnostics.
1. Rectal examination.
2. Complete blood count.
3. Urine and semen culture and sensitivity.
4. Screen for STDs.
5. Doppler ultrasonography or nuclear medicine scan for testicular torsion.

Treatment

A. Prostatitis.
1. Antibiotics.
2. Analgesics, stool softeners, and sitz baths.

B. Epididymitis.
1. Bed rest with elevation of the scrotum (scrotal support or scrotal bridge).
2. Antibiotics, if indicated.
3. Treatment of client's sexual partners (or gonorrhea infection).
4. Cold compresses; NSAIDs.

Complications

A. Chronic prostatitis can lead to recurrent UTIs and epididymitis.

B. May cause chronic reoccurring incapacitating infections.

Nursing Interventions

Goal: To assist client to understand measures to maintain health.

A. Encourage early treatment to prevent complications.

B. For chronic prostatitis, encourage activities that drain the prostate, including intercourse, masturbation, and prostatic massage.

C. Antibiotics may not be effective because it is difficult to obtain therapeutic levels in prostatic secretion.

D. Encourage treatment of sexual partners when epididymitis is caused by chlamydia or gonorrhea.

 Undescended Testes (Cryptorchidism)

Cryptorchidism is a condition of failure of one or both testes to descend into the scrotal sac.

Assessment

A. Inability to palpate the testes in the scrotal sac.

B. Cremasteric reflex is normal retraction of the testes when stimulated by stroking the thigh on affected side downward; may present a problem in attempting to determine whether there is an undescended testicle or if a testicle is retractable.

C. Testicle may be absent or small or may be located in the abdomen.

Treatment

A. Condition may be observed for 1 year; most cases descend spontaneously; if undescended after 1 year, surgery may be required.

B. Surgical intervention-orchiopexy: testis is brought into the scrotal sac and secured.
  1. Prevents damage to the undescended testicle by body heat.
  2. Decreases the incidence of tumor formation.
  3. Usually done between the ages of 6 and 24 months; fewer complications are encountered if repair is done before 5 years of age.
  4. Men with a history of cryptorchidism are at increased risk for fertility problems and development of testicular cancer in adulthood.

Nursing Interventions

 Home Care

A. Long-term follow-up regarding fertility.

B. Prevent infection by careful cleansing after defecation and urination because of the close proximity of the scrotum.

C. Teach parents to show the child how to do testicular self-examinations when he is old enough.

 Testicular Tumors (Cancer)

Tumors of the testicles are often malignant and tend to metastasize quickly.

Assessment

A. Most common cancer in men ages 15 to 35 years.

B. More common in clients who have had cryptorchidism and infections.

C. A painless lump (typically, pea-sized) is palpated in the scrotum.

D. Most men experience "heaviness" in the scrotum.

E. For clients ages 40 to 60 years old, if possible, determine if mother was given diethylstilbestrol (DES) during pregnancy There is a significant increase in the risk for testicular cancer among these clients.

F. A significant enlargement of or shrinking of one testicle.

G. Diagnostics.
  1. Levels of alpha-fetoprotein (AFP) and human chorionic gonadotropin (hCG) are increased.
  2. Computed tomography (CT) and magnetic resonance imaging (MRI).
  3. Ultrasound.
  4. Biopsy is not possible because of the risk for spreading cancer locally.

Treatment

A. Surgical intervention: orchiectomy (removal of the testicle) is performed as soon as possible to remove the tumor and make a definite diagnosis. If there is lymph node involvement, a retroperitoneal lymph node dissection, which is extensive radical abdominal surgery, is performed.

B. Medical.
  1. Postoperative irradiation to the lymphatic drainage pathways.
  2. Multiple chemotherapy medications.

Nursing Interventions

Goal: To detect any abnormality of the testes through self-examination by client (Box 22-2).

Box 22-2   TESTICULAR SELF-EXAMINATION

- Examine the testicles at same time every month, to help you remember to do it.
- Visually inspect scrotum in front of a mirror observing for swellings.
- Perform the examination after a bath or shower because this is when the scrotal sac is relaxed.
- Examine each testicle individually by placing index and middle fingers of both hands under one testicle at a time with thumbs on top of testicle. Roll the testicle between the thumbs and fingers. This should NOT cause pain. The tissue should feel smooth.
- Locate the epididymis which is a tubular sac behind the testicle. This sac should not be confused with a lump.
- Also assess for any "heaviness" or dull ache in the groin or abdomen or significant increase or decrease in size of either testicle.
- If there is any lump or irregularity on either testicle, report it to the doctor as soon as possible.

A. Teach clients, especially those between the ages 15 and 35 years, to self-examine monthly while showering or bathing to detect any abnormality of the testes.

B. Emphasize importance of follow-up for clients with a history of undescended testes or a previous testicular tumor.

Goal: To assist the client to understand the implications of surgery.

Hydrocele and Varicocele

A. Hydrocele: a collection of fluid around the testicle or along the spermatic cord. Client usually does not experience any pain. If circulation becomes impaired, then client experiences more discomfort.

B. Varicocele: a cluster of dilated veins in the scrotal sac, often just above the testes; occurs most often in young adults.
   1. Does not experience severe pain, but a chronic dull ache in the scrotal area.
   2. May contribute to infertility because sperm temperatures may be too high which affects sperm formation and motility.

C. Treatment.
   1. Hydrocele: needle aspiration or surgical aspiration and drainage.
   2. Varicocele: surgical intervention only if there are complications with fertility; otherwise, a scrotal support is used.

D. Nursing intervention: provide preoperative and postoperative care (see Chapter 3).

Erectile Dysfunction (ED)

Inability to attain or maintain an erect penis.

Assessment

A. Risk factors/etiology.
   1. Physiologic (organic): diabetes, hypertension, prostatectomy.
   2. Psychologic (functional): stress, depression, low self-esteem.

B. Clinical manifestations.
   1. Inability to attain or maintain an erection.
   2. Gradual onset with physiologic ED and abrupt onset with psychologic ED.

Treatment

A. Medical: ED medications (Figure 22-4 and Appendix 22-1).

B. Vacuum constriction devices (VCD): applying a suction device to the penis to pull blood up into the corporeal bodies, then placing a penile ring or constrictive band to trap the engorgement.

FIGURE 22-4 Erectile dysfunction drugs. (From Zerwekh J, Claborn J, Gaglione T: *Mosby's pharmacology memory notecards: visual, mnemonic, and memory aids for nurses,* ed 2, St. Louis, 2008, Mosby.)

C. Intraurethral devices: medicated urethral system for erection (MUSE)—administration of medications as a topical gel, injection into penis, or insertion of medication pellet into urethra.

D. Penile implants: surgical insertion of an implant.

Nursing Interventions

Goal: To help the client understand the implications of the medications or devices used to treat ED and assist to obtain counseling.

A. Teach client about how ED medications can potentiate hypotensive effects of nitrates and should not be taken at the same time.

B. Client should abstain from alcohol if taking ED medications.

Cystocele and Rectocele

Cystocele is a weakened support between the vagina and bladder allowing the bladder to bulge into the vagina. Rectocele is a weakened support between the vagina and rectum allowing the rectum to bulge into the vagina.

Assessment

A. Risk factors/etiology.
   1. Obesity and childbearing.
   2. Genital atrophy caused by aging.

B. Clinical manifestations.
   1. Cystocele: protrusion of the bladder into the vagina.
      a. Stress incontinence: occurs during coughing, lifting, or sneezing.

b. Frequency and urgency.

c. Difficulty emptying bladder.

2. Rectocele: protrusion of the rectum through the vaginal wall.

a. Constipation.

b. Incontinence of gas or liquid feces.

C. Diagnostics: bimanual pelvic examination.

Treatment

A. Medical: Kegel exercises for mild stress incontinence (tighten and release perineal muscles several times during the day); client can also practice stopping urination in midstream and holding it for a few seconds.

B. Surgical.

1. Cystocele: anterior colporrhaphy.

2. Rectocele: posterior colporrhaphy.

3. Procedure is usually called "A and P repair."

Nursing Interventions

Goal: To help the client understand the implications of, and be prepared for, surgery.

A. Preoperative teaching.

B. Postoperative period.

1. Prevent wound infection.

2. Warm compresses to abdomen may relieve discomfort.

3. Assess for urinary retention and excessive vaginal bleeding.

C. Frequent perineal care as well as after each voiding or defecation.

Home Care

A. Encourage the use of mild laxatives to prevent straining at stool.

B. Prevent constipation

C. Certain activities are restricted until area has healed: lifting objects heavier than 5 pounds; intercourse; prolonged standing, walking, and sitting.

D. Call the doctor if there is persistent pain or purulent, foul-smelling vaginal discharge.

Vaginal Inflammatory Conditions

Common Predisposing Factors

A. Excessive douching.

B. Oral contraceptives, steroids.

C. Antibiotics: especially broad-spectrum, which wipe out normal vaginal flora (vagina is protected by an acidic pH and the presence of Döderlein's bacilli).

D. Improper cleaning after voiding and defecating.

E. Assess for recurrent chronic infection; there may be an underlying condition (prediabetic state, HIV infection) that should be further evaluated.

Bacterial Vaginosis

A. Characteristics.

1. Causative organisms: E. coli, Haemophilus vaginalis, and Gardnerella vaginalis.

2. Profuse yellowish discharge, "fishy smell."

3. Itching, redness, burning, and edema, which are exacerbated by voiding and defecation.

B. Treatment: antibacterial/antiprotozoal medication.

C. Complications: bacterial vaginosis may increase susceptibility to STDs and HIV infection if woman is exposed to either.

D. Factors associated with bacterial vaginosis include multiple sex partners, douching, smoking but may occur in non-sexually active women.

Candidiasis

A. Characteristics.

1. Organism: *Candida albicans* (fungus).

2. Internal itching, beefy red irritation, inflammation of vaginal epithelium.

3. White, cheese-like, odorless discharge that clings to the vaginal mucosa.

4. Occurs frequently and is difficult to cure.

5. Increased risk in women with diabetes and women taking birth control pills, during pregnancy, and after treatment with antibiotics.

B. Treatment.

1. Antifungal vaginal medication.

2. Oral antifungals.

Trichomoniasis

A. Characteristics.

1. Organism: *Trichomonas vaginalis* (protozoan).

2. May be asymptomatic.

3. Itching, burning, dyspareunia (painful intercourse).

4. Frothy, green-yellow, copious, malodorous vaginal discharge; strawberry spot on cervix.

5. Sexual partners must be treated also because of cross-infection; men are usually asymptomatic.

B. Treatment: antibacterial/antiprotozoal medication.

C. Prevention: avoid extended time in synthetic or tight-fitting undergarments; use of condoms may reduce incidence of STDs.

Postmenopausal Vaginitis (Atrophic Vaginitis)

A. Characteristics.

1. Lack of estrogen (this is also the cause).

2. Itching and burning.

3. Loss of vaginal tissue folds and epithelial covering.

B. Treatment: estrogen vaginal cream.

Nursing Interventions

Goal: To teach client to prevent infection by performing appropriate personal hygiene, to decrease inflammation, and to promote comfort.

A. Appropriate cleansing from front of vulva to back of perineal area.

B. Frequently a postmenopausal problem.

C. Client should not douche; douching removes normal protective bacteria from vaginal cavity, and other bacteria are introduced.

D. If infection is chronic, it may be necessary to have sexual partner tested; partner may be reinfecting the woman.

E. Discourage use of feminine hygiene sprays because they cause increased irritation.

F. Discourage client from wearing constricting clothing and synthetic underwear (encourage use of cotton underwear).

Goal: To educate the woman regarding correct use of medication.

A. Vaginal suppositories, ointments, and creams are often used.
   1. Handwashing before and after insertion of suppository or application of cream.
   2. Remain recumbent for 30 minutes after application to promote absorption and prevent loss of the medication from the vaginal area.
   3. Wear a perineal pad to prevent soiling of clothing with vaginal drainage.

Dysfunctional Uterine Bleeding

Dysfunctional uterine bleeding is bleeding that is excessive or abnormal in amount or frequency without regard to systemic conditions; occurs when the hormonal events responsible for the balance of the cycle are interrupted.

Amenorrhea

A. Absence of menses.
   1. Primary: no menstruation has occurred by age 16 years.
   2. Secondary: woman previously had menses.
B. May be indicative of menopause.
C. May be first indication of pregnancy.
D. Occurs when woman has lost a critical fat percentage (e.g., athletes, clients with anorexia).

Menorrhagia

A. Excessive vaginal bleeding.
B. Single episode of heavy bleeding may indicate a spontaneous abortion.
C. May be associated with an intrauterine device (IUD).
D. Causes: hypothyroidism, uterine fibroids, hormone imbalance.

Metrorrhagia

A. Vaginal bleeding between periods.
B. May be normal menopause.
C. Ectopic pregnancy.
D. Breakthrough bleeding from oral contraceptives.
E. Cervical polyps.

> **! NURSING PRIORITY** Vaginal bleeding after menopause or surgical hysterectomy is a symptom of a problem that needs to be evaluated.

Nursing Interventions

A. Help determine most likely cause of problem.
B. Report excessive bleeding, abdominal pain, fever.
C. Treatment.
   1. Dilation and curettage (D&C) for diagnostic purposes in older women.
   2. Endometrial ablation.
   3. Removal of fibroids.
      a. Often done on outpatient basis with either general regional or local anesthesia.
      b. Spotting and vaginal drainage are common for several days; if amount is more than a normal period or if it lasts longer than 2 weeks, client should call the doctor.
      c. Client should report any signs of infection: fever; foul, purulent discharge; increasing abdominal pain.
      d. Nonsteroidal antiinflammatory drugs are often used for pain control.
      e. Client should avoid sexual intercourse and use of tampons for about 2 weeks.
D. Assess and treat for anemia.
   1. Encourage diet high in iron.
   2. Administer iron preparations, if required.

Endometriosis

Endometriosis is the presence of endometrial tissue outside of the uterus. The tissue responds to hormonal stimulation by bleeding into areas within the pelvis, causing pain and adhesions.

Assessment

A. Risk factors/etiology.
   1. Small pieces of endometrial tissue back up through the fallopian tubes into the abdomen during menstruation.
   2. Most common in women in their late 20s and early 30s who have never been pregnant.
B. Clinical manifestations.
   1. Dysmenorrhea: deep-seated aching pain in the lower abdomen, vagina, posterior pelvis, and back occurring 1 to 2 days before menses.
   2. Abnormal excessive uterine bleeding and dyspareunia; painful defecation.
C. Diagnostics.
   1. Laparoscopy.
   2. Ultrasonography.

Treatment

A. Medical: androgenic agents may be given over a 6- to 8-month period; or oral contraceptives may be prescribed; if a woman desires more children, she is encouraged to get pregnant, because the condition recedes during pregnancy.
B. Surgical intervention.
   1. Laser treatment of endometrial tissue in the extrauterine sites.

2. Hysterectomy (usually carried out in women close to menopause).

Nursing Interventions

Goal: To help client minimize the pain and discomfort associated with endometriosis.

A. Warm baths or moist heat packs may reduce discomfort.

B. Encourage client to explore alternative sexual positions that may minimize discomfort during intercourse.

C. Encourage client to discuss abstinence with partner if intercourse is painful.

Goal: To assist client to understand measures to maintain health.

A. Teach client about disease process; clarify any false ideas.

B. Provide emotional reassurance; discuss potential for infertility.

C. Initiate preoperative and postoperative teaching if surgery is elected.

Pelvic Inflammatory Disease

Pelvic inflammatory disease (PID) is an infectious condition of the pelvic cavity that involves the fallopian tubes, the ovaries, and/or the peritoneum.

Assessment

A. Risk factors/etiology.
1. Complication of gonorrhea and Chlamydia trachomatis.
2. IUDs are correlated with an increased incidence of PID.
3. Increased number of sexual partners increases incidence of PID.
4. Increases risk for repeat cases after previous episode of PID.

B. Clinical manifestations.
1. General malaise, fever, chills, nausea, and vomiting.
2. Leukocytosis and pain on urinating.
3. Dull tenderness or bilateral lower abdominal pain.
4. Vaginal discharge that is heavy and purulent.
5. Painful intercourse.
6. Chronic PID: persistent pelvic pain, secondary dysmenorrhea, dysfunctional uterine bleeding, and periodic episodes of acute symptoms.

C. Complications.
1. Sterility caused by adhesions and strictures within the fallopian tubes.
2. Ectopic pregnancy.
3. Pelvic abscess or generalized peritonitis.
4. Septic shock.

D. Diagnostics.
1. Abdominal pain on palpation.
2. Culture and sensitivity of drainage from the vagina, cervix, or cul-de-sac of Douglas.
3. Ultrasonography, laparoscopy, culdocentesis.

Treatment

A. Medical: broad-spectrum antibiotics, analgesics.

B. Surgical: incision and drainage of abscesses with or without a laparotomy.

Nursing Interventions

Goal: To prevent the spread and extension of the infection.

A. Maintain semi-Fowler's position to promote drainage of the pelvic cavity by gravity.

B. Strict medical asepsis when in contact with discharge; wound and skin precautions.

C. Encourage oral fluids and maintain adequate nutrition.

D. Client should avoid sexual activity and douching.

E. Strongly encourage sexual partner(s) to seek medical treatment.

Goal: To provide psychologic support.

A. Encourage expression of feelings related to guilt and possibility of sterility.

B. Explain factors relating to the long-term management of PID and the importance of medical supervision.

Sexually Transmitted Diseases

Infectious diseases transmitted most commonly through sexual contact.

A. Characteristics.
1. Transmitted by sexual activity, including oral and rectal activities between people of the same or opposite sex.
2. One person can have more than one STD at a time.
3. All sexual partners need to be evaluated.

B. Nursing role is to recognize and provide factual information.
1. Mode of transmission.
2. Prevention of transmission.
3. Importance of contacts being identified and treated.
4. Information provided in accepting, nonjudgmental manner.
5. Oral contraceptives do not provide any protection.

C. Incidence.
1. Nearly two thirds of STDs occur in people younger than 25 years.
2. The number of STDs continues to rise.

D. Clients with STDs should be tested for HIV.

E. Hepatitis B and HPV are considered STDs (see Chapter 19).

> **■ NURSING PRIORITY** Consider all oral, genital, and rectal lesions to contain pathologic organisms until documented otherwise.

Syphilis

Characteristics

A. Causative agent: spirochete *Treponema pallidum*.

B. Incubation period: 10 to 90 days; average is 20 to 30 days.

C. Transmission: direct contact with primary chancre lesion, body secretions (saliva, blood, vaginal discharge, semen); also transmitted transplacentally to the fetus.

D. Communicability: highly infectious during the primary stage; blood contains the spirochete during the secondary stage; usually noninfectious after 1 year during the latent stage; and noninfectious in the late (tertiary) stage.

Assessment

A. Primary stage.
   1. Chancre: small, hard, painless lesion found on the penis, vulva, lips, vagina, or rectum.
   2. Usually heals spontaneously within 2 to 3 weeks, with or without treatment.
   3. Regional lymphadenopathy.
   4. Will progress without treatment.

B. Secondary stage.
   1. Client may be asymptomatic; secondary stage usually begins anywhere from 2 weeks to 6 months after the chancre has healed.
   2. Maculopapular rash on the palms of the hands and soles of the feet, sore throat, and headache.
   3. Lymphadenopathy; gray mucous patches in the mouth.
   4. Condylomata lata: flat lesions that may appear in moist areas; are most infectious of any syphilitic lesion (not to be confused with condylomata acuminata in genital warts).
   5. Symptoms will disappear within 2 to 6 weeks.

C. Latent stage.
   1. Absence of clinical symptoms.
   2. Results of serologic tests for syphilis remain positive.
   3. Transmission can occur through blood contact.
   4. The majority of clients remain in this stage without further symptoms.

D. Congenital syphilis.
   1. Maculopapular rash over face, genital region, palms, and soles.
   2. Snuffles: a mucopurulent nasal discharge indicative of some degree of respiratory obstruction.
   3. After the age of 2 years: Hutchinson's teeth (notched central incisors with deformed molars and cusps).

E. Diagnostics.
   1. Serologic screening tests: Venereal Disease Research Laboratories (VDRL).
   2. Rapid plasma reagin test (PRP and RPR): may produce false-negative results in early stages.
   3. Fluorescent treponemal antibody absorption (FTA-ABS) test.
   4. VDRL and fluorescent treponemal antibody absorption tests are based on presence of antibodies, and results are not positive until about 4 weeks after the appearance of the chancre.

F. Complications: development of late (tertiary) syphilis and the resultant systemic involvement of the cardiovascular and central nervous systems.

Nursing Interventions

A. Administration of parenteral penicillin is treatment of choice. Tetracycline or doxycycline is administered if client is allergic to penicillin.

B. If pregnant mother is treated before the 18 weeks' gestation, the fetus will usually be born unaffected.

C. Preventive education regarding sexual exposure, adequate case finding, and treatment of contacts.

D. All cases are reported to local public health authorities.

 ## Gonorrhea

Characteristics

A. Most common venereal disease; an infection of the genitourinary tract; however, gonorrhea may also affect the rectum, pharynx, and eyes; caused by the bacteria Neisseria gonorrhoeae.

B. Incubation period: 3 to 4 days.

C. Transmission: direct contact with exudate via sexual contact or transmission to the neonate during passage through the birth canal.

D. Communicability: contagious as long as organisms are present.

Assessment

A. Men.
   1. Urethritis, epididymitis, dysuria, and purulent urethral discharge.
   2. Increased evidence of asymptomatic disease or a chronic carrier state in males.

B. Women.
   1. Initial urethritis or cervicitis that is often mild enough to remain undetected by client.
   2. Vulvovaginitis, vaginal discharge, dysuria.
   3. If untreated, may result in PID.

C. Both men and women; arthralgias, joint pain from disseminated gonococcus.

D. Neonate: ophthalmia neonatorum.

E. Diagnostics.
   1. Positive Gram stain smear of discharge or secretion.
   2. Positive culture.

F. Complications.
   1. Men: prostatitis, urethral strictures, urethritis, and sterility.
   2. Women: PID, Bartholin's abscess, ectopic pregnancy, infertility.

Nursing Interventions

A. Prophylactic antibiotic treatment for gonorrhea eye infection in the neonate (ophthalmia neonatorum).

B. Encourage follow-up cultures in 4 to 7 days after treatment and again at 6 months.

C. Teach importance of abstinence from sexual intercourse until cultures are negative.

D. Urge client to inform sexual partner so that he or she may be treated for infection.

E. Important to take the full course of antibiotics.

Herpes Genitalis

Characteristics

A. Infection caused primarily by herpes simplex virus 2 (HSV-2), which is characterized by painful vesicles surrounded by an erythematous area; progresses to shallow ulcers, pustules, and crusts; healing occurs spontaneously in about 2 to 4 weeks during the initial infection.

B. HSV-1 causes infection above the waist, involving the gingivae, dermis, and upper respiratory tract.

C. HSV-2 lesions characteristically occur below the waist, generally in the genital area and perineum; however, it is possible for HSV-2 to cause oral lesions and HSV-1 can cause genital lesions.

D. Virus enters a latent phase and may be harbored by the individual for an indefinite period of time; virus may be reactivated by stress, sunburn, sexual activity, and fever.

E. Recurrent outbreaks are usually less severe than the original outbreak of lesions.

F. Incubation period: unknown.

G. Transmission: by direct contact with the vesicles; asymptomatic shedding and transmission of virus are well documented.

H. Communicability: highly contagious.

Assessment

A. Initial sensation of tingling and itching before rupture of the lesion.

B. Signs of primary infection usually consist of local inflammation, pain, lymphadenopathy, and systemic symptoms.

C. Initial systemic malaise, fever, headache, and muscle aches.

D. Irritation of the genitals.

E. Genitals may become reddened with painful blisters, which burst into lesions that gradually heal.

F. Diagnostics: confirmed by using a tissue culture technique that identifies herpes type 2 virus; also by viral culture, serologic blood tests for antibodies for HSV-2, both IgG and IgA.

G. Complications.
   1. Increased incidence of cervical cancer in women possibly due to co-infection with human papilloma virus (HPV).
   2. Lesions or a positive viral tissue culture in a pregnant woman would be cause for concern. Client should be closely monitored to determine whether a problem with delivery is anticipated; cesarean delivery may be necessary.

Nursing Interventions

A. Teach importance of genital hygiene and avoidance of unprotected sexual contact.

B. Teach good hygiene practices. Explain that the fluid inside the lesions contains the virus. If a lesion breaks open, the virus can be spread by contact with the fluid and cause a lesion in any area of the body.

> **! NURSING PRIORITY** Always wear gloves when cleaning the perineal area of a client with HSV-2 to prevent herpetic whitlow, a herpes lesion around the nail bed. Nurses are at risk for developing this because of local contact with the HSV on broken skin areas around the nails.

C. If administration of oral antiviral agent is started at the first sign of a lesion, the duration of the outbreak may be decreased.

D. Symptomatic treatment: sitz baths, wet compresses, and analgesics for relief of pain.

Cytomegalovirus

Characteristics

A. Cytomegalovirus is a virus belonging to the herpes family, which leads to very mild illnesses but can cause a wide range of serious congenital deformities in the fetus or newborn (known as congenital cytomegalovirus).

B. Transmission: human contact.

C. Communicability: about four of five people older than 35 years have been infected with cytomegalovirus, usually sometime during childhood or young adulthood; symptoms are so mild that the diagnosis is frequently overlooked.

Assessment

A. The mother is usually asymptomatic or has mononucleosis-type symptoms.

B. Effect on the neonate: serious hematologic and central nervous system consequences; high mortality rate in severely affected neonates.

C. Diagnostics.
   1. **TORCH** screening: **T**oxoplasmosis, **O**ther (hepatitis), **R**ubella, **C**ytomegalovirus infection, **H**erpes simplex.
   2. Increased lymphocyte count and abnormal liver function test results.

Nursing Interventions

A. Prevention is the primary goal. Pregnant women should avoid being around affected individuals and congenitally infected infants.

B. Prevention of exposure is almost impossible, because the primary infection is asymptomatic.

Chlamydia Infection

Characteristics

A. An infectious disease caused by Chlamydia trachomatis (most common STD).

B. Incubation period: 1-3 weeks.

C. Transmission: direct contact; sexual contact.

Assessment

A. Males.
   1. Urethritis, epididymitis, proctitis.
   2. Primary reservoir is the male urethra.
B. Females.
   1. Mucopurulent cervicitis, postpartal endometritis, salpingitis, vaginitis.
   2. Primary reservoir is the cervix.
C. Newborns.
   1. Inclusion conjunctivitis.
   2. Pneumonia.
   3. Hepatomegaly and splenomegaly.
D. Both males and females are frequently asymptomatic and often do not seek medical attention until a complication arises (PID, epididymitis).
E. Diagnostics: isolation of the organism in a tissue culture or serologic complement fixation testing.
F. Complication: reactive arthritis (can also be a primary symptom).

Nursing Interventions

A. Urge client to have sexual partner treated.
B. Emphasize the importance of long-term drug therapy because of the pathogen's unique life cycle, which makes it difficult to eliminate.
   1. Antibiotics: doxycycline and azithromycin are primary antibiotics for treatment.
   2. Penicillin and its derivatives are not effective against these organisms; consequently, this usually explains the persistence of infection in clients who are treated for gonorrhea and do not respond.

Genital Warts

Characteristics

A. Characterized by cluster of warts caused by the human papilloma virus (HPV): condylomata acuminata.
B. HPV is continually shed from the surface, and reinfection may occur.

Assessment

A. Warts are found in areas subject to trauma during sexual activity: penis, urethra, perianal area, anal canal, vulva, cervix, vaginal canal.
B. Diagnosed by observation and biopsy of lesions.
C. The cervix and anal canal may be involved if there are lesions on the vaginal or anal area.
D. Lesions are raised, skin-toned, damp, cauliflower-like growths.
E. Genital itching.
F. May cause nonmenstrual bleeding after intercourse.

Nursing Interventions

A. Education regarding transmission.
B. Close follow-up with Pap smears in women; genital warts are associated with an increased incidence of cervical cancer.

C. Increased incidence of squamous cell cancer of penis in men.
D. Podophyllin, applied topically once or twice a week, and antimitotic preparations are the most common treatments.
E. Transmission is by direct contact with a person who has lesions present.
F. Vaccination with Gardasil may reduce or prevent genital warts.

Cervical Cancer

Assessment

A. Risk factors/etiology.
   1. Multiple sex partners.
   2. First intercourse at early age.
   3. History of STDs, HSV-2.
   4. Genital warts (HPV-positive), abnormal Pap smears.
B. Clinical manifestations.
   1. Clients are asymptomatic until late in disease state.
   2. Thin and watery drainage that becomes dark and foul smelling as the disease progresses.
   3. Abnormal vaginal bleeding or discharge.
   4. Low back pain.
   5. Painful sexual intercourse.
C. Diagnostics.
   1. Pap smear.
      a. Initial Pap smear at age 21 or after first sexual intercourse.
      b. Pap smears are continued after menopause and hysterectomy.
   2. Classification of Pap test results: Bethesda Classification System (2001) replaced older system, which had 5 classes.
      a. The adequacy is assessed as satisfactory or unsatisfactory.
      b. The findings are described as negative or having epithelial cell abnormalities (either squamous cell or glandular cell).

> **NURSING PRIORITY** If cancer of the cervix is identified before it becomes invasive (or in the in situ stage), there is virtually a 100% cure rate.

   3. Cervical biopsy (office procedure)—after the test, the client should:
      a. Avoid strenuous activity for 24 hours.
      b. Leave vaginal packing in for about 24 hours.
      c. Abstain from sexual intercourse for approximately 24 hours.
      d. Avoid using tampons and douching.

Treatment

A. Surgical intervention.
   1. Conization (cryosurgery): used for carcinoma in situ.
   2. As treatment for cervical cancer, the following procedures may be done:

a. Vaginal hysterectomy: removal of the uterus; fallopian tubes and ovaries remain intact.
b. Hysterectomy: total abdominal hysterectomy with bilateral salpingo-oophorectomy (TAH-BSO); includes removal of fallopian tubes and ovaries.
c. Radical hysterectomy: a panhysterectomy plus a partial vaginectomy and removal of lymph nodes.
d. Pelvic exoneration: radical hysterectomy plus total vaginectomy, removal of bladder with urinary diversion, bowel resection, and colostomy.
3. Radiation therapy, either internal (radium implant) or external for invasive cancer.
4. Gardasil vaccine for prevention of cervical cancer.

Nursing Interventions

Goal: To provide health teaching to help clients detect premalignant cervical dysplasia.
A. Warning signs of cancer.
B. Importance of yearly Pap smears.
C. Encourage verbalization of feelings related to the surgery and diagnosis of cancer.
Goal: To provide preoperative and postoperative teaching in preparation for a total abdominal hysterectomy.
A. General preoperative care.
B. After surgery, assess for complications, such as backache or decreased urine output, because these symptoms can indicate accidental ligation of the ureter.
C. Urinary retention may occur as a result of bladder atony and edema; explain to client the necessity for a urinary retention catheter.
D. Early ambulation is encouraged to prevent postoperative thrombophlebitis.
E. Determine whether hormone replacement therapy will be used and provide appropriate teaching.
F. If dyspareunia occurs, client should contact her doctor.
Goal: To provide psychologic support.
A. Encourage verbalization of concerns related to body image.
B. Teach that sexual activity should be avoided until checkup to determine wound healing (about 4 to 6 weeks).
C. Client should avoid heavy lifting.
D. Client who has had a pelvic exoneration will have many concerns regarding sexual function, because the vagina will be lost. Menopause will occur, and there may be a urinary or bowel diversion to the abdominal wall (an ileal conduit or colostomy).

Breast Carcinoma

Assessment

A. Risk factors/etiology.
1. Leading cause of cancer death in women ages 14 to 54 years.
2. Family history of breast cancer; however, 85% of women with breast cancer have a negative family history.
3. Nulliparity or parity after the age of 30 years.
4. Early menses, late menopause; removal of the ovaries before the age of 35 years significantly decreases the risk for breast cancer.
5. The incidence of recurrence of breast cancer is significant.
6. Presence of other cancer: endometrial, ovarian, colon, rectal.
B. Clinical manifestations.
1. Asymmetry of the breasts.
2. Skin dimpling, flattening, and nipple deviation are suggestive of a lesion.
3. Skin coloring and thickening, large pores, sometimes called peau d'orange (orange peel appearance).
4. Changes in the nipple; discharge from the nipple.
5. Mass is painless, nontender, hard, irregular in shape, and nonmobile.
6. Majority of malignant lesions are found in the upper outer quadrant of the breast (tail of Spence).
C. Diagnostics.
1. Mammography; ultrasound.
2. Breast biopsy.
3. Serum tumor markers: carcinoembryonic antigen (CEA), human chorionic gonadotropin (hCG).
D. Complications:
1. Metastases via the lymphatic system to bone, lungs, brain, and liver.
2. Postmastectomy pain syndrome: pain persisting past 3 months.
3. Sentinel lymph node dissection (SLND).

Treatment

A. Surgical.
1. Modified radical mastectomy (most common): removal of all breast tissue and axillary lymph nodes; the pectoralis major muscle remains intact; preservation of the muscle helps to prevent the arm edema frequently associated with mastectomy.
2. Local excision (lumpectomy): may be done to stage the malignancy and determine appropriate chemotherapy/radiation therapy, but the breast is preserved.
3. Radical mastectomy (less common): removal of all of the breast tissue, the pectoral muscles, and the axillary lymph nodes of the surrounding tissue.
4. Breast reconstruction: may be delayed until after radiation therapy is completed or may be done at the time of the mastectomy.
B. Radiation: combined with surgery and chemotherapy.
C. Hormonal therapy: breast cancers that are classified as "estrogen receptors" are less invasive tumors and respond to changes in estrogens; hormone therapy is being used in conjunction with surgical intervention to prevent/decrease recurrence.
D. Chemotherapy: a combination of drugs will be used to treat the malignancy.

Nursing Interventions

Goal: To promote early detection of breast cancer through mammography, clinical breast exam, and breast self-examination (BSE).

A. Screening mammography should begin at age 40.

B. Teach client how to perform breast self-examination. (see Box 22-3).

C. Clinical breast exam should begin with clients in their 20s and 30s, and every year for asymptomatic woman age 40 or older.

D. American Cancer Society recommends a yearly MRI and a mammography for women age 30 or older who have a family history of breast cancer.

Goal: To prepare the client physiologically and psychologically for surgery (normal preoperative and postoperative care; see Chapter 3).

A. Assist woman to decrease emotional stress and anxiety; encourage use of spiritual and social resources.

B. Provide emotional support; encourage verbalization.

C. Anticipate concerns related to sexuality and fear of rejection by husband or sex partner after the mastectomy (see the section on Body Image in Chapter 9).

ALERT Plan measures to assist client to cope with anxiety; assess client's response to illness; identify coping mechanisms of client and family.

D. Determine whether any plans for reconstructive surgery have been discussed.

Goal: To recognize and prevent postoperative complications (Figure 22-5).

A. There may be one or more drains in the incisional area. Jackson-Pratt drains are commonly used.

ALERT Empty and reestablish negative pressure of portable wound suction devices.

B. Assess wound for infection.

C. Position client in semi-Fowler's and arm on affected side so that each joint is elevated and positioned higher than the more proximal joint; this promotes gravity drainage via the lymphatic and venous circulations.

D. Do not take blood pressure or perform any injections or venipuncture on the arm of the affected side.

E. Arm exercises are usually started on the first postoperative day.

1. Assist/teach the woman to perform flexion and extension exercises with the wrist and elbow frequently throughout the day. Squeezing a ball is good exercise at this time.

2. The affected arm should not be abducted or externally rotated in initial exercises. Encourage movement of the arm in activities of daily living (brushing her hair, eating, washing her face).

F. Active exercises are begun after wound healing is well established.

G. Approximately 2 to 3 weeks after surgery and with good wound healing, more active exercises are initiated.

1. Pendulum arm swings.

2. Pulley-type rope exercise to promote forward and lateral movement of the arms.

3. "Wall climbing" with the fingers.

Box 22-3   BREAST SELF-EXAMINATION

- Evaluate risk factors; educate woman about increased risk factors.
- Woman should perform breast self-examination (BSE) on a regular basis; once a month about a week after her period or at the same time each month if the woman has no periods.
- It is important for the BSE to be done on a regular basis; this makes it easier to detect abnormalities when they occur.
- The BSE should include the following three steps:
  1. Step 1: Inspection before a mirror to determine asymmetry or changes in size. Breast should be evaluated from three positions: with the arms relaxed at the sides; with the arms over the head pressing on the back of the head; with the hands on the hips, palms pressing inward to flex the chest muscles. Look for dimpling, differences in sizes of the breast, ulcerations, nipple retraction, and increased vascularity.
  2. Step 2: Breast should be palpated while lying down; flatten the right breast by placing a pillow under the right shoulder. With the fingers flat, use the sensitive pads of the middle three fingers of the left hand. Feel for lumps or changes using a rubbing motion. Press firmly enough to feel the different breast tissues. Examine the entire breast from the collarbone to area on which the base of your bra rests and the axillary area. Pay particular attention to the upper outer quadrant of each breast. Gently squeeze the nipple to determine presence of any drainage.
  3. Step 3: In the shower or bath examine your breasts; hands glide easier over wet skin.
- Women older than 40 years should have a mammogram every year; women with increased risk factors should maintain regular follow-up with a physician.
- The American Cancer Society provides excellent teaching opportunities for nurses, as well as extensive information for women regarding early detection of breast cancer and rehabilitation after a mastectomy.

ALERT Questions regarding teaching women about breast cancer, risk factors, BSE, and preventive health care are common on the exam.

POST MASTECTOMY
NURSING CARE

• Elevate affected side with distal joint higher than proximal joint.

• No BP, injections or venipunctures on affected side.

• Watch for S & S of edema on affected arm.
(edema may occur post op or years later)

• Lymphedema can occur any time after
axillary node disection.

• Flexion and extension exercises of the hand in recovery

• Abduction and external rotation arm exercises
after wound has healed.

• Assess dressing for drainage.

• Assess wound drain for amount and color.

• Provide privacy when client looks at incision.

• Chemotherapy.

• Radiation therapy.

• Psychological concerns:
Altered body image
Altered sexuality
Fear of disease outcome

©2007 Nursing Education Consultants, Inc.

FIGURE 22-5 Postmastectomy nursing care. (From Zerwekh J, Claborn J: *Memory notebook of nursing,* vol 1, ed 4, Ingram, Texas, 2008, Nursing Education Consultants.)

ALERT Identify factors interfering with wound healing. The arm on the affected side will be at increased risk for developing problems of edema and infection. The arm should be protected throughout rehabilitation and during activities of daily living for an indefinite period of time.

Home Care

Goal: To promote the client's return to homeostasis and to help her understand implications of modified lifestyle; to identify measures to maintain health.

A. Discuss symptoms of recurrence and importance of making regular visits to the physician to monitor recovery and to detect changes.

B. Promote a positive self-image and reintegration with family and loved ones.

C. Discuss with client plans for obtaining a breast prosthesis.

D. Encourage the woman to participate in the Reach to Recovery program through the American Cancer Society. Check with the physician to see whether representatives may visit with the client before the surgery.

E. Compression arm sleeves used to minimize swelling from lymphedema.

Appendix 22-1   MEDICATIONS USED IN REPRODUCTIVE SYSTEM DISORDERS

MEDICATIONS	SIDE EFFECTS	NURSING IMPLICATIONS
Benign prostatic hyperplasia Medications that decrease the size of the prostate, therefore decreasing pressure on the urinary tract in clients with BPH or by promoting smooth muscle relaxation (alpha adrenergic blockers).		
Alpha Adrenergic Blocker (Nonselective) Doxazosin **(Cardura)**: PO Tamsulosin **(Flomax)**: PO Terazosin **(Hytrin)**: PO	Dizziness, fatigue, orthostatic hypotension, dyspnea, headache	1. Advise client of possible problems of decreased blood pressure and orthostatic hypotension. 2. Prostatic cancer should be ruled out before medications are started. 3. Medication should decrease problems of urination associated with BPH. 4. Monitor blood pressure closely if taking antihypertensive medications.
Finasteride **(Proscar)**: PO	Erectile dysfunction, decreased libido	1. Client should take contraceptive precautions or not have sexual intercourse with women who could become pregnant. 2. Women who may be or are pregnant should not handle the tablets.
Antifungal/Protozoal Medications Used to treat vaginal fungal infections.		
Clotrimazole **(Gyne-Lotrimin)**: intravaginally (OTC) Miconazole **(Monistat 3)**: intravaginally Fluconazole **(Diflucan)**: PO Terconazole **(Terazol)**: intravaginally Metronidazole **(Flagyl)**: PO	Nausea, vomiting, headache, vaginal irritation	1. Creams are not recommended to be used with tampons or diaphragms. 2. Not recommended for use during pregnancy or lactation. 3. **Flagyl** is used to treat trichomoniasis; instruct client *to avoid alcohol* because it can lead to serious side effects of throbbing headaches, nausea, excessive vomiting, hyperventilation, and tachycardia. 4. Suppositories or applicators are used to place medication in the vagina. 5. If client does not see improvement within 3 days, she should return to her health care provider. 6. **Diflucan** can be given as a single dose for vaginal candidiasis.
Erectile Dysfunction Medications Promote an increase in arterial pressure and inflow of blood into the penis and reduce the venous outflow causing engorgement and producing an erection.		
Sildenafil **(Viagra)**: PO Vardenafil **(Levitra)**: PO Tadalafil **(Cialis)**: PO	Hypotension can be a serious SE Headache, flushing, visual changes **■ NURSING PRIORITY** Always inquire if a client is taking an ED medication before treating chest pain with any nitrate medication.	1. Should not be taken concurrently with nitrates. 2. Alpha blockers (used for treatment of BPH) are contraindicated in the client taking tadalafil and vardenafil, should be used with caution in client taking **Viagra**. 3. Vardenafil can cause prolonged QT interval on ECG, should not be used in combination with antidysrhythmic medications. 4. Primary differences in the medications are the onset and duration of action. 5. Priapism, painful erection, or erection lasting over 4 hours may require medical intervention to prevent penile damage.

BPH, Benign prostatic hypertrophy; *IV,* intravenous; *OTC,* over the counter; *PO,* by mouth (oral).

Appendix 22-2 HORMONE REPLACEMENT

MEDICATIONS	SIDE EFFECTS	NURSING IMPLICATIONS
Conjugated estrogen **(Premarin, Ortho-est, Prempro):** PO, intravaginally	Nausea, vomiting, breakthrough bleeding, weight gain, swollen tender breasts, increased blood pressure	1. Should not be given unopposed to women who have a uterus. Estrogen compounds should be given with progesterone combinations.
Micronized estradiol **(Estrace):** PO, IM, intravaginally Estradiol **(Estraderm, Ortho Tri-Cyclen Lo):** transdermal patches	Increased risk for uterine cancer	2. Important for menopausal women to continue with 1200 to 1500 mg/day calcium intake and weight-bearing exercises along with estrogen replacement to prevent osteoporosis. 3. Should not be used by women who have known or suspected cancer of the breast, undiagnosed vaginal bleeding, or possible pregnancy. 4. Used with precaution—or not at all—in women with clotting disorders or history of DVT/PE. 5. Report any unusual bleeding to primary care provider. 6. Research data changed the practice of treating perimenopausal women's symptoms with HRT. It is their decision to take it or not, but use should be short-term and lowest effective dose with risks outlined. 7. *Use:* Replacement hormone to treat symptoms associated with menopause—hot flashes, atopic vaginitis (local vaginal application of low-dose estrogen—**Vagifem**) prevention of postmenopausal osteoporosis.
Medroxyprogesterone acetate **(Provera, Depo-Provera):** PO, IM	Menses may become more irregular	1. *Use:* **Provera**—for menopausal women who still have a uterus, significantly decreased risk for uterine cancer when used with estrogen therapy. **Depo-Provera**—birth control injection given every 3 months. 2. Women should continue with increased calcium intake and weight-bearing exercises to prevent osteoporosis; should have yearly Pap smears, mammograms, and cholesterol series.

IM, Intramuscular; *IV,* intravenous; *PO,* by mouth (oral).

Study Questions Reproductive System

More questions on companion CD!
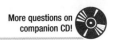

1. A client's Pap test reveals epithelial cells characteristic of adenocarcinoma of the cervix. The nurse understands that which of the following is a major risk factor for cervical cancer?
   1 Long-term use of oral contraceptives
   2 Recurrent outbreaks of human papilloma virus (HPV)
   3 Grand multiparity with history of preterm labor
   4 Alternative therapy for treatment of menopausal symptoms

2. A client has been diagnosed with genital herpes. The nurse would explain to the client that she is most contagious at what stage?
   1 When vesicles rupture and release transudate
   2 When superficial, painful ulcers appear
   3 When yellow vaginal drainage is present
   4 When pustules become inflamed and erythematous

3. What is important to include in the discharge teaching plan for a 38-year-old client who has had a vaginal hysterectomy?
   1 Do not douche with any type of solution.
   2 Refrain from sexual intercourse for 2 months.
   3 Take hormone replacement therapy.
   4 Anticipate heavy vaginal bleeding.

4. During a well-woman physical examination, a young woman is diagnosed with a primary genital herpes lesion. When completing the client's history, the nurse would anticipate the client to report:
   1 Anuria
   2 Pruritus
   3 Leukorrhea
   4 Dyspareunia

5. A client had a left modified radical mastectomy 48 hours ago. What would be important for the nurse to include in a discharge teaching plan for this client? Select all that apply.
   _____ 1 Massage wound site with essential oils once incision has healed.
   _____ 2 Avoid needle-sticks in the left arm.
   _____ 3 Begin active exercises, such as pendulum arm swings, immediately.
   _____ 4 Avoid abduction and external rotation of the upper arm.
   _____ 5 Elevate arm on pillows to prevent edema.
   _____ 6 Take blood pressure readings from the right arm.

6. What is an important nursing action when assisting the doctor with a pelvic examination?
   1 Instruct the client to douche before the exam.
   2 Explain to the client that she will not feel any pain.
   3 Have the client empty her bladder before the examination begins.
   4 Lubricate the speculum well before handing it to the doctor.

7. A teenage boy comes to the office complaining of intense burning while urinating and gray-green discharge coming from his penis. The nurse recognizes these as symptoms of what problem?
   1 Herpes (HSV-2) with open lesions
   2 Secondary stage syphilis
   3 Urinary tract infection
   4 Gonorrhea

8. After examining a painless sore on the penile shaft, the doctor asks the nurse to order a fluorescent treponemal antibody absorption (FTA-ABS) test. The nurse knows that the purpose of this test is to diagnose what condition?
   1 Herpes simplex virus type 2 (HSV-2)
   2 Trichomoniasis
   3 Cytomegalovirus
   4 Syphilis

9. The night shift nurse notes at the end of her shift that a client who had a mastectomy has a total of 90 mL of serosanguineous drainage after a 24-hour period. What is the best nursing action?
   1 Report amount of drainage to the physician.
   2 Start frequent blood pressure checks and observe for hemorrhage.
   3 Continue to monitor the drainage.
   4 Reinforce packing at the wound site.

10. The nurse is caring for a client who has had a mastectomy. What is important nursing care regarding the positioning of the affected arm?
    1 Hold the arm close against the side of her body.
    2 Secure the arm below the level of the heart.
    3 Wrap the arm in an Ace bandage and keep it below the heart.
    4 Elevate arm above heart level.

11. A client is admitted because of benign prostatic hypertrophy and is scheduled to have a transurethral prostate resection. What assessment data would indicate to the nurse that a complication is developing?
    1 The client has difficulty emptying his bladder.
    2 Client states he feels like he cannot empty his bladder.
    3 The client complains of frequency and nocturia.
    4 Increasing complaints of flank pain and hematuria.

12. The nurse is discussing the importance of breast self-examination with a client who is being discharged after a vaginal hysterectomy. What is important information for the nurse to give this client?
    1 Perform breast self-examination 1 week after her normal period.
    2 Examine her breasts on a regular basis about the same time every month.
    3 Breasts should be palpated while in the sitting position.
    4 Use the tips of the fingers to palpate deeply into the breast tissue.

13. The nurse is discussing testicular self-examination with a male client. What information is important for the nurse to include in the discussion?
    1. The best time to perform the examination is 24 hours after sexual intercourse.
    2. The examination should be conducted at the same time each month.
    3. The client should perform this self-examination every 3 to 4 months.
    4. When the scrotum is pulled up tight against the body, the testes are easier to palpate.

14. The nurse is assessing a client who had a transurethral resection of the prostate (TURP) 6 hours ago. He has a urinary catheter with continuous bladder irrigation running. What nursing observations would indicate a complication is developing?
    1. Catheter drainage of 50 mL in the past hour and increase in suprapubic pain
    2. Dark, grossly bloody catheter drainage with pieces of tissue
    3. Client states that he feels like he needs to void
    4. Moderate amount of bloody discharge from around the catheter

15. A client is diagnosed with epididymitis related to bladder outlet obstruction. The nurse teaches which intervention to assist the client in recovery?
    1. Walk briskly at least 30 minutes every day.
    2. Limit oral intake to minimize nausea and vomiting.
    3. Apply scrotal support to relieve edema and discomfort.
    4. Use warm baths and compresses during acute inflammation.

16. A sexually active 17-year-old female is diagnosed with trichomoniasis through vaginal discharge analysis. The nurse explains which pharmacologic intervention to minimize symptoms and the risk for reoccurrence?
    1. Return to clinic each week for intramuscular injection of penicillin.
    2. Perform a daily vaginal douche with a weak iodine solution.
    3. Oral administration of metronidazole three times a day to client and partner.
    4. Application of trichloroacetic acid to lesions daily for 6 to 8 weeks.

17. A client is scheduled for an abdominal hysterectomy. Preoperative teaching includes which of the following?
    1. A nasogastric tube will be left in to control vomiting after surgery.
    2. A douche and an enema may be done the evening before surgery.
    3. There will be a moderate amount of bloody vaginal drainage after surgery.
    4. Ambulation will be delayed for 48 hours because of the extensive nature of the procedure.

18. A woman has experienced an incomplete abortion. She is scheduled for a dilation and curettage (D&C). What is the purpose of this procedure?
    1. To protect the uterus and the ovaries for future pregnancies
    2. To provide a healthier uterine environment for future pregnancies
    3. To provide reinforcement for an incompetent cervix
    4. To scrape the uterine walls and remove the uterine contents

19. The nurse is teaching a client with a pelvic inflammatory disease. The nurse instructs the client to sleep with her head elevated about 45 degrees. What is the rationale behind instructing the client to sleep in this position?
    1. Assists to localize drainage in the lower abdomen
    2. Decreases abdominal muscle tension
    3. Makes coughing and deep breathing more effective
    4. Prevents scarring of the fallopian tubes

20. A young woman comes into the emergency department with menorrhagia. What is the priority concern for the nurse caring for this client?
    1. The chronic bleeding will cause anemia.
    2. The client is at a high risk for development of an infection.
    3. The woman may be pregnant and is aborting the fetus.
    4. The increased bleeding will promote later problems with infertility.

21. What is the immediate posthysterectomy priority nursing action?
    1. Assist with sitz baths three times daily.
    2. Provide a high-protein diet.
    3. Teach the client exercises to strengthen the abdomen.
    4. Observe the client for decreased urine output.

Answers and rationales to these questions are in the section at the end of the book titled Chapter Study Questions: Answers and Rationales.

CHAPTER TWENTY-THREE

Urinary-Renal System

PHYSIOLOGY OF THE KIDNEY AND URINARY TRACT

A. Kidney function.
1. Excretory.
   a. Rid the body of metabolic wastes.
      (1) Regulate fluid volume; normally, 125 mL of fluid is filtered each minute (glomerular filtration rate [GFR]); however, only 1 mL is excreted as urine; average urine output is about 1440 mL per day.
      (2) Regulate the composition of electrolytes.
      (3) Assist in maintaining acid-base balance.
   b. Regulation of blood pressure.
      (1) Juxtaglomerular cells are located in the afferent arteriole just before it enters the glomerulus.
      (2) The cells respond to a decrease in the blood flow (decrease in blood pressure) by increasing the secretion of renin.
      (3) Renin acts on angiotensin I and converts it to angiotensin II, which is a powerful vasoconstrictor. Peripheral resistance is increased; therefore, blood pressure is increased.
      (4) Kidneys receive 20% to 25% of total cardiac output with a renal blood flow rate of 600 to 1300 mL/min.
2. Endocrine.
   a. Aldosterone production is stimulated by the increase in angiotensin I; therefore sodium and water are retained to increase circulating volume and increase blood pressure.
   b. Regulates red blood cell production through synthesis of erythropoietin; released in response to hypoxia and reduced renal blood flow.
   c. Aids in calcium metabolism by activating vitamin D, which allows for absorption of calcium from the gastrointestinal tract.

B. Nephron function.
1. Filtration: occurs in the glomerulus via a semipermeable membrane. The membrane does not normally allow large protein molecules to be filtered out of the blood.
   a. GFR is the amount of blood filtered by the glomeruli in a given time (approximately 120 to 140 mL/min).

   b. Changes in GFR occur when the pressure gradients from the glomerular capillaries across the semipermeable membrane to the glomerulus are altered.
      (1) Pressure gradient changes occur when there is a variation in the systemic blood pressure (hypotension), a significant change in the pressure in Bowman's capsule in the glomerulus (edema) occurs, and when ureteral obstruction occurs.
      (2) The kidneys' response to changes in pressures is buffered by an autoregulatory mechanism to maintain a stable range of blood pressure. The autoregulatory mechanism maintains renal blood flow and the GFR within wide fluctuations of blood pressure. When the pressure range is outside the autoregulatory mechanism (hypotension/hypertension), the GFR will fluctuate with the systemic blood pressure.

> **NURSING PRIORITY** Determine whether client has a decreased urinary output (below 30 mL per hour in an adult, 20 mL per hour in a child, and 1 mL/kg/hr in an infant); urinary output should be carefully evaluated regarding blood pressure level; blood pressure must provide renal perfusion to maintain adequate urinary output. The level of blood pressure to maintain renal perfusion varies greatly from one client to another.

      (3) If the glomerular membrane is damaged, plasma proteins will escape. A decrease in serum proteins decreases the normal serum oncotic pressure; this results in water retention and edema formation.
2. Tubular reabsorption: after the glomerulus has filtered the blood, the tubules separate the water and solutes by osmosis and diffusion. Water moves across the semipermeable membrane and is reabsorbed or excreted in response to the concentration gradient of the solutes (sodium, potassium, chloride, urea, etc.). Only a small amount of the total water filtered out of the kidneys is excreted as urine. Solutes are also reabsorbed according to the concentration gradient.

479

3. Tubular secretion: regulates the potassium level and maintains the acid-base balance with other regulatory mechanisms.

C. Urinary tract.

1. Ureters.
   a. Muscular tubes through which urine flows from the kidneys to the bladder.
   b. Ureterovesical valve: located at the opening of the ureter into the bladder (ureterovesical junction); prevents backflow of urine into the ureters when the bladder contracts.

2. Bladder.
   a. As the bladder fills, the stretch receptors are stimulated. In the adult, the first urge to void will occur when 100 mL to 150 mL has collected; approximately 400 mL to 600 mL of urine will initiate a feeling of bladder fullness.
   b. Bladder capacity varies from 600 mL to 1000 mL.

3. Voiding: stimulation is sent to the sacral area of the spinal column where the micturition reflex, or voiding reflex, is initiated; after toilet training, the cerebral cortex (via the spinal column) allows for voluntary control of bladder contractions that initiate urination.

4. Urethra: a small, membranous tube that conveys urine from the bladder to the exterior of the body.
   a. Female urethra is 1 to 2 inches long.
   b. Male urethra is 8 to 10 inches.

System Assessment

A. External assessment.

1. Inspect skin for changes in color, turgor, texture (urate crystals), bruising, and excoriations.

2. Assess face, abdomen, and extremities for edema.

3. Determine weight gain or loss.

4. Palpate kidneys and bladder.
   a. Landmark: for kidney palpation, the landmark is the costovertebral angle, formed by the rib cage and the vertebral column.
   b. Bladder is palpated just above the suprapubic area (or symphysis pubis bone).
   c. Kidney and bladder should be nonpalpable with no discomfort on palpation.

5. General: fatigue, lethargy, level of alertness.

B. History.

1. Presence of renal or urologic congenital defect.

2. Determine whether client has ever been exposed to chemicals, especially carbon tetrachloride, phenol, and ethylene glycol, because these are nephrotoxic. Determine smoking history: cigarette smoking is a risk factor for bladder cancer.

3. Determine whether client has received antibiotics that may be nephrotoxic: aminoglycosides, amphotericin B, and sulfonamides.

4. Assess dietary intake: determine increased levels of calcium. Anorexia and nausea and vomiting may cause dehydration or be the result of altered renal function.

5. Determine level of activity: immobility leads to demineralization of the bones, which can predispose to infection and calculus formation.

6. Evaluate complaints of pain: dysuria; flank, costovertebral, or suprapubic pain.

7. Assess changes in pattern of urination: frequency, nocturia, urgency, enuresis, incontinence (Box 23-1 and Table 23-1).

8. Assess changes in urine output: polyuria, oliguria, anuria.

9. Assess changes in urine consistency: hematuria, pyuria, diluted, concentrated, change in color.

10. Determine whether client is taking any medications that may affect urinary or renal function.

11. Determine whether client has any chronic health care problems that affect renal and urinary tract structures (diabetes mellitus, hypertension, allergies, or multiple sclerosis).

DISORDERS OF THE URINARY-RENAL SYSTEM

 Urinary Tract Infections

Stasis of urine in the bladder and reflux of urine back into the original reservoir are the primary causes of urinary tract infections (UTIs). *Escherichia coli* **is the most common pathogen leading to UTIs (Figure 23-1).**

A. Upper UTIs: *pyelonephritis*, an inflammation of the renal pelvis and the parenchyma of the kidney(s).

B. Lower UTI.
   1. Cystitis: inflammation/infection of the bladder.
   2. Urethritis: inflammation of the urethra.

Box 23-1   OLDER ADULT CARE FOCUS

Dealing with Incontinence

Need to Determine:
- Does client have difficulty initiating urinary flow?
- Is client aware of need to void?
- Can client empty bladder completely, or is there residual urine?
- Is there bladder distention and overflow dribbling?
- Is stress incontinence present or urge incontinence?
- What are usual voiding times?
- Is the client constipated or is there an impaction? Is this a chronic problem?

Nursing Interventions
- Help the client determine when he or she needs to urinate before an accident occurs.
- Maintain adequate fluid intake but limit fluids before bedtime.
- Establish a voiding schedule: offer assistance and encourage voiding.
- Assess the client's access to the bathroom; determine need for a bedside commode.
- Assess for presence of urinary tract infection.
- Teach client how to perform Kegel exercises.

Table 23-1	**TYPES OF URINARY INCONTINENCE**		
Type of UI	*Definition*	*Pathophysiology*	*Symptoms and Signs*
Urge	Involuntary loss of urine associated with a strong sensation of urinary urgency	• Involuntary detrusor (bladder) contractions (DI), along with sphincter relaxation • Seen with CNS disorders (Parkinson's disease); bladder disorders (interstitial cystitis)	Loss of urine with an abrupt and strong desire to void; involuntary loss of urine (without symptoms); nocturia is common
Stress	Urethral sphincter failure, usually associated with increased intraabdominal pressure	• Urethral hypermobility caused by anatomic changes or defects such as fascial detachments, relaxed pelvic floor musculature, atrophy due to loss of estrogen • ISD: Failure of the sphincter at rest (prostate surgery for BPH or cancer)	Small amount of urine loss during coughing, sneezing, laughing, or other physical activities; continuous leak at rest or with minimal exertion (e.g., postural changes)
Mixed	Combination of urge and stress UI	• Combination of urge and stress features (as listed above) • Common in women, particularly postmenopausal women	Combinations of urge and stress UI symptoms (as listed above)
Overflow	Bladder overdistention	• A contractile detrusor • Hypotonic or underactive detrusor caused by drugs, fecal impaction, diabetes, lower spinal cord injury, or disruption of the motor innervation of the detrusor muscle • In men—secondary obstruction caused by prostatic hyperplasia, prostatic carcinoma, or urethral stricture • In women—obstruction caused by severe genital prolapse or surgical overcorrection of urethral detachment	Frequent or constant dribbling or urge or stress incontinence symptoms, as well as urgency and frequent urination Residual urine after voiding is common
Functional	Chronic impairment of physical and/or cognitive functioning	• Chronic functional and mental disabilities	Urge incontinence or functional limitations or environmental factors
Unconscious or reflex	Neurologic dysfunction secondary to nerve damage	• Decreased bladder compliance with risk for vesicoureteral reflux and hydronephrosis • Caused by radiation cystitis, inflammatory bladder conditions, radical pelvic surgery, or spinal cord lesions above S2 • In many non-neurogenic cases, no demonstrable DI	Postmicturitional or continual incontinence; severe urgency with bladder hypersensitivity (sensory urgency)

From Fantl J et al: *Managing acute and chronic incontinence: clinical practice guideline. quick reference guide for clinicians,* No. 2, Rockville, MD, 1996, U.S. Department of Health and Human Services, Public Health Service, Agency for Health Care Policy and Research, AHCPR Pub. No. 96-0686.; Lewis SL et al: *Medical-surgical nursing: assessment and management of clinical problems,* St. Louis, 2007, Mosby
DHIC, Detrusor hyperactivity with impaired bladder contractility; *DI,* detrusor instability; *ISD,* intrinsic urethral sphincter deficiency; *UI,* urinary incontinence.

C. UTIs occur in an ascending route up the urinary tract system.

ALERT Use alternative measures to promote voiding; promote bowel and bladder control.

Assessment

A. Factors contributing to UTI.
   1. Adult female urethra is short and close to the rectum and vagina, which predisposes it to contamination from fecal material.
   2. Ureterovesical reflux: the reflux of urine from the urethra into the bladder; this causes a constant residual of urine in the bladder after voiding and precipitates UTI.
   3. Vesicoureteral reflux (ureterovesical reflux): the reflux of urine from the bladder into one or both of the ureters and possibly into the renal pelvis.
   4. Instrumentation: catheterization or cystoscopic examination.
   5. Stasis of urine in the bladder leading to urinary retention for any reason (clients with prostate disease).
   6. Obstruction of urinary flow: congenital anomalies, urethral strictures, ureteral stones, contracture of the bladder neck, tumor, fibrosis, or fecal impaction (Figure 23-2).
   7. Bladder hypotonia: mechanical compression of the ureters; hormone changes predispose pregnant and postmenopausal women to more frequent UTIs.

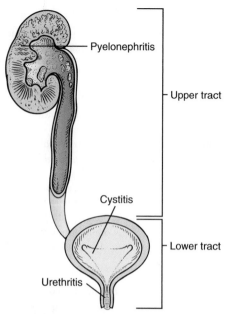

FIGURE 23-1 Urinary tract infections. (From Lewis SL et al: *Medical-surgical nursing: assessment and management of clinical problems*, ed 7, St. Louis, 2007, Mosby.)

FIGURE 23-2 Causes of urinary obstruction. (From Lewis SL et al: *Medical-surgical nursing: assessment and management of clinical problems*, ed 7, St. Louis, 2007, Mosby.)

   8. Metabolic disorders such as diabetes.
   9. Sexual intercourse promotes development of UTI.
 10. Fecal contamination of the urethral meatus.

ALERT Identify an infection and be able to assess and to identify pertinent data indicating a urinary tract and/or kidney infection.

B. Clinical manifestations.
   1. Cystitis (lower UTI).
      a. Frequency, urgency, dysuria (classic triad of symptoms).
      b. Hematuria.

      c. Nocturia, incontinence, hesitancy, weak stream.
      d. Often asymptomatic with bacteriuria.
      e. Low back pain or suprapubic pain.
   2. Pyelonephritis (upper UTI).
      a. Fever, chills, malaise, flank pain on affected side.
      b. Symptoms of cystitis.
      c. Older adults may not have a fever, and those older than 80 years may have a decrease in temperature and exhibit confusion (Box 23-2).
   3. Urosepsis: a urinary tract infection that has become systemic and is life threatening.
C. Diagnostics (see Appendix 23-1).
D. Complications.
   1. A lower UTI may progress to an upper UTI.
   2. Chronic pyelonephritis may develop after repeated bouts of acute pyelonephritis.

Treatment

A. Medical (see Appendix 23-2).
   1. Broad-spectrum antibiotics, especially the sulfonamides for lower urinary tract infections; fluoroquinolones for upper urinary tract infections.
   2. Urinary analgesics.
   3. Antispasmodics.
   4. Antipyretics.
B. Dietary.
   1. Encourage fluid intake of 3000 mL per day.
      a. Dilute urine causes less irritation.
      b. The increase in flow of urine through the urinary tract decreases the movement of bacteria up the urinary tract.
      c. Discourage consumption of carbonated beverages and foods or drinks containing baking powder or baking soda. Caffeine, alcohol, citrus fruits, and highly spiced foods can cause bladder irritation.
      d. Daily intake of cranberry juice or cranberry essence tablets is helpful for some clients, as it appears to decrease the ability of bacteria to adhere to the epithelial cells lining the urinary tract.

Nursing Interventions

Goal: To provide relief of pain, urgency, dysuria, and fever.

A. Antibiotics need to be taken as scheduled. Initially, therapy may be required for 1 to 3 days; if problem is recurrent, 10 to 14 days of therapy may be required. For pyelonephritis, antibiotics may be taken for 14 to 21 days; severe symptoms may require hospitalization.

B. Encourage consumption of 8 to 10 glasses of fluids daily (3000 mL).

C. Teach client importance of voiding every 2 to 3 hours during the day to completely empty the bladder.

D. Sitz baths may be taken to decrease irritation of urethra.

Goal: To prevent recurrence of infection.

A. Avoid sitting in a bathtub with added bubble bath products or other bath oils and fragrances; a warm bath will decrease symptoms, but nothing should be added to the water.

B. Explain importance of cleansing the perineal area from front to back after voiding and after each bowel movement. Avoid use of perineal sprays and powders.

C. If intercourse seems to predispose to infection, encourage voiding immediately before and after intercourse. A female client with recurrent UTIs may need to temporarily stop using a diaphragm and spermicidal creams/jelly.

D. Teach importance of long-term therapy if recurrent infections are a problem.

E. Encourage and explain the need for follow-up care to prevent complications of chronic UTIs.

F. Caffeine, alcohol, citrus juices, and carbonated beverages should be avoided.

Urinary Calculi

Stones may form anywhere in the urinary tract; the most common location for stones is in the pelvis of the kidney. If the stones are small, they may be passed into the bladder (see Figure 23-2).

A. Stones in the bladder may increase in size if urinary stasis and alkaline pH are present.

B. Types of urinary calculi.
1. Calcium oxalate or phosphate stones: tend to be small; account for 40% to 50% of all upper urinary tract calculi.
2. Struvite stones: contain bacteria and tend to be large; more common in women than men.
3. Uric acid stones: occur most often in clients with primary or secondary problems of uric acid metabolism (gout); high incidence in men, particularly Jewish men.

Assessment

Regardless of the type of stone formed, the clinical manifestations, diagnostics, and treatment are essentially the same.

A. Risk factors/etiology.
1. Infection, urinary stasis, immobility.
2. Hypercalcemia and hypercalciuria (hyperparathyroidism, renal tubular acidosis).
3. Excessive intake of dietary proteins, which increases uric acid production.
4. Excessive consumption of tea or fruit juice, which elevates urinary oxalate levels.
5. Low fluid intake.
6. Majority of clients are between the ages of 20 and 55. Stones occur more often in the summer months.
7. Increased incidence of family history with stone formation due to inherited metabolic risk factors.

B. Clinical manifestations.
1. Sharp, sudden, severe abdominal or flank pain.
   a. May be described as "colic," either ureteral or renal.
   b. Pain may be intermittent, depending on the movement of the stone; spasm in the ureter occurs as it attempts to move the stone toward the bladder.
   c. Pain may radiate around the flank area, down into the bladder, the genitalia, and the thigh.
2. Hematuria may be present as a result of the traumatic effects of the stone on the ureter and the bladder.
3. Oliguria or anuria suggest urinary obstruction and must be treated immediately.
4. Nausea and vomiting are common.
5. May be associated with fever and infection.

C. Diagnostics (see Appendix 23-1).

D. Complications.
1. Recurrent stone formation.
2. Infection.
3. Renal failure.

Treatment

A. Medical.
1. Increase fluid intake to 3000 mL/day to decrease urine concentration.
2. Medications that prevent the absorption of calcium (thiazide diuretics and phosphates).
3. Spasmolytic agents (anticholinergics).
4. For uric acid stones, allopurinol (Zyloprim).
5. Opioids for pain relief.
6. Dietary.
   a. Sodium may also be restricted, because sodium increases the excretion of calcium in the urine.
   b. Decrease in protein intake or an alkaline-ash diet for clients with uric acid stones.
   c. Decrease intake of cola, coffee, and tea, which tends to increase the risk for calculi formation.

B. Surgical.
1. Nephrolithotomy: incision into the kidney and removal of the stone.
2. Ureterolithotomy: incision into the ureter to locate a stone and remove it.

3. Stenting: insertion of a small tube (stent) into ureter via ureteroscopy to dilate ureter to enlarge passageway for expulsion of stone or stone fragments.

C. Lithotripsy: cystoscopic, percutaneous ultrasonic, laser, or extracorporeal shock-wave litohtripsy (ESWL).

1. For ESWL, client is anesthetized and placed in a water bath. Some lithotripters do not require submersion.

   a. Sound waves travel through the water and are directed to the stone. The force of the sound wave shatters the stone, and the remains are excreted in the urine.

   b. It is essential that the client remain absolutely motionless during the procedure, which lasts about 30 to 45 minutes. Therefore some form of sedation or analgesia is necessary during the procedure.

   c. A ureteral stent is often placed after lithotripsy procedures to promote passage of stone fragments and left in place for 2 weeks.

2. Hematuria is common after the procedure.

Nursing Interventions

Goal: To relieve pain.

A. Administer analgesics as prescribed: morphine or hydromorphone (Dilaudid).

B. Hot baths or moist heat applied to flank area.

C. Encourage increased fluid intake (3000 mL/day) to prevent dehydration.

D. Strain all urine and inspect for blood clots and passage of stone.

E. If stone is passed, it should be saved and sent to the lab for analysis to determine the type of stone so appropriate therapy can be maintained.

Goal: To promote understanding of health care regimen.

A. Dietary restrictions, depending on type of stone.

B. Discuss rationale, dose, frequency, and important information relating to medication administration.

C. Teach symptoms of recurring stone formation, such as hematuria, flank pain, and signs of infection.

D. Instruct client to continue high fluid intake.

E. Promote periodic medical follow-up visits to evaluate for symptoms of infection and recurring stone formation.

 Hypospadias and Epispadias

A. Hypospadias: the urethral opening is located behind the glans penis or along the penile shaft; this is a common anomaly.

B. Epispadias: the urethral opening is located on the dorsal or upper side of the penis; this is a rare problem.

Assessment

A. Clinical manifestations.

1. Visualization of defect.

2. Chordee: ventral curvature of the penis, which gives it a crooked appearance (hypospadias).

3. Stream of urine does not come out the end of the penis.

4. Hypospadias is associated with cryptorchidism in severe cases.

5. Bladder exstrophy is a severe form of epispadias.

Treatment

A. Surgical correction of the defect.

1. Hypospadias: recommended repair by 6 to 18 months of age.

2. Epispadias is much more complex and frequently associated with other genitourinary system defects; repair may be very involved and require multiple staged surgical procedures.

Nursing Interventions

Goal: To provide emotional support and to promote normal growth and development.

A. Frequently the infant is not circumcised until the repair of the hypospadias.

B. The infant with epispadias may be discharged home before repair is done.

C. The preferred time for repair is between 6 and 12 months; it is important not to delay repair of hypospadias beyond the time for toilet training.

D. A diaper and a sterile nonadherent dressing are applied over the exposed bladder when the infant has a bladder defect.

E. Teach parents signs of UTI.

F. Help parents understand realistic expectations of the outcome of surgery (epispadias and/or bladder exstrophy).

 Nephrotic Syndrome

A problem with glomerular permeability to plasma proteins results in massive urinary protein loss. The most common type is a primary condition, minimal change nephrotic syndrome.

A. Changes occur in the basement membrane of the glomeruli that allow the large protein molecules to pass through the membrane and be excreted. The loss of albumin from the serum decreases the oncotic pressure in the capillary bed and allows fluid to pass into the interstitial tissues and the abdominal cavity (ascites) and interstitial spaces (edema).

B. The interstitial fluid shift causes hypovolemia. The renin-angiotensin response is stimulated. Aldosterone secretion is increased, and the tubules begin to conserve sodium and water to increase the circulating volume.

C. In the majority of children with the syndrome, the cause is unknown; it may be congenital, idiopathic, or secondary to another disease; frequently, there is no evidence of renal dysfunction or systemic disease.

Assessment

A. Risk factors/etiology.

1. Usual history is a well child who begins to gain weight and exhibits pallor and fatigue.

2. Majority of children affected are male and between the ages of 2 and 4 years; uncommon in infants younger than 1 year.

3. May occur in adults secondary to systemic disease (e.g., SLE, diabetes) or may be idiopathic.

B. Clinical manifestations.

  1. Hallmarks: edema, proteinuria, hypoalbuminemia, and hyperlipidemia in the absence of hypertension and hematuria in children.

    a. Facial edema, especially periorbital edema; may be more pronounced in the morning and subside during the day.

    b. Generalized edema of the lower extremities; may increase during the day.

    c. Labia or scrotum may become very edematous.

    d. Edema may progress to the level of severe generalized edema (anasarca).

    e. Ascites and pleural effusion.

  2. Gradual increase in weight.

  3. Volume of urine is decreased, and urine may be foamy and tea colored.

  4. Irritability, fatigue, lethargy.

  5. Malnourishment: child is malnourished as a result of decreased intake and loss of protein in the urine but may not appear so because of edema.

  6. Infection can result in significant morbidity or mortality.

C. Diagnostics (see Appendix 23-1).

  1. Decreased serum protein levels: hypoalbuminemia.

  2. Urinalysis: increased specific gravity, massive proteinuria (>3+ as determined by dipstick test).

  3. Creatinine clearance may be decreased, with normal serum creatinine levels.

D. Potential complications.

  1. Compromised immune system leading to an increase in infections (e.g., pneumonia, bronchitis, peritonitis).

  2. Circulatory insufficiency caused by hypovolemia, with severe edema.

  3. Thromboembolism secondary to hypercoagulability.

Treatment

A. Medical.

  1. Corticosteroids: prednisone/prednisolone.

  2. Diuretics: used when edema progresses despite sodium restriction.

  3. Salt-poor human albumin is used for treatment of vascular insufficiency and severe edema.

  4. Prophylactic broad-spectrum antimicrobial agents.

  5. Immunosuppressant therapy is prescribed for children who are not responsive to steroid therapy.

B. Dietary.

  1. Decreased sodium intake.

  2. Proteins consumed should have high biologic value (low to moderate protein diet).

  3. Usually, fluid is not restricted.

Nursing Interventions

Goal: To monitor disease progress and reduce edema.

A. Support edematous areas such as scrotum.

B. Provide and encourage a salt-restricted diet.

C. Administer salt-poor albumin; monitor closely for circulatory overload during and after administration.

D. Provide meticulous skin care and keep opposing skin surfaces dry; change position frequently, and monitor good body alignment.

E. Determine weight daily, maintain accurate intake and output record, measure abdominal girth daily.

F. Test urine with dipstick for protein; check specific gravity.

G. Monitor cardiac function for complications of fluid balance (marked edema but hypovolemic).

Goal: To prevent infection.

A. Child is susceptible to infection because of a compromised immune state, as well as steroid therapy.

B. Protect child from upper respiratory tract infections; provide good pulmonary hygiene; check breath sounds.

C. Prevent skin excoriation and breakdown; assess carefully for indications of infection.

Goal: To promote nutrition.

A. Encourage low to moderate protein intake of high biologic value.

B. Serve frequent small quantities of food to child.

C. Encourage input from child in selection of foods from prescribed diet.

Home Care

A. Inform child and parents about medical regimen: steroids, diuretics, antibiotics.

B. Reassure parents that the prognosis is good; there may be relapses that will require therapy, but few children progress to chronic disease.

C. Obtain medical assistance if relapse occurs; relapse is indicated by edema, proteinuria, fever.

D. Encourage normal growth and development activities; try to prevent social isolation.

E. Teach parents how to perform dipstick urine test for protein; may need to keep a daily diary to evaluate level of proteinuria.

Glomerulonephritis

Glomerulonephritis is an inflammatory reaction in the glomerulus most commonly as a result of an antigen-antibody response to beta-hemolytic streptococci. An immune complex is formed as a result of the antigen-antibody formation; the complex becomes trapped in the glomerulus. As a result of the edema in the glomeruli, the GFR is significantly decreased. It is the third leading cause of renal failure in the United States.

Assessment

A. Risk factors/etiology.

  1. The stimulus of the antigen-antibody reaction is most often group A beta-hemolytic Streptococcus infection of the throat (tonsillitis, pharyngitis) or skin (impetigo), which ordinarily precedes the onset of the condition by about 10 to 21 days.

  2. Most common in children, but all age groups can be affected; males are more frequently affected than females.

B. Clinical manifestations (Figure 23-3).
1. Acute glomerulonephritis.
   a. Disease may be mild with proteinuria and/or asymptomatic hematuria.
   b. Tea- or cola-colored urine caused by hematuria.
   c. Facial and periorbital edema.
   d. Decrease in urine output (oliguria).
   e. Mild to moderate increase in blood pressure; hypertension is more severe in adults.
   f. Azotemia: presence of nitrogenous waste products in the blood.
2. Chronic glomerulonephritis: symptoms reflect progressive renal failure; more common in adults.
C. Diagnostics (see Appendix 23-1): reduced complement (C3) levels in early stages and elevated antistreptolysin O titer.
D. Complications.
1. Chronic renal failure.
2. Circulatory overload (pulmonary edema) and congestive heart failure (CHF).
3. Hypertensive episodes.

Treatment

A. Medical.
1. Diuretics for severe edema and fluid overload.
2. Antihypertensives.
3. Antibiotics, if the streptococcal infection is still present.
4. Plasmapheresis for filtering out immune complexes (antigens and antibodies).
B. Dietary.
1. Decrease sodium intake.
2. Protein restriction if client is azotemic; however, the anorexia that a child experiences frequently limits protein intake sufficiently.
3. Foods containing large amounts of potassium are often restricted during the oliguric phase.

GLOMERULONEPHRITIS

Antigen-Antibody Complex From Recent Strep Infection

Antigen-Antibody Complex in Glomeruli Causing:
- Inflammation
- ↓ Glomerular Filtration Rate

- Headache
- ↑ BP
- Facial / Periorbital Edema
- Lethargic
- Low Grade Fever
- Weight Gain (Edema)
- Proteinuria
- Hematuria
- Oliguria
- Dysuria

©2007 Nursing Education Consultants, Inc.

FIGURE 23-3 Glomerulonephritis. (From Zerwekh J, Claborn J: *Memory notebook of nursing,* vol 2, ed 3, Ingram, Texas, 2007, Nursing Education Consultants.)

C. Children with normal blood pressure, adequate urine output, and mild symptoms are cared for at home.
D. Fluid restriction may be implemented if urinary output is decreased.

Nursing Interventions

Goal: To protect client's kidneys by preventing secondary infections.
A. Antibiotic therapy if cultures are positive.
B. Child usually experiences fatigue and malaise and will voluntarily restrict activity.
C. Avoid medications that are nephrotoxic.
Goal: To maintain fluid balance.
A. Monitor intake and output; maintain diet and fluid restrictions.
B. Monitor renal function: check proteinuria, specific gravity, and color of urine; weigh client daily; if client has hypertension, check blood pressure every 2 to 4 hours.
C. Monitor serum potassium levels.
D. Frequently, the first sign of improvement is an increase in the urine output, which may progress to profuse diuresis.
Goal: To prevent complications and promote comfort.
A. Encourage verbalization of fears.
B. Decrease anxiety by explaining treatments and reassuring client and family that the majority of clients recover fully.
C. Most children recover spontaneously, and recurrences are uncommon.

Home Care

A. Teach parent or client symptoms to be reported to physician: nausea, fatigue, vomiting, decrease in urinary output, and symptoms of infection.
B. Explain the need for rest, good nutrition, and avoidance of people with respiratory tract infections.
C. Teach measures to prevent UTIs.
D. Instruct client in regard to diet, fluid needs, and medication therapy.
E. Teach client to perform dipstick urine test to monitor for protein.

Wilms' Tumor (Nephroblastoma)

Nephroblastoma (Wilms' tumor) is one of the most common intraabdominal tumors of childhood and is associated with congenital anomalies, especially those of the genitourinary tract. The treatment and survival rate are based on the stage of the tumor at the time it is diagnosed.
A. Risk factors/etiology.
1. Associated with genitourinary anomalies.
2. Majority of children (80%) are younger than 5 years; peak incidence at 3 years.
B. Clinical manifestations.
1. Swelling or mass within the abdomen: firm, confined to one side of the abdomen, causing vague or no pain.
2. Abdominal pain as tumor enlarges.

3. Hematuria, pallor, anorexia, weight loss, and malaise occur as condition progresses.
4. Hypertension (63%).
C. Diagnostics (see Appendix 23-1).

Treatment

The survival rate greatly depends on the stage of the tumor at the time of diagnosis. If the tumor is diagnosed and treated in the early stages, there is a high survival rate (see Chapter 8).
A. Surgery.
   1. Surgery is frequently scheduled within 24 to 48 hours after the diagnosis.
   2. Nephrectomy: kidney is removed, but the adrenal gland may be spared, depending on the invasiveness of the tumor.
   3. If both kidneys are involved, the less affected kidney is retained, and the more involved one is removed. Bilateral nephrectomy is a last resort.
B. Medical.
   1. Preoperative and postoperative radiation therapy for large tumors.
   2. Postoperative chemotherapy.

Nursing Interventions

Goal: To provide safe preoperative care.

> **! NURSING PRIORITY** Post a sign above the bed that reads "Do Not Palpate Abdomen."

A. Handle child carefully to prevent trauma to the tumor site.
B. Prepare child and family for the surgery, including anticipation of a large incision and dressing. ICU care immediately after surgery.
C. Assess vital signs, especially blood pressure, for indications of hypertension. If adrenal gland is removed, blood pressure may be labile.

Goal: To assess kidney function and to prevent infection.
A. Usual postoperative care for abdominal surgery.
B. Monitor for GI complications.
C. Provide good pulmonary hygiene because child is at increased risk for pulmonary infections postoperatively.
D. Vincristine is frequently used in chemotherapy; closely observe the child for the development of a paralytic ileus.
E. Child is at risk for intestinal obstruction from the vincristine-induced adynamic ileus, edema caused by radiation, or postsurgical adhesions.

Home Care

A. Teach parents effects of chemotherapy.
B. Child has only one kidney; teach parents how to protect renal function.
   1. Signs and symptoms of UTI.
   2. Methods to prevent UTIs.
   3. Advise all health care providers of compromised renal function.
   4. Prompt treatment of other infections.

Acute Renal Failure

A clinical syndrome with abrupt loss of renal function that may occur over several hours or days, characterized by uremia. The most common cause is hypotension and prerenal hypovolemia or exposure to a nephrotoxin.

Phases of Acute Renal Failure

A. Oliguric phase.
   1. Urinary output decreases to less than 400 mL per 24 hours.
   2. Increase in BUN, creatinine, uric acid, potassium, and magnesium levels and presence of metabolic acidosis.
   3. Duration is 1 to 3 weeks; the longer it lasts, the less favorable the recovery.

> **! OLDER ADULT PRIORITY** The older adult client loses the ability to concentrate urine; therefore urinary output may not be significantly reduced in this stage of renal failure.

   4. Nonoliguric renal failure: referred to as *high output failure;* urine is dilute and renal disease is present. These clients usually recover quicker and have fewer complications.
B. Diuretic phase.
   1. Often has a sudden onset within 2 to 6 weeks after oliguric phase. Diuresis up to 10 L/day; urine is very dilute.
   2. Hypovolemia and hypotension may occur due to massive fluid losses.
   3. BUN level stops increasing. Urinary creatinine clearance stabilizes.
   4. Client must be monitored for hypokalemia and hyponatremia.
   5. May last for 1 to 3 weeks.
C. Recovery (convalescent) phase.
   1. Begins when the GFR increases. May take up to 12 months for renal function to stabilize.
   2. There is usually some permanent loss of renal function, but remaining renal function is sufficient to maintain healthy life. The older adult is less likely to experience a return to full kidney function.
   3. Complications: secondary infection, which is the most common cause of death.

Assessment

A. Risk factors/etiology.
   1. Prerenal (renal ischemia).
      a. Circulatory volume depletion: caused by hemorrhage, dehydration.
      b. Decreased cardiac output: pump failure and/or CHF, especially in older adults.
      c. Decreased peripheral resistance: caused by septic shock, anaphylaxis, antihypertensives.
      d. Volume shifts: third spacing of fluid, gram-negative sepsis, hypoalbuminemia.
      e. Vascular obstruction: renal artery occlusion, dissection abdominal aneurysm.

2. Intrarenal (kidney tissue disease).
   a. Acute tubular necrosis: caused by hemolytic blood transfusion reaction, nephrotoxic chemicals (carbon tetrachloride, arsenic, lead, mercury), nephrotoxic medication (aminoglycoside antibiotics, amphotericin B, and streptomycin), radiology contrast material.
   b. Infections: acute glomerulonephritis, pyelonephritis, CMV, candidiasis.
   c. Diseases that precipitate vascular changes (e.g., atherosclerosis, diabetes mellitus, hypertension).
3. Postrenal (obstructive problems).
   a. Urinary and renal calculi.
   b. Benign prostatic hypertrophy.
   c. Urethral stricture.
   d. Trauma resulting in obstruction.
   e. Bladder cancer, neuromuscular disorders.

! NURSING PRIORITY Many disorders across the life span can precipitate acute renal failure. It is important to know who is at increased risk for developing renal failure and the initial symptoms. Renal failure is frequently incorporated into a test question as a complication of a variety of conditions.

B. Clinical manifestations (multiple body systems affected).
   1. Urinary: decreased urinary output (oliguria, less than 400 mL/day; in older adults, may be 600 to 700 mL/day).
      a. Intrarenal and postrenal failure: fixed specific gravity, increased sodium in the urine; proteinuria with glomerular membrane alteration, "muddy brown" casts.
      b. Prerenal failure: history of precipitating event; urine specific gravity may be high; high urinary sodium concentration and proteinuria.
      c. High output renal failure: the kidney no longer filters the urine; high urinary output, but the urine is dilute and does not contain waste products from filtering.
   2. Cardiovascular.
      a. Pericarditis, pericardial effusion.
      b. Arrhythmias caused by acidosis or hyperkalemia.
      c. CHF, hypotension followed by hypertension.
   3. Respiratory.
      a. Pulmonary edema caused by fluid overload.
      b. Kussmaul respiration caused by metabolic acidosis.
      c. Pleural effusions.
   4. Hematologic.
      a. Anemia caused by impaired erythropoietin.
      b. Leukocytosis, increased susceptibility to infection.
      c. Altered platelet function leading to bleeding tendencies.
   5. Neurologic.
      a. Decreased seizure threshold caused by uremia.
      b. Altered mentation, memory impairment, lethargy.
   6. Fluid and electrolyte imbalances.
      a. Fluid retention.
      b. Hyperkalemia.
      c. Hyponatremia (usually dilution).
      d. Metabolic acidosis from accumulation of acid waste products.
C. Diagnostics (see Appendix 23-1).

Treatment

A. Medical.
   1. Identify and treat precipitating cause of acute renal failure (management varies according to whether disorder is prerenal, intrarenal, or postrenal).
   2. Diuretic therapy may be used with fluid challenges.
   3. Decrease serum potassium level.
      a. Sodium polystyrene sulfonate (Kayexalate): a cation exchange resin given by mouth or retention enema.
      b. Sorbitol: an osmotic cathartic; may be given with exchange resins to induce diarrhea to eliminate potassium ions.
      c. IV hypertonic glucose and regular insulin may be administered to move potassium into the intracellular space; used for severe hyperkalemia.
   4. IV administration of sodium bicarbonate: corrects metabolic acidosis and causes electrolyte shift.
   5. IV dopamine to enhance renal perfusion. **Caution**: always check for correct concentration before beginning infusion (see Appendix 16-7).
B. Dietary.
   1. Fluid restriction; intake may be carefully calculated with output.
   2. Intake of protein, potassium, and sodium is regulated according to serum plasma levels.
   3. Increased intake of carbohydrates and protein of high biologic value.
C. Dialysis (see Box 23-3): indications are volume overload, BUN level greater than 120 mg/dL, metabolic acidosis, increased potassium with electrocardiographic changes, pericardial effusion, and cardiac tamponade.

Nursing Interventions

Goal: To maintain client in functional homeostasis and monitor renal function.
A. Identify and monitor high-risk clients (any client with a transient or significant decrease in blood pressure, regardless of the precipitating cause).
B. Maintain accurate intake and output record.
C. Determine weight daily (client may lose 0.2 to 0.3 kg/day during oliguric phase).
D. Assess fluid balance (hypervolemia or hypovolemia), urine specific gravity, pulmonary status, cardiac output, mental status changes.
E. Assess status of electrolytes and renal parameters: serum potassium, BUN, creatinine, phosphate levels; evaluate fluctuations of serum sodium levels.
F. Evaluate for hypertension or hypotension.

Box 23-3   TYPES OF DIALYSIS

Hemodialysis
Circulation of the client's blood through a compartment that contains an artificial semipermeable membrane surrounded by dialysate fluid, which removes excess body fluid by creating a pressure differential between the blood and the dialysate solution.

Continuous Renal Replacement Therapy (CRRT)
An alternative measure for treating acute renal failure. The uremic toxins are removed slowly and continuously. This allows for constant maintenance of acid-base and electrolyte balance in an unstable client. Can be used in conjunction with hemodialysis. There are two types: continuous arteriovenous hemofiltration (CAVH) and continuous venovenous hemofiltration (CVVH).

Peritoneal Dialysis
Utilization of the peritoneal cavity and the peritoneum as the semipermeable membrane that removes excess fluid.

Continuous Ambulatory Peritoneal Dialysis
The dialysate is infused into the abdomen and remains there for a specified time (2 to 6 hours). The dialysate is removed by gravity drainage after the prescribed time.

Automated Peritoneal Dialysis
Uses a peritoneal dialysis cycling machine. It can be done continuously, intermittently, or nightly. Most clients prefer to have the dialysis done at night.

G. Support involved body systems.
  1. Cardiac dysrhythmias.
  2. Pulmonary function.
H. Avoid nephrotoxic medications, including NSAIDs.
Goal: To maintain nutrition.
A. Maintain dietary restrictions on sodium, potassium, and protein.
B. Encourage intake of carbohydrates and fats for energy source. Caloric needs are 30 to 35 kcal/kg.
C. Offer small frequent feedings; limit fluids.
D. Total parenteral or enteral nutrition may be necessary to promote healing if caloric intake cannot be maintained.
Goal: To prevent infection.
A. Avoid use of indwelling urinary catheter, if possible.
B. Assess for development of infectious processes (local or systemic). Client is at increased risk because of compromised immune system; may not have an elevated temperature.
C. Assess for and prevent UTI.
Goal: To prevent skin breakdown.
A. Frequent turning and positioning; inspect the skin for problem areas.
B. Beds and protective devices are used to prevent pressure areas (see Pressure Ulcers section in Chapter 11).
C. Frequent range of motion and activities to increase circulation.

Goal: To provide emotional support.
A. Always explain procedures.
B. Provide honest information regarding progress of condition.
C. May take 3 to 12 months for recovery.
D. Encourage client to express fears and concerns regarding condition.

Chronic Renal Failure

Chronic renal failure is a progressive, irreversible reduction in renal function such that the kidneys are no longer able to maintain the body environment. The GFR gradually decreases as the nephrons are destroyed. The nephrons left intact are subjected to an increased workload, resulting in hypertrophy and inability to concentrate urine.

Stages of Chronic Renal Failure
A. Diminished renal reserve.
  1. Normal BUN and serum creatinine levels.
  2. Absence of symptoms.
  3. The healthier kidney tissue compensates for the diseased tissue.
  4. GFR 60% to 89% of normal.
B. Renal insufficiency.
  1. GFR is 25% of normal.
  2. BUN and serum creatinine levels are increased (azotemia); decreased urinary creatinine clearance.
  3. Mild anemia.
  4. Impaired urine concentration leading to nocturia, then polyuria.
  5. Headaches.
C. End-stage renal failure (uremia).
  1. GFR is less than 10% of normal.
    a. Severe azotemia.
    b. Hyperkalemia, hypernatremia, and hyperphosphatemia.
    c. Metabolic acidosis.
    d. Altered renin-angiotension system.
    e. Decreased erythropoietin production.
  2. Urinary system: specific gravity of urine fixed at 1.010; proteinuria, casts, pyuria, hematuria; oliguria eventually leads to anuria less than 100 mL/24 hr.
  3. Endocrine system.
    a. Hyperparathyroidism causes hypocalcemia and hyperphosphatemia resulting in demineralization of the bones (renal osteodystrophy).
    b. Hypothyroidism.
  4. Hematologic system: anemia and bleeding, infection.
  5. Cardiovascular system: hypertension, CHF, uremic pericarditis, pericardial effusion, atherosclerotic heart disease.
  6. Gastrointestinal system: anorexia, nausea, vomiting, ammonia odor (uremic fetor) to the breath,

gastrointestinal bleeding, peptic ulcer disease, gastritis.

7. Metabolic system: hyperglycemia, hyperlipidemia, gout, hypoproteinemia, carbohydrate intolerance.
8. Neurologic system: general central nervous system depression and peripheral neuropathy, headaches, seizures, sleep disturbances.
9. Musculoskeletal system: renal osteodystrophy, tissue calcification.
10. Integumentary system: yellow/gray discoloration, pruritus, uremic frost, ecchymosis.
11. Psychologic changes: emotional lability, withdrawal, depression, and psychosis, personality and behavioral changes.

Assessment

A. Risk factors/etiology.
1. Chronic hypertension and poorly controlled diabetes account for about 70% of cases of chronic renal failure.
2. Chronic glomerulonephritis and pyelonephritis.
3. Nephrosclerosis and renal artery disease.
4. Polycystic kidney disease.
5. Renal disease caused by nephrotoxic drugs or chemicals.
6. Systemic lupus erythematosus (SLE).
7. Chronic kidney disease (CKD) is more common in African Americans and Native Americans.
B. Diagnostics (see Appendix 23-1).
1. Elevated blood sugar and triglyceride levels.
2. Increased serum potassium level.
3. Decreased hemoglobin and hematocrit.

Treatment

A. Medical.
1. Measures to reduce serum potassium level (see discussion under acute renal failure).
2. Antihypertensives (see Appendix 16-5).
3. Diuretics: thiazide and loop diuretics may be used early in the course of disease.
4. Erythropoietin **(Epogen, Procrit, Aranesp)** for treatment of anemia.
5. Phosphate binders and supplemental vitamin D for renal osteodystrophy.
B. Dietary.
1. Problems with the client losing body weight, both adipose tissue and muscle mass.
2. Restricted protein intake; may vary from just a decrease in protein intake to a specific restriction of 20 to 40 g/day.
3. Protein should be of a high biologic value (1.2 to 1.3 g/kg); this enhances the utilization of the amino acids and results in formation of fewer nitrogen waste products.
4. Fluid restriction: 600 to 1000 mL, adjusted according to urinary output and/or dialysis.
5. Sodium and potassium restriction: based on laboratory values.

C. Dialysis (see Box 23-3).
D. Surgical: kidney transplantation—the primary limiting factor in the number of transplantations done is the availability of kidneys; the average wait is 18 months to 4 years; clients with blood types B and O have the longest wait.
1. Recipient criteria: candidates are evaluated on an individual basis as to how well they would benefit from transplantation.
   a. Candidates are usually younger than 70 years, have a life expectancy of at least 2 more years, and have reasonable expectations that the transplantation will improve the quality of life.
   b. Infection, disseminated malignancy, refractory cardiac disease, chronic respiratory failure, and unresolved psychologic disorders are contraindications to transplantation; the presence of hepatitis B or C is not contraindicated if controlled.
2. Donor criteria: living related donors provide the best possible match with a 95% 1-year graft survival; when they are not available, cadaver donors are considered; these have a 90% 1-year graft survival.

Nursing Interventions

Goal: To assist the client to maintain homeostasis in early chronic renal failure.

A. Evaluate adequacy of fluid balance.
1. Determine weight daily.
2. Control hypertension.
3. Discuss with the client how to monitor fluid intake and plan for the allocated amount to be distributed over the day.

ALERT Monitor hydration status, identify signs of fluid and electrolyte imbalance, and identify interventions to correct any imbalance.

B. Encourage nutritional intake within dietary guidelines.
1. Relieve gastrointestinal dysfunctions before serving meals.
2. Plan diet according to client's preferences, if possible.
3. Advise client that most salt substitutes contain potassium and should not be used.
C. Prevent problem of constipation.
1. Include bran/fiber in diet.
2. Stool softeners.
D. Avoid use of sedatives and hypnotics; increased sensitivity to these medications is caused by decreased ability of kidney to metabolize and excrete them.
E. Monitor electrolyte balance, especially levels of potassium and calcium.

! **NURSING PRIORITY** Hypocalcemia and hyperkalemia are critical problems and may cause fatal dysrhythmias.

F. Assess cardiovascular status to determine how effectively the client's cardiovascular system is compensating for the increased fluid load and increased workload from the chronic anemic state.

G. Assess client for bleeding tendencies initially related to a decrease in production of erythropoietin and decreased platelet adhesiveness. Encourage intake of folic acid (1 mg daily) for red blood cell production and integrity.

H. Evaluate client for pruritus and assist with measures to decrease skin irritation and itching.

I. Avoid products containing magnesium (antacids).

J. Assess client's activity tolerance in relation to anemia.

Goal: To provide emotional support and to promote psychologic equilibrium.

A. Encourage client to express concerns.

B. Recognize that the long-term management of a chronic disease may lead to anxiety and depression.

C. Encourage ventilation of feelings regarding lifestyle changes.

D. Encourage client and family members to seek out support groups and community resources, as well as other clients with renal failure who are undergoing the same types of treatment.

 Renal Transplant

The transplantation of a kidney from a compatible-blood-typed deceased donor, blood relative, or a live donor. Transplanted kidney is usually placed extraperitoneally in the iliac fossa (usually right side to facilitate anastomoses and decrease occurrence of ileus).

Assessment

A. Recipient selection: based on a variety of factors—history of disseminated malignancies, untreated cardiac disease, chronic respiratory failure, extensive vascular disease, chronic infection, and noncompliance with medical regimens would contraindicate a transplant.

B. Rejection.
   1. Hyperacute (antibody-mediated): not common.
      a. Occurs within minutes to hours after transplant.
      b. No treatment; transplanted kidney removed.
   2. Acute rejection: mediated by cytotoxic T lymphocytes.
      a. Can occur within days; 3 months is most common time, but can be as late as 2 years; it is common to have at least one rejection episode.
      b. Increased white blood cell count, fever.
      c. Deteriorating renal function: increasing serum creatinine and BUN levels, increasing blood pressure.
      d. Tenderness over graft site—often an early sign, along with malaise.
      e. Hypertension.
      f. Treatment is increased immunosuppressive therapy: usually high-dose steroids, polyclonal or monoclonal antibody therapy.
   3. Chronic rejection: mediated by B cells and some T cells.
      a. Occurs over months or years and is due to gradual occlusion of the renal vasculature. It is irreversible, and the client will again require dialysis and/or be placed back on the transplant list.
      b. Hypertension, increasing serum creatinine and BUN levels, and proteinuria.
      c. Graft tenderness, malaise, and signs of early end-stage renal disease.
      d. Treatment is supportive.
         (1) Change immunosuppressive therapy or increase doses.
         (2) Add tacrolimus **(Prograf)** or mycophenolate mofetil **(CellCept).**

Treatment

A. Immunosuppressant medications (Appendix 23-3).

B. Steroids (Appendix 6-7).

Nursing Interventions

Goal: To provide preoperative care for client scheduled for kidney transplantation.

A. Maintain client's metabolic state as close to homeostasis as possible; continue with dialysis.

B. Tissue typing and antibody screening are conducted to determine histocompatibility of the donor and recipient.

C. Immunosuppressant drugs: may be started prior to surgery.

D. Conduct routine preoperative procedures, including labeling the arm with vascular access for dialysis, because the client may require dialysis in the immediate postoperative period.

Goal: To provide postoperative care for the kidney transplant recipient.

A. Immunosuppressant therapy is continued indefinitely; the most frequent combination of maintenance therapy consists of azathioprine, cyclosporine, and prednisone.

B. Assess for renal graft function.
   1. Maintain fluid and electrolyte balances because of early diuresis. Avoid dehydration.
   2. Cadaveric transplant recipients may need dialysis because of acute tubular necrosis until the transplanted kidney begins to function.
   3. A sudden decrease or change in urine output should be reported.

C. Monitor for rejection.

D. Prevent and monitor for infection (UTI, pneumonia, and sepsis are biggest threats in the early posttransplantation period; fungal and viral infections are also common).
   1. It is important to make a distinction between infection and rejection, because impaired renal function and fever occur in both.
   2. Symptoms of septicemia: infection, shaking, chills, fever, tachycardia, leukocytosis, and tachypnea.

E. Atherosclerotic cardiovascular disease is common in transplant recipients. It is the leading cause of death in these clients.

F. Promote adaptation and psychologic support for the client who has undergone successful transplantation.
   1. Often, there is a continual fear of possible rejection.
   2. A major concern of the client and the family is related to long-term use of immunosuppressant medication, which puts tremendous psychologic and financial stress on the family.
   3. Refer client to community and national agencies: National Association of Patients of Hemodialysis and Transplantation, Inc. and the National Kidney Foundation.

Dialysis

Dialysis is the passage of particles (ions) from an area of high concentration to an area of low concentration across a semipermeable membrane.

A. Water, by osmosis, will move toward the solution in which the ion concentration is the greatest.
B. When hemodialysis is performed, the semipermeable membrane used has pores that are large enough for waste products and water to move through but too small for blood cells and protein molecules to pass through. In peritoneal dialysis, the same process occurs, except that the client's own intraabdominal peritoneal membrane is used and protein is lost due to the pore size.
C. Indications.
   1. GFR less than 15 mL/min.
   2. Fluid volume overload.
   3. Serum potassium level greater than 6 mEq/L.
   4. BUN level greater than 120 mg/dL.
   5. Uremia, uncontrolled hypertension, and metabolic acidosis.
D. Types of dialysis (Box 23-3). Note that dialysis solutions are High-Alert Medications.

Nursing Interventions

Goal: To remove waste products of metabolism and excess fluid; to maintain a safe concentration of blood components.

A. Peritoneal dialysis.
   1. Prepare client for procedure: establish baseline criteria of lab values, weight, and vital signs; bowel and bladder should be empty.
   2. Provide support and information to the client when the peritoneal catheter is first inserted.
      a. Permanent peritoneal catheters are fitted with a device to keep them in place; types of catheters—bent neck, curl, and disc.
      b. Temporary peritoneal catheters are inserted, and usually, a purse-string suture holds them in place; this usually occurs in the intensive care unit.
   3. Type of peritoneal dialysis being used and the physical stability of the client determine how long each cycle of dialysis will take.
      a. Cycle is initiated with the inflow of the dialysate by gravity into the abdominal cavity. The client should be carefully observed during the initial infusion to determine how well he or she will tolerate the additional fluid in the abdominal cavity. Initial infusion is usually 1 to 2 L over 10 to 20 minutes (fill time).
      b. The dialysate remains in the abdomen (dwell time) and is allowed to drain by gravity (drain time). The dwell time and drain time are specified in the doctor's orders. Seriously ill clients may receive up to 24 exchanges in a day.
      c. One exchange constitutes infusion, dwell time, and drainage.
      d. The dialysate should be warmed to body temperature before it is infused (do not use a microwave oven) to increase clearance.
      e. The procedure should be considered sterile in that masks and sterile gloves should be used when accessing the catheter to change the tubing. Remember the catheter is an open conduit to the peritoneal cavity.
   4. Insufficient outflow.
      a. Constipation is the primary cause of inflow and outflow problems.
      b. Check the tubing for patency and keep drainage bag below the level of the abdomen.
      c. Turn client from side to side or put client in semi-Fowler's position to increase abdominal pressure.
      d. Gently massaging the abdomen can also help.
   5. Complications: possible bowel perforation from catheter insertion, peritonitis, bleeding, hypoalbuminemia, hyperglycemia in clients with diabetes.

> **NURSING PRIORITY** If dialysate is left in the peritoneal cavity too long, then hyperglycemia may occur. Heparinization is not required for peritoneal dialysis, as it is for hemodialysis.

B. Hemodialysis.
   1. Vascular access site must be established; access may be temporary or permanent (Figure 23-4).
      a. External arteriovenous shunts: temporary catheters are inserted into an artery and into a vein and are connected together on the outside of the arm in a U pattern.
      b. Internal arteriovenous fistula or graft: an artery and a vein in the arm are anastomosed either directly or via a synthetic graft; access is achieved via two 14- to 16-gauge needles inserted into the access site.
      c. After an internal access site is created, it must heal before it can be used for dialysis.
   2. Evaluate access site for patency: the appropriate method to determine patency depends on the type of vascular access used; auscultate for bruit or palpate for a thrill over site.
   3. Do not take blood pressure, obtain blood samples, or infuse fluids or medications in the access site or the extremity that has a vascular access site.
   4. Assess the patency of the pulses distal to the access site.

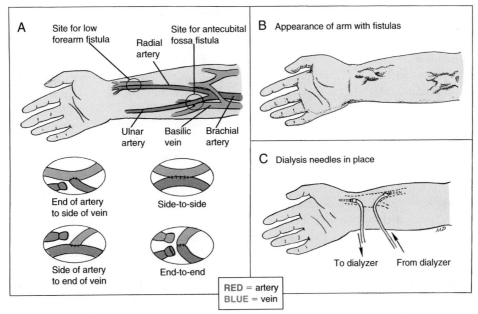

FIGURE 23-4 Internal Arteriovenous Fistula. Surgical creation of an arteriovenous anastomosis provides easy access to blood for hemodialysis. This method reduces the risk for infection and makes external shunts unnecessary except during hemodialysis. The internal fistula must be created 2 to 6 weeks before it can be used. A, Types of fistulas. B, Appearance of arm with fistulas. C, Dialysis needles in place. (From Black JM, Hawks JH: *Medical-surgical nursing: clinical management for positive outcomes,* ed 8, Philadelphia, 2009, Saunders.)

ALERT Provide care for client with a vascular access site before and after hemodialysis.

Goal: To maintain homeostasis after hemodialysis.

A. Determine whether medications need to be withheld before dialysis (antihypertensives); in hospitalized clients there are often standing orders for these situations.

B. Assess weight, blood pressure, peripheral edema, lung and heart sounds, and vascular access site before and after dialysis.

C. Most common side effects are hypotension, headache, muscle cramps, and bleeding from access site; monitor client for postural hypotension. If client has bleeding from the access site, apply pressure evenly and notify the dialysis unit.

D. Complications.
   1. Dialysis disequilibrium syndrome: cerebral edema and neurologic complications (headache, nausea, vomiting, seizures); may be minimized by slower dialysis.
   2. Sepsis, hepatitis B and C.

Goal: To maintain homeostasis during and after peritoneal dialysis.

A. Pain is common during first few exchanges; should gradually decrease.

B. Assess for development of peritonitis; antibiotics may be added to dialysate.

C. Dialysate should return clear to slightly yellow tinged; should not be cloudy or opaque.

D. Closely monitor blood pressure and activity after dialysis.

E. Increase protein in diet to compensate for removal of protein in dialysis; low protein level will impair tissue healing.

Goal: To provide emotional support and to promote psychologic equilibrium.

A. Encourage client to express feelings of anger and depression. An increased rate of suicide exists among clients undergoing dialysis.

B. Encourage appropriate coping skills.

C. Clients undergoing chronic dialysis are in limbo; they know they are probably not going to get better and that they may or may not receive a transplant. Frequently, they have ambivalent feelings about dialysis; it maintains life but severely restricts lifestyle.

Renal Tumors

The majority of renal tumors are malignant and occur more frequently in men between the ages of 50 and 70 years. Most often, the tumor begins in the renal cortex, where it can actually become quite large before it begins to compress the adjacent renal tissue. The most common areas of metastasis are the liver, lungs, and bone, especially the mediastinum.

Risk Factors

A. Cigarette smoking is one of the most significant risk factors.

B. Obesity.

C. Exposure to asbestos, cadmium, and gasoline.

Assessment

A. Clinical manifestations.
  1. Palpable abdominal mass.
  2. Hematuria, flank pain.
  3. Weight loss, weakness, anemia, hypertension.
B. Diagnostics (see Appendix 23-1).

Treatment

A. Medical.
  1. Palliative radiation therapy.
  2. Biologic therapy with alpha interferon and interleukin-2.
B. Surgical: radical nephrectomy (includes kidney, adrenal gland, ureter, lymph nodes, and surrounding fascia).

Nursing Interventions

Goal: To provide preoperative nursing care (see Chapter 3).
A. Inform client that flank incision will be on affected side and that surgery will be performed in a hyperextended, side-lying position.
B. Often, client experiences postoperative muscle aches and discomfort as a result of surgical positioning.
C. Radiation, biologic therapy, or both after surgery.

Goal: To provide postoperative care.
A. Urinary output is important to assess; catheters should be labeled, and drainage should be recorded accurately.
B. Because of the level of the incision, respiratory complications are common; encourage coughing and deep breathing, as well as incentive spirometry, every 2 hours while client is awake.
C. Assess for abdominal distention and paralytic ileus.
D. Monitor for unstable blood pressure after surgery; may be caused by removal of adrenal gland.
E. Provide adequate pain control.

Goal: To provide supportive nursing care in relation to malignancy.
See Chapter 8 for detailed nursing management.

Appendix 23-1 DIAGNOSTICS OF THE URINARY-RENAL SYSTEM

LABORATORY TESTS	NORMAL	CLINICAL AND NURSING IMPLICATIONS
BUN level	10-20 mg/dL	Common test used to diagnose renal problems; may be affected by an increase in protein intake or tissue breakdown.
Creatinine level	0.5-1.5 mg/dL	End product of protein and muscle catabolism; more accurate determinate of renal function than the BUN level; values are higher in males. Elevated in renal disease.
Calcium level	9-11 mg/dL	Provides the matrix for bone and is important in muscle contraction, neurotransmission, and clotting; in chronic renal failure, low levels of calcium lead to renal osteodystrophy.
Phosphorus level	2.5-4.8 mg/dL	Phosphorus and calcium balances are inversely related; when phosphorus level is elevated, calcium level is decreased, which is seen in renal disease.
Urinalysis		Obtain first-voided specimen in the morning. Presence of protein, WBC, RBC, glucose, bacteria, and hyaline casts indicate problems. Dipstick urinalysis is initially performed to determine levels of nitrites and leukocyte esterase related to infections.
Urine culture and sensitivity		Colony count of at least 100,000 colonies/mL of urine indicates infection.
Urinary creatinine clearance	Males: 21-26 mg/kg/24 hr Females: 16-22 mg/kg/24 hr	Measure of GFR; 24-hour urine collection must be done; have client void and discard the first specimen and then begin timing the test; specimens should be kept cool or refrigerated. Decreased in renal disease.
Urine specific gravity	Adults: 1.003-1.030 Children: 1.001-1.030	May be increased when the client is dehydrated and with glomerulonephritis. A decrease is associated with decreased tubular absorption. In renal failure it may be fixed at 1.000 to 1.012. Proteinuria will increase the specific gravity.

Appendix 23-1   DIAGNOSTICS OF THE URINARY-RENAL SYSTEM—cont'd

Laboratory Diagnostics

PROCEDURE

KUB x-ray exam: A flat plate x-ray film of the abdomen and pelvis.

Intravenous urography (IVP or excretory urogram): IV injection of radiopaque dye to visualize the urinary tract system.

Retrograde pyelogram: An x-ray study of the urinary tract conducted during a cystoscopic exam; ureteral catheters are inserted into the renal pelvis, and dye is injected (retrograde) into the catheters.

Renal arteriogram (angiogram): An IV injection of radiopaque dye into the renal artery (catheter is inserted into femoral artery) to visualize the renal blood vessels.

Renogram (renal scan): An IV injection of a radioactive nuclide (isotope) followed by use of a scanning device to detect radioactive emissions from the kidney(s); identifies renal blood flow, tubular functions, and renal excretion.

Cystoscopy: A direct method to visualize the urethra and bladder by use of a tubular lighted scope (cystoscope). Scope may be inserted via the urethra or percutaneously.

Bladder scan: A portable ultrasound scanner used to estimate residual urine in the bladder.

Urodynamic studies

Cystometrogram (CMG): A procedure to determine the pressure exerted against the bladder wall by inserting a catheter and instilling water or saline solution; used to evaluate bladder capacity, bladder pressure, and voiding reflexes.

Urethral pressure profile or urethral pressure profilometry (UPP): Evaluates for urinary incontinence and retention by recording variations of pressure in the urethra.

Urine stream testing: Evaluates pelvic floor muscle strength.

CLINICAL AND NURSING IMPLICATIONS

Bowel preparation may or may not be indicated.

1. Client's status is NPO for 8 hours before procedure.
2. Cathartic or enema given the evening before procedure.
3. Radiocontrast medium may cause an allergic (hypersensitivity) reaction in iodine-sensitive clients.
4. Instruct client that he or she will need to lie still on table while serial x-ray films are taken.
5. Evaluate for iodine reaction after test and force fluids after test to flush out the dye.
6. Be sure the older adult client is not dehydrated before the procedure; the contrast medium is nephrotoxic and can precipitate renal failure.

1. Client's status is NPO for 8 hours before test.
2. Assess for sensitivity to iodine.
3. Explain that there may be discomfort on insertion of the cystoscope.
4. General anesthesia may be indicated for procedure.

1. Client's status is NPO after midnight.
2. Preoperative medication is administered.
3. Client should be assessed for sensitivity to iodine before the procedure.
4. Evaluate venipuncture insertion site every 15 to 30 min after the procedure to assess for bleeding.
5. Assess pulses distal to the injection site to detect occluded blood flow. Compare pre- and postprocedure pulses.
6. Sandbag or pressure dressing may be applied to groin.

1. No specific activity or dietary restrictions.
2. Explain procedure to client.

1. Force fluids or administer fluids intravenously.
2. Explain lithotomy position that will be used.
3. Client may have general anesthesia or conscious sedation.
4. Preoperative medication is given.
5. Evaluate urine output after procedure; check for frequency, pink-tinged urine, and burning on urination (these are expected effects and will decrease with time).
6. Evaluate for orthostatic hypotension and thrombus formation after the procedure.
7. Provide warm sitz baths and mild analgesics to alleviate urethral discomfort.

1. No specific preparation.
2. After client voids, apply gel to the suprapubic area, and use scanner to visualize bladder and possible retained urine.
3. Make certain that the crosshairs on the aiming icon on the scanner are centered on or over the bladder; if crosshairs are offset then the reading may not be accurate.

1. Assess and evaluate for UTI after procedure.
2. Test is often indicated for clients having difficulty with urinary control (e.g., those with spinal cord traumatic injuries, stroke, etc.).

Continued

Appendix 23-1   DIAGNOSTICS OF THE URINARY-RENAL SYSTEM—cont'd

PROCEDURE	CLINICAL AND NURSING IMPLICATIONS
Renal biopsy: A percutaneous needle biopsy to evaluate renal disease by obtaining a specimen of renal tissue for pathologic examination. Rarely done if client has only one kidney.	1. Results of blood coagulation studies should be available on the chart before the biopsy procedure. 2. Results of IVP or ultrasound studies should be available before the biopsy. 3. Immediately after the procedure, pressure dressing is applied to biopsy site and checked frequently for bleeding. Right kidney is the usual biopsy site. 4. Assess for gross hematuria, flank pain, or a rise or fall in blood pressure. 5. Report pain radiating from the flank area to the abdomen. 6. Encourage intake of fluids: 3000 mL per day unless the client has renal insufficiency. 7. Assess for complication of hemorrhage; may necessitate emergency surgical drainage or nephrectomy.
Renal ultrasound exam: A noninvasive procedure in which ultrasound waves are used, with the aid of a computer, to record images related to tissue density.	1. Encourage fluids because test requires a full bladder. 2. Place in prone position. 3. Skin care to remove sonographic gel after procedure.

BUN, Blood urea nitrogen; *GFR,* glomerular filtration rate; *IV,* intravenous; *IVP,* intravenous pyelogram; *KUB,* kidneys, ureters, and bladder; *NPO,* nothing by mouth; *UTI,* urinary tract infection.

Appendix 23-2   RENAL MEDICATIONS

℞

General Nursing Implications

— Encourage intake of 2000-3000 mL of fluid per day during treatment.
— Continue medication therapy until all medication has been taken.
— Most medications are better absorbed on an empty stomach; however, if GI distress occurs, they may be taken with food.
— Monitor intake and output, as well as symptoms of increasing renal problems.
— Check drug package insert for interactions with anticoagulants.
— See Appendix 6-9 for sulfonamide medications for UTI.

MEDICATIONS	SIDE EFFECTS	NURSING IMPLICATIONS
Urinary Tract Antiseptics These drugs concentrate in the urine and are active against common urinary tract pathogens; they do not affect infections in blood or tissue.		
Nitrofurantoin **(Furadantin, Macrodantin, APO-Nitrofurantoin, Nitrofan):** PO, IM	GI upset, blood dyscrasia, pulmonary reactions	1. Requires adequate renal function to concentrate medication in urine. 2. Should not be administered to renal transplant recipients. 3. Will turn the urine brownish-orange.
Urinary Analgesics Pain relievers typically used on urinary tract mucosa.		
Phenazopyridine hydrochloride **(AZO-Standard, Pyridium, Urodine, Urogesic):** PO Available OTC	Headache, GI disturbances	1. Contraindicated in renal and liver dysfunction. 2. Advise client to report any yellow discoloration of skin or eyes. 3. Urine will turn orange. 4. Administer with caution in clients with impaired renal function. 5. Can alter dipstick urine results.

Appendix 23-2 **RENAL MEDICATIONS—cont'd**

MEDICATIONS	SIDE EFFECTS	NURSING IMPLICATIONS
Bladder Relaxants Suppress detrusor contractions and enhance bladder storage (drugs with anticholinergic activity).		
Oxybutynin (**Ditropan, Ditropan XL**): PO, transdermal	Drowsiness, dizziness, weakness, blurred vision, dry mouth, constipation	1. Contraindicated in glaucoma, myasthenia gravis, or GI obstruction. 2. Used cautiously in older adults. 3. Can relieve bladder spasms in surgical clients. 4. Monitor intraocular pressure.
Tolterodine (**Detrol, Detrol LA**): PO Solifenacin succinate (**Vesicare**): PO	Fatigue, headache, dry mouth, dry eyes, constipation	1. Grapefruit juice can increase blood levels. 2. Caution client to avoid use of alcohol or OTC antihistamines.
Glycoprotein Hormones Stimulate bone marrow production of RBCs.		
Epoetin alfa (**Epogen, Procrit**): IV, subQ	Hypertension, thromboembolic problems, headaches, GI disturbances	1. Closely evaluate hemodialysis access ports for clotting. 2. Evaluate client for adequate serum iron level, hematocrit, and blood pressure; adequate levels are required for medication to be effective. 3. Uses: Maintain hemoglobin and hematocrit values in client with renal failure and those who are HIV+ or on chemotherapy. Do not administer if Hgb is 12 or greater.

GI, Gastrointestinal; *HIV+*, human immunodeficiency virus–positive; *IV*, intravenously; *PO*, by mouth (orally); *subQ*, subcutaneously; *UTI*, urinary tract infection.

Appendix 23-3 **IMMUNOSUPPRESSIVE MEDICATIONS**

General Nursing Implications
— Avoid exposure to infection; wash hands frequently.
— Wear protective clothing; use sunscreen.
— Report any sore throat, fever, or other signs of infection to health care provider.
— Take medication at the same time each day to maintain consistent blood levels.
— No live virus vaccines or immunity-conferring agents should be administered while client is immunosuppressed.
— Depending on level of immunosuppression, client may need protective isolation.

MEDICATIONS	ACTION	SIDE EFFECTS	NURSING IMPLICATIONS
Immunosuppressive Medications Inhibit the immunologic response.			
Azathioprine (**Imuran**): PO, IV	Inhibits RNA and DNA protein synthesis Suppresses T-cell (cell-mediated) production Antiinflammatory properties Used to suppress kidney transplant rejection and treat IBS and RA	Dose- and duration-dependent Bone marrow suppression: leukopenia, thrombocytopenia, anemia Nausea, vomiting, anorexia Alopecia, rash	1. Interacts with allopurinol, causing an increase in **Imuran** toxicity. 2. Avoid use in pregnancy. 3. Take with food or milk to decrease GI upset. 4. Should not be given to client with active infection. 5. Follow-up CBCs should be done at least monthly while client is taking medication. 6. Closely monitor client for development of infections.

Continued

Appendix 23-3   IMMUNOSUPPRESSIVE MEDICATIONS—cont'd

MEDICATIONS	ACTION	SIDE EFFECTS	NURSING IMPLICATIONS
Cyclosporine **(Sandimmune, Neoral):** PO, IV	Inhibits T-lymphocyte proliferation and function	Dose- and duration-dependent Infections, nephrotoxicity, hepatotoxicity, hypertension, hirsutism, gum hyperplasia, tremors, blood dyscrasias	1. Monitor renal function because nephrotoxicity occurs frequently. 2. Avoid use in pregnancy. 3. Use the pipette supplied by manufacturer to measure dose; mix with 4-8 oz. of water, milk, or juice. 4. Evaluate blood pressure and report elevations (especially occurs with heart transplants). 5. Monitor liver function studies. 6. Good oral hygiene should be practiced to reduce gum problems. 7. Teach client that he/she should not stop taking the medication or change dosage without physician's order. 8. Serum blood levels and CBC are monitored at regular intervals. 9. Hirsutism that occurs is reversible.
Methotrexate **(Mexate)** Cyclophosphamide **(Cytoxan)**	See Appendix 8-1 See Appendix 8-1		
Antilymphocyte globulin **(ALG)** Murine monoclonal anti-lymphocyte therapy **(OKT3)** Daclizumab **(Zenapax)**	Polyclonal antibody that blocks function of T cell by reacting with T_3 antigen Monoclonal antibody that binds to CD3 receptors and inhibits T-cell proliferation	Fever, chills, tachycardia, hypotension, bronchospasm Aseptic meningitis **(OKT3)** GI toxicity (diarrhea, nausea, abdominal pain)	1. More than 50% of clients experience a fever. 2. Have epinephrine and supportive emergency care available, because an allergic reaction can occur at any time during therapy. 3. Administer slowly over 4-6 hr. 4. Client may be premedicated with acetaminophen, diphenhydramine HCl, or methylprednisolone.
Methylprednisolone sodium **(Solu-Medrol)**	See Appendix 6-7		
Tacrolimus **(Prograf, FK506)**	Inhibits T-lymphocyte production	Hepatotoxicity, nephrotoxicity, neurotoxicity, hyperglycemia, seizures, hypertension, GI effects	1. Monitor blood pressure closely. 2. Increases risk for infection.
Sirolimus **(Rapamune)**	Suppresses lymphocyte proliferation; inhibits B cells from synthesizing antibodies	GI toxicity (diarrhea, nausea, vomiting, abdominal pain)	1. Has synergistic effect with cyclosporine and corticosteroids. 2. Increases risk for infection. 3. Increases cholesterol levels.
Mycophenolate mofetil **(CellCept)**	Antimetabolite that inhibits DNA and RNA synthesis	Leukopenia, thrombocytopenia, GI (diarrhea, nausea, vomiting), UTI, hypertension, peripheral edema	1. Usually used in combination with cyclosporine, tacrolimus, sirolimus, or glucocorticoids. 2. Give on an empty stomach.

CBCs, Complete blood counts; *GI,* gastrointestinal; *IL-2,* interleukin 2; *IV,* intravenous; *PO,* by mouth (orally); *RA,* rheumatoid arthritis; *UTI,* urinary tract infection.

Appendix 23-4 URINARY DIVERSION

A urinary diversion is a means of diverting urinary output from the bladder to an external device or via a new avenue (Figure 23-5).

Temporary Urinary Diversion

Nephrostomy tubes (catheters): Insertion of catheters into the renal pelvis by surgical incision or percutaneous puncture. A small catheter is inserted into the renal pelvis and attached via connecting tubing to a closed-system drainage. Nephrostomy tubes may be temporary or permanent.

Nursing Implications
1. Catheter should never be clamped or irrigated (renal pelvis capacity is 3 to 5 mL).
2. Complications: Infection and secondary renal calculus formation; erosion of the duct by the catheter.

Ureteral catheters: Small, narrow catheters placed through the ureters into the renal pelvis; drain each renal pelvis individually. Often client also has a urinary retention catheter draining the urinary bladder. The catheter splints the ureters during healing and prevents edema from occluding the ureter.

Nursing Implications
1. Check frequently for placement of ureteral catheters; tension should be avoided.
2. Ureteral catheter should not be clamped or irrigated.
3. Maintain accurate intake and output records and label all catheters.

Permanent Urinary Diversion

Ileal conduit (ileal loop): Transplantation of ureters into a segment of ileum or colon, which is then brought to the abdomen; a stoma is then constructed.

Nursing Implications
1. Stoma site is marked before surgery, because a device must be worn continuously.
2. Mucus is present in the urine after surgery when ileum segment is used; encourage a high fluid intake to "flush the ileal conduit."
3. Maintain meticulous skin care and changing of appliances.
4. Provide discharge instructions in regard to symptoms of obstruction, infection, and care of the ostomy; client needs information relating to purchase of supplies, ostomy clubs, follow-up visits, enterostomal therapists, and the importance of not irrigating the ileal conduit.

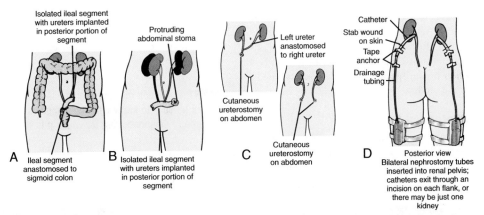

FIGURE 23-5 Urinary Diversions. A, Ureteroileosigmoidostomy. B, Ileal loop (or ileal conduit). C, Ureterostomy (transcutaneous ureterostomy and bilateral cutaneous ureterostomies). D, Nephrostomy. (From Lewis SL et al: *Medical-surgical nursing: assessment and management of clinical problems,* ed 7, St. Louis, 2007, Mosby.)

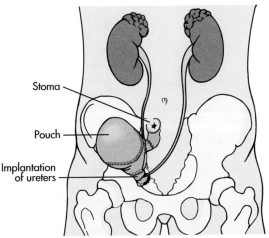

FIGURE 23-6 Creation of a Kock pouch with implantation of ureters into one intussuscepted portion of the pouch and creation of a stoma with the other intussuscepted portion. (From Lewis SL et al: *Medical-surgical nursing: assessment and management of clinical problems,* ed 7, St. Louis, 2007, Mosby.)

Continued

Appendix 23-4 URINARY DIVERSION—cont'd

Continent Urinary Diversion

Kock, Mainz, Indiana, or Florida pouch: A segment of the bowel is made into a reservoir; client is taught to use a catheter to drain the pouch and maintain continence (Figure 23-6). The main difference among the diversions is the segment of intestine utilized (ileum, ileocecal segment, or colon).

Nursing Implications

1. Client will not need to wear an appliance but will need to self-catheterize every 4 to 6 hours.
2. A small bandage/pouch may be worn to collect any mucus drainage or small leaks.

3. Continuous assessment of status of skin around stoma.
4. Client should understand how to care for the stoma before he or she leaves the hospital:
   - Know how continent diversion functions and how to prevent complications.
   - Increase fluid intake.
   - Contact health care provider if there are changes in the color of the stoma or if urine becomes dark and foul smelling.
5. A catheter will be inserted into the reservoir every 4 to 6 hours to drain urine.

Appendix 23-5 NURSING PROCEDURE: URINE SPECIMEN COLLECTION

✓ KEY POINTS: Random Sample

- May be collected at any time.
- Client may be specifically ordered to collect first voided specimen or to collect sample on second voiding.

✓ KEY POINTS: Clean Catch and Midstream

- Specimen is collected for culture.
- Cleanse urinary meatus before specimen collection.
- For midstream collection, tell client to start the urinary stream and collect the specimen after voiding has begun. Regardless of how well the urinary meatus is cleansed, the specimen must be a midstream collection or the specimen will be contaminated with the bacteria in the urethra.

✓ KEY POINTS: Catheterized Specimen

- Straight in-and-out catheterization to obtain sample for culture.
- Procedure is discouraged because of introduction of bacteria and irritation producing a urinary tract infection. More common in

 infants and children and those unable to provide a midstream specimen.

✓ KEY POINTS: 12- to 24-Hour Collection

- When the collection time is started, have the client void, discard the urine, and start the collection with the next voiding.
- Mark the collection container and collect the urine over the prescribed time frame.
- When the time frame is completed, have the client void again, add it to the specimen collection, and send to lab for evaluation.

ALERT Collection of urine specimens is a common nursing action; be sure to know why the sample is being obtained and the type of diagnostic test for which it is being collected.

Appendix 23-6 NURSING PROCEDURE: URINARY CATHETERIZATION

✓ KEY POINTS: Insertion of a Retention Catheter

- A sterile procedure.
- Lubricate catheter with sterile lubricant provided in tray.

ALERT Insert a urinary catheter.

- Cleanse the meatus:
  For a Female
  1. Cleanse the meatus with sterile cotton ball held in forceps; use one downward stroke of the forceps.
  2. Repeat at least three to four times using new sterile cotton ball each time.
  3. Continue to hold the labia apart until you insert the catheter.
  4. When urine appears, advance the catheter another 1 to 2 inches.
  For a Male
  1. Hold the penis upright. Hold the sides of the penis to prevent closing the urethra.
  2. Cleanse the meatus in a circular motion from urinary meatus to glans with sterile cotton ball held in forceps; use one downward stroke of the forceps.
  3. Repeat at least three to four times.

4. Continue to hold the penis until you insert the catheter.
5. Insert the catheter 1 to 2 inches beyond the point at which urine begins to flow. Inserting the catheter farther into the bladder ensures it is beyond the neck of the bladder.
6. Instill sterile water into balloon after catheter is inserted.
- Anchor the catheter.
  For a female: Anchor or tape catheter to the side of the leg.
  For a male: Anchor or tape catheter to the abdomen to prevent pressure on the penoscrotal angle.
- Attach drainage bag to bed frame (not side rails), so that it hangs freely, and below the level of the catheter.

✓ KEY POINTS: Providing Catheter Care

- Maintain external cleanliness around the catheter; wash thoroughly with mild soap and water when soiled—or at least once every 24 hours.
- Maintain closed system. Do not allow urine to flow from the bag or tubing back into the bladder.
- Encourage high fluid intake to maintain constant flow of urine. Increased flow of urine inhibits the upward movement of bacteria.

Appendix 23-6 NURSING PROCEDURE: URINARY CATHETERIZATION—cont'd

✓ KEY POINTS: Removal of a Catheter
- Clamp catheter.
- Do not cut the catheter with a scissors. Balloon may not totally deflate if cut.
- Withdraw fluid from balloon (usually 5 to 10 mL water in balloon.)
- Pull gently on catheter to ensure balloon is deflated before attempting to remove. Damage to the urethra can occur if balloon is not totally deflated. If the catheter has been in place for longer than 10 days, reinflate the balloon after removal to assess for degradation.
- Record output on intake and output (I&O) bedside record.
- Wash perineum with soap and water. Dry thoroughly.
- Instruct client to drink fluids as tolerated and observe for signs and symptoms of urinary tract infection (burning, frequency, urgency).
- Offer bedpan or urinal at least every 2 to 4 hours after removing catheter, until voiding occurs. Keep accurate I&O record.

Clinical Tips for Problem Solving
1. If catheter is inserted in the vagina of female client:
   - Leave the catheter in place so you do not reintroduce a new catheter into the vaginal area. Obtain a new catheter and sterile gloves.
   - If sterile field has been contaminated, obtain a whole new kit.

2. If unable to insert catheter into male client:
   - Obtain a new catheter kit.
   a. Hold penis vertical to the body.
   b. Insert catheter while applying slight traction by gently pulling upward on the shaft of the penis.
   c. If you encounter resistance, rotate the catheter, increase the traction, and change the angle of the penis slightly.
   d. When urine begins to flow, lower the penis.
3. If pain occurs during inflation of balloon:
   - Remove any injected water and insert the catheter farther into the bladder.
4. If urine exceeds 1000 mL with catheterization:
   - Clamp catheter for 20 to 30 minutes and then unclamp.
5. If catheter comes out with balloon still inserted:
   - Assess client for signs of urethral trauma (i.e., bleeding, pain).
   - Obtain a new catheter and repeat the catheterization procedure, making sure that the balloon is inflated with at least 10 mL water.
   - Monitor urine output for bleeding.

Study Questions Urinary-Renal System

More questions on companion CD!

1. The client has had a right nephrostomy tube placed after a nephrolithotomy for removal of a kidney stone. When the client returns to the room, what is a priority nursing action?
   1. Irrigate the tube with 30 mL of normal saline solution four times a day.
   2. Clamp the tube if drainage is excessive.
   3. Advance the tube 1 inch every 8 hours.
   4. Ensure that the tube is draining freely.
2. The nurse is infusing dialysate during peritoneal dialysis. What is a nursing action to make the client more comfortable at this time?
   1. Increase the rate of flow.
   2. Raise the head of the bed.
   3. Turn the client from side to side.
   4. Refrigerate the fluid before infusion.
3. A client has had a kidney stone removed, and the nurse instructs him in measures to decrease kidney stone formation in the future. Which statement by the client indicates to the nurse that he understood the teaching?
   1. "I can continue to drink soda if it is sugar free."
   2. "I should consume at least 3000 mL of fluid daily."
   3. "I should report nocturia that occurs once a night."
   4. "I will ingest megadoses of vitamins C and D daily."

4. The nurse understands that the following clinical findings are indications for dialysis. Select all that apply:
   _____ 1. Volume overload
   _____ 2. Blood urea nitrogen level of 18 mg/dL
   _____ 3. Potassium level of 5.2 mEq/L
   _____ 4. Decreased creatinine clearance
   _____ 5. Metabolic acidosis
   _____ 6. Creatinine level of 5.0 mg/dL
5. A client in renal failure is to have a serum blood urea nitrogen level determined. What will this diagnostic test measure?
   1. Concentration of the urine osmolarity and electrolytes
   2. Serum level of the end products of protein metabolism
   3. Ability of the kidneys to concentrate urine
   4. Levels of C-reactive protein to determine inflammation
6. A client with chronic renal failure has an internal venous access site for hemodialysis on her left forearm. What action will the nurse take to protect this access site?
   1. Irrigate with heparin and normal saline solution every 8 hours.
   2. Apply warm moist packs to the area after hemodialysis.
   3. Do not use the left arm to take blood pressure readings.
   4. Keep the arm elevated above the level of the heart.

7. What nursing measure would be included in the plan of care for a client with acute renal failure?
   1 Observe for signs of a secondary infection.
   2 Provide a high-protein, low-carbohydrate diet.
   3 In and out catheterization for residual urine
   4 Encourage fluids to 2000 mL in 24 hours.

8. What will the nurse identify as the goal of treatment for a client with chronic renal insufficiency?
   1 Increase the urine output by increasing liver and renal perfusion.
   2 Prevent the loss of electrolytes across the basement membrane.
   3 Increase the concentration of electrolytes in the urine.
   4 Maintain present renal function and decrease renal workload.

9. The nurse is discussing the prevention of urinary tract infections with a female client. What would be important to include in the discussion?
   1 Decrease fluid intake to decrease burning on urination.
   2 Take warm sitz baths with a mild bubble bath.
   3 Avoid spermicides with nonoxynol-9.
   4 Drink only acidic fluids such as orange juice.

10. At 9:00 a.m. a 24-hour urine collection is started. What instructions will the nurse provide to the client?
    1 Place the first voided specimen in the container and continue to collect the urine until 9:00 a.m. the following day.
    2 Discard the first morning specimen, collect urine for the next 24 hours, and make sure to void before the collection is completed at 9:00 a.m. the following day.
    3 Discard the first morning specimen because it may contain concentrated abnormal components.
    4 Collect all urine from 9:00 a.m. onward in separate containers that are labeled for time and amount of voiding.

11. Which nursing observations indicate that a male client with a kidney stone is experiencing renal colic?
    1 Severe flank pain radiating toward the testicles
    2 Stress incontinence with full bladder
    3 Hematuria and severe burning on urination
    4 Enuresis with hyperalbuminuria

12. The nurse is evaluating a client's response to hemodialysis. The laboratory values reflect that dialysis is achieving positive results. Which lab values would not reflect changes resulting from the hemodialysis?
    1 Serum creatinine levels
    2 Sedimentation rate
    3 Serum potassium levels
    4 Hemoglobin levels

13. Which of the following are the signs and symptoms of cystitis? Select all that apply:
    _____ 1 Increased bladder capacity
    _____ 2 Frequency
    _____ 3 Dysuria
    _____ 4 Nocturia
    _____ 5 Urgency
    _____ 6 Polydipsia

14. A client with chronic renal failure has been prescribed calcium carbonate. What is the rationale for this particular medication?
    1 Diminishes incidence of gastric ulcer formation
    2 Alleviates constipation
    3 Binds with phosphorus to lower concentrations
    4 Increases tubular reabsorption of sodium

15. Which of the following is an appropriate nursing action for a child with glomerulonephritis?
    1 Initiating contact isolation precautions
    2 Encouraging increased fluid intake
    3 Encouraging ambulation, as tolerated
    4 Providing a high-calorie, low-protein diet

16. The nurse understands that a client may experience pain during peritoneal dialysis because of which of the following? Select all that apply:
    _____ 1 Warming the dialysate solution before administration
    _____ 2 Too-rapid instillation of the dialysate
    _____ 3 Infiltration of solution into the bloodstream
    _____ 4 Accumulation of dialysate solution under the diaphragm
    _____ 5 Too-rapid outflow rate of the dialysate solution

17. What is significant about the development of proteinuria in a client with type 1 diabetes mellitus?
    1 Renal failure will develop in approximately 10 years.
    2 It indicates that the client's diabetes is uncontrolled.
    3 Serum creatinine will diminish as albuminuria increases.
    4 Insulin maintenance dose should be lowered.

18. A client with acute renal failure develops severe hyperkalemia. What would the nurse anticipate to be used to treat this imbalance?
    1 Furosemide (**Lasix**)
    2 Amphojel (aluminum hydroxide)
    3 50% glucose and regular insulin
    4 Epoetin (**Procrit**)

Answers and rationales to these questions are in the section at the end of the book titled Chapter Study Questions: Answers and Rationales.

CHAPTER TWENTY-FOUR

Antepartum

FAMILY PLANNING

 Infertility

Infertility is the inability to conceive a child after a year or more of regular unprotected intercourse or the inability to carry a pregnancy to live birth (recurrent miscarriages).

Assessment

A. Causes of infertility.
1. Male.
   a. Coital difficulties, testicular abnormalities.
   b. Semen factors.
      (1) Sperm abnormalities: small ejaculatory volume (less than 2 mL); low sperm count (less than 20 million/mL); poor motility of sperm.
      (2) Sperm autoantibodies caused by trauma, infection, or surgical occlusion (found after a re-anastomosis of the vas deferens).
   c. Structural abnormalities.
2. Female.
   a. Hormonal dysfunction, structural abnormalities.
   b. Coital factors: use of lubricants or douches that change the pH and may cause infection.
   c. Chronic pelvic and vaginal infections.
   d. Isoimmunization to sperm: development of antibodies.
B. Diagnostics.
1. Male.
   a. Complete history and physical examination; laboratory studies such as thyroid function tests and other endocrine tests may be ordered.
   b. Complete semen analysis.
      (1) Collection of specimen: client should avoid ejaculation for 2 to 3 days; collect a masturbated specimen in a glass jar; and transport specimen to physician's office no later than 2 hours after collection (should not be warmed or chilled); sterile, unlubricated condoms can be used for collection when clients have religious or cultural objections to masturbation.

> **❗ NURSING PRIORITY** Two or more abnormal samples must be obtained before a definitive diagnosis is made. Semen collections should be repeated at least 72 hours apart to allow for new germ cell maturation.

      (2) Normal values of semen: volume 2 to 6 mL; pH 7.2 to 8.0; density of sperm 20 to 200 million/mL *(preferably);* motility greater than 50%; forward progression greater than 2+ (on a scale from 0 to 4); morphology of sperm greater than 60% normal.
2. Female.
   a. Complete history and physical examination: includes routine complete blood count, urinalysis, serologic studies, thyroid function studies, sedimentation rate, chest x-ray film, and Papanicolaou (Pap) smear.
      (1) Hormonal assay of luteinizing hormone (LH; value is greatest at midcycle) or progesterone (peaks 8 days after the LH surge).
   b. Recording of basal body temperature (BBT) and cervical mucus to document ovulation.
      (1) BBT drops and then rises about 1° after ovulation.

> **❗ NURSING PRIORITY** Actual release of ovum occurs around 24 to 36 hours before the first temperature elevation; BBT does not predict ovulation; it only indicates that it has occurred.

      (2) A suggestion to couples for intercourse based on serial BBTs might be to recommend sexual intercourse every other day in the period of time beginning 3 to 4 days before and continuing for 2 to 3 days after the expected time of ovulation.
   c. Cervical mucus method.
      (1) Cervical mucus is thin, clear, profuse, watery, alkaline, and stringy at the time of ovulation.
      (2) Estrogen secretion is often inadequate for the development of receptive cervical mucus.
      (3) Supplemental estrogen therapy 6 days before ovulation enhances the development of *spinnbarkeit,* which means elasticity of the cervical mucus.
      (4) *Ferning* is noted on a microscopic slide and is caused by an increase in sodium chloride that crystallizes when the mucus dries on the slide.
   d. Postcoital test.
      (1) Conducted at time of ovulation, from 1 to 12 hours after coitus, to obtain a cervical mucus specimen.

(2) Purpose is to determine sperm survival and motility along with the characteristics of cervical mucus.

e. Tubal patency tests.
   (1) Hysterosalpingography or hysterogram.
      (a) Instillation of a radiopaque substance into the uterine cavity.
      (b) Reveals tubal patency and any distortions of the endometrial cavity.
      (c) Scheduled during the proliferative phase, usually 6 days after menstrual flow.
      (d) Antibiotics may be prescribed if there is a history of pelvic inflammatory disease or blocked tubes.
   (2) Laparoscopy.
      (a) Direct visualization of the pelvic organs via an incision into the abdomen (around umbilicus).
      (b) General anesthesia is used.
      (c) Discomfort from organ displacement and shoulder and chest pain caused by carbon dioxide gas in the abdomen lasting 24 to 48 hours after procedure may occur.

f. Endometrial biopsy.
   (1) A sample of the endometrium is obtained during days 1 to 2 before menstruation.
   (2) Assesses the adequacy of the endometrium for implantation, presence of polyps, and inflammatory conditions.

C. Treatment.
   1. Male.
      a. Autoimmune sperm antibodies: administration of immunosuppressants, and sperm washing-dilution insemination techniques.
      b. Poor quality or immotile sperm: artificial insemination.
   2. Female.
      a. Vaginal-cervical factors.
         (1) Vaginal fluid is acidic; cervical mucus is alkalotic.
         (2) Vaginal/cervical infections change the pH, which often destroys sperm.
         (3) Treat infections with antibiotics.
      b. Tubal factors.
         (1) Tubal infection: treated with antibiotics.
         (2) Surgery may be indicated to drain an abscess or to correct obstruction.
         (3) Tubal flushing: both diagnostic and treatment by flushing fallopian tubes with either an oil contrast media (OSCM) or a water-based contrast media (WSCM).
      c. Ovarian factors: administration of fertility medications.
         (1) Clomiphene citrate **(Clomid)**.
            (a) Indicated when ovaries are normal and pituitary gland is intact.
            (b) Increases the secretion of follicle-stimulating hormone and LH, which stimulates follicle growth.

(c) Administration: client takes it daily for 5 days, beginning on day 5 of the menstrual cycle; supplemental low-dose estrogen is usually given concurrently.
(d) Side effects: vasomotor flushes, visual spots, nausea, vomiting, headache, and hair loss.
(2) Human menopausal gonadotropin **(Pergonal)**: used when **Clomid** fails to stimulate ovulation.
   (a) Potent hormone, combination of LH and follicle-stimulating hormone obtained from postmenopausal women's urine.
   (b) Administration: given intramuscularly every day for varying periods of time during the first half of the cycle.
   (c) Couple advised to have intercourse on the day the woman receives human menopausal gonadotropin and for the next 2 days.

> **⚠ NURSING PRIORITY** The use of fertility drugs may lead to a multiple birth rate.

Nursing Interventions

Goal: To assist with the assessment and treatment of the couple's specific infertility problem.
A. Provide information regarding the normal functioning of the male and female reproductive systems.
B. Thoroughly explain specific examinations and diagnostic procedures to decrease anxiety and fear.

Goal: To provide emotional support and encourage expression of feelings connected with infertility.
A. Promote expression of feelings related to sexuality, self-esteem, and body image.
B. Assess for common reactions of surprise, denial, anger, and guilt.
C. Promote a variety of coping strategies to help deal with the uncomfortable feelings.
D. Explore alternatives such as adoption.
E. Refer to supportive community agencies.

Contraception

Contraception is the voluntary prevention of pregnancy. Two important factors influence the selection of the particular type of contraceptive method: acceptability and effectiveness.

> **ALERT** Determine client's attitude toward and use of birth control methods and consider contraindications to chosen contraceptive method.

Assessment

A. Types of contraception.
   1. Temporary contraception: methods used to delay or avoid pregnancy.
   2. Permanent: voluntary sterilization.
B. Contraceptive methods (see Appendix 24-1).

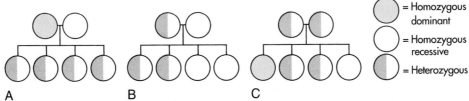

FIGURE 24-1. Possible Offspring in Three Types of Matings. A, Homozygous-dominant parent and homozygous-recessive parent. Children all heterozygous, displaying dominant trait. **B,** Heterozygous parent and homozygous-recessive parent. Children 50% heterozygous, displaying dominant trait; 50% homozygous, displaying recessive trait. **C,** Both parents heterozygous. Children 25% homozygous, displaying dominant trait; 25% homozygous, displaying recessive trait; 50% heterozygous, displaying dominant trait. (From Lowdermilk DL, Perry SE: *Maternity and women's health care,* ed 9, St. Louis, 2007, Mosby.)

Genetic Counseling

A. Definitions.
  1. Genetic (hereditary): describes any disorder or disease that is transmitted from generation to generation.
  2. Congenital: describes any disorder present at birth or existing before birth that is caused by genetic or environmental factors or both.
B. Patterns of inheritance (Figure 24-1).
  1. Autosomal recessive: examples are cystic fibrosis, phenylketonuria (PKU), sickle cell anemia, Tay-Sachs disease.
  2. Autosomal dominant: examples are Huntington's disease, Marfan syndrome, neurofibromatosis.
  3. X-linked recessive: examples are hemophilia, Duchenne muscular dystrophy, color blindness.
  4. X-linked dominant: examples are vitamin D-resistant rickets and fragile X syndrome (FXS).

Assessment

A. Families at risk.
  1. Maternal factors.
    a. Increased age.
    b. Presence of disease (e.g., diabetes mellitus, epilepsy).
    c. Reproductive history of spontaneous abortions, stillbirths, or birth defects in previous children.
  2. Family history (e.g., Huntington's chorea, hemophilia, spina bifida).
  3. Ethnicity/racial background (e.g., sickle cell trait, Tay-Sachs disease).
B. Diagnostics.
  1. Prenatal detection: amniocentesis, chorionic villus sampling (CVS), percutaneous umbilical blood sampling (PUBS), maternal alpha-fetoprotein.
  2. Postdelivery detection.
    a. Most institutions screen for inborn errors of metabolism; these tests all use the same dried blood spot. Many states screen for inborn errors in metabolism. Examples include phenylketonuria (PKU) testing, galactosemia, hypothyroidism, sickle cell anemia, maple syrup urine disease, homocystinuria, biotinidase deficiency. The list of "screenable" tests will certainly increase as technology improves.
    b. Cytologic studies.
      (1) Detect chromosomal abnormalities.
      (2) Cells from the bone marrow, skin, or blood are obtained to prepare a karyotype.
    c. Dermatoglyphics.
      (1) The assessment of the dermal ridges in the palm, toes, or soles of feet.
      (2) Characteristic palm creases: simian line (Down syndrome).

Nursing Interventions

Goal: To allow families to make informed decisions about reproduction.
A. Assist with detailed family history and pedigree chart.
B. Determine family's understanding of the information.
Goal: To provide information about available diagnostic tests and treatment.
A. Be precise and give detailed information.
B. Use familiar examples to illustrate probability of specific risks (e.g., flipping coins).
C. Emphasize the importance of the couple making an informed decision.
Goal: To reduce incidence and impact of genetic disease by identifying families at risk and making appropriate referrals.
A. Refer to specific agencies (e.g., Cystic Fibrosis Foundation, Muscular Dystrophy Association) or a genetic counseling service.
B. Provide alternatives to childbearing such as adoption and artificial insemination.

FETAL AND MATERNAL ASSESSMENT TESTING

Amniocentesis

An invasive procedure performed on the mother to obtain amniotic fluid.
A. An outpatient procedure performed at 14 to 16 weeks of pregnancy.
B. Procedure: placenta is located by ultrasound examination; a needle is inserted through the abdomen (puncture site has been anesthetized); amniotic fluid is aspirated and sent to the laboratory for testing.

Table 24-1	GENETIC TESTING EXAMPLES
Disease	*Test (Amniotic Fluid Sample)*
Cystic fibrosis	Decreased amounts of 4-methylumbelliferyl guanidinobenzoate (MUGB) reactive proteases
Neural tube defects: Anencephaly Spina bifida	Elevated maternal alpha-fetoprotein (MSAFP) level; decreased level may indicate Down syndrome

1. Indications for amniocentesis: increased maternal age, history of child with a genetic defect, mother carrying an X-linked disease, or history of either parent carrying a chromosomal abnormality (Table 24-1).
2. Complications: unlikely (less than 1% of the cases), though possible; some mild discomfort at the needle site, or rarely, abdominal wall hematoma; risk for miscarriage.
3. Maturity studies.
   a. Lecithin/sphingomyelin (L/S) ratio: the components of phospholipid protein substance that comprise surfactant; L/S ratio of 2:1 or greater is indicative of sufficient surfactant (occurs around 35 weeks' gestation).

> ⚠ **NURSING PRIORITY** The fetal heart rate (FHR) is assessed before and after amniocentesis.

Ultrasonography

Ultrasonography is a noninvasive technique in which high-frequency pulse sound waves are transmitted by a transducer applied directly to the woman's abdomen or transvaginally.
A. Purpose.
   1. Identifies placental location for amniocentesis or to determine placenta previa.
   2. Determines gestational age by crown-rump length (first trimester); later, gestational age is determined by biparietal diameter.
   3. Detects fetal anomalies: hydrocephalus, myelomeningocele, anencephaly.
   4. Detects multiple gestations.
   5. Monitors fetal growth to assess for intrauterine growth retardation.
   6. Evaluates volume of amniotic fluid.
B. Procedure (abdominal).
   1. Procedure may be done anytime during pregnancy.
   2. Performed with a full bladder, except when ultrasonography is used to localize the placenta before amniocentesis.
   3. Requires approximately 20 to 30 minutes to perform; client must lie flat on back, which may be uncomfortable.
C. Transvaginal is better tolerated because client is in lithotomy position and full bladder is not required.

Chorionic Villus Sampling

Chorionic villus sampling is a method of obtaining fetal tissue for genetic testing.
A. Purpose: to obtain fetal tissue to establish a genetic profile as a first trimester alternative to amniocentesis; use is declining due to noninvasive screening techniques.
B. Procedure.
   1. An invasive procedure performed with the use of ultrasound guidance between 10 and 12 weeks' gestation; technique may be transcervical or transabdominal.
   2. Allows for earlier diagnosis of genetic defects than does amniocentesis.
   3. Early sampling (8 to 9 weeks' gestation) has been associated with an increased incidence of limb defects.
   4. Administer RhoGAM to Rh-negative mothers because of possibility of fetal-maternal hemorrhage.

Percutaneous Umbilical Blood Sampling (PUBS)

An invasive procedure, also called cordocentesis, PUBS is fetal blood sampling performed during the second and third trimester.
A. Purpose: most widely used method for fetal blood sampling and transfusion.
B. Procedure.
   1. Insertion of a needle directly into a fetal umbilical vessel under ultrasound guidance.
   2. Umbilical cord is punctured 1 to 2 cm from its insertion into the placenta.
   3. Continuous FHR monitoring for up to an hour and a repeated ultrasound an hour later to ensure that bleeding or hematoma formation did not occur.

Daily Fetal Movement Count

A simple activity performed by the mother is to count daily fetal movement, also called "kick counts."
A. Purpose: to monitor the fetus when there may be complications affecting fetal oxygenation (e.g., preeclampsia, diabetes).
B. Procedure.
   1. Count all fetal movements within a 12-hour period until a minimum of 10 movements are counted or count fetal activity 2 to 3 times daily (after meals and before bed) for 2 hours until 10 movements are counted.
   2. Any change in fetal activity, either an increase or a decrease, should be reported to the health care provider.
   3. *Fetal alarm signal:* no fetal movements during a 12 hour period.

> ⚠ **NURSING PRIORITY** Alcohol, depressant medications, and smoking temporarily reduce fetal movement, and obesity decreases the woman's ability to assess fetal movement. Fetal movement is not felt during fetal sleep cycle, and the movements *do not* decrease as the woman nears term.

Nonstress Test (NST)

A. Purpose: to observe the response of the FHR to the stress of activity.

B. Procedure.
1. Requires approximately 20 minutes; client is placed in semi-Fowler's position; external monitor is applied to document fetal activity; mother activates the "mark button" on the electronic fetal monitor when she feels fetal movement.
2. If no fetal movement is detected, client may gently rub or palpate abdomen to stimulate movement or may be asked to eat a light meal, because an increased blood glucose level may increase fetal activity.

C. Interpretation.
1. Reactive: shows two or more fetal heart rate accelerations of 15 beats/min or more lasting at least 15 seconds for each acceleration within 20 minutes of beginning the test; indicates a healthy fetus; test may be rescheduled, as indicated by condition (the 15 × 15 criteria is for a fetus at least 32 weeks' gestation).
2. Nonreactive: reactive criteria are not met. The accelerations are less than two in number, the accelerations are less than 15 beats/min, or there are no accelerations. If nonreactive, then the test is extended another 20 minutes; if the tracing becomes reactive, the NST is concluded. If the NST is still nonreactive after a second 20-minute trial (total of 40 minutes), then additional testing, such as a biophysical profile, is considered. If gestation is near term, a contraction stress test (CST) may be done.

> **! NURSING PRIORITY** Appearance of any decelerations of the FHR during an NST should be immediately evaluated by the physician.

D. Advantages of NST.
1. Simple; easy to perform.
2. Does not require hospitalization.
3. Has no contraindications.

Biophysical Profile

Noninvasive dynamic assessment of a fetus that is based on acute and chronic markers of fetal disease. Is an accurate indicator of impending fetal death.

A. First choice for follow-up fetal evaluation.

B. Assesses *five* fetal variables: breathing movement, fetal body movement (FBM), muscle tone, amniotic fluid volume (AFV), and FHR—the first four are assessed by ultrasonography; the fifth is assessed by NST.

C. Each area has a possible score of 2, with a maximum score of 10. A score of 4 or below indicates need for immediate delivery.

Contraction Stress Test or Oxytocin Challenge Test and the Breast Self-Stimulation Contraction Stress Test

A. Purpose: to observe the response of FHR to the stress of oxytocin-induced uterine contractions; means of evaluating respiratory function (oxygen and carbon dioxide exchange) of the placenta as an indicator of fetal health.

> **! NURSING PRIORITY** Many facilities now use the breast self-stimulation contraction stress test, because endogenous oxytocin is produced in response to stimulation of the breasts or nipples.

B. Indications.
1. Preexisting maternal medical conditions: diabetes mellitus, heart disease, hypertension, sickle cell disease, hyperthyroidism, renal disease.
2. Postmaturity, intrauterine growth retardation, nonreactive NST results, preeclampsia.

C. Contraindications.
1. Third-trimester bleeding.
2. Previous cesarean delivery.
3. Risk for preterm labor because of premature rupture of the membranes, incompetent cervical os, or multiple gestation.

D. Procedure: breast self-stimulation contraction stress test.
1. Semi-Fowler's position, with fetal monitor in place.
2. Nipple stimulation begins with woman brushing her palm across one nipple through her shirt or gown for 2 to 3 minutes. If contractions start, nipple stimulation should stop. If contractions do not occur, one nipple should be massaged for 10 minutes.
3. Advantages: takes less time to perform, is less expensive, and causes less discomfort because no intravenous line is used.

E. Procedure: oxytocin challenge test.
1. Client must be NPO and be closely observed, either hospitalized or as an outpatient.
2. Place client in semi-Fowler's position to avoid supine hypotension.
3. Intravenous (IV) administration of oxytocin stimulates uterine contractions; uterine activity and FHR are recorded by means of external monitoring.
4. Hypoxia is reflected in late deceleration on monitor, which indicates a diminished fetal-placental reserve.
5. IV oxytocin is delivered at a rate of 0.5 mU/minute with the rate increased every 15 to 30 minutes until contractions occur at a rate of three per 10 minutes; then oxytocin is discontinued, and the woman is observed until contractions stop.

F. Interpretation: oxytocin challenge test.
1. Negative (reassuring): shows no late decelerations after any contraction; implies that placental support is adequate.
2. Positive (nonreassuring; abnormal): shows late decelerations with at least two of the three contractions; may indicate the possibility of insufficient placental respiratory reserve.

> **! NURSING PRIORITY** If the CST result is positive and there is no acceleration of FHR with fetal movement (nonreactive NST result), the positive CST result is an ominous sign, often indicating late fetal hypoxia. **A negative CST result with a reactive NST result is desirable.**

NORMAL PREGNANCY CYCLE: PHYSIOLOGIC CHANGES

Uterus

A. Increase in size caused by hypertrophy of the myometrial cells (increase 17 to 40 times their prepregnant state) as a result of the stimulating influence of estrogen and the distention caused by the growing fetus.
B. Weight of uterus increases from 50 to 1000 g.
C. Increased fibrous and connective tissues, which strengthen the elasticity of the uterine muscle wall.
D. Irregular, painless uterine contractions (Braxton-Hicks) may begin in the early weeks of pregnancy; contraction and relaxation assist in accommodating the growing fetus.

> **! NURSING PRIORITY** Multigravidas tend to report a greater incidence of Braxton-Hicks contractions than primigravidas.

E. Cervical changes.
  1. Softening of the lower uterine segment (Hegar sign).
  2. Softening of the cervical tip caused by increased vascularity, edema, and hyperplasia of cervical glands (Goodell sign).
  3. Formation of the mucous plug to prevent bacterial contamination from the vagina.

Vagina

A. Influence of estrogen leads to hypertrophy and hyperplasia of the lining along with an increase in vaginal secretions.

> **! NURSING PRIORITY** A blue-purple hue of the vaginal walls is seen very early (Chadwick sign).

B. Vaginal secretions: acidic (pH is 3.5 to 6.0), thick, and white.

Breasts

A. Increase in breast size accompanied by feelings of fullness, tingling, and heaviness.
B. Superficial veins prominent; nipples erect; darkening and increase in diameter of the areolae.
C. Thin, watery secretion, precursor to colostrum, can be expressed from the nipples by the end of the 10th week of pregnancy.

Cardiovascular System

A. Blood volume.
  1. Increases progressively throughout pregnancy, beginning in the first trimester and peaking in the middle of the third trimester at about 40% to 50% above prepregnant levels.
  2. Normal blood pressure is maintained by peripheral vasodilation.
  3. Extra volume of blood acts as a reserve for blood loss during delivery.
B. Heart.
  1. Slight cardiac hypertrophy and systolic murmurs.
  2. Increase in heart rate by 10 to 15 beats/minute by the end of the first trimester.

> **! NURSING PRIORITY** Blood pressure falls during the second trimester and rises slightly (no more than 15 mm in either systolic or diastolic) during the last trimester.

  3. Cardiac output increases 30% to 50%.
  4. Palpitations of the heart are usually due to sympathetic nervous system disturbance; later in pregnancy, palpitations are due to intraabdominal pressure of the growing uterus.
C. Red blood cells.
  1. Stimulation of the bone marrow leads to a 20% to 30% increase in total red blood cell volume.
  2. The plasma volume increase is greater than the red blood cell increase, which leads to hemodilution, typically referred to as *physiologic anemia of pregnancy* (pseudoanemia).
  3. The hematocrit, the proportion of erythrocytes in whole blood, decreases by 7%.
D. White blood cells: 10 to 11,000/mm³; may increase up to 15,000/mm³ during labor and after delivery.

Respiratory System

A. **pH** slightly increases, P_{CO_2} decreases, and HCO_3^- decreases.
B. Tidal volume increases steadily throughout pregnancy.
C. Oxygen consumption is increased by 15% to 20% between the 16th and 40th weeks.
D. Diaphragm is elevated; change from abdominal to thoracic breathing occurs around the 24th week.
E. Vital capacity increases slightly, while pulmonary compliance and diffusion remain constant.
F. Common complaints of nasal stuffiness and epistaxis are due to estrogen influence on nasal mucosa.

Urinary-Renal System

A. Ureter and renal pelvis dilate (especially on the right side) as a result of the growing uterus.
B. Frequency of urination increases (first and last trimester).
C. Decreased bladder tone (effect of progesterone); bladder capacity increases: 1300 to 1500 mL.
D. Reduced renal threshold for sugar leads to glycosuria.
E. Because of an increased glomerular filtration rate, as much as 50%, serum blood urea nitrogen, creatinine, and uric acid levels are decreased.

Gastrointestinal System

A. Pregnancy gingivitis: gums redden, swell, and bleed easily.
B. Increased saliva (ptyalism); decreased gastric acidity.
C. Nausea and vomiting caused by elevated human chorionic gonadotropin (HCG) level.
D. Cravings due to change in sense of taste: pica (craving for nonfood, which is not a normal change).
E. Decreased tone and motility of smooth muscles; decreased emptying time of stomach; slowed peristalsis caused by increased progesterone level leads to complaints of bloating, heartburn (pyrosis), and constipation.
F. Pressure of expanding uterus leads to hemorrhoidal varicosities and contributes to continuing constipation.
G. Gall bladder: decreased emptying time, slight hypercholesterolemia, and increased progesterone level may contribute to the development of gallstones during pregnancy.
H. Liver: minor changes.

Musculoskeletal System

A. Increase in the normal lumbosacral curve leads to backward tilt of the torso.
B. Center of gravity is changed, which often leads to leg and back strain and predisposition to falling.
C. Pelvis relaxes as a result of the effects of the hormone relaxin; leads to the characteristic "duck waddling" gait.
D. Abdominal wall stretches and looses tone.

Integumentary System

A. Increased skin pigmentation in various areas of the body.
1. Facial: mask of pregnancy (chloasma).
2. Abdomen: striae (red or purple stretch marks) and linea nigra (darkened vertical line from umbilicus to symphysis pubis).
B. Appearance of vascular spider nevi, especially on the neck, arms, and legs.
C. Acne vulgaris, dermatitis, and psoriasis usually improve during pregnancy.
D. Pruritus may occur and is common in pregnancy due to cholestasis of pregnancy.

Endocrine

Endocrine system is needed for maintenance of pregnancy, fetal growth, and postpartum recovery.
A. Placenta.
1. Functions include transport of nutrients and removal of waste products from the fetus.
2. Produces HCG and human placental lactogen.
3. Produces estrogen and progesterone after 2 months of gestation.
B. Thyroid gland.
1. May increase in size and activity.
2. Increase in basal metabolic rate.
3. Parathyroid glands: increase in activity (especially in the last half of the pregnancy) because of increased requirements for calcium and vitamin D.

C. Pituitary gland.
1. Enlargement greatest during the last month of gestation.
2. Production of anterior pituitary hormones: follicle-stimulating hormone, LH, thyrotropin, adrenotropin, and prolactin.

NURSING PRIORITY Production of posterior pituitary hormones: oxytocin promotes uterine contractility and stimulation of milk let-down reflex, which are essential changes for postpartum lactation and uterine involution.

D. Adrenal glands.
1. Hypertrophy of the adrenal cortex.
2. Increase in aldosterone, which retains sodium, results in a decreased ability of the kidneys to excrete salt during pregnancy; consequently, improper control of dietary sodium can lead to increased fluid retention and edema.

Metabolism

A. Weight gain: determined by prepregnancy weight-for-height calculated by using the body mass index (BMI); BMI of 19.8 to 26 is considered normal.
1. Normal weight gain: recommended 11.5 to 16 kg (about 26 to 28 lb).
a. Underweight: 12.5 to 18 kg.
b. Overweight: 7 to 11 kg.
c. Normal for multiple gestations: 21 to 28 kg.

NURSING PRIORITY The pattern of weight gain is important. Approximately 0.4 kg per week for normal weight; 0.5 kg/week for underweight; 0.3 kg/week for overweight. Inadequate weight gain for a normal-weight woman would be less than 1 kg/month. Excessive weight gain is considered more than 3 kg/month and should be evaluated, because this can indicate preeclampsia if it occurs after the 20th week of gestation.

2. Total weight gain is accounted for as follows:
a. Fetus: 7 to 8.5 lb.
b. Placenta and membranes: 2 to 2.5 lb.
c. Amniotic fluid: 2 lb.
d. Uterus: 2 lb.
e. Breasts: 1 to 4 lb.
f. Increased blood volume: 4 to 5 lb.
g. Remaining 4 to 9 lb is extravascular fluid and fat reserves.
B. Nutrient metabolism.
1. Protein: positive nitrogen balance; fetus makes greatest demands during the second half of gestation, as it doubles weight in the last 6 to 8 weeks.
2. Carbohydrate: increases, especially during the last two trimesters; ketosis and glycosuria occur, along with lipidemia.

3. Fat: more completely absorbed; increase in serum lipid, lipoprotein, cholesterol, and phospholipid levels.
4. Increased intake of folic acid: 600 mcg daily (to prevent neural tube defects).

C. Mineral metabolism.
1. Increased need for calcium and phosphorus, especially during the last 1 to 2 months of gestation.
2. Iron: approximately 30 mg daily.

D. Water metabolism.
1. Increased need for water (i.e., 3 L/day): normal is 2.3 L/day, so an increase of 700 mL/day is needed.
2. Increased water retention is frequently seen as a result of the effects of hormones and the decreased plasma protein level.
3. Dehydration increases risk for cramping, contractions, and preterm labor.

> ⚠ **NURSING PRIORITY** High levels of mercury can possibly harm the fetus' developing nervous system. Certain fish contain high mercury levels.

PRENATAL CARE

Assessment

A. Initial visit.
1. Complete history and physical exam.
2. Obstetric history.
    a. Past pregnancies (date, course of pregnancy, labor and postpartum period; information about infant and neonatal course).
    b. Present pregnancy.

B. Schedule of return prenatal visits.
1. Frequency of return visits.
    a. Monthly for first 32 weeks.
    b. Every 2 weeks to the 36th week.
    c. After the 36th week, weekly until delivery.
    d. If a high-risk pregnancy, prenatal visits may be more often.

2. Subsequent assessment data follow-up.
    a. Vital signs.
    b. Urinalysis: check for protein and sugar.
    c. Monitor weight.
    d. Measurement of height of uterine fundus.
    e. Auscultation of FHR.

C. Definitions of common terms (Table 24-2).
D. Signs and symptoms of pregnancy (Table 24-3).
E. Summary of the antepartum period (Table 24-4).

Diagnostics

A. Pregnancy tests: all tests, including over-the-counter "home pregnancy" tests are based on the presence of human chorionic gonadotropin (hCG) as the biologic marker. A false-negative test result may be due to testing too early. Whenever there is doubt about the results, further evaluation or retesting in a few days is appropriate.

B. Laboratory tests.
1. Urinalysis and/or urine culture.
2. Complete blood count, electrolytes, BUN, creatinine.
3. Venereal Disease Research Laboratory (VDRL) test, rapid plasmin reagin (RPR) test, or fluorescent treponemal antibody-absorption (FTA-ABS) test: serologic screening for syphilis.
4. Rubella antibody titer.

> ⚠ **NURSING PRIORITY** It is important to understand the rubella titer and its significance to pregnancy. The rubella vaccination is not given during pregnancy, and pregnancy should be prevented for at least a month after receiving the vaccination.

    a. Titer of 1:8 or less is considered serologically negative; titer 1:8 or greater indicates that woman is immune.
    b. Vaccination can be given 4 to 6 weeks after delivery.
    c. Teach pregnant woman who has not had rubella or a vaccination or who has a titer less than 1:10

Table 24-2	DEFINITIONS OF COMMON TERMS
Common Term	**Definition**
Gravida*	The number of pregnancies regardless of the duration; includes the present pregnancy.
Para*	The number of pregnancies in which the fetuses have reached 20 weeks of gestation when they are born.
Primigravida	Woman who is pregnant for the first time.
Multigravida	Woman who is pregnant for the second or subsequent time.
Nullipara (para 0)	Woman who has not had children.
Primipara (para 1)	Woman who has completed one pregnancy with a fetus who has reached 20 weeks of gestation.
Multipara (para II, para III, para IV, etc.)	Woman who has given birth to two or more children.
Parturient	A woman in labor.

*The terms *gravida* and *para* refer to the number of pregnancies, not the number of fetuses. The woman who delivers twins on her first pregnancy remains a para 1, in spite of having two infants. She is also a para 1 if the fetus was stillborn or died soon after birth. The most common system used to describe reproductive status is the five-digit identification system characterized by the acronym GTPAL: G = total number of pregnancies, T = number of term infants (at least 37 weeks' gestation), P = number of preterm infants (before 37 weeks' gestation), A = number of spontaneous or therapeutic abortions, L = number of living children.

Table 24-3	SIGNS AND SYMPTOMS OF PREGNANCY	
Presumptive/Subjective	*Probable/Objective*	*Positive/Diagnostic*
1. Amenorrhea	1. Positive pregnancy test result	1. Fetal heart rate—10th to 12th week: Doppler ultrasonography; 18th to 20th week: fetal stethoscope
2. Nausea and vomiting	2. Enlarged abdomen	2. Fetal movements
3. Excessive fatigue	3. Hegar sign: softening of lower uterine segment	3. Fetal sonography (after 16th week)
4. Urinary frequency	4. Chadwick sign: bluish discoloration of vagina	4. Fetal skeleton on x-ray film (not used often)
5. Breast changes: tenderness, fullness, increased pigmentation of areola, precolostrum discharge	5. Goodell sign: softening of cervical lip	
6. Quickening: active movements of the fetus felt by the mother	6. Ballottement: pushing on fetus (fourth to fifth month) and feeling it rebound back	
7. Increased pigmentation of skin and abdominal striae	7. Fetal outline distinguished by palpation	
	8. Braxton-Hicks contractions	

ALERT Be sure you are able to differentiate between presumptive, probable, and positive signs.

to avoid contact with children who have rubella or who have received a recent vaccination.
5. Blood type and Rh status.
  a. Administration of Rh$_o$(D) immune globulin, such as RhoGAM, to prevent Rh sensitization in the pregnant woman.
    (1) Rh$_o$(D) immune globulin is given at 28 weeks' gestation to an Rh-negative mother, as a prophylaxis measure.
    (2) A second dose of Rh$_o$(D) immune globulin is given within the first 72 hours after delivery to prevent the mother from producing antibodies to the fetal blood cells that may have entered her bloodstream during labor and delivery, if the infant is Rh positive.
      (a) Has no effect against antibodies already present in maternal bloodstream.
      (b) Provides passive immunity.
      (c) Not a treatment for women who are already sensitized; recommended only for nonsensitized Rh-negative women at risk for developing Rh isoimmunization.
      (d) Administered after abortion (13+ weeks' gestation), amniocentesis, blood transfusion, trauma, abruptio placentae, or placenta previa.
    (3) A minidose of Rh$_o$(D) immune globulin is administered after pregnancies that terminate before 13 weeks' gestation, after chorionic villus sampling, and after ectopic pregnancy.
6. Tuberculin skin testing.
7. Hepatitis B surface antigen (HBsAg).
8. HIV antibody with client permission.
9. Maternal serum alpha-fetoprotein (MSAFP) at 15 to 22 weeks.

C. Pelvic examination.
  1. Papanicolaou smear (Pap smear) of the cervix.
  2. Pelvic measurements (pelvimetry).
D. Calculation of estimated date of birth (EDB).
  1. Nägele's rule: count back 3 calendar months from the first day of the last menstrual period (LMP) and add 7 days.
  2. Examples.
    a. LMP, April 10: EDB, January 17.
    b. LMP, September 25: EDB, July 2.

High-Risk Pregnancy

A. Maternal factors.
  1. Age: younger than 16 years or older than 35 years.
  2. Parity: primigravida or greater than gravida 5.

NURSING PRIORITY Pregnant adolescents are at risk both physiologically and psychologically. Often, they do not receive prenatal care, or care is delayed because of late recognition of pregnancy. Physiologic risks include preeclampsia, iron deficiency anemia, sexually transmitted diseases (15- to 19-year-old teens have second highest incidence of sexually transmitted diseases), and low-birth-weight neonates. Psychologic risks include interruption of normal growth and development for both partners; adolescent parents may drop out of school.

  3. Unusual stress or anxiety, single parenthood, teenage pregnancy, abusive environment.
  4. Environmental and occupational hazards: excessive exposure to radiation, handling of teratogenic chemicals.
  5. Drug use: alcohol, nicotine, cocaine, heroin, marijuana, and other addictive drugs.

| Table 24-4 | SUMMARY OF NURSING MANAGEMENT DURING THE ANTEPARTUM PERIOD | | |

Weeks' Gestation	Physical Signs and Symptoms	Characteristic Behaviors	Nursing Interventions
0-16	Amenorrhea Fatigue Nausea, vomiting Increased breast size and tenderness Urinary frequency Increased appetite	Ambivalence with mood swings. Anxiety related to confirmation of pregnancy. Telling selected close persons of pregnancy. *Couvade syndrome* refers to the presence of physical discomforts in the father during the pregnancy that mimic his partner's symptoms.	1. Obtain complete history, including gynecologic and obstetric histories. 2. Ascertain any maternal high-risk problems such as maternal age (greater than 35 years or less than 16 years), heart disease, diabetes or potential neonatal high-risk problems such as history of congenital defects, premature births, etc. (See complete discussion in this chapter on high-risk problems.) 3. Identify maternal nutritional status by assessing height and weight and comparing with BMI chart. 4. Complete a diet history and instruction. Important to teach about necessary changes, rather than all the concepts of good nutrition. 5. Food cravings are usually benign and may be indulged, providing a well-balanced diet is maintained. Pica is an abnormal eating pattern and requires treatment. 6. Encourage client to express feelings or ambivalence about pregnancy. 7. Anticipatory guidance and teaching (including family) related to: OTC drugs, normal signs and symptoms of pregnancy, reportable signs of possible complications, and the normality of her mood swings.
16-30	Quickening "Pregnant figure" Increased energy Feeling of well-being Round ligament pain	Wears maternity clothes. Tells the world she's pregnant; begins to notice other pregnant women. Interested in learning about birth and babies: reads books, seeks out and questions friends and family, attends classes. Increased dependency as time goes on. Promote father's involvement by allowing him to watch and feel fetal movement. Father needs to confront and resolve his own conflicts about the fathering he received as a child. Father will make decisions about what he does or does not want to imitate based on his own father as role model.	1. Ongoing assessment of maternal and fetal status: FHR; vital signs; fundal height. 2. Urine test for glucose (mild glycosuria is usually benign), and protein. 3. Finger-stick for hemoglobin analysis (12-14 g/dL normal). 4. Balanced diet. 5. Prevent or minimize activity intolerance and promote adequate rest by: Encouraging 8 hours sleep each day, plus one nap. Scheduling rest periods at place of employment. Napping at home while other small children are sleeping. Using left lateral position while resting or sleeping. 6. Promote adequate exercise (e.g., Kegel, pelvic rocking, modified sit ups), sitting tailor-fashion (lotus position). 7. Anticipatory guidance/teaching (including family) related to: libido changes, mood swings, increasing dependency, introversion, and reportable signs of possible complications.
30-40	Dependent edema Pressure in lower abdomen Frequent urination Round ligament pain Backache Insomnia Clumsiness Fatigue	Introversion. Increased dependency (craves attention and tenderness). Altered responsiveness and spontaneity, as well as abdominal bulk and fatigue, may decrease interest in genital sex. Intensifies study of labor and delivery. Increasingly feeling more vulnerable. Prepares nursery; buys baby things. Decides on feeding method for baby.	1. Ongoing continued physical assessment at more frequent intervals. 2. Reassure: provide emotional support related to attractiveness and self-worth. 3. Anticipatory guidance and teaching (including family) related to: signs and symptoms of labor, environmental modification for coming infant, providing rest for mother, teaching associated with either breastfeeding or bottle-feeding, advising client concerning birthing and anesthesia options, promoting the developing parent/child attachment (encourage family to verbalize mental picture of infant and concepts of selves as parents).

ALERT Plan anticipatory guidance for developmental transitions. Pregnancy is considered a normal maturational crisis and developmental stage for the expectant couple.

6. Delayed or absent prenatal care.
7. Prolonged infertility or hormone treatment.
8. Group B streptococcus (GBS) infection in previous pregnancy, GBS bacteruria.

B. Preexisting medical problems.
1. Diabetes mellitus, renal disease.
2. Hypertension and cardiovascular disease.
3. Seropositivity for syphilis.
4. Viral infections: rubella, cytomegalovirus, herpes virus type 2, human immunodeficiency virus.
5. Urinary tract infections, anemia.
6. Psychiatric disorders.

C. Obstetric factors.
1. History of a previous high-risk pregnancy (premature labor, small-for-gestational-age or large-for-gestational-age infants, abortion, stillbirth, or maternal complications).
2. Present pregnancy (exposure to teratogens, hyperemesis gravidarum, bleeding, preeclampsia, oligohydramnios, polyhydramnios, multiple gestation, abnormal presentation, premature labor, and isoimmune disease).

D. Nutritional factors.
1. Underweight: 10% below for height.
2. Overweight: 20% over normal for height.
3. Inappropriate weight gain during pregnancy—either too little or too much.
4. Adolescents: need additional nutrition for their own growth and development (approximately 1.5 to 1.7 g of protein per kilogram of body weight and as many as 50 calories per kilogram of body weight).

E. Genetic factors.
1. History of an inheritable disorder (e.g., Down syndrome).
2. Previous infant with a congenital anomaly.
3. Parents with recessive disorders (hemophilia, cystic fibrosis).

Nursing Interventions

> **ALERT** Instruct client about antepartal care; modify approaches to care in accordance with client's developmental stage (adolescence).

Goal: To educate families regarding general health practices.
A. Hygiene: tub baths permitted, but may be awkward during latter weeks of gestation.
B. Clothing: loose, comfortable clothing with supportive brassiere; low-heeled shoes.
C. Breast and nipple care: client should avoid using excessive amounts of soap or rubbing the nipples with a towel because this dries the nipple area and removes natural secretions; creams, lotions, and ointments are not needed on the nipple or areola and should be avoided.
D. Employment: no severe physical straining, heavy lifting, or prolonged periods of sitting or standing.

E. Travel: client should avoid travel during the last month of pregnancy; when client is traveling by car or airplane, frequent walking and stretching are advised; seat belts (both lap and shoulder) should be used, with the lap belt positioned under the abdomen.
F. Rest and exercise: adequate amounts of exercise such as walking or swimming; client should stop exercising when she begins to feel tired; moderation is key.
G. Sexual activity: coital position may need to be altered to provide greater comfort; there is no contraindication to intercourse or any activity leading to orgasm, providing that membranes are intact, no vaginal bleeding exists, and there is no history of threatened abortion or premature labor.
H. Smoking: not advised; associated with infants who are small for gestational age.
I. Alcohol: recommended that the pregnant woman not consume any alcohol; the more consumed, the greater the risk for fetal alcohol syndrome.
J. Dental care: regular prophylactic care is encouraged; a soft-bristled toothbrush may be needed because of bleeding gums; x-ray exams should be postponed, if possible.
K. Immunization: live, attenuated virus immunizations (e.g., measles-mumps-rubella vaccine) are contraindicated during pregnancy; client is cautioned against getting pregnant for at least 3 months after receiving this type of immunization.
L. Medications: client advised to avoid medications, especially during the first trimester, because of possible teratogenic effects.

Goal: To promote relief of common discomforts through client education regarding self-care measures (Table 24-5).

Goal: To promote adequate nutrition.
A. Obtain a complete diet history (see Chapter 3).
1. Assess normal food intake.
2. Determine prepregnant nutritional status (existence of deficiency state; severity and time at gestation in which it occurs).

B. Identify nutritional risk factors.
1. Age: adolescents and older gravidas.
2. Maternal weight variations.
3. Abnormal dietary patterns: pica; fad diets; excessive use of alcohol, drugs, or tobacco.
4. Socioeconomic status: low income, insufficient money to buy food.
5. Preexisting medical problems: diabetes mellitus, anemia.

C. Dietary instructions and nutrient requirements.
1. Increase calories for pregnancy (an additional 300 calories per day).
2. Increase calories for lactation (an additional 500 calories per day over prepregnant intake).
3. Increase protein (an additional 10 g per day for pregnancy; an additional 5 g per day for lactation); because the protein intake of many nonpregnant women is quite high, there may be little or no need to increase the protein intake during pregnancy.

Table 24-5	SUMMARY OF COMMON DISCOMFORTS AND RELIEF MEASURES
Discomfort	*Relief Measures*
First Trimester	
Nausea and vomiting (morning sickness)	Frequent small meals; avoid empty stomach; between meals eat crackers without fluid; take vitamin B_6 supplement.
Urinary frequency and urgency	Void frequently; decrease fluids before bedtime; avoid caffeinated or carbonated beverages; use perineal pads for leakage; perform Kegel exercises; report any pain or burning.
Breast tenderness	Wear a well-fitting supportive bra; alter sleep positions; avoid using soap on the nipple and areola area.
Increased vaginal discharge	Good hygiene; use perineal or panty liner pads; cotton underwear; no douching unless prescribed; report any pruritus, foul odor, or change in character or color.
Second and Third Trimesters	
Heartburn (pyrosis or acid indigestion)	Avoid fat and fried, spicy foods; eat small, frequent meals; maintain good posture; sit upright.
Ankle edema	Need ample fluid intake; avoid prolonged sitting or standing; support stockings should be applied before rising; elevate feet while sitting.
Varicose veins	Avoid prolonged periods of standing; apply support hose before rising; elevate feet while sitting; do not cross legs at knees.
Hemorrhoids	Avoid constipation, do not strain; use ointments, bulk-producing laxatives, anesthetic suppositories as prescribed.
Constipation	Increase fluid intake (6 to 8 glasses/day); eat food and fruits high in roughage; exercise moderately; use bulk-producing laxatives as prescribed.
Backache	Maintain correct posture; wear low-heeled shoes; perform pelvic tilt exercises.
Leg cramps	Stretch affected muscle and hold till it subsides; apply warm packs; maintain adequate calcium intake.
Faintness	Sit or lie down; avoid sudden changes in position; avoid prolonged standing.
Shortness of breath	Maintain correct posture; sleep with head elevated by several pillows.

ALERT Instruct client on antepartal care.

4. Increase vitamins (generally, intake of all vitamins is increased, especially folic acid).
5. Increase amount of minerals (especially iron, calcium, and phosphorous).
6. Additional calories and protein may be recommended for the pregnant adolescent.

Goal: To educate expectant family with regard to danger signs and symptoms requiring immediate attention.
A. Vaginal discharge: blood or amniotic fluid.
B. Visual disturbances: dimness or blurring of vision, flashes of light or dots before the eyes.
C. Swelling of the face or fingers.
D. Fever and chills.
E. Severe or continuous headache.
F. Pain in the abdomen.
G. Persistent vomiting.
H. Absence of fetal movement after quickening.

Goal: To provide education and preparation for childbirth.
A. Childbirth programs aim to erase previous negative impressions of pregnancy, labor, and delivery; promote a positive, healthy attitude; and teach students physical exercises and relaxation techniques.

B. Points about breathing recommendations during labor.
1. Slow abdominal breathing or chest breathing is practiced for the first stage of labor; woman concentrates on making abdominal muscles rise.
2. Rapid shallow chest breathing is for the active and transitional phases of labor.
3. Panting is used to prevent pushing.

FETAL DEVELOPMENT

Developmental Stages
A. Preembryonic stage: stage of the ovum.
1. Fertilization to the first 3 weeks.
2. Fertilized ovum grows and differentiates.
3. Formation of the three primary germ layers: endoderm, mesoderm, ectoderm.
4. Implantation in the endometrial tissue.
B. Embryonic stage.
1. Fourth to eighth weeks of development.
2. Period of organogenesis: differentiation of cells, organs, and organ systems.
3. Highly vulnerable time; congenital anomalies are likely to occur during this period.

4. At the end of this period of development, embryo has features of the human body.

C. Fetal stage.
1. Nine weeks to the time of birth.
2. Characterized by growth and development of organs and organ systems.

Summary of Growth and Development

A. 6 weeks: heart begins beating.

B. 8 weeks: brain activity begins; fetus moves in response to touch; 1 inch long.

C. 16 weeks: sucking response begins; fetus is 3½ inches long; sex clearly identifiable.

D. 20 weeks: hearing begins to develop; fetus can respond to external sounds in environment; 10 inches long.

E. 28 weeks: fetus can perceive light; senses are functional; sleep-wake periods; brown fat has formed; 16 inches long; viable.

F. 30 to 40 weeks: increase in subcutaneous fat and weight.

> **! NURSING PRIORITY** At week 34 or 35, surfactant production is sufficient.

Multifetal Pregnancy

A. Incidence.
1. One in 430 pregnancies results in twins.
2. Steady rise in multifetal pregnancies since 1973 due to delayed childbearing and use of ovulation-enhancing drugs.

B. Dizygotic or fraternal twins.
1. Fertilization of two separate ova.
2. There are two placentas; however, they may be fused.
3. Fraternal twin can be either the same sex or a different sex; fraternal twins may also have different gestational ages.
4. Increased incidence in African-American women.

C. Monozygotic or identical twins.
1. One ovum and one sperm; cells of the zygote separate and form two embryos.
2. Same sex: resemble each other in appearance and structure.
3. Usually one placenta, one chorion, and two amnions are present; however, two placentas may be present, if cell division occurs soon after fertilization.

Placenta

A. Function.
1. Transfer of oxygen, nutrients, and metabolites.
2. Elimination of waste products from the fetus.
3. Production of hormones: HCG, human placental lactogen, estrogen, and progesterone.

B. Development of the placenta.
1. Formed from the chorionic villi lying over the decidua basalis.
2. Formed by the end of the third month of gestation.
3. Separated by 15 to 30 sections: cotyledons.

4. At term, the placenta weighs one-sixth of the weight of the fetus (e.g., 6-lb fetus: 1-lb placenta).
5. Fetal surface is shiny and slightly grayish: *Schultze*.
6. Maternal side is rough and beefy red: *Duncan*.

C. Placental circulation.
1. Maternal and fetal bloodstreams are in close relationship to each other, but the circulations do not mix.
2. Approximately 500 to 700 mL of maternal blood circulates through the placenta every minute.

Fetal Circulation

A. Fetal lungs do not participate in respiratory gas exchange.

B. There are special fetal structures to bypass blood supply to the lungs.
1. Placenta.
2. Umbilical cord: length, 55 cm (22 inches); diameter, 1.25 to 2.5 cm (½ to 1 inch).
    a. One umbilical vein carries oxygenated blood from maternal circulation to fetus.
    b. Two umbilical arteries carry unoxygenated (venous) blood from fetus to placenta.
    c. Wharton's jelly is a gelatinous substance that surrounds the three blood vessels, providing support.
3. Foramen ovale: an opening between the right atrium and the left atrium of the heart.
4. Ductus arteriosus: connects the pulmonary artery and the aorta.
5. Ductus venosus: connects the umbilical vein and the inferior vena cava.

C. At the time of birth, fetal circulation begins the transition to the adult pattern of circulation; a functional closure occurs within a few days; however, anatomic closure of the fetal vessels is not complete for several weeks or months.

> **! NURSING PRIORITY** A newborn heart murmur may not be significant because of incomplete closure of the ductus arteriosus.

COMPLICATIONS ASSOCIATED WITH PREGNANCY

High-Risk Pregnancy

A. Preexisting medical problems complicate pregnancy.

B. Often, these problems affect the mother quite mildly; however, the effect on the fetus is severe, as evidenced by developmental anomalies and even death.

C. The medical and obstetric treatment of these conditions is described in the chapter under the appropriate body system.

> **ALERT** Identify signs of potential prenatal complications.

Abortion

Abortion is termination of pregnancy before 20 weeks of gestation; abortions can be spontaneous (miscarriage) or induced (therapeutic or elective); approximately 75% to

80% of all spontaneous abortions occur during the second and third months of gestation.

Assessment

A. Risk factors.
  1. Maternal: chronic infections, fibroid tumors, structural uterine anomalies.
  2. Acute infection.
  3. Endocrine disturbance: progesterone and thyroid hormone (hypothyroidism) dysfunction.
  4. Exposure to teratogens, evidence of malnutrition, and psychologic factors.
B. Diagnostics.
  1. Decreased hemoglobin (less than 10.5 mg/dL if bleeding has been significant).
C. Clinical manifestations (types of spontaneous abortions).
  1. Threatened abortion: slight bleeding, mild back and lower abdominal cramping, no cervical dilation, no passage of the products of conception.
  2. Inevitable abortion: moderate amount of bleeding and cramping; internal cervical os dilates, and membranes may rupture.
  3. Incomplete abortion: only some of the products of conception are expelled.
  4. Complete abortion: all the products of conception are expelled.
  5. Missed abortion: fetus dies in utero, and the products of conception are retained from 4 to 8 weeks; symptoms of pregnancy subside; if fetus is retained past 6 weeks, complications of disseminated intravascular coagulation (DIC) may develop as a result of the release of thromboplastin from the fetal autolysis process.
  6. Recurrent or habitual abortion: three or more successive, spontaneous abortions.

Treatment

Treatment varies according to type of abortion.
A. Threatened abortion: bed rest and sedation; sometimes progesterone therapy is tried (may cause congenital anomalies).
B. Inevitable and incomplete abortion.
  1. Fluid replacement: IVs, type and cross-match for possible blood transfusion.
  2. Administration of oxytocin.
  3. Dilation and curettage (D&C) or suction evacuation to remove products of conception.
  4. Administration of $Rh_o(D)$ immune globulin (RhoGAM) if mother is Rh negative (given within 72 hours).
C. Missed abortion.
  1. If abortion does not occur spontaneously after 6 weeks, suction evacuation or D&C will be performed.
  2. Pregnancy beyond 12 weeks' gestation: induction of labor by IV Pitocin, prostaglandin.

D. Recurrent or habitual abortion: determination of cause, then specific therapy to correct.

Nursing Interventions

Goal: To assess or control hemorrhage.
A. Monitoring of vital signs.
B. Accurate determination of number of pads used to assess bleeding.
C. Assist in medical treatment: IV therapy, preparation for D&C.
Goal: To prevent complications.
A. Observe for shock, hypofibrinogenemia, and DIC.
B. Prevent isoimmunization by administration of $Rh_o(D)$ immune globulin.
C. Assess for infection and anemia.
Goal: To provide emotional support to the couple experiencing the loss of pregnancy.
A. Encourage verbalization of feelings.
B. Often, verbal expression of the experience helps couple cope with the situation.
C. Be available and actively listen.

Ectopic Pregnancy

Any pregnancy where the gestational sac is implanted outside of the uterine cavity. Most (95%) of ectopic pregnancies are tubal; they are more common on the right side.

Assessment

A. Risk factors: any condition that causes scarring or obstruction of the fallopian tubes (e.g., pelvic inflammatory disease, gonorrheal infections, postabortion salpingitis).
B. Diagnostics.
  1. Ultrasonography.
  2. Culdocentesis: assesses intraperitoneal bleeding by needle puncture of the cul-de-sac of Douglas.
  3. Laparoscope: an instrument that provides visualization of the pelvic organs via a small external incision on the abdomen; if affected tube is found, a laparotomy can be performed for treatment.
C. Clinical manifestations.
  1. If tube is unruptured, slow, chronic bleeding usually occurs, and the abdomen gradually becomes rigid and very tender.
  2. If a tube ruptures, sudden excruciating pain is felt in the lower abdomen, usually over the mass; referred shoulder pain is possible as the abdomen fills with blood; vaginal bleeding and shock may also occur.

NURSING PRIORITY When a woman of child bearing age has extreme sudden abdominal pain, an ectopic pregnancy should be considered, even if the woman reports that there is no risk of her being pregnant.

Treatment
A. Surgical: laparoscopy, laparotomy, salpingectomy.
B. Medical: methotrexate used to dissolve residual tissue or as a one-time treatment for unruptured pregnancies.

Nursing Interventions
Goal: To prevent and detect early complications.
A. Provision of nursing care for shock, as indicated.
B. Prepare for surgery (IVs, oxygen, blood, etc.).
C. Administer Rh₀(D) immune globulin, if mother is Rh negative.
Goal: To provide emotional support (loss of pregnancy and reproductive organ).

 Incompetent Cervical Os (Recurrent Premature Dilation of the Cervix)

An incompetent cervical os is a defect related to trauma of the cervix or a congenitally short cervix, which leads to habitual abortion and premature labor.

Assessment
A. Risk factors: cervical trauma related to D&C, conization, cervical lacerations from previous deliveries.
B. Clinical manifestations.
   1. Cervical dilation or cervical effacement without painful uterine contractions.
   2. Membranes rupture, labor begins, and premature fetus is delivered.

Treatment
A. Medical.
   1. Bed rest, hydration, and tocolytic agents.
B. Surgical.
   1. Reinforcement of the weakened cervix by a purse-string suture, which encircles the internal os.
   2. McDonald cerclage: left in place until term, then removed around 37 weeks or left in place if a cesarean birth is anticipated.

Nursing Interventions
Goal: To provide client education regarding presence of purse-string suture or cerclage.
A. Advise client that some vaginal spotting may occur for several days after placement of suture.
B. Client should abstain from intercourse and douching and should reduce activity level for 2 weeks after surgery.
C. Stress the importance of monitoring signs and symptoms of preterm labor.
D. During labor, the suture will be removed for a vaginal delivery, or it may be left in place for a cesarean delivery.

 Hydatidiform Mole (Molar Pregnancy)

Gestational trophoblastic disease is a spectrum of diseases resulting from abnormal proliferation of the placenta— for example, hydatidiform moles, gestational trophoblastic neoplasia, choriocarcinoma.

Assessment
A. Risk factors.
   1. Found more commonly in women of Asian descent.
   2. A molar pregnancy creates a 20 to 40 times higher risk for having it again.
   3. Increased incidence with advanced maternal age.
B. Diagnostics.
   1. Ultrasonography reveals no fetal skeleton.
   2. Elevated hCG level.
C. Clinical manifestations.
   1. Exaggerated symptoms of pregnancy: uterus too enlarged for pregnancy, excessive nausea and vomiting, early symptoms of preeclampsia.
   2. Discharge of brownish-red fluid (like prune juice) from vagina around the 12 weeks; fluid may contain vesicles.
   3. Anemia caused by loss of blood, absence of FHR.
D. Complications.
   1. Infection, DIC.
   2. Trophoblastic embolization occurring after evacuation of molar pregnancy.
   3. Possible choriocarcinoma.

Treatment
A. Surgical: D&C to empty uterus.
B. Medical: follow-up supervision for 1 year.
   1. Obtain hCG levels at 2-week intervals for the first 3 months of remission followed by screening at 1-month intervals until hCG levels have been normal for 1 year.
   2. Rising titers of hCG indicate disease: choriocarcinoma.

⚠ NURSING PRIORITY For the treatment of increasing or rising hCG levels, which often indicate choriocarcinoma, the chemotherapeutic agent methotrexate is given.

   3. Pregnancy should be avoided for at least 1 year.
   4. Oral contraceptive is preferred for birth control—no IUD.

Nursing Interventions
Goal: To assess for complications associated with hemorrhage and the possibility of uterine rupture.
Goal: To provide emotional support and assist in selection of a contraceptive method.
A. Provide simple explanations and determine understanding of course of treatment.
B. Encourage ventilation of fears associated with molar pregnancy and increased incidence of choriocarcinoma.

ALERT Molar pregnancy and ectopic pregnancy are situations in which nurses must integrate care of the client with an obstetric problem and use of chemotherapeutic medications.

Hyperemesis Gravidarum

Hyperemesis gravidarum is intractable vomiting during pregnancy that results in dehydration, electrolyte imbalance, and weight loss of at least 5% of prepregnancy weight. It occurs in approximately 70% of all pregnancies; the cause is uncertain.

Assessment

A. Risk factors: none known.
B. Diagnostic: by symptoms.
C. Clinical manifestations.
   1. Severe, persistent vomiting that leads to dehydration, weight loss, and nutritional deficiency; progresses to fluid electrolyte imbalance and alkalosis from loss of hydrochloric acid.
   2. If untreated, ketoacidosis (from loss of intestinal juices), hypovolemia, hypokalemia, jaundice, and hemorrhage may occur.
   3. Hypothrombinemia and decreased urine output.

Treatment

A. Medical: replacement of fluids, electrolytes, and vitamin B_6 (pyridoxine), along with a tranquilizer or an antiemetic.
B. Dietary: client receives nothing by mouth (NPO status) for first 48 hours; after condition improves, six small feedings are alternated with liquid nourishment in small amounts every 1 to 2 hours; if vomiting recurs, NPO status is resumed, and administration IV fluids is restarted.
C. May require placement of central line for extended nutritional delivery of total parenteral nutrition.

Nursing Interventions

Goal: To assist with medical and dietary management.
A. Accurate recording of volume of vomitus.
B. Daily weight checks and maintenance of intake and output.
C. Desired urine output is 1000 mL in 24 hours; usually, administration of IV fluids at 3000 mL/hr in first 24 hours after admission to correct hypovolemia.
D. Oral hygiene measures.
E. Clear liquids with gradual progression to small meals that are low-fat and high protein.
Goal: To detect and treat complications.
   1. Initial acid-base imbalance is alkalosis from the loss of hydrochloric acid; however, with prolonged vomiting and loss of alkaline intestinal juices, a ketoacidotic state occurs.
   2. Esophageal rupture and deficiencies of vitamin K and thiamine resulting in Wernicke encephalopathy can occur in severe cases.

Hypertensive Disorders

Hypertensive disorders are a common medical complication of pregnancy occurring in about 6% to 8% of pregnancies and the second leading cause of maternal and perinatal morbidity and mortality. Cause is unknown.

Pathophysiology

A. Synthesis of prostaglandin E_2 and prostacyclin is decreased. Both prostaglandin E_2 and prostacyclin are potent vasodilators. Possible decreases in these factors may lead to increased sensitivity to angiotensin II and may be responsible for most of the pathophysiology associated with preeclampsia.
B. Arteriolar vasospasm and hypovolemia: renal glomerular lesions lead to loss of serum protein, (e.g., albumin and globulin); sodium reabsorption is elevated, and water is retained.
C. Oliguria results from decreased glomerular filtration rate and renal blood flow.
D. Coagulation disorder: decreased platelet count, increased intravascular coagulation, and fibrinogen deposits.
E. Central nervous system effects (hyperactivity): headaches, cerebral edema, hyperreflexia, and convulsions.

Assessment

A. Risk factors.
   1. Diabetes mellitus, hypertension.
   2. Renal disease, hydatidiform mole.
   3. Multiple gestation, polyhydramnios.
   4. Age (younger than 20 or older than 40 years).
   5. Primarily a disease of the primigravida.
   6. Preeclampsia most often occurs after 20 weeks of gestation.
B. Clinical manifestations of preeclampsia (Table 24-6).

> **NURSING PRIORITY** The common symptoms of preeclampsia are hypertension and proteinuria.

C. Complications (severe preeclampsia): *maternal.*
   1. Retinal arteriolar spasm leads to scotoma (blind spots) and blurring.
   2. Cerebral edema and hemorrhages with increased irritability (headache, hyperreflexia, positive ankle clonus, and seizures).
   3. **HELLP** (**H**emolysis, **E**levated **L**iver function tests, **L**ow **P**latelet count) syndrome.
      a. Associated with severe preeclampsia and with hepatic dysfunction: epigastric pain, right upper quadrant pain.
      b. Complications of HELLP syndrome include renal failure, pulmonary edema, ruptured liver hematoma, placental abruption, DIC.
   4. Thrombocytopenia, hemolytic anemia, pulmonary edema.
D. Complications: *fetal.*
   1. Usually small for gestational age; born prematurely.
   2. Newborn may be born oversedated because of medications given to mother.
   3. May have hypermagnesemia because of maternal treatment with magnesium sulfate.

Table 24-6	CLINICAL MANIFESTATIONS OF PREECLAMPSIA AND ECLAMPSIA	
Mild Preeclampsia	*Severe Preeclampsia*	*Eclampsia*
Elevated BP: systolic increase to 140 mm Hg and diastolic increase of 90 mm Hg × 2 readings, 4 to 6 hours apart, no more than 1 week apart	Increased hypertension: systolic at 160 mm Hg; diastolic at 110 mm Hg or more on 2 separate occasions	Convulsions appear suddenly and without warning. Increased hypertension and tonic contraction of all body muscles (arms flexed, hands clenched, legs inverted) precede the tonic-clonic convulsions. Hypotension follows and then coma. Nystagmus and muscular twitching persist for a time.
Proteinuria: greater than 0.3 g/24 hour (1+ proteinuria)	Proteinuria: greater than 2 g/24 hour (3+ to 4+ proteinuria)	Coma (lasts from few minutes to several hours).
	Elevated BUN, serum creatinine, uric acid levels, LDH, ALT, AST Oliguria: less than 500 mL/ 24 hour Cerebral or visual disturbances Severe headache Vomiting Epigastric pain (due to edema of liver capsule, usually indicative of impending seizure)	

BP, Blood pressure; *BUN*, blood urea nitrogen.

Treatment
A. Medical.
   1. Mild preeclampsia: bed rest lateral recumbent position.
   2. Severe preeclampsia or HELLP syndrome: admitted to hospital, complete bed rest, antihypertensives (hydralazine [**Apresoline**]), anticonvulsants (magnesium sulfate); prepare for preterm delivery via cesarean section if HELLP syndrome begins.

> ❗ **NURSING PRIORITY** Monitor for magnesium toxicity characterized by loss of patellar reflexes, respiratory depression, oliguria, decreased level of consciousness. Magnesium may increase the duration of labor requiring the client to have oxytocin to augment labor; usually requires more than a client not receiving magnesium. When administering antihypertensives in preeclampsia that is associated with a contracted intravascular volume, give medications with caution and monitor client closely.

   3. Eclampsia: seizure precautions (vital signs, oxygen, suction, positioning).
B. Dietary: high-protein diet, no added salt intake, and fluid intake of 6 to 8 glasses of water per day.

Nursing Interventions
Goal (mild preeclampsia): To initiate preventative measures.

A. Instruction for home care: encourage bed rest, provide dietary instruction, schedule regular prenatal checkups, teach symptoms of worsening of condition, provide meaningful activities to prevent boredom while on bed rest.
B. Tests to evaluate fetal status (e.g., fetal movement record, ultrasonography, NST, determination of estriol and creatinine levels).
C. Goals and nursing intervention for clients with severe preeclampsia and eclampsia are outlined in Box 24-1.

 Hydramnios

Polyhydramnios is an excessive amount of amniotic fluid. Any amount over 2000 mL is considered excessive. Oligohydramnios is having less than 300 mL of amniotic fluid. A normal amount of fluid is 500 to 1200 mL.

Assessment
A. Risk factors (increased incidence occurs).
   1. Diabetes, erythroblastosis fetalis.
   2. Presence of congenital anomalies.
   3. Twins, preeclampsia.
B. Diagnostics.
   1. Observation of abdomen (excessive enlargement).
   2. Ultrasonography for measurement of amniotic fluid index.

Box 24-1 NURSING MANAGEMENT OF CLIENTS WITH GESTATIONAL HYPERTENSION AND PREECLAMPSIA

Goal: To recognize the early signs of gestational hypertension and increased BP.
1. Check BP and record Korotkoff phase V (disappearance of sound) for diastolic reading. Take BP in left lateral recumbent position or seated. Allow 10 minutes of quiet rest before taking BP to encourage relaxation. No caffeine or nicotine use 30 minutes prior to taking BP.
2. Monitor urine for proteinuria.
3. Monitor for nondependent pathologic edema (e.g., periorbital area and hands).

⬛ NURSING PRIORITY Systolic increase of 30 mm Hg and a diastolic BP increase of 15 mm Hg warrant close observation if the BP elevation occurs with proteinuria.

Goal: To recognize progression of gestational hypertension symptoms and minimize or control their sequelae.
1. Institute weight controls. Check for sudden increases of 2 lb/week or 6 lb/month.
2. Increase protein intake in the diet. Maintain normal sodium intake; avoid use of diuretics.
3. Institute bed rest.
4. Monitor for ominous signs of deteriorating condition: headache, visual disturbances, hyperreflexia, markedly decreased urine output, epigastric or right upper quadrant pain, dyspnea,

vaginal bleeding (abruptio placentae), or any change in fetal activity.
5. Administer antihypertensives, as ordered, check maternal BP, pulse and fetal heart rate.

Goal: To prevent or control seizures.
1. Administer IV MgSO₄. (Have calcium gluconate available as antidote for possible respiratory/neurologic depression.)
2. Have emergency equipment readily available (e.g., oxygen, suction, airway, sedatives).
3. Modify environment to ensure rest and quiet.
   a. Eliminate noise, bright lights, and other harsh stimuli.
   b. Minimize number of personnel giving care.
   c. Initiate painful and/or intrusive procedures after sedation.
   d. Promote comfort and total bed rest.
4. Monitor I&O, edema, and weight for evidence of vasodilation and increased tissue perfusion.

Goal: To recognize alterations in fetal well-being and promote safe delivery of the infant.
1. Auscultate and record FHR pattern, noting presence of variability or accelerations, and report decelerations.
2. Instruct and support client during amniocentesis.
3. Collect specimen for estriol determination.
4. Assist with NST and/or oxytocin challenge test.
5. Give instructions about induction of labor and electronic FHR monitoring.

BP, Blood pressure; *FHR,* fetal heart rate; *IV,* intravenous; *MgSO₄,* magnesium sulfate; *NST,* nonstress test; *OCT,* oxytocin challenge test.

C. Clinical manifestations.
   1. Shortness of breath, pedal edema.
   2. Generalized abdominal discomfort.

Treatment
A. Amniocentesis.

Nursing Interventions
Goal: To anticipate, detect, and prevent complications associated with polyhydramnios.
A. Assess for history of risk factors.
B. Anticipate premature labor.
C. Provide comfort measures.

Appendix 24-1 CONTRACEPTIVE METHODS

| METHODS/DESCRIPTION | NURSING IMPLICATIONS/CLIENT TEACHING |

Family Awareness Methods

Calendar (rhythm)
BBT
Ovulation (Billings)
Cervical mucus
Symptothermal
Fertility awareness

Client Teaching
1. Calendar (rhythm) method: calculate the days of fertility; considered to be days 10 to 17 of a 28-day menstrual cycle.
2. BBT method: a slight decrease, then an increase of about 0.4° to 0.8° in temperature when ovulation occurs; fertile period ends 3 days after temperature elevation; need a special BBT thermometer.
3. Cervical mucus method: before ovulation, mucus becomes clear and stringy; nonfertile period occurs when mucus becomes thick, cloudy, and sticky or when no mucus is apparent.
4. Symptothermal method: combines two methods, usually cervical mucus and BBT.

IUD

Progesterone **(Progestasert)** IUD;
  Copper T 380A **(ParaGard)** IUD

Client Teaching
1. Discuss the technique and the experience of IUD insertion and removal.
2. Emphasize the need for yearly Pap smears; failure rate is less than 1%.
3. Encourage client to check IUD string, especially after each period.
4. Make sure the woman understands which type of IUD she has and when to return to have it checked or replaced. Copper IUD is approved for 10 years. The progesterone IUD is effective for up to 5 years, and uterine cramping and bleeding are diminished as compared with the copper IUD.
5. Review common side effects and serious complications. Report any of the following symptoms (**PAINS**): **P**eriod late, abnormal spotting or bleeding; **A**bdominal pain, pain with intercourse; **I**nfection exposure, abnormal vaginal discharge; **N**ot feeling well, fever or chills; **S**tring missing; shorter or longer.

Hormonal Methods

Combined oral contraceptive: the "pill" is a combination of estrogen and progestin
Progestin only **(Minipill):**
  norethindrone;
  medroxyprogesterone
Transdermal contraceptive patch: applied once a week; has both hormones
Vaginal contraceptive ring: a ring inserted into the vaginal for 3 weeks; removed for 1 week, then new ring inserted

Client Teaching
1. Instruct as to correct use of medication, the need for follow-up in 3 months, and importance of taking the pill at same time each day; effectiveness is close to 100% when used correctly.
2. Explain that if a pill is forgotten one day, she should take it when she remembers; then take the next pill as scheduled the following day.
3. If two pills are missed, she should take them as above and use some other form of contraception for the remainder of the month.
4. Review common side effects and serious complications. Report any of the following symptoms (**ACHES**): **A**bdominal pain, **C**hest pain or shortness of breath, **H**eadaches, **E**ye problems, and **S**evere leg pain.
5. Progestin only pill causes more menstrual irregularity (breakthrough bleeding, variation in blood flow, etc.).

Injectable/Implantable Progestins

Injectable **(DMPA, Depo-Provera)**

Client Teaching
1. Requires injections only 4 times per year (every 11-13 weeks).

> **! NURSING PRIORITY** Do not massage the site after the injection because it may speed up absorption and decrease duration of effectiveness; effectiveness rate is comparable to that of oral contraceptives.

2. Disadvantages include weight gain, prolonged amenorrhea, and breakthrough uterine bleeding. Long-term use may decrease bone density; need to encourage calcium intake and exercise.

Implantable: single rod implant **(Implanon)**

1. Requires a small incision in the inner aspect of the nondominant upper arm with a local anesthetic; provides up to 3 years of contraception.
2. The most common side effect is irregular menstrual bleeding.

Continued

Appendix 24-1   CONTRACEPTIVE METHODS—cont'd

METHODS/DESCRIPTION	NURSING IMPLICATIONS/CLIENT TEACHING

Barrier Methods

Diaphragm: a dome-shaped rubber device that fits over the cervix

Client Teaching
1. Should be refitted after every pregnancy or when there is a weight gain or loss of 20 lb; failure rate in the first year of use may be 20%.
2. Instruct client to use spermicidal jelly or cream around diaphragm rim and in the dome.
3. Instruct client to leave diaphragm in place 6 to 8 hours after intercourse.
4. Explain the proper method for cleansing (use mild soap only), storing (dry thoroughly and dust with cornstarch, not baby powder), and checking for defects or holes in the diaphragm.
5. Allow for sufficient practice of insertion/removal techniques and use with a spermicide, such as nonoxynol-9 (N-9).

Condoms: "rubbers" are thin sheaths of rubber that fit over an erect penis

1. Advise client to apply condom to erect penis by rolling the sheath along the entire shaft and leaving enough slack at the end of the penis to receive the semen.
2. Explain importance of holding the condom in place while withdrawing the penis to prevent emptying of sperm into the vagina.
3. Condom should be applied before any penetration because the preejaculatory seminal fluid may contain sperm; failure rate in the first year is 14%.
4. Ask client about allergy to latex.

> **❗ NURSING PRIORITY** Use of nonoxynol-9 with diaphragms or condoms is not a recommended method for preventing STDs or HIV.

Unreliable Practices

Withdrawal (coitus interruptus): withdrawal of penis before ejaculation

Nursing Implications
1. Requires absolute cooperation and control of partner.
2. Good choice for couples who do not have any other contraceptive methods available.
3. Douching may actually move the sperm upward in the vagina.

Douching: the act of cleansing washing the semen out of the vagina

Client Teaching
1. Encourage use of a more reliable contraceptive practice.

Emergency Contraception

Plan B: 2 doses of progestin

Client Teaching
1. Available without a prescription; prescription required if under age 18.
2. Should be taken within 120 hours of unprotected intercourse.
3. Is ineffective if the woman is pregnant, since pills do not disturb an implanted pregnancy.

Permanent Sterilization

Tubal ligation (minilaparotomy)

Client Teaching
1. Discuss the permanence of the sterilization procedure with the couple—informed consent required for all procedures.
2. Explain that the woman may experience sensation of tugging, but not pain during procedure, which is carried out via local anesthetic.

Essure system

1. Insertion of an occlusive agent (small metallic implants) into the uterine tubes, which stimulate scar tissue formation that occludes the tubes.
2. Procedure does not provide immediate contraception—need to use another form of contraception until tubal blockage is proven, which may take up to 3 months.

Vasectomy: surgical ligation and resection bilaterally of the vas deferens

Client Teaching
1. Discuss with couple the permanence of vasectomy (informed consent required); even if the vas deferens is reconnected, the fertility varies between 5% and 60%.
2. Activity level should be moderate for 2 days; skin sutures are usually removed within a week.
3. Encourage the use of a scrotal support and application of ice for pain or swelling.
4. Follow-up visit for sperm sample is usually done in 4 to 6 weeks.
5. Advise couple to use another form of birth control until it is verified that two ejaculate sperm counts contain no sperm.

BBT, Basal body temperature; *CO₂*, carbon dioxide; *IUD*, intrauterine device.

Study Questions Antepartum

More questions on companion CD!

1. How can a primigravida client most readily meet her increased daily iron requirements?
   1 By consuming at least four glasses of milk daily
   2 By adding an extra source of red meat to her daily diet
   3 By taking an iron supplement with a vitamin C source
   4 By including an extra source of fruits or vegetables

2. A primigravida client is experiencing Braxton-Hicks contractions. Which statement is true concerning these contractions?
   1 They are intensified by walking about.
   2 They are confined to the low back.
   3 They do not increase in intensity or frequency.
   4 They result in cervical effacement and dilation.

3. A primigravida client at 26 weeks' gestation has been administered a glucose tolerance test. What would the nurse expect the results considered within a normal range to be?
   1 Glycosylated hemoglobin A_{1c} of 5.0%
   2 Blood glucose of 200 mg/L at 60 minutes
   3 24-hour urine glucose level of 5 mg/dL
   4 Blood glucose level of 110 mg/L at 3 hours

4. Which statement about the results of a stress test (oxytocin challenge test) is considered accurate?
   1 Negative if no fetal heart rate accelerations occur with accompanying fetal movements
   2 Nonreactive if no late decelerations occur in more than half of the contractions
   3 Positive if late decelerations occur in more than half of the contractions
   4 Reactive if the fetal heart rate accelerates with accompanying fetal movement

5. At the beginning of her third trimester, a client reports she is having some discomfort in her lower back. What would the nurse check?
   1 The client's posture and the type of shoes she usually wears
   2 The client's bowel habits
   3 Advice of health care professional
   4 The amount of milk the client drinks

6. The nurse is encouraging the pregnant woman to eat a diet rich in folic acid. Which of the following food sources would provide the most folic acid?
   1 Meat and dark green, leafy vegetables
   2 Dairy products
   3 Carrots and raisins
   4 Shellfish

7. A young woman calls the clinic and reports missing her period. She states that she used a home pregnancy test last night and the results were negative. She tells the nurse that her breasts are tender and that she feels nauseated most of the day. What does the nurse understand about home pregnancy tests?
   1 They are radioimmunoassay-type tests, which are quick and most accurate.
   2 Home pregnancy tests are more reliable if used on a randomly collected specimen.
   3 The test is accurate, and she is not pregnant.
   4 False-negative results should be followed up in the presence of pregnancy symptoms.

8. The nurse is preparing a teaching plan for a client who has just had her pregnancy confirmed. What will be important for the nurse to include in the teaching plan? Select all that apply:.
   _____ 1 Change position frequently and participate in aerobic exercise three times a week.
   _____ 2 Prevent constipation with a stool softener.
   _____ 3 Sexual activity is permitted as long as membranes are intact.
   _____ 4 Showers are preferred to prevent contamination of vaginal area.
   _____ 5 Tetanus and measles, mumps, and rubella vaccinations will be given now.
   _____ 6 Encourage a balanced dietary intake with approximately 300 to 500 additional calories.

9. The nurse is assessing a primigravida client who is at 26 weeks' gestation; the client's blood type is AB negative, her serology is negative, and she has a history of one miscarriage at 20 weeks. Based on this information, what will the nurse anticipate being ordered for this client?
   1 An amniocentesis at 30 weeks' gestation
   2 Administration of $Rh_o(D)$ (RhIG or RhoGAM) at 28 weeks' gestation
   3 A blood test on the father to determine his blood type
   4 Fetal blood sampling to determine fetal blood type

10. A client reports that her last menstrual period was November 10. She asks the nurse, "When will my baby be due?" What is the best answer?
   1 "July 3"
   2 "August 30"
   3 "Around the middle of September"
   4 "The first or second week of August"

11. A lecithin-sphingomyelin (L/S) ratio is ordered for a primigravida client at 35 weeks' gestation. What is the goal of this test?
   1 To determine fetal lung maturity
   2 To evaluate the level of maternal-fetal estriol production
   3 To check the position of the fetal head
   4 To test the intrauterine fetal-placental circulation

12. The nurse is conducting prenatal teaching with a 16-year-old primigravida client during her first prenatal visit. What is the most important information for the nurse to discuss with the client during this visit?
    1. Components of a balanced diet, with increased intake of meat and poultry, as well as increased intake of whole-grain products
    2. The importance of attending the childbirth programs and understanding the growth of the fetus and normal changes in pregnancy
    3. The importance of understanding measures to decrease risks associated with pregnancy since she is at an increased risk for complications during pregnancy and delivery
    4. The importance of reporting any problems with swelling of her hands and face or any increase in vaginal discharge

13. A client is at 30 weeks' gestation when she comes in for her regular prenatal checkup. What nursing assessment findings would cause the most concern?
    1. Increased vaginal discharge, weight gain of 3 lb, and decreased activity tolerance
    2. Presence of 2 g of protein in a 24-hour urine collection, swelling of the face and hands, weight gain of 7 lb
    3. Complaints of backache and contractions that occur randomly and are uncomfortable
    4. States she is dizzy when she stands up from sitting and has leg cramps and her feet are swelling

14. A 26-year-old client comes into the emergency department and tells the nurse she has severe lower left side abdominal pain. The client says that the pain began suddenly and has gotten worse over the past few hours. What is the most important information for the nurse to obtain?
    1. Whether she has had an appendectomy or a cholecystectomy
    2. What she has had to eat over the last 24 hours
    3. Whether she has recently been diagnosed with a sexually transmitted disease
    4. The date of her last menstrual period and whether she could be pregnant

15. A client is admitted to the hospital after experiencing a miscarriage at 16 weeks. When the nurse enters her room, the client is crying. What would be appropriate for the nurse to do at this time?
    1. Explain to her the infant was probably not healthy and this was the reason for the miscarriage.
    2. Reassure her that everything happens for a reason and this was probably the best for her.
    3. Acknowledge that losing a pregnancy is very difficult time and sit with her for awhile.
    4. Ask her how many children she already has and if she is going to get pregnant again.

16. The nurse is assessing a client who is at 36 weeks' gestation; this client has type 2 diabetes. The client says she is extremely upset by the fact that she will not be able to breastfeed her infant. The best nursing response would be based on what information?
    1. There are no contraindications to diabetic mothers breastfeeding their infants; it will be important for the mother to carefully monitor her blood glucose levels and insulin needs.
    2. Because the mother's blood sugar level will be controlled by oral hypoglycemics, the medications are excreted in breast milk and would not be good for the baby.
    3. Breastfeeding puts increased carbohydrate metabolism demands on the mother and makes it unrealistic to control her blood glucose level.
    4. Offer the mother reassurance that there are some very good, nutritious infant formulas that are very close to breast milk and her infant should do well with them.

17. A positive pregnancy test result is related to the presence of which hormone?
    1. Chorionic gonadotropin
    2. Progesterone
    3. Lactogen
    4. Estrogen

18. When providing teaching to a pregnant client, the nurse knows that striae gravidarum:
    1. Occur in 100% of pregnancies
    2. Are silvery streaks that appear especially during the last trimester
    3. Can be decreased by a local application of cocoa butter or other types of emollient creams
    4. Will fade from their initial reddish appearance

19. The nurse is caring for a client who is not pregnant but who is considering pregnancy. A rubella titer has been done, and the titer was negative. What will be important for the nurse to tell this client?
    1. The client should get a rubella vaccine now and not get pregnant for at least a month.
    2. Because the rubella titer was negative, there should be no problems with getting pregnant.
    3. It is important for the client to get pregnant as soon as possible because the titer was negative.
    4. The client can get pregnant now, but she should receive the rubella vaccine during the first trimester.

Answers and rationales to these questions are in the section at the end of the book titled Chapter Study Questions: Answers and Rationales.

CHAPTER TWENTY-FIVE

Intrapartum and Postpartum

LABOR AND DELIVERY

Intrapartal Factors

A. The passenger (fetus).
  1. Fetal head.
    a. Bones of the skull: two frontal, two parietal, two temporal, and one occipital.
    b. Suture: membranous tissues between the bones.
    c. Fontanel.
      (1) Anterior, large fontanel (bregma) is located at the juncture of the coronal suture, sagittal suture, and frontal suture; diamond-shaped; closes by 18 months.
      (2) Posterior, or small, fontanel: triangular space located at the junction of the sagittal and lambdoidal sutures; closes at approximately 6-8 weeks after birth.
    d. Areas of the skull.
      (1) Occiput: lies behind small fontanel.
      (2) Vertex: lies between the anterior and posterior fontanels.
      (3) Bregma: area of the large fontanel.
      (4) Sinciput: the brow area.
  2. Fetal attitude: relationship of the various parts of the fetal body to one another in utero; characteristic uterine posture is one of moderate flexion of the head, extremities on the abdomen and chest.
  3. Fetal lie: relationship of the fetal axis to the maternal axis—longitudinal or transverse.
  4. Presentation and presenting parts: that part of the fetus that lies close to or has entered the true pelvis (Figure 25-1).
    a. Cephalic: most common (96%).
    b. Breech: buttocks or feet first.
    c. Shoulder: most commonly seen with transverse lie.
  5. Position: relationship of the landmark on the presenting part to a specific part of the maternal pelvis.
    a. Maternal pelvis divided into six segments: anterior, transverse, and posterior segments on the right side; anterior, transverse, and posterior segments on the left side.
    b. Fetal landmarks: occipital (O) vertex presentation, mentum (M) in a face presentation, sacrum (S) in breech presentation, acromion process of the scapula (SC) in a shoulder presentation.
      Example: LOA, left occiput anterior (very common); LSP, left sacrum posterior (frank breech); LSCA, left scapula anterior (shoulder presentation, transverse lie).
  6. Station of the presenting part: the relationship between the presenting part and the maternal ischial spines (Figure 25-2).

> **⚠ NURSING PRIORITY** If presenting part is higher than the ischial spines (floating), a negative number is assigned, indicating the number of centimeters above 0 station. As labor progresses, the presenting part moves from the negative stations to the midpelvis at 0 station (engagement) into the positive stations (sequence as follows: −5, −4, −3, −2, −1, 0, +1, +2, +3, +4, +5).

B. The passage.
  1. Types of pelvis.
    a. Gynecoid: normal female pelvis; inlet is rounded.
    b. Android: normal male pelvis; inlet is heart shaped.
    c. Anthropoid: Inlet is oval.
    d. Platypelloid: flat female pelvis; inlet is transverse oval.
  2. Soft tissues.
    a. Ability of the lower uterine segment to dilate and efface.
    b. Ability of the vaginal canal to distend for delivery.
C. The powers: involuntary, intermittent contractions of the uterine muscle (Figure 25-3).
  1. **Duration** of the contraction: the time between the first tightening sensation of the muscle and its subsequent complete relaxation.
  2. **Frequency** of the contraction: time interval from the beginning of one contraction to the beginning of the next.
  3. **Intensity** of the contraction: firmness of the uterine muscle during the contraction.
    a. Mild: slightly tense; easy to indent with fingertips (feels like touching finger to tip of nose).
    b. Moderate: firm fundus; difficult to indent with fingertips (feels like touching finger to chin).

525

Frank breech

Lie: Longitudinal or vertical
Presentation: Breech (incomplete)
Presenting part: Sacrum
A   *Attitude:* Flexion, except for legs at knees

Single footling breech

Lie: Longitudinal or vertical
Presentation: Breech (incomplete)
Presenting part: Sacrum
Attitude: Flexion, except for one leg extended
B   at hip and knee

Complete breech

Lie: Longitudinal or vertical
Presentation: Breech (sacrum and feet presenting)
Presenting part: Sacrum (with feet)
C   *Attitude:* General flexion

Shoulder presentation

Lie: Transverse or horizontal
Presentation: Shoulder
Presenting part: Scapula
D   *Attitude:* Flexion

FIGURE 25-1 Fetal presentations. (From Lowdermilk DL, Perry SE, *Maternity & women's health care*, ed 9, St. Louis, 2007, Mosby.)

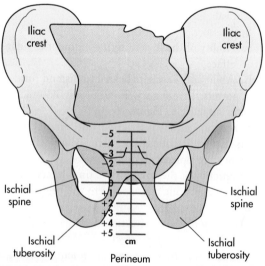

FIGURE 25-2 Stations of presenting part, or degree of descent. (From Lowdermilk DL, Perry SE: *Maternity & women's health care*, ed 9, St. Louis, 2007, Mosby.)

c. Strong: rigid, board-like fundus; almost impossible to indent with fingertips (feels like touching finger to forehead).

4. **Resting tone:** tension in the uterine muscle between contractions.

5. Abdominal muscle contractions are the second power; during the second stage of labor, they push the fetus to the outside.

Assessment of the Labor Process

Maternal Assessment

A. Differentiate *true* labor from *false* labor (Box 25-1; Figure 25-4).

B. Mechanism of labor: sequence of passive movements of the presenting part as it moves through the birth canal.
Engagement → Descent → Flexion → Internal rotation → Extension → External rotation (*restitution*) → Expulsion

C. Stages of labor (Table 25-1).

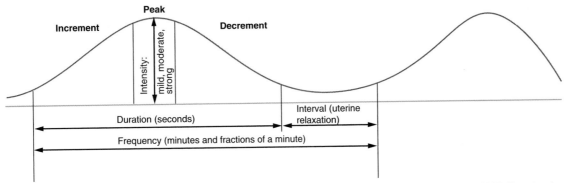

FIGURE 25-3 Labor contraction cycle. (From McKinney ES et al: *Maternal-child nursing,* ed 3, St. Louis, 2009, Saunders.)

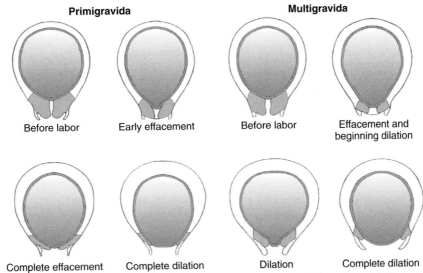

FIGURE 25-4 Cervical dilation and effacement. (From McKinney ES et al: *Maternal-child nursing,* ed 3, St. Louis, 2009, Saunders.)

Box 25-1   DIFFERENCE BETWEEN *TRUE* LABOR AND *FALSE* LABOR

True Labor
- Cervical dilation and effacement.
- Contractions occur at regular intervals and increase in duration and intensity; intensity usually increases with walking.
- Pain in the back that radiates around to the abdomen.
- Bloody show: expulsion of the mucus plug: bloody show may be observed at the onset of labor.

🛑 **NURSING PRIORITY** The two most important signs of **true labor** are cervical dilation and effacement (see Figure 25-4).

False Labor
- Lightening: descent of the fetal head into the pelvis; experienced as "dropping" of the baby.
- Increased vaginal mucus discharge.

- Softening of the cervix.
- Braxton-Hicks contractions may become uncomfortable, especially at night; discomfort is usually located in the abdomen.
- Sudden burst of energy.
- Weight loss of 1 to 3 lb; sometimes client has diarrhea, indigestion, or nausea and vomiting.
- Rupture of membranes.
  - If rupture occurs before onset of labor, it is called *premature rupture of the membranes.*
  - Delivery should occur within 24 hours to decrease incidence of infection.
  - Test with phenaphthazine (Nitrazine) paper; amniotic fluid is alkaline; phenaphthazine paper turns blue; normal vaginal and urinary secretions are acidic and turn the paper yellow.

Table 25-1	SUMMARY OF OBSERVATIONS AND NURSING CARE DURING LABOR

Physical Findings	*Nursing Interventions*

Stage 1—Cervical Dilation: Begins with onset of regular contractions and ends with complete cervical dilation and effacement; divided into phases—latent, active, and transition.

Latent Phase	
Cervical dilation: 0 to 3 cm	1. Orient to hospital environment and personnel.
Cervical effacement in primipara is usually complete before dilation; in multipara, it occurs with dilation	2. Assess history and physical status. 3. Assess attitudes, past experiences, expectations.
Duration of latent phase: 6 to 8 hours	4. Teach about labor.
Uterine contractions are mild to moderate, 5 to 30 minutes apart, and last 30 to 45 seconds	5. Practice breathing and relaxation techniques. 6. Monitor physical status: obtain vital signs including FHR.
Membranes ruptured or intact	7. Monitor urine output.
Scant brown or pink vaginal discharge or mucous plug	8. Amount and character of vaginal discharge.
Station: primipara, usually 0; multipara, 0 to −2	9. Provide comfort measures, oral hygiene.
FHR: clearest at level of or below umbilicus, dependent on fetal position	

Active Phase	
Cervical dilation: 4 to 7 cm	1. Anticipate needs:
Duration of active phase: approximately 3 to 6 hours	• Sponge face.
Uterine contractions are moderate to strong, 3 to 5 minutes apart, and last 40 to 70 seconds	• Keep bed clean and dry. • Care for dry, cracked mouth.
Scant to moderate bloody mucus	• Check bladder for fullness.
Station: +1 to +2	2. Stay at bedside, working through each contraction with client; praise woman's efforts; point out progress.
FHR: heard slightly below umbilicus or lower abdomen	3. Reinforce supportive efforts of the father.
	4. Use touch to soothe, relax, comfort.
	5. Check FHR every 15 minutes and BP every 30 minutes.
	6. Observe for hyperventilation.
	7. Client may need analgesia to enhance coping.
	8. Monitor IV and fluid status: increased risk for hypervolemia as a result of fluid retention.
	9. Encourage ambulation if membranes intact. Lateral position preferred when in bed as it increases uteroplacental blood flow.

Transition Phase	
Cervical dilation: 8 to 10 cm	1. Continue physical and supportive care.
Duration of transition phase: 1 to 2 hours	2. Use palpation or uterine contraction monitor to help client define contractions and rest periods.
Uterine contractions of transition phase: strong, 2 to 3 minutes apart, and last 45 to 90 seconds	3. Observe perineum for bulging.
Copious bloody mucus	
Station: +2 to +3	
FHR: clearest directly about symphysis pubis	

Stage 2—Expulsion of Fetus: Begins with complete cervical dilation and ends with delivery of the fetus.

Cervical dilation complete at 10 cm	1. Direct pushing efforts with assistance and support from father or birthing coach for each contraction.
Cervical effacement 100%	2. Provide comfort measures and facilitate rest between contractions:
Duration of stage 2: 20 to 50 minutes	• Apply cool cloth to face.
Uterine contractions are strong, 2 to 3 minutes apart and last 60 to 90 seconds; fetal bradycardia may occur during contraction	• Keep perineum clean and dry. 3. Encourage efforts; point out progress.
Membranes may rupture; copious bloody mucus	4. Explain preparations being made for delivery.
Station: fetal descent continues at a rate of 1 cm/hour in primiparas and 2 cm/hour or more in multiparas until perineal floor is reached	5. Check FHR with each contraction. 6. Help with panting for delivery of head and shoulders.
Urge to push begins	
Perineum flattens, bulges	**ALERT** Monitor client in labor.
Crowning occurs	
Infant is born	

Table 25-1	SUMMARY OF OBSERVATIONS AND NURSING CARE DURING LABOR—cont'd
Physical Findings	*Nursing Interventions*

Stage 3—Expulsion of Placenta: Begins immediately after the infant is delivered and ends when the placenta is delivered.

Usually within 5 to 10 min of delivery Uterine shape is globular, usually firmer; fundus rises Dark vaginal bleeding: gush or trickle Umbilical cord protrudes further from introitus Placenta intact: Shiny presentation of fetal side of placental separation occurs from inner to outer margins (Schultze mechanism); rough presentation of maternal side of placental separation occurs from outer margins inward (Duncan mechanism)	1. Congratulate. 2. Initiate maternal contact with infant. 3. Coach in relaxation for delivery of placenta and perineal repair. 4. Watch for signs of placental separation: discoid to globular shape of uterus, gush of blood, lengthening of umbilical cord, and rise of uterine fundus. 5. May administer oxytocics after placenta has been delivered (see Appendix 25-2).

Stage 4—Maternal Homeostatic Stabilization: Begins after the delivery of the placenta and continues for 1 to 4 hours after delivery.

Fundus firm or becomes firm when massaged, in midline at level of umbilicus Moderate lochia rubra Episiotomy or laceration repair clean without ecchymosis or discharge, minimal edema; tenderness commensurate with analgesia, usually mild; edges well approximated Possible extrusion of hemorrhoids	1. Facilitation of attachment: Ensure that parents have time with newborn; mother may initiate breastfeeding. 2. Ongoing assessment (every 15 minutes for 1 hour, then every 30 minutes for 2 hours) of vital signs, fundus, lochia, episiotomy, and bladder function. 3. Encourage rest for both parents.

BP, Blood pressure; *FHR,* fetal heart rate.

A   B   C   D

FIGURE 25-5 Leopold maneuver. (From Lowdermilk DL, Perry SE: *Maternity & women's health care,* ed 9, St. Louis, 2007, Mosby.)

Fetal Assessment

A. Determining fetal position by performing Leopold's maneuvers (Figure 25-5).
   1. First maneuver: upper abdominal palpation to discover contents of uterine fundus.
   2. Second maneuver: location of fetal back in relationship to right and left sides of mother; accomplished by sliding the hands down to a slightly lower position on sides of the abdomen. *FHR heard best through fetal back.*
   3. Third maneuver: location of presenting part at pelvic inlet and determination as to whether the presenting part is floating or has engaged; spread hand is applied to the abdomen above the symphysis pubis; gentle palpation of the part of the fetus that lies between thumb and fingers.
   4. Fourth maneuver: palpation in a downward and slightly inward direction, toward the pelvic inlet; done to determine how far the presenting part has descended into the pelvis.

B. Fetal heart rate monitoring.

ALERT Monitor fetal heart rate pattern.

   1. Intermittent auscultation (IA).
      a. Very common, inexpensive, easy-to-use method using either a fetoscope or ultrasound fetoscope by counting the FHR for 30-60 seconds between contractions to obtain the baseline rate.
      b. Auscultate the FHR during a contraction and for 30 seconds after a contraction to identify any increases or decreases in FHR in response to the contraction.
      c. If ultrasound device is used; FHR can be heard as early as 10 to 12 weeks.

2. Electronic fetal monitoring (EFM).
   a. **External monitoring:** noninvasive procedure that uses two external transducers placed on the maternal abdomen—the *ultrasound transducer* uses high-frequency sound waves to detect FHR and the *tocotransducer* monitors frequency and duration of contractions by a pressure-sensing device.
      (1) Advantage is its noninvasiveness.
      (2) Does not require rupture of the membranes or cervical dilation.
   b. **Internal monitoring:** invasive procedure that provides accurate, continuous information through use of a *spiral electrode* applied to the fetal presenting part to assess FHR and an *intrauterine pressure catheter (IUPC)* to assess uterine activity (frequency, duration, and intensity of contractions) and pressure.
      (1) Spiral electrode picks up electrical impulses from the fetal ECG.
      (2) Membranes must be ruptured and cervix sufficiently dilated.
C. Fetal scalp sampling: blood sample is drawn from fetal scalp to assess acid-base status; pH 7.25 or above is considered normal.

Nursing Interventions During Labor and Delivery

Maternal

Goal: To monitor changes during each stage of labor (see Table 25-1).
Goal: To provide relief from pain and discomfort.
A. Administer analgesic medication.
   1. Butorphanol tartrate **(Stadol)** or nalbuphine hydrochloride **(Nubain).**
      a. Widely used and results in good analgesia.
      b. Has less respiratory depression and nausea and vomiting.
      c. Should not be given to women with opioid dependency as may cause withdrawal symptoms.
   2. Fentanyl **(Sublimaze):** used with local anesthetic for induction of spinal block or epidural anesthesia.
   3. Sedatives: diazepam **(Valium),** hydroxyzine **(Vistaril),** and promethazine **(Phenergan).**
      a. Are often given as adjuncts to analgesia to relieve tension and anxiety.
B. Assist with regional or general anesthesia (see Table 3-7 for nursing care).
   1. Pudendal: administered late in second stage of labor.
      a. Perineal anesthesia of short duration (30 minutes).
      b. Does not cause central nervous system depression in the fetus.
      c. May eliminate bearing-down reflex.
   2. Epidural.
      a. Given in first and second stages of labor (can be administered with dilation of 4 to 6 cm in active phase); intermittent or continuous administration.
      b. May cause maternal hypotension, labor dysfunction, and inability to push effectively.
   c. Patient-controlled epidural anesthesia (PCEA): enables mother to have sense of control of pain management.
   3. Spinal anesthesia (block).
      a. Used for delivery (vaginal or cesarean), not suitable for labor pain control.
      b. May cause marked hypotension, impaired placental perfusion, and ineffective breathing pattern.
      c. Postdural puncture headache (PDPH) can occur due to leakage of CSF from site of puncture of the dura mater.
      d. Epidural blood patch: most rapid way to relieve a PDPH; inject 10-20 mL of woman's blood into lumbar epidural space, creating a clot.

Fetal

Goal: To monitor fetal status and detect early complications (Table 25-2).
Goal: To provide immediate care to the healthy newborn.

ALERT Assess a newborn.

A. Airway: clear air passages to establish respirations.
B. Body temperature.
   1. Maintain warmth with a radiant heater or warm environment during initial newborn assessment.
   2. Snuggly wrap the newborn in warm blankets for the mother and father to hold the infant; if infant is placed on mother's chest for skin contact, cover infant with a warm blanket.
   3. Place a stocking cap on the infant to decrease loss of heat by evaporation from infant's head.
C. Apgar scoring: immediate appraisal of newborn's condition taken at 1 minute and again at 5 minutes (Table 25-3).

ALERT Determine Apgar score of newborn.

D. Care of the umbilical cord: clamped after pulsation ceases; examine for number of vessels and record (one umbilical artery indicates increased incidence of congenital anomalies, especially renal and genitourinary); no dressing is applied to cord.
E. Care of the eyes: prophylaxis against ophthalmia neonatorum (gonorrhea and chlamydia); ophthalmic tetracycline or erythromycin; silver nitrate is not effective against chlamydia.
F. Identification: wristbands fastened to both infant and mother; appropriate footprints and fingerprints are obtained.
G. Administration of vitamin K (Aqua-Mephyton): 0.5 mg to 1.0 mg injected intramuscularly for prevention of neonatal hemorrhagic disease caused by lack of *Escherichia coli*, necessary for the synthesis of vitamin K in the intestines.
H. Inspection for gross abnormalities: clubfoot, imperforate anus, birthmarks, etc.
I. Attachment: ensure contact between newborn and mother as soon as possible after birth.

| Table 25-2 | SUMMARY OF FETAL HEART RATE: CHARACTERISTICS AND PATTERNS |

Term	Definition	Therapeutic Interventions

Baseline rate: Approximate mean FHR rounded to increments of 5 bpm during a 10-minute segment, excluding periodic and episodic changes, periods of marked variability, and segments of baseline that differ by greater than 25 bpm. During the 10-minute time frame, the minimum baseline duration must be at least 2 minutes; otherwise, the baseline for that period is undetermined. Normal range at term is 110-160 bpm.

Variability: Irregular fluctuations in the baseline FHR of two cycles per minute or greater. It is considered *reassuring* to have variability.

Baseline Changes

Term	Definition	Therapeutic Interventions
Tachycardia	Baseline rate greater than 160 beats/minutes for 10 minutes or more ***Pathophysiology***: Mild fetal hypoxia Maternal fever Maternal tachycardia Fetal neurologic immaturity	1. Monitor maternal vital signs. 2. Change maternal position. 3. Continue to watch closely.
Bradycardia	Baseline less than 110 beats/minute ***Pathophysiology***: Later sign of fetal hypoxia Known to occur before fetal death	1. Inform neonatal personnel. 2. Change maternal position. 3. Administer oxygen to mother. 4. Prepare for immediate delivery.
Loss of variability	Smooth baseline as recorded by fetal monitor Can be: Absent—amplitude range undetectable Minimal—amplitude range detectable but ≤5 bpm Moderate—amplitude range 6-25 bpm Marked—amplitude range greater than 25 bpm ***Pathophysiology***: Maternal medication Fetal acidosis (especially if accompanied by late decelerations) Fetal neurologic immaturity	1. Note time and dose of medication on record. 2. See Late Deceleration below. 3. Change maternal position. 4. Temporary decrease in variability can occur when fetus is in a sleep state.

Periodic Changes

Term	Definition	Therapeutic Interventions
Acceleration	Abrupt increase in FHR above the baseline rate of 15 bpm or greater and lasting 15 seconds or more Pathophysiology: Breech presentations; occur during fetal movement and are indications of fetal well-being	1. No specific intervention required.
Early deceleration	Visually apparent gradual decrease of the FHR with return to baseline associated with contractions Onset, maximal fall, and recovery coincide with onset, peak, and end of contraction, respectively ***Pathophysiology***: Head compression	1. Distinguish from late deceleration. 2. Observe mother for progress in labor, because these changes are usually indicative of cervical dilation of 4 to 6 cm or more. 3. Considered a reassuring pattern not associated with fetal hypoxemia, acidosis, or low Apgar.
Late deceleration	Visually apparent gradual decrease (onset to lowest point [nadir] greater than or equal to 30 seconds) of FHR below the baseline Generally, the onset, nadir, and recovery of the deceleration occur after the onset, peak, and recovery of the contractions ***Pathophysiology***: Uteroplacental insufficiency	1. Correct underlying cause—examples: • Supine hypotension—change maternal position. • Conduction anesthesia—elevate legs, increase hydration with IV fluids. • Uterine hyperactivity—reduce or discontinue dosage of oxytocin. 2. Considered a nonreassuring pattern. 3. Left lateral position during labor. 4. Administer oxygen to mother. 5. Fetal scalp sampling. 6. Be prepared for operative delivery if fetal condition warrants.
Variable deceleration	Visually apparent abrupt decrease (onset of nadir less than 30 seconds) of the FHR below baseline Decrease is greater than or equal to 15 seconds and less than 2 minutes ***Pathophysiology***: Umbilical cord compression	1. Change maternal position. 2. If severe, lasting more than 1 min, attempt upward displacement of presenting part; help mother into knee-chest or Trendelenburg position; prepare for immediate delivery if pattern does not improve. 3. Administer oxygen to mother.

⚠ NURSING PRIORITY Reassuring FHR characterized by 110-160 beats/min with no periodic decelerations and moderate baseline variability; accelerations with fetal movement. Nonreassuring FHR are associated with fetal hypoxemia and include increase or decrease in baseline rate, tachycardia (greater than160 beats/min), decrease in baseline variability, severe variable decelerations, late decelerations, absence of FHR variability, prolonged deceleration (greater than 60-90 seconds) and severe bradycardia (less than 70 beats/minute).

FHR, Fetal heart rate; *IV*, intravenous, bpm, beats per minute.

Table 25-3	APGAR SCORING SYSTEM		
Sign	**0**	**1**	**2**
Heart rate	Not detectable	Slow (below 100)	Over 100
Respiratory effort	Absent	Slow, weak cry	Good crying
Muscle tone	Flaccid, limp	Some flexion of extremities	Well flexed
Reflex irritability	No response	Grimace	Cough, sneeze, or cry
Color	Blue, pale	Body pink, extremities blue	Completely pink

Induction of Labor

Indications

A. Presence of preexisting maternal disease (e.g., diabetes mellitus, hypertension, and renal disease).

B. Premature rupture of membranes, postterm pregnancy.

C. Hemolytic disease, fetal death, congenital anomaly (e.g., anencephaly).

D. Elective.

Procedure

A. Prostaglandin E_2 gel is inserted vaginally to soften the cervix.

B. Amniotomy: artificial rupture of membranes ("bag of water"); labor often begins spontaneously.

> **!** **NURSING PRIORITY** FHR is assessed before and immediately after an amniotomy.

▲ C. Oxytocin **(Pitocin)** is administered intravenously with a physician in attendance and a physician order. **High-Alert Medication.**

1. Oxytocin is always piggybacked and hooked up to an infusion pump along with a primary intravenous (IV) line in case it needs to be discontinued.

2. Nursing management and information regarding **Pitocin** is covered in Appendix 25-2.

Assessment

A. Careful assessment of uterine contractions is a priority; tetanic contractions could result in uterine rupture, premature separation of the placenta, and fetal hypoxia.

B. FHR: check every 15 minutes along with mother's vital signs.

Nursing Interventions

Goal: To monitor and evaluate uterine response and fetal response to induction of labor.

A. Frequent vital sign checks and determination of FHR (every 15 minutes); electronic fetal monitoring may be used.

B. Discontinue **Pitocin** infusion if:

1. Contractions are more frequent than every 2 minutes.

2. Contraction duration lasting greater than 90 seconds.

3. Uterus does not relax; remains contracted and tetanic.

4. Nonreassuring FHR pattern occurs; absent variability; abnormal baseline rate.

5. Repeated late decelerations or prolonged decelerations.

Goal: To provide basic intrapartal nursing care as outlined in Table 25-1.

Emergency Delivery by the Nurse

A. The most important aspect of nursing care is for the nurse to remain calm and support the mother; the delivery process *cannot* be stopped.

B. *Never* force or hold back the oncoming fetal head.

C. As the head appears in the vaginal introitus, the nurse should apply gentle, even pressure with the hand on the emerging head to slow down the baby's process through the birth canal and to protect the mother's perineum from lacerations.

D. If the membranes have not ruptured when the head is delivered, they should be broken immediately to minimize aspiration of amniotic fluid.

E. Support the head after it is delivered; it will drop toward the mother's rectum, and external rotation (restitution) will take place.

F. Check around the infant's neck for the umbilical cord; if it is found around the infant's neck, gently slip it over the head.

G. Hold infant's head between the palms of both hands and, with a gentle downward motion, bring the anterior shoulder under the symphysis pubis. Then with a gentle upward motion, the posterior shoulder can be delivered.

H. The rest of the body follows easily.

I. Immediately position with head dependent to facilitate clearing of the airway passages, if there is no spontaneous cry or respirations.

J. Keep infant warm by placing on mother's abdomen, skin to skin; then cover both with a warm dry blanket.

K. Palpate the uterus and assist in the delivery of the placenta.

L. Transfer both mother and infant as soon as possible to a hospital facility; it is *not* necessary to cut and tie the umbilical cord, although it may be done if sterile equipment is available.

OPERATIVE OBSTETRICS

 ## Episiotomy

An episiotomy is an incision through the perineal body to facilitate delivery by enlarging the vaginal orifice. Episiotomy is no longer routinely performed because of evidence regarding harmful effects related to postpartum pain, blood loss, and risk for infection. Practice now is to support perineum and allow the perineum to tear rather than perform an episiotomy.

Types

A. Median: midline.
   1. Easy to repair; heals well.
   2. Increased chance of extension through the rectal sphincter muscle (third-, fourth-degree laceration).
B. Mediolateral: made at a 45-degree angle on either right or left side.
   1. More painful healing; increased blood loss.
   2. Less risk for extension into sphincter ani muscle.

Assessment

A. Observe perineal site for bleeding, swelling, redness, or any discharge.
B. Evaluate for pain and discomfort; should be minimal discomfort related to episiotomy; pain may indicate hematoma or abscess formation.

Nursing Interventions

Goal: To alleviate pain and swelling and to promote comfort.
A. Ice pack (first 2 hours, then PRN for pain relief); later followed by sitz baths, application of dry heat lamp (heat lamp treatment for 20 minutes, three to four times per day).
B. Analgesic sprays, ointments, or foam, as ordered.
C. Teach importance of perineal cleansing (i.e., use of the squeeze spray bottle; direct flow from front to back; and change perineal pad after each elimination—apply peripad from front to back to avoid contamination).

 ## Forceps Delivery

Forceps delivery is the use of an instrument (forceps) with two curved blades to extract the fetal head during delivery.

Types

A. Outlet forceps: used if fetal scalp is visible on the perineum without manually separating the labia.
B. Low forceps: application of forceps to the fetal head that is at least +2 cm station.
C. Midforceps: fetal head is at or below the level of the ischial spine.
D. Piper forceps: used in breech deliveries.

Indications

A. Fetal conditions: nonreassuring fetal heart rate pattern, abnormal presentation.
B. Maternal conditions: to prevent worsening of dangerous conditions (e.g., heart disease), exhaustion, infection and dystocia.

Assessment

A. Determine criteria for forceps delivery.
   1. Head fully engaged.
   2. Complete dilation of the cervix.
   3. Membranes have ruptured.
   4. Bowel and bladder should be empty.
   5. Arrest of rotation or delivery of head in a breech position.
B. Monitor FHR because forceps may compress umbilical cord.

Nursing Interventions

Goal: To assist with forceps delivery.
A. Provide physician with type of forceps required.
B. Assess for conditions necessitating forceps application.
Goal: To briefly explain procedure to couple.
A. Monitor FHR.
B. Provide emotional support.
Goal: To detect complications from forceps application.
A. Maternal: lacerations to birth canal and rectum.
B. Fetal: cephalhematoma, lacerations and bruising to face, facial paralysis, skull fracture, umbilical cord compression, brain damage.

 ## Vacuum-Assisted Birth or Vacuum Extraction

Birth method involving the attachment of a vacuum cup to fetal head using negative pressure to assist in the birth of the fetal head.

Indications

A. Fetal: nonreassuring fetal heart rate pattern; abnormal presentation.
B. Maternal: prevent worsening of dangerous condition (e.g., heart disease), exhaustion, infection.

Assessment

Same as forceps delivery.
A. Determine criteria for vacuum delivery.
   1. Head fully engaged.
   2. Complete dilation of the cervix.
   3. Membranes have ruptured.
   4. Bowel and bladder should be empty.
   5. Arrest of rotation.

Nursing Interventions

Goal: To assist with vacuum delivery.
A. Provide physician with vacuum and vacuum cup.
B. Assess for conditions necessitating vacuum application.

Goal: To briefly explain procedure to couple.
A. Monitor FHR.
B. Provide emotional support.
Goal: To detect complications from vacuum application.
A. Maternal: lacerations to birth canal and rectum.
B. Fetal: cephalhematoma, scalp lacerations, and subdural hematoma.

 Cesarean Delivery

In cesarean delivery, an incision is made in the abdominal and uterine walls to remove the fetus.

Types

A. Low-segment transverse incision.
 1. Preferred and most common method.
 2. Decreased blood loss; less chance of uterine rupture with subsequent pregnancy because incision is made into lower uterine segment.
 3. Fewer complications (e.g., peritonitis and postoperative adhesions).
B. Classic cesarean incision: rarely performed.
 1. Used in cases of placenta previa when there are adhesions in the lower uterine segment transverse fetal lie or in cases of severe prematurity.
 2. Vertical incision is made between the umbilicus and symphysis pubis.

Indications

A. Maternal.
 1. Uterine dystocia.
 2. Preexisting maternal disease: heart disease, diabetes, genital herpes, gonorrhea.
 3. Severe preeclampsia and eclampsia.
 4. Previous cesarean delivery or surgery on the uterus.
 5. Tumors of the uterus; postterm pregnancy.
 6. Placenta previa and abruptio placentae.
B. Fetal.
 1. Nonreassuring fetal heart rate pattern.
 2. Prolapsed cord; placental abnormalities.
 3. Fetal abnormalities (e.g., hydrocephalus).
 4. Malpresentation; multiple gestation.

Assessment

A. Assess for possible indication for cesarean delivery.
B. Trend is that once a cesarean birth occurs, it is highly likely that subsequent births will also be cesarean.
C. Cesarean delivery may be planned for a specific date or may occur as an emergency procedure; common elective reasons are previous cesarean delivery, breech presentation, and cephalopelvic disproportion, along with medical risk factors of hypertension, active genital herpes, positive HIV status, and diabetes.

Nursing Interventions

Goal: To provide preoperative care.
 Preparation is similar to that for any abdominal operation (see Chapter 3).

Goal: To provide postoperative care.
 Cesarean delivery includes both normal abdominal postoperative care and postpartum care (see Chapter 3).

COMPLICATIONS ASSOCIATED WITH LABOR AND DELIVERY

Preterm Labor

Preterm labor is defined as cervical changes and uterine contractions occurring between 20 and 37 weeks' gestation.

Assessment

A. Risk factors.
 1. Maternal infection; multiple gestations.
 2. Hydramnios; third-trimester bleeding.
 3. Premature rupture of the membranes: bag of water ruptures before the onset of labor.
 4. Incompetent cervical os; previous preterm labor or birth.
 5. Medical complications (e.g., diabetes, hypertension, anemia, periodontal disease).
B. Clinical manifestations.
 1. Contractions occurring in increasing frequency and intensity.
 2. Premature rupture of the membranes.
 3. Cervical dilation; cervical effacement.
 4. Cervical shortening in length.

Treatment

A. Medications (see Appendix 25-3).
 1. Tocolytics.
 2. Prostaglandin synthetase inhibitors: indomethacin **(Indocin).**
 3. Antenatal corticosteroids.

Nursing Interventions

Goal: To assist in delivery if maternal complications are present.
A. Maternal complications: diabetes, pregnancy-induced hypertension, hemorrhage.
B. Prepare for delivery of premature infant: if indicated, administer betamethasone **(Celestone)** or dexamethasone **(Decadron)** to minimize/prevent respiratory distress syndrome in the newborn.

> **! NURSING PRIORITY** Any woman admitted to the hospital who is 24 to 34 weeks' pregnant should receive antenatal glucocorticoids to promote fetal lung maturity, unless she has chorioamnionitis. The drug requires a 24- to 48-hour period to become effective.

 1. Most effective if delivery is delayed 48 hours after administration.
 2. Do not administer if lecithin/sphingomyelin ratio is adequate; if the mother has diabetes, an infection, or

hypertension; or if gestational age is greater than 34 weeks.

3. Administered intramuscularly; watch for pulmonary edema.

Goal: To provide emotional support.

A. Encourage expression of feelings related to anxiety and guilt.

B. Identify and support coping mechanisms for couple.

Goal: To minimize fetal complications.

A. Promote fetal oxygenation.

1. Avoid supine position during labor: associated with risk for vena caval syndrome.

> **! NURSING PRIORITY** Encourage lateral Sims' position, as it promotes placental perfusion.

2. Avoid maternal hyperventilation: leads to maternal alkalosis, which may decrease oxygen to fetus.

B. Avoid respiratory distress in the newborn.

1. Conduct labor with minimal analgesia or anesthesia.

2. Assist with breathing techniques and provide support to the laboring woman.

Dystocia

Dystocia is a long, difficult, or abnormal labor.

Assessment

A. Dysfunctional labor.

1. Hypotonic contractions: slow, infrequent, weak contractions occurring more than 3 minutes apart and lasting less than 40 seconds.

   a. Causes: uterine overdistention caused by large fetus or twins, polyhydramnios, and grandmultiparity.

   b. Complications: relate to prolonged or arrested labor.

2. Hypertonic contractions: frequent, strong, painful contractions occurring 2 to 3 minutes apart, lasting 60 seconds or more.

   a. Occur more frequently in latent phase of labor.

   b. Cause: cephalopelvic disproportion (CPD) or abnormal fetal position.

   c. Tetanic contractions: uterus stays contracted for more than 90 seconds; may be caused by misuse of oxytocin or mechanical obstruction.

   d. Maternal complications: exhaustion, excessive pain, and uterine rupture.

   e. Fetal complications: fetal distress.

B. Abnormal labor patterns.

1. Cephalopelvic disproportion (CPD): also called fetopelvic disproportion (FPD); related to excessive fetal size (>4000 g or more).

   a. Fetal macrosomia occurring in women with diabetes and cases of postmaturity.

   b. Hydrocephalus.

   c. Fetal malformations: abdominal distention, incomplete twinning.

   d. Maternal pelvis may be too small or abnormally shaped.

2. Abnormal fetal presentation: breech is most common.

3. Prolonged or arrested labor: labor lasting for more than 24 hours after onset of regular contractions.

   a. Maternal complications: intrauterine infection, postpartum hemorrhage, fatigue, exhaustion, and dehydration.

   b. Fetal complications: fetal distress and infection.

4. Precipitous delivery: a very rapid, intense labor lasting less than 3 hours from onset of contraction to time of birth.

   a. Maternal complications: trauma to the soft tissues of the cervix, vagina, and perineum; hemorrhage; loss of self-control.

   b. Fetal complications: fetal hypoxia.

Treatment

A. Dystocia relating to CPD or faulty presentation may be treated by a cesarean delivery.

B. Prolonged labor or hypotonic uterine contractions are treated by IV administration of **Pitocin.**

C. Hypertonic uterine contractions are treated by sedation and rest.

Nursing Interventions

Goal: To monitor level of fatigue and ability to cope with pain.

A. Provide basic comfort measures, back rubs, change of position, clean dry linen.

B. Provide emotional support to mother and significant other.

C. Give reassurance and stay with client continually.

Goal: To assist in the medical management of dystocia.

A. Explain procedures used to rule out cause of dystocia: sonogram, x-ray studies, etc.

B. Monitor **Pitocin** administration, if indicated for hypotonic dysfunction or prolonged labor.

C. Prepare client for cesarean delivery (indicated in cases of CPD and/or faulty presentation).

D. Administer broad-spectrum antibiotics to decrease incidence of infection.

E. Maintain hydration, monitor intake and output, and administer oxygen as needed.

Goal: To detect early complications associated with dystocia.

A. Monitor maternal vital signs.

B. Assess mother for signs of exhaustion, dehydration, increasing temperature, and acidosis.

C. Assess fetal heart tones frequently through fetal electronic monitoring.

Supine Hypotensive Syndrome

Supine hypotensive syndrome, or vena caval syndrome, occurs when the weight of the uterus causes partial

occlusion of the vena cava, leading to decreased venous return to the heart.

Assessment

A. Shock-like symptoms seen when pregnant woman assumes a supine position.
B. Clients at greatest risk: nulliparas with strong abdominal muscles, gravidas with polyhydramnios or multiple gestations, and obese women.

Nursing Interventions

Goal: To decrease the duration of an episode of supine hypotensive syndrome.

A. Educate mother to turn to either right or left side; preferred position because pressure is removed from vena cava.
B. Administer oxygen as necessary.
C. Assess FHR.

Placenta Previa

Placenta previa is the abnormal implantation of placenta in the lower uterine segment near or over the internal cervical os.

Assessment

A. Types of placenta previa.
  1. Complete: placenta totally covers internal cervical os.
  2. Partial: placenta only partially covers internal cervical os.
  3. Marginal: only an edge of the placenta extends to the margin of the internal os.
  4. Low-lying: placenta is implanted in the lower uterine segment but does not reach the cervical os.
B. Diagnostics.
  1. Ultrasonography: ascertains position of placenta.
  2. Ultrasonography is usually repeated during the third trimester because of the so-called migrating placenta phenomenon: the placenta gives the illusion of moving up in the uterus.
C. Clinical manifestations.
  1. Painless, bright red vaginal bleeding, occurring after 24 weeks' gestation.
  2. Bleeding may stop spontaneously and reoccur without warning during labor and delivery.

Treatment

A. Medical: if gestation is less than 37 weeks, conservative management of rest and monitoring of hematocrit and hemoglobin values.
B. Surgical: if fetus is mature, delivery via cesarean section (possible vaginal delivery for marginal placenta previa if bleeding is not excessive).

Nursing Interventions

Goal: To provide nursing care associated with hemorrhage (Table 25-4).
Goal: To detect complications associated with placenta previa: hemorrhage, preterm labor.

ALERT Recognize occurrence of a hemorrhage. It is important to be able to plan nursing management for the pregnant client who has bleeding, or hemorrhage (see Table 25-4). General nursing diagnoses for the hemorrhaging client are included.

Abruptio Placentae

Abruptio placentae is the premature separation of part or all of a normally implanted placenta, leading to hemorrhage.

Assessment

A. Types of abruptio placentae.
  1. External: blood escapes from the vagina with separation of the placenta.
  2. Concealed or internal: hemorrhage occurs within the uterine cavity.
  3. Partial separation: may occur with external bleeding or be associated with concealed bleeding.
  4. Complete separation: most severe, with profound symptoms of shock.
B. Risk factors.
  1. Maternal hypertension; previous abruptio.
  2. Cocaine use; blunt trauma to abdomen.
  3. Multiple gestations.
C. Clinical manifestations.
  1. Hemorrhage; hypovolemic shock.
  2. Board-like abdomen.
  3. Cramp-like abdominal pain.
  4. Coagulation problems: hypofibrinogenemia.

Treatment

A. Medical: treatment of blood loss and shock; before surgery, type and cross-match for blood transfusion.
B. Surgical: emergency cesarean delivery.

Nursing Interventions

Goal: To provide nursing management associated with hemorrhage (see Table 25-4).
Goal: To detect early complications.

A. Disseminated intravascular coagulation (DIC): may occur as a result of concealed uterine hemorrhage and damage to the uterine wall, leading to large amounts of thromboplastin released into the maternal bloodstream, which leads to hypofibrinogenemia.
  1. Assess for indications of DIC: bleeding from injection sites, epistaxis, bleeding gums, purpura, and petechiae.
  2. For decreased platelet and fibrinogen levels: administer packed red cells, frozen plasma, and cryoprecipitate.
B. Hypovolemic shock: fluid volume loss caused by hemorrhage, concealed or apparent; monitor vital signs and perineal area.
C. Couvelaire uterus: bleeding into the myometrium, which causes the uterine muscle to lose its power to contract; hysterectomy may be indicated.

Table 25-4	NURSING MANAGEMENT OF HEMORRHAGE IN THE PREGNANT CLIENT	
Causes and Sources	*Symptoms*	*Nursing Interventions*
Antepartal Period		
Abortion	Vaginal bleeding Intermittent uterine contractions	1. Obtain history of onset, duration, amount of bleeding, and associated symptoms.
Placenta previa	Rupture of the membranes Painless vaginal bleeding	2. Observe perineal pads for amount of bleeding (blood loss can be measured by weighing perineal pads, approximately 1 g = 1 mL of blood). 3. Monitor vital signs of mother and fetus (frequency is determined by severity of clinical symptoms).
Abruptio placentae	Vaginal bleeding Extreme tenderness in abdomen Rigid, board-like abdomen Increase in size of abdomen	**ALERT** Recognize the occurrence of hemorrhage and assess mother for complications.
Intrapartal Period		
Placenta previa Abruptio placentae Uterine atony in stage 3	Bright, painless vaginal bleeding Bright, red vaginal bleeding Ineffectual contractility	1. Start IV and provide volume replacement. 2. Request type and cross-match for blood. 3. Administer fluids and blood as prescribed. 4. Monitor intake and output. 5. Minimize chances for further bleeding. 6. *NO* vaginal or rectal exams. 7. Bed rest in position of comfort. 8. Anticipate delivery by cesarean section.
Postpartal Period		
Uterine atony Retained placental fragments Lacerations of cervix or vagina	Boggy uterus Dark vaginal bleeding Presence of clots Firm uterus Bright red blood	1. Massage fundus of uterus. 2. Anticipate administration of oxytocin for client with uterine atony. 3. Reduce anxiety. 4. Keep woman and family advised of treatment plan. 5. Record amount of bleeding in a specific amount of time. 6. Monitor vital signs: Overt hypotension and shock will not be seen until the woman has lost almost one third of her blood volume (1500-2000 mL); watch for tachycardia and orthostatic BP changes first. **! NURSING PRIORITY** Frequent, accurate assessment and documentation of blood loss are a priority in postpartum care; two-thirds of cases of postpartum hemorrhage occur without any predisposing risk factors.

BP, Blood pressure; *IV*, intravenous.

 Ruptured Uterus

A ruptured uterus is characterized by a tearing or splitting of the uterine wall during labor; it is usually a result of a thinned or weakened area that cannot withstand the strain and force of uterine contractions.

Assessment

A. Risk factors.
 1. Multiparity; large fetus.
 2. Obstructive labor; multifetal gestation.
 3. Excessive use of **Pitocin.**
 4. Weakened, old cesarean section scar.
 5. External forces such as trauma.
B. Clinical manifestations.

! NURSING PRIORITY Monitor the following warning signs of impending uterine rupture: restlessness and anxiety, no indication of labor progress, ballooning out of the lower uterine segment (which simulates a full bladder), appearance of a pathologic retraction ring (an indentation across the lower abdominal wall with acute tenderness above the symphysis pubis).

 1. Pain above the symphysis pubis.
 2. Sudden, acute abdominal pain during a contraction.
 3. Vaginal bleeding, shock; fetal distress.

Treatment

A. Surgical: laparotomy to remove fetus, possibly followed by a hysterectomy.

B. Medical.
   1. Blood transfusions.
   2. Prophylactic antibiotics.

Nursing Interventions

Goal: To provide nursing management associated with hemorrhage (see Table 25-4).

Goal: To assess for early diagnosis.

A. Maternal mortality rate is high.

B. Prognosis for fetus is poor; fetus usually dies as a result of anoxia caused by placental separation.

Amniotic Fluid Embolism

An amniotic fluid embolism occurs when amniotic fluid, which contains fetal debris (e.g., hair, vernix, or meconium), enters the maternal circulation through open venous sinuses in the placenta, at an area of placental separation, or through cervical tears under pressure from the contracting uterus. The fluid travels to the maternal pulmonary arterioles, and the pulmonary vessels become obstructed; prognosis is poor, and the maternal mortality rate is high.

Assessment

A. Risk factors.
   1. Increased incidence in multiparas.
   2. Increased incidence in a difficult, rapid labor.

B. Clinical manifestations.
   1. Sudden respiratory distress (dyspnea, cyanosis, pulmonary edema).
   2. Profound shock and vascular collapse.
   3. Decreased fibrinogen (hypofibrinogenemia) and DIC.

Treatment

A. Medical: management is similar to that for pulmonary embolism or respiratory distress.
   1. Medications: fibrinogen replacement and IV heparin.
   2. Insertion of central venous pressure line, blood transfusions, and cardiopulmonary resuscitation, as indicated.

Nursing Management

> ❗ **NURSING PRIORITY** The nurse needs to be particularly observant for symptoms of amniotic fluid embolism in any client who has had a short or difficult labor.

Goal: To assist in emergency resuscitation and provide critical care.

A. Assist with ventilation.

B. Prepare for central venous pressure line insertion.

C. Administer medications and blood to treat DIC and shock.

Goal: To provide emotional support to father and significant others.

Abnormal Fetal Position

Assessment

A. Occiput: posterior position (most common).
   1. Dysfunctional labor pattern.
   2. Prolonged active phase of labor.
   3. Intense back pain.

B. Breech presentation.
   1. Increased incidence with premature birth, placenta previa, polyhydramnios, multiple pregnancies, and grand multiparity.
   2. FHR is usually auscultated above the umbilicus.
   3. Often, passage of meconium is seen.
   4. Increased danger of prolapsed umbilical cord, especially in incomplete breech presentation.

C. Transverse lie (shoulder presentation).
   1. Increased incidence with placenta previa, neoplasms, fetal anomalies, and preterm labor.
   2. Dysfunctional labor patterns are seen.

Treatment

A. Occiput: posterior position.
   1. Vaginal delivery is possible; forceps may be needed.
   2. If CPD is present, cesarean delivery is necessary.

B. Breech presentation.
   1. Cesarean delivery is most often performed.
   2. Vaginal delivery: for a frank breech presentation, Piper forceps are used to assist in the extraction of the after-coming head.

C. Transverse lie (shoulder presentation).
   1. Cesarean delivery is the treatment of choice.
   2. External version and extraction may be attempted.
      a. No presence of CPD.
      b. Bag of waters is intact.
      c. Fetus is moveable and contractions are mild.

Nursing Interventions

Goal: To provide reassurance and explanations of procedures, as indicated.

A. Explanation of possible cesarean delivery.

B. When fetus is in occiput-posterior position, encourage positioning of mother on the side or in a modified knee-chest position to decrease pressure on the sacral nerves.

C. Assess for complications related to prolonged labor and possible infection.

Multiple Pregnancy

Assessment

A. Risk factors.
   1. Increased incidence of dizygotic twins (fraternal twins) is dependent on race, heredity, advanced maternal age, use of fertility drugs, and parity.
   2. Maternal risks.
      a. Spontaneous abortions are more common.
      b. Anemia occurs.

c. Increased incidence of pregnancy-induced hypertension, abruptio placentae, placenta previa, and polyhydramnios.

B. Diagnostics.
1. Auscultation of two or more fetal heart rates.
2. Measurement of fundal height exceeds gestational age.
3. Ultrasound.

C. Clinical manifestations.
1. Increased experience of more physical discomfort: shortness of breath, dyspnea on exertion, backaches, and leg edema caused by excessive size of uterus.
2. Complications occurring during labor include:
   a. Uterine dysfunction caused by overstretched uterus.
   b. Abnormal fetal presentations.
   c. Preterm labor.

Treatment

A. Medical.
1. Bed rest in lateral position to promote uteroplacental perfusion.
2. Antiemetic for nausea and vomiting after the first trimester.

B. Dietary: increase of 300 calories, along with increased protein, iron, folic acid, and vitamin supplements.

C. Serial ultrasound exams to evaluate for intrauterine growth retardation.

D. Nonstress tests, starting at 30 to 34 weeks' gestation; usually done every 3 to 7 days until delivery.

Nursing Interventions

Goal: To provide anticipatory guidance during the antepartal period.

A. Second trimester: prenatal visits every 2 weeks.

B. Third trimester: weekly visits if there are no complications.

C. Discourage travel, because labor may begin without warning.

Goal: To provide psychologic support.

A. Provide assistance and advice regarding care of twins at home.

B. Because twins are apt to be small, anticipate nursing care for premature neonates.

C. Assess for maternal complications (e.g., postpartum hemorrhage).

D. Ensure correct identification: Baby A and Baby B.

Prolapsed Cord

A prolapsed cord occurs when the cord is washed down in front of the presenting part.

Assessment

A. Risk factors.
1. Malpresentations: breech.
2. Transverse lie; unengaged presenting part.

3. Increased incidence with prematurity (because of small size of fetus).

B. Clinical manifestations.
1. Commonly occurs after rupture of the membranes.
2. Cord is washed through the birth canal with a gush of amniotic fluid.
3. Visualization of the cord: FHR is decreased, with variable decelerations noted.

Treatment

A. Surgical.
1. If dilation is incomplete, cesarean delivery is necessary.
2. Occasionally, if dilation is complete, vaginal delivery is possible.

Nursing Interventions

Goal: To maintain fetal oxygenation and assist with immediate delivery.

A. Continuing assessment of FHR.

B. Insert a gloved finger into the vagina and lift the fetal head off the cord to relieve the pressure.

C. Administer oxygen to the mother; start an IV.

D. Place mother in modified Sims' position, knee-chest position, or in Trendelenburg position (head of bed or table is lowered).

E. Any prolapsed cord outside the vagina should be kept moistened with gauze soaked in saline solution.

F. Offer emotional support to the couple.

Severely Depressed Neonate

A neonate with hypoxia and significant acidosis is a severely depressed neonate (Apgar score is 0 to 6).

Assessment

A. Risk factors.
1. Preexisting maternal disease: diabetes, hypertension, preeclampsia.
2. Placental insufficiency caused by:
   a. Maternal hypotension, hypertension, or hemorrhage.
   b. Umbilical cord compression.
   c. Polyhydramnios.
   d. Postmaturity.
3. Rh isoimmunization disease.
4. Uterine dystocia.

B. Clinical manifestations.

> **! NURSING PRIORITY** Initiate actions in response to signs and symptoms of fetal distress. During fetal monitoring, indications of fetal distress are often late or severe variable decelerations, lack of variability, and increase in baseline rate.

1. Severe hypoxia and acidosis.
2. Pale, flaccid, apneic neonate.
3. Heart rate less than 100 beats/min.
4. Slightly reactive or unresponsive to stimulation.

Treatment

A. Medical.
   1. Administration of oxygen, and possibly **Narcan,** to reverse narcotic respiratory depression.
   2. Laryngoscopy and airway suctioning; administration of oxygen.
   3. Cardiopulmonary resuscitation, as indicated.
   4. Insertion of an umbilical artery catheter; administration of glucose to alleviate hypoglycemia and calcium gluconate to alleviate hypocalcemia.

Nursing Interventions

Goal: To identify appropriate treatment and initiate it quickly for the severely depressed neonate.

A. Assess for fetus at risk and be prepared for emergency measures at birth.
B. Initiate resuscitation procedures.

Intrauterine Fetal Death

Intrauterine fetal death is also called *fetal demise.*

Assessment

A. Absence of FHR and fetal movement.
B. Decreased maternal estriol level.
C. Diagnosis: ultrasound examination determines absence of FHR and occurrence of fetal skull collapse.
D. Monitor for complications: hypofibrinogenemia from fetal breakdown products.

Nursing Interventions

Goal: To support the couple through the grieving process.

A. Objectively listen; encourage expression of feelings; do not minimize the situation or event.
B. Anticipate the steps of the grieving process (denial, anger, bargaining, depression, and acceptance).
C. Provide an opportunity for the couple to spend time with the stillborn infant, if they so desire.
D. Prepare the parents to return home by providing ways to inform the siblings, other family members, and friends about the death.
E. Offer information regarding resource or support groups for parents who have lost an infant.
F. Monitor for complications.

POSTPARTAL ASSESSMENT

> **ALERT** Assess client for postpartal complications. The puerperium is the period of time spanning the first 6 weeks after delivery. It is the period of time in which the body adjusts both physically and psychologically to the process of childbearing.

Physiologic Changes

A. Uterus.
   1. Uterine involution: process by which the uterus returns to its normal prepregnant condition.
   2. Immediately after delivery, top of fundus is several finger breadths above the umbilicus.
   3. At 12 hours after delivery, the fundus of the uterus is one finger breadth above the umbilicus.
   4. Fundus recedes/descends into the pelvis approximately one finger breadth per day.
   5. The uterus should not be palpable abdominally after 2 weeks.
   6. Afterpains: alternating contractions and relaxations of the uterine muscle.
      a. Occur primarily in multiparas.
      b. May be severe, requiring analgesics.
      c. Usually subside in 48 hours.
   7. Lochia.

> **NURSING PRIORITY** Always chart the amount first, followed by the character (e.g., moderate amount of lochia rubra).

   a. Lochia rubra: dark red discharge; occurs the first 3 days.
   b. Lochia serosa: pinkish, serosanguineous discharge; lasts approximately 3 to 10 days.
   c. Lochia alba: creamy or yellowish discharge; occurs after day 10 and may last a week or two.
   d. When lochia subsides, uterus is considered closed; postpartal infection is less likely.

B. Cervix.
   1. May be stretched and swollen.
   2. Small lacerations may be apparent.
   3. External os closes slowly; at the end of the first week after delivery, the opening is fingertip size.

C. Vagina.
   1. Does not return to its original prepregnant state.
   2. Rugae reappear in 3 weeks but not as prominent.
   3. Labia majora and minora are more flabby.

D. Perineum.
   1. May be bruised and tender.
   2. Pelvic floor and ligaments are stretched.
   3. Muscle tone is restored by Kegel exercises.

E. Ovulation and menstruation.
   1. Non-breastfeeding women.
      a. Menstruation resumes in 6 weeks.
      b. Ovulation: 50% may ovulate during the first cycle.
   2. Lactating women.
      a. Varies.
      b. 45% resume menstruation within 12 weeks after delivery.

F. Abdomen.
   1. Soft and flabby.
   2. Possible separation of the abdominal wall: diastasis recti.
   3. Muscle tone can be restored within 2 to 3 months with exercise.

G. Breasts.
   1. Anterior pituitary releases prolactin, which stimulates secretion of milk.
   2. Engorgement may occur approximately 36 to 48 hours after delivery.

3. Colostrum (thin, yellowish fluid) is released.
   a. Contains antibodies (immunoglobulin A is 90% of the immunoglobulin present) along with more protein, fat-soluble vitamins (E, A, K), and more minerals such as sodium and zinc.
   b. Colostrum has a laxative effect on the newborn; promotes expulsion of bilirubin-laden meconium.
   c. Also encourages the colonization of the intestine with *Lactobacillus bifidus*, bacteria that inhibit the growth of pathogenic bacteria, fungi, and parasites.
H. Gastrointestinal system.
   1. Immediately after delivery, hunger is common.
   2. Gastrointestinal tract is sluggish and hypoactive because of decreased muscle tone and peristalsis.
   3. Constipation may be a problem.
I. Urinary tract.
   1. Risk for urinary tract infection is increased, if client was catheterized during labor and delivery.
   2. May have bruising and swelling caused by trauma around the urinary meatus.
   3. Increased bladder capacity, along with decreased sensitivity to pressure, leads to urinary retention.
   4. Diuresis occurs during the first 2 days after delivery.
   5. Bladder distention may displace the uterus, leading to a "boggy" uterus and increased bleeding.
J. Integumentary system.
   1. Chloasma usually disappears at the end of pregnancy.
   2. Spider nevi, darker pigmentation of areolae and linea nigra may persist. Gradual fading of dark red stitch lines.
   3. Fingernails return to normal.
   4. Profuse diaphoresis occurs immediate postpartum.
K. Vital signs.
   1. Temperature may be slightly elevated (100.4° F) after a long labor; should return to normal within 24 hours.
   2. Blood pressure may be slightly decreased after delivery; however, it should remain stable.
   3. Pulse rate slows after delivery.
L. Blood values.
   1. Leukocytosis is present: white blood cell count of 20 to 25,000/mm³ are common.
   2. Hemoglobin and hematocrit values and red blood cell count return to normal within 2 to 6 weeks.
   3. Rule of thumb: 4-point drop in hematocrit equals 1 pint of blood loss.
   4. Pregnancy-induced increase in coagulation factors during the first week after delivery leads to increased risk for development of thrombophlebitis and thromboembolism.
M. Weight loss.
   1. Initial 10- to 12-lb loss is from the weight of the infant, placenta, and amniotic fluid.
   2. Diuresis leads to an additional 5-lb weight loss.
   3. Six to eight weeks after delivery: return to pre-pregnant weight if an average of 25 to 30 lb was gained.

Attachment: Psychosocial Response
A. Phases.
   1. Taking-in phase.
      a. First few days after delivery.
      b. Characterized by passiveness and dependency.
      c. Mother is preoccupied with own needs: food, attention, and physical comforts and care.
      d. Talkative.
   2. Taking-hold phase.
      a. Occurs about 2 to 3 days after delivery; characterized by increase in physical well-being.
      b. Emphasis on the present; woman takes hold of the task of mothering; requires reassurance.
      c. Very receptive to teaching.
B. Attachment behaviors.
   1. Exploration and identification pattern.
      a. Touch: begins by stroking the extremities and the outline of the head with the fingertips; gradually moves toward using the entire surface of the hand; touches and observes first at arm's length, then on lap, or slightly away from the body; finally enfolds infant close to body with both arms.
      b. Eye-to-eye contact: *en face position* (gazing into the eyes of the infant).
   2. Factors influencing maternal-infant attachment.
      a. Relationship with own parents.
      b. Previous experience with infants.
      c. Social, economic, and developmental level of mother.
      d. Acceptance of pregnancy as a positive event.
      e. Anesthetic/analgesic used in labor; type of delivery.
      f. Support of significant others.
      g. Amount of time of initial contact between mother and infant.
      h. Health and responsiveness of infant.
C. Postpartum blues.
   1. Transient period of depression (occurring during the puerperium).
   2. Complaints of anorexia; insomnia; tearfulness; a general let-down, sad feeling.
   3. Thought to be caused by fatigue, discomfort, sensory overload or deprivation, and hormonal changes.
   4. Woman needs support and reassurance that it is a transient and self-limiting experience.
   5. A very small percentage of new mothers are at risk for developing severe postpartum depression, leading in the extreme to postpartum psychosis, both of which require hospitalization. Safety of both the mother and baby is critically important priority if either of these conditions develop.

POSTPARTUM NURSING CARE

ALERT Perform postpartum assessments and instruct client on postpartum care.

Goal: To initiate routine postpartum assessment.

A. General observations of mood, activity level, and feelings of wellness; routine vital sign assessment.

B. Inspection of breasts: check for beginning engorgement and presence of cracks in nipples, any pain or tenderness, and progress of breastfeeding.

C. Check uterine fundus: determine height of fundus in relation to umbilicus; should feel firm and globular (Figure 25-6).

D. Assess for bladder distention, especially during the first 24 to 48 hours after delivery.

E. Perineal area.
1. Observe episiotomy site.
   a. Evaluate healing status of episiotomy.
   b. Apply anesthetic sprays or ointments to decrease pain.
2. Determine whether hemorrhoids are present, and if so, provide relief measures.

F. Lochia: record color, odor, and amount of discharge.

G. Lower extremities: assess for thrombophlebitis; encourage ambulation as soon as possible to decrease venous stasis.

H. Abdomen and perineum.
1. Initiate strengthening exercises for both abdominal wall and perineum (e.g., leg lifts and isometric Kegel exercises for strengthening pelvic floor).
2. Kegel exercises: practice trying to stop the passing of gas or the flow of urine midstream, which replicates the sensation of the pelvic muscles drawing upward and inward.

Goal: To provide comfort and relief of pain.

A. Episiotomy: ice packs for first few hours; followed by dry heat lamp, sitz baths.

B. Perineal care: use of "Peri bottles" to squirt warm water over perineum (front to back) to prevent contamination and avoid use of toilet tissue.

C. Afterpains: use of analgesics (preferably 1 hour before feeding, especially for breastfeeding mothers).

D. Hemorrhoidal pain.
1. Sitz baths, anesthetic ointments, rectal suppositories, astringent wipes.

One hand remains cupped against the uterus at the level of the symphysis pubis to support the uterus.

The other hand is cupped to massage and gently compress the fundus toward the lower uterine segment.

FIGURE 25-6 Fundal massage technique. (From McKinney ES et al: *Maternal-child nursing*, ed 3, St. Louis, 2009, Saunders.)

2. Encourage lying on side and avoidance of prolonged sitting.

3. Stool softeners or laxatives may be indicated; client usually has normal bowel movement by second or third day after delivery.

E. Breast engorgement (during lactation): well-fitting bra should be worn to provide support.

F. Lactation suppression: well-fitting bra or breast binder, ice packs to breasts; application of fresh cold cabbage leaves inside of bra.

Goal: To promote maternal-infant attachment and facilitate integration of the newborn into the family unit.

ALERT Facilitate parental bonding with newborn.

A. Use infant's name when talking about him or her.

B. Serve as a role model; be cautious not to appear too expert in handling the infant because it may lead to feelings of discouragement in the mother.

C. Assist parents in problem solving and meeting their infant's needs. Explain ways to distinguish different types of cries—those related to hunger, illness, discomfort, etc.

D. Encourage parents to provide as much of the care to the infant as possible while still in the hospital.

E. Accept parents' emotions; encourage expression of feelings.

F. Help parents in understanding sibling behavior and planning for the arrival of the new family member.

Goal: To establish successful infant feeding patterns.

A. Nonlactating mother.
1. Provide supportive bra.
2. Explain and demonstrate proper position for feeding.
3. Formulas: review formula recommended and how it is supplied.

B. Lactating mothers.
1. Teach mother to refrain from using sunlamps or hair dryers to dry nipples or apply breast creams.
2. Application of expressed breast milk to nipples after each feeding has a bacteriostatic effect and may provide protection to damaged skin.
3. On first post partum checkup, assess breasts for engorgement, nipple inversion, cracking, inflammation, or pain.
4. Explain process of lactation and refer mother to community resources such as La Leche League.

Goal: To prevent infection and detect potential complications.

A. Recognition of significant postpartum risk factors in the new mother (Box 25-2).

B. Encourage a postpartum checkup visit to take place 4 to 6 weeks after delivery.

C. If symptoms of excessive bleeding, temperature elevation, pain in the calves, foul-smelling vaginal discharge, swollen breasts, or general feelings of malaise and illness occur, woman should contact her health care provider immediately.

Box 25-2 POSTPARTUM HIGH-RISK FACTORS

Preeclampsia
Diabetes
Cardiac disease
Cesarean delivery
Overdistention of uterus (multiple gestations)
Abruptio placentae and placenta previa
Precipitous or prolonged labor
Difficult delivery
Extended period of time in lithotomy position (legs in stirrups)
Retained placenta

FIGURE 25-7 Correct attachment (latch on) of infant at breast. (From Wong D et al: *Maternal child nursing care*, ed 3, St. Louis, 2006, Mosby.)

Box 25-3 BREASTFEEDING

Types of Feeding Positions
• Cradle position, side-lying, football or clutch position, and modified clutch position.

Teach Mother to
• Bring infant to level of the breast: do not lean over.
• Turn infant completely on side with arms embracing the breast on either side.
• Bring infant in as close as possible with legs wrapped around the mother's waist and the tip of the nose touching the breast.
• Bring infant's lips to nipple; when infant opens mouth to its widest point, draw the infant the rest of the way on to the nipple for him or her to latch on (see Figure 25-7).
• Break the suction by placing a clean finger in the side of the infant's mouth before removing the infant from the breast.
• Put infant to breast 8 to 12 times per day.
• Avoid the use of nipple shields or bottle nipples.

Box 25-4 EVALUATING BREASTFEEDING

How do you know that an infant is getting enough breast milk?
• Hear infant swallow and make soft "ka" or "ah" sounds.
• Observe for smooth nutritive suckling—the smooth series of sucking and swallowing with occasional rest periods (not the short, choppy sucks that occur when the baby is falling asleep).
• Breast gets softer during the feeding.
• Infant is breastfeeding 8 to 12 times per day; more milk is produced with frequent breastfeeding.
• Infant has at least two to six wet diapers per day for first 2 days after birth; six to eight diapers per day by the fifth day.
• Infant has at least three bowel movements daily during the first month and often more.
• Infant is gaining weight and is satisfied after feedings.

Goal: To prepare and plan for discharge.

ALERT Assist client with infant feeding.

A. Determine whether mother will need household help (especially important in birth of twins or after cesarean delivery).
B. Explain and teach the following infant care skills.
   1. Infant feeding (Box 25-3 and Figure 25-7).
      a. Hold bottle so that air does not get into nipple.
      b. Method of making or preparing formula.
      c. How to break the infant's suction on the nipple.
      d. Positioning for burping and bubbling.
      e. Teach how to determine whether infant is getting enough milk (Box 25-4).
   2. Diapering.
      a. Frequent changing to prevent diaper rash.
      b. Protective ointment can be used to prevent irritation.
      c. Keep diaper below umbilical area.
   3. Bathing.
      a. Use of a mild soap.
      b. Kitchen sink is often a good place to bathe infant.
      c. Lotions can be applied; best advice is to avoid use of powders.
   4. Umbilical cord.
      a. Apply alcohol or wash with soap daily and after every diaper change.
      b. Stump usually falls off in a week to 10 days.
   5. Pacifiers.
      a. May be used to meet infant's sucking need.
      b. Should be discontinued around 4 to 6 months, or when infant shows lack of interest.
   6. Sleeping.
      a. Usually sleeps through the night at around 2 to 3 months of age.
      b. Encourage mother to sleep while infant is sleeping to avoid sleep deprivation.

7. Illness.
   a. Common behavior changes are irritability, crying, loss of appetite, and fever.
   b. Explain how to take an infant's temperature.
8. Taking the infant outside.
   a. Dress infant as you would dress yourself; do not overdress infant or "bundle up."
   b. Traveling: use a car seat.
9. Explain importance of follow-up well-baby checkup visits with health care provider, usually scheduled within a week of discharge.

ALERT Assess new mother for postpartum complications.

COMPLICATIONS OF THE PUERPERIUM

Hemorrhage

Assessment

A. Risk factors.
   1. Precipitous labor.
   2. Dystocia.
   3. Premature separation of placenta.
      a. Abruptio placentae.
      b. Placenta previa.
   4. Forceps delivery.
   5. Multiple pregnancy.
   6. Large fetus.
   7. Polyhydramnios.
   8. Prolonged labor.
B. Causes.
   1. Uterine atony.
   2. Lacerations.
   3. Retained placental tissue.
C. Clinical manifestations.
   1. Early postpartal hemorrhage: blood loss greater than 500 mL within the first 24 hours after delivery.
   2. Late postpartal hemorrhage: blood loss greater than 500 mL after the first 24 hours.
   3. Symptoms of shock: weak, rapid pulse; low blood pressure; pallor; restlessness; etc.

Treatment

A. Medical.
   1. Uterine atony.
      a. Oxytocic medications.
      b. Bimanual compression of the uterus.
      c. Fluid and blood replacement.

NURSING PRIORITY The key to successful management of hemorrhage is prevention, which includes adequate nutrition, good prenatal care, early diagnosis and management of any complications as they arise, and avoidance of traumatic procedures.

B. Surgical.
   1. Lacerations: suturing the bleeding edges.
   2. Retained placenta: dilation and curettage (D&C) to remove retained fragment(s).

Nursing Interventions

Goal: To control and correct the cause of the hemorrhage.
A. Uterine atony.
   1. Massage uterus to stimulate contractions.
   2. Administer oxytocic medications.
B. Lacerations.
   1. Inspect perineal area.
   2. Hematoma formation.
      a. Vulvar hematoma may appear as a discoloration of the perineal area.
      b. Any complaint of pain in the perineal area should prompt careful inspection.

NURSING PRIORITY Careful observation of vaginal bleeding, by doing a pad count or weighing the perineal pads, is very important. Always check under client's buttocks, as blood may flow between buttocks onto linens under the client.

C. Retained placenta.
   1. Inspect placenta at the time of delivery for intactness.
   2. Never force the expulsion of the placenta.
Goal: To maintain adequate circulating blood volume to prevent shock and anemia.
A. Type and cross-match blood for women at high risk for development of postpartum hemorrhage.
B. Anticipate replacement of IV fluids and blood.
C. Check hematocrit and hemoglobin values.
D. Monitor for development of hypovolemic shock.
E. Monitor vital signs and amount of lochia.
Goal: To prevent postpartal infection.
A. Maintain aseptic technique.
B. Administer prophylactic antibiotics.
C. Monitor vital signs.
Goal: To prevent postpartal hemorrhage.
A. Identify women at increased risk.
B. Monitor hematocrit levels throughout pregnancy.
C. Encourage use of supplemental iron to prevent anemia.
D. Promote good nutrition.
E. Instruct client to palpate uterus for firmness, and teach client how to massage fundus.

Puerperal Infection

Puerperal infection is any clinical infection of the genital canal that occurs within 28 days after miscarriage, abortion, or childbirth.

Assessment

A. Predisposing factors.
   1. Antepartal infection.
   2. Premature rupture of the membranes.
   3. Prolonged labor.
   4. Laceration.
   5. Anemia; postpartum hemorrhage.
   6. Poor aseptic technique.
B. Clinical manifestations.
   1. Temperature elevation 38°C (100.4°F), if taken at least four times daily on any 2 of the first 10

postpartum days, with the exception of the first 24 hours.

2. Symptoms vary depending on the system involved.
3. Area of involvement is characterized by five cardinal symptoms of inflammation (redness, pain, heat, edema, and loss of function).
4. Tachycardia, chills, and abdominal tenderness are common.
5. Headache, malaise, deep pelvic pain.
6. Profuse, foul-smelling lochia.

C. Area involved.
1. Uterus is most often affected: endometritis.
2. May have localized infection of the perineum, vulva, and vagina.
3. Local infection may extend via the lymphatics into the pelvic organs resulting in:
   a. Salpingitis.
   b. Oophoritis.
   c. Peritonitis.
   d. Septicemia.
4. Urinary system.
   a. Pyelitis.
   b. Cystitis.

Treatment

A. Medications.
1. Antibiotics.
2. Antipyretics.
3. Oxytocics.

B. Dietary.
1. High-protein, high-calorie, high-vitamin diet.
2. Encourage intake of 3000 to 4000 mL of fluid per day.

Nursing Interventions

Goal: To prevent puerperal infection.

A. Maintain meticulous aseptic technique during labor and delivery.
B. Assess and treat antepartal infection.
C. Detect anemia: check hematocrit during prenatal visits.
D. Avoid prolonged labor.

Goal: To promote mother's resistance to infection.

> **! NURSING PRIORITY** The pathophysiology related to maintaining semi-Fowler's position to localize infection is important to remember, not only for clients with obstetric complications, but also for others with contaminated drainage.

A. Administer antibiotic, antipyretic, and oxytocic medications.
B. Encourage good nutrition.
C. Isolate client from other maternity clients.
D. Use semi-Fowler's position to promote free drainage of lochia and prevent upward extension of infection into pelvis.

Mastitis

Mastitis is the invasion of the breast tissue by pathogenic organisms.

Assessment

A. Predisposing factors.
1. Fissured nipples.
2. Erosion of the areola.
3. Mastitis is most frequently caused by staphylococci, which are transmitted from the nasopharynx of the nursing infant.

B. Clinical manifestations.
1. Occurs most often between the first and fourth weeks of the postpartal period.
2. Chills and tachycardia.
3. Red, swollen, painful breast(s).
4. Fever of 39.4° C (103° F) or 40° C (104° F).

Treatment

A. Medication.
1. Antibiotics for 10 to 14 days.
2. Antipyretics.
3. Analgesics.

Nursing Interventions

Goal: To prevent the complication of mastitis.
A. Teach mother how to care for breasts and nipples.

> **! NURSING PRIORITY** Mother should continue to breastfeed on the affected side, because failure to do so increases the risk for abscess formation and relapse.

B. Explain the importance of wearing a bra that provides adequate support.

Goal: To promote comfort and maintain lactation.
A. Frequent breastfeeding, starting on the affected side.
B. Breast massage before and during each feeding to thoroughly drain any blockages (a breast pump may be used if the infant is unable to do this).
C. Encourage good nutrition and adequate rest.
D. Application of moist heat; increased intake of fluids and vitamin C.
E. Administer antibiotics, as ordered.

Postpartum Psychosis

A. Assessment.
1. Psychotic complication is uncommon.
2. Most mothers who experience postpartum psychosis have a history of psychiatric disturbance.
3. Pregnancy is usually the precipitating event that leads to the crisis.
4. Depression is the most common type of psychiatric disorder seen after childbirth.

B. Treatment and nursing interventions are outlined in Chapter 11.

Thrombophlebitis

There is an increased risk (five times) for thrombophlebitis and pulmonary embolism during the puerperium. The reason for the increased incidence is a change in blood coagulation during pregnancy and a decrease in partial thromboplastin time, along with engorgement of the veins of the lower extremities and pelvis, which leads to pooling of blood and venous stasis. Assessment and nursing interventions are discussed in Chapter 16.

Cystitis and Pyelitis

Cystitis and pyelitis occur as a result of trauma to the bladder mucosa, the temporary loss of bladder tone, and an increased bladder capacity. All three lead to distention and incomplete emptying of urine, predisposing the postpartum client to cystitis and pyelitis (see Chapter 23).

Parents' Reaction to Preterm Infant, Ill Newborn, or Infant With Congenital Anomaly

Assessment

A. Period of disorganization.
   1. Grief reaction characterized by guilt, anger, and sorrow.
   2. Feelings of exhaustion, emptiness, and frequent crying.
B. Period of information seeking and resource utilization.
   1. Anxiety decreases; problem-solving begins.
   2. Begins to resolve the crisis.
   3. Often information seeking leads to further anger and sorrow, followed by a period of denial or disbelief.
C. Resolution of the crisis situation.
   1. Development of new coping strategies.
   2. Acceptance and coming to terms with the situation.

Nursing Interventions

Goal: To provide emotional support to the parents.
A. Encourage verbalization of feelings and expression of grief.
B. Promote maternal-infant contact; point out normal characteristics.
C. Encourage parents to visit, touch, and care for their infant as much as possible.
D. Refer parents to social and community agencies.

 Appendix 25-1 MAGNESIUM SULFATE

MEDICATIONS	SIDE EFFECTS	NURSING IMPLICATIONS
Anticonvulsant IV: Given via an IV pump, piggybacked to primary infusion. A bolus dose (4 to 6 g over 15 to 20 minutes) is routinely given, followed by a maintenance infusion (1 to 4 g/hour).	***Maternal:*** Sweating, flushing, muscle weakness, depressed or absent reflexes, oliguria, respiratory paralysis ***Fetal:*** Crosses placenta; lethargy, hypotonia, and weakness ***Contraindications:*** Maternal—impaired renal function	1. Criteria for continuing administration: a. Respirations: greater than 12 breaths/minute. b. Presence of patellar knee-jerk movement. c. Urinary output: greater than 30 mL/hour. 2. Check BP frequently for symptoms of hypotension. 3. Antidote for magnesium sulfate is *calcium gluconate*; should be available at bedside in case of respiratory paralysis. 4. Monitor FHR and serum magnesium levels. 5. Administration of magnesium sulfate is continued at least 24 hour after delivery to reduce risk for seizure activity. 6. ***Uses:*** Prevention or control of eclampsia and as a tocolytic.

BP, Blood pressure; *FHR,* fetal heart rate; *IV,* intravenous.
 High-Alert Medication.

Appendix 25-2 OXYTOCIC MEDICATIONS AND PROSTAGLANDINS TO CAUSE UTERINE CONTRACTIONS

MEDICATIONS	SIDE EFFECTS	NURSING IMPLICATIONS
Oxytocic Medications Stimulate contraction of uterine muscle fibers; have a mild antidiuretic effect; stimulate postpartum milk flow but do not affect amount.		

▲ Oxytocin **(Pitocin)**: IM, IV, intranasal
Ergonovine **(Ergotrate)**: PO, IM, IV
Methylergonovine **(Methergine)**: PO, IM, IV
	Maternal: Tetanic uterine contractions, hypertension, tachycardia
	Fetal: Hypoxia, irregularity and decrease in FHR, possible hyperbilirubinemia
	Contraindications:
	Severe preeclampsia or eclampsia
	Predisposition to uterine rupture or CPD
	Preterm infant or presence of fetal distress
		1. Apply fetal monitor: assess FHR pattern throughout oxytocin administration.
		2. Assess maternal vital signs before increasing oxytocin infusion rate.
		3. Discontinue IV oxytocin and turn on primary IV solution, if any of the following occur:
		  a. Nonreassuring fetal heart rate pattern; absent variability; abnormal baseline rate.
		  b. Sustained uterine contractions lasting more than 90 seconds.
		  c. Insufficient relaxation of the uterus between contractions.
		  d. Contractions occurring more often than every 2 minutes.
		  e. Repeated late decelerations or prolonged decelerations.
		4. **Pitocin** is the only oxytocic used to induce labor; others (**Ergotrate** and **Methergine**) are used after delivery to control bleeding.
		5. *Uses:* Uterine dystocia; induction of labor, control of hemorrhage and uterine atony: uterine involution.

Prostaglandin F2a **(Hemabate)**: IM	*Contraindications:* Asthma	1. Used to contract the uterus in situations of postpartum hemorrhage.

CPD, Cephalopelvic disproportion; *FHR*, fetal heart rate; *IM*, intramuscularly; *IV*, intravenously; *PO*, by mouth (orally).
▲ High-Alert Medication.

Appendix 25-3 TOCOLYTIC AGENTS TO SUPPRESS LABOR

MEDICATIONS	SIDE EFFECTS	NURSING IMPLICATIONS
Tocolytic Agents Relax myometrial cells of the uterus leading to inhibition of labor. Also result in bronchial dilation and cardiac output.		
Beta-adrenergic agonists (Betamimetics) Terbutaline **(Brethine)**: IV, subQ, PO	*Maternal:* Tachycardia (very little effect on BP), nervousness and tremors, headache, and possible pulmonary edema *Fetal:* Tachycardia, hypoglycemia	1. Assess maternal (especially pulse) and fetal vital signs frequently; fetal monitoring is necessary; notify physician if maternal pulse is greater than 120 beats/minute or FHR is greater than *180 beats/minute.* 2. Strict I&O, daily weight. 3. Encourage lateral position (Sims') to decrease hypotension and increase placental perfusion. 4. IV: Use a pump for continuous infusion; infusion is continued for 12 hours after labor has stopped. 5. *Use:* Premature labor.
		NURSING PRIORITY Watch carefully when administering IV fluids to women in preterm labor, because there is an increased risk for tocolytic-induced pulmonary edema, especially when a beta-adrenergic agonist or magnesium sulfate is used. It is recommended that infusion be restricted to 1500 to 2400 mL in 24 hours.

Continued

MEDICATIONS	SIDE EFFECTS	NURSING IMPLICATIONS
Ritodrine **(Yutopar):** IV, PO	*Maternal:* Altered pulse and BP (dose-related), tachycardia, palpitations, hypotension, nausea and vomiting, hyperglycemia, nervousness and tremors *Fetal:* Altered FHR (dose-related), increased serum glucose, acidosis, hypoxia, and hypotension at birth *Contraindications:* Severe preeclampsia, hypovolemia, cardiac disease; used with caution in mothers with diabetes	1. Obtain baseline maternal ECG. 2. Assess maternal (especially pulse) and fetal vital signs frequently; fetal monitoring is necessary; notify physician if maternal pulse is greater than 120 beats/minute or FHR is less than *180 beats/minute.* 3. Strict I&O, daily weight. 4. Encourage lateral position (Sims') to decrease hypotension and increase placental perfusion. 5. IV: Use a pump for continuous infusion; infusion is continued for 12 hours after labor has stopped. 6. Anticipate use of propranolol **(Inderal)** to reverse cardiac effects. 7. Watch for signs of pulmonary edema, assess blood glucose with IV ritodrine administration, and do not give in presence of an infection. 8. *Use:* Premature labor. **!** **NURSING PRIORITY** Terbutaline is usually preferred over ritodrine because of minimal effects on BP and on maternal and fetal heart rates.
Calcium channel blockers Nifedipine **(Procardia):** PO, sublingual	*Maternal:* Facial flushing, mild hypotension, reflex tachycardia, headache, nausea *Fetal:* rare problems	1. No reported fetal side effects. 2. Not commonly used as a tocolytic agent. 3. Monitor blood pressure for hypotension. 4. Do not use sublingual route.
Prostaglandin synthesis inhibitors Indomethacin **(Indocin):** PO or rectally	*Maternal:* Nausea, vomiting, dyspepsia *Fetal:* Oligohydramnios, premature closure of the ductus arteriosus in utero syndrome, respiratory distress syndrome	1. Used when other methods fail and gestational age is less than 30 weeks. 2. Administer for 48-72 hours or less as may close the fetal patent ductus. 3. Administer with food or use rectal route to decrease gastrointestinal distress.
Magnesium sulfate	*Maternal:* Promotes relaxation of smooth muscles Watch for other maternal and fetal side effects listed in Appendix 25-1	1. ***Most commonly used tocolytic agent,*** because maternal and fetal/neonatal adverse reactions are less common than with the other tocolytic agents, especially the beta-adrenergic agonists (ritodrine and terbutaline). 2. Monitor serum magnesium levels. 3. Have antidote of calcium gluconate available. (See Appendix 25-1 for additional nursing implications.)

BP, Blood pressure; *FHR,* fetal heart rate; *I&O,* intake and output; *IM,* intramuscularly; *IV,* intravenously; *NSAIDs,* nonsteroidal anti-inflammatory drugs; *PO,* by mouth (orally); *subQ,* subcutaneously.

Study Questions Intrapartum and Postpartum

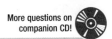

More questions on companion CD!

1. The nurse is caring for a 20-year-old primigravida who has been in the first stage of labor for about 8 hours. What assessment findings would indicate the client is progressing into the second stage of labor?
   1 Uterine contractions about 10 minutes apart, cervical dilation of 6 cm
   2 Cervical effacement at 100%, dilation at 10 cm
   3 Scant to moderate bloody mucus showing, station +2
   4 Fetal station at −2 and fetal heart rate noted at level of umbilicus

2. The labor monitor tracing shows variable decelerations. What complication would the nurse anticipate is occurring?
   1 Cord compression
   2 Fetal hypoxia
   3 Placental insufficiency
   4 Head compression

3. The nurse is assessing a client 12 hours after a prolonged labor and delivery. What assessment data would cause the nurse the most concern?
   1 Oral temperature of 100.6° F
   2 Moderate amount of dark red lochia
   3 Episiotomy area bruised with small amount of dark bloody drainage
   4 Uterine fundus palpated to the right of the umbilicus

4. The nurse is caring for a client in labor. How are contractions timed?
   1 End of one to the beginning of the next
   2 Beginning of one to the end of the next
   3 End of one to the end of the next
   4 Beginning of one to the beginning of the next

5. The nurse assesses the psychologic status of the mother and promotes bonding during delivery and after delivery. Which of the following maternal observations would cause the nurse to be concerned regarding the bonding process?
   1 Mother is not interested in breastfeeding after birth.
   2 Mother hands the infant to the father to hold immediately after delivery.
   3 Mother is tired and does not want to see the infant at birth.
   4 Mother is concerned regarding the newborn's acrocyanosis and molding of the head.

6. The nurse is monitoring a client during labor and observes an erratic fetal heart rate (FHR) pattern on the monitor at the height of the contraction. What is the first action of the nurse?
   1 Position the mother on her right side.
   2 Check the monitor leads for placement.
   3 Begin oxygen administration at 4 L/min and check fetal heart rate.
   4 Determine whether contractions are increasing in duration, intensity, and frequency.

7. A client is 38 weeks' pregnant and is admitted with bright red vaginal bleeding. She complains of abdominal discomfort, but she is not having contractions. After assessing the client's vital signs and the FHR, what is the most important information to obtain?
   1 The amount of cervical dilation
   2 The exact location of abdominal discomfort
   3 The station of the presenting part
   4 At what time the client last ate

8. The pelvic examination reveals the fetus to be at −1 station. What information does this indicate to the nurse about the presenting part of the fetus?
   1 Is visible on the perineum
   2 Has not yet entered the true pelvis
   3 Is above the ischial spines
   4 Is too large to fit through the opening into the true pelvis

9. A client complains to the nurse of abdominal cramping and pain after breastfeeding. What should the nurse explain to the client about this type of pain?
   1 All women experience abdominal discomfort during the postpartum period.
   2 Breastfeeding causes the release of oxytocin, which causes uterine contractions.
   3 Abdominal cramping is frequently associated with endometriosis.
   4 Abdominal discomfort is a sign of subinvolution and may occur for 3 to 4 weeks.

10. What is the usual length of time of the second stage of labor in a woman who is a primipara?
    1 20 to 30 minutes
    2 50 to 60 minutes
    3 2 hours
    4 3 hours

11. A mother delivers a healthy term infant and has decided she wants to bottle-feed her baby. What will be important to teach the mother regarding the care of her breasts?
    1 She should wear a tight bra and apply ice packs to both breasts to decrease engorgement.
    2 She will need to pump her breast every 3 hours to prevent engorgement.
    3 She will be given medication to prevent formation of milk and breast engorgement.
    4 She can take warm showers and decrease her fluid intake to decrease milk formation.

12. During the first stage of labor, the cervix becomes thin and indistinct from the body of the uterus. What is the term the nurse would use to describe this observation?
    1 Dilation
    2 Attitude
    3 Effacement
    4 Transition

13. The client complains of severe perineal pain the first hour after delivery. What should the nurse assess for?
    1 A soft boggy uterus
    2 Swollen, discolored area on the perineum
    3 Presence of a cervical laceration
    4 Increase in vaginal flow

14. The nurse is checking a laboring client. Her assessment reveals the head at +3 station. The nurse should:
    1 Prepare for the delivery of the infant.
    2 Begin administration of oxygen at 6 L/min.
    3 Determine whether contractions are increasing.
    4 Determine the FHR.

15. A woman who gave birth 3 weeks ago calls the nurse to ask what she should do for her sore, cracked nipples. What should the nurse tell her to do?
    1 Stop breastfeeding the infant until the nipples heal.
    2 Make sure all of the areola is in the infant's mouth when she breastfeeds.
    3 Cleanse the nipples with half-strength peroxide and air dry.
    4 Place a cool compress on the nipples after breastfeeding.

16. The nurse is caring for a woman in the afternoon who delivered at 8 a.m. The client complains to the nurse about the big blue veins on her legs. The nurse observes the mother's legs and notes multiple varicosities on her lower legs. What will be most important for the nurse to teach the mother regarding the varicosities?
    1 Wear elastic support stockings when out of bed and avoid prolonged sitting.
    2 Rest in bed for at least 1 hour three times during the day.
    3 Elevate the legs and apply warm moist soaks four times a day.
    4 Notify health care provider if moist lesions begin to form around the ankles.

17. The nurse is caring for a client who is at 38 weeks' gestation and is scheduled for an elective cesarean delivery. Which assessment finding would indicate a need for the nurse to contact the health care provider?
    1 Urinary output of 75 mL/hour
    2 Contractions occurring 3 minutes apart and lasting 2 minutes
    3 Complaints of burning and bloody urine on voiding
    4 Maternal heart rate regular at 98 beats/minute

18. A multigravida client comes to the emergency department complaining of abdominal pain. She is at 30 weeks' gestation. On assessment, the nurse observes complete dilation and effacement of the cervix with the perineal area bulging and the infant's head crowning. The mother states she is feeling a strong urge to push. What is the best nursing action?
    1 Prepare the client for an emergency cesarean delivery.
    2 Place even gentle pressure on infant's head and support it through the birth canal.
    3 Have the client hold her legs together and take her to the labor and delivery unit.
    4 Have the client take two deep breaths and push hard with next contraction.

19. The nurse is assisting a new mother to breastfeed her infant. The mother says "I am so afraid my baby is not getting enough to eat. I can't see how much she is getting." What information would be important for the nurse to discuss with this client? Select all that apply:
    _____ 1 The breast will begin to get softer as the infant feeds.
    _____ 2 The infant is satisfied for about 2 to 3 hours after breastfeeding.
    _____ 3 The infant latches on and feeds for a total of 10 minutes.
    _____ 4 The infant should be on a schedule of breastfeeding every 3 hours.
    _____ 5 The infant should have about five to eight wet diapers a day.
    _____ 6 The infant should regain his or her birth weight within the first month.

20. A woman is in labor with contractions 3 minutes apart. Her membranes have ruptured, and the umbilical cord is visibly protruding from the vagina. Rank the following nursing actions in order of importance (with 1 being the first action and 4 being the last).
    _____ 1 Wrap the exposed cord loosely in sterile saline soaks.
    _____ 2 Place an emergency call to the physician or health care provider.
    _____ 3 Initiate an IV or increase the rate of flow on the existing IV.
    _____ 4 Begin administering oxygen to the mother and have her assume a knee-chest position.

Answers and rationales to these questions are in the section at the end of the book titled Chapter Study Questions: Answers and Rationales.

CHAPTER TWENTY-SIX

Newborn

HEALTHY NEWBORN

Biologic Adaptations in the Neonatal Period

Assessment

A. Respiratory system.
1. Lung maturation process.
   a. Development of functioning lungs does not occur until at least 26 weeks' gestation.
   b. Pulmonary surfactant is usually of sufficient quantity at 35 weeks' gestation; acts to stabilize respirations and prevent atelectasis.
2. Respiratory effort.
   a. Respirations are usually established within 1 minute after birth, often within the first few seconds.
   b. Lusty cry usually accompanies good respiratory effort.
   c. Newborn respiration should be quiet; no dyspnea or cyanosis.
   d. Cyanosis may be apparent in the hands and feet (acrocyanosis); circumoral cyanosis (around the mouth) may persist for an hour or two after birth but should subside.
   e. Average respiratory rate: 30 to 60 breaths/minute.
   f. Respiratory movements: diaphragmatic and abdominal muscles are used; very little thoracic movement.
   g. Neonate breathes through the nose (obligate nose-breather); consequently, nasal obstruction with mucus will lead to respiratory distress.

> **! NURSING PRIORITY** Oxygen transport in the newborn is significantly affected by the presence of greater amounts of HbF (fetal hemoglobin) than HbA (adult hemoglobin), which holds oxygen easier but releases it to the body tissues only at low Po_2 levels.

B. Circulatory system.
1. Cessation of blood flow through the umbilical vessels and placenta.
2. Closure of the ductus arteriosus, the foramen ovale, and the ductus venosus.
3. Increase in and shift to pulmonary circulation.
4. Circulatory changes are not always immediate and complete: usually complete in a few days; often this period is called *transitional circulation*.

5. Anatomic closing of the fetal blood vessels may not be complete for weeks or months; functional closure is usually adequate to produce normal circulation.
6. Heart.
   a. May hear transitory heart murmurs.
   b. Assess for dextrocardia: auscultated heart sounds are louder on the right side of the chest.
   c. Pulse rate: 100 to 160 beats/minute.
7. Blood pressure.
   a. Measured using Doppler ultrasonography: need correctly sized cuff.
   b. Blood pressure varies with size and age.
   c. Recognition of hypotension.
      (1) Neonates are considered hypotensive if the mean BP is less than the gestational age.
      (2) Decrease in systolic of 15 mm Hg during first hour of life is common.
      (3) Normal BP is systolic 60 to 80 mm Hg and diastolic 40 to 50 mm Hg.
      (4) Any infant: systolic blood pressure less than 40 mm Hg.
C. Body temperature and heat production.
1. Loss of body heat.
   a. Evaporation: heat loss as water evaporates from skin and from lungs; occurs when infant's body is wet with amniotic fluid at birth.
   b. Convection: movement of body heat to flow of cool air; infant loses heat to the cool air in the delivery room.
   c. Conduction: direct transfer of heat to a surface on which the infant is lying; infant loses heat to a cool sheet or blanket.
   d. Radiation: heat is lost from the infant's warm body as it travels through the air to cooler objects in the room; heat loss often occurs during the days after birth, especially when an unclothed infant is placed in an open crib or isolette.

> **! NURSING PRIORITY** Excessive heat loss occurs from radiation and convection because of the newborn's larger surface area as compared with body weight. It is important to remember that conduction loss occurs as a result of the marked difference between core body temperature and skin temperature.

   e. Body temperature changes.
      (1) Body temperature at birth is 0.5° C higher than mother's.

(2) Body temperature may drop to 94°F (34.4°C) or even as low as 92°F (33.3°C) after birth unless the infant is adequately protected.

2. Production of body heat.
   a. Heat is generated immediately by *shivering*; infant shivering is characterized by increased muscular activity, restlessness, and crying.
   b. Infant shivering activity is not as apparent as adult shivering activity.
   c. Metabolism of brown fat (brown adipose tissue).
      (1) Functions to produce heat under the stress of cooling.
      (2) Brown fat is located in the intrascapular region, in the posterior triangle of the neck, in the axillae, behind the sternum, and around the kidneys.
      (3) Brown fat is metabolized and utilized within several weeks after birth.
   d. Increase in metabolic rate.
      (1) Stimulation of the thyroid gland leads to increased general metabolism; usually takes 12 to 24 hours.
      (2) Metabolic rate remains elevated for 7 to 10 days, even after warming.
      (3) Effect of chilling on the neonate.
         (a) Increased heat production leads to increased oxygen consumption.
         (b) Increased oxygen consumption utilizes glucose and brown fat.
         (c) When heat production is high, caloric need is high.
         (d) Tendency to develop metabolic acidosis occurs.
         (e) Production of surfactant is inhibited by cooling, and respiratory distress syndrome may occur.
         (f) Increased risk with smaller infants, because they have low reserve of glycogen and low reserve for increasing ventilation; leads to tendency to become more acidotic.

General Characteristics

> ❗ **NURSING PRIORITY** Assess a newborn; monitor a newborn for complications.

A. Length.
   1. Average length of term neonate: 45 to 55 cm (18 to 22 inches).
   2. To measure: infant is placed flat on the back on paper; a pencil is used to mark the locations of the infant's head and heels; after infant is removed from the paper, the distance between the two pencil marks is measured.
B. Weight.
   1. Average birth weight for a term neonate: 3400 g (7 lb 8 oz).
   2. Low birth weight: 2500 g (5 lb 8 oz).
   3. Excessive weight: 4000 g (9 lb).
   4. Weight loss: between 5% and 10% of birth weight within the first few days of life; infant usually regains weight within 10 to 14 days.
C. Head.
   1. Molding.
      a. Head may appear elongated at birth; molding usually disappears within 24 to 48 hours.
      b. Occurs as a result of abnormal fetal posture in utero and pressure during passage through the birth canal.
   2. Caput succedaneum (Figure 26-1).
      a. Edema of the scalp caused by the pressure occurring at the time of delivery.
      b. Disappears within 3 to 4 days.
      c. Edema goes across the cranial suture lines.
   3. Cephalhematoma (see Figure 26-1).
      a. A collection of blood between the periosteum and the skull.
      b. Usually results from trauma during labor and delivery.
      c. Absorbed in a few weeks.
      d. Does not cross cranial suture lines.

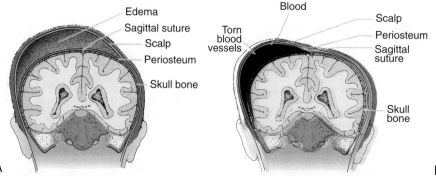

FIGURE 26-1 A, Caput succedaneum. **B,** Cephalhematoma. (From Lowdermilk D, Perry S: *Maternity and women's health care,* ed 9, St. Louis, 2007, Mosby.)

4. Head measurement.
   a. Average head circumference of the term neonate: 34.2 cm; usual variation ranges from 33 to 35 cm (13 to 14 inches).
   b. Head circumference is approximately 2 to 3 cm greater than the chest circumference; extremes in size may indicate microcephaly, hydrocephaly, or increased intracranial pressure.
5. Fontanels.
   a. Anterior: diamond shape about 5 cm, will increase as molding resolves.
   b. Posterior: smaller than anterior.
   c. Palpate for size and tension.
   d. Increase in tension may indicate tumor, hemorrhage, infection, or congenital anomaly.
   e. Decrease in tension (sunken fontanel) may indicate dehydration.
   f. Anterior will close in about 12 to 18 months; posterior will close in 2 to 3 months.
D. Umbilical cord.
   1. Determine number of blood vessels; there should be two arteries and one vein surrounded by Wharton's jelly.
   2. Cord atrophies and sloughs off in about 10 to 14 days.
   3. Should be no bleeding or oozing.

Behavioral Characteristics

A. Sleep and awake states.
   1. Newborn sleeps an average of 16 to 20 hours a day during the first 2 weeks of life, with an average of 4 hours at a time.
   2. May vary from a drowsy or semi-dozing state to an alert state to a crying state.

B. Infants vary a great deal in how they respond to stimuli.
   1. Infants move easily from one state of sleep to another state of consciousness.
   2. As the infant develops, he or she will reduce the total amount of sleeping time; wakeful periods will lengthen; sleeping will shift from daytime to nighttime.

Specific Body System Clinical Findings

A. Nervous system.
   1. Nervous system is relatively immature and characterized by the following:
      a. Poor nervous control; easily startled.
      b. Quivering chin.
      c. Tremors of the lower extremities of short duration.
   2. Reflex activity: the presence or absence of certain reflexes is indicative of ongoing normal development.
   3. Presence of positive Babinski sign.
      a. Normal finding until the age of 1 year.
      b. Dorsiflexion of big toe and fanning of the other toes.
   4. Neonatal reflexes (Table 26-1).

> **! NURSING PRIORITY** Intactness of the neonate's nervous system is indicated by the state of alertness, resting posture, cry, and quality of muscle tone and motor activity.

B. Hematologic system.
   1. Initially at birth.
      a. Increased number of red blood cells (RBCs): 4,800,000/mm^3 of blood.
      b. Hemoglobin: 14 to 24 g/dL of blood.
      c. Hematocrit: 44% to 64%.

Table 26-1	MAJOR NEONATAL REFLEXES		
Reflex	**Disappears**	**How to Elicit**	**Response**
Rooting	3 to 4 months; may persist during sleep until 7 to 8 months	Stroke cheek.	Head turns toward side that is touched.
Babinski	1 year	Lightly stroke lateral side of foot from heel to toe across the foot.	Infant's toes fan, with dorsiflexion of great toe.
Sucking	10 to 12 months	Touch or stroke lips.	Infant sucks.
Moro (startle)	3 to 4 months	Make a loud noise or suddenly disturb infant's equilibrium.	Infant stiffens, briskly abducts, and extends arms with hands open and fingers extended to C shape. Infant's legs flex and abduct, and arms return to an embracing posture. Crying is usual.
Grasp palmar	3 to 4 months	Press a finger against infant's palm.	Infant's fingers momentarily close around object.
Asymmetric tonic neck (fencer's position)	3 to 4 months	Turn supine infant's head over the shoulder to one side.	Infant's arm and leg partially or completely extend on side to which head is turned; opposite arm and leg flex.

2. Leukocytosis is present at birth (white blood cell count of 9000 to 30,000 mm³).
   a. Considerable decrease in white blood cell count occurs within a few days after birth.
   b. Shift in the type of cells occurs: neutrophils decrease, and lymphocytes increase until they predominate by the end of the first week.
3. Anemia.
   a. Erythropoiesis slows down during the first 6 to 8 weeks of life; RBCs break down, and their life span ends with resultant anemia.
   b. This drop in hemoglobin and RBC count is termed *physiologic anemia of the newborn*.
   c. After the third month, a slow rise begins.
4. Jaundice.
   a. Physiologic jaundice; increased incidence in breastfed infants; occurs on the second or third day of life as a result of an increase in the serum bilirubin level.
   b. Pathologic jaundice occurs within 24 hours of birth (see hemolytic disease of the newborn).
   c. Pathophysiology (physiologic).
      (1) Inability of the liver to clear bilirubin from the plasma.
      (2) Increased level of RBCs from the maternal circulation at birth leads to increased breakdown and bilirubin production.
   d. Criteria for physiologic jaundice.
      (1) Does not appear until *after* 24 hours following birth.
      (2) Total serum bilirubin level is less than 12 mg/100 mL.
      (3) Infant does not show any sign of illness or cardiac decompensation.
      (4) Total serum bilirubin level does not increase more than 5 mg/100 mL per 24 hours.
      (5) Clinical evidence of jaundice disappears within 1 week in the term infant and by the end of the second week in the premature infant. Bilirubin peaks around day 3, plateaus for 12 to 14 days, and then steadily decreases.
   e. Treatment: phototherapy.
      (1) Converts unconjugated bilirubin into conjugated (water-soluble) form, which can be excreted.
      (2) Indication for phototherapy varies according to the maturity of the fetus and presence of disease; treatment may be started earlier for premature infants.
      (3) If bili lights are used, expose all areas to the light except for eyes and genitalia; cover infant's eyes with an opaque mask or eye patch and cover genitalia with a diaper or a disposable face mask (string bikini to expose more skin).
      (4) Hour specific serum bilirubin levels are recommended to predict rapid rising levels in the high risk newborn.
      (5) Noninvasive transcutaneous bilirubinometry (TcB): allows for repetitive estimation of bilirubin level; cannot be used after phototherapy has been initiated.

> **⚠ NURSING PRIORITY** If a face mask is used to cover genitalia, remove the metal nose strip to prevent burning the infant.

      (6) If a fiberoptic blanket is used, infant's eyes do not need to be covered; should have a covering pad between the infant's skin and the fiberoptic blanket; with this method, the infant may remain in the room with the mother or the fiberoptic blanket may be used at home.
      (7) Monitor skin temperature: treatment may increase temperature.
      (8) Reposition infant every 2 hours to expose as much body surface as possible.
      (9) Chart pertinent information: time phototherapy was started and stopped, maintenance of shielding of the eyes from bili light, type and intensity of lamp used, distance of light from infant, whether used in combination with an isolette or an open bassinet, and any side effects.
      (10) Remove infant from light treatment for feedings; encourage parents to hold and feed infant.
      (11) Effects.
         (a) Vasodilation of the skin.
         (b) Increased insensible water loss: encourage intake of fluids to maintain adequate hydration.
         (c) Decreased gastrointestinal (GI) transit time: frequent loose, green stools.
         (d) Skin discoloration: skin may become grayish brown; color is transient with no complications.
      (12) Phototherapy may be used as an adjunct to treatment of pathologic jaundice.
      (13) Effectiveness is determined by:
         (a) A decrease of 3 to 4 mg/100 mL of blood in the serum bilirubin after 8 to 12 hours of therapy.
         (b) A gradual diminishing of jaundice.
5. Transitory coagulation defects.
   a. Occur between the second and fifth postnatal days.
   b. Result from the lack of intestinal synthesis of vitamin K because of insufficient bacterial flora in the GI tract.
   c. Vitamin K (0.5 to 1.0 mg) is administered intramuscularly to prevent complications.
C. GI tract.
   1. Able to absorb proteins and simple carbohydrates.
   2. Stomach produces hydrochloric acid immediately after birth.

3. Digestive enzymes are present except for pancreatic amylase and lipase; this results in the inability to absorb fat adequately.
4. Stools.

> **⚠ NURSING PRIORITY** Monitor the passage of the first meconium stool.

   a. Meconium: sticky, black, odorless, sterile stool that is passed within the first 24 to 48 hours after birth; if no stool is passed, further assessment is needed.
   b. Stools change according to type and amount of feedings.
      (1) Transitional stools: occur during period between second and fourth day; consist of meconium and milk; greenish brown or greenish yellow; loose and often contain mucus.
      (2) Milk stools: usually occur by the fourth day; stools of formula-fed infant are drier, more formed, paler, and occur once or twice daily or 1 stool every 2 to 3 days.
      (3) Stools of breastfed infants are golden yellow, have a pasty consistency, and occur more frequently than stools of formula-fed infants, 3 to 4 stools in 24 hours.

D. Genitourinary system.
   1. Urinary.
      a. Urinary output is low during the first few days of life or until fluid intake increases.

> **⚠ NURSING PRIORITY** Most newborns void within the first 24 to 48 hours after birth. Weigh dry diaper before applying; then weigh wet diaper after infant voiding. Each gram of added weight equals 1 mL of urine.

      b. About 30 to 60 mL are voided per day during the first 2 days of life; followed by 200 mL per day by the end of the first week.
      c. Frequency of voiding: average of two to six times per day, increasing up to 10 to 15 times per day.
   2. Genitalia.
      a. Female: labia majora are underdeveloped; small amount of bloody discharge from the vagina may be seen as a result of the presence of maternal hormones.
      b. Male: scrotum may be edematous; testes should have descended; assess the urethral opening.

E. Integumentary system.
   1. Vernix caseosa: a white cheesy-like material covers the skin at birth, particularly noted in the folds and creases.
   2. Petechiae: pinpoint bluish discolorations primarily on the skin and face as a result of pressure from delivery; bruising of tissues may be seen.
   3. Lanugo: downy, fine covering of hair that may be present on the shoulders, back, earlobes, and forehead; disappears during the first week.

4. Milia: pinpoint white bumps seen over the bridge of the nose and on the cheeks during the first 2 weeks of life.
5. Erythema toxicum: splotchy pink papular rash appearing anywhere on the body; disappears within the first few days of life; no treatment is necessary.
6. Mongolian spots: dark bluish pigmented areas seen on the back or buttocks of dark-skinned infants (African-American and Asian American infants and those of Mediterranean descent); usually disappear by school age.

F. Endocrine system.
   1. Because of the presence of maternal hormones in the bloodstream, neonate may have breast enlargement or vulvar or prostatic enlargement.
   2. Thymus gland is normally large; grows rapidly until age of 5 years; remains the same until about age of 10 years, then finally diminishes.

G. Sensory system.
   1. Vision: visual acuity of 20/100 to 20/400; retinal development is advanced.
      a. Eyes appear large, and pupils appear small.
      b. All infants' eyes are blue or slate blue at birth; become their permanent color at age 3 months.
      c. Tears do not develop until 2 to 4 weeks of age.
      d. Eyes close in response to bright light; red reflex is present; pupils react to light.
      e. Visual preferences: yellow, green, pink, and black and white patterns.
   2. Hearing.
      a. Sudden loud noises may elicit startle response.
      b. Usually able to locate the general direction of sounds.
   3. Sense of smell is present at birth; infants react to strong odors.
   4. Taste.
      a. Differentiates between pleasant and unpleasant tastes.
      b. Rejects especially salty, sour, or bitter tastes by grimacing; also stops sucking.
   5. Tactile senses.
      a. Most sensitive area is around the mouth.
      b. Searches for food when cheek is touched or begins sucking movement when lips are touched.

H. Musculoskeletal system.
   1. Assumes the position of comfort, which is usually the position assumed in utero.
   2. Normal palmar crease is present (simian crease is indicative of Down syndrome).
   3. Spine is straight and flat when in prone position.
   4. Creases and fat pads are present on the soles of the feet.
   5. All digits are present on hands and feet; fingernails are present.

Nursing Interventions

> **ALERT** Provide newborn care and education.

Goal: To establish and maintain a patent airway and promote oxygenation.
A. Position infant with head slightly lower than chest; may use postural drainage or side-lying position.
B. Suction nostrils and oropharynx with bulb syringe.
C. Observe for apnea, cyanosis, and mucus collection and be ready to use oropharyngeal suctioning, stimulation, oxygen administration, or resuscitative procedures, if necessary.

> **! NURSING PRIORITY** During first 4 hours after birth, the priority nursing goals are to maintain a clear airway, prevent heat loss, prevent hemorrhage and infection, and monitor transition. Bathing will be initiated when infant's temperature is stabilized; feeding may begin immediately if infant is interested.

Goal: To protect against heat loss (Figure 26-2).
A. Immediately after birth, wrap infant in warm blanket and dry off amniotic fluid.
B. Replace wet blanket with warm dry blanket.
C. Cover wet hair and head with a blanket or cap.
D. Immediately after birth, may provide for skin-to-skin contact with the mother; cover infant with warm blanket.
E. For initial physical assessment, place baby on a warm padded surface, preferably under a radiant heater.
F. Wrap infant securely in a warm blanket and give him or her to parents to cuddle and observe.
G. Avoid any unnecessary procedures until body temperature is stable.

Goal: To perform a newborn physical assessment and collect data on behavior (Box 26-1).
A. Determine Apgar score at 1 minute and again at 5 minutes (see Table 25-3 for Apgar scoring).

> **! NURSING PRIORITY** Assess a newborn and determine Apgar scores.

Cold → ↑O₂ consumption → ↑Respiratory rate
↓O₂ uptake by lungs ← Pulmonary vasoconstriction
↓O₂ to tissues ← Peripheral vasoconstriction
↑Anaerobic glycolysis → ↓in Po₂ and pH
Metabolic acidosis

FIGURE 26-2 Effects of cold stress. (From Lowdermilk D, Perry S: *Maternity and women's health care*, ed 7, St. Louis, 2007, Mosby.)

> **Box 26-1   GUIDELINES FOR PHYSICAL ASSESSMENT OF THE NEWBORN**
>
> - Perform procedures that require quiet first, such as auscultating the lungs, heart, and abdomen.
> - Perform procedures that may causing crying last, such as testing reflexes.
> - Measure head, chest, and length at the same time to compare results.
> - Obtain an axillary temperature (rectal thermometer may perforate mucosa).
> - Monitor vital signs every 15 minutes to 1 hour until infant's temperature stabilizes (usually in about 4 hours).
> - Perform glucose checks for hypoglycemia on an infant of a mother with diabetes or on a newborn with complications.

1. The 1-minute Apgar score is a rapid evaluation of the status of the neonate's intrauterine oxygenation.
2. The 5-minute Apgar score is an evaluation of the neonate's response to cardiorespiratory adaptation after birth.
B. Gestational age assessment within 2 hours of birth.
C. Comprehensive physical assessment completed within 24 hours of birth.
D. Determine special needs and whether any significant risk factors are present.

Goal: To assess periods of reactivity.
A. First period of reactivity.
1. Lasts approximately 30 minutes.
2. Newborn is alert, awake, and usually hungry.

> **! NURSING PRIORITY** Periods of reactivity are excellent opportunities for promoting attachment response.

B. Sleep phase.
1. First sleep usually occurs an average of 3 to 4 hours after birth and may last from a few minutes to several hours.
2. Newborn is difficult to awaken during this phase.
C. Second period of reactivity.
1. Infant is alert and awake.
2. Lasts approximately 4 to 6 hours.

> **! NURSING PRIORITY** It is important to monitor the infant closely because apnea, decreased heart rate, gagging, choking, and regurgitation may occur and require nursing intervention.

Goal: To protect against infection.
A. Follow guidelines for proper hand hygiene before handling infant.
B. Prevent ophthalmia neonatorum.
1. Administer prophylactic treatment to eyes soon after birth.
2. Place ophthalmic ointment or solution in the conjunctival sac.
C. Avoid exposure to people with possible upper respiratory tract, skin, or GI infections.

Goal: To prevent hypofibrinogenemia.

A. Administer 0.5 to 1.0 mg of vitamin K, intramuscularly into the upper third of the lateral aspect of the thigh.

Goal: To properly identify infant.

A. Secure identification bands to wrist or ankle of infant and wrist of mother in the delivery room.

B. Prints of infant's foot, palms, or fingers may be obtained according to hospital policy; mother's palm prints or fingerprints may also be obtained.

C. Advise parents not to release the infant to anyone who does not have proper unit identification.

> **⬛ NURSING PRIORITY** Always check the infant's ID band with the mother's ID band every time the infant and mother have been separated; monitor area for anyone who does not have a security clearance to be in the newborn area; security of the newborn is a priority!

Goal: To promote parental attachment to infant immediately after birth.

A. Wrap infant snugly in warm blanket and encourage parents to hold infant. Do not allow chilling to occur.

B. Encourage touching and holding during periods of reactivity.

Goal: To initiate feeding and to evaluate parents' ability to feed infant and provide nutrition.

A. Encourage breastfeeding, if desired, immediately after delivery or in recovery area; breast milk is bacteriologically safe.

B. Assess infant's ability to feed; assess for active bowel sounds, absence of abdominal distention; rooting, sucking, swallowing reflexes and alertness.

C. First formula feeding or test feeding: administer 10 to 15 mL of sterile water to assist GI tract patency followed by formula.

D. Considerations in infant feeding.

1. An infant should always be placed on the right side after feeding to avoid aspiration and prevent regurgitation and distention.

2. Infant will require more frequent feedings initially; will generally establish a routine of feeding every 3 to 4 hours.

E. Infant needs approximately 50 kcal/lb or 108 kcal/kg of body weight for first 6 months.

Example: An infant weighing 8 lb 8 oz would need 50 kcal × 8 lb = 400 kcal plus 25 cal for 8 oz (½ lb) = 425 kcal. Most formulas contain 20 kcal/oz. Divide 425 kcal by 20 = 21.25 oz of formula per day.

Goal: To provide daily general care.

A. Ongoing assessment and observation of vital signs, activity, appearance, color, and bowel and bladder function.

B. Care of the umbilical cord stump.

1. Hospital protocol directs routine cord care, which may include using a drying solution of alcohol and triple dye that is applied to the cord.

2. Clean the umbilical cord stump several times a day with soap and water, especially after infant voids (for a male infant).

3. To encourage drying of the cord, expose umbilical area to air frequently and position diaper below umbilicus.

4. Observe for bleeding, oozing, or foul odor.

C. Circumcision care.

1. Keep area clean; change diaper frequently.

2. Observe for bleeding: check site hourly for 12 hours postprocedure.

3. A small sterile petrolatum gauze dressing may be applied to the area during the first 2 to 3 days (Gomco and Mogen clamp).

4. If a PlastiBell was used, keep area clean; application of petrolatum jelly is not necessary; plastic ring will dislodge when area has healed (5 to 7 days).

> **⬛ NURSING PRIORITY** Teach the parents that a whitish-yellow exudate around the glans is granulation tissue and is normal and not indicative of infection. It may be observed for 2 to 3 days and should not be removed.

D. Neonate's bath.

1. Bath is delayed until vital signs and temperature stabilize.

2. Warm water is used for the first 4 days; do not immerse infant in water until umbilical cord stump has been released.

3. When bathing neonate, apply principles of clean-to-dirty areas; wash areas in the following order: eyes, face, ears, head, body, genitals, buttocks.

4. Head is an area of significant heat loss; keep it covered.

E. Determine weight loss over first 24 hours after birth—monitor wet diapers.

F. Assess stools.

1. Meconium stools.

2. Transitional stools.

Goal: To detect complications and provide early treatment.

A. If infant is discharged before 24 hours; explain to parents the importance of returning to health care provider for newborn checkup and screening tests. A newborn screen for PKU should be done after the first 24 hours for a formula-fed infant; if mother is breastfeeding, the newborn screen should be done when infant is 1 week old. National newborn screening requires PKU and thyroid screens. Many states require additional newborn screens.

B. Administration of first hepatitis B vaccine before discharge; also, if mother is a hepatitis B carrier, hepatitis B immune globulin is given intramuscularly.

1. Encourage follow-up visits for second and third doses of hepatitis B vaccine and other immunizations.

2. Infants are tested at 9 months for hepatitis B surface antigen (HBsAg) and anti-HBsAg.

> **⬛ NURSING PRIORITY** Explain to parents the importance of returning for a well-baby check when the infant is 2 to 4 weeks old.

Goal: To promote infant feeding.

A. Breastfeeding.
1. First feeding should occur immediately or within a few hours after birth.
2. Stimulates release of prolactin to initiate milk production.
3. Assess the mother's knowledge of breastfeeding during the first feeding and provide teaching (see Chapter 25 for further discussion of breastfeeding).
4. Frequent feedings are important initially to establish milk production, often every 1½ to 2 hours.
5. One of the primary reasons mothers stop breastfeeding is the perception that their milk supply is not sufficient.
6. Encourage mother to not offer the infant a bottle until lactation is well established, generally after about 4 weeks.
7. Engorgement and nipple soreness are the most common problems the mother experiences.

B. Bottle-feeding.
1. It is not necessary to sterilize the water used to reconstitute infant's formula.
2. The infant should be placed in a semi-upright position for feeding.
3. Never prop the bottle; always hold the infant.
4. Mother should not coax infant to finish all of the bottle every time; any unused formula should be discarded.
5. Do not warm bottles or any food for infants in the microwave because formula or food gets excessively hot and the temperature is not uniform.

> ❗ **NURSING PRIORITY** Proportions of formula must not be altered. Teach mother to not dilute or expand the amount of formula or concentrate it to provide more calories.

🔦 HIGH-RISK NEWBORN

Gestational Age Variation

Assessment

A. Gestational age assessment (Table 26-2).
B. Clinical estimation of gestational age assessed by using visual Ballard scale.
C. Respiratory parameters.
1. Observe respiratory rate, rhythm, and depth.
   a. Initially, rate increases without a change in rhythm.
   b. Flaring of nares and expiratory grunting are early signs of respiratory distress.
2. Increase in apical pulse rate.
3. Subcostal and xiphoid retractions progress to intercostal, substernal, and clavicular retractions.
4. Color.
   a. Progresses from pink to circumoral pallor to circumoral cyanosis to generalized cyanosis.
   b. Increased intensity of acrocyanosis.
5. Progressive respiratory distress.

Table 26-2	GESTATIONAL AGE ASSESSMENT	
By Weight	*By Age*
Large for gestational age (LGA): Above the 90th percentile for estimated weeks of gestation; weight of 4000 g or more at birth.	Postmature: Born after completion of 42 weeks' gestation and demonstrating progressive placental insufficiency.
Appropriate for gestational age (AGA): Weight between 10th and 90th percentile for infant's age.	Postterm (postdate): Born after completion of 42 weeks' gestation.
Small for gestational age (SGA): Weight below the 10th percentile for estimated weeks of gestation.	Term: Born between the beginning of week 38 and the end of week 42 of gestation.
Very low birth weight (VLBW): Weight of 1500 g or less at birth.	Later preterm or near term: Born between 34 and 37 weeks' gestation.
Intrauterine growth restriction (IUGR): Growth of fetus does not meet expected norms.	Preterm or premature: Born before completion of 37 weeks' gestation, regardless of birth weight.

   a. Chin tug: chin pulled down and in with mouth opening wider; auxiliary muscles of respiration are used.
   b. Abdominal seesaw breathing patterns.
   c. Distinguish between apneic episodes (15 seconds or longer) and irregular breathing (cessation of breathing for 5 to 10 seconds).
6. Progressing anoxia leading to cardiac decompensation and failure.
7. Increased muscle flaccidity: frog-like position.

D. Nutrition.
1. Assess readiness and ability to feed: swallowing, gag reflexes.
2. Screen for hypoglycemia.
3. Observe for congenital dysfunction and anomalies related to tracheoesophageal fistula, anal atresia, and metabolic disorders.
4. Check amount and frequency of elimination.
5. Assess for vomiting or regurgitation; a preterm infant's stomach capacity is small, and overfeeding can occur.
6. Check mucous membranes, urine output, and skin turgor to identify fluid and electrolyte imbalances.
   a. Skin turgor over abdomen and inner thighs.
   b. Sunken fontanel.
   c. Urinary output of less than 30 mL/day.

E. Temperature regulation (see Figure 26-2).
1. Assess infant's temperature: frequently done with a skin probe for continuous monitoring of temperature in infants at high risk for complications.
2. Check coolness or warmth of body and extremities.

3. Detect early signs of cold stress.
    a. Increased physical activity and crying.
    b. Increased respiratory rate.
    c. Increased acrocyanosis or generalized cyanosis along with mottling of the skin (cutis marmorata).
    d. Male with descended testes: presence of cremasteric reflex (testes are pulled back up into the inguinal canal on exposure to cold).
4. Monitor infant's temperature.
    a. Axillary temperature: 36.5° C (97.7° F).
    b. Place a temperature skin probe on infant while he or she is in the radiant warmer or isolette.

> **! NURSING PRIORITY** Maintain desired temperature of newborn by using external devices.

Nursing Interventions for the High-Risk Newborn

Goal: To maintain respiratory functioning.
A. Provide gentle physical stimulation to remind infant to breathe.
    1. Gently rub the infant's back.
    2. Lightly tap the infant's feet.

> **! NURSING PRIORITY** Physically stimulate a newborn to breathe; administer oxygen; monitor newborn's gas exchange by obtaining arterial blood gas values, pulse oximetry readings, etc.

B. Ensure patency of respiratory tract.
    1. Maintain open airway by means of nasal, oral, or pharyngeal suctioning.
    2. Position to promote oxygenation.
        a. Elevate head 10 degrees with neck slightly extended by placement of a small folded towel under the shoulders.
        b. Flex and abduct infant's arms and place at sides.
        c. Avoid diapers or adhere them loosely.
        d. Turn side to side every 1 to 2 hours.
        e. Do not place in prone position.
C. Assist infant's respiratory efforts.
    1. Monitor oxygen pressure.
        a. Anywhere from 21% to 100% oxygen is administered to maintain the Po_2 around 50 to 80 mm Hg.
        b. Avoid high concentrations of oxygen for prolonged periods; may lead to complication of bronchopulmonary dysplasia.
    2. Positive end-expiratory pressure helps keep alveoli open at the end of expiration by providing positive pressure.
    3. Continuous positive airway pressure (CPAP) counteracts the tendency of the alveoli to collapse by providing continuous distending airway pressure.
        a. CPAP is administered either by endotracheal tube or nasal prongs.
        b. CPAP must be regulated with regard to humidification, temperature, and pressure; 6 to 10 cm of

water pressure is the therapeutic range for keeping the alveoli open.
D. Monitor oxygen therapy.
    1. Transcutaneous oxygen tension monitoring: measures oxygen diffusion across the skin.
    2. Pulse oximeter: monitors beat-to-beat arterial saturation; less dependent on perfusion than transcutaneous oxygen tension or carbon dioxide tension monitoring; gives a more rapid "real time" reading.

Goal: To provide adequate nutrition.
A. Detect hypoglycemia and treat immediately: administer 5% dextrose in water intravenously if infant is unable to tolerate oral feeding.
B. Oral feeding: initial feeding.
    1. Use sterile water: 1 to 2 mL for a small infant.
    2. Use preemie nipple to conserve infant's energy.
    3. Because of small size of infant's stomach, feedings are small in amount and increased in frequency.
C. Orogastric tube feedings.
    1. Usually administered by continuous flow of formula with an infusion pump (kangaroo pump) when the infant is:
        a. Having severe respiratory distress.
        b. Too immature and weak to suck.
        c. Tired and fatigues easily when a preemie nipple is used.
    2. Placement and insertion of orogastric feeding tube.
        a. Position infant on the back or toward the right side with the head and chest slightly elevated.
        b. Measure correct length of insertion by marking on the catheter the distance from the tip of the nose to the ear lobe to the tip of the sternum.
        c. Lubricate tube with sterile water and slowly insert catheter into mouth and down the esophagus into the stomach.
        d. Test for placement of the tube by aspirating stomach contents or injecting 0.5 to 1.0 mL of air for the premature infant (up to 5 mL for larger infants) and auscultating the abdomen for the sound.
        e. Before infusing a feeding by gravity into the stomach, check for residual; this is done by aspirating and measuring amount left in stomach from previous feeding; often, the residual amount is subtracted from the current feeding so that overfeeding does not occur.
        f. If feeding is not continuous, remove tubing by pinching or clamping it and withdrawing it rapidly.
        g. Burp infant after feeding by turning head or positioning him or her on the right side.
        h. Check to see whether mother wants to pump her breast to provide the milk supply to the infant for gavage.
D. Total parenteral nutrition may be ordered to provide complete nutrition through an indwelling catheter threaded into the vena cava.

E. Detect complications that arise with feeding the preterm infant as a result of:
1. Weak or absent sucking and swallowing reflexes.
2. A very small stomach capacity, which necessitates the use of high-calorie food.
3. Poor gag reflex, leading to aspiration.
4. Incompetent esophageal cardiac sphincter.
5. Increased incidence of vomiting and development of abdominal distention.
6. Inability to absorb essential nutrients.
7. Excessive loss of water through evaporation from the skin and respiratory tract.

Goal: To maintain warmth and temperature control (see maintaining temperature of healthy newborn).
A. Oxygen and air should be warmed and humidified.
B. Maintain abdominal skin temperature at 36.1° to 36.7° C (97° to 98° F); axillary temperature 36.5° C (97.8° F).
C. Monitor infant's temperature continuously; make sure that temperature probe is set on control panel, probe is in contact with infant's skin, and all safety precautions are maintained.
D. Prevent rapid warming or cooling, because this may cause apnea and acidosis; warming process is increased gradually over a period of 2 to 4 hours.
E. Infant may need extra clothing or need to be wrapped in an extra blanket for additional warmth.

> **ALERT** Provide care and education that meets the special needs of the infant client 1 month to 1 year.

 Respiratory Distress

A. Types of respiratory distress.
1. Respiratory distress syndrome: occurs as a result of the deficiency of surfactant, which lines the alveoli; alveoli collapse at the end of each expiration, retaining little or no residual air, leading to generalized atelectasis.
2. Meconium aspiration syndrome.
   a. A fetus may pass meconium in utero.
   b. Associated with fetal growth retardation (small for gestational age) and postmaturity.
   c. Meconium can enter the lungs in utero and plug small air passages; this leads to inflammation of the lung tissues; areas of atelectasis occur because of obstruction and consolidation of the meconium; secondary infection frequently occurs in the lungs.
3. Pneumonia: often associated with premature rupture of the membranes or a prolonged labor.
4. Central nervous system depression: often associated with excessive maternal analgesia or anesthesia.

Diagnostics
A. Chest x-ray film.
B. Blood gas values and pulse oximetry.
C. Echocardiogram.

D. Possible lumbar puncture (to rule out central nervous system problems).
E. Determine the lecithin/sphingomyelin ratio.

Clinical Manifestations
A. Tachypnea: more than 60 breaths/minute.
B. Apneic spells (in excess of 15 seconds).
C. Abnormal breath sounds: rales and rhonchi.
D. Chest retraction.
1. Indicative of increased respiratory work.
2. Begins as a mild sinking of the intercostal spaces or xiphoid retraction on each inspiration.
3. Severe distress characterized by seesaw breathing: abdomen rises and chest sinks on inspiration; abdomen falls and chest expands on expiration.
E. Chin tug: noticed on inspiration; mouth open, lips apart.
F. Flaring of the nares.
G. Expiratory grunting.

> **! NURSING PRIORITY** Grunting is an ominous sign and indicates impending need for respiratory assistance; most often, mucus needs to be cleared from airway.

1. Protective reflex mechanism that prolongs end expiration, which increases oxygenation.
2. Grunting sound occurs as a result of air pushing past a partially closed glottis.
3. Often, it is accompanied by a whining or moaning sound.
H. Prolonged expiration: air flows in easier than it flows out.
I. Cough caused by excessive secretions in the respiratory tract.
J. Generalized cyanosis: usually not observed until Po_2 is less than 42 mm Hg.

Complications
A. Hypoxia continues to increase, leading to decreased lung compliance.
B. Respiratory acidosis caused by alveolar hypoventilation.
C. Metabolic acidosis occurs as a result of hypoxia, which leads to anaerobic metabolism, which leads to increased lactate levels and results in base deficit.
D. Retrolental fibroplasia caused by high levels of oxygen.
E. Bronchopulmonary dysplasia: chronic stiff, noncompliant lungs.

Treatment
A. Respiratory distress syndrome.
1. Lack of surfactant and poor lung functioning lead to decreased Po_2, increased Pco_2, and a decreased pH.
2. As condition worsens, metabolic acidosis may be superimposed on respiratory acidosis and lead to a severe decrease in pH.
3. Constant passive airway pressure (CPAP) is the primary treatment (see Appendix 15-8).
4. Administration of surfactant through the airway into the infant's lungs.

B. Meconium aspiration.
1. Administration of oxygen with humidification.
2. Postural drainage and percussion.
3. Antibiotic therapy.
4. Correction of acid-base imbalance.

Nursing Interventions

Goal: To promote oxygenation and respiratory functioning.
A. Administer a steroid to mother at least 48 hours before delivery and administer surfactant to neonate after delivery to stimulate surfactant production.
B. Refer to nursing intervention for the high-risk newborn.

Goal: To prevent respiratory distress.
A. Assess for infants at high risk because of gestational age and predisposing factors.
B. Monitor lecithin/sphingomyelin ratio of infants at risk.

 ## Cleft Lip

Pathophysiology

A. A fissure of the upper lip to the side of the midline, which may vary from a slight notch to a complete separation extending into the nostril; may be unilateral or bilateral.
B. Caused by failure of the maxillary process to close in early fetal life; usually occurs during the sixth week of gestation.
C. Increased incidence in males; occurs in about 1:800 live births.

Assessment

Visible at birth on an incompletely formed lip.

Treatment

Surgical: closure of lip defect is usually done within a few weeks of birth.

Nursing Interventions

Goal: To provide preoperative care.
A. Maintain nutrition.
1. Use a large-holed nipple or a modified nipple to increase infant's ability to obtain milk without sucking.
2. Feed slowly.
3. Bubble and burp frequently (after every 15 to 30 mL).
4. Rinse cleft with water after each feeding to help prevent infection.
5. Feed with infant's head in an upright position.
B. Prepare parents for newborn's surgery.
1. Encourage parents to position infant flat on back in upright position or on side to accustom infant to the postoperative positioning.
2. Encourage parents to place infant in arm restraints periodically before hospital admission, so they become familiar with the necessary restriction of arm motion after surgery.
3. Encourage parents to feed infant with the same method that will be used after surgery.

Goal: To provide postoperative care.
A. Prevent trauma to suture line.
1. Position infant on back or side and elevate head (infant seat).
2. Restrain arms with soft elbow restraints.
3. Cleanse suture line gently after each feeding; use cotton-tipped applicator with prescribed solution and roll along the suture line; may apply antibiotic ointment.
4. Prevent any crust or scab formation on lip and suture line.
5. May use protective lip device.
B. Maintain a patent airway and facilitate breathing.
1. Assess for respiratory distress.
2. Observe for swelling of the nose, tongue, and lips.
C. Provide adequate nutrition.
1. Feed in an upright, sitting position.
2. Feed slowly and burp/bubble at frequent intervals.
D. Provide discharge teaching to parents.
1. Encourage parents to cuddle and play with infant to decrease crying and prevent trauma to suture line.
2. Teach feeding, cleansing, and restraining procedures.
3. Refer to local community agencies for continued support.

 ## Cleft Palate

Pathophysiology

A. Failure of fusion of the secondary palate; may involve the soft and hard palates along with the alveolar (dental) ridge.
B. Generally associated with a low-birth-weight infant; important to determine if defect is isolated or if it is part of a broader syndrome. Problem is associated with increased incidence of other malformations, especially GI tract defects.

Assessment

A. Opening in roof of mouth; usually associated with a cleft lip.
B. Sucking difficulties.
C. Breathing problems.
D. Later problems include increased incidence of upper respiratory tract infection and otitis media.
E. Later problems are related to speech and hearing difficulties and self-esteem issues.

Treatment

A. Surgical.
1. Surgery may be done in stages; closure of palate defect may begin in neonatal period.
B. Long-term care management.
1. Extensive orthodontics to correct problems of malpositioned teeth and maxillary arches.
2. Speech therapy.
3. Hearing problems related to chronic, recurrent otitis media; varying degrees of hearing loss may occur.

Nursing Interventions

Goal: To provide preoperative care.

A. Maintain nutrition.
1. Use a modified nipple for feeding.
2. Encourage toddler to drink from a cup.
3. Feed child in upright position.
4. Cleanse mouth with water after feeding.

B. Prevent infection.
1. Teach parents symptoms of otitis media.

C. Provide support and teaching to parents.
1. Determine type of restraints that may be used postoperatively; parents may begin to use restraints preoperatively to promote adaptation postoperatively.
2. Teach about various methods to meet infant's sucking needs.

Goal: To provide postoperative care.

A. Maintain patent airway.
1. Observe for respiratory distress and have emergency equipment available at bedside (endotracheal tube, suction, and laryngoscope).
2. Immediate postoperatively position on side to provide for drainage of mucus.

B. Prevent injury and trauma to the suture line.
1. Maintain age-appropriate restraints: elbow restraints for infants, jackets for older children.
2. Avoid use of any objects in the mouth (e.g., straws, suction catheters, tongue depressors, pacifiers, or spoons).
3. Decrease crying by providing attention and affection or diversional activities if child is older.

C. Maintain nutrition.
1. Give fluids initially; then advance to appropriate diet based on age.
2. Child (even an older child) is not allowed to eat hard items such as toast, crackers, potato chips, etc.
3. Cleanse suture line after each feeding by rinsing mouth with water.

D. Provide guidance to parents regarding long-term rehabilitation.
1. Provide for emotional support.
2. Encourage verbalization of feelings regarding infant with defect.
3. Refer to appropriate community resources.

> ❗ **NURSING PRIORITY** Provide surgical wound care.

 Esophageal Atresia With Tracheoesophageal Fistula

Assessment

A. Risk factors.
1. Prematurity.
2. History of maternal hydramnios.
3. Associated with other anomalies, especially congenital heart defects, anorectal problems (imperforate anus), and genital anomalies (extrophy of the bladder).
4. Incidence 1:4000 births; occurs equally in both sexes.

B. Types.
1. Esophageal atresia and tracheoesophageal fistula.
   a. Most common form of cases.
   b. Proximal end of esophagus ends in a blind pouch, and the lower segment connects to the trachea.
   c. Characterized by the classic 3 *C*s: *choking, coughing*, and *cyanosis*.
   d. Excessive frothy saliva and constant drooling.
   e. Aspiration is a complication, especially during feeding.

C. Diagnostics.
1. Inability to pass a catheter into the stomach.
2. Chest x-ray films with use of radiopaque catheter.

Treatment

A. Surgical correction (for esophageal atresia with tracheoesophageal fistula).
1. Thoracotomy with ligation of the tracheoesophageal fistula and an end-to-end anastomosis of the esophagus.
2. If infant is in poor condition or premature, a temporary gastrostomy may be performed to allow for adequate nutrition, and the defect will be repaired at a later date.
3. A colon transplant may be done if a segment of the esophagus is too short for anastomosis.
4. Surgical repair is done in stages.

Nursing Interventions

> ❗ **NURSING PRIORITY** When there is any suspicion of possible esophageal problems, infant should receive nothing by mouth (have NPO status) until further evaluation can be done.

Goal: To provide preoperative care.

A. Maintain patent airway.
1. Supine position with head elevated on an inclined plane of at least 30 degrees.
2. Suction nasopharynx.
3. Observe for symptoms of respiratory distress.
4. Maintain NPO status.

B. Early recognition of defect is important.
1. Assess for the classic 3 *C*s: choking, coughing, cyanosis.
2. Excessive salivation and drooling may occur along with gastric distention.

C. Prepare parents for infant's surgery.

Goal: To provide postoperative care.

A. Maintain respirations and prevent respiratory complications.
1. Pneumonia, atelectasis, pneumothorax, and laryngeal edema are common complications.
2. Administer oxygen.

3. Oral suction of secretions and position for optimum ventilation.
4. Maintain care of chest tubes.
5. Administer antibiotics.
6. Place in warm, high-humidity isolette.
7. Maintain nasogastric suctioning.
B. Provide adequate nutrition.
1. Gastrostomy feedings may be started on the second or third postoperative day.
2. Oral feedings are frequently delayed after surgery or until the esophageal anastomosis is healed.
3. Meet oral sucking needs by offering infant a pacifier.
C. Prepare parents for discharge.
1. Teach techniques such as suctioning, gastrostomy tube feeding, and progression of diet.
2. Explain signs of respiratory difficulty and indicators of esophageal constriction (e.g., difficulty in swallowing, coughing).

 Imperforate Anus

Assessment

A. More common in males; often associated with neurologic defects.
B. Types.
1. A membrane over the anal opening, with a normal anus just above the membrane.
2. Complete absence of anus (anal agenesis), with the rectal pouch ending some distance above.
3. Rectum may end blindly or have a fistula connection to the perineum, urethra, bladder, or vagina.

Diagnostics

A. Visual examination revealing absence of anal opening.
B. Abdominal ultrasound examination.
C. Voiding cystourethrogram: identifies any urinary fistula malformation.

Clinical Manifestations

A. Absence of meconium.
B. No anal opening.
C. Gradual increase in abdominal distention.

Treatment

A. Surgery.
1. Anoplasty: reconstruction of the anus.
2. Abdominal-perineal pull-through.
3. Colostomy.

Nursing Interventions

Goal: To identify anal malformation.
A. Detect increasing abdominal distention.
B. Inspect anal area for opening.

> **⚠ NURSING PRIORITY** Record the first passage of meconium stool. If infant does not pass stool within 24 hours, further assessment is required.

Goal: To provide postoperative care.
A. Prevent infection by maintaining good perineal care and keeping operative site clean and dry, especially after passage of stool and urine.
B. Place infant in side-lying prone position.
C. Instruct parents in care of colostomy (e.g., frequent dressing changes, meticulous skin care, placement of collection device, avoidance of tight diapers and clothes around stoma).

 Neural Tube Defects

Assessment

A. A neural tube defect (spina bifida) results in midline defects and closure of the spinal cord (may be noncystic or cystic); most common site is lumbosacral area.
B. Types.
1. Spina bifida occulta.
   a. Noncystic spina bifida, which results in failure of the spinous processes to join posteriorly in the lumbosacral area, usually around L5 and S1.
   b. Neuromuscular disturbances may be apparent with lower extremity weakness, bowel and bladder sphincter disturbance, and numbness and tingling of the extremities.
   c. Infant may have no apparent clinical manifestations.
2. Spina bifida cystica.
   a. Meningocele: a sac-like cyst of meninges filled with spinal fluid that protrudes through a defect in the bony part of the spine.
   b. Myelomeningocele: a sac-like cyst containing meninges, spinal fluid, and a portion of the spinal cord with its nerves that protrudes through a defect in the vertebral column; other defect most frequently associated with this is hydrocephalus.
C. Diagnostics.
1. Ultrasound examination.
2. Computed tomography; magnetic resonance imaging.
3. Prenatal diagnosis: ultrasound examination and elevated alpha-fetoprotein level (determined from amniotic fluid sample).

Treatment

A. Surgical: closure of defect with 24 to 48 hours to decrease risk for infection, relieve pressure, repair sac, and possibly insert a shunt.
B. Prophylactic: a decrease in the incidence of neural tube defects is associated with an increase in folic acid intake during pregnancy.

Nursing Interventions

> **⚠ NURSING PRIORITY** Correct positioning of the infant is critical in preventing damage to the sac, as well as in providing nursing care after surgery.

Goal: To provide preoperative care.

A. Prevent and protect sac from drying, rupturing, and infection.
   1. Position infant prone on abdomen.
   2. Avoid touching sac.
   3. Provide meticulous skin care after voiding and bowel movements.
   4. Often, sterile, normal saline soaks on a nonadherent dressing may be used to prevent drying.
B. Detect early development of hydrocephalus.
   1. Measure head and check circumference frequently.
   2. Check fontanels for bulging and separation of suture line.
C. Monitor elimination function.
   1. Note whether urine is dripping or is retained.
   2. Indwelling catheter may be inserted or intermittent catheterization may be used at regular intervals to ensure regular bladder emptying.
   3. Assess for bowel function: glycerin suppository may be ordered to stimulate meconium passage.

Goal: To provide postoperative care.

A. Prevent trauma and infection at the surgical site.
   1. Place infant in same position (prone on abdomen) as before surgery.
   2. Continue to provide scrupulous skin care as described under preoperative goal.
   3. Good perineal care because there is frequent continuous urinary drainage.
B. Assess neurologic status frequently for indications of increasing intracranial pressure, development of hydrocephalus, or early signs of infection.
   1. Continue to measure head circumference daily.
   2. Perform frequent neurologic checks.
C. Provide parents with education in regard to positioning, feeding, skin care, elimination procedures, and range-of-motion exercises.
   1. Encourage and facilitate parental bonding.
   2. Refer to community and social agencies for financial and social support.
   3. Encourage long-range planning and support of parents for long-term rehabilitation of infant.

Necrotizing Enterocolitis

Pathophysiology

A. Usually occurs in the first week of life of a full-term infant; increased incidence in preterm infants; cause is unknown.
B. Characterized by ischemic necrosis of the GI tract, which leads to perforation.
   1. Bowel is often dilated, and surface is hemorrhagic.
   2. Ileus often develops, and bowel may perforate.
   3. Peritonitis and neonatal sepsis ensue.

Assessment

A. Problems occur within 4 to 10 days of initiating feeding and in preterm infants may be delayed for up to 30 days.
B. Abdominal distention and rigidity may be seen.

C. Bowel sounds may be absent.
D. Bile-stained emesis and blood-streaked diarrhea or guaiac-positive stool.
E. Other symptoms include episodes of apnea, temperature instability, jaundice, and shock-like symptoms.
F. Diagnostics: abdominal x-ray film.

Treatment

A. Medical.
   1. All enteric feedings are discontinued.
   2. Nasogastric suctioning is initiated.
   3. Intravenous therapy and total parenteral nutrition.
B. Medications: antibiotics.
C. Abdominal x-ray films to check for peritonitis, obstruction, or pneumoperitoneum (free air in peritoneum).
D. If condition is severe, surgery is indicated for intestinal perforation, obstruction, and peritonitis; temporary or permanent colostomy may be required.

Nursing Interventions

Goal: To assist with the medical and surgical management.

A. Maintain nasogastric suctioning; keep infant NPO.
B. Administer antibiotics, IV fluids, and total parenteral nutrition.
C. Promote ventilation; prevent respiratory complications.

Goal: To detect early complications.

A. Assess vital signs.
B. Check for bowel sounds; absence may indicate obstruction.
C. Measure abdominal girth at regular intervals to detect abdominal distention.
D. Avoid pressure on abdomen by not diapering the infant; do not place in prone position.

Goal: To provide support and education to the family.

A. Explanation of treatment and, if surgery is done, postoperative management.
B. Assist in teaching parents how to care for infant's ileostomy or colostomy, as necessary.

Neonatal Sepsis

Cause

A. Predisposing factors are prematurity, invasive procedures, and nosocomial exposure to infection.
B. Immature immunologic system.
C. Maternal antepartal infection: toxoplasmosis, cytomegalic inclusion disease (cytomegalovirus).
D. Intrapartal maternal infections: amnionitis, premature rupture of membranes, bacterial (beta-hemolytic streptococci, gonococci, staphylococci), fungal (*Candida albicans*), or direct contact with maternal GI or urinary tract organisms.

Assessment

🛈 NURSING PRIORITY Neonate often has very subtle behavioral changes, which make it more difficult to assess a gradual onset of sepsis.

A. Clinical manifestations.
1. Apathy, lethargy, poor temperature control.
2. Poor feeding, abdominal distention, diarrhea.
3. Cyanosis, irregular respirations, apnea.
4. Hyperbilirubinemia.
5. Infant often described as "not acting right"; may be irritable.
B. Diagnostics.
1. Cultures of blood, urine, feces, and mucosa.
2. Lumbar puncture and spinal fluid for culture and sensitivity.
3. Complete blood count, chest x-ray film, and viral studies (Table 26-3).

Treatment

A. Medications.
1. Antibiotics.
2. Antiviral.
3. Antifungal.
B. Supportive: may include oxygen, IV therapy, regulation of fluids and electrolytes.

Nursing Interventions

Goal: To prevent neonatal sepsis by prenatal prevention; maternal screening for sexually transmitted diseases and assessment of rubella titers.

A. TORCH (toxoplasmosis, other [congenital syphilis and viruses], rubella, cytomegalovirus, and herpes simplex virus) syndrome is discussed in Chapter 8 and in Table 26-3.

Goal: To prevent infection during the intrapartal period.
A. Maintenance of sterile technique.
B. Prophylactic antibiotic treatment.

 Phenylketonuria

Pathophysiology

A. Inherited as an autosomal recessive trait.
B. Inborn error of metabolism; an absence of the enzyme necessary to metabolize phenylalanine (an essential amino acid).
C. Excessive phenylalanine leads to mental retardation.

Diagnostics

1. Screening is mandatory in all states.
2. Guthrie blood test, blood obtained via heel stick.
   a. Done as close to discharge as possible and no later than 7 days after birth.
   b. Obtain an additional blood sample at 2 weeks if original sample was collected before infant was 24 hours old.

Table 26-3	DISORDERS ACQUIRED DURING AND AFTER BIRTH		
	Trauma	*Peripheral Nerve Injuries*	*Neonatal Sepsis*
Assessment	Soft tissue injury Caput succedaneum Cephalhematoma	Temporary paralysis of the facial nerve is the most common. Affected side of the face is smooth.	Apathy, lethargy, low-grade temperature Poor feeding, abdominal distention, diarrhea
	Injury to bone: Fractured clavicle is the most common; often occurs with a large-sized infant	Eye may stay open. Mouth droops at the corner. Forehead cannot be wrinkled. Possible difficulty sucking. Brachial palsy: A partial or complete paralysis of the nerve fibers of the brachial plexus. Cannot elevate or abduct the arm. Abnormal arm position or diminished arm movements.	Cyanosis, irregular respirations, apnea Hyperbilirubinemia Infant often described as "not acting right." CBC, chest x-ray film, and viral studies TORCH syndrome blood screening
Nursing interventions	1. Place affected arm against chest wall with hand lying across chest. 2. Position is held by a figure 8 stockinette around the arm and chest. 3. Pick infant up carefully; shoulder should not be pressed toward middle of body. 4. Affected side should not be placed in gown or undershirt.	*Facial nerve palsy* 1. Apply eye patch; may use artificial tears to prevent corneal irritation. 2. Provide support during feeding; infant may not latch on to nipple well. *Brachial nerve palsy* 1. Keep arm abducted and externally rotated with elbow flexed. 2. Arm is raised to shoulder height, and elbow is flexed 90 degrees.	1. Prenatal prevention, maternal screening for STDs, and assessment of rubella titers 2. Maintenance of sterile technique 3. Prophylactic antibiotic treatment 4. Possible cesarean delivery for mother with genital herpes

CBC, Complete blood count; *TORCH, t*oxoplasmosis, *o*ther (congenital syphilis and viruses) *r*ubella, *c*ytomegalovirus, and *h*erpes virus.

c. Concern that all infants are not rescreened for PKU after early discharge.

> **! NURSING PRIORITY** The newborn must be fed protein (breast milk or formula) before screening test.

Assessment
A. Musty urine odor.
B. Typical physical characteristics: blond hair, blue eyes, fair skin (caused by a lack of melanin).
C. Vomiting, irritability.

Treatment
A. Dietary: initiated no later than 3 weeks of age.
B. Breastfeeding is preferred, but formula with low phenyl-alanine content may be used.

Nursing Interventions
Goal: To identify infants at risk.
A. Assess newborns for clinical manifestations.
B. Proper use of the Guthrie blood test (avoid layering of blood).
C. Discuss importance of returning for a second blood test.
Goal: To prevent mental retardation.
A. Teach parents the dietary restrictions.
B. Encourage breastfeeding.
C. Provide family support.

DISORDERS OF MATERNAL ORIGIN

 Isoimmune Hemolytic Disease of the Newborn

Pathophysiology
A. An antigen-antibody response causing destruction of fetal RBCs as a result of maternal sensitization of fetal RBC antigens and subsequent transfer of the resulting antibodies to the fetus.
B. Types.
  1. ABO incompatibility: most frequently occurs when the mother's blood group is type O (contains anti-A and anti-B antibodies) and the fetus's blood group is type A, B, or AB.
    a. Milder form of hemolytic disease.
    b. Can occur in the first pregnancy.
    c. Does not necessarily increase in severity with each subsequent pregnancy.
  2. Rh incompatibility: Rh antigens from an Rh-positive fetus enter the blood of an Rh-negative mother, and she produces Rh antibodies; these cross the placenta back into the fetal circulation; if the fetus is Rh posi-tive, the antibodies destroy the fetal RBCs.
    a. Occurs with an Rh-negative mother who is carry-ing an Rh-positive fetus.
    b. Affects the second or subsequent pregnancies; rarely affects the first pregnancy.
    c. Severity of disorder progresses with each preg-nancy if prophylactic treatment with $Rh_o(D)$ immune globulin is not administered.

d. The hemolysis of fetal RBCs can vary in severity from anemia to erythroblastosis fetalis; the most severe form is hydrops fetalis.

Assessment
A. Clinical manifestations: ABO incompatibility.
  1. Hyperbilirubinemia.
  2. Rarely causes hemolysis that results in severe anemia of the newborn.
B. Clinical manifestations: Rh incompatibility.
  1. Hyperbilirubinemia and usually jaundice within first 24 hours.
    a. Jaundice occurs in a cephalocaudal direction: begins at the face, advances downward on the body to trunk and extremities, and finally reaches the palms and the soles of the feet.

> **! NURSING PRIORITY** Press skin against a bony prominence (e.g., chin, nose) to detect early color change.

    b. Bilirubin level rises above 12 mg/100 mL of blood; may reach 30 to 40 mg/100 mL within a few days if treatment is not initiated immediately.
  2. Anemia: usually evident within 12 hours; increased number of immature RBCs.
  3. Placental enlargement.
  4. Enlarged liver and spleen.
C. Diagnostics.
  1. Prenatal screening and prevention: Rh incompat-ibility.
    a. Administration of $Rh_o(D)$ immune globulin to prevent Rh sensitization in first pregnancy of Rh-negative mother (see prenatal care).
      (1) Has no effect against antibodies already present in maternal bloodstream.
      (2) Provides passive immunity.
      (3) Not a treatment for women who are already sensitized; recommended only for nonsensi-tized Rh-negative women at risk for develop-ment of Rh isoimmunization complications.
    b. Indirect Coombs test: performed on the mother's serum to measure the number of Rh-positive anti-bodies; critical level is usually defined as a titer greater than 1:8.
    c. Antibody rescreening is usually done at 24, 28, and 34 weeks' gestation to detect any developing sen-sitization during pregnancy.
  2. Obtain prenatal history regarding Rh incompatibility.
    a. Check to see whether mother has been pregnant before or has received a blood transfusion.
    b. Determine whether mother received $Rh_o(D)$ immune globulin after previous pregnancies or blood transfusions.
  3. Postdelivery detection (Rh incompatibility).
    a. Direct Coombs test on cord blood: reveals pres-ence of maternal antibodies attached to the RBCs of an Rh-positive infant.

b. Rh$_o$(D) immune globulin is administered within 72 hours of an Rh-negative mother's delivery of an Rh-positive infant.
4. Other tests.
a. Hemoglobin and hematocrit values may be decreased.
b. Increased reticulocyte count.
c. Elevated bilirubin level.

Treatment (of Affected Infants)

A. Phototherapy for hyperbilirubinemia (see previous discussion of healthy newborn and hyperbilirubinemia).
B. Intrauterine blood transfusion (Rh incompatibility).
1. Fetus transfused with Rh-negative type O packed RBCs to improve oxygenation and decrease anemia.
2. May be done until fetal lung maturity is achieved and delivery can occur.
3. Rarely done because problem is usually prevented by administration Rh$_o$(D) immune globulin.
C. Exchange transfusion.
1. Purpose.
a. Decrease serum bilirubin levels.
b. Correct anemia.
c. Remove the antibodies that are responsible for hemolysis.
d. Prevent cardiac failure and erythroblastosis fetalis.
2. Not a common procedure because of decreased incidence of condition with prophylactic administration of Rh$_o$(D) immune globulin.

Nursing Interventions

> **! NURSING PRIORITY** It is important for the nurse to differentiate between pathologic and physiologic jaundice to detect early problems.

Goal: To recognize jaundice and distinguish the physiologic type (which occurs within 48 to 72 hours) from the pathologic type (which occurs within 24 hours).
A. Prenatal monitoring of maternal-fetal status.
B. Identify high-risk mother.
C. Monitor bilirubin levels in the newborn.
Goal: To assist with medical treatment.
A. Phototherapy (see discussion of healthy newborn).
B. Exchange transfusion.

Infant of a Mother With Diabetes

> **ALERT** Identify signs of hyperglycemia and hypoglycemia.

Assessment

A. Perinatal hazards.
1. Infant may be large for gestational age as a result of receiving a great deal of glucose (maternal hyperglycemia), or infant may be small for gestational age because of insufficient placental perfusion.
2. Size is inconsistent with gestational age; usually less mature.

3. Maternal hyperglycemia stimulates increased fetal insulin production. Because insulin does not cross the placental barrier freely, whereas glucose does, the fetus is left with excessive insulin during the neonatal period after maternal blood glucose has been withdrawn.
B. Clinical manifestations.
1. Puffy, cushingoid appearance, with round cheeks and stocky neck.
2. Enlarged heart, liver, and spleen.
3. Rapid, irregular respirations.
4. Increased Moro reflex and irritability on slight stimulation or lethargy at times.
C. Common complications.
1. Hypoglycemia: blood glucose level of below 36 mg/dL within 1½ to 4 hours after birth.
a. Lethargy, irritability, hypocalcemia.
b. High-pitched cry.
c. Twitching, jitteriness, seizures.
d. Apneic spells and abdominal distention.
2. Respiratory distress syndrome.
3. Polycythemia.
4. Birth trauma caused by excessive size.
5. Congenital defects, specifically cardiac (patent ductus arteriosus is most common) and central nervous system defects (anencephaly, myelomeningocele, and hydrocephalus).

> **! NURSING PRIORITY** Prolonged hypoglycemia can cause irreversible brain damage.

Treatment

A. Administration of glucose intravenously or 10% dextrose solution orally, depending on severity of hypoglycemia.

> **! NURSING PRIORITY** A rapid infusion of 25% to 50% glucose is contraindicated because it may lead to profound rebound hypoglycemia after an initial brief increase in the blood glucose level.

B. Hydration.
C. Blood glucose determinations on cord blood are done on samples obtained from infant at 30 minutes, 1 hour, 2 hours, and 4 hours after birth.
D. Maintaining glucose levels above 45 mg/dL.

Nursing Interventions

Goal: To identify infant at risk.
A. Careful antepartal assessment of maternal diabetic status.
B. Treat infant as high risk and monitor continuously.
Goal: To monitor glucose levels.
A. Blood glucose levels.
B. Minimize trauma to heel site by performing heel stick correctly (Figure 26-3).
1. Warm heel for 5 to 10 minutes before sticking.
2. Cleanse site with alcohol and dry before sticking.
3. The lateral heel is the site of choice.

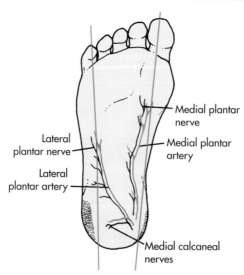

Medial plantar nerve

Lateral plantar nerve

Medial plantar artery

Lateral plantar artery

Medial calcaneal nerves

FIGURE 26-3 Heel stick sites. (From Lowdermilk D, Perry S: *Maternity and women's health care*, ed 7, St. Louis, 2007, Mosby.)

Study Questions Newborn

More questions on companion CD!

1. The nursing assessment of an infant reveals expiratory grunting, substernal retractions, and a temperature of 99° F. What is the first nursing action?
   1. Place the infant in Trendelenburg position.
   2. Begin administration of 40% humidified oxygen via hood.
   3. Increase the temperature of the environment.
   4. Perform a complete assessment for congenital anomalies.

2. To meet the goal of promoting infant feeding in a breastfed baby, the nurse should teach the mother to do which of the following? Select all that apply:
   _____ 1. Feed the baby on a 3- to 4-hour schedule.
   _____ 2. Alternate breast milk and formula for each feeding.
   _____ 3. Stop breastfeeding if her nipples get sore.
   _____ 4. Maintain on-demand breastfeeding for the first 4 weeks.
   _____ 5. Drink lots of fluids and get adequate rest.
   _____ 6. Offer a pacifier between feedings to meet sucking needs.

3. Which statement best describes the problem of regulation of body temperature in a 3-lb premature infant?
   1. The surface area of the premature infant is relatively smaller than that of a healthy term infant.
   2. There is a lack of subcutaneous fat, which furnishes insulation.
   3. There are frequent episodes of diaphoresis causing loss of body heat.
   4. There is a limited ability to produce body proteins.

4. The nurse is caring for an infant with an unrepaired tracheoesophageal fistula. In planning care, the nurse will identify what priority nursing goal?
   1. To promote oxygen exchange
   2. To prevent lung infection
   3. To promote bonding
   4. To replace fluids and electrolytes

5. The nurse would identify which situation as an indication for the administration of RhoGAM?
   1. A woman who has been Rh-sensitized in the past two pregnancies
   2. An infant with increased hemolysis of red blood cells because of ABO incompatibility
   3. An infant with an increase in serum bilirubin levels as a result of the presence of Rh factor antibodies
   4. A primigravida who is Rh negative is pregnant with an infant who is Rh positive

6. In the recovery room, the *best* immediate postoperative position for an infant who has had a cleft lip repair is:
   1. Prone with the head turned to one side
   2. Left Sims' position
   3. Supine with the head turned to the side
   4. Trendelenburg position to facilitate drainage

7. An infant born at 28 weeks' gestation weighs 4 lb 3 oz. What does the initial nursing care of this infant include?
   1. Place the infant in protective isolation because of the underdeveloped immune system.
   2. Feed him a low-phenylalanine formula to increase digestion and utilization of calories.
   3. Provide gavage feedings every 2 hours because of an inadequate sucking and swallow reflex.
   4. Place the infant under a radiant heater to maintain regulation of body temperature.

Answers and rationales to these questions are in the section at the end of the book titled Chapter Study Questions: Answers and Rationales.

NORMAL LABORATORY DATA

TEST	NORMAL ADULT VALUES
Blood Serum Values	
Red blood cell (RBC) count	Men: 4.5-6.0 10^6/mcl
	Women: 4.0-5.0 10^6/mcl
Hemoglobin	Men: 13.5-18 g/dL
	Women: 12-16 g/dL
Hematocrit	Men: 40%-54%
	Women: 38%-47%
Complete white blood cell (WBC) count	4.0-11 10^3/mcl
Differential WBC count	Expressed as a percentage of total WBCs
Granulocytes	
Segmented neutrophils	50%-70%
Eosinophils	0%-4%
Basophils	0%-2
Nongranular leukocytes	
Monocytes	4%-8%
Lymphocytes	20%-40%
Sodium (serum or plasma)	135-145 mEq/L
Potassium (plasma)	3.5-5.0 mEq/L
Chloride (serum)	95-105 mEq/L
Magnesium (serum)	1.5-2.5 mEq/L
Iron, total serum	50-150 mcg/dL
Iron binding capacity	250-410 mcg/dL
Calcium (ionized) serum	4.5-5.5 mg/dL
Calcium, total serum	9-11 mg/dL
Phosphorus serum	2.8-4.5 mg/dL
Alkaline phosphatase	30-120 units/L
Blood urea nitrogen (BUN)	10-30 mg/dL
Creatinine (serum)	0.2-1.0 mg/dL
Uric acid (serum)	Men: 4.0-8.5 mg/dL
	Women: 2.7-7.3 mg/dL
Creatinine kinase (CK)	Men: 15-105 units/L
	Women: 10-80 units/L
Alanine aminotransferase (ALT)	5-36 units/L
Aspartate aminotransferase (AST)	7-40 units/L
C-reactive protein (highly sensitive-hs-CRP)	less than 1.0 mg/dL
Erythrocyte sedimentation rate (ESR)	Men over 50: less than 20 mm/hr
	Women over 50: less than 30 mm/hr
Blood platelets	150-400 X 10^3 units/L
Serum osmolarity	285-295 mOsm/kg
Prostate specific antigen	less than 4 ng/mL
Prothrombin time	11-12.5 sec
Activated partial thromboplastin time (aPTT)	30-45 sec
Partial thromboplastin time (PTT)	60-70 sec
Bleeding time	Ivy: 1-9 minutes
International normalizing ratio (INR)	2-3 prophylaxis for deep venous thrombosis
	2.5-3.5 prosthetic cardiac valves

TEST	NORMAL ADULT VALUES
Carbon dioxide (venous CO_2)	20-30 mEq/L
Fibrin split-products (FSP)	Less than 10 mcg/mL
Fibrinogen	Quantitative: 200-400 mg/dL
Lactic acid dehydrogenase (LDH)	100-190 units/L
Serum albumin	3.5-5.0 g/dL
Glucose (baseline fasting)	70-100 mg/dL
Glycosylated hemoglobin assay	4%-6%
Glucose 2-hour postprandial	Less than 140 mg/dL
Ammonia	30-70 mcg/dL
Indirect bilirubin	0.1-1 mg/dL
Direct bilirubin	0.1-0.3 mg/dL
Total bilirubin	0.2-1.3 mg/dL

Normal Arterial Blood Gas Values

Acidity index (pH)	7.35-7.45
Partial pressure of dissolved oxygen (Pao_2)	80-100 mm Hg
Percentage of hemoglobin saturated with oxygen (O_2 saturation)	95% or above
Partial pressure of dissolved carbon dioxide ($Paco_2$)	35-45 mm Hg
Bicarbonate (HCO_3)	22-26 mEq/L

Urine Values

Urinalysis	
Microalbumin	0.2-1.9 mg/dL
Bilirubin	Negative
Color	Clear, golden yellow
Glucose	Negative
Specific gravity	Adult:1.005-1.030
	Older adult: values decrease
Ketones	24 hr specimen—20-50 mg/dL
Microscopic urinalysis	
Bacteria	Negative
Casts	None present
Crystals	Negative
RBCs	less than 2
WBCs	0-4 per low-power field
Uric acid (urine)	250-750 mg/24 hr
Urine electrolytes (24 hour urine collection)	
Sodium	40-250 mEq/24 hr (varies with dietary intake)
Calcium	100-250 mg/day
Urine osmolarity	50-1200 mOsm/kg H_2O (random sample)
Creatinine clearance (24-hour urine collection)	Men 107-139 ml/minite
	Female: 87-107 ml/minute
	Values decrease with age

Cerebral Spinal Fluid (CSF) Analysis

Color	Clear and colorless
Blood	None
White blood cells	Adults: 0-5
	Children: 0-10
Enzymes (LDH)	Less than 40 units/L
Glucose	50-75 mg/dL or 60%-70% of blood glucose level
Protein	15-45 mg/dL (higher in older adults and children)
Albumin	56%-76%
Immunoglobulin G (IgG)	0-4.5 mg/dL
Pressure	less than 20 cm H_2O

Chapter Study Questions: Answers and Rationales

CHAPTER 2: HEALTH IMPLICATIONS ACROSS THE LIFE SPAN

1. **2** Usually, the toddler clings to the mother. As separation anxiety becomes intolerable, the child ignores the parent. At this stage the child relates better to the staff and doesn't mind the absence of the parent. Eating with his fingers and afraid of the dark are normal for this age infant.

2. **3** While the infant is quiet, it is important to auscultate the heart and lungs. Placing a tape measure on the infant's head, shining a light in the eyes, or undressing the infant before weighing may cause distress, which could make auscultating the heart and lungs, as well as the rest of the examination, more difficult.

3. **2** When interviewing an older client, auditory acuity is the most common age-related aspect to take into consideration. It is important to make sure the client hears and understands the questions. If the client does not hear the question correctly, the response time cannot be determined. The IQ may decline with dementia.

4. **2** Children at this age are prone to anemia, especially when milk is offered frequently. Therefore holding liquids until after solid food is offered prevents the child from filling up on liquids.

5. **2** Stacking rings are a good toy to promote fine motor skills for a toddler and will not be adversely affected by the humid environment. 18-month-old infants tend to put objects in their mouth, so crayons and soap bubbles would not be appropriate.

6. **2** Since the woman is perimenopausal, she needs increased calcium intake (1500 mg/day). With a diagnosis of hypertension, she also needs a decreased-sodium diet. Foods high in calcium include milk products, leafy green vegetables, and dried beans. Yellow vegetables are not high in calcium. Pasta and breads are a source of sodium.

7. **2** The increased potassium found in dried peaches and apricots is contraindicated for a client with increased potassium and blood urea nitrogen (BUN) levels. Dried fruit is high in potassium.

8. **3** Having medications and other dangerous cleaning materials and chemicals locked away in secure areas is an important safety issue for toddlers. It is not advisable to induce vomiting (giving Syrup of Ipecac) without calling the local poison control center first to be sure that it is okay to do so. Ingested materials may be corrosive, and inducing vomiting would not be an appropriate nursing action.

9. **4** Immunizations are started as early as 1 month (first dose of hepatitis B vaccine is recommended to be given before discharge from the hospital). The diphtheria, tetanus, and pertussis (DTaP) vaccine and inactivated poliovirus vaccine (IPV) series, pneumococcal vaccine (PCV), *Haemophilus influenzae* (Hib) series are started at 2 months. The completion of the series of childhood immunizations generally occurs when the infant is around 12 to 15 months old.

10. **4** The varicella vaccine (chicken pox) can be administered any time after 12 months of age. It is not given before this age because the infant's immune system has not yet matured.

11. **3** Varicella is an acute viral disease characterized by a maculopapular rash with vesicular scabs in multiple stages of healing. Most erythematous rashes start on the face and progress to the rest of the body.

12. **4** Deep, penetrating wounds that are contaminated by soil, dust, or excreta containing *Clostridium tetani* are the cause of tetanus, or lockjaw. First, the wound should be thoroughly cleansed, but not with antibiotic solution. The nurse should determine when the client received his last tetanus immunization. As a rule, clients will receive a tetanus booster as a safeguard.

13. **4** Nutrition is the key to adequate growth and development for an infant who is immunocompromised. Supplements will support normal nutrition and should be considered as part of the care for an infant with this nursing diagnosis. The family should be encouraged to participate in care, but that does not necessarily promote nutrition.

14. **3** The older adult finds meaning in life and adjusts to the death of a spouse or loved one. He or she is aware of death as an inevitable part of living and often reacts to dying as a time of reflection, rest, and peace.

15. **3** Ice cream is not a clear liquid. The gelatins are okay; however, red-colored gelatin is often prohibited. Coffee and tea are both acceptable with sugar, but no cream is allowed.

CHAPTER 3: CONCEPTS OF NURSING PRACTICE

1. **3** To obtain an accurate reading on any client, the blood pressure cuff should cover the upper two-thirds of the client's arm; it should be positioned approximately 2 inches above the antecubital space. This is applicable to the very thin client as well as the obese client. The blood pressure cuff should be about 20% wider than the arm or leg. If it is too large or too small, it will affect the accuracy of the reading. The systolic reading is obtained with the first of the Korotkoff sounds.

2. **1** The family should be encouraged to sit with the dying client, touch him, and talk to him. This is a method of saying goodbye and acknowledging the impending death. Several members of the family can be present at the same time, and if the client is comfortable, no pain medication is necessary.

3. **4** The hemoglobin level is low, and the nurse needs to make sure the surgeon has the most recent laboratory values before surgery. This client may need a transfusion before surgery. The cholesterol is elevated but is not a concern before surgery. The platelets and the BUN are within normal limits.

4. **2** An initial focused assessment should be conducted to determine the client's current status with regard to his primary health care needs. Does the assessment correlate with the information received in the shift report? Is the client experiencing any difficulties? Does the nursing care plan need to be changed? Other options presented do not reflect an evaluation of the current status of the client at the time the nurse begins the initial care for that shift.

5. **1** The man with the fractured femur is in traction, which means he is immobilized. The immobilization is necessary to prevent rotation and/or further movement of the fracture site after the repair. The client who is immobilized is at highest risk for venous stasis, particularly in the large pelvic veins in the abdomen. The other clients listed are all mobile—the client with the fractured hip is in physical therapy, postpartum client is going home, and the postthoracotomy client should be out of bed 2 or 3 times a day. Clients with chest tubes should be ambulated, when possible, to enhance pulmonary expansion.

6. **3** It is important to determine whether the airway is patent and whether the client is breathing. If a significant amount of mucus and gurgling are noted in the upper airway, the client should be suctioned. Insertion of an oral airway may be necessary to maintain an open airway, but the airway must be assessed before determining a course of action. Inserting an airway will not solve the problem if the client is not breathing.

7. **2** Children may withdraw and sleep as a way to deal with pain. Frequently, the parent is the best judge of the young child's pain. Six hours have passed since the last dose, it would be very appropriate to awaken the child and administer the medication.

8. **2, 3, 4** Options 2, 3, and 4 indicate a correct understanding of the preoperative teaching. The pneumatic compression device is worn during bed rest and is removed when the client is out of bed or ambulating. The informed consent document should be signed before preoperative medication administration and before the client enters the operating room. Part of safety standards is to initiate a timeout in the operating room before the surgery is started.

9. **1, 3** Parents should be included in the teaching of the pediatric client, and separation anxiety should be minimized. If the client is younger than 4 years, he or she will generally not benefit from anatomy and physiology information; simple explanations are better. A "no" response from a toddler is usually an assertion of independence, rather than an indication that the child is not ready to learn. Learning moves from concrete to abstract.

10. **4** Consent forms must be signed by the client, family, or guardian with medical power of attorney before any procedure can be done. Consent forms must also be signed before the client receives any narcotics or medications that would affect his reasoning. These medications are frequently in the preoperative medications ordered.

11. **2** Relief of pain in the client with terminal cancer is palliative. Medications should be given around the clock, and the client should be evaluated frequently to determine the level of pain control. The nurse should not wait until the client complains of pain but should assess the level of pain control frequently. The medication should not be administered every 3 hours; it is to be given on an as-needed basis. The nurse should anticipate administering the medication every 3 hours. If the client is not resting comfortably with this schedule, the health care provider should be notified.

12. **2, 3, 1, 4**
    1 __3__ Desired diet progression then advances to full liquid.
    2 __1__ The client's status is NPO immediately after surgery.
    3 __2__ Desired diet progression advances next to clear liquid.
    4 __4__ Desired diet progression next advances to a soft diet and then finally to a regular diet as tolerated by the client.

13. **2** The best approach to a good interview is to start with the easy, less personal questions while building a rapport. Waiting for the client to initiate the conversation is not an efficient use of time; furthermore, the client will not know what information the nurse needs. Assume the client can provide an accurate health history unless there are indications that he or she cannot give accurate information.

14. **1470 mL** All of the listed IV fluids should be infused within the nurse's 8-hour shift. The nasogastric tube will have been irrigated four times.
    IV @ 125 mL/hr × 8 hours = 1000 mL
    Vancomycin IVPB = 50 mL
    Reglan IVPB = 50 mL
    PRBCs = 250 mL
    NG irrigation = 30 mL × 4 = 120 mL
    Total = 1470 mL

15. **3** A full liquid diet includes liquids, as well as foods that are liquid at room temperature.

16. **4** It is important to create a comprehensive picture of the client's medical history by placing events in their proper chronologic order.

17. **2** When the nurse conducts a teaching session, it is most important to determine physical comfort at the beginning of the session. A client cannot focus on learning if he or she needs to go to the bathroom, is too cold, or is experiencing pain. The other options are important to teaching, but physiologic needs must be addressed before continuing with the teaching session.

18. **2** Weight bearing increases the vascular tone and decreases venous stasis, thereby preventing thrombi from developing; the increase in activity increases respiratory expansion and quality of breathing. Passive range of motion maintains joint mobility but is not as effective as weight bearing to prevent venous stasis and the complications of immobility. Turning and coughing every 30 minutes around the clock is too often—it would disrupt effective rest and sleep. Every 2 hours is the standard. Prevention of complications of immobility begins when the client becomes immobilized.

19. **4** The first step in the nursing process is to assess the client. Assessment must occur before planning and implementation. It is important to assess the client to determine whether the pain is abdominal and is appropriate pain for the client to be experiencing at this stage of his recovery from surgery.

CHAPTER 4: CONTROL FUNCTIONS AND MANAGEMENT

1. **3** Errors in charting on a paper chart should never be obliterated, recopied, or covered with correction fluid. When the erroneous information is not legible, it raises questions as to what the person was trying to cover up.

2. **4** Legal reporting laws include exceptions for the invasion of privacy (including suicide attempts). Communicable diseases, gunshot and knife wounds, and child abuse must be reported.

3. **3** Many institutions provide a specific code word to identify individuals who are allowed to have access to the client care information. The nurse should not assume that any individual is truly a family member—this must be verified. Copies of client's charts or records should not be made by anyone. The chart should not be reviewed by anyone who does not have

a need to know in order to provide care. The CEO does not provide care.

4. **3** The client needs to show an understanding of the informed consent document by giving an explanation in his own words. He should also be able to tell you what he expects to happen regarding the procedure, as well as the possible complications. It is the physician's responsibility to provide the client with this information.

5. **2** The physical characteristics and the child's emotional response to the father are suspicious. Any suspected child abuse situation should be reported to the nursing supervisor, who is obligated to report it through the facilities channels to the appropriate agencies.

6. **3** The nurse needs to keep skills and nursing knowledge current to deliver competent, safe care. A contract and current license are not protection against negligence. It is important to follow hospital policy; however, if the nurse feels the hospital policy is inadequate and/or incomplete, she should follow the established competencies for nursing practice.

7. **1** The chart is considered a legal document. Any illegal alterations can be considered fraud. Arguing and withholding information are not wise and will certainly not benefit the case; however, making illegal changes in the chart would be the most damaging error since this is a clear violation of the law.

8. **4** The nurse was in violation of the Good Samaritan Act. Allowing the family to replace the soiled clothes was a form of compensation, which is in direct violation of the Good Samaritan Act. None of the other choices is applicable to the situation. The ANA Code of Ethics provides principles to facilitate ethical problem solving. HIPAA is a law providing confidentiality for the client to protect written and verbal communication about the client. The Patient Self-Determination Act requires that hospitalized patients indicate whether they have an advanced directive.

9. **4** Suggesting that the physician meet with the nursing supervisor would be the most appropriate approach, giving the physician enough time to rethink his position. Giving the medication would place the nurse in a position of liability, and not signing for it would increase the legal liability. Arguing with the physician would only escalate the issue.

10. **3, 1, 5, 2, 4, 6** Use the acronym RACE—**R**escue, **A**ctivate, **C**ontain, **E**xtinguish—to remember the emergency fire response. Fire extinguisher safety can be remembered by another acronym: PASS—**P**ull the pin, **A**im at the base of the fire, **S**queeze the trigger, and **S**weep from side to side.
    1 ___2___ Activate the alarm.
    2 ___4___ Pull the pin on the extinguisher.
    3 ___1___ Remove any victims from the fire.
    4 ___5___ Aim the extinguisher to the base of the fire.
    5 ___3___ Contain the fire.
    6 ___6___ Extinguish the fire from side to side.

11. **1** In option 1, the nurse has threatened the client with physical restraint if he does not quit being verbally abusive; the threat is considered an assault. Option 2 is a situation of battery or abuse, as well as nonconsensual touching, when the nurse gives a medication the client does not want. In option 3 the nurse is committing false imprisonment when she threatens the client with physical restraint to prevent him from leaving. Option 4 describes a breach of confidentiality and invasion of privacy; the nurse did not check to see whether the pastor had permission from the client to receive this information.

12. **4** The client is scheduled for surgery and is beginning to exhibit symptoms of a urinary tract infection. The client needs to be assessed immediately for an infection, and the doctor must be notified. If an infection is present, the surgery may be postponed or canceled. The other clients are not unstable, and their needs do not have to be addressed immediately.

13. **2** A child with RSV involves contact with ribavirin, a teratogenic medication that is classified as Pregnancy Risk Category X. The nurse who is pregnant should not come in contact with this medication. The other clients do not pose any particular risk to the pregnant nurse.

14. **4** Option 4 represents the most stable client who could be discharged. Clients in options 1 and 3 are showing signs of being unstable with their diagnoses. The client in option 2 is stable, but because of the extensiveness of his surgery and because he had surgery only 3 days ago, he is a less likely candidate to move than the client in option 4.

15. **2** The Joint Commission (TJC) requires two points of objective identification. For a client with an armband, it is recommended that the nurse check the chart against the name and hospital number on the client's armband. Options 1 and 3 are incorrect because in the hospital environment the client should not participate in his identification. Option 4 should have been done to verify the correct order, not the client's identity.

16. **1** The assignment of obtaining a stool specimen in option 1 has the most specific guidelines for performance. The other procedures require nursing assessment and judgment and should not be assigned to a nursing assistant.

17. **4** The client with cardiac disease is the most unstable and is beginning to exhibit symptoms that could be warning signs of increasing cardiac irritation; the client needs to be assessed immediately, and the nurse should anticipate administration of IV medication. The client in option 1 may be developing hypostatic pneumonia, but the situation does not require immediate attention. The client in option 2 is also not in an unstable situation, even though she is uncomfortable. The client with dehydration in option 3 is exhibiting symptoms of his dehydration but is not unstable at this time.

CHAPTER 5: PHARMACOLOGY

1. **3** The vastus lateralis is the preferred site for an infant because the muscle is not located near any vital nerves or blood vessels. It is the best choice for intramuscular injections for children younger than 3 years. The deltoid muscle has too little muscle mass in a young infant or toddler and is unable to hold large injected volumes of medication. The ventrogluteal muscle is safe for intramuscular injections for older children. The safety of using the ventrogluteal site for infants and young children is currently being researched.

2. **2** Only one antibiotic should be administered at a time; therefore if the medications are given during the same hour, the IV tubing will need to be flushed between administrations. Both drugs should be administered at the time ordered.

3. **1** Tolerance occurs when there is a decrease in the response to a drug after repeated drug administration. More of the analgesic is needed to maintain the same level of pain control. Requiring pain medication around the clock for adequate pain relief is not tolerance because the client is obtaining proper pain relief. Option 2 may be an adverse reaction to the medication, or another problem may be occurring. Options 4 may indicate that the client is overmedicated.

4. **1** An older adult client receiving multiple medications simultaneously is at risk for drug interactions that could be harmful. More than one physician may be ordering medications without knowledge or consideration of medications the client is already taking. Older adult clients do not metabolize or excrete drugs differently than younger clients do, just less effectively. Medications do not have an increased effect in the morning, nor do they specifically affect the respiratory system of the older adult.

5. **3** The first step in drug delivery to a client is to check the order with the medication administration sheet for possible discontinuance or a change in dose, route, or time. The question asks for steps to ensure the right medication is being given, not for client identification.

6. **3** The dose should be recorded as "not taken," and the poured dose should be discarded. If the dose is a controlled substance, the discarded dose must be witnessed. Checking the medication administration record or the medication order for changes before preparing the medication helps to eliminate waste and/or mistakes.

7. **1** Administer the medication as ordered.
   Ordered: 1 g every 8 hours = 1 g × 3 doses = 3 g per day.
   Highest safe dose: 150 mg × 40 kg = 6000 mg or 6 g per day.

8. **1, 4, 6** Garlic, ginkgo, and vitamin E may interfere with platelet aggregation and increase the risk for bleeding in clients who are taking Coumadin.

9. **4 mL**

1 g = 1000 mg; therefore 0.1 g = 100 mg

125 mg : 5 mL :: 100 mg : × mL

Formula: 125 × X = 125X (Note: multiply the two outside numbers of the ratio equation together, then the two inside numbers; solve for X by dividing the total of the inside numbers with the outside numbers.)

5 × 100 = 500

X = 500/125 = 4 mL

10. **1.5 mL**

500 mg : 1 mL :: 750 mg : X

Formula: 500 × X = 500X

1 × 750 = 750

X = 750/500 = 1.5

The dosage calculation cannot be made from the amount of solution added to the vial. The ratio of mg per mL after reconstitution is 500 mg per mL.

11. **4** The medication administration record should be reviewed for current physician's orders. Medication administration records are routinely reviewed to determine the currency of medication orders. The client's name and hospital number are checked to validate client identification before administration of the medication. The nurse should check the medication for the expiration date when she prepares the medication, and the physician will order the route of administration.

12. **2** The Z track method of administering medications requires the tissue be pulled to one side before injection and then released after the needle is removed. This allows the tissue to occlude the needle track and prevents the medication from tracking out the site. This will decrease tissue irritation. A 19-gauge, 2-inch needle is too large for any IM injection. Option 3 describes an IM injection without consideration of the irritating medication. Option 4 is incorrect because the deltoid site is not appropriate for a deep IM injection of irritating medications.

13. **4** The nurse administered a narcotic without a doctor's order and is liable for the action. The nurse's license is jeopardized because this action is a violation of the nurse practice act, as well as the Controlled Substance Act of 1970.

14. **3** It is important for the nurse to be familiar with the safe dose range. 10 kg × 0.2 mg/kg (maximum dose) = 2 mg. Therefore the medication dose would be within the safe range. Dose range for a 10-kg infant would be from 1 mg to 2 mg. Multiply each end range by the infant's weight to determine the safe range. Morphine is supplied in 2 mg/mL solutions. It is important to check the infant's respirations before administering the morphine; however, the safe dose should be calculated before the preparation of the medication.

15. **4** The client has the right to know what he is receiving and why he is receiving it, and he has the right to decline the medication. It is not appropriate to refer this problem to the charge nurse unless further complications develop. The doctor should not be called unless the situation escalates and the anxiety increases.

16. **3** The first step in drug delivery to a client is to check the order against the medication administration sheet for possible discontinuance or a change in dose, route, or time. The question asks for steps to ensure the right medication is being given, not for client identification.

17. **10 mL**

25 mg : 5 mL :: 50 mg : x mL

Formula: 25 × X = 25X

5 × 50 = 250

X = 250/25 = 10 mL (Remember, only enter numerals [no units of measure] in the blank.)

18. **2 tablets**

0.25 = 250 mcg; 0.25 mg : 1 tablet :: 0.5 mg : x tablet

Formula: 0.25 x = 0.5 × 1 = x = 2 (tablets)

CHAPTER 6: HOMEOSTASIS

1. **4** The nurse would expect to see a decreased pH and increased Pco_2 in a client with respiratory acidosis. Normal pH is 7.35 to 7.45, and normal Pco_2 is 35 to 45 mm Hg.

2. **3** The priority assessment for a client with fluid problems is to obtain the daily weight. Weight gain and loss are the most accurate measurements of fluid gain and loss. Checking tissue turgor on an older adult is not very accurate since many older adults have poor turgor. Thirst is too nonspecific. The I&O is important, but this is not as objective in evaluating the amount of fluid retained as is the daily weight.

3. **1** The cost-effective and safest decision is to finish the current liter of fluid. The second and fourth answers are not relevant to the ordered fluid. The third answer does not indicate whether the client has voided and is least cost effective. The liter of Ringer's lactate has already been considered in the replacement of client fluids from the OR.

4. **1** Potassium should *never* be administered IV push. It is extremely irritating and painful at the catheter site, as well as very dangerous to the client. It should be diluted in an IV solution and run over the time of the total infusion (1000 mL D_5W with 40 mEq potassium over 8 hours), or small amounts should be given in less solution (potassium 10 mEq in 250 mL D_5W to run over 3 hours). The other orders listed are all within acceptable limits for a postoperative client.

5. **3** With dehydration or fluid deficit, orthostatic hypotension may occur. The nurse should assess for other symptoms of fluid volume deficit: decreased blood pressure, weight loss, imbalance of urine output and fluid intake, dry skin and mucous membranes.

6. **3** Long-term steroids will suppress the production of glucocorticoids from the adrenal glands. Glucocorticoids are responsible for vascular stability; abrupt withdrawal will precipitate hypotension. The client should also monitor his or her weight for excessive gain; however, option 3 is more important. The dose of steroids should never be increased unless ordered by a health care provider.

7. **3** The client with renal problems is more likely to experience problems with electrolyte balance, especially potassium balance. The kidneys control the excretion of sodium and potassium through the countercurrent mechanism. The liver is involved in metabolism. The client with a peripheral edema and heart failure may or may not experience problems with electrolyte balance. Frequently, the fluid overload is a problem with the client in heart failure. A client with obstructive lung disease may or may not experience electrolyte imbalance.

8. **4** In infants, validation of renal function must be established before the delivery of IV KCl. This is necessary to prevent hyperkalemia and possible death.

9. **1** Daily weights are a very accurate indicator of fluid retained or lost. 2.2 pounds (1 kg) is equal to 1 L of fluid. Measuring the intake and output does not take into consideration insensible fluid loss and is not as accurate an evaluation as is the daily weight. Changes in vital signs are less reliable because they do not reflect subtle changes in retention of fluid. Although adventitious sounds may be present if the client is overhydrated, the daily weights would have increased before the pulmonary changes occurred.

10. **4** With a continuous flow at 75 mL/hour, a small-gauge IV catheter (intercath) is appropriate. IVs should be started in the lowest vein possible and progress upward. The antecubital area is not a preferred area.

11. **3** Headache and dizziness in a client receiving IV fluid are frequently signs of fluid overload from the increase in circulating volume, which increases cerebral vascular pressure. After decreasing the IV rate, the nurse should continue with the assessment of the vital signs. If other assessment findings (increased blood pressure, lethargy, bounding pulse, weight gain, adventitious breath sounds) confirm the problem, the physician needs to be notified. If the increase in circulating volume continues, it can cause pulmonary edema.

12. **1, 2, 5** Contact precautions would require the nurse to wear clean gloves to remove the old dressing, put on a gown when entering the room, and leave all extra dressing supplies in the room. A face shield is not necessary unless splattering of fluids is anticipated. The gown and mask should be disposed of in the client's room; they should not be removed from the room. The stethoscope and scissors should not be taken into the client's room.

13. **4** The client is losing fluids, but the replacement fluid only contains sodium. The laboratory value of 155 mEq/L indicates that the client has hypernatremia. This increases retention of fluids and subsequently increases the cardiac workload. The glucose level is elevated, but that is not unusual in clients in the immediate postoperative period. The hemoglobin and hematocrit values are within the normal ranges. The blood urea nitrogen (BUN) level is elevated, and this needs to be investigated and correlated with the serum creatinine level. However, it is not alarmingly high and could be an indication of decreased fluids—and it is not the priority concern.

14. **4** The client is lethargic from the anesthetic and needs to be stimulated to deep-breathe to facilitate ventilation. The client is at increased risk for development of respiratory acidosis. Stimulation should be done before suctioning to determine whether it relieves the problem. Increasing the oxygen flow does not address the problem of hypoventilation. Neurologic checks can be done but are not a priority at this time.

15. **4** This series of values best represents metabolic acidosis, a complication of type 1 diabetes. Option 1 reflects respiratory alkalosis, option 2 reflects respiratory acidosis, and option 3 reflects metabolic alkalosis.

16. **1** The IV is infiltrated and should be discontinued. A warm, moist pack can be applied for client comfort. The IV should be discontinued but not restarted distal to the previous site; it should be started proximal to or above the current infiltrated site or in the other extremity.

17. **4** The client is experiencing acute respiratory alkalosis from hyperventilation caused by anxiety. Rebreathing in a paper sack will help to reestablish normal Pco_2 levels. The other options do not address the origin of the problem and may further increase his anxiety.

18. **1, 2, 4** The specific name of the vein is not necessary; however, the general location of the site is important. Standard precautions are used for everyone, and it is not necessary to chart that they were used. The order and time for the IV should be on the client's chart; it is not necessary to repeat it in the documentation. The question did not ask for *all* the information that could be charted.

19. **1** Phlebitis has developed at the site, and the catheter should be removed. A warm, moist pack can be applied to the affected area. If continued administration of fluids is necessary, the catheter should be moved to another vein. It does not make any difference whether the catheter is still in the vein: the catheter must be removed because of the inflammation. Assessment of medications causing the problem can be done at a later time after the current problem is resolved. The rate of infusion should remain the same.

CHAPTER 7: IMMUNE SYSTEM

1. **2** The ESR and the CRP are indicators of inflammation in the body. Neither is diagnostic of SLE; however, the level of inflammation is a index to the progress of the condition. Presence of ANA is a characteristic of SLE, but it does not indicate progression. Complement fixation does not indicate progression, nor does absence or presence of the butterfly rash.

2. **3** Live viruses are usually not administered when a client is immunosuppressed. Frequently, measles-mumps-rubella vaccine and varicella vaccine are not given to the immunocompromised client; they may be administered when the client has a more competent immune system. Childhood vaccinations are encouraged when the client is not immunocompromised (in remission or not on immunosuppressant medications).

3. **2** Type IV (cell-mediated; delayed hypersensitivity) reaction is a delayed response that occurs 24 to 72 hours after exposure to the allergen (e.g., PPD). The client has been sensitized to tuberculosis. There is no indication of active TB, and it is not a type II reaction. The client's immune system has not been compromised; rather, it has responded normally with the production of antibodies after exposure to the allergen. This does not represent an autoimmune response.

4. **1** This situation best describes an anaphylactic reaction to the penicillin injection. This is a rapidly occurring response that may result in a life-threatening occlusion of the airway (laryngeal edema, bronchospasm). The client may require an emergency tracheotomy or endotracheal intubation. Time should not be wasted on checking the chart or further assessment. The client is obviously in distress, and the presence of breath sounds will not be significant in determining the nursing actions. The chin lift is not an effective method for opening an airway that is occluded from edema or bronchospasm. Epinephrine is the drug of choice for a serious anaphylactic reaction.

5. **2** Even though there is no allergy band, if the client provides information that may indicate a previous reaction to a medication (especially penicillin), hold the medication. With each exposure to an allergen, the reaction could become worse (type I reaction). Notifying the supervisor is not necessary; there is enough information for the nurse to make this decision.

6. **4** Systemic lupus erythematosus is characterized as an autoimmune disorder in which the body begins to invade and destroy normal tissue. Option 1 is a type IV response that is characteristic of a transplant rejection or reaction to tuberculin skin testing. Option 2 describes a type I reaction characterized by a prior exposure to antigen. This occurs with atopic reactions and anaphylaxis. Option 3 is a type III response, which occurs with acute glomerulonephritis.

7. **1** Immunodeficiency is the condition when the immune system is depressed, weak, or compromised and is unable to defend the body from invading microorganisms. Option 2 describes an anaphylactic reaction; option 3 reflects phagocytosis as the white cells destroy the foreign protein; option 4 is an autoimmune condition, in which the body no longer recognizes health tissue. Immunodeficiency may be primary if it is caused by an absence or by poorly developed immune cells. It is secondary if it is caused by illnesses or treatment.

8. **1** Active acquired immunity occurs when a client (infant, child, or adult) receives an immunization against a specific disease. Natural active immunity occurs when the client has had the disease. Natural passive immunity occurs with transfer of antibodies from the mother to the infant at birth or through breast milk. Passive artificial immunity occurs with injection of gamma globulins; the response is immediate but short term.

9. **1, 3, 5, 6** The client with systemic lupus erythematosus is photosensitive and needs protection from sunlight. The client needs to keep joints mobilized because of the invasion of the lupus erythematosus cells into the joints. This condition also affects the circulation in the fingertips, and Raynaud's phenomenon is characteristic of the disease. Fatigue is a problem, and the client needs to prioritize activities of daily living. Nonsteroidal antiinflammatory drugs (NSAIDs) are frequently used to reduce the musculoskeletal discomforts. There is no specific contraindication to pregnancy, except for the medications that may be used in her treatment. The woman should be advised regarding progress of her disease and implications for pregnancy, but she can carry and deliver a healthy infant.

10. **4** *Pneumocystis jirovecii* pneumonia (PCP) is not easily transmitted from an infected person to a healthy person. The pathogen is frequently dormant in the body and is reactivated when the client's immune system is significantly depressed. There is no need for airborne or droplet precautions, but standard precautions must be strictly adhered to with this client.

11. **4** Clients usually have symptoms within 6 to 12 weeks of exposure; however, symptoms may not develop until 6 months after exposure. This is the period of seroconversion. Although the client may remain asymptomatic for an undetermined period of time, option 4 is a more specific answer to the question. The client may be HIV-positive for years before he is diagnosed as having AIDS.

12. **1** An acute infection occurs when the primary condition is identified or the client has recently been infected. He may be asymptomatic at this time, or he may have symptoms of early nonspecific changes characterized by fatigue, weight loss, persistent fever, diarrhea, night sweats, and generalized lymphadenopathy.

13. **2** After initial infection, there is a window of sero-conversion in which the virus begins to replicate and produce antibodies. The client may have a negative test result early in the window; when the body begins to produce antibodies against the virus, the test result will convert to a positive. She should not get pregnant, but contraceptives (oral birth control) do not protect her against human immunodeficiency virus (HIV). Abstaining from sexual activity is frequently unrealistic, and counseling would be beneficial but is not the priority.

14. **4** Epinephrine, given subcutaneously or intravenously, is the drug of choice for anaphylactic reactions. The reaction described is a mild to moderate anaphylactic reaction. The other medications listed may be used in treatment of the reaction, but epinephrine is the immediate drug of choice.

15. **4** The CDC recommends standard precautions for all clients; this is particularly important for the client with AIDS. Although strict handwashing is not an incorrect response, this should be performed when caring for *all* clients and is a part of standard precautions. Airborne precautions are not indicated for clients with opportunistic infections such as *Pneumocystis* pneumonia. Protective isolation is indicated for clients who are severely immunocompromised—for example, clients who have undergone transplants.

16. **1** It is important to identify the client's routines and discuss how he can adapt those routines to take his medications as prescribed. Discussing with the client the importance of taking the medications does not assist him to identify ways in which he can incorporate the medications into his daily routines. Talking to and working with another client is positive, but it still does not incorporate the medication routine into his own daily living routines.

17. **2** Shock is a common problem in anaphylactic reactions; therefore it is important to establish an IV for fluid and medication administration. There should be no pain, and there is no reason the client cannot void on his or her own. A history can be taken at a later time.

18. **1** There is no specific nursing care required for Kaposi's sarcoma lesions. Gentle cleansing of the area and protecting it from abrasive trauma, which could open the lesions, would be appropriate. Dressings, steroid cream, and antibiotic ointment are not indicated.

CHAPTER 8: ABNORMAL CELL GROWTH

1. **2** The nadir refers to the point in the chemotherapy when the leukocytes or neutrophils are at the lowest level. The client's ability to resist infections is at the lowest point, and the client is at the highest risk for developing an infection. Bleeding precautions are implemented with thrombocytopenia or decreased platelets. Nutritional problems are a common problem throughout chemotherapy, and there is no increased risk for development of problem with fluid balance.

2. **2** Abnormal skin pigmentation, erythema, and dry desquamation may develop within a few days of beginning the radiation treatment. Wet desquamation may occur with progression of the radiation treatment; however, the skin does not have blisters. Vertigo may be a sign of orthostatic hypotension associated with hypovolemia. The weight loss occurs, but it is not due to the radiation, it is most often due to the malignancy.

3. **4** Once the implant is in place, keeping it in the exact measured position without disruption is a primary goal of care. Strict bed rest is maintained. The head of the bed should be raised only slightly to accomplish this. A urinary retention catheter is placed to gravity drainage. The client should be in a private room. Constipation should be avoided, but a high-residue diet will increase the bulk of the stool and possibly dislodge the implant.

4. **4** Skin markings are used by the radiotherapist to delineate the exact area of the body to be irradiated. Treatments are completed in a series depending on the location of the malignancy, as well as the level of radiation being administered. The treatments do not require fasting or any form of activity restriction.

5. **3** A common side effect of chemotherapy is stomatitis. It may be manifested as inflammation of the gums and ulcerations in the mouth. There is a decrease in the leukocytes making the client less resistive to infection. Dysrhythmias are not common in cancer therapy; they may occur with electrolyte imbalances secondary to chemotherapy. The slowed speech may occur with hypercalcemia as a complication involving the parathyroid gland.

6. **2** The client should avoid swimming during the treatment period because of the irritating chemicals in swimming pools. The other options are correct for external radiation—showering with a mild soap, eating small nutritious meals, and using an emollient cream.

7. **3** Irritation at the insertion site is a problem in a client who is immunocompromised. Checking the IV site and surrounding area for signs of infection is a priority nursing action. Frequently, the central lines are long and narrow, and withdrawing blood does confirm the location. Transparent dressings are changed on a need-to basis. Opaque (gauze) dressings are usually change every 48 hours.

8. **3, 4, 6** Adverse effects of antineoplastic drugs can be classified as acute, delayed, or chronic. Acute toxicity includes nausea, vomiting, arrhythmias, and allergic reactions. Delayed side effects include stomatitis, alopecia, and bone marrow depression. Chronic toxicity involves organ damage. Common urinary problems include cystitis and nephrotoxicity. Extravasation is not an adverse effect but a complication of an infiltrated IV running a chemotherapy medication that is a vesicant.

9. **4** One of the most common, as well as most severe, toxicities of doxorubicin is cardiotoxicity. After months of treatment, this can be manifested as heart failure (dyspnea, tachycardia, peripheral edema). Early side effects include dysrhythmias and ECG changes. These can occur within hours of receiving the medication.

10. **1** Pulmonary toxicity (dry nonproductive cough, crackles, dyspnea, tachypnea) is an adverse affect of busulfan (Myleran). It can lead to pulmonary fibrosis. Hemoglobin is within normal limits. The nausea and vomiting may be a side effect of the chemotherapy, and the client would be treated for this. Problems occur with a high (not low) serum acid level.

11. **3** Combination drug therapy is important, because different drugs inhibit cancer cell growth at various phases of cellular replication. This makes each of the medications more effective. Medications are given together because this is a more effective method of treatment, not because of cost or to reduce the side effects.

12. **2** Ulcerations in the mouth (stomatitis) can occur when a client is receiving chemotherapy medication. Alleviation of the pain can be achieved by administering systemic analgesics, as well as coating agents such as antacids. Frequent saline rinses are encouraged. Lemon-glycerin swabs may irritate the mucosa and lead to further pain, as would trying to remove oral plaques.

13. **3** A general body or system effect is fatigue, because it occurs as a result of changes in cell cycle patterns and toxic effects from cell destruction. The other problems occur when radiation is directed at specific parts of the body.

CHAPTER 9: PSYCHIATRIC NURSING CONCEPTS

1. **3** Toddlers react very strongly to separation. Nurses frequently must act as surrogate mothers. Option 1 would leave the mother with feeling guilty. Option 4 is giving advice, which is not appropriate. Option 2 does not address her concerns about leaving, nor does it offer reassurance that the toddler will be cared for.

2. **2** The child usually has a fairly accurate evaluation of the situation, and the nurse needs to respond to his questions about dying in a way that allows him a chance to express his concerns. The other options do not answering the child's question.

3. **4** The dying of a child places an intense emotional strain on the parents, and they may use the nurse as a target for their anger. The nurse can become an ally of the parents by allowing them to express their emotions and by assisting them in understanding what is happening.

4. **2** Studies show that terminally ill children they may experience anxiety in relationship to loneliness, separation, and death more frequently than do children who are well.

5. **1** Parents whose children are diagnosed with pyloric stenosis often feel that the problem was in some way related to inadequate parenting or feeding skills. An open-ended comment will encourage discussion and conversation around these issues. Option 2 is false reassurance. Although option 3 is open-ended, it does not address the woman's feeling like a bad mother. Option 4 is comforting, but it does not address the issue.

6. **2** Continued presence of the same helping person enables the dying person to avoid experiencing a sense of abandonment and allows the client and the family to establish the necessary trust for a comfortable working relationship.

7. **1, 2, 3** The client is demonstrating paranoid behavior, which necessitates a matter-of-fact approach that is nonjudgmental and accepting of the client's statements and shows the nurse's willingness to listen attentively to the issue. Options 4, 5, and 6 do not help the paranoid client gain trust to talk with the nurse.

8. **2** Obtaining informed consent for examination is a priority before any other action is taken, including obtaining laboratory specimens and notifying the police.

9. **2** Although anxiety, fear, and guilt all play a part in the reaction to abuse, the hostage response occurs when victims assume responsibility for the violence inflicted on them. In this response, victims tend to blame themselves for the abuse and develop a sense of unworthiness.

10. **3** Indicators of neglect include poor hygiene, poor nutrition, poor skin integrity, contractures, urine burns/excoriation, pressure ulcers, and dehydration. A hip fracture may be due to osteoporosis. Confusion and disorientation are associated with dementia.

CHAPTER 10: PSYCHIATRIC DISORDERS

1. **3** The client is at particular risk for suicide when she appears to be coming out of her depression because she may have the energy and opportunity to kill herself.

2. **1** For the client's protection, he should be moved into a quiet environment away from others. This will help him regain some control and will not produce unneeded stimuli. Setting firm limits would be appropriate for manipulative behavior. Until the manic behavior is under control, including a client in group activities (physical or otherwise) would not be therapeutic for him and would more than likely be disruptive to others.

3. **4** Affective changes in the schizophrenic are self-protective, because they enable the client to deny the painful emotional impact of the external world.

4. **2** The priority nursing action is to determine the suicidal lethality. Ask clients whether they plan to hurt themselves, what the method would be, and what factors might interfere with the rescue. The more

detailed the plan, the more lethal and accessible the method. The more effort that is exerted to block rescue, the greater the likelihood will be of the suicidal effort being successful. Although the other three options are definitely plausible, they are not the priority.

5. **3** Lithium toxicity is a serious problem for clients with bipolar disorder. Symptoms include diarrhea, confusion, ataxia, slurred speech, hypotension, seizures, oliguria, coma, and death.

6. **4** The nurse, by his or her attitude and approach, conveys interest and caring. If the nurse is repulsed by the client's incontinence, this will be conveyed to the client nonverbally, if not verbally.

7. **4** During a manic phase in bipolar disorder, all the body systems speed up, as described in the situation.

8. **1** Detoxification or controlled withdrawal from alcohol via a medical protocol includes regular assessment for withdrawal signs and symptoms and administration of prescribed medications. Signs and symptoms of alcohol withdrawal include anorexia, irritability, nausea, tremulousness, insomnia, nightmares, hyperalertness, tachycardia, increased blood pressure, diaphoresis, and anxiety.

9. **2** Babies with Down syndrome have a high incidence of congenital heart disease, especially atrial defects.

10. **1** The withdrawn client with schizophrenia maintains emotional distance until the barrier of fear of rejection can be broken through contact with another person in a therapeutic relationship. Making emotional contact with the client is one strategy to assist in developing a therapeutic relationship. The other options do not focus on the building of trust, which is the foundation for the care of this type of client.

11. **2** One of the common side effects of antipsychotic medications is drowsiness. The effect usually diminishes after the client has taken the medication for a few days.

12. **3** When the parents can verbalize the need to change the plans that they had made for their infant, it usually signifies that they are beginning to face reality. Although option 2 is correct, it is incorporated into a more comprehensive response (caring and anticipated changes) in option 3. Option 1 focuses outside the family and needs of the child with Down syndrome. Understanding the causative factors of Down syndrome is important but not a priority in the new parents' adjustment to the child.

13. **1** When assisting in the medical treatment of alcohol withdrawal, the nurse should encourage intake of fluids. Alcohol depletes the body of fluid, and detoxification is usually smoother if the client takes fluids readily. A high protein and high carbohydrate diet would be encouraged, because alcoholic clients often have poor nutrition and become debilitated.

14. **3** Bizarre ideas that focus on the body being incapacitated are known as somatic delusions and are sometimes observed in schizophrenia. Grandiose delusions

are beliefs of being important. Ideas of reference or delusions of reference occur when a person having a belief or perception that irrelevant, unrelated or innocuous things in the world are referring to them directly or have special personal significance. Persecutory delusions are when a person believes (wrongly) that they are being picked on, or threatened by someone/something else.

15. **3** To prepare a client for ECT, the nurse must do the following: check the client's record for routine preoperative information; institute and maintain NPO status for 6 hours before the treatment since the client will be receiving a general anesthetic agent—short-acting barbiturate (methohexital [Brevital]) and muscle paralyzing agent (succinylcholine); have the client remove dentures; and administer preoperative medication.

16. **4** According to Eugene Bleuler's classic symptoms of schizophrenia, associative looseness is a lack of logical thought progression, resulting in disorganized and chaotic thinking. Grandiose delusions are beliefs of being important. Ideas of reference or delusions of reference occur when a person believes or perceives that irrelevant, unrelated, or innocuous things in the world are referring to him or her directly or have special personal significance. Depersonalization is characterized by a change in how an affected individual perceives or experiences his or her sense of self. The usual sense of one's own reality is temporarily lost or changed. A feeling of detachment from, or being an outside observer of, one's mental processes or body occurs such as the sensation of being in a dream.

17. **1** The nurse needs to monitor lithium blood levels. There is a high incidence of increased thirst and increased urination. The nurse must assess clients at high risk for developing toxicity and report polyuria, prolonged vomiting, diarrhea, or fever.

18. **2** The client receiving monoamine oxidase inhibitors must avoid coffee, tea, cola beverages, aged cheeses, beer and wine, pickled foods, avocados, figs, and many over-the-counter cold-relief preparations.

19. **4** In disturbance of thought processes, the individual has irrational thoughts. The nurse must initiate interaction by seeking out the client at every opportunity. Avoid denying or arguing with the client when he or she is experiencing hallucinations. Do not give attention to the content of hallucinations. Acknowledge the client's experience but point out that you do not share the experience. Direct the client's attention to real situations.

20. **1, 2** The client with borderline personality disorder expresses problems through behavior rather than as a physical symptom of stress. The pleasure principle is dominant with inadequate superego control. This client is unable to develop meaningful relationships with others and communicates ineffectively. He or she rarely acknowledges that there is

a problem. The client with borderline personality disorder experiences unstable interpersonal relationships and moods. This disorder is characterized by impulsiveness and unpredictability. There is recurrent suicidal behavior, including suicidal gestures and threats. This client engages in self-mutilation, experiences intense anger, and has chronic feelings of emptiness.

CHAPTER 11: INTEGUMENTARY SYSTEM

1. **2** The burns are on the anterior trunk and do not involve extremities; hence the problem would be watching for infection because the eschar makes it difficult to visually examine the healing skin. Removal of the eschar enhances healing and prevents infection, which occurs because of the moist, enclosed area under the eschar.

2. **3** Impetigo is caused by *Streptococcus* or *Staphylococcus* species. Ointments are applied if the lesion is not on the face. For facial lesions, a systemic antibiotic is given.

3. **2** Pediculosis capitis (head lice) is characterized by tiny white nits (eggs) that attach to the base of the hair shaft and are highly contagious. Scabies form burrows, and the itching is often more intense at night. Acne is characterized by pustules. Tinea capitis is characterized by a red, scaly, rash with central clearing in the well-defined margins.

4. **4** An allergic reaction to ampicillin would be the most life threatening; hence patch skin testing is often done before administration of the antibiotic for the first time to determine whether or not the client is allergic. Electromyography measures muscle nerve potential, and there is no pretest screening associated with the test. A child with cystic fibrosis may have a sweat test, which is performed on the skin.

5. **2** Malignant melanoma is the most difficult to treat; it involves extensive full-thickness skin resections, and hence, has the poorest prognosis. Basal cell epithelioma and squamous cell epithelioma are easier to treat and do not metastasize as does melanoma. An Oats cell tumor is a tumor of the lung.

6. **3** This is classified as a stage III pressure ulcer because of the full-thickness tissue loss extending to the deep fascia. Subcutaneous fat may be visible, but bone, tendon, or muscle are not exposed. Slough may be present but does not obscure the depth of tissue loss. There may be undermining and tunneling. A stage I pressure ulcer is characterized by intact skin with nonblanchable redness of a localized area usually over a bony prominence. Darkly pigmented skin may not have visible blanching; its color may differ from the surrounding area. A stage II pressure ulcer is characterized by partial-thickness loss of dermis presenting as a shallow, open ulcer with a red-pink wound bed without slough, which may also present as an intact or open/ruptured serum-filled blister. A stage IV pressure ulcer is characterized by full-thickness tissue loss with exposed bone, tendon, or muscle. Slough or eschar may be present on some parts of the wound bed and often includes undermining and tunneling.

7. **3** Scaling, itching, and redness are common signs of tinea pedis or athlete's foot. Eczema or atopic dermatitis in adults is characterized by reddened lesions in antecubital and popliteal space with pruritus or in children on cheeks, arms, and legs. Pediculosis corporis is body lice and is a parasitic infection.

8. **1** People with light to pale skin and who are excessively exposed to sunlight are most at risk for development of malignant melanoma. Dark-skinned individuals have more melanin in their skin, which provides a measure of protection from UV exposure.

9. **2** Herpes zoster is considered infectious and contact precautions should be used with an older adult client who has a temperature of 102.4°F. Antiviral medications would be given instead of antifungal agents. Lesions are usually along the sensory dermatomes (waist, neck, face) and not in the perineal area. A herpes zoster vaccination should be administered providing the client is not moderately or severely ill, or has a temperature of 101.3°F, as they should usually wait until they recover before getting the vaccine.

10. **2, 4, 5, 6** Elevating the head of the bed to 30° or less will decrease the chance of pressure ulcer development from shearing forces. When placing the client in side-lying position, use the 30° lateral inclined position. Do not place the client directly on the trochanter, which can create pressure over the bony prominence. Avoid the use of donut-shaped cushions because they reduce blood supply to the area, which can lead to extension of the area of ischemia. Bony prominences should not be massaged, because this increases the risk for capillary breakage and injury to underlying tissue leading to pressure ulcer formation.

11. **1** Dry skin should be moisturized daily and as needed, especially after client takes a bath. The number of baths and showers should be limited.

12. **2** When there is evidence of burns around the face, the airway should be carefully assessed. Increased respiratory rate and hoarseness may be the first sign of respiratory complications.

CHAPTER 12: SENSORY SYSTEM

1. **1** Atropine causes mydriasis or pupillary dilation, which can precipitate an attack of acute glaucoma. It should be questioned if it is ordered for a client with glaucoma. The other drugs would be safe for a client with glaucoma.

2. **2** Blindness from glaucoma is preventable; a comprehensive eye examination should be done around age 40, then every 2 to 3 years until 64 years, and then every 1 to 2 years after age 65. There is a familial tendency and a significantly higher incidence in African Americans.

3. **1** Medications must be evaluated in terms of their potential for increasing the intraocular pressure. An

increase in intraocular pressure could cause further damage to the eye in the client with glaucoma. The question states the client has already been diagnosed; glaucoma is painless and is not correlated with the blood pressure.

4. **4** The goal of a myringotomy is to relieve pressure on the tympanic membrane by draining the fluid behind the membrane. Relieving the pressure will relieve pain and prevent eardrum perforation and possible hearing loss. The procedure will drain any purulent fluid behind the membrane and help prevent further infections.

5. **2** The use of warm normal saline solution or hydrogen peroxide irrigation, along with instillation of mineral oil, would soften the wax to help remove the cerumen from the ear canal.

6. **3** The client's cranial nerve IX (glossopharyngeal nerve) may have been damaged during the removal of the tumor and may affect his ability to swallow; prevention of aspiration is a safety issue. The tumor is benign; therefore the client will not begin chemotherapy. The nurse will need to evaluate the hearing loss in the affected ear as well as the impact of hearing loss on the client's body image and ability to perform ADLs; however, these are secondary to the safety problem of aspiration.

7. **2** The eye has been anesthetized; therefore there is no feeling or sensation in it. It would be very easy to rub the eye and cause damage. Option 1, not watching television, would have no impact on the safety; option 3 is not necessary. Because there is no impact on the client's tolerance of direct sunlight, sunglasses would be optional.

8. **4** Conjunctivitis is contagious through physical contact. The child should be directed not to touch the eye, if possible. Handwashing should be stressed after any contact with the eye, and the child should not share any items that might be contaminated.

9. **1** When an unknown solution has been splashed into the eyes, it is most important to remove as much of the solution as possible by rinsing the eyes with large amounts of water or normal saline solution, if available. Options 2, 3, and 4 do not address removing the excess solution from the eye to prevent further damage.

10. **2** Participating in physical contact sports puts this person at the highest risk for retinal detachment because trauma is a leading cause. The other pathologies will affect eye function but have minimal likelihood of causing retinal detachment.

CHAPTER 13: ENDOCRINE SYSTEM

1. **1** When clients are sleeping, the only observable symptom of hypoglycemia is diaphoresis. Options 2 and 3 are indicative of hyperglycemia.

2. **3** If bleeding occurs, the blood will drain posteriorly or behind the client's neck. Serum levels of calcium are important to monitor because of possible damage to the parathyroids during surgery. Oral intake of calcium is not immediately significant. The client is often hoarse; it is important to monitor for increasing hoarseness that would be indicative of edema but not every 5 to 10 minutes. A cervical collar is not indicated.

3. **1** Symptoms of acute pancreatitis are steatorrhea (fatty stools), hyperglycemia, elevated lipase and amylase levels, abdominal pain with muscle guarding, nausea, vomiting, and fever. Hypotension, jaundice, tachycardia may also be present. Bowel sounds are most often hyperactive, and there is no melena present.

4. **2** The unconscious, hypoglycemic client needs immediate treatment with 50% intravenous glucose (highly concentrated). 1000 mL of D_5W over 12 hours does not provide enough glucose to treat the problem. Trying to give oral fluids to an unconscious client should never be done, because it increases the risk for aspiration. Urine sugar does not need to be evaluated if the serum blood glucose is available.

5. **4, 5** Addison's disease is due to a hypofunctioning of the adrenal cortex. The clinical manifestations have a very slow onset, and skin hyperpigmentation (melanosis) is a classic sign. This bronze coloring of the skin is seen primarily in those areas exposed to the sun, pressure points, joints, and in skin creases (especially on the palms). Fatigue, weight loss, hypotension, hyponatremia, and hyperkalemia are other findings associated with the condition.

6. **3** Levothyroxine (Synthroid) increases the metabolic rate of body tissues. Some serious side effects include cardiovascular collapse, dysrhythmias, and tachycardias. Because of these side effects, clients should be instructed not to take the medication if their pulse is greater than 100 beats/min and to notify their physician of headaches, nervousness, chest pain, palpitations, or any unusual symptoms.

7. **1** As carbohydrates are used for energy, insulin needs decrease. Therefore during exercise, carbohydrate intake should be increased to cover the increased energy requirements. The beneficial effects of regular exercise may result in a decreased need for diabetic medications in order to reach target blood glucose levels. Furthermore, it may help to reduce triglycerides, LDL cholesterol levels, increase HDLs, reduce blood pressure, and improve circulation.

8. **1** Impaired venous drainage from the orbit of the eye causes fluid and fat accumulation in the areas behind the eyeballs, which forces the eyes forward and out of their sockets. It is the increased pressure in the area that causes the eyeballs to be forced outward and protrude.

9. **1** Diaphoresis and a shaky feeling are early signs of hypoglycemia. Severe thirst is a sign of hyperglycemia, whereas drowsiness and coma are late symptoms of hypoglycemia.

10. **4** Glucose attaches to the hemoglobin molecule of the red blood cell. A glycosylated hemoglobin test gives an average of blood glucose over the past 3 months, and a blood sample can be obtained at any time during the day. It is not used in the diagnosis of diabetes and does not need to be a fasting specimen.

11. **1** Vasopressin alleviates polyuria by increasing antidiuretic hormone (ADH) secretion. Urine specific gravity will return to a normal level of 1.010 to 1.030.

12. **1** An adverse reaction to corticosteroids is hyperglycemia. A client with type 2 diabetes must monitor her blood glucose level closely while taking steroids. Creatinine clearance measures renal function. Platelets aggregation is associated with hematologic disorders. Ketones are elevated in ketoacidosis.

13. **4** Cushing's syndrome develops because of an excess of cortisol, in this case from prolonged exogenous steroid administration. This syndrome may be diagnosed from truncal (central) obesity, hypertension, weakness, hirsutism, abdominal striae, edema, and glucosuria. Flank pain is associated with kidney problems. Bulging eyes are found in hyperthyroidism. Jaundice is associated with liver and gallbladder problems.

14. **3** Metformin (Glucophage) is administered with meals to minimize gastrointestinal effects. These adverse effects are abdominal bloating, diarrhea, nausea, vomiting, and an unpleasant metallic taste.

15. **3** SIADH occurs when excessive antidiuretic hormone (ADH) is released, even when the plasma (serum) osmolality is normal. The excess ADH increases the permeability of the renal tubules, causing reabsorption of water into the circulation. As a result of extracellular fluid expansion, serum osmolality decreases. Also, sodium levels decline (as a result of being diluted), leading to hyponatremia.

16. **1** Diabetes insipidus (DI) is associated with a decrease (or deficiency) in the secretion of antidiuretic hormone (ADH). Lack of ADH leads to increased urinary output (as much as 5 to 20 L/day). Clients with DI become very fatigued from nocturia. Fluid volume deficit can occur due to the excess urine output. There is no edema or muscle weakness.

17. **4** Pheochromocytoma is a tumor in the adrenal medulla that produces excess catecholamines (epinephrine and norepinephrine). An excess of these catecholamines can cause severe hypertension. Surgery (an adrenalectomy) alleviates the elevated blood pressure most of the time. In 10% to 30% of clients, hypertension remains and must be monitored and treated.

18. **4** Fever is a symptom of thyroid storm. The correct treatment would be a *hypo*thermia blanket to cool the client. All other choices are appropriate interventions for this diagnosis.

19. **1** Calcium chloride or calcium gluconate should be available to treat tetany caused by accidental removal of the parathyroid glands during surgery. This condition may be caused by accidental removal or damage to the parathyroid glands during surgery. Sodium bicarbonate replaces lost base in the body. Potassium chloride replaces the electrolyte potassium. Magnesium sulfate is used in the treatment of eclampsia.

20. **2** Regular insulin (a short-acting insulin) peaks in 2 to 4 hours, and NPH (an intermediate-acting insulin) peaks in 6 to 12 hours. Hypoglycemia would most likely occur between 11 a.m. and 5 p.m. (1100 to 1700 hours).

CHAPTER 14: HEMATOLOGIC SYSTEM

1. **3** In autosomal recessive traits, when both parents have the trait, there is a 25% chance with each pregnancy that the child will have the disease. When only males are affected, it is an X-linked recessive disease, such as hemophilia (option 2). Options 1 and 4 are too specific—because there is a 1 in 4 *chance* of transmitting the trait, it is possible that none of the children would be affected. Frequently, there is a negative family history of the disease.

2. **2, 3, 5** Because clients who are anemic experience chronic fatigue, it is important to balance rest and activities to avoid problems with tachycardia and dyspnea. If a client has a problem with dyspnea during activities, supplemental oxygen may be necessary. The health care provider should be notified if bruising occurs, because this could indicate further problems in the hematologic system. Iron should be taken on an empty stomach; all alcoholic beverages should be avoided; and there is no indication to increase the intake of dairy products and protein. A balanced diet should be followed.

3. **1** Adequate hydration is critical during stress periods for the client with sickle cell disease, and this is particularly true of a client in labor. Oxygen may or may not be ordered in low concentrations. A urinary retention catheter is not necessary at this time and would be a potential cause of infection. Although pain relief is important for both the sickling issues and the labor pains, continuous sedation would not be indicated, as this would be detrimental to the fetus.

4. **2** When there is inadequate hydration, the sickled cells begin to clump together, which leads to vascular occlusion. Tissue hypoxia occurs as a result of the decreased oxygen-carrying capacity of the sickled red blood cells, as well as from the vascular occlusion.

5. **2** Iron deficiency anemia is characterized by fatigue, dizziness, weakness, increased pulse, palpitations, and increased sensitivity to cold. The adult female often becomes anemic for a variety of reasons, such as poor nutrition and heavy menses.

6. **2** Fresh fruits and vegetables harbor microorganisms, which can cause infections in the immunosuppressed client. Fruits and vegetables should either be peeled

or cooked. The doctor should be notified of a temperature above 100°F. A diet low in protein is not indicated, and humidifiers harbor fungi in the water containers.

7. **2** The toddler will need to eat a balanced diet and may require an iron supplement. A diet based primarily on milk products will not cover the iron needs of a toddler. A client in sickle cell crisis may experience anemia, but it is due to the increased destruction of red blood cells, not poor iron intake. The client receiving radiation therapy may also develop anemia, but it is not due to poor nutritional intake. The client who has had surgery may develop anemia as a result of a lack of adequate utilization of vitamin B_{12}.

8. **4** Rest, ice, compression, and elevation (RICE) are the immediate treatments to reduce the swelling and bleeding into the joint. These are the priority actions for bleeding into the joint, regardless of the cause. The other options may be done, but they are not the priority actions.

9. **2** The whole blood must be given within the first 30 minutes to prevent hemolysis and growth of bacteria in the blood. Vital signs are to be checked after administration of the first 50 mL and after the first 15 minutes.

10. **2** Stop the blood infusion and disconnect the line to decrease the further infusion of red blood cells. Begin administration of normal saline solution with new tubing. The remainder of the blood should be returned to the blood bank for evaluation regarding the reaction.

CHAPTER 15: RESPIRATORY SYSTEM

1. **3** Retained secretions may cause hypoventilation; this results in an increase in the $Paco_2$. The other options do not as effectively reflect a problem with clearing mucus. Pleural fluid is not removed via coughing; the fluid is in the pleural space, not in the lung. Although the $Paco_2$ is within the normal limits, there is still an increase noted, which is due to the hypoventilation. The nurse cannot easily measure the forced vital capacity at the bedside.

2. **2** A leak in the cuff would allow air to pass through the trachea and vocal cords, allowing the client to make a noise—or to speak. The nurse may also hear the air leak. An air leak may occur when there are changes in the pressure on the ventilator, but this is not the most common cause or the best response from the nurse. Increased swallowing is indicative of irritation in the throat. Increase in adventitious sounds indicates excessive mucus in the lungs.

3. **4** The primary purpose of oxygen therapy is to decrease the workload of the heart in clients with chronic pulmonary diseases and to assist in preventing right-sided heart failure. Use of oxygen may help to relieve shortness of breath but will not eliminate it. Oxygen supports combustion but is not explosive; supplemen-

tal oxygen will allow more activity for the client, not less.

4. **2, 1, 3, 4**
   1 ___2___ Because oxygen is a priority, begin administration of oxygen.
   2 ___1___ The first action is to place the client in semi-Fowler's position. Oxygen or inhalation therapy cannot be effective with severe orthopnea if the client is not in a sitting or upright position.
   3 ___3___ Then administer the nebulizer treatment, which would include bronchodilators.
   4 ___4___ Physiologic needs must be addressed before teaching or psychosocial needs are considered.

5. **4** Physical conditioning is important for clients with COPD. Activity needs to be paced so that undue fatigue does not occur. Some increase in shortness of breath with exercise is to be expected but will not damage the lungs. If the client stops exercising before an increase in shortness of breath, he will not experience a training effect.

6. **4** The catheter must be advanced to an adequate depth (to prevent secretion buildup at the end of the tube and to clear the airway as much as possible). To minimize trauma, suction is applied only during catheter withdrawal. If the upper airway is suctioned, another sterile catheter must be obtained to suction the ET tube.

7. **3** This is important information to explain to the client's wife regarding the bloody drainage in the chest tube collection system. After the nurse has explained the reason for the drainage, it would then be appropriate to sit down and talk with the wife (option 1). Options 2 and 4 do not answer the question or address the wife's concern.

8. **2** CPAP only works when the infant is breathing on his own. When the airway is opened for a breath, the CPAP increases the pressure in the airway, which increases airflow to the lungs and oxygenation. CPAP is not used when a child requires controlled ventilation. Option 3 may be appropriate, but the child must be able to breathe spontaneously for this to be effective. The child is not suctioned unless an excessive amount of mucus must be removed.

9. **1** An endotracheal tube that is inserted too far—beyond the carina—is most likely to enter the right main stem bronchus. The volume of air from the ventilator is only delivered to the right lung; breath sounds are decreased or absent over the left lung. The pressure alarm indicates that the current pressure is not adequate to deliver the tidal volume prescribed. This may occur but does not confirm the migration of the tube.

10. **4** Before the child is fully awake, he or she should be placed on the abdomen with the head turned to one side to facilitate the drainage of secretions and to prevent aspiration. When alert, the child may sit up or assume a position of comfort. The other options

are not appropriate because they do not allow for drainage of secretions from the mouth and throat after a tonsillectomy.

11. **2** An autosomal recessive inheritance pattern occurs with cystic fibrosis. The parents are not affected, but each parent carries the trait. With each pregnancy, there is a 25% chance that the child will have the condition. If children do not have the disease, there is a 50% chance that they will be carriers and a 25% chance that they will not have the disease or be carriers. The other options do not describe an autosomal recessive inheritance pattern.

12. **2** Tension pneumothorax occurs when air enters the pleural space with each inspiration, becomes trapped there, and is not expelled during expiration (i.e., one-way valve effect). Pressure builds in the chest as the accumulation of air in the pleural space increases. This can lead to a mediastinal shift. Atelectasis occurs when the atmospheric pressure enters the pleural cavity. This procedure has nothing to do with an infection or pulmonary consolidation.

13. **3** The wheezing is due to narrowing of the airway caused by bronchospasm. Increased mucus production hinders the airway as well; this also results in trapping of air in the alveoli. Increased pulmonary compliance indicates the lungs have good recoil and expansion.

14. **1** Diminished breath sounds are typically noted over the consolidated area. The cough is generally productive. The breathing is rapid and shallow without the use of accessory muscles. Hemoptysis may occur, but not hematemesis (blood from the GI tract).

15. **1** The respiratory rate is within normal limits at 18 breaths/min. The option for the pulse oximetry is too low. The pulse rate is too high, and the productive cough with rapid breathing is not as significant as the decrease in respiratory rate.

16. **3** In clients with chronic high Pco_2 levels (COPD), the administration of oxygen at a flow rate that increases the PaO_2 may cause apnea and require the use of a bag valve mask resuscitator to ventilate the client. When the PaO_2 increases significantly, it can decrease the client's stimulus to breath and may cause carbon dioxide narcosis.

17. **2** Positioning over the bedside table allows the ribs to separate, which assists the physician in positioning the needle into the pleural cavity. If the client is unable to assume a sitting position, he or she is placed on the affected side with head of bed slightly elevated. The area containing the fluid should be dependent.

18. **2** The ineffective clearing of secretions with resultant pooling can lead to an increased risk for infection. The client's appetite is usually decreased. The client has an increased anteroposterior diameter of the chest.

19. **3** Decongestants should be avoided by clients with hypertension, because these medications often contain pseudoephedrine and phenylephrine, which cause central nervous system stimulation with vasoconstriction and increased blood pressure. They also precipitate anxiety and insomnia.

20. **1** Because croup causes upper airway obstruction, inspiratory stridor is a predominant symptom. Expiratory wheezing is heard in the asthmatic client, paroxysmal coughing occurs more with spasmodic laryngitis, and hemoptysis is not common with croup syndromes.

CHAPTER 16: VASCULAR SYSTEM

1. **2** The level of the right atrium must be determined, and each successive reading must be determined from the same point of reference on the client. This area is also called the phlebostatic axis.

2. **4** Medication should be administered with a small-gauge (25-gauge) needle into the subcutaneous tissue without aspirating or massaging the area. Partial thromboplastin time (PTT) is used to monitor the effects of heparin. Heparin is most often not infused by IVPB.

3. **3** Noncompliance with blood pressure medications is a common problem in the treatment of hypertension. The client must understand that the only way to keep her blood pressure under control is to continue to take her medications. She will not be able to discontinue the medications unless there is a significant change in her condition as a result of weight loss, an exercise program, and/or decreased stress.

4. **2, 3, 4** Healing of venous stasis ulcers is dependent on relieving the venous congestion in the extremity. Compression devices and elevation of the extremity are the most effective methods. The client should avoid standing for long periods since this increases venous stasis. Moist cool and/or warm packs are not used, but moist environment dressings are utilized. Dressings need to be changed as frequently as necessary, because there may be excessive drainage.

5. **1** Early ambulation is the most effective and safe way to prevent thrombophlebitis with any type of client. This promotes venous return and prevents venous stasis. Anticoagulants are not routinely given postpartum unless there is another pathologic condition present. The legs should be elevated when the client is in a sitting position.

6. **1** Aldactone is a potassium-sparing diuretic. The client's potassium level is high; therefore the medication should be held, and the doctor should be notified. The other options are not affected by this medication.

7. **4** The postoperative client has decreased mobility, which may create an environment in which clotting can be caused by venous stasis. Active exercise, such as having the client ambulate as soon as possible, will stimulate circulation and venous return. This reduces the possibility of clot formation. The lower extremities should not be massaged, because this may disrupt a clot and cause a pulmonary embolism.

8. **1** The client should be referred for further evaluation of blood pressure. The blood pressure is definitely

elevated, the client is overweight, and she has an increased level of cholesterol. A multifocus approach is necessary to control the blood pressure.

9. **3** Occlusion to the aortic/femoral bypass graft is considered a medical emergency, and physician notification is imperative. No other nursing options would alleviate the problem. Massaging the leg and having the client ambulate would be contraindicated. If the pulses cannot be palpated and the client is experiencing pain, the nurse should not wait to call the physician.

CHAPTER 17: CARDIAC SYSTEM

1. **2** The treatment of choice is lidocaine IV push to attempt to convert the dysrhythmia before it progresses to ventricular fibrillation. Adenosine is given for supraventricular tachycardia. Transvenous pacing is initiated for symptomatic bradycardia or asystole. Defibrillation will be necessary if the client loses consciousness.

2. **1** Jugular vein distention with the client in a sitting position, or with a 45-degree head elevation, is indicative of an increase in the central venous pressure. Many clients experience jugular vein distention when in a supine position, and this is not indicative of an increase in central venous pressure. Adventitious breath sounds, bradycardia, restlessness, and tachypnea are not directly associated with increased jugular vein distention but may occur if the client develops right-sided heart failure.

3. **4** Nitroglycerin is a vasodilator. It dilates the coronary arteries, thereby increasing myocardial blood supply; vasodilation of the peripheral circulation decreases the pressure against which the heart must pump, thereby decreasing the afterload. Glomerular filtration may increase from an increased cardiac output, but the primary purpose is to increase blood supply to the myocardium. The vasodilation will also assist to relieve chest pain, but it does so through increased blood supply to myocardium.

4. **4** To help decrease pulmonary congestion and dyspnea, the nurse should encourage adequate rest to decrease cardiac workload; the client should not exert himself to the point of fatigue. Bed rest does promote venous return, but that is not the purpose of bed rest in the client with heart failure. A hospital bed is not necessary, and a quiet room is important if that is what promotes rest for the client.

5. **3** A sustained low cardiac output decreases renal perfusion and results in oliguria and impaired renal function. Oliguria is marked by output of less than 30 mL/hour. Increased BUN, changes in specific gravity (osmolarity), and creatinine clearance will be affected if the client develops renal failure.

6. **2** Nitro-Dur is used to prevent angina so that the client can perform the normal activities of daily living without chest pain. Sublingual nitroglycerin, or translingual spray, is used to treat immediate chest pain.

7. **1, 3, 4, 5** A focused cardiac assessment is directed toward assessing physiologic symptoms that provide immediate information regarding the client's condition, which is appropriate for the nurse to do at the beginning of each shift. After the physiologic parameters have been evaluated, the nurse can determine any history of difficulty breathing and a list of medications the client was taking before admission.

8. **3** Restlessness and diaphoresis may be indicative of decreased cardiac output, frequently originating from a dysrhythmia. Checking temperature and blood glucose levels is not a priority. Option 2 will be done when all physical problems are resolved. Physiologic needs must be addressed first. It is important to obtain critical assessment data before calling the doctor.

9. **3** The rhythm is premature ventricular beats or contractions (PVCs). The nurse should immediately prepare and administer lidocaine by IV push. The PVCs indicate an increased irritability of the ventricles and frequently precede ventricular tachycardia. This is a 6-second tracing, and the PVCs are frequent and multifocal. It is not necessary to call a code at this time. Options 1 and 4 do not address the problem.

10. **1** It is important to perform a thorough nursing assessment before the surgery. This provides a baseline for comparison of physiologic assessment data after surgery. Physiologic needs come first. The client and family do need to know about the chest drainage; however, this is client education. Options 2 and 3 are not important information to discuss with the client.

11. **4** A low potassium level can precipitate digitalis toxicity. The client has been taking her medications and not eating regularly. She also has an irregular heartbeat and increased lethargy along with nausea, all of which can be signs of digitalis toxicity. She is taking a diuretic, which increases the excretion of potassium, and a low potassium level can cause digitalis toxicity.

12. **3** First-degree heart block can only be evaluated with an ECG or monitor tracing because the distinguishing factor is a prolonged P-R interval; all beats are being conducted. Other options are appropriate for this client; however, they do not assess first-degree block.

13. **3** In cardiac catheterization with angiography, contrast dye is injected into the coronary arteries, which allows visualization of the coronary arteries and provides information on their patency. Exercise tolerance is a stress test, and an electrocardiogram (ECG) is a study of the conduction system. Myocardial contractility can be evaluated during a catheterization, but the question specifically asked about cardiac angiography, which is a study of cardiac vessels.

14. **4** Most demand pacemakers are set somewhere between 60 and 72. If the client's pulse rate falls below the preset pacemaker rate, the pacemaker should take over the pacing. With bradycardia, ventricular escape

beats occur. Option 1 is normal, and options 2 and 3 are not indicative of pacemaker problems.

15. **4** The nurse needs to auscultate the apical pulse when a client is in atrial fibrillation. The point of maximal impulse is the correct location for auscultation of the apical pulse. It is located at the fifth intercostal space, at the midclavicular line. This is the apex of the heart. It is noted with a black dot on the correct area in the illustration.

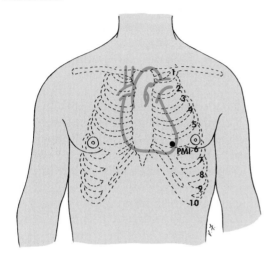

16. **1** Atropine is administered for symptomatic bradycardia. An increase in pulse rate is the therapeutic response for this client. All other options are characteristic of atropine but are not desired actions for this client.

17. **1** Dyspnea on exertion is a classic sign of left ventricular problems, regardless of the precipitating cause. Lower extremity edema is also characteristic, but it is not as significant as dyspnea on exertion. Dizziness and fainting on standing are indicative of postural (orthostatic) hypotension.

18. **4** An echocardiogram provides information regarding flow of blood through the mitral valve and left ventricular performance. An angiogram is done to determine coronary artery blood flow. A stress test is done to evaluate exercise tolerance. An ECG is done to evaluate cardiac conduction.

19. **3** Antibiotics (usually administered by IVPB) are indicated for bacterial endocarditis. This may continue at home with the assistance of a home care nurse to administer the IVPBs, or the client may be changed to oral antibiotics. The continued antibiotic is critical to the prevention of vegetation growth on the valves. Other options are not specific to bacterial endocarditis.

CHAPTER 18: GASTROINTESTINAL SYSTEM

1. **1** Coffee-ground material is old blood. This is a normal occurrence on the third postoperative day and should be correlated with the vital signs. The tube is in the correct position since it is draining gastric secretions. There is no indication to notify anyone or to irrigate the nasogastric tube.

2. **1** Nasogastric tubes are left in place for several days after gastric resection. It is important to prevent the stomach from becoming distended and putting pressure on the suture line. A diet will be started after there is evidence of good bowel function. Diet will be clear liquids until client tolerance is determined. It is not a nursing responsibility to advise the client regarding prognosis and status of malignancy. A urinary retention catheter may or may not be in place; preferably, the client will be voiding.

3. **1** NPO status before a barium swallow and a gastroduodenoscopy and a low-residue diet the evening before the procedures are routine orders for these tests. There is no general anesthesia. The client can eat or drink as tolerated after procedure, and there is no routine placement of nasogastric tubes.

4. **3** Enemas or laxatives are not administered before surgery in clients with an acute abdomen. If gastric motility is stimulated, there is an increased danger of appendiceal rupture. All other orders are appropriate before an appendectomy.

5. **1, 3, 6** The characteristic position of comfort for the client with appendicitis is on the side with the legs flexed against the abdomen; the head of the bed should remain slightly elevated to decrease the upward spread of infection in case the appendix ruptures. Keep the client NPO because of the impending surgery; initiate IV fluid replacement. Maintain the client on bed rest. Do not apply any type of heat to the abdomen. Narcotics are given with caution, if at all, since the analgesic may mask the symptoms of rupture.

6. **2** Dumping syndrome is not uncommon after a combination bariatric surgery. Precautions such as limiting the amount of fluids taken with a meal should be implemented. The intake of foods high in iron, calcium, and B_{12} may not prevent the vitamin or mineral deficiencies since the problem is with the *absorption* of these elements; supplements may be necessary. The surgery frequently prevents or corrects the problem with gastroesophageal reflux. The client should plan to eat 6 small meals a day to decrease distention of the remaining stomach.

7. **2** Dumping syndrome is self-limiting; it is not a permanent problem. Decreasing fluid intake with and after meals, eating small meals, and decreasing carbohydrate and salt intake will decrease the dumping effect. Activity does not play an essential role in preventing dumping syndrome.

8. **1** Rebound pain is elicited by pressing firmly over the area known as McBurney's point; pain occurs when pressure is released. The rebound pain, decreased bowel sounds, fever, and tender abdomen are all characteristic of the clinical picture of appendicitis. Gastric distention, diarrhea, and gnawing radiating pain are not common signs of appendicitis. Remember, all the items in an option have to be correct if it is the correct answer.

9. **1** Perforation is characterized by increasing distention and board-like abdomen. There is frequently increasing pain with fever and guarding of the abdomen. Peritonitis occurs rapidly. The nurse should maintain the client NPO, keep the client on bed rest, and immediately notify the physician. Decreasing hemoglobin and hematocrit and decreasing blood pressure are associated with hemorrhage rather than perforation. Remember to select an answer that reflects what the question is specifically asking.

10. **4** Topical sedation during endoscopy helps to block the gag reflex and numbs the esophagus, eliminating the discomfort of the tube. The nurse would know the dangers of allowing the client to eat or drink before the sedation has lost its effect. The nurse will test for the return of the client's gag reflex before allowing sips of water to be taken to avoid aspiration.

11. **3** Duodenal ulcers are characterized by high gastric acid secretion and rapid gastric emptying. Food buffers the effect of the acid; consequently, pain increases when the stomach is empty. Pain does not characteristically occur after eating, and the client does not usually have bouts with nausea unless bleeding or obstruction is a problem.

12. **1, 2, 3, 5** Each of these actions will help either to neutralize the acid in the stomach or to decrease the physiologic reflux. Increased fluids with meals will exacerbate the problem, as will eating before going to bed.

13. **2** Constipation increases problems with diverticula. A diet high in fiber is recommended. The other options do not have any specific relevance to diverticula disease.

14. **1** Evaluate the nasogastric tube patency; it is important to prevent the nausea and vomiting. The next action would be to put the client in semi-Fowler's position. It is very important to assess the client and take nursing measures to determine the source of the nausea and to decrease the nausea before calling the doctor.

15. **2** Sims' lateral position is most commonly used for best access and visualization during the procedure, as well as for the client's comfort.

16. **1** Stool samples should be taken from different areas of the stool to more accurately reflect the presence of occult blood. The nurse only needs to collect a small sample of stool for the test. The test is done on the nursing unit and is not sent to the laboratory for further evaluation. Three separate samples will more accurately validate the presence of blood, but it is not required. Diets rich in red meat may cause a false-positive result.

17. **4** The child with celiac disease will need a gluten-free diet, eliminating foods such as pastas and breads that are made from wheat or dessert foods made from malt whey. Remember ROW—rye, oats, and wheat. Barley is also to be avoided. Foods that would be appropriate include rice and corn cereals, milk, corn and potato breads, tapioca, peanut butter, and honey.

18. **3 cans**

     55 mL/hr × 24 hours/day = 1320 total mL for 24 hours or 5.28 cans ÷ 2 (half-strength) = 2.64 cans, or 3 cans.

CHAPTER 19: HEPATIC AND BILIARY SYSTEM

1. **4** Accurate intake and output measurements are essential for clients receiving diuretics. Hypokalemia, not hyperkalemia, is a frequent occurrence with diuretic therapy. Hypovolemia is a greater risk with an increased urine output. Clients should be weighed daily.

2. **1, 2, 3** Acetaminophen is metabolized by the liver and is contraindicated in clients with liver disease. Morphine and Demerol are very potent narcotic analgesics and would not be ordered for a headache. The other medications (aspirin, naproxen, and ibuprofen) may be allowed for the treatment of headache in an individual with cirrhosis.

3. **4** Vitamin K is necessary for normal clotting. Cholecystitis can decrease the absorption of fat-soluble vitamins (A, D, E, and K) by interfering with fat metabolism, which can lead to potential difficulties with clotting.

4. **3** Neomycin sulfate decreases bacterial flora in the bowel, thus decreasing ammonia. Proton pump inhibitors and H_2 blockers decrease gastric acidity in the treatment of cirrhosis. Lactulose acidifies feces in the bowel and traps ammonia, causing its elimination in the feces. Propranolol (Inderal) reduces portal venous pressure.

5. **3** Daily weight measurement is essential to monitor for volume overload. Clients with cirrhosis need increased vitamin B, especially B_6. Tylenol is hepatotoxic. The diet should be high in carbohydrates, include adequate amounts of protein to build tissue, and be moderate to low in fat intake.

6. **1** HBV is spread by sexual contact. The client should not be sexually active until the laboratory test determines that the hepatitis is no longer contagious, which usually occurs when the anti-HBs or HBsAB (antibodies to antigen) are present. There will be no bilirubin in the urine or stools; clay-colored stools are expected, so they would not be reported.

7. **1** Vital signs must be assessed first if the nurse is monitoring the client for bleeding or shock.

8. **3** IV salt-poor albumin is given to replace protein lost in the ascites fluid and to restore oncotic pressure in the vascular bed. $D_{10}W$ is an IV fluid, not a medication. Lasix will diminish the ascitic fluid. The client has respiratory compromise and would not be given a narcotic pain medication (Demerol).

9. **3** Hepatitis A is transmitted via fecal contamination and oral ingestion. Paper towels are used to create a clean area surface. Alcohol preps are not effective.

The mask is not appropriate because hepatitis is not spread by respiratory secretions.

10. **3** In end-stage liver disease, the liver cannot break down ammonia by-products of protein metabolism. The increased ammonia levels in the serum cross the blood-brain barrier, causing uncontrolled drowsiness and confusion. Hyperglycemia is characterized by polyphagia, polydipsia, and polyuria, along with fatigue, weight loss, excessive thirst, and abdominal pain. Hypocalcemia is characterized by tetany symptoms. Increased bile production does not cause neurologic symptoms; it is related more to digestion.

11. **3** In a client with end-stage liver disease, lactulose is used to decrease ammonia levels in the blood, thus improving cognition and alertness. The ammonia is eliminated through the regular bowel movements that the medication promotes, preventing obstructions. Lactulose is not involved in blood clotting.

12. **2** A semi-Fowler's position improves lung expansion. The incision for a cholecystectomy is high and may interfere with respiratory exchange. The other positions would probably interfere with respirations.

13. **3** Continue monitoring, as T-tube drainage decreases after day 2 and may stop between days 3 and 5. T-tubes are not irrigated. Placement is not checked. Repositioning will not change the drainage.

14. **1** Standard precautions are the appropriate type of infection precautions for all clients with hepatitis. Droplet precautions are not necessary for clients with hepatitis. Because hepatitis A is transmitted by the oral-fecal route, contact precautions are not necessary, except for the methods provided by standard precautions. Bloodborne precautions (part of standard precautions) are necessary for clients with hepatitis B and C (which are bloodborne), as well as for clients with hepatitis D and G.

15. **3** The hepatitis vaccine is used to protect health care workers and other individuals from hepatitis B. The series consists of three intramuscular injections, the first two given at least 1 month apart and the third given 4 to 6 months later to provide long-lasting protection from hepatitis B only.

16. **2** The function of the gallbladder is the concentration and storage of bile. With the gallbladder absent, the liver will continue to produce bile to emulsify fats, but there will not be an excess of bile available. Clients who have undergone a cholecystectomy should eat a low-fat diet but do not need to make any other dietary adjustments.

17. **3** Increased levels of bilirubin (greater than 2.0 mg/dL) cause a discoloration of the skin called jaundice. The bilirubin value needs to be two to three times the normal level for jaundice to be manifested. Normal value of total bilirubin is 0.2 to 1.3 mg/dL. Jaundice occurs because of an alteration in normal bilirubin metabolism or flow of bile into the hepatic or biliary system. Increased ammonia and ALT levels do not cause jaundice; they are problems associated with the malfunctioning liver.

18. **3** A T-tube is used after a common bile duct exploration to drain bile and maintain patency of the duct until healing can occur. A T-tube should never be irrigated by the nurse.

19. **3** The altered clotting mechanisms in a client with hepatic cirrhosis mean that the client has fewer clotting factors available to assist in the clotting process. Bleeding precautions should be in place. Although the client may be able to be independent in ADLs, for reasons of safety, supervision should be provided. Antibiotics and increased nutritional intake will not speed clotting times.

20. **2** Sexual contact should be avoided by clients with hepatitis B. All activities that result in contact with the blood should be avoided. Bathroom sanitization and droplet precautions are not necessary with hepatitis B. Vaccinations are administered to prevent hepatitis B infections.

CHAPTER 20: NEUROLOGIC SYSTEM

1. **3** Open-ended questions are most helpful in obtaining accurate health history information because they elicit more detailed descriptions of the symptoms. Although the other options are applicable to the presenting symptom, they result in "yes" or "no" responses; this does not encourage the client to provide detailed information about the problem.

2. **3** Recurrent headaches that increase in frequency and severity are frequently the first complaint of a client with a brain tumor; the headaches usually correlate with the area of the brain involved. The other options are not relevant to a brain tumor.

3. **1** The rehabilitation program for a client who has had a stroke includes actions that prevent deformity (passive range of motion on affected side and active ROM on the unaffected side) and prevent complications that may be associated with immobility. The client's affected side should be protected, and food should be placed on the unaffected side so that the client can control it. The client should be turned to his right (affected side) but for shorter periods of time.

4. **4** An electroencephalogram measures the brain's electrical activity. There are no ultrasonic waves in the brain. An electroencephalogram determines the electrical activity but not the brain activity; it has no relevance to skeletal muscle activity.

5. **3** When a stroke occurs in the dominant hemisphere, the client experiences communication difficulties, or aphasia. Speech retraining cannot begin until the client understands and can follow directions. The question is focusing on the client's ability to speak and his current problem with aphasia.

6. **2** Straining at defecation or the use of the Valsalva maneuver may exacerbate increased intracranial pressure. The nurse promotes normal bowel movements

that prevent straining by encouraging a high-fiber diet and stool softeners when needed. Enemas are discouraged, and it is important to prevent constipation so that an impaction does not occur.

7. **2** The priority after a grand mal seizure is to maintain a patent airway. The question is asking for a nursing intervention after the seizure is over. The clothes should be loosened so that they do not constrict the client. The nurse may need to remain with the client, and the events of the seizure need to be recorded, but the priority of this question is the airway.

8. **4** The first side effect to be noticed may be gastrointestinal problems. Taking medication with meals may alleviate these symptoms. The client may continue to take the medication, and attempts should be made to minimize the side effects. The client's food preferences and his blood pressure are not relevant to the situation.

9. **3** Most CSF leaks resolve spontaneously. The child should be maintained on bed rest until drainage ends. NSAIDs are not contraindicated. The child may turn and assume a position of comfort, and there are usually no dietary restrictions.

10. **2** An early symptom of Parkinson's disease is slowness of movements in all normal activities of daily living. Tremors and weight loss may occur but are not commonly the first symptoms.

11. **3** Because of the emotional stress of Parkinson's disease, mood disturbances often occur. Problems with communication, intellectual skills, and diversional interest are usually not as common as mood disturbance in the early stages.

12. **3** Decreased mobility over an extended period leads to stasis of secretions. There is no associated dysfunction in the CNS regarding the respiratory system; the immune response is mature but may become impaired as a result of the chronic illness.

CHAPTER 21: MUSCULOSKELETAL SYSTEM

1. **2** After surgery, edema may cause compression of structures in the operative area, resulting in pain similar to that experienced before surgery. Twisting will cause pain, but it is usually a different type of pain than the pain the client had before surgery. Limitation of movement will decrease pain.

2. **2, 3, 5** The paresthesia, edema, and leg pain unrelieved by analgesics are classic indicators of the development of compartmental syndrome. The decrease in pulse rate is not important; the *quality* of the pulse is the important observation. The pins usually do not cause undue pain, and frequently, the client is angry regarding the immobility and does not use effective coping measures.

3. **1** Osteoarthritis has a gradual onset and affects weight-bearing joints with pain that is more pronounced after exercise. The client will usually complain of morning stiffness.

4. **4** For any client in traction, a nursing priority is to determine the correct amount of weight and to assess for effectiveness of countertraction. Weights must hang freely for countertraction to be effective. In Buck's traction, the entire foot of the bed is elevated to prevent the client from moving toward the end of the bed, and the weights hang freely from the end of the bed with the client serving as the countertraction.

5. **2** Client should lie on the abdomen for 30 minutes 3 to 4 times/day and position the hip in extension while prone. The residual limb is wrapped from distal to proximal. Ice packs are not used on the residual limb after surgery, and antiinflammatory medications may be used for pain relief but not to prevent edema.

6. **3** The cast should be supported on a pillow that will not absorb the moisture and will not keep the cast wet (e.g., plastic-covered pillow). Palms of the hand should be used in turning the client. Heat should not be applied to a damp cast.

7. **4** Always check the weight amounts and make sure they are not lodged against the bed or another area. There are no pin sites, and the boot does not need to be removed that often.

8. **1** Physical therapy relaxes muscles and relieves the aching and stiffness of the involved joints. It usually does not restore lost range of motion, and it does not prevent inflammation. Physical therapy does make the client more comfortable, but it does not assist in coping with pain.

9. **1** Heparin is administered prophylactically to prevent thromboembolic complications in clients who are immobilized for prolonged periods. It is not effective in preventing fat emboli or venous stasis or promoting vascular perfusion.

10. **1** Circulation and neurosensory status distal to the fracture are always priorities for clients with fractures. The amount of swelling is important; however, the primary concern regarding swelling is circulatory and neurosensory deficits. The amount of bone healing cannot be assessed. There is concern regarding pain, but circulatory and neurologic checks are the priority actions.

11. **1** The movement and sensation should be evaluated before surgery to serve as a baseline for comparison during the postoperative recovery period. Radiating leg pain is diagnostic of the condition, and assessing it before surgery is not as beneficial as determining movement and sensation.

12. **2** A hip spica cast is used for the treatment of congenital hip dysplasia. Check the cast to make sure it is not too tight and constricting circulation by inserting a finger between the skin and cast. The child is not in traction with a hip spica cast, and the arms are not being treated. The circulation is checked distal, not proximal, to the cast.

13. **2** The priority of care is to check the status of circulation distal to the area of injury. The client is generally

kept in the supine position to promote straight pull on the traction; the client is not out of bed. Deep breathing is encouraged, but the semi-Fowler's position does not facilitate the traction.

14. **2** Compartmental syndrome is characterized by consistent pain and loss of sensation distal to the area of injury. The client can have an adequate peripheral pulse and still have a problem with compartmental syndrome. The client in balanced suspension traction has pins or wires exerting traction on the bone, and pin site care is important, but evaluating for compartmental syndrome is the priority. Maintaining good fluid intake is also important, but assessing neurocirculatory status is the higher priority.

15. **1** Balanced suspension traction with a Thomas splint requires checking the groin area where the thigh is supported. The leg of the affected side is suspended off the bed, and the heel is usually not a problem.

16. **2** Conservative treatment would not involve surgical intervention. The most common conservative therapy includes bed rest and a muscle relaxant.

17. **4** Phantom limb pain is real pain for the client and is common in amputees. Phantom pain can best be controlled by pain medication. It is important to respect a client's interpretation of the experience of pain.

18. **2** Lab work will need to be done periodically during administration to monitor for the development of anemia, leukopenia, thrombocytopenia, and/or hepatic toxicity.

19. **2** Clients with total hip replacement should not bring their operative leg across midline, which may result in prosthesis dislocation. Crossing the legs is abduction, which is contraindicated for this client.

20. **2** Greenstick fracture is a splintering of the bone, not a complete fracture. The name comes from the splintering effect that would occur in an attempt to break a "green" (young) stick. It is a common fracture in children. A comminuted fracture has multiple bone fragments and is more common in adults (option 4). Greenstick fractures do not affect the growth plate, and there is no bone separation.

CHAPTER 22: REPRODUCTIVE SYSTEM

1. **2** Increased risk for cervical cancer is associated with a history of HPV (genital warts) infection, STDs, HSV-2, multiple sex partners, first intercourse at early age, and abnormal Pap tests. The use of alternative therapy and estrogen therapy for menopause, oral contraceptive use, and multiple pregnancies do not increase the risk.

2. **1** The herpes simplex virus (HSV-2) is concentrated in the vesicles, and therefore the infection is highly contagious when this clear fluid is released. The lesions rupture and form shallow, moist ulcerations (not pustules) that eventually crust, allowing epithelialization of the erosions to occur. There is no yellow drainage. The primary infection is associated with local inflam-

mation and pain and often accompanied by systemic symptoms of fever, headache, malaise, myalgia, and regional lymphadenopathy.

3. **1** Before discharge, the client should be instructed to avoid douching. On her postoperative visit to the doctor, he will evaluate the healing of the cervical area and will advise her regarding sexual intercourse. There is no mention in the question that the client had her ovaries removed, so hormone replacement therapy is not necessary. Heavy vaginal bleeding might indicate hemorrhage. The client may experience a moderate amount of serosanguineous drainage immediately postoperative; once healed, she will not experience menses.

4. **4** The client usually seeks treatment for a variety of symptoms, including dyspareunia (painful intercourse) due to the pain from the ulcerations caused by HSV-2. Anuria would be a complication of renal failure, as would pruritus. Leukorrhea is a thick, whitish, vaginal discharge that is common during pregnancy and at other times during a woman's reproductive years.

5. **2, 5, 6** Important teaching to include in the discharge plan of care for a client who has undergone a mastectomy includes the avoidance of needle-sticks in the arm on the side of the mastectomy and having blood pressure readings taken from the opposite arm. These measures are done to avoid any type of trauma, which could lead to the development of lymphedema. Begin finger, wrist, and hand exercises to facilitate muscle contraction and to help prevent edema. Active exercises, such as pendulum swings and wall-climbing, are started *after* the incision has healed. As the area heals, abduction and external rotation will help to improve the range of motion.

6. **3** Having the client void before the examination will make the procedure less painful and more accurate. Lubricant on the speculum may interfere with the Pap smear. The client should not douche or have intercourse before a pelvic exam, especially if any specimens are to be obtained, because changes in the normal flora and pH could occur from douching and the presence of semen.

7. **4** Gonorrhea in men is the most symptomatic, with urethritis, dysuria, and purulent drainage; however, the disease can be asymptomatic. The purulent secretion should be cultured to identify the microorganism. HSV-2 infections are characterized by painful vesicles surrounded by an erythematous base that progress to shallow ulcers, which eventually crust and epithelialize as they heal. In the secondary stage of syphilis the client is often asymptomatic; however, a maculopapular rash on the palms of the hands and soles of the feet may be noted with lymphadenopathy, sore throat, headache, and condylomata lata (flat lesions appearing in moist areas—not to be confused with condylomata acuminata in genital warts). A lower urinary tract infection would be characterized

by dysuria, urgency, frequency, hematuria, and possible low back pain.

8. **4** The fluorescent treponemal antibody absorption test is a serum blood test used to identify the spirochete *Treponema pallidum*, which causes syphilis. HSV-2 is diagnosed by tissue culture from a specimen obtained from an active lesion and by a serologic blood test. Trichomoniasis is diagnosed by a wet mount slide obtained from vaginal or penile secretions. Cytomegalovirus is diagnosed by blood test, but also by urine and tissue culture.

9. **3** Up to 100 mL of serosanguineous fluid would be an acceptable amount of drainage over a 24-hour period in a client who has had a mastectomy. There is no indication of hemorrhage or the need to perform frequent BP checks. If the nurse observes a greater amount of fluid in the drains, then it would be important to notify the physician.

10. **4** Elevating the affected arm promotes drainage of lymph from the extremity and decreases fluid from the wound site, which reduces swelling. An elastic wrap may be applied to the affected arm to reduce swelling, but it would not be positioned below the heart level.

11. **4** Flank pain may be indicative of an infection or a ureteral obstruction causing increased pressure on the renal pelvis. Other options are symptoms of benign prostatic hypertrophy, for which he will be treated while he is in the hospital.

12. **2** Because she no longer has regular periods, the client should pick a date and perform breast self-examination at the same time each month. Self-examination of the breast a week after the normal period is the best time for a woman who still has menstrual periods, because the breast tissue is less glandular a week after the normal period. Breasts are examined lying down and standing, not sitting. The pads of the fingers are used to examine the breast using small circular motions in a spiral pattern or in an up-and-down motion.

13. **2** The examination should be done at the same time each month to develop a regular routine. After a shower, when the scrotum is warm and the testicles are descended away from the body, is a good time to perform the examination.

14. **1** The primary complication is the obstruction of the urinary catheter with clots or tissue. There should be a large amount of drainage from the catheter because the irrigating fluid is infusing into the bladder. The catheter drainage should be closer to 300 to 400 mL/hr. It is not unusual for the drainage to be grossly bloody on the operative day, but it should begin to clear over the next 24 hours. It is common to have a feeling of needing to void with a catheter in place.

15. **3** To facilitate lymphatic drainage from the inflamed epididymis, the client should be taught to use a towel roll to act as a "scrotal bridge." Cool compresses

should be used in acute phase. There is no reason to limit oral intake.

16. **3** Trichomoniasis is a protozoal infection transmitted through sexual intercourse. All sexual partners need to be treated with the oral administration of metronidazole (Flagyl), a systemic antiprotozoal. Males may be asymptomatic. Intramuscular injection of penicillin is prescribed for syphilis. Douching should be avoided because it destroys the normal vaginal flora and increases the risk for developing the problem. Trichloroacetic acid (TCA) or podophyllin is topically applied to genital warts.

17. **2** Douching and some method of bowel preparation are part of the preoperative measure to cleanse the field of bacteria and pathogens. Vaginal drainage occurs with a vaginal, not an abdominal hysterectomy. Ambulation is encouraged to prevent venous stasis.

18. **4** D&C is the dilation (opening) of the cervix and curettage (scraping) of the inner walls of the uterus to remove the uterine contents in order to control bleeding and in this instance remove any products of conception that were not expelled. It does not protect the uterus or the ovaries. It is not recommended for incompetent cervical os, nor does it promote health of future pregnancies.

19. **1** The nurse teaches the client to maintain a semi-Fowler's position to prevent or decrease movement of the contaminated fluid to the upper abdomen and the area of the diaphragm.

20. **3** The nurse must rule out pregnancy/aborting first because of the potential for shock or damage to a fetus. Once aborting is ruled out or treated, the nurse addresses the issues of anemia and infection. Infertility would be the last concern, although it should be assessed.

21. **4** Low back pain and decreased urine output are serious symptoms that may indicate accidental intraoperative cutting of the ureter and should be reported immediately to the surgeon. Following an abdominal hysterectomy, the client would not be taking sitz baths. Leg exercises should be encouraged to promote circulation and prevent DVT. Abdominal exercises would be restricted during the immediate postoperative period to avoid disruption of the suture line.

CHAPTER 23: URINARY-RENAL SYSTEM

1. **4** Failure of the tube to drain freely can result in pain, trauma, wound dehiscence, and infection. Nephrostomy tubes should not be irrigated or adjusted.

2. **3** Movement of the client will help disseminate the fluid throughout the abdomen. The fluid should be instilled within the prescribed period of time; therefore the dialysate flow should not be decreased. Raising the head of the bed will make the client more uncomfortable and increase intra-abdominal pressure. The solutions should be infused at body temperature.

3. **2** A high fluid intake will help keep solutes diluted, thus preventing kidney stone formation. Drinking soda (diet or otherwise) is not the best method of increasing urine output. Nocturia and vitamins C and D are not relevant to renal stones.

4. **1, 3, 5, 6** Indications for dialysis include volume overload, weight gain, hyperkalemia, metabolic acidosis, and rising BUN (10 to 20 mg/dL) and serum creatinine (0.5 to 1.5 mg/dL) levels, along with decreased urinary creatinine clearance. A potassium of 5.2 is hyperkalemia, and a BUN of 18 mg/dL is within normal range.

5. **2** Urea is an end product of protein metabolism. In renal failure, the kidneys cannot clear all of the urea from the blood, and the creatinine and BUN level will be elevated. The C-reactive protein is a diagnostic test used in assessing clients with inflammatory bowel disease, rheumatoid arthritis, autoimmune diseases, and pelvic inflammatory disease (PID). A specific gravity test of the urine would assess the ability of the kidneys to concentrate urine. The urine osmolarity (concentration of particles in urine) and electrolytes assess fluid balance. The kidneys play an important role in the balance of electrolytes and fluids.

6. **3** Protect the arm with the functioning shunt. No blood pressure readings should be taken from that arm, and there should be no needle-sticks. The access is not irrigated with heparin.

7. **1** Secondary infections are the cause of death in 50% to 90% of clients with acute renal failure. A low-protein diet is most often offered. Catheterizations are avoided. Fluids may be limited if the client is in acute renal failure.

8. **4** The goal in chronic renal failure is to prevent acute failure and maintain whatever function is left. This is best done by minimizing stress and the workload on the kidneys. Increasing liver perfusion does not affect renal function. Until the renal function improves, there will be increased permeability in the basement membrane and electrolyte concentration in the urine will be diminished, because solutes are being retrained rather than excreted.

9. **3** The use of nonoxynol-9 spermicides can be irritating to the urinary tract and lead to infections. Urinary tract infections in women can be prevented by urination before and after sexual intercourse. Fluid intake should be increased, and no soap should be added to the sitz bath.

10. **2** The first specimen is discarded before the collection is started. Collection will continue until the completed time frame; the client should void before the collection is completed.

11. **1** The most characteristic symptom of renal colic is sudden, severe pain. The client may also exhibit nausea and vomiting, pallor, and diaphoresis during the acute pain episode. Hematuria and burning on urination are associated with UTIs, although there may be some bleeding with the passage of the renal stone.

12. **4** Removal of excess fluids and clearing of nitrogenous waste products of metabolism (urea, lactic acid) are the primary actions of hemodialysis. Evaluating the level of creatinine and BUN provides a measure of how effective the dialysate was in removing the waste products. The electrolyte components of the blood (sodium, potassium, calcium) are altered by the dialysis, but not hemoglobin, white blood cells, sedimentation rate, or plasma proteins—these cells are too large to diffuse through the pores of the dialysate membrane.

13. **2, 3, 4, 5** Classic signs of a cystitis include frequency, urgency, decreased bladder capacity, nocturia, and dysuria caused by the inflammatory process. Polydipsia (excessive thirst) is associated with diabetes mellitus.

14. **3** Clients with acute renal failure have hyperphosphatemia. Clients are prescribed calcium-based phosphate binders (such as calcium acetate, aluminum hydroxide gel, or calcium carbonate) to improve excretion of phosphorus.

15. **4** Because of the decreased ability to handle proteins as a result of the autoimmune process affecting the glomerulus, the diet should be high in calories and low in protein. A low-protein diet allows the kidney to rest, because they will handle fewer protein molecules and nitrogenous waste products. Fluid intake should be normal, provided that hypertension is under control. Isolation is not required because this is an autoimmune problem. Although ambulation is not incorrect for the child, it is best to encourage rest periods and focus on ways to allow the kidneys to repair and restore themselves.

16. **2, 4** Rapid instillation of dialysate fluid, as well as accumulation of the fluid under the diaphragm, can lead to pain and discomfort. Warming the dialysate solution helps in the clearance and may diminish any cold sensation of fluid entering the body. It will also assist to diminish any cold sensation of fluid entering the body. The dialysate fluid does not infiltrate and enter the circulatory system. Rapid outflow of dialysate does not cause pain.

17. **1** Diabetic nephropathy is the primary cause of end-stage renal failure. Laboratory findings of early proteinuria do not occur until 10 years or more after the onset of type 1 diabetes, but they may be present in persons with type 2 diabetes. A microscopic amount of albumin in the urine is one of the earliest indications of renal abnormality and is asymptomatic.

18. **3** Hyperkalemia can develop into an emergency situation (cardiac arrest). It is important to quickly move the potassium back into the cells by administering 50% glucose and regular insulin, usually in

conjunction with some type of base to correct the acidosis, such as sodium bicarbonate or calcium gluconate given intravenously. Insulin assists in the movement of potassium into the cells and helps to reduce the serum potassium level. Amphojel is used for the treatment of hyperphosphatemia that occurs with acute renal failure. Procrit is used for the treatment of anemia caused by a decrease in erythropoietin production by the kidneys. A diuretic, such as Lasix, may lead to a loss of potassium, but the rate is too slow.

CHAPTER 24: ANTEPARTUM

1. **3** Iron needs during pregnancy can most readily be met by taking iron supplements.

2. **3** False labor contractions decrease when the client is walking, are not concentrated in one part of the uterus, do not increase in intensity and frequency, and do not result in cervical effacement or dilation.

3. **4** In the glucose tolerance test, the blood glucose level is evaluated before the test (a fasting blood glucose), 1 hour after a 100-g glucose load, 2 hours after the glucose load, and 3 hours after the glucose load. The normal value for 1 hour is less than 180 mg/L, the normal value for 2 hours is less than 155 mg/L, and the normal value for 3 hours is less than 140 mg/L. The glycosylated hemoglobin value reflects blood glucose control for the past 120 days, and the urine glucose level is not as reliable an indicator of control as the serum glucose level.

4. **3** An oxytocin challenge test, or stress test, is conducted by giving an infusion of oxytocin to the mother and evaluating the fetal response to subsequent uterine contractions as plotted on a fetal monitor. The test result is negative if there are no late decelerations; it is positive if there are late decelerations in more than one half of the contractions. If the CST result is positive and there is no acceleration of FHR with fetal movement (nonreactive NST result), the positive CST (nonreassuring; abnormal) result is an ominous sign, often indicating late fetal hypoxia. A negative CST (reassuring) result with a reactive NST result is desirable.

5. **1** Pregnant women should be advised about the importance of good posture and body mechanics to prevent back strain, especially during the last trimester with the increase in size of the growing uterus. Low-heeled shoes help to maintain the body's center of gravity and prevent backaches. Constipation would not necessarily cause lower back discomfort.

6. **1** Rich dietary sources of folate are dark green, leafy vegetables, whole wheat bread, lightly cooked beans and peas, nuts and seeds, sprouts, oranges and grapefruits, liver and other organ meats, poultry, fortified breakfast cereals, and enriched grain products. Shellfish is rich in iodine. Dairy products are rich in calcium.

7. **4** All pregnancy tests, including over-the-counter "home pregnancy" tests, are based on the presence of human chorionic gonadotropin (hCG) as the biologic marker. A false-negative test result may be caused by testing too early. Whenever there is doubt about the results, further evaluation or retesting in a few days is appropriate. Results are most accurate when the first-voided specimen of the day is used, and the result may be positive within the first few days after a missed period. If symptoms of pregnancy are present, then the home pregnancy test may have produced a false-negative and the woman needs to be further evaluated.

8. **1, 3, 6** Changing position, moderate exercise, normal sexual activity as long as membranes are intact, and increasing calories by 300 calories for pregnancy and 500 calories for lactation are all included in the teaching plan. Constipation should be controlled first by dietary intake. Showers are okay, and tub baths are not contraindicated; however, safety (falling) is a concern during the last trimester. Live virus vaccines should not be administered during pregnancy.

9. **2** Rh$_o$(D) is given to all Rh-negative women in the 28th week of gestation. The blood type of the father may be determined, but paternity is not an important issue in this situation. An amniocentesis is not necessary at this time, and obtaining fetal blood to determine blood type is more risky than administering the medication to the mother.

10. **4** According to Nägele's rule, count back 3 months from the date of the last menstrual period and add 7 days to determine the estimated date of conception. About 35% of all women deliver within 5 days of (either before or after) this date.

11. **1** An L/S ratio (converts 2:1 at approximately 34 to 35 weeks' gestation) determines the relationship of two components of the fetal lung (lecithin and sphingomyelin) known as surfactant. Adequate surfactant must be present at birth for the alveoli to maintain expansion.

12. **1** All women who are pregnant need an increase in protein, as well as increased intake of foods that contain folic acid. This option would provide those nutrients. It is especially important to discuss this as early as possible with the adolescent client because it will affect fetal development. The other options are important to discuss but can be planned for future prenatal visits. Swelling of the hands and face could be an indication of preeclampsia or fluid retention, but this does not usually develop until the last trimester. A normal increase in vaginal discharge, called leukorrhea, occurs in response to cervical stimulation by estrogen and progesterone during pregnancy.

13. **2** Preeclampsia occurs most often after 20 weeks' gestation and is characterized by hypertension and proteinuria. Presence of swelling of the face and hands and a weight gain of 5 pounds would cause concern. The other options describe the normal discomforts of

pregnancy, especially at this time in the pregnancy. In option 3, Braxton-Hicks contractions occur randomly, and there is no cervical dilation. The contractions are uncomfortable but not particularly painful.

14. **4** In women of childbearing age who complain of sudden, sustained abdominal pain, an ectopic pregnancy must be ruled out immediately. The pain is on the wrong side of the abdomen for appendicitis, and gallbladder problems do not characteristically present with sudden, sustained pain. A sexually transmitted disease may have caused scarring of the fallopian tubes but would not cause the current immediate pain problem.

15. **3** It is important to acknowledge that this is a difficult time for her. Sitting with the client establishes contact, reinforces the nurse-client relationship, and offers support for the client. Telling her that this is the best thing that could happen is not acknowledging her feelings of loss, and asking about her other children is changing the subject.

16. **1** Mothers with diabetes can breastfeed; however, they must frequently check their blood glucose levels, and insulin is recommended to maintain good blood glucose control. Oral hypoglycemics are not usually recommended for breastfeeding mothers. Breastfeeding does put an increased demand on the mother's metabolism, but this can be controlled with careful monitoring of blood glucose levels. Multiple formulas are available, but if mother can breastfeed, that option should be made available to her.

17. **1** Human chorionic gonadotropin (hCG) is a placental hormone that, when present, indicates pregnancy. It can be detected in the serum and urine as early as 7 to 10 days after conception.

18. **4** Striae gravidarum are caused by the stretching and separation and atrophy of the deep connective tissue of the skin during the second half of pregnancy. They are pink or reddish during pregnancy and fade to silvery white (scars) after delivery.

19. **1** A negative rubella titer (serologically a titer of 1:8 or enzyme immunoassay [EIA] level of 0.8) is an indication that the woman needs to be vaccinated. Women must understand the importance of using reliable contraception to avoid pregnancy for at least a month after being vaccinated because of the potential for teratogenic effects.

CHAPTER 25: INTRAPARTUM AND POSTPARTUM

1. **2** Characteristics of the second stage of labor are complete cervical effacement and dilation and delivery of the infant. The characteristics in the other options all occur in the first stage of labor.

2. **1** Variable decelerations may be evidence of cord compression if they do not change. It would be appropriate to encourage the mother not to push with every contraction, because this would provide more time for the infant to recover between contractions. Fetal hypoxia and uteroplacental insufficiency are associated with late decelerations. Head compression is associated with early decelerations.

3. **4** Uterus palpated to right of umbilicus may indicate a full bladder. The fundus should be at the level of the midline. The temperature, lochia, and episiotomy assessment findings are within normal limits.

4. **4** The correct method of timing contractions is from the beginning of one contraction to the beginning of the next. The point at which the contraction ends is of concern only when the nurse needs to know the *duration* of the contraction, not the frequency or timing of the contractions.

5. **3** When a woman does not want to view her infant at birth, inadequate bonding may be occurring, which requires further evaluation by the nurse. Most mothers ask questions about their infant's bluish color and molding of the head. Sharing in the holding of the infant immediately after birth is a positive action.

6. **2** The erratic pattern on the fetal monitor is due to faulty lead placement. Although positioning on the side is an excellent nursing measure, it does not address the cause of the erratic pattern. Options 3 and 4 would possibly be done after the leads were checked.

7. **4** The bright red bleeding may be an indication of placenta previa or abruptio placentae, and the nurse should anticipate and plan for an emergency cesarean delivery. Because of the anesthesia and potential for aspiration, it is important to know when the client last ate. The other options are appropriate to check, but they are not of any assistance in the woman's current situation, which could progress to hemorrhage and the need for emergency surgery.

8. **3** *Station* refers to the relationship of the biparietal diameter of the fetal head to the ischial spine of the mother. When this diameter reaches the ischial spine, the station is zero (0) or engagement. A station of −1 indicates that the fetus is 1 cm above the ischial spine or floating.

9. **2** The release of oxytocin from the posterior pituitary during the infant's suckling increases the contractions of the uterus and gives rise to abdominal cramping. It is not associated with endometriosis or subinvolution of the uterus, and all women do not experience the contractions.

10. **2** The second stage of labor for a primigravida is about 1 hour; for a multipara client, it may be as little as several minutes.

11. **1** Wearing a breast binder or tight bra and applying ice packs are the best ways to decrease milk production and relieve the discomfort of engorgement. Medication is not recommended. Pumping the breast will stimulate and increase the milk production. A warm shower will also stimulate milk production. The mother should not decrease her fluid intake. Her fluid intake needs to be increased

to help prevent urinary tract infections and to keep the urine dilute.

12. **3** *Effacement* is the term used to indicate thinning of the cervix. *Dilation* refers to cervical opening, *attitude* refers to fetal posture, and *transition* refers to the last phase of the first stage of labor.

13. **2** A mother's complaint of excruciating perineal pain after birth is frequently related to the development of a perineal hematoma. A soft, boggy uterus will cause an increase in the bloody flow but is usually not associated with pain. A cervical laceration may be painful at the time it occurs but not after delivery.

14. **1** When a laboring client is at +3, delivery is imminent. The + stations are noted after the neonate has engaged and is moving through the birth canal. The sequence is as follows: −4, −3, −2, −1, 0, +1, +2, +3, +4, and delivery.

15. **2** If the entire areola is in the infant's mouth, the infant will not suck on the end of the nipple and traumatize it. Mothers should begin breastfeeding on the least affected nipple to initiate the let-down reflex, which occurs only with stronger sucking. The breast should not be cleaned with peroxide. Application of cool compresses may feel good after breastfeeding, but this does not prevent the problem.

16. **1** Activities that decrease venous stasis should be encouraged: wearing elastic stockings, walking, and general increased activity. The legs should also be elevated when the client is in the sitting position, but warm, moist packs are used to treat thrombophlebitis and are not necessary at this time. The health care provider would need to be notified if vascular lesions began to form, but the priority here is to prevent venous stasis and decrease the risk for formation of pulmonary emboli.

17. **3** Since this is a scheduled cesarean delivery, any signs of urinary tract infection before the surgery would be of concern and should be investigated further. A cesarean delivery is scheduled before the woman goes into labor; therefore she would not be well into the labor process. Urinary output is normal, as is the maternal heart rate in this situation.

18. **2** The birth of this infant is imminent. The infant is probably small because of prematurity. The mother is multigravida, and she has not received any analgesics. The nurse should firmly support the infant's head and prepare to deliver. The infant will probably be delivered with one or two more contractions; therefore an attempt to take the mother to labor and delivery should not be made. If the mother pushes hard with the next contraction, the infant may progress too rapidly and tear the vaginal orifice. There is no need for a cesarean delivery. No attempt should be made to slow or prevent the delivery, because this would put the infant in further jeopardy.

19. **1, 2, 5** The breast will get softer as the infant drains the breast, the infant is usually satisfied for 2 to 3 hours after breastfeeding, and adequate fluid intake is demonstrated by adequate urine output. Initially, the infant should suck for about 15 minutes on each breast, for a total breastfeeding time of about 30 minutes. The infant should regain her lost birth weight sooner than a month (in about a week to 10 days after delivery). The infant should be on a "demand" schedule until she begins to feed well; then a routine can be established.

20. **4, 2, 3, 1**
    1 ___4___ The exposed cord should be kept moist, but the other options take priority.
    2 ___2___ After position has been changed and oxygen administration has been started, an emergency call to the health care provider should be made.
    3 ___3___ An IV should be in place, and emergency vaginal delivery or cesarean delivery should be anticipated.
    4 ___1___ The most important action is to immediately attempt to relieve the pressure on the umbilical cord and increase the amount of oxygen being delivered to the infant. Placing the woman in a modified Sims', Trendelenburg, or knee-chest position will assist in relieving some of the pressure. The other important action is to insert sterile, gloved fingers into the vagina on either side of the cord and apply gentle manual pressure to relieve the pressure of the presenting part on the cord.

CHAPTER 26: NEWBORN

1. **2** The priority here is the respiratory distress. The first nursing action is to increase the inspired oxygen; it would be appropriate to determine whether the infant has any mucus in the airway. Do a quick but thorough assessment of the infant and advise the supervisor or doctor regarding the infant's status.

2. **4, 5, 6** The mother should be taught to feed the baby on demand for at least the first 4 weeks, until lactation is well established. Feeding only breast milk frequently stimulates milk production. Nipple soreness is one of the most common problems; however, the use of a cream to soften the nipples is often helpful, as well as offering a pacifier to meet sucking needs of the newborn between feedings. Adequate rest and good fluid intake help promote milk production.

3. **2** The premature infant's temperature-regulating mechanism is poorly developed at birth. Heat production is low, and heat loss is high because of the greater body surface area relative to weight and the infant's lack of subcutaneous fat. No diaphoresis should be occurring, and the question has nothing to do with protein metabolism. The first option describes the body surface area of the infant. This is a true statement but does not have any implication for maintaining temperature.

4. **1** Promoting lifesaving oxygen exchange is a priority measure at this time. Prevention of infection will be appropriate after surgical repair. It is important to

prevent pulmonary infection, especially aspiration, but oxygen exchange is still a priority.

5. **4** The medication is given to prevent maternal sensitization to the Rh antibodies to women who are Rh negative. It will not prevent or treat the problem if it has already occurred; it is not given to the infant.

6. **3** It is important that the child be positioned in such a manner that he does not traumatize the incisional area and that the airway is maintained. Trendelenburg position would compromise respiration, the prone position would cause trauma to the incisional area, and the Sims' position is not appropriate for an infant.

7. **4** The premature infant is at greater risk for chilling. A premature infant has less brown fat than does a term neonate, as well as a lower reserve of glycogen and lower reserve for breathing. A lower body temperature leads to greater oxygen consumption, a decrease in surfactant production, and a tendency to develop acidosis.

Index